WOMEN'S HEALTH
A Primary Care Clinical Guide

WOMEN'S HEALTH
A Primary Care Clinical Guide

FOURTH EDITION

Ellis Quinn Youngkin, PhD, WHNP-BC, ARNP
Retired Professor and Associate Dean
Christine E. Lynn College of Nursing
Women's Health Care Nurse Practitioner
University Student Health Services
Florida Atlantic University
Boca Raton, Florida
Faculty Emeritus
School of Nursing
Virginia Commonwealth University
Richmond, Virginia

Marcia Szmania Davis, MS, MS ED, RNC, WHCNP-BC, ANP-BC
Women's Health Care Nurse Practitioner
Commonwealth OB/GYN Specialists
Richmond, Virginia

Diane Marie Schadewald, DNP, MSN, RNC, WHNP-BC, FNP-BC
Clinical Assistant Professor
School of Nursing
University of Minnesota
Minneapolis, Minnesota

Catherine Juve, PhD, MSPH, RNC, WHNP-BC
Clinical Associate Professor
School of Nursing
University of Minnesota
Minneapolis, Minnesota

PEARSON

Boston Columbus Indianapolis New York San Francisco Upper Saddle River
Amsterdam Cape Town Dubai London Madrid Milan Munich Paris Montréal Toronto
Delhi Mexico City São Paulo Sydney Hong Kong Seoul Singapore Taipei Tokyo

Publisher: Julie Levin Alexander
Assistant to Publisher: Regina Bruno
Design Director: Maria Guglielmo
Senior Editor: Kim Norbuta
Editorial Assistant: Erin Rafferty
Marketing Coordinator: Michaeal Sirinides
Senior Marketing Manager: Phoenix Harvey
Production Manager: Fran Russello
Full Service Production: Murugesh Rajkumar/PreMediaGlobal
Printer/Binder: Edwards Brothers Malloy
Art Director: Jayne Conte
Cover Designer: Suzanne Behnke
Cover Printer: Lehigh/Phoenix

Notice: This volume is intended to educate students and health care providers, not to be a guide for any individual therapy. The authors and the publisher of this volume have taken care to make certain that the doses of drugs and schedules of treatments are correct and compatible with the standards generally accepted at the time of publication. Nevertheless, as new information becomes available, changes in treatment and in the use of drugs, devices, and other therapies become necessary. The reader is advised to carefully consult the instruction and information material included in the package insert of each drug, device, or therapy agent, as well as appropriate, current references before administration. This advice is especially important when using, administering, or recommending new or infrequently used drugs/devices/agents. The authors and publisher advise that an individual with a particular problem consult a primary care provider or a specialist in obstetrics, gynecology, or the field of medicine or advanced practice nursing appropriate for that problem. Under no circumstances should the reader use this volume in lieu of or to substitute for the judgment of the treating provider. The authors and the publisher disclaim all responsibility for any liability, loss, injury, or damage incurred as a consequence, directly or indirectly, of the use and application of any of the contents of this volume.

Library of Congress Cataloging-in-Publication Data

Women's health: a primary care clinical guide / [edited by] Ellis Quinn
Youngkin . . . [et al.].—4th ed.
p. ; cm.
Includes bibliographical references and index.
ISBN-13: 978-0-13-257673-4 (alk. paper)
ISBN-10: 0-13-257673-2 (alk. paper)
I. Youngkin, Ellis Quinn.
[DNLM: 1. Women's Health—United States. 2. Primary Health Care—United States. WA 309 AA1]
LC Classification not assigned
613'.04244—dc23

2012005805

10 9 8 7 6 5 4 3 2 1

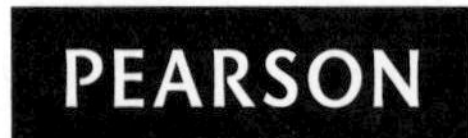

ISBN 10: 0-13-257673-2
ISBN 13: 978-0-13-257673-4

CONTENTS

CONTRIBUTORS

Kristine Alswager, MS, RNC, WHNP
Women's Health Care Nurse Practitioner
Women's Health Consultants
Minneapolis, Minnesota

Anne Bateman, EdD, APRN, BC
Assistant Professor, School of Nursing
University of Massachusetts Medical School
Worchester, Massachusetts

Mary Benbenek, PhD, RNC, FNP, PNP
Clinical Assistant Professor, School of Nursing
University of Minnesota
Minneapolis, Minnesota

Linda Christinsen-Rengel, MS, RNC, CNP
Nurse Practitioner
United Hospital Breast Center
St Paul, MN

Michele R. Davidson, PhD, RN, CNM, CFN
Associate Professor, School of Nursing
Prince William Campus
George Mason University
Manassas, Virginia

Jennifer M. Demma, MSN, RN, CNM
Assistant Professor
Minnesota State University
Mankato, Minnesota Associate Director

Mary Dierich, PhD, RN, CNP
Adjunct Faculty, School of Nursing
University of Minnesota
Minneapolis, Minnesota

Christine Durler, MS, BSN, RN, CNP
Women's Health Care Nurse Practitioner
Women's Health Consultants
Minneapolis, Minnesota

Melissa A. Feldhaus Dahir, APRN, NP-C
Nurse Practitioner, Pelvic Pain and Sexual Medicine Clinic
Methodist Physicians Clinic
Omaha, Nebraska

Cheri Friedrich, DNP, MS, RN, CNP
Clinical Assistant Professor, School of Nursing
University of Minnesota
Minneapolis, Minnesota

Melissa Frisvold, PhD, RN, CNM
Clinical Assistant Professor, School of Nursing
University of Minnesota
Minneapolis, Minnesota

Karen Trister Grace, MSN, CNM
Adjunct Instructor
Georgetown University
Washington, DC

Debra J. Hain , PhD, APRN, GNP-BC
Assistant Professor, Christine E Lynn College of Nursing
Florida Atlantic University
Boca Raton, Florida

Jane Houston, DNP, CNM
Clinical Assistant Professor, College of Nursing
University of Florida
Gainesville, Florida

Jennifer M. Laubach, MS, BSN, RN, CNP
Obstetrics and Gynecology
Fairview Health Services, Blaine Clinic
Blaine, Minnesota

Reena Lorntson, MS, RNC, WHNP
Obstetrics and Gynecology
Fairview Health Services, Andover Clinic
Andover, Minnesota

Coralie Pederson, MSN, RN, WHNP
Nurse Practitioner
Family Tree Clinic
St. Paul, Minnesota

Debbie Ringdahl, DNP, RN, CNM
Clinical Assistant Professor, School of Nursing
University of Minnesota
Minneapolis, Minnesota

Jo Lynne W. Robins, PhD, RN, ANP-BC
Assistant Professor, School of Nursing
Virginia Commonwealth University
Richmond, Virginia

Susan D. Schaffer, PhD, RN, CFNP
Associate Professor, College of Nursing
University of Florida
Gainesville, Florida

Gwendolyn Short, DNP, MSN, MPH, APRN, FNP
Faculty
Frontier Nursing University
Hyden, Kentucky

Renee Sieving, PhD, MSN, RN
Associate Professor, School of Nursing
University of Minnesota
Minneapolis, Minnesota

Sarah Stoddard, PhD, RN, CNP
Research Assistant Professor
Health Education & Health Behavior
School of Public Health, University of Michigan
Ann Arbor, Michigan

Debera Jane Thomas, DNS, FNP/ANP, APRN
Dean and Professor, School of Nursing
Northern Arizona University
Flagstaff, Arizona

Donna Treloar, PhD, ARNP
Associate Professor, College of Nursing
University of Florida
Gainesville, Florida

Michelle J. Valentine, RN, WHNP-BC
Nurse Practitioner
Allina Hospitals and Clinics
Minneapolis, Minnesota

Elizabeth Walcker, MSN, RN, WHNP
Nurse Practitioner
Family Tree Clinic
St. Paul, Minnesota

Susan Wysocki, RN, WHNP
Past President and CEO
Nurse Practitioners in Women's Health
Washington, DC

Eugenia H. Zelanko, PhD, RN, CNS-BC
Urshel Recovery Science Institute
Dallas, Texas

CONTRIBUTORS TO THIRD EDITION

A special thank you and recognition go to those who contributed to the third edition of this book:

Kathleen M. Akridge
Postpartum and Lactation

Lynette Galloway Branch
Breast Health

Joan Corder-Mabe, RNC, MS, WHCNP
Complications of Pregnancy

Valerie T. Cotter, MSN, CRNP
The Climacteric, Menopause, and the Process of Aging

Leslie Fehan, MS, CNM, WHNP
Integrating Wellness: Complementary Therapies and Women's Health

Elaine Ferrary, MS, RN, CFNP
Common Medical Problems: Cardiovascular Through Hematological Disorders
Common Medical Problems: Musculoskeletal Injuries Through Urinary Tract Disorders

Donna E. Forrest, RNC, MS, FNP, WHCNP
Common Gynecologic Pelvic Disorders

Marion Herndon Fuqua, MS, RNC, WHCNP
Assessing Fetal Well-Being

Jennifer R. Gardella, RNC, MSN
Infertility

Deborah Griswold, MSN, CFNP, ARNP
Menstruation and Related Problems and Concerns

Janet C. Horton, MS, RN, APRN-BC
Health Care Concerns for Women With Physical Disability and Chronic Illness

Rita A. Seeger Jablonski, PhD, RN, ANP-BC
Common Medical Problems: Cardiovascular Through Hematological Disorders
Common Medical Problems: Musculoskeletal Injuries Through Urinary Tract Disorders

Angela Carter Martin, MS, RN, CFNP, CS
Psychosocial Health Concerns

Deborah A. Raines, PhD, RNC, CNS
Assessing Adolescent Women's Health

Maryellen C. Remich, RNC, MS(N), OGNP
Promoting a Healthy Pregnancy

Kathleen J. Sawin, DNS, RN, CS, FAAN
Health Care Concerns for Women With Physical Disability and Chronic Illness

Barbara Peterson Sinclair, MN, OGNP, FAAN
Women and the Health Care System

Rachel Effolia Smith, MSN, FNP-CS
Women and HIV

Kelly L. Cokely Yeong, MS, WHNP
Assessing Health During Pregnancy

CONTRIBUTORS TO SECOND EDITION

A special thank you and recognition go to those who contributed to the second edition of this book:

Brenda T. Brickhouse
Emergency Childbirth

Cynthia W. Bailey
Assessing Health During Pregnancy

Sharon Baker
Menstruation and Related Problems and Concerns

Judith B. Collins
Women and the Health Care System

Judy Parker-Falzoi
Common Medical Problems

Martha Edwards Hart
Immediate Assessment of the Newborn

Judith A. Lewis
Legal Issues in Primary Care of Women

Cathy James
Infertility

Mary Beth Bryant McGurin
Emergency Childbirth

Nancy Sharp
Women and the Health Care System

REVIEWERS

Dr. Kathryn Deitch, WHNP-BC
Director, WHNP Program
California State University, Long Beach,
School of Nursing
Long Beach, California

Julie Koch, DNP, MSN, RN, FNP-BC
Assistant Professor of Nursing
Valparaiso University, College of Nursing
Valparaiso, Indiana

Michele Bracken, Ph.D., RN
Assistant Professor
Salisbury University
Salisbury, Maryland

Karen Crowley, DNP, MSN, BSN
Associate Professor, Nursing Department
Regis College
Weston, Massachusetts

Barbara Cannella, Ph.D., RN
Clinical Associate Professor
Rutgers University, College of Nursing
Newark, New Jersey

PREFACE

Many women, by choice or by necessity, will seek out the women's health care provider as their source of primary care. This fourth edition of *Women's Health: A Primary Care Clinical Guide* is designed to help meet the needs of providers who offer women more than basic reproductive health care. It covers the traditional reproductive and gynecologic content as well as selected common medical, psychosocial, developmental, and political problems, issues, and needs. We have updated every chapter, and added the *Assessing Older Women's Health* chapter. We also took material from the *Assessing Adult Women's Health* chapter and created a separate chapter, *Epidemiology, Diagnostic Methods, and Procedures for Women's Health.* We combined the chapters on prenatal care into one chapter and made major revisions to the chapter on breast health. In addition, the chapter on complementary therapies has been significantly expanded.

Part I, Women, Health, and the Health Care System, begins with a chapter on the major historical and contemporary changes in the education of women's health care nurse practitioners, focusing on the important societal, economic, and political factors that will affect the profession at the beginning of this century. Chapter 2 discusses women's growth and development, followed by Chapter 3, the new epidemiology and diagnostic test and procedures chapter. Chapter 4 deals with adolescent health issues. Chapter 5 includes general guidelines for health care screening, and interventions for adult women. Chapter 6 is new chapter on older women's health. We thought this new chapter was important to include given our aging population.

Part II, Promotion of Wellness for Women, includes Chapter 7 on sexuality, Chapter 8 on the health needs of lesbians and other sexual minority women, Chapter 9 on health needs of women with disabilities, and Chapter 10 on complementary therapies in women's health.

Part III, Promotion of Gynecologic Health Care, delves into the more traditional health problems and needs of women related to the reproductive system. Chapters 11 through 18 cover menstrual concerns; fertility management; infertility; sexually transmitted infections (STIs) and vaginitis, including the 2010 STI guidelines from the CDC; special needs of women with HIV; pelvic and abdominal diseases; breast concerns; and health concerns related to the menopausal transition.

Part IV, Promotion of Women's Health Care During Pregnancy, details uncomplicated and complicated pregnancy care, postpartum needs and problems, lactation issues, and fetal surveillance.

Part V, Primary Care Conditions Affecting Women's Health, addresses medical problems frequently encountered in primary care of women such as headaches, anemia, hypertension, asthma, and dermatologic conditions. Chapters 23 and 24 are dedicated to current information on common medical problems. Selected psychosocial problems, such as violence, depression, eating disorders, and their impacts on women, with insights into related health care needs and therapies, are discussed in Chapter 25.

The appendixes address emergency childbirth and assessment of the newborn (Appendix A), selected screening tools for women's health (Appendix B), billing and coding in women's health (Appendix C), laboratory values commonly referenced in women's health (Appendix D), and federal agencies in the United States that are concerned with women's health (Appendix E).

We particularly intend this book to be a handbook, a resource that allows students and any primary health care provider to retrieve basic information easily. We see it as a reference with enough depth to be useful in a clinical setting, serving as a source of teaching advice for clients, including differential medical diagnoses, screening and early intervention measures, and guidelines for referral. Some of the chapters fit more easily into an outline format for diseases or other conditions, whereas many chapters conform to a more traditional text format or a combination format for presentation of issues.

We wish to remind the reader that the scope of advanced practice nursing varies from state to state, and the individual practitioner is responsible for knowing his or her legal limits of practice. Also, recognizing the rapidity with which new knowledge becomes available and standards change, the practitioner must stay ever alert.

Women's health care providers are continuously challenged to expand their knowledge and ability to help women fulfill a wide spectrum of needs, both physical and psychosocial. Women's health has not been limited to reproductive organs for some time now. The broadening scope of women's health care is a critically important issue in this period of rapidly changing health care systems. The Patient Protection and Affordable Care Act of 2010 along with the Institute of Medicine's 2011 broad recommendations for essential services to be included for woman have the potential to greatly expand opportunities for women as well as providers of women's health care services. With these changes, hopefully, the struggle to attain holistic health care services for women will be relieved. That is, as long as the Patient Protection and Affordable Care Act is not overturned by the Supreme Court in the United States. If the act is overturned, it is not clear what will happen with the recommend essential services for women identified in 2011 by the Institute of Medicine. Resources are burgeoning, empowering women to become more informed consumers in the health care arena. We, with the contributing authors, hope that you as students and primary care providers in a rapidly changing world of health care will find this book a useful and effective resource in your endeavors to provide women with the health care they need and deserve.

Our sincere thanks go to our excellent contributing authors. Their outstanding expertise and effort have made this book the useful clinical reference we envisioned. We also wish to thank the fine editors and staff at Pearson Publishing Company for their support and many hours of work on this project. Last, our deep appreciation goes to our families who encouraged us during the months of preparation and work. A special thanks to Matt for his technical assistance. Last, a note goes to our inspiring "little women," Hanna, Abby, Cassidy, Michelle, Debbie, Taylor, and Emmy Lou, who join the women of the 21st century in deserving the best health care of the new millennium.

We would also like to thank our co-editors Ellis Quinn Youngkin and Marcia Szmania Davis for the opportunity to work with them on this new edition of their well known and widely used women's health text. We hope that this new edition continues to contribute to excellence in women's health care and remains the go to text for educators and clinicians.

Diane Marie Schadewald
Catherine Juve

I ❖ Women, Health, and the Health Care System

CHAPTER ❖ 1

NURSE PRACTITIONERS IN WOMEN'S HEALTH: WHERE IS THE FUTURE HEADING?

Susan Wysocki

Highlights

- Humble Beginnings
- WHNP Practice Today
- WHNP Programs of the Future
- Questions for the Future

HUMBLE BEGINNINGS

In the 1960s, a set of domestic programs promoted by President Lyndon Johnson and a liberal Democratic Congress were initiated. Known as the Great Society programs, the programs were aimed at decreasing poverty and racial injustice. These new programs included education and housing programs as well as the health programs Medicare and Medicaid. The programs also created a demand for primary care providers that could not be met by physicians alone (Way, 1995).

As a public health nurse, Loretta Ford, RN, EdD, PNP, FAAN, FAANP, found pediatric care lacking in her state of Colorado and seized the opportunity to do something about the lack of primary care providers to create a new role for nursing. In 1965, together with Dr. Henry Silver, she created the first pediatric certificate nurse practitioner program at the University of Colorado. By expanding the skills of experienced registered nurses to include physical assessment, diagnosis, and management, this new nurse specialty was able to address the demands for care that were found to be so lacking. It was a sentinel change for the nursing profession (Ford, 2009). However, it was not accepted as a positive change by the profession. In fact, many in the nursing profession regarded the nurse practitioner (NP) role as a sellout to medicine (Way, 1995).

This model of care provided by NPs in pediatrics was recognized as a model of care that could also serve women's contraceptive and reproductive needs for the family planning programs that were created as Title X of the Public Health Service Act of 1970. Pioneers such as Miriam Manisoff at the Planned Parenthood Federation of America, Frances Way at Planned Parenthood of Wisconsin, and John Marshall, MD, at Harbor-UCLA Medical Center spearheaded new programs to create what was then called Family Planning Nurse Practitioners (FPNPs). In 1972, the Department of Health Education and Welfare authorized funds to support these and other programs to educate experienced registered nurses to provide family planning and reproductive health care in Title X clinics and programs. Over the years, over $20 million were invested in educating these clinicians (Way, 1995).

EARLY PROGRAMS

These early programs were closely allied with medical schools, as many of the skills taught were borrowed from medicine. NP faculty did not exist. The affiliation with schools of medicine led to some additional criticism of the role. When the Nurse Training Act was passed in 1975, funds were earmarked for schools of nursing for NP education through the Division of Nursing (DON). The objection to the NP role began to subside. Almost all the early programs for all types of NPs were certificate programs. Once the DON funds became available, the NP programs were integrated into graduate nursing programs and conferred master's degrees. Certificate programs and NP programs supported by federal Title X funds were eventually phased out completely in the early 1990s (Way, 1995).

Certification of Women's Health Nurse Practitioners (WHNPs) by the National Certification Corporation (NCC) became available in 1980. Prior to that, the FPNP programs added components to include obstetrics, general physical assessment, primary care topics, and male exam in order to make their graduates qualified to take the exam. The name of the specialty then changed to OB/GYN NP. The specialty name changed once more to WHNP as the concept that women's health care meant more than care of reproductive function became popularized.

IMPACT OF TITLE X

With the phasing out of the Title X–funded programs, there was considerable concern about the availability of qualified NPs to practice in family-planning programs. The concern remains even today. The vast majority of clinicians in family planning clinics (Title X, health departments, and Planned Parenthood) are NPs. For example, of the approximately 2,000 clinicians employed in Planned Parenthood clinics, only one-third are physicians, and many of those physicians do not provide direct care on a regular basis. Finding an NP specifically qualified to provide contraceptive services and deal with the complex and sensitive topics surrounding reproductive and sexual health issues has become increasingly more difficult (Bednash, Worthington, & Wysocki, 2009). Many NP education programs that are not specific to women's health provide little content or clinical experience in these areas.

In addition to specific clinical skills, the graduates of the Title X programs were community based and had often been the registered nurses in the clinics they returned to after they became NPs. This meant, for example, that on average, there were double the number of minority graduates from the Title X programs. Practically speaking, these NPs were "culturally competent" because they were from the culture in which they practiced. The structure and length of the certificate programs was such that it allowed for community-based nurses to attend the programs. Further, the programs offered full scholarships and housing (Way, 1995).

As certificate programs decreased, the number of master's programs offering tracks in women's health increased. That number of programs has waxed and waned over the years. The absence of the certificate programs has had an impact on the number of NPs entering the specialty because they tended to have larger classes than the WHNP tracks in master's programs. In fact, certificate program graduates made up close to 60 percent of the graduates of WHNP programs in the 1990s (Way, 1995).

According to statistics from NCC, the body that certifies WHNPs, the number of certified WHNPs in the past 3 years was between 350 and 450 a year. Compared to the estimated 140,000 NPs in the United States, the NCC (2011) has certified approximately 13,000 WHNPs. Family nurse practitioners (FNPs) are seen as having more employment options, particularly in some areas of the country. Many FNPs either prefer providing women's health care or find themselves providing care to women in their practice by default because of the nature of the mix of providers in a family practice setting.

WHNP PRACTICE TODAY

The 2009 NCC WHNP exam content analysis surveyed approximately 10 percent of currently certified WHNPs. Among those surveyed, 33 percent identified their practice setting as a physician's office, 3 percent as an independent practice, 15 percent as a public health clinic, 4 percent as an academic clinical practice, and the rest as a variety of clinic settings (from the hospital and ambulatory care setting to prenatal clinics). The respondents of the survey saw women from adolescence past the age of menopause. Not surprisingly, the largest concentration of patients seen was in the prime reproductive years. Thirty-four percent of WHNPs see men in their practice primarily focused on reproductive health issues.

WHNPs provide a wide range of services, with a concentration on issues related to female health—contraception, management of menopausal symptoms, pregnancy, reproductive-related infections, and pathology. WHNPs also provide a wide range of preventive care such as depression screening, addiction screening, preconception counseling, and smoking cessation advice. Fifty percent or more of WHNPs prescribe antidepressants, for example (NCC, 2009).

AGING OUT

A 2011 survey of NPs practicing women's health care by the National Association of Nurse Practitioners in Women's Health (NPWH) and the RAND Corporation identified that 25 percent of those NPs are 60 years of age or older. Those 50 years of age and older make up 55 percent of this group of NPs. These percentages are in line with other NPWH surveys in the past several years. It also reflects the percentage of WHNPs certified for 16 or more years by NCC.

A key concern about the aging out of the WHNP is not only the number of NPs with this expertise for clinical practice, but also the availability of faculty with this expertise whether for faculty in the university setting, for continuing education programs, or for being a mentor or resource for other NPs.

GENERALIST VERSUS SPECIALIST

The concept of women's health has changed dramatically over the past 20 years. Prior to the 1990s, women's health was almost entirely focused on reproductive functions. There is now great recognition that, with regard to health, women are not just little men who can have babies. Whether regarding reproduction, heart disease, immunological function and disease, as well as many other issues, care for women is, and should be, different from that for men. In an era in which medical science is recognizing the importance of gender-based differences, the NP profession is becoming more and more generalized.

WHNP PROGRAMS OF THE FUTURE

Some WHNP programs have addressed the desire of students to have job flexibility with a more generalized NP educational background (i.e., FNPs and adult nurse practitioners [ANPs]) by combining WHNP and ANP tracks. This has worked well in several universities. However, the recent combining of gerontology into the ANP exam has added challenges of having courses that meet the requirements for the adult/gerontology exam as well as the WHNP certification exam in a combined course. These types of program adaptations have some promise for the future. Other programs offer the WHNP/certified nurse midwife (CNM) course work so that graduates will qualify for both the CNM and the WHNP exam (NPWH, 2011).

By 2015, the proposed entry degree for practice as an NP is the Doctor of Nursing Practice (DNP). The course work to become a DNP can vary, but the overarching principle is to educate NPs to be leaders in the health care field (Bednash et al., 2009). The impact this will have on the WHNP as a specialty is unknown. The proposed date of 2015 for the DNP is a suggested target date. In reality, each state will have to adopt this requirement in order for this entry-level degree to be broadly implemented. What is apparent is that more and more universities are converting their master's degree programs into DNP programs. Therefore, the availability of master of science in nursing (MSN) programs is shrinking. However, the total conversion of programs is highly dependent on the availability of doctoral-prepared faculty and, in other instances, whether an MSN program is in an institution or a school of nursing that has doctoral-level programs of any type. Nevertheless, the trend toward doctoral education of NPs is the future path.

QUESTIONS FOR THE FUTURE

In an article in the *Harvard Business Review,* Harvard business professor Clayton Christensen writes about innovations that take root in their simplicity and often take over a market. For example, he describes how less complex personal computers (PCs) overwhelmed the need for mainframe computers. PCs are accessible to everyone, easy to operate, and affordable. Further, PCs perform almost all the tasks any user would need (from word processing to data processing). The availability of mainframe computers, however, is still needed for certain tasks requiring large amounts of memory and other specialized functionality (Christensen, Bohmer, & Kenagy, 2000).

In his article, "Will Disruptive Innovations Cure Health Care," Professor Christensen analyzes the NP role from the perspective of innovation. NPs, he notes, make for accessible health care, delivering health care in a way that people/patients understand. Further, NPs can deliver most of what patients need to remain healthy or manage a chronic illness. The health care system, he suggests, should be designed so that care is done by the appropriate professionals. A highly specialized physician is not the appropriate primary care giver for basically healthy individuals. When patients require a high level of specialization, they should be able to access it (Christensen et al., 2000).

Christensen offers a note of caution about all disruptive innovations whether in health care or in any other business. His caution is that when a disruptive innovation is "improved upon," those improvements can make the price increase until the innovation is no longer competitive (Christensen et al., 2000). The same caution might apply to the NP profession. From being rooted in the simple concept of access to those without care, the entire profession was birthed by Loretta Ford. It worked. It did what it was intended to. Will requiring a DNP as entry into practice "improve" the profession?

It is important to ask what people want out of the profession when they become NPs. Most people become NPs because they want to do direct patient care. They want to be competent providers of health care. Not all want to be in leadership positions in the health care system. This is not to argue that NPs should not be leaders in their own settings whether advocating for patient services or for themselves with regard to things like parity in reimbursement for the same services. The profession needs leaders who can argue for what NPs do that is unique and how the nursing aspects of NP care are as important as the medical aspects we bring. We need people who can quantify these unique qualities to advocate for the profession and most of all our patients.

There is a perception that WHNPs are a less employable specialty versus FNPs (NPWH, 2011). That may be true to some degree because a community may have a limited number of OB/GYN or women's specialty practice compared to family practice settings. However, every community needs competent providers of women's health services. WHNP jobs may not be listed in the "Help Wanted" column as much as ads for FNPs. However, finding employment as an NP should not be dependent on seeing an ad in the paper. The pioneers of the NP movement know this. There were no ads in the paper when the NP profession was barely known. Then it was about selling a unique set of skills to an employer or developing a niche in which to practice. In many ways, it was not that different than it is today, although the expectations are different now that the NP profession is widely known.

The following are a few things to consider for the future:

> Should the WHNP education model be more like the ANP/WHNP model? Should that dual role be achieved in DNP programs where the additional hours of education can be dedicated toward additional clinical competencies versus issues like leadership skills? Who should then certify these dual providers now that the ANP certification is a dual exam of ANP/gerontology nurse practitioner (GNP)?
>
> Given that the geriatric population is predominantly women, should there be even more attention to the

primary care of geriatric-aged women such that the WHNP/ANP/GNP would be a model for the future needs of our aging population?

Are perceptions about the limitations of practice opportunities for the WHNP a reality or a lack of creativity? For example, WHNPs specializing in sexuality counseling, incontinence, and other niches make sense in the current marketplace. There are a number of niche markets that WHNPs could nicely fill that any practice could use. Should there be an examination of what those niche markets might be with attention to educating NPs to fill those niches?

What will the future bring to the NP profession in terms of minimally invasive surgery such as tubal sterilization, hysteroscopic surgery to remove fibroids, or ablation? It isn't out of the question. NPs graduating in the 1970s never envisioned NPs doing coloposcopy or even endometrial biopsy.

Is there a need in educational programs for exploring more and more "disruptive innovations" for the profession/specialty rather than looking to "improve upon" the existing model of the NP?

What will the role of the WHNP be like when we are truly sophisticated in predicting future illness and disease through genotyping? What can we do to prepare for that eventuality? Can we position the profession as the best health educators to keep people healthy?

Women are the cog in the wheel for health care for their families. How can women's health care be revolutionized to take this fact into consideration?

The future for NPs is far brighter than Loretta Ford and the other pioneers of the profession ever imagined. Like the Great Society programs, the Affordable Care Act will provide access to many more people. It also promises to emphasize the importance of health promotion and disease prevention—the very thing that is at the foundation of the NP profession. We should heed Christensen's warning about over-"improvement" of the profession that may increase costs without comparable benefit to the consumer. We should meet the future by continuing to innovate and be creative in order to provide the best and most accessible care for the women to whom we provide care.

CARPE DIEM!

REFERENCES

Bednash, P., Worthington, S., & Wysocki, S. (2009). Nurse practitioner education: Keeping the academic pipeline open to meet family planning needs in the United States. *Contraception, 80*(5), 409–411.

Christensen, C., Bohmer, R., & Kenagy, J. (2000). Will disruptive innovations cure health care? *Harvard Business Review*. Retrieved February 9, 2012, from http://hbr.org/web/extras/insight-center/health-care/will-disruptive-innovations-cure-health-care

Ford, L. C. (2009). *Excerpts from pivotal moments in nursing: Leaders who changed the path of a profession*. Indianapolis, IN: Sigma Theta Tau International.

National Association of Nurse Practitioners in Women's Health (NPWH). (2011, October). *Stakeholder conference call convened by Susan Wysocki*. Washington, DC: Author.

National Association of Nurse Practitioners in Women's Health & Rand Corporation. (2011, July). *Internal survey*. Washington, DC: Author.

National Certification Corporation. (2009). *WHNP content validation task analysis study*. Retrieved February 9, 2012, from http://www.nccwebsite.org/resources/docs/09whnpcvfinal.pdf

National Certification Corporation. (2011). Retrieved from http://www.NCCnet.org

Way, F. (1995, Fall). *The education and utilization of nurse practitioners in women's health care*. Washington, DC: National Association of Nurse Practitioners in Reproductive Health (NANPRH).

CHAPTER ❖ **2**

GROWTH AND DEVELOPMENT OF WOMEN

Diane Marie Schadewald ◆ *Marcia Szmania Davis* ◆ *Ellis Quinn Youngkin*

Perhaps as more emphasis is given to female perspectives, society can move toward acceptance of power-with, rather than power-over, which would help facilitate a more peaceful environment on a larger scale. (Lewis & Bernstein, 1996)

Highlights

- Growth and Development
- Adult Developmental Theories
- Views on Women's Development
- Major Periods and Tasks: The Women's Perspective
- Women's Growth and Development and Family Theory

❖ INTRODUCTION

In order to define and understand women's development, one must consider the societal norms that prevail over time. One important change during the late 1960s and early 1970s was women's realization that many individual concerns they had previously been hesitant to discuss were actually widespread and political in nature. "The personal is political" slogan reflected an energy borne out in consciousness-raising groups where women talked about their lived experiences, learning that their innermost feelings were shared by women in general. A period of self-discovery ensued as women began to break out of socially constrictive stereotypes.

Earlier, in the 1950s, remarkable changes in women's lives were associated with fewer births, extended longevity, greater acceptance of lifestyle options in marriage and family formation, and attachment to the labor force (O'Rand & Henrette, 1982). Affirmative action movements eventually developed into academic programs in women's studies beginning in the 1960s (Grosskurth, 1991). These courses addressed limitations set on women by patriarchal societies and encouraged women to contemplate the reasons. The concept of *her*story versus *his*tory was introduced (Morgan, 1970). In the 21st century, a higher percentage of women, compared with their mother's generation, are better educated, spend more of their adult life living alone, and bear their first child at a later age or choose to remain childless (Cain, 2001). Women also participate more consistently in the labor force (Lyndon-Rochelle & Woods, 2008). In addition, there is a group between age 45 and 56 who are married, out of the workforce, and caring for both young children and elderly parents (Pierret, 2006).

Is the contemporary view of society toward women indeed different, however, from the past? The answer must be an equivocal yes, in part because traditional sex role stereotypes continue to pervade the thinking of many men and women. Women who do not marry and reproduce still may be viewed as having failed to develop their fullest potential. Moreover, femininity has long been, and to a great extent continues to be, equated with passivity, looking attractive, making relationships work, and being unselfish and of service while being competent without complaint (Levine, 2005; Pipher, 1994). As the 21st century progresses, women continue in a state of flux, where old role-restricting expectations have broken down but unfortunately have been replaced with new ideas that seem fragmentary, unrealistic, and often contradictory.

GROWTH AND DEVELOPMENT

Growth and development are often viewed according to a person's stage in the life cycle. Whereas *growth* refers to quantitative physical and physiological changes, *development* encompasses more qualitative changes, including functional, psychosocial, and cognitive behaviors. Both areas need to be assessed by health care providers in order to offer anticipatory guidance to women as they adapt to personal and environmental changes. Providers must understand contemporary women's roles and expectations as well as their stressors within a social context in order to assist women in developing health promotion behaviors (Lyndon-Rochelle & Woods, 2008). The developmental theories most closely linked to sequential ages and life stages have frequently been used for clinical evaluation. Controversy exists, however, about the applicability of such theories to women, particularly because cultural biases may be a problem. Also, developmental norms may not apply to all cultural backgrounds, and stage theories could promote ageism if one does not fulfill expectations, such as marriage, by a given point in life (Erikson, 1968; Norman, McCluskey-Fawcett, & Ashcroft, 2002). In the 21st century, the concept that one must achieve certain goals by a given age has become more fluid (Stassen Berger, 2010). Nevertheless, familiarity with these theories is helpful.

A growing body of knowledge is emerging regarding the impact of adverse childhood experiences (ACEs) both emotionally and physically later in life. Physical changes are thought to possibly extend to the epigenome and, therefore, to future generations. Assessment by clinicians to determine the presence and number of ACEs may become routine in order to evaluate potential problems with growth and development and plan appropriate intervention (Anda, Butchart, Felitti, & Brown, 2010). See Chapter 5 for more information about an assessment of ACEs and Appendix B for an assessment tool.

Today, women's lives are very complex. Numbers of different life cycles and lines of development exist, overlap, conflict, and perhaps enhance each other. Seiden (1989) whimsically referred to a "life pretzel" where the biologic-reproductive circle, the family-marital circle, and the educational-vocational circle are all bound together. Considering women's lives as a simple circle tied to a reproductive life cycle simply no longer suffices (if it ever did).

STAGE THEORIES OF DEVELOPMENT

Investigation of developmental change across the life span has gained prominence over the past 60 years, largely as a result of psychoanalytic influence. The resulting developmental theories emerged from the body of knowledge in child psychology. Although the life span developmental framework focused primarily on men, the resulting theories were generalized to apply to both sexes. Women's development, which was seldom alluded to, was viewed narrowly and judged aberrant if gender development did not conform to the accepted male pattern (Kaschak, 1981).

Characteristics commonly attributed to women, such as being less aggressive, more emotional, and less independent, were seen to be less healthy. Although the majority of psychoanalytic clients were women, little was known about their experiences as women. Virtually no attention was directed toward the effects of the societal environment on women. Feminists thus came to view traditional psychotherapy as an agent of social control, reinforcing traditional sex roles and traditional values and devaluing women.

HISTORICAL PSYCHOANALYTIC INFLUENCE

Freudian psychosexual theory and practice—the largest influence on psychotherapeutic knowledge—gave therapists a largely antifeminine orientation (Benjamin, 2004; Gilligan, 1982a; Hyde, 2007). Freud espoused that biological drives influence a person's psychological and personality development. In his view, superiority of men was largely derived from the possession of a penis. Penis envy purportedly led to feminine aggression. According to Freud, limitations of women inherent in their biology ("anatomy is destiny") included women's innate dependency, passivity, and masochism, which were required for their primary fulfilling role, successful motherhood. Compared with men, women were viewed as more narcissistic, more prone to jealousy, and having a weaker sense of justice (Strachey, 1961). Women were labeled "frigid" if they were incapable of mature (phallocentric) vaginal orgasm versus clitoral orgasm. The studies of Masters and Johnson proved this concept incorrect (Kaschak, 1981).

FEMINIST VIEWS ON PSYCHOANALYSIS

Critics condemned Freud for deriding women who displayed qualities that would be lauded in men, primarily boldness and independence (Grosskurth, 1991). Many women also voiced resentment toward the implied foreclosure on women's opportunities.

- Karen Horney (1920s and 1930s) proposed that if penis envy existed, it was because the penis symbolized the social and political power of men (Hyde, 2007).
- Simone de Beauvoir (*The Second Sex*, 1949) caused a great deal of controversy by challenging the ideation of biological and psychological determination of roles for women.
- Betty Friedan (*The Feminine Mystique*, 1963) attempted to broaden society's narrow role of women's place being in the home.
- Kate Millet (*Sexual Politics*, 1969) continued to scorn Freud for upholding the male body as the norm and questioned the validity of Freud's concept of female fear of castration while ignoring issues such as rape.
- Jessica Benjamin (*The Shadow of the Other*, 1998) argued that Freud's dichotomous view of passivity (feminine) versus activity (masculine) presents a false choice, leaves no room for coexistence of feminine and masculine traits within individuals, and devalues the strength of femininity.

ADULT DEVELOPMENTAL THEORIES

Although developmental changes during childhood and adolescence have been studied, Levinson (1986) maintained that relatively little attention had been paid to the adult years. The study of women's development to this day remains in its infancy, and the climate exists for an interdisciplinary approach to the study of human development.

ERIKSON'S STAGES OF PSYCHOSOCIAL DEVELOPMENT (1950S TO 1960S)

One of the earliest contributors to the study of adult development, Erikson (1950, 1968) suggested the normalcy and necessity of growth and change during adult years and not just in childhood. His theories, grounded in conceptions of the life cycle and the life course, addressed stages in ego development. According to Erikson,

- Each stage is primary at a particular age level, or segment of the life cycle, from infancy to old age.
- If a task that is appropriate to a given phase of life is not resolved, then development in subsequent phases of life may be impaired.
- A patterned sequence of stages occurs, each with appropriate physical, emotional, and cognitive tasks.
- A person who successfully passes through each stage eventually attains ego integrity, which is associated with high self-esteem and a positive outlook on life.
- A major difference for a woman is that her identity is enmeshed in a married state, wherein the task of her mate is to provide her with an adult identity, a necessary step in her mature integration of personality.

Erikson's eight stages of development, composed of bipolar tasks at various stages of life, include trust versus mistrust (infancy), autonomy versus shame and doubt (early childhood), initiative versus guilt (preschool age), industry versus inferiority (school age), identity versus identity diffusion (adolescence), intimacy versus isolation or self-absorption (young adulthood), generativity versus stagnation (middle adulthood), and integrity versus despair and disdain (late adulthood).

Erikson takes into account how biopsychosocial environment and culture impact development of the individual (Hoare, 2005). Slater (2003) further developed Erikson's stage of middle adulthood to illustrate how the stages before and after generativity versus stagnation can be operationalized within that stage. That is, trust versus mistrust reveals itself as inclusivity versus exclusivity, autonomy versus shame and doubt becomes pride versus embarrassment, initiative versus guilt changes to responsibility versus ambivalence, industry versus inferiority is career productivity versus inadequacy, identity versus identity diffusion appears as parenthood versus self-absorption, intimacy versus isolation becomes being needed versus alienation, and finally, ego integrity versus despair is honesty versus denial. These features, along with how development in Erikson's theory can be determined by life review or storytelling (Haber, 2006), were utilized as the framework for a study that examined middle-aged and older women of Amish, Appalachian, and Mormon cultures' expression of generativity versus stagnation through quilting (Cheek & Piercy, 2008). The women, through semistructured interview, shared how quilting was a way to pass something of meaning down, express caring, give back to the community, and feel a sense of belonging and value. The importance of interconnectivity in these women is noted.

The economic climate of the Great Recession, which began in 2007, posed many challenges in Erikson's developmental pathway, as reflected in adulthood. Loss of employment may have caused feelings of embarrassment and inadequacy for women or their spouses. Adding the challenges of caring for children and possibly elderly parents to the mix, as done by many women in the "sandwich generation" (Pierret, 2006), very likely further increased the potential for difficulties in successful completion of Erikson's developmental tasks. Utilizing Slater's (2003) adult operationalization of Erikson's categories may be helpful in reaching an understanding of how growth and development has been affected in these women. Time will reveal if there is a long-term impact and what the impact, if indeed it exists, will be on the various cohorts of women who experienced the challenges of the psychosocial environment of the Great Recession.

LEVINSON'S MODEL OF ADULT DEVELOPMENT (1970S TO 1990S)

This well-known model of adult development, grounded in psychoanalytic theory, is applied in research and psychotherapy (Levinson, 1978). Levinson proposed a single human life cycle through which both men and women evolve (the life structure). Tremendous variation exists related to gender, class, race, culture, historical epoch, specific circumstances, and genetics (Levinson, 1996). Levinson expanded on Erikson's notion of development and characterized each segment of adulthood in terms of intrinsic tasks (Erikson, 1950; Levinson, 1978, 1996). This theory contains an underlying set of developmental periods and tasks along with transition crises that involve reassessment of one's life. Adult development is seen as an evolving process of mutual interaction between self and the world, of which family and work are central components. Career choice and work are paramount in terms of goals, social roles, ethical standards and values, and development of self-concept. The assumption is that we desire self-actualization, which requires psychological and realistic changes in controllable measures. To this extent, men and women are similar.

Levinson uses a central concept of gender splitting, which views a sharp division between feminine and masculine permeating every aspect of human life from cultural to individual. Levinson (1996) also described the early stages of a vast historical transition where traditional patterns are eroding but satisfactory new ones have not been discovered and legitimized. (Women's adult development is addressed later in this chapter in Major Periods and Tasks: The Women's Perspective.) Levinson's stages are as follows.

Early Adult Transition (Ages 17 to 22)

The shaky start toward maturity involves taking new steps in individuation. Choices are made concerning career, lifestyle, and modification of existing family and social relationships. This is an era of greatest energy and abundance—and of greatest contradiction and stress.

Entering Adult World (Ages 22 to 28)

Through the establishment of an independent living situation, exploration, and commitment to adult roles, the 20s reflect structure building.

Age 30 Transition (Ages 28 to 33)

During the transition period, the sense of being young, especially in terms of options, is given up. Current lifestyles, values, family situations, and career choices are evaluated. Biologically, the 20s and 30s are the peak years of life.

Settling Down (Ages 33 to 40)

Affirming personal integrity, realizing oneself as a full-fledged adult, and goal achievement are characteristics of this period.

Midlife Transition (Ages 40 to 45)

Lifestyle is critically examined, and the need arises to recognize time limitations for goal achievement. Polarities, including young–old and destruction–creation, are integrated. Levinson believed that the character of living always changes appreciably between early and middle adulthood.

Entering Middle Adulthood (Ages 45 to 50)

Undergoing restabilization after midlife transition, individuals in middle adulthood have biological capacities below earlier years but normally are still sufficiently fit for energetic, personally satisfying, and socially valuable lives.

Age 50 Transition (Ages 50 to 55)

Once more, lifestyle and major goals are reevaluated.

Middle Adulthood Culmination (Ages 55 to 60)

Work continues toward achieving life goals and contributing to society.

Late Adulthood (Ages 60 and above) and Late Adult Transition (Ages 60 to 65)

Although the character of one's life is fundamentally altered as a result of biological, psychological, and social changes, the individual recognizes that this period can be distinctive and fulfilling.

Mitchell (2009) proposes that Levinson's developmental theory can be well utilized in counseling women who are seeking help during stressful times in their lives. In order to do this for older women, Mitchell has further developed the theory into the periods from 60 to 80 and 80 on. These later periods were never fully developed by Levinson. Late adulthood is the period from 60 to 80, and old age is the term proposed for the developmental period from 80 on. As during the transitions in other stages of life in Levinson's theory, during the transition to late adulthood, lifestyle and goals are reevaluated. Reflection on life's accomplishments along with a freedom to pursue an interest that was set aside because of other life responsibilities, such as childrearing and career development in the previous stage, can now occur. Spirituality, introspection, and new awareness of self arise (Levine, 2005; Mitchell, 2009). A woman in late adulthood may also find expression of herself in her home. The period from 80 on is less fully developed by Mitchell, but roughly consists of an active life review and a passing of the baton to younger generations.

VIEWS ON WOMEN'S DEVELOPMENT

WOMEN'S CONTRIBUTIONS

Women's influence has been less acknowledged in many areas, including art, literature, social sciences, and psychological research. Even though many women have devoted their lives to supporting the development of others, their development experiences are still essentially untold. Women's life experiences and viewpoints may indeed be different from men's as a result of complex factors such as social status, power, and reproductive biology (Gilligan, 1982a, 2002; Miller, 1986). Indeed, the lives of women make up a complex web of economic, psychological, and social contradictions. Opportunities in one area have been linked to constraints in others so that choices in one can have unexpected consequences (or benefits) many years later in another (Coogan & Chen, 2007; Orenstein, 2000).

Gilligan's Theory of Moral Development

Gilligan (1982a), a clinical psychologist, traced women's voices as she studied the development of morality. She found that existing psychological accounts failed to describe the progression of relationships toward a maturity of interdependence or trace the evolution of the capacity for responsible care. Gilligan (1982b) challenged Freud, Piaget, and Kohlberg, who studied boys and men and then assumed that women's ability to make moral judgments was inferior. Gilligan's (1982a) work asserts that

- Women have learned, from their early socialization, to place priority on responsibility toward others in important relationships (the ethics of care) rather than on individual welfare and concerns. Identity and intimacy are not separate stages of development for women.
- When faced with a dilemma, women are interested in understanding individual circumstances and in obtaining the best possible solution for all concerned, rather than using more abstract universal justice principles employed by men.
- The standard of moral judgment that women use for self-assessment also has to do with relationships: the ability to nurture, to care for others, and to bear responsibility.
- Women's differing modes of moral reasoning lead to different forms of self-definition and different views of relationships.

Gilligan's work was criticized as perpetuating gender stereotypes during the socially conservative 1980s (Mednick, 1989).

Bardwick's Model of Human Development

Bardwick's model addresses women's adult development while incorporating much of Levinson's model of adult maturation. Bardwick (1980) maintains that psychological growth and change are intertwined and never cease. Moreover, the goals and values of one's life reflect changing societal and cultural values. The transition from one developmental stage to the next includes a process of self-evaluation. For women, transitions to new values and lifestyles are likely to be more extreme and more emotionally volatile than in previous generations, as options provided to women become more numerous.

Bardwick defines the self in terms of dependent, interdependent, and egocentric mental stances. A woman may maintain a *dependent* sense of self, which is basically relational, or move toward a more *interdependent* stance, in which a sense of self exists simultaneously with a keen awareness of being a contributing and receiving member of an affectional relationship. Bardwick, however, contends that for a woman, developing a permanent *egocentric* stance is rare, because socialization of women in our society and the definition of femininity tend much more toward an interdependent or dependent sense of self.

A NEW PSYCHOLOGY OF WOMEN

Equality

In 1986, a new psychology of women was proposed by Miller based on the observation that caring for others is valued less in our society than individuation and individual achievement, leading to women's concern with relationships often being viewed as a weakness. Individuation and individual achievement remain greatly valued in our society. The need for social equality is reflected in problems that arise when affiliation and relationships are molded by domination and subordination. Miller advised that a new language in psychology should describe the structuring of women's sense of self, that is, the need to make and then maintain relationships. Caring and connection must be separated from the resulting inequality and oppression. A few decades past, women judged themselves in terms of their ability to care, so much so that professional and academic endeavors had the potential to be seen as jeopardizing their own sense of themselves (Gilligan, 1982a). Now, as women have increased their presence in many professional fields, their healthy sense of self is generally enhanced by such endeavors (Hyde, 2007). However, personal conflict may still arise when women have to choose between achievement and caring, especially if being successful is at the expense of another's failure.

Valuing Self

The psychology of women has been seen as distinct in relationships of temporary and permanent inequality (Gilligan, 1982b). Women are often seen as subordinate in social position to men, yet at the same time they are entwined with them in the intimate and intense relationships of adult sexuality and family life. Feminist therapy promotes the individual's recognition of restrictive social binds that have influenced many women, including an overdependence on men for self-esteem and financial, psychological, and social needs. In a small study, Hollis (1998) found that women, but not men, expressed regret and sometimes frustration toward perceived missed opportunities in life (e.g., career) due to confining social roles of wife and mother in decades ranging from the 1920s to the 1960s.

Today's women have many career opportunities open to them, and they are taking full advantage of such opportunities often by delaying childbearing in order to develop their career (Hyde, 2007; Shulman, 2006). Women traditionally have taken care of men, and men have tended to assume or devalue that care (Coogan & Chen, 2007; Gilligan, 1982a). More and more, men have begun to take on these caregiving roles, thus increasing their understanding of the value of such roles (Shulman, 2006). Women's psychology has reflected and continues to reflect both sides of relationships of interdependence.

Empowerment

Despite Hillary Clinton's 36 million cracks in the glass ceiling, the ceiling does continue to exist with women representing less than 1 percent of CEOs (Hyde, 2007). Miller (1986) maintained that women need power to advance their own development and to maintain an identity characterized by self-determination and a diminished need for continuous approval. To this day, too often women find their lives being dominated by prevalent societal values. Often, women and men experience enormous differences in access to power and control of resources (Lott, 1987), and for women, a stance of less power may result in an emphasis on relatedness to others and compassion (Mednick, 1989). Powerlessness, or learned helplessness, in femininity has been thought to be exhibited in relationships of battering and more subtly as depression (Friedan, 1993; Kaschak, 1981; Tolman, Impett, Tracy, & Michael, 2006). Perhaps as more emphasis is given to female perspectives, society can move toward a focus of power-with rather than power-over, which would help facilitate a more peaceful environment on a larger scale (Lewis & Bernstein, 1996). Mutuality in relationships may help foster efforts toward elimination of many social maladies such as violence against women and discrimination based on ethnicity and gender. Women could take significant steps toward healthier lives as stressors compromising many intimate affiliations diminish.

Many women have learned to demystify aspects of their lives, finding strength in the shared experiences of other women. Their strength is reflected in greater self-sufficiency, assertiveness, and self-knowledge (Levine, 2005). Consider the example of violence against women. Issues such as rape, battering of women, child sexual abuse, and incest were largely ignored, or their existence disbelieved, before the collected efforts of enraged women brought these issues into the public policy arena (Miller, 1986). Women have effected changes in medical/gynecologic care and no longer accept care that is limited to their reproductive organs to the exclusion of concerns such as cardiac disease or to the discounting of entities such as premenstrual syndrome (PMS), as was the case in the not-so-distant past.

A Different Starting Point in Defining Women's Development/Tend and Befriend

Women's development has often been described as related to their attachment to others. The cornerstone of one proposed new psychology of women is the appreciation of the power of relationship and connection in women's lives (Lewis & Bernstein, 1996). Women's sense of self, as well as their perceived strength, has been considered as based on the ability to form affiliations and relationships (Gilligan, 1982a; Lewis & Bernstein, 1996). Although experience of attachment to others provides women with more opportunities for interpersonal pleasure, there can be concurrent fear of separation. Many women perceive the threat of a disrupted affiliation as a total loss of self.

Along a similar vein, findings of a landmark study out of UCLA (Taylor et al., 2000) strengthen women's sense of value of friendship and affiliation. Women's response to stress may not be well characterized by the fight-or-flight response. Women's stress responses have developed to enhance survival of themselves and their offspring. Females create, maintain, and utilize social groups (befriend), particularly their female friends, in order to manage stressful situations, building on the attachment–caregiving process. Women also nurture their offspring (tend), while in turn reducing neuroendocrine responses that may compromise their health.

The tend-and-befriend behavior is thought to be oxytocin mediated, moderated by sex hormones and endogenous opioid peptide mechanisms. It is well known that animals as well as humans derive health benefits from social contact. Positive physical contact such as touching or hugging is known to release oxytocin, which further counters stress and produces a calming effect. The fact that men and women respond differently to stress has significant implication for health. Perhaps women need to find more time to partake of each other's nurturance and healing talk, rather than let other responsibilities close those ties (Apter & Josselson, 2000; Levine, 2005).

THE WAYS THAT WOMEN KNOW

In the 1980s, the intellectual development of women became another topic of study (Belenky & Field, 1985; Belenky, Clinchy, Goldberger, & Tarule, 1997). Inability of women to gain a voice may be seen as reflective of being powerless, subjugated, and inadequate. More women than men pose questions, listen to others, and refrain from speaking out (Jack, 1991). For example, a mother may refrain from sharing ideas too quickly with her child in order to foster the child's own ability to form ideas. This mode of discourse, similar to Socratic thinking, was thought to serve as a model for promoting development (Rosenblatt, 1995).

Women today are in general more assertive than in the 1980s. However, the findings of Belenky and colleagues may still be reflective of an approach to thinking and communication by women that is different than the approach taken by men and not in fact reflective of lack of power. Hyde (2007) maintains that such gender differences in communication style are small when they exist and possibly not interrupting reflects more politeness in women's communication tendencies rather than a lack of power.

WOMEN'S ISSUES AND CONFLICTING VALUES

Value Changes

The value changes that occurred most dramatically during the 1970s redefined and expanded choices for women in their roles related to work and family (Bardwick, 1980). Many women now address both modern and traditional patterns of lifestyle in their decision making. Facing conflicting life choices, societal norms, and changing economies, women continue to grapple with cultural ambiguity and personal uncertainty. Traditional norms regarding femininity prevail in many instances, even for women in less traditional roles. For example, despite reduced gender separation of work and family roles, couples still tend to make decisions concerning geographical locations and timing of major family events according to the husband's career needs. On the other hand, women are choosing to have fewer children. This fact, combined with increasing longevity, means that a substantially shorter percentage of women's lives are spent childrearing. Also, with a lower marriage rate, later marriage, divorce, and widowhood, today's women spend more of their lives alone than in any previous era (Orenstein, 2000; Trimberger, 2005).

Cultural Ambiguity and Personal Uncertainty

Although choices women face can create ambiguity and uncertainty, the freedom of choice is perhaps less frustrating than the restrictions of the past (Bardwick, 1980). Often, however, change may be an illusion for women; the reality of the social foundation of power still leans strongly toward enhanced status for traditional feminine values (Mednick, 1989; Orenstein, 2000). Modern women also face significant challenges to have it all because the social changes necessary to allow for ample choices have not been resolved. Although passage of the Lilly Ledbetter law regarding pay equity has been helpful, barriers still exist to equitable pay, adequate childcare, and breaking through old boy networks. Women may have adequate drive to achieve; however, they may feel limited to a level of achievement that society deems appropriate for their gender difference or, some would argue, their social status. Conflict may arise between the need for affiliation or the desire for approval from other people and the pursuit of achievement for its own sake. Competition may be viewed as contrary to the traditional feminine ideal and may lead to social rejection. Although women and men tend to be compared favorably in neutral situations, women tend to have less internal hope for success in more competitive situations (Orenstein, 2000). A particular dilemma for women has been to achieve success in a traditionally male occupation or to achieve career success when contemplating motherhood. Economic and logistical demands (e.g., childcare and eldercare) often find women slipping into more traditional roles (Hewlett, 2007; Orenstein, 2000).

Gender Issues

Levinson (1986, 1996) maintained that the timing of developmental periods and tasks is similar for women and men, while giving weight to how men's and women's lives are affected by gender-splitting issues, creating in human life a rigid division between male and female, masculine and feminine. Though the concept that women and men have lived in different social worlds with very different social roles, identities, and psychological attributes persists, the dramatic socioeconomic changes of the 2000s have created constrictions for men, which have increased the opportunities for both genders to move into the other's sphere or social role.

The historical process within postindustrial conditions has included a gender revolution. Many social changes reduced women's involvement in the family and increased involvement in outside work. Some of these changes include (1) the sharp rise in human longevity; (2) the decreasing demand for women's work in the family, concomitant with smaller family size (contraception options); and (3) the growing incidence of divorce. Nearly 60 percent of all U.S. women are now in the labor force—part-time or full-time, paid or volunteer, continuously or sporadically (Bureau of Labor Statistics [BLS], 2009).

Other developmental themes hold that gender differences exist in movement through developmental periods (Bardwick, 1980; Caffarella & Olson, 1993; Hyde, 2007; Mercer, Nichols, & Doyle, 1989). Women's self-esteem and identity have also been described as dependent more heavily on validation by others (Bardwick, 1980).

Life Events, Options, and Stress

Along with more options, women may also experience discontent and/or stress, as it may be less clear what is expected of them. Stressors occur in traditional homemaker choices, in career options, in childcare, in eldercare, and in attempts to combine or juggle it all. In addition, women may experience developmental periods at later ages and in more irregular sequences, while focusing on different aspects of their life structure (Mercer et al., 1989; Stassen Berger, 2010). Moreover, developmental tasks may be dealt with very differently at different times, as women themselves may change psychologically over time.

MAJOR PERIODS AND TASKS: THE WOMEN'S PERSPECTIVE

A body of knowledge on women's development has been presented and continues to evolve, although it is not as well formed as some other developmental areas. Issues in women's development are discussed here, using Levinson's framework, where feasible, and other authors' contributions that have remained valid over time, including those of Bardwick (1980). The novice phase of early adulthood—individuals as apprentice adults, ages 17 to 33—encompasses several large tasks, including forming a dream, a mentor relationship, an occupation, and an enduring relationship. Women and men may have significant differences in accomplishing these tasks (Roberts & Newton, 1987). Timing of major life events is not as important as understanding the importance in forming the life structure. A discussion of key transition periods follows. Newer data is added where relevant to the discussion.

EARLY ADULT TRANSITION/ EMERGING ADULTHOOD (AGES 17 TO 22/25)

Major tasks for women in this period include value assessment; goal setting for education and work; formation of important peer relationships that focus on sex, love, and commitment; formation of relationships to occupation; and separation from parents. However, today's emerging adults are more likely to receive help from their parents for educational expenses or rent (Pew Research Center, 2007). Pipher (1994) described young women's need to reject the person they most closely identify with as they grow up. They have a tremendous fear of becoming like their mothers, and yet, in a way if a young woman hates her mother, she hates herself. Strong girls may manage to stay close to their families and maintain some family loyalty, usually having someone in the family whom they love and trust. The task is not to end the relationship, but rather to reject certain aspects (e.g., submission and defiance), sustain more valued aspects, and build in new qualities such as mutual respect (Levinson, 1996). Individuation may be reflected in great differences in values between parents and young adults in areas such as politics and career choices. Values may more strongly reflect identification with peer groups, however, than true individuation or autonomy. Pipher noted girls may stay in adolescence longer now, taking about 12 years to make it through the crucible (age 22). Economics may be one reason; however, home may seem a safe haven in an increasingly dangerous world.

A major conflict exists between making commitments and avoiding them in order to keep options open (Erikson, 1968). Commitments are more easily made if one's peers are doing so. The early adult is often egocentric as she progresses through rapid emotional and physical changes.

Gender Identity

A crucial task is to internalize a sense of gender, which encompasses a sense of one's body in relation to sexuality. A great deal of psychological fluidity exists with some sense of egocentrism. Today's emerging adult women have been found to identify with more masculine traits of self-reliance, assertiveness, and ambition than their predecessors who came of age at the dawning of the second wave of the women's movement. Their identification with feminine traits, however, remains unchanged (Strough, Leszczynski, Neely, Flinn, & Margrett, 2007). Therefore, masculine traits have been added to gender identity for the emerging adult woman but not at the diminution of feminine traits. The need to form relationships continues to dominate. For example, a woman may fear that her own ambitions will cost a relationship. A conflict exists between fulfillment of egocentric, self-reliant, and interpersonal/dependent priorities as the early adult tries to define the sense of self.

Identity and Adult Commitments

Erikson (1968) describes the male adolescent as developing an autonomous, initiating, and industrious self through the forging of an identity based on the ideal image—ability to support and justify adult commitments. He describes the female adolescent as holding her identity in abeyance while preparing to attract the man she will marry and by whose status she will be defined. Such attitudes predominated well into the 1960s. Pipher (1994) describes our culture as look obsessed. Body objectification by female adolescents has been associated with increased risks for problems with self-esteem and depression (Tolman et al., 2006). Despite advances of feminism, escalating levels of sexism and violence against women and girls exist. Sexual harassment can begin in elementary school. Girls face undervaluement of their intelligence and low self-esteem. Girls remain prey to depression/suicide attempts and eating disorders as well as addictions now more than ever (Orenstein, 2011). Media images of thin bodies as the ideal may play a role in this (Grabe, Ward, & Hyde, 2008). Many women, however, have emerged as breadwinners in their own right, often choosing professions once thought of as strictly in the man's domain (Hyde, 2007; Orenstein, 2000).

Identity and Intimacy

For men, identity precedes intimacy and generativity in the traditional view of the optimum cycle of human separation and attachment. For women, these tasks have been seen as fused, developing together as the woman comes to know herself as she is known, primarily through her relationships with others (Gilligan, 1982a). Vocation or career identity is often in an exploration phase with young women of today either changing jobs frequently or if in college taking time to settle on a major (Stassen Berger, 2010). Many emerging adults satisfy their needs for intimacy outside of marriage with friendships, family, or lovers. Cohabitation is much more common than marriage for this age group (Hyde, 2007; Stassen Berger, 2010).

Factors Influencing Identity

For women, identity and intimacy are developed at the same time (Gilligan, 1982a). Identity development in women is influenced by communion, connection, relation (to friends and all significant others), embeddedness, spirituality, and affiliation (Josselson, 1987). In addition, in order to keep their true selves and grow into healthy adults, girls need the above as well as meaningful work, respect, challenges, and physical and psychological safety (Pipher, 1994). Online social media began to play a role in identity development with the debut of MySpace and Facebook. Research regarding the impact of these social media sites on self-esteem has to date revealed both positive and negative outcomes for both emerging adult women and men (Gonzales & Hancock, 2011; Mehdizadeh, 2010; Rosen, 2011). Exactly what impact online media will have on identity over time is not entirely clear.

Identity and Parenthood

Motherhood is perceived by some as central to women's sense of femininity, far more so than marriage (Orenstein, 2000). Whereas the choice to remain childless is being intentionally made by many at this stage of life, single parenthood is chosen by others (Cain, 2001; Maier, 2007). Safer (1996), a psychologist, found most women see children as a source of fulfillment and not as an obstacle to it. Yet large studies show childless couples can be as happy as parents who have good relationships with their children and certainly happier than those whose relationships have distanced.

ENTRY LIFE STRUCTURE FOR EARLY ADULTHOOD (AGES 22/25 TO 28)

Life structures for women tend to be less stable than those for men, essentially because of more diverse concerns involving marriage, motherhood, and career. The primary tasks of this period are to build and maintain a first adult life structure and to enrich one's life within that structure.

Women, especially working women or those with difficult infants, experience appreciably more change than men if in the transition to parenthood (McBride, 1990). They also experience the contagion of stress as they internalize the distress experienced by those to whom they are closest, particularly family members. During this period, however, if work serves as a visible marker of achievement, it may lessen stress. Indeed, women with multiple roles may be the most well adjusted. A supportive family buffers a woman from endless demands of childcare and other family responsibilities.

AGE 30 TRANSITION AND THE SETTLING DOWN PERIOD OF EARLY ADULTHOOD (AGES 28 TO 39)

Both sexes in settling down must give up the idea that involvements are tentative. Priorities of the 20s may be reversed; choices and their consequences may be reassessed, and options regarding marriage and especially childbearing may be considered more pressing or not to exist much longer at the later stages of early adulthood (Hewlett, 2002; Levinson, 1986). A bewildering discovery occurring at about age 30 is that the life one has arduously constructed has major imperfections and that there is still some growing up to do (Levinson, 1996).

- *Men's Success.* Success in work is imperative to men's timetable. A shift in centrality by men—from work to family—may be a reaction to a combination of stress, age, or failure in work. Men sever ties with mentors in order to be seen as knowledgeable and successful in their own right of becoming one's own man (Levinson, 1986).
- *Women's Success.* In contrast, few women would define becoming one's own woman primarily through success in their work (Bardwick, 1980). Those who are successful in their careers may be anxious about their femininity unless they are also involved in significant relationships and have experienced motherhood. Women previously sacrificed success in careers and financial status as they compromised to maintain relationships while slipping into traditional roles (Orenstein, 2000). However, this sacrificial choice is now being addressed by changes in the corporate world that are designed to make reentry into the workforce easier and, hopefully, this compromise obsolete (Hewlett, 2007). Sadness and depression may develop from self-silencing if women suppress their authentic selves and make repeated compromises (Jack, 1991). A woman's success includes becoming more fully adult by dealing with the child in herself and with the old cultural assumption that an adult female is still a girl (Levinson, 1996).
- *Prolonged Transition.* Women in their 30s are likely to experience a more prolonged and profound transition period than men are, perhaps most importantly linked to the age limits for childbearing (the biological clock). Technology may permit some women to become pregnant well beyond their earlier expectations; however, these expectations may be unrealistic (Hewlett, 2002). During the period of evaluation and reappraisal (ages 28 to 33), married women may demand that husbands recognize and accommodate their aspirations and interests outside of the home (Orenstein, 2000; Roberts & Newton, 1987).
- *Career Versus Family.* Women reappraise the relative importance of career and family, often adding the missing component rather than reversing priorities (e.g., a mother may begin a career). A second-guessing of priorities is frequently present (Hewlett, 2007; Orenstein, 2000). Women may attempt to lead a life in which they do it all. The mental health stressors of women's multiple roles may be influenced more by marital factors than by work factors. Work often buffers some marital stress, but parenthood exacerbates occupational stress, especially if responsibilities are not shared in the home (McBride, 1990).

Hewlett (2002) warned that when women embrace a male model of single-minded career focus, they may encounter a "creeping nonchoice" in future motherhood. Unfortunately, many women do not realize that after age 30 their chances of becoming pregnant begin to decline. Women in the past feared that by slowing down their careers to have children, they would run the risk of never catching up. As mentioned previously, this fear has a realistic historical basis, but is being addressed by the Center for Work-Life Policy with some recommendations for greater flexibility for workforce reentry being brought forward (Hewlett, 2007). However, time to form meaningful relationships can be limited by work factors when a focus on productivity predominates over balance.

Recent census data shows childlessness doubling in the past several years so that one in five women between the ages of 40 and 44 is childless. Twenty-four percent of those of the same age with professional degrees are childless. This is an increase in the fertility rate for professional women as compared in 1994, when the childless rate for professional women was 47 percent. Certainly, many of these women choose not to have children (Cain, 2001; Maier, 2007). Hewlett's figures from 2002 showed that 14 percent made this choice, while the others had the choice made for them by delaying attempting to conceive until they became too old to conceive.

- *Multiple Roles.* Having multiple roles may counterbalance some negative effects of a particular role. Thus, the healthiest women and men may be those with multiple roles, including having a career, a spouse, and often children (Barnett & Hyde, 2001). Employment status accounted for most of the variance in psychological well-being for women aged 35 to 55. Married women with children and high prestige jobs reported the greatest well-being. However, "having it all" may mean "doing it all," and women may experience strain in attempting to fulfill multiple role obligations. Women's ability to cope with the stresses has been associated with having a high income and job satisfaction, marrying later, and arranging time for family activities (McBride, 1990).
- *American Values and Women's Sexuality.* The U.S. culture values youth and beauty, and often by age 35, a woman is no longer considered young. However, as the percentage of the population in the United States over the age of 30 has begun to increase and midlife women have begun to see themselves as more vibrant (Shulman, 2006), a decreased emphasis on these cultural values of youth and beauty may be emerging.
- *Confusing Choices.* Women in their 30s and 40s have grown up with mothers and other role models who have experienced the growing influence of feminist thinking and more egalitarian life patterns. The demands and needs of motherhood in this half-changed world are extremely complicated whether a woman works full-time or part-time, or stays at home.
- *Readjustment in the 30s.* Demographically, many women now in their 30s have never married. The percentage of never-married women between the ages of 25 and 34 was around 46 in 2009. However, that does not mean that these women are childless because 41 percent of births are now to single women (Mather & Lavery, 2010). As married women reach ages 35 to 40, their husbands' tremendous involvement in their own careers and children's decreasing dependence on them may provide the opportunity for personal change. Women may return to work or school or look for other relationships in the community. Family members may initially agree to change their lifestyles in order to accommodate the women's needs; however, when changes impact them directly, they may become resentful or confused.
- *Stress.* Stress is inherent in the reality or the illusion of choice. Some women may sacrifice personal relationships to achieve career success; others may be doing it all with very little support from their partners. Partners' expectations of each other in their relationship are not always clear. For married women, responsibilities outside the home—community and career involvement—may help them become less dependent economically, socially, and psychologically. Most women in this age group tend toward interdependence.

MIDLIFE TRANSITION AND MIDDLE ADULTHOOD (AGES 39 TO 60)

An appreciable change in the character of living occurs between early and middle adulthood. The main tasks of entering middle adulthood are making crucial choices, giving those choices meaning and commitment, and building a life structure around them (Levinson, 1986).

Midlife Transitions

- Assessment for both men and women may have a sense of urgency as they wish to accomplish their life goals. Those who do not assess their lives at this point may feel frightened and unable to make changes in their lifestyles or careers. Men assess what they receive and what they give to work, family, friends, and community as they reach the symbolically powerful age of 40 (Levinson, 1978, 1986). Their established autonomy now allows greater compassion, more reflection, less tyranny by inner conflicts and external demands, and more genuine love of self and others. Middle-aged men may experience this as their fullest and most creative period.

  By the end of middle adulthood, problems may include declining health, aging or death of parents, spousal death, and stagnation at work with no viable options. Although the relationship with one's spouse may only be comfortable, the option of ending it means losing crucial roots. Nonetheless, divorce has increased markedly for both men and women in their 40s. One may see a partner as a reason for discontent or as someone to blame for perceived losses. A new relationship may be viewed as a way to recoup the feelings and pleasure of youth.

- Women and men become more autonomous as they age, but women gain in larger increments (Goode, 1999; Levine, 2005). Becoming involved in a career after 40 can be an opportunity for real beginnings, but it also can be frightening. This may be a time for women to generate new values internally, reflecting who they are rather than what they do.
- Losses or adjustments in relationships may cause depression in women beginning the midlife phase; they may experience loneliness as children leave home or they become widowed or divorced. Women, but not men, tend to define their age status in terms of the timing of events within their family; even unmarried career women may discuss middle age in terms of the family they might have had (Orenstein, 2000). Women with more complex lives may experience sadness and joy in this time of readjustment as they face losses along with new beginnings. Many more men than women remarry at this age. The past four decades have seen a 40 percent decline in women's remarrying after divorce. They are now more economically independent and may no longer see marriage as their best option (Orenstein, 2000).
- Although women may feel dismay over excessive value placed on their appearance, including its damaging impact on young girls, they may also feel invisible as their looks change, and men may not notice them as they did in the past. Use of cosmetic surgery and other methods to look younger is on the rise (Lachman, 2004). Yet as women reach their 40s, they reach more toward something deeper: an authentic personal voice. At this time, women start viewing their life by how much is left to live (Lachman, 2004; Lachman & James, 1997; Levine, 2005).

A majority of women have made a reality transition, as evidenced by a high employment rate. The expansion of activities, as well as maturing and increased self-confidence, leads many of these women to be more interdependent rather than dependent.

Middle Adulthood

Although Levinson's studies ended with men and women in their 40s, he believed that a major transition phase occurs from ages 50 to 55. According to Levinson (1978, 1986), a stable period follows from ages 55 to 60, during which rejuvenation in some can result in achieving significant fulfillment and enrichment. This period of fulfillment and enrichment has all but disappeared for many women and men in this age group during the economic uncertainty, high unemployment, and shrinkage of the middle class that began to occur in the United States in the beginning of the 21st century. For men, especially whose connection with others depends largely on their jobs, job loss or forced early retirement may be associated with a loss of prestige and decreased self-esteem. During the Great Recession, women in this age range may have experienced fewer problems with unemployment and forced retirement than men, similar to what occurred in the Great Depression of the 1930s, when women at times became the only breadwinner in the family (Boehm, 2004). However, women faced and continue to face concerns about job loss, decrease in wages, loss of health benefits, and whether they will have Social Security (National Economic Council [NEC], 2010). As the economic climate improves, such concerns will hopefully diminish.

Over past decades, middle adulthood women tended to face loss much earlier than men of this age group if their primary role in life was that of mother, their secondary role that of homemaker, and their tertiary role that of sexual partner. As family becomes less central to women's lives, other sources of satisfaction can become significant. Often, the marital relationship has to be modified as women strive to create better lives for themselves. Accomplishments in careers may not bring the same satisfaction or sense of accomplishment as in earlier years (Belenky, Clinchy, Goldberger, & Tarule, 1986; Orenstein, 2000).

- The aging process traditionally has been symbolized as retirement for men and menopause for women, although the formerly predominant all negative views regarding menopause have been challenged (Friedan, 1993; Sheehy, 2006). Anticipating menopause is often more dreadful than the difficulty experienced with its actual occurrence. Women often feel relief with the loss of menses as well as the loss of tasks associated with rearing young children. The real difficulty may be adjusting to the aging process—a continuum that does not just begin after menses ends. Other changes associated with aging are socially more apparent, such as graying hair and wrinkles. Bifocal glasses and hearing aids may be a threat to self-esteem and a visible admission of aging, which may cause problems in intimate relationships. Yet physical changes may be a liberating process, allowing women to reclaim lost parts of themselves, reviving connections to family, work, and community and, finally, to a more authentic sense of self (Levine, 2005; Orenstein, 2000). Interestingly, another change that occurs around menopause is a growth spurt of myelination of cells in the hippocampus similar to, but to a lesser extent than, the spurt that occurs in adolescence, possibly promoting further maturation and integration of emotional and cognitive processes in the menopausal woman (Benes, 1998; Levine, 2005). Perhaps the wisdom of aging!

- "The sandwich generation" refers to the women who are caregivers for their children as well as for their aging parents. Depression, anxiety, and fatigue may result as women may neglect their own needs (Murray & Bachman, 2000; Pierret, 2006).

Aging is a gradual process, and changes of aging are adaptive across the life span. During middle age, women may to some extent lose their roles of mother and sex partner, especially through divorce or death. A partner's retirement may force another adaptation. Distancing from parents in the middle years is replaced by establishing a commitment for parents' care, which allows some women who see themselves primarily as homemakers to reestablish that lifestyle.

- Women in middle adulthood years may feel the need to change or reassess values or direction at this stage in their lives; others will reject new values, believing themselves incapable of achieving different goals. Women most at risk for psychological dependence are traditional housewives who lack involvement or outside commitments. Interdependence is more likely to occur among older women who have found fulfillment in their traditional roles and who have assumed varied roles, whether through employment or other options. Some older women are egocentric as a result of being widows, divorced, or displaced homemakers, or having never married.
- Societal views of aging women include negative stereotypes such as being inactive, unhealthy, asexual, unattractive, and ineffective—despite the diversity of older women who lead interesting, productive lives (Lott, 1987). The baby boomers are determined to refute these views. Friedan (1993) addressed our denial of the personhood of age, with its definition ensuring the blackout of people over 50 as sexual beings, especially women. Widowed or divorced women may yearn for an intimate, sexual relationship. They may be hampered in moving beyond sexual measures of themselves in their youth. In fact, there may be an intimacy that may be possible only as we age. Health care providers need to recognize the diversity among women as they age. Older women receive messages that growing older is a process to be prevented (with face lifts or antiaging facial creams) rather than to be enjoyed. Even professional women view aging as a serious impairment. Discrimination in employment is particularly harmful for women reentering the workforce after their children leave home or when the loss of a spouse decreases their income and security (see information about the Center for Work-Life Policy) (Hewlett, 2007). Throughout adulthood, women are increasingly threatened by poverty as a result of greater numbers of female-headed households and the continuing disparity in salaries between men and women. Older women are particularly affected by inadequate spousal retirement plans, especially if they themselves have a history of unemployment. As women live longer, they have more opportunity to develop illness, another stress on their finances.

YOUNG-OLD TRANSITION (AGES 60 TO 70)

Ages 60 to 65 mark the end of middle life and entry into the late adult transition (Levinson, 1996). Overall, women feel good about themselves and what they are accomplishing as they use time freed by retirement or other life changes to pursue creative activities, community work, and self-development (Mercer et al., 1989). Many older women are beginning to embrace what they can't change in regard to their aging bodies and balance this by employing health-promoting exercise to increase vitality (Levine, 2005). Women's presence in the labor force has increased dramatically. In 2009, about 12.6 percent of women over age 65 were working (BLS, 2009). Yet higher poverty rates exist among older women. Women have substantial involvement in unpaid work, specifically caregiving and home labor, and suffer from discriminatory retirement policies. When women outlive their husbands, creativity may develop as a response to loss and loneliness, including social and emotional isolation. Women may also return to creative activities they enjoyed in earlier years. During their 60s, women are most likely to experience transitions relating to their own illness and the illness and death of significant others.

OLD-OLD ADULT AND OLDEST-OLD ADULT WOMEN

Women can expect to live well into their 70s and 80s. Ages 76 to 80 may represent a transition toward wisdom as women are challenged to adapt to a number of changes, including loss of health, friends, and family (Mercer et al., 1989). Women are more likely than men to experience chronic illness in later life. Bodily restrictions may impede social and personal activities leading to lowered self-esteem. Yet the importance of body image may decrease with age as women accept natural changes with aging (Hurd, 2000). A surge of creativity may continue as women find pleasurable ways to enrich their lives. Relationships and affiliation with others remain important for women, and their creativity may take the form of altruistic responses to the needs of others. Successful or creative aging may be associated with maintaining meaningful activities, keeping close relationships with persons of all ages, and remaining flexible and adaptable. Nonconformists who are willing to take risks and who sustain a positive outlook on life perhaps experience the greatest success in aging. Psychological development never ends as long as the individual engages in reality; thus, the potential for growth and change is always present.

WOMEN'S GROWTH AND DEVELOPMENT AND FAMILY THEORY

Family developmental theory is important to consider when discussing women's growth and development. Family theory takes fully into account how interpersonal relationships with changing structures, roles, and processes impact an individual's growth and development over time. Bioecological theories, such as Bronfenbrenner's Bioecological Systems, or systems theories, such as Family Systems Theory, based on von Bertalanffy's work, have been useful in development of family assessment tools. Carter and McGoldrick have revised the original work of Duvall and Duvall and Miller's Developmental and Family Life Cycle to better reflect the modern family's stages of development (Kaakinen, Gedaly-Duff, Coehlo, & Hanson, 2010). This updated theory, along with Family Systems Theory, has influenced the continued evolution of Wright and Leahy's Calgary Family Assessment Model (CFAM) (2009) described in Chapter 5. CFAM has been widely used as a tool for family assessment both nationally and internationally.

A woman's growth and development cannot be considered in isolation. Inclusion of family assessment with a fluid definition of family is a way to avoid this isolation. Evolution to a more interconnected world demands this broader consideration.

REFERENCES

Anda, R.F., Butchart, A., Felitti, V.J., & Brown, D.W. (2010). Building a framework for global surveillance of the public health implications of adverse childhood experiences. *American Journal of Preventive Medicine, 39*(1), 93–98.

Apter, T.E., & Josselson, R. (2000). *Best friends: The pleasures and perils of girls' and women's friendships.* New York: Crown Publishing.

Bardwick, J.M. (1980). The seasons of a woman's life. In D.G. McGuigan (Ed.), *Women's lives: New theory, research, and policy.* Ann Arbor: University of Michigan, Center for Continuing Education of Women.

Barnett, R.C., & Hyde, J.S. (2001). Women, men, work, and family: An expansionist theory. *American Psychologist, 56*(10), 781–796.

Belenky, M.F., & Field, M. (1985). Epistemological development and the politics of talk in family life. *Journal of Education, 167*(3), 9–27.

Belenky, M.F., Clinchy, B., Goldberger, N., & Tarule, J. (1986). *Women's ways of knowing. The development of self, voice, and mind.* New York: Basic Books.

Belenky, M.F., Clinchy, B., Goldberger, N., & Tarule, J. (1997). *Women's ways of knowing: The development of self, voice, and mind.* Tenth Anniversary Edition. New York: Basic Books.

Benes, F.M. (1998). Brain development, VII human brain growth spans decades. *American Journal of Psychiatry, 155*(11), 1480.

Benjamin, J. (1998). *The shadow of the other: Intersubjectivity and gender in psychoanalysis.* New York: Routledge.

Benjamin, J. (2004). Deconstructing femininity: Understanding "passivity" and the daughter position. *Annual of Psychoanalysis, 32*, 45–57.

Boehm, L.K. (2004). Women, impact of the great depression on. In R.S. McElvaine (Ed.), *Encyclopedia of the great depression.* Farmington Hill, MI: Macmillan Reference USA.

Bureau of Labor Statistics (BLS). (2009). Table 1. In *Women in the labor force: A databook.* Retrieved August 10, 2011, from http://www.bls.gov/cps/wlf-databook-2010.pdf

Caffarella, R.S., & Olson, S.K. (1993). Psychosocial development of women: A critical review of the literature. *Adult Education Quarterly, 43*(3), 125–151.

Cain, M. (2001). *The childless revolution: What it means to be childless today.* Cambridge, MA: Perseus Publishing.

Cheek, C., & Piercy, K.W. (2008). Quilting as a tool in resolving Erikson's adult stage of human development. *Journal of Adult Development, 15*, 13–24.

Coogan, P.A., & Chen, C.P. (2007). Career development and counselling for women: Connecting theories to practice. *Counselling Psychology Quarterly, 20*(2), 191–204.

de Beauvoir, S. (1949). *The second sex.* New York: Random House.

Erikson, E.H. (1950). *Childhood and society.* New York: Norton.

Erikson, E.H. (1968). *Identity, youth and crises.* New York: Norton.

Friedan, B. (1963). *The feminine mystique.* New York: Norton.

Friedan, B. (1993). *The fountain of age.* New York: Simon & Shuster.

Gilligan, C. (1982a). *In a different voice: Psychological theory and women's development.* Cambridge, MA: Harvard University Press.

Gilligan, C. (1982b). New maps of development: New visions of maturity. *American Journal of Orthopsychiatry, 52*(2), 199–212.

Gilligan, C. (2002). *The birth of pleasure.* New York: Alfred A. Knopf.

Gonzales, A.L., & Hancock, J.T. (2011). Mirror, mirror on my Facebook wall: Effects of exposure to Facebook on self-esteem. *Cyberpsychology, Behavior, and Social Networking, 14*(1–2), 79–83.

Goode, E. (1999, February 16). New study finds middle age is prime of life. *New York Times*, p. D6.

Grabe, S., Ward, L.M., & Hyde, J.S. (2008). The role of the media in body image concerns among women: A meta-analysis of experimental and correlational studies. *Psychological Bulletin, 134*(3), 460–476.

Grosskurth, P. (1991). The new psychology of women. *New York Review of Books, 38*(17), 25–32.

Haber, D. (2006). Life review: Implementation, theory, research, and therapy. *International Journal on Aging and Human Development, 63*(2), 153–171.

Hewlett, S.A. (2002). *Creating a life: Professional women and the quest for children.* New York: Talk Miramax Books.

Hewlett, S.A. (2007). *Off-ramps and on-ramps: Keeping talented women on the road to success.* Boston: Harvard Business School Press.

Hoare, C.H. (2005). Erikson's general and adult developmental revisions of Freudian thought: "Outward, forward, upward." *Journal of Adult Development, 12*(1), 19–31.

Hollis, L.A. (1998). Sex comparisons in life satisfaction and psychosocial adjustment scores with an older adult sample: Examining the effect of sex role differences in older cohorts. *Journal of Women and Aging, 10*(3), 59–77.

Hurd, L.C. (2000). Older women's body image and embodied experience: An exploration. *Journal of Women and Aging, 12*(3/4), 77–97.

Hyde, J.S. (2007). *Half the human experience: The psychology of women* (7th ed.). Florence, KY: Cengage Learning.

Jack, D. (1991). *Silencing the self: Women and depression.* Cambridge, MA: Harvard University Press.

Josselson, R. (1987). *Finding herself: Pathways to identity development in women.* San Francisco: Jossey-Bass.

Kaakinen, J.R., Gedaly-Duff, V., Coehlo, S.P., & Hanson, S.M.H. (2010). *Family health care nursing: Theory, practice and research* (4th ed.). Philadelphia: F. A. Davis Company.

Kaschak, E. (1981). Feminist psychotherapy: The first decade. In S. Cox (Ed.), *Female psychology* (pp. 387–401). New York: St. Martin's Press.

Lachman, M.E. (2004). Development in midlife. *Annual Reviews in Psychology, 55,* 305–331.

Lachman, M.E., & James, J.B. (Eds.). (1997). *Multiple paths to midlife development.* Chicago: University of Chicago.

Levine, S.B. (2005). *Inventing the rest of our lives: Women in second adulthood.* New York: Viking.

Levinson, D.J. (1978). *The seasons of a man's life.* New York: Alfred A. Knopf.

Levinson, D.J. (1986). A conception of adult development. *American Psychologist, 41*(1), 3–13.

Levinson, D.J. (1996). *The seasons of a woman's life.* New York: Alfred A. Knopf.

Lewis, J.A., & Bernstein, J. (1996). *Women's health: A relational perspective across the life cycle.* Sudbury, MA: Jones & Bartlett.

Lott, B. (1987). *Women's lives: Themes and variations in gender learning.* Pacific Grove, CA: Brooks/Cole.

Lyndon-Rochelle, M., & Woods, N.F. (2008). Women and their health. In C.I. Fogel & N.F. Woods (Eds.), *Women's health care in advanced practice nursing.* New York: Springer Publishing Company, LLC.

Maier, C. (2007). *No kids.* Toronto, Ontario: McClelland & Stewart Ltd.

Mather, M., & Lavery, D. (2010). *In U.S., proportion married at lowest recorded levels.* Retrieved August 11, 2011, from http://www.prb.org/Articles/2010/usmarriagedecline.aspx

McBride, A.B. (1990). Mental health effects of women's multiple roles. *American Psychologist, 45*(3), 381–384.

Mednick, M.T. (1989). On the politics of psychological constructs: Stop the bandwagon, I want to get off. *American Psychologist, 44*(8), 1118–1123.

Mehdizadeh, S. (2010). Self-presentation 2.0: Narcissism and self-esteem on Facebook. *Cyberpsychology, Behavior, and Social Networking, 13*(4), 357–364.

Mercer, R.T., Nichols, E.G., & Doyle, G.C. (1989). *Transitions in a woman's life: Major life events in developmental context.* New York: Springer.

Miller, J.B. (1986). *Toward a new psychology of women* (2nd ed.). Boston: Beacon Press.

Millet, K. (1969). *Sexual politics.* Chicago: University of Illinois Press.

Mitchell, V. (2009). Who am I now? Using life span theories in psychotherapy in late adulthood. *Women & Therapy, 32,* 298–312.

Morgan, R. (1970). *Sisterhood is powerful: An anthology of writings from the women's liberation movement.* New York: Random House.

Murray, J.L., & Bachman, G.E. (2000). Sandwich generation. In B.E. Johnson, C.A. Johnson, J.L. Murray, & B.S. Apgar (Eds.), *Women's health care handbook* (2nd ed.). Philadelphia: Hanley & Belfus, Inc.

National Economic Council (NEC). (2010). *Jobs and economic security for America's women.* Retrieved September 17, 2011, from http://www.whitehouse.gov/the-press-office/2010/10/21/jobs-and-economic-security-americas-women-report

Norman, S.M., McCluskey-Fawcett, K., & Ashcroft, L. (2002). Older women's development: A comparison of women in their 60s and 80s on a measure of Erikson's developmental tasks. *International Journal of Aging and Human Development, 54*(1), 31–41.

O'Rand, A.M., & Henrette, J.C. (1982). Women at middle age: Development and transitions. In *Annals of the American Academy of Political and Social Sciences.* Beverly Hills, CA: Sage.

Orenstein, P. (2000). *FLUX: Women on sex, work, love, kids and life in a self-changed world.* New York: Anchor Books.

Orenstein, P. (2011). *Cinderella ate my daughter: Dispatches from the front lines of the new girlie girl culture.* New York: HarperCollins.

Pew Research Center. (2007). *A portrait of "generation next": How young people view their lives, futures and politics.* Pew Research Center. Retrieved August 10, 2011, from http://pewsocialtrends.org/2007/01/09/a-portrait-of-generation-next/

Pierret, C.R. (2006, September 3–9). The "sandwich generation": Women caring for parents and children. *Monthly Labor Review.*

Pipher, M. (1994). *Reviving Ophelia: Saving the selves of adolescent girls.* New York: Ballantine Books.

Roberts, P., & Newton, P.M. (1987). Levinsonian studies of women's adult development. *Psychology and Aging, 2*(2), 154–163.

Rosen, L. (2011, September 6). *Poke me: How social networks can both help and harm our kids.* Presentation at American Psychological Association 119th Annual Convention in Washington, DC.

Rosenblatt, E.A. (1995). Emerging concept of women's development: Implications for psychotherapy. *Psychiatric Clinics of North America, 18*(1), 95–106.

Safer, J. (1996). *Beyond motherhood: Choosing a life without children.* New York: Pocket Books.

Seiden, A.M. (1989). Psychological issues affecting women throughout the life cycle. *Psychiatric Clinics of North America, 12*(1), 1–24.

Sheehy, G. (2006). *Passages: Predictable crises of adult life.* New York: Ballantine Books.

Shulman, L. (2006). Celebrating women: Leaping into the future with energy. *Alive: Canada's Natural Health & Wellness Magazine, 285*, 42–46.

Slater, C.S. (2003). Generativity versus stagnation: An elaboration of Erikson's adult stage of human development. *Journal of Adult Development, 10*(1), 53–65.

Stassen Berger, K. (2010). *Invitation to the life span.* New York: Worth Publishers.

Strachey, J. (Ed. & Trans.). (1961). *The standard edition of the complete psychological works of Sigmund Freud.* London: Hogarth Press.

Strough, J., Leszczynski, J.P., Neely, T.L., Flinn, J.A., & Margrett, J. (2007). From adolescence to later adulthood: Femininity, masculinity, and androgyny in six age groups. *Sex Roles, 57*, 385–396.

Taylor, S.E., Klein, L.C., Lewis, B.P., Gruenewald, T.L., Gurung, R.A., & Updegraff, J.A. (2000). Biobehavioral responses to stress in females: Tend-and-befriend, not fight-or-flight. *Psychological Review, 107*(3), 411–429.

Tolman, D., Impett, E.A., Tracy, A.J., & Michael, A. (2006). Looking good, sounding good: Femininity ideology and adolescent girls' mental health. *Psychology of Women Quarterly, 30*, 85–95.

Trimberger, E.K. (2005). *The new single woman.* Boston: Beacon Press.

Wright, L., & Leahy, M. (2009). *Nurses and families: A guide to family assessment and intervention* (5th ed.). Philadelphia: F. A. Davis Company.

SELECTED BIBLIOGRAPHY

Bem, S.L. (1993). *The lenses of gender: Transforming the debate on sexual inequality.* New Haven, CT: Yale University Press.

Brown, L., & Gilligan, C. (1992). *Meeting at the crossroads: Women's psychology and girls' development.* Cambridge, MA: Harvard University Press.

Eisler, R. (1988). *The chalice and the blade.* San Francisco: Harper.

Gilligan, C. (2002). *The birth of pleasure.* New York: Alfred A. Knopf.

Gilligan, C., & Richards, D.A.J. (2008). *The deepening darkness: Patriarch, resistance, and democracy's future.* Boston: Cambridge University Press.

Goodman, E., & O'Brien, P. (2001). *I know just what you mean: The power of friendship in women's lives.* New York: Simon & Schuster.

Sheehy, G. (1998). *Menopause: The silent passage.* New York: Pocket Books.

Sheehy, G. (2006). *Passages: Predictable crises of adult life.* New York: Ballantine Books Random House.

Simmons, R. (2002). *Odd girl out: The hidden culture of aggression in girls.* New York: Harcourt.

Wiseman, R. (2002). *Queen bees and wannabes: Helping your daughter survive cliques, gossip, boyfriends and other realities of adolescence.* New York: Crown Publishers.

CHAPTER ❖ 3

EPIDEMIOLOGY, DIAGNOSTIC METHODS, AND PROCEDURES FOR WOMEN'S HEALTH

Catherine Juve ◆ *Diane Marie Schadewald* ◆
Ellis Quinn Youngkin ◆ *Marcia Szmania Davis*

Highlights

- Mortality and Morbidity in U.S. Women
- Sensitivity, Specificity, and Predictive Value of Tests
- Overview of Commonly Indicated Laboratory Tests
- Overview of Commonly Used Procedures and Diagnostic Imaging

MORTALITY AND MORBIDITY IN U.S. WOMEN

LEADING CAUSES OF MORTALITY IN U.S. WOMEN

The average life expectancy for U.S. women increased from 48.3 years in 1900 to 80.4 years in 2007 (Bernstein, Makuc, & Bilheimer, 2010). From 1900 through the late 1970s, the sex gap in life expectancy widened from 2.0 years to 7.8 years. Since its peak in the 1970s, the gap has been narrowing. The difference in life expectancy between the sexes was only 5.0 years in 2007 (Xu, Kochanek, Murphy, & Tejada-Vera, 2010). The discrepancy in life expectancy between white and black women continues to be significant: 80.8 years for white women in 2007 compared to 76.8 years for black women (Bernstein et al., 2010). In 2007, diseases of the heart, cancer, and stroke led the way as the top three causes of death for both women and men, with chronic lower respiratory diseases in fourth place and continuing to increase (Xu et al., 2010). However, causes of death do differ for U.S. women, depending on age and race (see Tables 3–1, 3–2, and 3–3). Heart disease is the leading cause of death for all groups except American Indian/Alaskan Native (AI/AN) and Asian women. Among these women, cancer is the overall leading cause of death. Cancer is the second leading cause of death among all other women and the number one cause of death among women aged 40 to 79. Among females, leukemia is the leading cause of cancer death before age 20, breast cancer at age 20 to 59, and lung cancer at age 60 and older (Jemal et al., 2007). Cancer prevalence rates had increased among women 45 years of age and older between 1999 and 2009 (Xu et al., 2010). The three most commonly diagnosed types of cancer among women in 2007 were cancers of the breast, lung and bronchus, and colon and rectum, accounting for about 52 percent of estimated cancer cases in women. Breast cancer alone accounts for 26 percent (178,480) of all new cancer cases among women (Jemal et al., 2007). Better screening and diagnostic technologies are partially responsible for this trend. Smoking is a major contributor to cancer deaths and chronic obstructive pulmonary disease (COPD) in women. Women smokers are more than 13 times more likely to die of lung cancer than nonsmoking women (Centers for Disease Control and Prevention [CDC], Cancer Prevention and Control, 2011). Kidney disease became a top 10 cause of death for all U.S. women in 1999. For white women, Alzheimer's disease is the fifth leading cause of death, and pneumonia/influenza remained in the top 10 (Xu et al., 2010). Other ethnic variations include the higher prevalence of diabetes among all women other than white women. Although the 20th century, by and large, saw declines in infectious diseases, influenza and pneumonia remain among the top 10 leading causes of death for all ethnic groups. Unintentional injuries also remain in the top 10. These injuries include motor vehicle accidents (MVAs), falls, poisonings, and others that were determined not to be self-inflicted. Suicide is the 15th leading cause of death among women. Four times as many males as females die by suicide. Females are more likely to commit suicide by poisoning (40% drug related) compared to men who are more likely to use firearms (56%) (National Institute of Mental Health [NIMH], 2010).

Adolescence to Young Adulthood (Ages 15 to 24)

The number of adolescents and young adults in this country has steadily increased since the 1990s. By 2020, 43 million teenagers, up from 35 million in 1990, will live in the United States. Adolescent and young adult women are at the greatest risk for death from accidents and violence. More than one in three unintentional fatal injuries among this age group is from motor vehicle fatalities. In adolescents, alcohol is a major contributing factor. In 2007, 26 percent of adolescent accident fatalities occurred among those who were alcohol impaired (blood alcohol level > 0.08). Alcohol use is associated with lack of use of auto safety restraints, which further increases the risk of fatalities (National Highway Traffic Safety Administration [NHTSA], 2009). Females are less likely to drink and drive and more likely to use safety restraints than their male counterparts. The under-20 age group had the highest proportion of distracted drivers involved in fatal crashes (16%). Sources of distraction include things such as conversation with passengers, use of media, grooming, and eating/drinking. Cell phone usage and texting have been implicated as a contributing factor to MVA deaths and injuries, especially among young people. The Transportation Safety Group at the National Safety Council found that distracted drivers account for nearly 80 percent of car crashes. The survey also found that teenagers and those between the ages 18 and 30 are more likely to send text messages while driving (National Transportation Safety Board, U.S. Department of Transportation, 2009).

Homicide and suicide are the second and third leading causes of death, respectively, among teens ages 15 to 19,

TABLE 3–1. Death Rates for U.S. Women by Selected Cause and Age (Per 100,000 Population)

Age	Heart Disease[a]	Cancer[a]	Accidents[a,b]	Cerebv. Dis.[a]	CLRD[a]	Pneumonia[c]	Suicide[a]	Liver Disease	DM	Homicide[a]
10–14	0.7	2.0	4.4	0.2	NA	NA	0.6	NA	NA	0.7
15–19	1.2	2.5	18.9	0.4	NA	0.4	2.8	NA	NA	2.9
20–24	2.4	3.7	19.9	0.6	NA	NA	3.6	NA	0.5	4.2
25–34	5.1	9.5	17.6	1.2	NA	NA	4.7	NA	1.5	3.7
35–44	17.0	36.4	23.4	4.8	2.0	NA	7.0	4.1	3.7	3.4
45–54	48.5	113.7	26.6	13.0	8.9	NA	8.4	10.0	9.9	NA
55–64	124.1	281.8	22.0	28.2	36.6	7.8	NA	13.0	29.1	NA
65–74	346.3	605.9	31.3	86.5	137.5	26.3	NA	NA	69.7	NA
75–84	1,136.7	1,012.5	84.1	328.0	312.8	107.8	NA	NA	148.1	NA
85 and older	4,322.1	1,305.5	245.8	1,089.8	508.7	NA	NA	NA	268.4	NA
Total for women[d]	154.0	151.3	25.8	41.3	36.0	14.2	4.7	5.9	19.5	2.5
Total for men[d]	237.7	217.5	55.2	42.5	48.0	19.3	18.4	12.7	26.4	9.6

Cerebv. Dis.—cerebrovascular diseases
CLRD—chronic lower respiratory diseases
DM—diabetes mellitus
NA—not available
[a]Heron, 2010, Tables 1 and 2
[b]Unintentional injuries
[c]Pneumonia and influenza
[d]Bernstein et al., 2010, Table 22, 2007 data

TABLE 3–2. Differences in Death Rates for U.S. Women by Selected Cause for All Ages and Detailed Race/Hispanic Origin (Per 100,000 Population)

Disease/Cause	White Females	Black Females	AI/AN Females	Asian/PI Females	Hispanic Females	White Non-Hispanic Females
Heart disease	224.2	174.3	75.1	64.9	62.6	254.7
Cerebrovascular diseases	57.9	46.5	19.8	26.7	17.5	65.5
Malignant neoplasms	190.1	147.7	76.8	77.8	59.7	214.7
Nephritis	14.8	22.2	9.5	5.8	6.1	16.4
Accidents	30.3	20.9	32.5	10.9	13.8	33.3
Alzheimer's disease	38.8	15.8	NA	6.4	7.4	44.8
Chronic lower respiratory diseases	49.9	17.4	17.1	6.8	7.5	58.0

AI/AN—American Indian/Alaskan Native
NA—not available
PI—Pacific Islander
Source: Heron, 2010, Table 2

TABLE 3–3. Leading Causes of Death in U.S. Females According to Detailed Race and Hispanic Origin in 2007

Disease	White	Black	American Indian/Alaskan Native	Asian/Pacific Islander	Hispanic
Heart disease	1	1	2	2	1
Malignant neoplasms	2	2	1	1	2
Cerebrovascular diseases	3	3	5	3	3
Chronic lower respiratory diseases	4	7	6	7	7
Alzheimer's disease	5	9		8	6
Unintentional injuries	6	6	3	5	5
Diabetes mellitus	7	4	4	4	4
Influenza and pneumonia	8	9	9	6	8
Nephritis/nephrotic syndrome/nephrosis	9	5	8	9	9
Septicemia	10	8	10		
Perinatal conditions					10
Chronic liver disease			7		
Essential hypertension and hypertensive renal disease		10		10	

Source: National Center for Health Statistics, 2010

after unintentional injury (Childtrends Data Bank, 2011). Homicide is the second most prevalent cause of death among young women between 15 and 24 years of age. However, when rates are examined by ethnicity, suicide is ranked number two for Asian/Pacific Islander, AI/AN, and white females in this age group (CDC, 2011a). In 2006, black females were four times as likely to die as a result of interpersonal violence than white females between the ages of 15 and 19 (21.2% vs. 5.2%). In contrast, AI/AN females were more than three times as likely as black females to die from suicide (13.5% vs. 3.4%). Female Hispanic students are more likely to attempt suicide than all other students. The suicide attempt rate also varies by race/ethnicity: Attempts are slightly higher for Hispanic students (11.3%) than for black non-Hispanic and white non-Hispanic students (7.6% and 7.3%, respectively) (National Adolescent Health Information Center, 2006). Gay youth may be two to three times more likely to attempt suicide as compared to their peers. This is more prevalent in homosexual/bisexual males, who in some studies have been found to be seven times more likely to attempt suicide. Overall, adolescent males are four times more likely than females to die from suicide, while adolescent females are more likely to attempt suicide. Whereas firearms are the most prevalent method among males, females are more likely to use poisoning (overdose) as a method. The incidence of attempted or completed suicides by hanging has increased in the past several years. Between 2000 and 2008, the rates of suicide for those between 15 and 24 years of age have remained essentially unchanged, indicating a need for providers to be alert to risks and signs of depression and suicidal intentions among young people (CDC, 2011a).

In 2009, females accounted for an estimated 23 percent of adolescents aged 13 to 19 diagnosed with HIV infection, compared with 19 percent of young adult females aged 20 to 24. Heterosexual contact (90%) followed by injection drug use (10%) are the most common routes of transmission of HIV among adolescent females between the ages of 13 and 24. African American (AA) youth have a disproportionate burden of HIV, representing over 60 percent of the HIV diagnoses for those between 13 and 24 years of age (CDC, 2011b). These data provide guidance regarding preventive measures and screening among young people.

Young Adulthood to Mid-Adulthood (Ages 25 to 44)

In 2006, among females aged 25 to 34, unintentional injury, primarily MVAs, ranked as the number one cause of death, while malignant neoplasms ranked number two (CDC, Cancer Prevention and Control, 2011). These causes were reversed for women in the 35 to 44 age group. Heart disease is the third leading cause of death for females in this age group. Suicide remained fourth. It has remained at number four since 1997, when it tied with HIV infection (which was not a major cause of death in 1999). Homicide deaths were fifth and ninth, respectively, in 2008 for 25- to 34-year-olds and 35- to 44-year-olds. Motor vehicle deaths accounted for 37 percent of deaths for AI/AN women between the ages of 25 and 44 in contrast to 27 percent of all females.

Mid-Adulthood to Older Adulthood (Ages 45 to 64)

In mid-adulthood, cancer and heart disease emerge as the primary causes of death among women of all ethnic backgrounds. Stroke and unintentional injuries are third and fourth, respectively, with chronic liver disease and diabetes following. Among black women, HIV deaths are the fourth most common cause of death in this age group (CDC, 2011c).

Maturity (Ages 65 and Older)

Heart disease increases dramatically with age, as do cancer, cerebrovascular diseases, chronic lower respiratory diseases, pneumonia/influenza, and diabetes. Alzheimer's disease ranked as the fifth or sixth leading cause of death among all ethnic groups. Chronic lower respiratory diseases, influenza and pneumonia, kidney disease, and diabetes were also important causes of death for older women. In 2008, there were 82 percent fall-related deaths among people aged 65 and older. Rates of fall-related fractures among older women are more than twice those among men. White women have significantly higher hip fracture rates than black women. Among older adults (those aged 65 or older), falls are the leading cause of injury death rather than MVAs. Impaired vision, poor balance, and side effects of medication are a few of the risk factors that contribute to increased fall rates in this age group (CDC, 2011a). See Chapter 6 for more information on falls.

Differences in Causes of Death for Women by Race

Heart disease and cancer are the number one and two causes of death, respectively, for women regardless of ethnic background or Hispanic origin. For women younger than age 64, cancer is the primary cause of death, with deaths from MVAs being significantly higher among AI/AN women than in any other race/origin. Deaths from HIV infection are significantly higher in black women, with Hispanic women much lower but higher than other races. Although the overall incidence of breast cancer among AA women is lower than in white American women, this cancer is more common in young premenopausal AA women, and AA breast cancer patients of all ages are more likely to have advanced disease at diagnosis, higher risk of recurrence, and poorer overall prognosis (Rose, Haffner, & Baillargeon, 2007) (see Table 3–3).

Although the risk of dying from pregnancy and childbirth-related causes in the United States is low, the rate has doubled since 1987, when it reached an all-time low of 6.6 deaths per 100,000 live births. This rate was maintained until about 2000, when the rates began to rise. Between 2003 and 2007, the maternal mortality rate rose from 12 to 15 per 100,000 women in the United States. Currently the United States is ranked 50th in the world by the United Nations for maternal mortality. The leading complications causing maternal deaths in the United States overlap with the main global causes; hemorrhage, pregnancy-related hypertensive disorders, and infection are among the top causes of death in both the United States and the developing world. Other leading causes of maternal death in the United States are thrombotic pulmonary embolism, cardiomyopathy, cardiovascular conditions, and other medical conditions, whereas in developing countries, obstructed labor and unsafe abortions lead. Black women are four times more likely to die of maternal complications than white women. Likewise, a study comparing maternal outcomes for Mexican-born women and white non-Latina women in California found that while Mexican-born women were less likely to suffer complications overall, they did face a greater risk of particular obstetric complications such as postpartum hemorrhage, major puerperal infections, and third- and fourth-degree lacerations, suggesting that the intrapartum care they received may have been of poorer quality (Guendelman, Thornton, Gould, & Hosang, 2005). Ethnic differences cannot be accounted for by an increased prevalence in health conditions related to maternal mortality. Access to care and quality of care are contributing factors (Tucker, Berg, Callaghan, & Hsia, 2007; World Health Organization [WHO], 2005, 2007).

Cancer

In 2006, cancer was the second leading cause of deaths in the United States (CDC, Cancer Prevention and Control, 2011). The most common sites for cancer regardless of race/ethnicity were the lung, trachea, and bronchus. Lung cancer was the number one cause of cancer death for all women with the exception of women of Hispanic origin, in whom breast cancer was the number one cause. Note that the Hispanic group, by definition, overlaps with all other groups. Although lung cancer is the number one cause of cancer death, female breast cancer is by far the most common cancer to occur among women. Over twice as many females have breast cancer than lung cancer, although the mortality prevalence is reversed for all but women of Hispanic origin. Colon rectal cancer is the third most common cause of cancer mortality among women of all ethnic backgrounds. Deaths from cancer of the pancreas and ovary are also ranked in the top 10 causes of cancer deaths among women. Although the incidence rate of breast cancer for black women is less than for white women, the mortality rate is significantly higher for black women (U.S. Cancer Statistics Working Group, 2010). It is estimated that the cost of cancer care in the United States in 2020 will be $158 billion per year, with a little over $19 billion going for breast cancer (Mariotto, Yabroff, Shao, Feuer, & Brown, 2011). The incidence and mortality rates for lung/bronchial cancer have remained the same between 1999 and 2007. However, the incidence and mortality rates for breast cancer have declined, due to better screening. In addition, breast cancer incidence rates decrease with the cessation of estrogen-progestin hormone therapy. Following the release of the 2002 report of the Women's Health Initiative (WHI) trial of estrogen plus progestin, the use of menopausal hormone therapy in the United States decreased substantially. Subsequently, the incidence of breast cancer also dropped, suggesting a cause-and-effect relation between hormone treatment and breast cancer. However, the cause of this decrease remains controversial (Chlebowski et al., 2009).

Lung cancer incidence is beginning to decrease among women and is continuing to decrease among men in most states. Lung cancer incidence is influenced by variations in smoking behavior (Henley et al., 2011).

Colorectal cancer deaths, the third leading overall cancer death cause, are higher in black women, indicating a need for earlier detection (CDC, Cancer Prevention and Control, 2011). Ovarian cancer rates are higher among white women, but mortality rates are similar for all ethnic groups. A 1.7 percent decrease in incidence rates was observed between 2002 and 2007, perhaps due to the use of hormonal contraception. Survival rate is tied directly to the stage of ovarian cancer (Howlader et al., 2010). New cases of cervical cancer in U.S. women in 2007 were 12,280; approximately 4,021 women died from this cancer in 2007. The U.S. incidence for cervical cancer in 2007 was highest in Hispanic and black women (U.S. Cancer Statistics Working Group, 2010). Some geographical areas of the United States also have higher incidences of cervical cancer. These higher incidences are thought to be related to lack of availability of screening (National Cancer Institute [NCI], 2010a) (see Figures 3–1 and 3–2).

HIV/AIDS

Between the ages of 20 and 54, HIV continues to be ranked among the top 10 causes of death for women, peaking at number five among women in the 35- to 44-year age group. For black women in this age group, HIV is the third leading cause of death. Among adult and adolescent females in the 40 states, the overall rate of diagnosis of HIV infection in 2009 was 9.8 per 100,000 persons. By race/ethnicity, the rate for blacks/AAs (47.8) was nearly 20 times as high as the rate for whites and more than four times as high as the rate for Hispanics/Latinos (11.9). Relatively few cases were diagnosed among Asian, AI/AN, Native Hawaiian/other Pacific Islander females and females reporting multiple races, although the rates of diagnoses of HIV infection among females in all these races/ethnicities were higher than that for white females. CDC (2011c) recommends routine HIV screening in health care settings for all adults, aged 13 to 64, and repeat screening at least annually for those at high risk.

Cardiovascular Diseases

More than one in three female adults has some form of cardiovascular disease (CVD), and it is the leading cause of death for all races and ethnicities except for Asian/Pacific Islanders (CDC, Office of Women's Health, 2010). Since 1984, the rate of CVD among women has been greater than among men, and in 2007, females represented 51.8 percent of deaths from heart disease. About 7.5 million living women have a history of a myocardial infarction (MI) or angina pectoris, with 3.5 million having had an MI. Despite a lower incidence rate, black women are more likely than white women to die of CVD. Women are more likely than men to die: 26 percent of women with a recognized MI die within 1 year of diagnosis compared to 19 percent of men over the age of 45 with a recognized MI. This is, in part, because women have heart disease, on average, at an older age than men. A total of 64 percent of women with CVD had no previous symptoms. Black women also are more likely to have a stroke (also known as cerebrovascular accident [CVA]) and to die from a stroke. Of all stroke deaths, 60.2 percent were among women. Hypertension (HTN) is a primary contributor to CVD. Again, black women are much more likely to have this condition than others, with

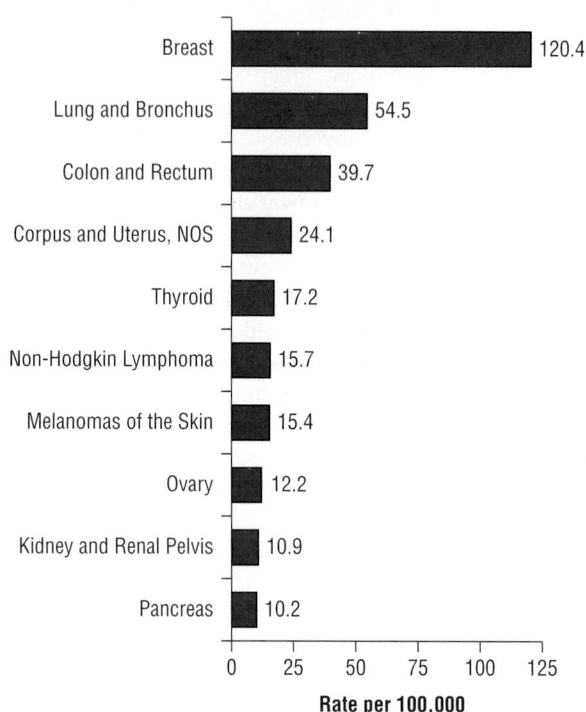

FIGURE 3–2. Top 10 Cancer Sites in Women. *Source:* U.S. Cancer Statistics Working Group, 2010.

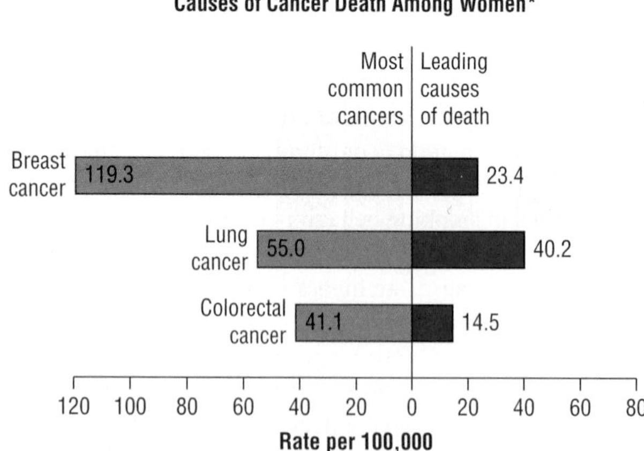

FIGURE 3–1. Most Common Cancers for Women. Source: United States Cancer Statistics: 2006 Incidence and Mortality Web-Based Report.

45.7 percent of black women over the age of 20 having HTN. After the age of 65, women are more likely than men to be diagnosed with HTN. Smoking, obesity, and cholesterol levels all contribute to the risks for CVD. A study comparing AA, Asian Indian American (AIA), and Caucasian American women found that AA and AIA women 30 years of age or older had more lifestyle, dietary, hemodynamic, anthropometric, and laboratory identified risk factors than Caucasian women, including higher apolipoprotein A-1, lipoprotein (a) (Lp(a)), fibrinogen, and fasting insulin levels in AA women, and higher Lp(a) and fibrinogen levels in AIA and Asian American/Pacific Islander women. Unfortunately, adopting a Western lifestyle, including more dietary fat and decreased exercise, further increases the risk for CVD (Banerjee, Wong, Shin, Fortmann, & Palaniappan, 2011; Guerra et al., 2005; Narayan et al., 2010; Velásquez-Mieyer et al., 2008). Data published by the American Heart Association confirms that women's risks for CVD are steadily increasing with the rise of obesity rates and metabolic syndrome and the subsequent increase in the incidence of diabetes mellitus, type II (DMII) and chronic kidney disease (CKD) (Véronique et al., 2011) (see Figure 3–3).

Many lifestyle risk factors are modifiable, such as eating too much fat and being sedentary. Smoking only four or fewer cigarettes per day increases the risk of MI by two times. Better screening for and management of diabetes, HTN, smoking, overweight, inactivity, and high cholesterol can significantly improve one in every three women's risk for coronary heart disease. Obesity is now one of the major preventive health dilemmas in the United States. As obesity and overweight grow as public health problems, efforts to begin to change the trajectory in childhood become critical.

LEADING CAUSES OF MORBIDITY IN U.S. WOMEN

Conditions Requiring Emergency Department or Hospital Visits

Between 1997 and 2007, the annual number of emergency department (ED) visits increased by 23 percent. Overall ED utilization rates were 26 percent higher for women than for men (476.5 visits per 1,000 women versus 377.6 visits per 1,000 men) (Owens & Mutter, 2010). Women made 57.1 percent of all ED visits in 2008. A new national

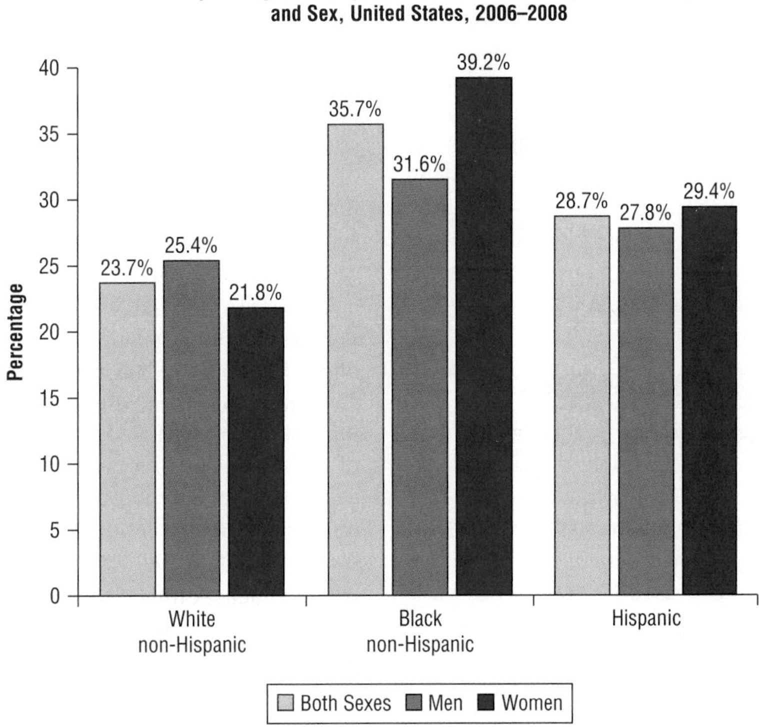

FIGURE 3–3. Obesity Among Adults. Source: Centers for Disease Control and Prevention at http://www.cdc.gov/Features/dsObesityAdults.

study showed that from 2005 to 2009 (the most recent year with available figures), there was a 49 percent increase in ED visits for drug-related suicide attempts by women aged 50 and older (from 11,235 visits in 2005 to 16,757 in 2009). This increase reflects the overall population growth of women aged 50 and older (Substance Abuse and Mental Health Services Administration, 2011).

Rates of ED visits varied by demographic characteristics, with rates highest among women, individuals 65 years and older, those from the lowest income areas, and those from rural areas. Falls led the list in 1999 as the major cause of unintentional injuries for all ages, except 18- to 24-year-old women, and increased dramatically in the 65-and-older age group. MVAs were the major reason for ED visits for those ages 18 to 24 and were the second major reason in all other age groups. Intentional injuries were highest in the 25- to 44-year-old age group. Females accounted for 59 percent of all hospital stays in 2006, mostly due to hospitalization for childbirth. Other major reasons for female hospitalizations were related to the circulatory system (13 percent), respiratory system (9 percent), and digestive system (8 percent). If pregnancy and childbirth are excluded, the major differences in hospitalizations between males and females are circulatory and digestive conditions. More men were hospitalized for circulatory problems and more women for digestive issues. Five heart-related diagnoses—coronary artery disease, congestive heart failure, heart attacks, nonspecific chest pain, and cardiac dysrhythmias—were among the 10 most common principal diagnoses for both male and female hospitalizations. Other conditions causing many more hospitalizations for females than males included mood disorders (57% female), degenerative joint disease (62% female), and urinary tract infections (72% female) (Levit, Stranges, Ryan, & Elixhauser, 2008).

Chronic Conditions

Most women in the United States are in good health, with 8 in 10 reporting excellent, very good, or good health. However, nearly one in five (19%) women reports that she is in fair or poor health. Not surprisingly, this proportion increases with age, to nearly one-third of women ages 65 and older. Nearly 4 in 10 women (38%) have a chronic condition that requires ongoing medical attention, compared to 30 percent of men. The incidence of chronic conditions increases with age with nearly 6 in 10 women in their senior years (65 and older) dealing with HTN (58%) and arthritis (61%), and almost half with high cholesterol (45%).

Many younger women also have chronic health problems. By the time women reach their middle years (45 to 64), 3 in 10 already have high cholesterol and arthritis, and even 1 in 10 women of reproductive age (18 to 44) says she has arthritis, HTN, high cholesterol, and asthma or another respiratory condition. Women are also more likely to experience pain (in the form of migraines, neck pain, lower back pain, or face or jaw pain) than men. Women were twice as likely to experience migraines or severe headaches, or pain in the face or jaw, than men (USDHHS, 2009). The increase in obesity, poor nutrition, and sedentary lifestyle contributes significantly to chronic illness. Overweight (BMI = 25–30) and obesity (BMI ≥ 30) are epidemic in the United States, with 78.6 percent of black African/American women and 59.6 percent of non-Hispanic white women falling into these categories (USDHHS, Office of Minority Health, 2010). One in every four women (23%) reports she has been diagnosed with depression or anxiety, over twice the rate for men (Kaiser Women's Health Survey, 2005).

Arthritis is reported to affect 26 percent of all women compared to just over 18 percent of men. A diagnosis of arthritis is associated with aging, female gender, obesity, physical inactivity, a history of smoking, and less than a high school education (Cheng, Hootman, Murphy, Langmaid, & Helmick, 2010). It is estimated that by 2020, 18 percent of all Americans will develop arthritis. It is the leading chronic condition in whites and greatly affects AAs, Hispanics, AIs, and ANs as a leading cause of activity limitation. Arthritis is the number one cause of work disability for women (24.3%) followed by back problems (16.8%) and heart conditions (5.3%) (U.S. Census Bureau, 2009).

The number of women age 50 and older who have osteoporosis or are at risk for developing the disease has increased from almost 30 million in 2002 to more than 35 million in 2010 and is projected to be approximately 41 million in 2020. Non-Hispanic white women are disproportionately afflicted with this disease, but the number of women of other races and ethnic groups is also significant (National Osteoporosis Foundation, 2011). Although more commonly seen in women (80% of those who have osteoporosis), the burden of osteoporosis in men remains underdiagnosed and underreported. Each year, 1.5 million fractures are attributed to osteoporosis, including 350,000 hip fractures (American Academy of Orthopaedic Surgeons, 2009; Mauck & Clarke, 2006). Seventy percent of those suffering from osteoporosis do not return to previous preinjury status. The acute and long-term medical care expenses associated with these fractures cost the nation an estimated $17 billion in 2005.The cumulative cost over the next two decades is estimated to be $474 billion. In addition to a financial burden, osteoporosis-related fractures bring a burden of pain and disability (National Osteoporosis Foundation, 2011).

Among older adults (those 65 years or older), falls are the leading cause of injury death. They are also the most common cause of nonfatal injuries and hospital admissions for trauma. The chances of falling and of being seriously injured in a fall increase with age. In 2009, the rate of fall injuries for adults 85 years and older was almost four times that for adults 65 to 74.3 years. Women are more likely than men to be injured in a fall. In 2009, women were 58 percent more likely than men to suffer a nonfatal fall injury. Over 90 percent of hip fractures are caused by falls. In 2007, there were 264,000 hip fractures and the rate for women was almost three times the rate for men. White women have significantly higher hip fracture rates than black women (CDC, 2011d). See Chapter 6 for more information on falls.

AAs, AIs, and ANs have a greater incidence of kidney disease than whites or Asians, with some of the disproportionate effect explained by higher numbers of these races with HTN and diabetes (CDC, 2010a). More women than men are affected. Other risk factors for developing CKD include CVD, obesity, elevated cholesterol, and a family history of CKD. The risk of developing CKD increases with age largely because risk factors for kidney disease become more common as one ages. Those most at risk are AAs, Hispanics, AIs, ANs, Asian/Pacific Islanders, older people (older than 60 years), and the poor.

Other serious chronic diseases that occur most often in women are autoimmune diseases, systemic lupus erythematosus (90%), multiple sclerosis, scleroderma, Hashimoto's thyroiditis, and Graves' disease. Lupus is two to three times more prevalent among women of color—AAs, Hispanics/Latinos, Asians, Native Americans, ANs, Native Hawaiians, and other Pacific Islanders—than among Caucasian women (Fairweather & Rose, 2004; Sacks, Helmick, Langmaid, & Sniezek, 2002). Alzheimer's disease, urinary incontinence, major depression, dysthymia, and anxiety disorders are also more prevalent in women.

Women's health needs are reflected in their provider choices. Virtually all older adult women (95%) have a regular provider, compared to three quarters of women ages 18 to 44 and 90 percent of women ages 45 to 64. As they age, women are also less likely to visit a reproductive health specialty provider. Only one quarter (26%) of senior women report a gynecological visit in the past year, and only 12 percent count a reproductive health provider among their regular providers, compared to 47 percent of women in their reproductive years (Kaiser Women's Health Survey, 2005).

SENSITIVITY, SPECIFICITY, AND PREDICTIVE VALUE OF TESTS

Clinicians must understand the concepts of sensitivity, specificity, and predictive value to use and interpret test results effectively. Two articles sequentially published in 2009 provide excellent explanations of these terms as well as guidelines for the use of likelihood ratios and receiver operating characteristic (ROC) curves (Tripepi, Jager, Dekker, & Zoccali, 2009; van Stralen et al., 2009). These articles are highly recommended to readers seeking further information.

Sensitivity is the percentage of people with a disease or condition who have a positive test. A sensitive test is used when the goal is to detect all people with the disease because nondetection consequences can be disastrous. An example is the initial enzyme-linked immunosorbent assay (ELISA) test for HIV antibodies. The test is designed to miss the lowest number of those exposed to the virus, though some nonexposed people are expected to have a positive test.

Specificity is the percentage of people with no disease who have a negative test. It takes the number of people without disease and a negative test and divides it by the total number of nondiseased people. An example is the Western blot test, which is very specific for HIV antibodies, the follow-up test for those with a positive ELISA, and is quite unlikely to be positive if HIV antibodies are absent.

Predictive value helps predict disease status. Positive predictive value (PPV) is the probability of disease if a test is positive, and negative predictive value (NPV) is the probability if the test is negative. The predictive value of a test utilizes disease prevalence in a particular site along with sensitivity and specificity. For example, a positive ELISA for HIV is more likely to be a false-positive result in a setting where prevalence of HIV disease is low.

OVERVIEW OF COMMONLY INDICATED LABORATORY TESTS

Performance of the tests discussed next requires the following rules and regulations established by the Clinical Laboratory Improvement Amendments (CLIA). Some tests are waived from regulation as long as the quality control tests recommended by the manufacturer are followed and the results of those tests are documented. Clinicians need to familiarize themselves with these rules and maintain knowledge of updates.

CERVICAL CYTOLOGY/CANCER SCREENING

Papanicolaou Smear

Purpose. The Papanicolaou (Pap) smear is a screening test for abnormal/atypical cells suggesting actual or possible preinvasive cervical neoplastic changes (Davey et al., 2002; Solomon et al., 2002). Cervical cancer deaths have decreased 70 percent since the Pap smear use began in 1950 (Jemal et al., 2008; Tierney, Westin, Schlumbrecht, & Ramirez, 2010). Cervical cancer is a major solid tumor that is virally induced in nearly all cases by human papillomavirus (HPV) DNA. There are more than 150 types of HPV, more than 40 of which infect the genital area (CDC, 2008; NCI, 2010b). The most common types (16 and 18) account for more than 70 percent of all invasive cancers of the cervix (NCI, 2010b). There are 13 known HPV types associated with cervical cancer. Selected other high-risk types associated with cervical cancer in order of frequency are 45, 31, 33, 52, 58, and 35 (Tierney et al., 2010). That is, some form of HPV genotype is present in more than 99 percent of Pap specimens evaluated as positive for cervical cancer. Preinvasive lesions are categorized in a variety of ways. Squamous intraepithelial lesions (SIL), either low grade (LSIL) or high grade (HSIL), encompass terminology of cervical intraepithelial neoplasia (CIN) grades 1, 2, or 3 (more serious neoplastic changes are indicated with the increasing numeral), and dysplasia (mild, moderate, or severe). This varied terminology can be confusing, but the 2001 Bethesda System for reporting cervical cytology results is helpful in interpretation (see Table 3–4) (Solomon et al., 2002; Wright et al., 2007a). (See Chapter 16 for more information on management of cervical cancer.)

Thirty-three percent of SIL regress, 41 percent stay the same, and 25 percent become more advanced. Ten percent of these latter lesions become carcinoma in situ (CIS); 1 percent becomes invasive cervical cancer. Viral transmission is through sexual intercourse. Prevalence of HPV infection decreases with age. The peak incidence is between 22 and 25 years (Koutsky, 2009).

Because it has a long preclinical phase, squamous cervical cancer is ideal for screening. Although the Pap smear can identify some infections of the cervix and vagina, other more definitive tests are needed for diagnosis (see later and Chapter 14). The Pap smear may also be used to evaluate the hormonal status of squamous cells, but modern serum hormone levels are more precise. New research and consensus of experts indicate that routine screening from age 21 until 65 or 70, with Pap and reflex to HPV tests as indicated for those over 30, may provide the most savings in lives lost to cervical cancer (Tierney et al., 2010). Recommendations for frequency of testing vary based both on age and on previous Pap test results (see Table 3–4). However, when considering discontinuing testing, risk factors for an individual woman should dictate the need to continue screening beyond age 65 or 70. Pap tests alone carry a 24 to 50 percent false-negative rate, have poor reproducibility, and have the potential for misclassification of the results (Apgar, Brotzman, & Spitzer, 2008; Cong, Cox, & Cantor, 2007; Fahey, Irwig, & Macaskill, 1995). Liquid-based Pap testing with reflex HPV testing may be more cost-effective because years of life would be saved at an acceptable increase in cost. HPV testing alone has been considered for a future screening method, but as HPV can clear on its own, unnecessary further screening might result (Tierney et al., 2010). That is, HPV testing has a high sensitivity for detection of presence of the virus but a low specificity for detection of cervical cancer.

General Principles for Pap Specimen Collection. Prepare all collection materials prior to positioning the patient in the stirrups. Collect *before* the bimanual. Collect the Pap smear *before* other tests, such as gonorrhea (GC) and chlamydia (CT) tests. This order of collection is clearly supported by the American College of Obstetricians and Gynecologists (ACOG); the rationale is to ensure the best sample with suspicious cells for the Pap smear. If a wet mount is to be done, collect the specimen from the vaginal fornices before the Pap or any test is done to avoid blood from the Pap obscuring cells on the wet mount (ACOG Practice Bulletin, 2009).

To obtain the best possible specimen for liquid-based cervical cytology (LBCC) or the conventional Pap test (CPT), be precise. It is essential to get samples from the transformation zone (TZ) (the squamocolumnar junction [SCJ]), the usual site of abnormal changes (Solomon et al., 2002). Sampling error is a major factor in false-negative results. Be sure that the entire cervix is visible prior to attempting to obtain the sample. Factors associated with unsatisfactory Pap results for CPT specimens include postpartum status, vaginal bleeding, and presence of endocervical polyps (Lu et al., 2010). Factors that have

TABLE 3–4. Cervical Cytology Results, Interpretation, and Recommended Actions for the Primary Care Provider (Don't Screen Before Age 21)

Cervical Cytology Results	Interpretation	Recommended Actions
Negative for intraepithelial lesions or malignancy	See Recommended Actions. The optional or organism findings should be interpreted in light of the history, the physical findings, and other appropriate laboratory findings.	Repeat in 3 years for women 21–29 years of age who are not at risk.[a]
Optional to report nonneoplastic findings other than organisms. These include but are not limited to reactive cellular changes associated with inflammation (includes typical repair), radiation, intrauterine device, glandular cells post hysterectomy, atrophy.		For women 30–65 years of age who are not at risk and also have a negative human papillomavirus (HPV) co-test,[a] repeat in 5 years. If no HPV co-testing is used, repeat in 3 years as done for women 21–29 years of age. If positive HPV co-test, then repeat Pap in 1 year, *or* if positive HPV type 16 or 18, refer for colposcopy. For women > 65 years of age who are not at risk,[a] do not screen if previous adequate results are negative.
Organisms that may be reported include organisms such as *Trichomonas vaginalis*, fungal organisms consistent with Candida species, shift in flora suggestive of bacterial vaginosis, bacteria morphologically consistent with *Actinomyces* species, cellular changes consistent with herpes simplex virus. Endometrial cells in women > 40 years of age.	Endometrial cells present in women > 40 years of age who are not currently menstruating requires further evaluation.	If there is a nonneoplastic finding reported, management should be specific to the cause. Treatment of organisms depends on other findings. The woman should be reexamined and tested for the specific problem and then treated appropriately if indicated.
No endocervical cells The presence or absence of endocervical cells is provided if adequate squamous cells are present. Ten well-preserved endocervical cells should be present.	The specimen contained no endocervical cells, hence may have missed the squamocolumnar junction in the transformation zone.	If judged "satisfactory for evaluation," repeat cytology is not necessary for 1 year if the woman is not at high risk and had negative cytology a year past. If judged "unsatisfactory for evaluation," repeat in 3–4 months. If the woman is at risk for cervical cancer, repeat the cervical cytology in 8–12 weeks.
ASC-US (atypical squamous cells of undetermined significance)	The cellular abnormalities are more marked than can be attributed to reactive change, but cannot be definitively called squamous intraepithelial lesions (SIL). They fall short of being SIL in quantity or quality. All ASC suggest SIL, and some ASC-US are associated with CIN 2,3, but the risk of invasive cancer is low.	Two options available: (If CIN 2,3 or cancer, management follows ASCCP guidelines.) 1. Repeat cervical cytology in 6–12 months. If positive, refer for colposcopy. If negative, move to routine screening. 2. If liquid-based cytology, perform reflex HPV DNA testing. If positive, refer for colposcopy. If negative, repeat cytology in 12 months at preferred management.
ASC-US in special circumstances *Postmenopausal and immunosuppressed*		Manage same as ASC-US result for general population.
Pregnancy	Endocervical curettage is unacceptable.	Manage same as ASC-US result for general population. Except may defer colposcopy until 6 weeks postpartum.

(continued)

TABLE 3–4. Cervical Cytology Results, Interpretation, and Recommended Actions for the Primary Care Provider (Don't Screen Before Age 21) (CONTINUED)

Cervical Cytology Results	Interpretation	Recommended Actions
Adolescence		Repeat cytology in 12 months. If HSIL on repeat or remains ASC-US or higher for 24 months, refer for colposcopy.
ASC-H (atypical squamous cells, cannot exclude high-grade SIL)	5–10% of ASC cases are in this category. It contains a mixture of real HSIL and cells that mimic. It is positively predictive (50%) for CIN 2,3 that falls between ASC-US and HSIL.	Refer for colposcopy. If biopsy confirms CIN 2,3, manage by ASCCP guidelines. If no CIN 2,3 found, repeat cytology in 6 and 12 months or perform HPV DNA testing in 12 months. If negative, return to routine screening. If positive ($\geq$ ASC or HPV+), repeat colposcopy.
AGC (atypical glandular cells) (include categories of endocervical or glandular cells) (see next if atypical endometrial cells present)	Only about 0.2% of smears have this finding. However, this result can represent a squamous or glandular abnormality in over one third of the cases.	All AGC results require colposcopy referral with HPV DNA testing and endocervical sampling; add endometrial sampling (if $\geq$ 35 or at risk for endometrial cancer).
AGC, atypical endometrial cells	Reflex HPV DNA testing or repeat cytology is unacceptable management.	Requires endometrial sampling and endocervical sampling. If no endometrial pathology, then need referral for colposcopy.
AGC, favor neoplasia	Reflex HPV DNA testing or repeat cytology is unacceptable management. This result indicates a higher risk of having high-grade CIN lesions upon biopsy.	If no invasive disease, requires diagnostic excisional procedure.
AIS (endocervical adenocarcinoma in situ)	AIS result is associated with a very high risk of having AIS or invasive cervical adenocarinoma.	If no invasive disease, requires diagnostic excisional procedure.
Low-grade SIL (LSIL)	Squamous cervical abnormalities are considered to be noninvasive; with no lesion or CIN 1. However, women with LSIL are considered at higher risk for developing CIN 2,3 (28% will develop in 2 years).	Refer for colposcopy. With satisfactory colposcopy and lesion, endocervical biopsy is considered acceptable. With satisfactory colposcopy and no lesion and nonpregnant, endometrial biopsy is preferred, or with unsatisfactory colposcopy, endocervical biopsy is preferred. Management is dependent upon findings. Follow ASCCP guidelines.
LSIL in special circumstances *Postmenopause*	Initial colposcopy may not be necessary. Important to evaluate for atrophy and contraindication to vaginal estrogen use.	Perform repeat cytology with reflex HPV DNA testing in 6 and 12 months or colposcopy. If HPV+ or ASC-US or greater, refer for colposcopy. If HPV negative, repeat cytology in 12 months. If two consecutive repeat cytologies are negative, return to routine screening.
Pregnancy		Colposcopy is the preferred approach for nonadolescent; however, may choose to defer colposcopy until 6 weeks postpartum. Endocervical curettage is not acceptable during pregnancy.

Adolescence		Repeat cytology in 12 months; refer for colposcopy if HSIL develops or if cytologic abnormality persists for 24 months. HPV DNA testing is not useful.
HSIL	Not a common diagnosis. Predicts a 70–75% chance of having CIN 2,3 (biopsy confirmed) or a 1–2% chance of invasive cervical cancer.	May choose immediate loop electrical excision procedure (LEEP) or refer for colposcopy with endocervical assessment. If colposcopy satisfactory without CIN 2,3 may repeat colposcopy and cytology every 6 months for 1 year (if negative at both screenings return to routine screening), proceed with LEEP, or review colposcopy findings with management based on revised results. If colposcopy satisfactory with CIN 2,3 confirmed, managed by ASCCP guidelines. If colposcopy unsatisfactory, diagnostic excisional procedure is recommended.
HSIL in special circumstances		
Pregnancy	Colposcopic evaluation indicated by experienced clinicians who are experienced in evaluating pregnancy-induced colposcopic changes. Pregnancy contraindicates endocervical curettage.	If HSIL on cytology confirmed but no CIN 2,3 confirmed with biopsy, colposcopy and cytology are recommended no earlier than 6 weeks postpartum. If CIN 2,3, repeat cytology and colposcopy every 12 weeks with repeat biopsy as indicated.
Adolescence	Performance of immediate LEEP is unacceptable.	Refer for colposcopy. If no CIN 2,3, observe with cytology and colposcopy every 6 months for up to 24 months. If HSIL or CIN 2,3 persists for 24 months, then diagnostic excisional procedure. If two consecutive negative Paps or no HSIL, then return to routine screening.

ASCCP—American Society for Colposcopy and Cervical Pathology

[a]Risk factors that may indicate need for more frequent screening include those infected with HIV, those who are immunosuppressed, those exposed to diethylstilbestrol in utero, and those previously treated for cervical intraepithelial neoplasia (CIN) 2, CIN 3, or cancer.

Sources: ACOG Practice Bulletin, 2009; Apgar et al., 2009; ASCCP, 2007; Saslow et al., 2012; Solomon et al., 2002; Wright et al., 2007a, 2007b

been identified to impact sample quality for either CPT or LBCC include bleeding, vaginal inflammation/infection, intercourse within past 24 hours, genital atrophy, history of cervical radiation, pregnancy, postpartum, lactation, or recent physical manipulation or chemical irritation of the cervix (Arbyn et al., 2008).

For CPT, the speculum can be warmed and lubricated with water prior to insertion. For LBCC, in addition to use of water for warming, the posterior blade of the speculum may also be lubricated with a small amount of water-based lubricant prior to insertion (Arbyn et al., 2007; Hathaway, Pathak, & Maney, 2006). Do not routinely clean or swab the cervix prior to sampling (Arbyn et al., 2007). Excessive amounts of mucus can be gently teased off the cervix by use of a large cotton swab placed either near the vaginal sidewall next to the cervix or in the posterior fornix; then rotate the swab gently to capture and tease the mucus away from the cervix. Be sure all collection containers or slides are labeled correctly with name, date, and source, and that the containers or slides match the paperwork.

The TZ may be quite different in different age groups. The TZ at the SCJ where the cells from the ectocervix and endocervix meet is the area most vulnerable to HPV DNA effects. In an older woman, a clinician must be sure to obtain the specimen from higher in the endocervix where the SCJ is likely to be found.

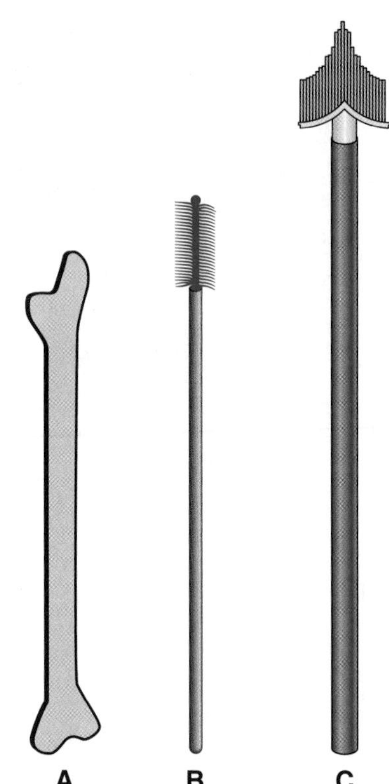

FIGURE 3–4. Sampling Devices for Pap Smears. Source: Adapted from Arbyn et al., 2007, p. 136.

Technique for Liquid-Based Cervical Cell Collection. A number of cytological cell collection systems that use a liquid-based or liquid-fixed method are on the market. The brand names of two that predominate in the United States are ThinPrep™ and SurePath™.

For sample collection with SurePath™, a detachable broom implement is used to sweep the cervix. The central portion of the broom implement is inserted in the cervical os and rotated. The detachable end of the broom implement used to collect the cervical sample is placed in the provided fixative container, and the container is then labeled and sent to the laboratory. An endocervical brush may be used in addition to the broom in order to obtain better sampling from the endocervical canal, or the company also has a plastic spatula with a removable end that can be used with the endocervical brush in place of the broom implement (BD, 2011). The additional use of an endocervical brush is particularly helpful for the nulliparous patient or a patient with a somewhat stenotic cervix in order to increase the probability of obtaining a sample from the TZ (see Figure 3–4).

Samples are collected when using ThinPrep™ following either a brush/spatula protocol or a broom protocol described by the company. The plastic spatula is to be rotated 360° around the exocervix while maintaining tight contact. The endocervical brush is to be inserted into the cervical os to a depth where only the bottommost fibers of the brush are exposed and then rotated ¼ to ½ turn in one direction. A warning to not overrotate is included in the company's protocol. The broom protocol advises to make sure that the longer central bristles are inserted into the cervical os to a depth that allows the shorter bristles to have full contact with the exocervix. The implements are rinsed by swishing them in the PreservCyt® liquid in the collection vial in order to remove the cervical cells from the implements. The brush is to be pushed against the container walls and rotated 10 times during the rinsing process (Hologic, 2011) (see Figure 3–5).

Technique for Conventional Slide Pap Smear. This technique for collecting a Pap specimen is now rarely used in the United States. For CPT, use the endocervical cytobrush instead of a cotton-tipped applicator and the plastic spatula instead of a wooden spatula. This is because the cotton-tipped applicator and wooden spatula may hold the best cells in porous material, and therefore, not transfer

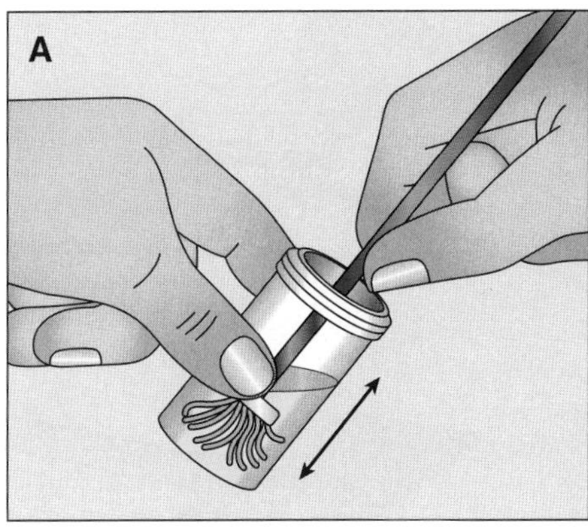

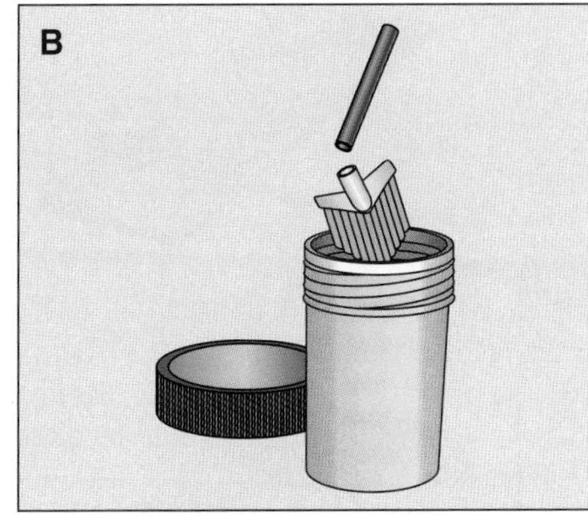

FIGURE 3–5. Collection of Liquid-Based Cervical Cytology using ThinPrep™ or SurePath™. Source: Adapted from Arbyn et al., 2007, p. 138.

the best cells to the slide. Use of an endocervical brush has been found to increase the endocervical cells obtained by sevenfold (Taylor et al., 1987). If a cotton-tipped applicator must be used, wet in normal saline first so that the cells will be released from the fibers onto the slide. The cytobrush may be used for pregnant women. However, many providers choose not to use the cytobrush during pregnancy. If used, warn patients that spotting may occur; in fact, this is true for many nonpregnant women. Do not use the long pointed end of the spatula for pregnant women.

Steps in obtaining the Pap smear sample using CPT include the following:

- Prepare slides and cytology fixative for use.
- Do not take the sample if large amounts of menses are present because it will obscure the cytologic field. A partially obscured specimen means 50 to 75 percent of cells cannot be visualized. An unsatisfactory specimen means that more than 75 percent of cells cannot be visualized (Solomon et al., 2002).
- Obtain portio (exocervix) sample first with the spatula, and then the endocervical brush sample because bleeding occurs frequently with the latter. If cervical shape/characteristics are not configured to ease of rotating the spatula, gently scrape it over the surface of the cervix. Remember, you want to get as complete a specimen from the TZ as possible.
- Rotate the brush 360° gently to minimize bleeding if possible. Be prepared to apply pressure with a large cotton-tipped applicator should bleeding occur after all specimens are obtained and before removing the speculum.
- Apply smear material evenly on the slide without clumping and fix rapidly (within 10 seconds); drying will significantly alter the sample. If using one slide, material must be collected very quickly to prevent drying effects. Ideally, two slides are desirable but seldom used.
- Be sure to rotate brush or paint cells with spatula onto the slide with slight pressure (see Figure 3–6).
- Use the more rounded end of the spatula to collect cells if the SCJ is out on the ectocervix.
- Rotate the broom implement several times in the os to get an adequate number of cells if it is used to collect the SCJ specimen.

These LBCC methods use an automated processor that concentrates epithelial cells and screens out blood cells, inflammatory cells, and other extraneous material to prepare a thin-layer slide that is read with computer-assisted screening (Apgar et al., 2008). Comparisons of CPT with LBCC have yielded conflicting results. Strander, Andersson-Ellström, Milsom, Rådberg, and Ryd (2007) found the percentage of satisfactory Pap tests significantly higher for LBCC and the percentage of unsatisfactory or limited satisfactory tests significantly lower for CPT. Others have found no difference in satisfactory results between CPT and LBCC (ACOG Practice Bulletin, 2009; Arbyn et al., 2008; Wright, Marchall, & Desai, 2010).

HPV TESTING

HPV testing is recommended for routine use in combination with cervical cytology screening for those over 30 years old (Apgar, Kittendorf, Bettcher, Wong, & Kaufman,

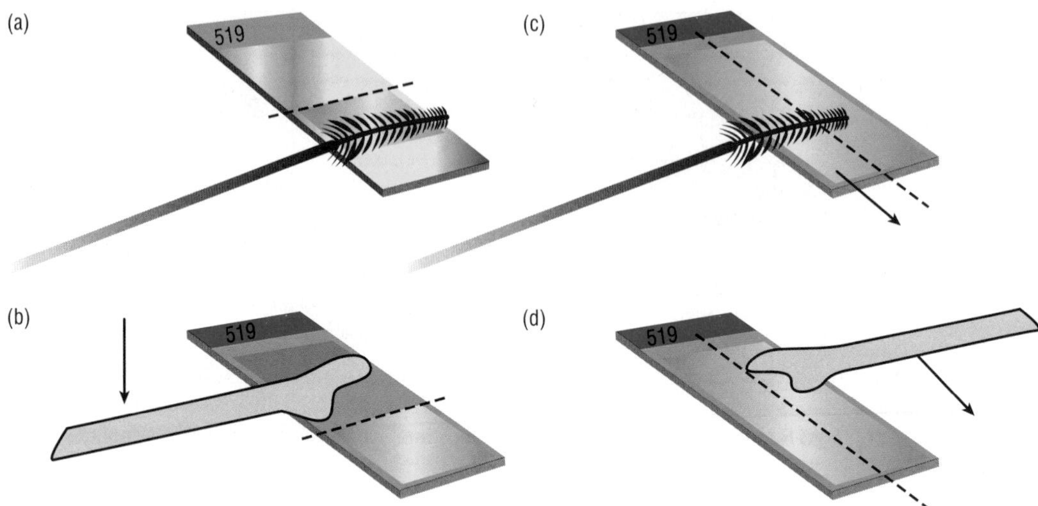

FIGURE 3–6. Method for Placing Sample on Slide for Conventional Pap Test. Source: Adapted from Arbyn et al., 2007, p. 137.

2009). It is not recommended for use in adolescents even as a reflex test for atypical squamous cells of undetermined significance (ASC-US). Pap results in adolescents as HPV is prevalent in adolescents and clears spontaneously in most cases (Wright et al., 2007b). HPV testing can be done with polymerase chain reaction testing or DNA testing (Juckett & Hartman-Adams, 2010). Sensitivity for finding CIN 2,3 confirmed by biopsy in women who have ASC is very high: 0.83 to 1.0. The NCI conducted a study to compare sensitivity and specificity of methods to detect CIN 3 in ASC-US–diagnosed women (Solomon, Schiffman, Tarone, & ALTS Study Group, 2001). Women were randomized for colposcopy, repeat Pap smear every 6 months, or HPV testing using Hybrid Capture 2™. HPV testing was 96 percent sensitive in accurately indicating a need for colposcopy as opposed to repeat Pap testing being only 86 percent sensitive (even less so with only one repeat Pap). Other studies have supported similar findings, leading the 2006 Consensus Guidelines group to include HPV testing in combination with a cervical cytology test in its recommendations for ASC results for those over 30 years old. Reflex HPV DNA testing is an advantage for women with ASC, eliminating a visit for a return pelvic exam to collect the specimen and sparing the need for colposcopy in 40 to 60 percent (Wright et al., 2007b). The reflex test can be performed with a small amount of the liquid from both of the LBCC methods described in this chapter. The test can also be performed stand-alone using the same collection method as used for a liquid-based Pap. Follow instructions for maintaining the specimen until transport.

Screening for cervical cancer with the use of self-collected vaginal samples for HPV testing (SC-HPV) has been proposed as potentially useful for those with little access to health care in clinic settings because it has greater sensitivity than Pap smears and the potential for a patient to collect the specimen herself. However, as HPV positivity does not directly correlate with cervical disease severity, and appropriate resources and methods for treating those screened are unclear, these proposals are still in the study phase (Gravitt, Belinson, Salmeron, & Shah, 2011). Others have proposed stand-alone HPV screening, along with visual inspection of the cervix with acetic acid (VIA), for use in developing countries. Its future use for high-risk populations may be preferred (Mandelblatt et al., 2002).

Interpretation of Results and Action

The 2001 Bethesda System is the test reporting system used nationwide that tells the provider the category of the findings and the recommended action (Wright et al., 2007a, 2007b). The categories have been modified from the original Bethesda System to include ASC with subcategories (ASC-US and ASC-H) and recommendations. Recommendations include those for special circumstances such as pregnancy and atypical glandular cells (AGC) with subcategories less severe than adenocarcinoma, but including endocervical adenocarcinoma in situ (AIS), and recommendations for follow-up. Action needed for categories of LSIL with recommendations for management with and without cervical lesions and in special circumstances such as postmenopause, as well as HSIL with recommendations for management with colposcopy and in special circumstances, is also included (see Table 3–4). The information in this table is from the most current management recommendations at the time of this writing (Apgar et al., 2009; Wright et al., 2007a, 2007b). See Chapter 16 for more information.

PREGNANCY TESTING

Pregnancy can be confirmed using urine sample or serum sample testing. There is both an α and a β subunit to human chorionic gonadotropin similar to other glycoproteins; the β subunit is measured for a pregnancy test. βhCG is present in the urine 5 to 7 days after conception. It is best to test on a first morning void as the hormonal level is most concentrated in the urine at that time. Serum testing can be done on a qualitative level, sensitivity is at 25 to 50 mIU/mL, or a quantitative level, sensitivity is as low as 1 to 3 mIU/mL. A serum level of 5 mIU/mL or above is considered to indicate pregnancy in women of childbearing age. In most instances, the urine pregnancy test is sufficient. Serum pregnancy testing is always used at the quantitative level to follow βhCG levels when ectopic pregnancy is suspected or to confirm resolution of an ectopic or molar pregnancy. Serum testing may also be used to evaluate bleeding in early pregnancy. The level of βhCG should nearly double in 48 hours during the first 6 weeks of gestation for those with a normally progressing pregnancy. Note that βhCG may also be elevated in some cancers (Fischbach & Dunning, 2009). In these cases, total hCG levels including measurement of both an α and a β subunit may be helpful (see Chapters 16, 19, and 20).

GC AND CT TESTS

Purpose

Testing is done if the woman is at high risk and/or under the age of 25 years, to diagnose both GC and CT (see Chapter 14 for further information on these diseases) (CDC, 2010b). In many instances, if CT is present, GC is also present. In 2007, the U.S. Preventive Services Task Force (USPSTF) lowered their recommended age for screening for CT to all women aged 24 and younger (Meyers, Halvorson, & Luckhaupt, 2007). The CDC has kept their age recommendation for CT screening for sexually active women aged 25 and younger. Cultures were the gold standard for years to diagnose both *Neisseria gonorrhoeae* diplococci and the *Chlamydia trachomatis* intracellular parasite. However, the use of culture has nearly disappeared since RNA hybridization assay probe testing became available. The Gen-Probe DNA test can diagnose GC and CT simultaneously. Target RNA is extracted from a woman's specimen; labeled DNA probe sequences specific for GC and for CT are added to the specimen; if the RNA of the organism is present, a tight helix forms on the probe that is measured by an optical scanner. The test has all the components needed for screening: high sensitivity and specificity, fairly low cost, ease of use, and ease of handling. Nucleic acid amplification testing (NAAT) is recommended by the CDC for testing for CT (CDC, 2010b). For screening large numbers of people and for screening men, NAAT using a urine sample has become standard. These researchers suggested that all young adults be tested using NAAT. NAAT can also be used for screening using endocervical or vaginal samples (Spigarelli, 2006; Turner et al., 2002). (See Chapter 14 for more information on diagnosis of GC and CT.)

Techniques for Specimen Collection

Prepare the woman for an exam requiring a speculum insertion. Collect the specimen after the cervical cytology. Use one of the two sterile swabs to clean off excess mucus from the cervical os and portio around the os. Be sure to discard this swab. Insert the second swab 1 to 1.5 cm into endocervical canal, rotate 10 to 30 seconds, withdraw without touching the vaginal walls or any other area, and place in the transport medium. Break the swab shaft where scored and place the cap securely. The specimen may be kept at room temperature or refrigerated for up to 7 days (Chapin, 1999).

The vaginal sample can be self-collected or collected by the clinician in the clinic setting. The sample is obtained by inserting a sterile Dacron-tipped swab to a depth of approximately 2.5 cm into the vagina and then rotating the swab for 15 to 30 seconds; upon removal the swab is placed in the same collection device as is used for endocervical samples (Smith et al., 2001).

The urine sample is obtained using a first catch collection method when used for CT screening. The patient is instructed to begin specimen collection immediately at the start of voiding. The urine specimen should be refrigerated and testing is recommended to occur within 4 days (Toye, Wood, Bobrowska, & Ramotar, 1998).

Results

Results are reported as positive or negative for both GC and CT. A small number of samples do not provide definitive results and retesting is needed (0.5% to 1.0%). The lab normally repeats the test, but if it continues to be indefinite, the woman may need to return for another specimen to be collected. In the presence of excessive gross blood, a false-positive result could occur with some of the older DNA tests; therefore, it was recommended to avoid collecting specimens during menses. This problem has not been found to be significant with the newer testing methods (Toye et al., 1998). Women at risk for GC or CT are also at risk for HPV. All three have negative consequences. Follow the policy of the site where the client is being seen for guidance. If the woman has recently taken an antibiotic, a false-negative result may occur. For positive results, it is crucial to treat the partner. Presumptive treatment may be given if signs and symptoms indicate infection. Retesting is indicated if the woman does not improve with treatment or if an area where resistant GC is known to occur. Three to four weeks after treatment is completed, a test of cure is indicated in women who are pregnant. For others, it is recommended to wait for 3 months to evaluate for test of cure (CDC, 2010b).

WET MOUNTS: NORMAL SALINE AND POTASSIUM HYDROXIDE

Purpose

Wet mounts (or preps) are done primarily to diagnose selected vaginal infections and to assist in determining causes of bleeding. A normal saline wet mount of vaginal secretions from a normal childbearing age nonpregnant woman shows lactobacilli and epithelial cells.

Technique

Wear gloves to collect and while handling specimens. Dip cotton swab into vaginal/cervical discharge pooled under the cervix in the posterior and lateral fornices. Depending on protocols at the clinic site, this sample may be placed in a tube with 1 mL saline and sent to the laboratory for testing or the wet prep may be performed in the clinic by the clinician. The next step that is done either in the laboratory or by the clinician in the clinic is to drop one drop of the saline solution on a clean slide and cover with coverslip. Drop another drop on a clean side and add a drop of 10 percent potassium hydroxide (KOH), assess for "fishy" odor, and cover with coverslip. Rather than this last step, the clinician who performs the wet prep in the clinic could obtain a second swab and dip it into the discharge; place it in a tube with 1 mL of 10 percent KOH and mix; drop one drop on a clean slide and cover. Placing a drop of vaginal discharge in a drop of 10 percent KOH may give off a fishy odor if amines are released. This is called a positive whiff test and indicates possible bacterial vaginosis (BV) or trichomoniasis. Evaluate the prepared slide(s) with low (10×) and high (40×) power microscope objectives. The value of the specimen is proportional to the effectiveness of the collection techniques and the quality of the clinician's interpretation. Vaginal/cervical discharge specimens may also be placed directly on a slide with a drop of solution, rather than placed in a tube. KOH is used to disrupt the epithelial cells (though not totally destroy them) and get rid of debris that may obscure hyphae and bacteria that are resistant to KOH. Obtaining the specimen(s) prior to cervical cytology or other tests is advised to avoid red blood cells (RBCs) obscuring the field.

Results

The following may be analyzed from a saline wet mount (Iglesias, Alderman, & Fox, 2000; Monif, 2002):

- Normal squamous epithelial cells—have smooth borders, few bacteria visible inside the cell, single central nuclei
- "Clue cells"—squamous epithelial cells with irregular, obscured border from multiple cocci adhered to outer cell membrane; have stippled appearance; indicative of BV
- Lactobacilli—rod-shaped bacteria evidencing acidity of normal vaginal environment; not found or decreased significantly in BV
- Polymorphonuclear leukocytes (PMNs)—in great numbers (more than 10 per high power field) indicate infection, such as GC or CT
- RBCs—indicate obvious or microscopic bleeding; may indicate need for diagnosis if cause unknown
- Trichomonads—motile protozoa indicative of trichomoniasis vaginitis
- Spores and/or hyphae—indicate fungal infection, such as with *Candida albicans*

If the wet mount is prepared with 10 percent KOH, the epithelial cells are lysed, and fungal spores and hyphae are easier to visualize (Iglesias et al., 2000). Management of the findings of any wet mount depends on the problem (see Chapter 14 for diagnosis and treatment of selected vaginitis and sexually transmitted diseases [STDs]).

Various office-based DNA/RNA tests have been developed to assist clinicians in diagnosing vaginitis. Two such tests, Affirm VP® and FemExam®, when used in combination, have a sensitivity of 91.0 percent and a specificity of 61.5 percent for the diagnosis of BV. Microscopy using established criteria, such as Amsel's (three or more of the following factors need to be present: clue cells, adherent homogenous vaginal discharge, pH of the vaginal fluid is > 4.5, and/or positive whiff test), has a sensitivity of 90 to 100 percent and a specificity of 86 to 97 percent. Culture for diagnosis of BV is not reliable. Microscopy for diagnosis of trichomonas has a specificity of 100 percent but a sensitivity of only about 61 percent. The product manufacturer of OSOM Trichmonas Rapid Test®, a rapid test, reports a sensitivity of 83 percent and a specificity of 99 percent. Culture techniques for diagnosis of trichomonas have a lower range of sensitivity and specificity (Spigarelli & Biro, 2005). Providers who use microscopy for diagnosis should gain depth in this area through special study and practice. They must also follow current CLIA rules and regulations for provider-performed microscopy.

EVALUATING VAGINAL pH

Purpose

This evaluation is done as part of the wet prep/mount or can be done as a stand-alone evaluation. A pH level of 3.8 to 4.2 is normal in the vagina and must be maintained to help keep the vaginal environment stable (ACOG Practice Bulletin, 2006). *Lactobacillus acidophilus* bacteria keep the vaginal ecosystem healthy by production of lactic acid that suppresses gram-negative and gram-positive anaerobes. Lactobacilli also produce hydrogen peroxide, which is toxic to anaerobes. If the lactobacilli growth is suppressed, pH level rises, hydrogen ion concentration falls, and pathogen growth is favored. Testing pH level helps in determining imbalances.

Technique and Results

Special pH paper is placed on the lateral vaginal wall or in vaginal secretions. If the pH is > 4.5, an increase in gram-negative facultative anaerobes and gram-positive and gram-negative obligate anaerobes is the probable cause, as is seen with BV (ACOG Practice Bulletin, 2006).

URINALYSIS

Purpose

A urinalysis provides supportive data in diagnosing urinary complaints; however, it should not be used alone if results are negative but other findings indicate that a problem exists. Urine culture is the gold standard for diagnosing urinary tract infections. Dipstick reagent strip findings of nitrites, leukocytes, and blood plus microscopic urinalysis data are usually adequate to indicate need for treatment in simple cystitis. Culture and sensitivity should be used with persistent bacteriuria (Mata, 1998). As few as two bacteria seen in a high-power field when the specimen has been centrifuged have a 90 percent sensitivity and specificity for diagnosing significant bacteriuria. Urinalysis can also be useful in assessing for renal and metabolic diseases.

Technique for Urine Specimen

The test procedure first involves obtaining the best specimen. Instruct the client to wash her hands well and collect a midstream urine specimen. A clean-catch specimen is not necessary. Studies indicate that a midstream collection is adequate (Leisure, Dudley, & Donowitz, 1993). The client should start to urinate in the commode, then catch a small amount of urine midstream in a sterile cup, and finish urinating in the commode. Replace the lid on the cup tightly without touching the inside or top edge. Client teaching should stress that failing to follow this procedure jeopardizes the accuracy of the test. Use a tampon or cotton ball in the introitus during collection of urine if heavy vaginal discharge or bleeding is present. Test or culture the specimen within a few minutes, or refrigerate it with a tight cover and test within a few hours. If collecting the specimen for CT screening, obtain a first void urine as described in the section on CT and GC testing.

- If screening for nitrite and normal pH, a dipstick test is done on a first morning urine specimen. Keep dipsticks in a cool, dark, tightly closed container. Assess glucose, ketones, blood, leukocytes, protein, and specific gravity.
- Microscopic examination should be done on centrifuged sediment, or a specimen may be sent out for analysis. Look for white blood cells (WBCs, or leukocytes), RBCs (or erythrocytes), crystals, bacteria, epithelial cells, and casts. Use low light to see casts better.
- Culture and sensitivity tests are indicated when the number of WBCs is greater than five per high power field or when dipstick results indicate infection.

Results

All findings should be within normal limits (see standard laboratory testing text or manual).

HERPES CULTURE AND TYPE-SPECIFIC TESTS

Purpose

Culture is done to definitively diagnose herpes simplex genitalis (ACOG Practice Bulletin, 2004). However, sensitivity decreases the longer the lesion is present (Spigarelli & Biro, 2005). Serologic testing can be done to confirm presence of antibodies to the virus and typing of virus, but it doesn't provide information regarding the site of outbreak. Serum testing can be useful for those who are aware of a previous outbreak for counseling guidance regarding use of suppressive therapy. Those who are infected with herpes simplex virus type 2 (HSV-2) have a higher incidence of recurrent outbreaks than those infected with HSV type 1 (HSV-1). Site of outbreak is not necessarily correlated with viral typing (see Chapter 14).

Technique

For obtaining a sample for culture, the following is recommended: Wear glasses to protect eyes and cover unclothed skin with a mask, gloves, gown, and/or lab coat. Carefully puncture (unroof) intact vesicle with sterile tuberculin needle or rub open lesion vigorously (if vesicle already draining) with saline-moistened Dacron-tipped swab to get viral sample (ACOG Practice Bulletin, 2004). Vesicular fluid is needed for testing; it is high in viral particles. Place specimen in culture medium immediately. Do not swab to dry. If obtaining a cervical culture, the swab is inserted in the endocervix and rotated, and then rubbed over the ectocervix. Refrigerate and transport within 12 hours or follow directions for transport and storage.

HSV-1 and HSV-2 can be detected using type-specific serologic assays. There are a number of type-specific serologic assays. The CDC recommends using assays that are based upon glycoprotein G (gG). These assays have a sensitivity of 80 to 98 percent and a specificity of 96 percent or greater. Examples of assays are BioKit HSV-2, HerpeSelect-1 and -2 ELISA IgG, and HerpeSelect 1 and 2 Immunoblot IgG. All three are FDA approved (Spigarelli & Biro, 2005).

Results

Positive culture growth of HSV-1 and HSV-2 takes 2 to 3 days for results, but laboratories wait 7 to 14 days to be sure results are negative.

HIV TESTING

Testing for presence of the human immunodeficiency virus (HIV) is most often performed with a serum sample. ELISA is used as a screening test. If the results are positive for ELISA, it is confirmed with the Western blot, which is a more specific test (Spigarelli & Biro, 2005). Use of an immunofluorescent assay as a rapid screen prior to Western blot is another option. There are other rapid screening tests available: OraQuick Rapid HIV-1 Antibody Test™ uses a finger stick sample. Various saliva screening tests are also available. If either of these screening tests is positive, the result should be confirmed with the Western blot (Fischbach & Dunning, 2009) (see Chapter 15).

SYPHILIS TESTING AND SCREENING

Dark-field microscopy performed on fluid obtained from a chancre or condyloma lata is the definitive test for syphilis. But in order to be considered negative, the exam must be performed and must remain negative for identification of *Treponema pallidum* on three different days (Brown & Frank, 2003).

Two nontreponemal tests are recommended by the CDC for screening for syphilis: the Venereal Disease Research Laboratory (VDRL) test and the rapid plasma reagin (RPR). These screening tests can have a false-positive result from a number of conditions, including pregnancy. Therefore, both of these tests must be confirmed with either the fluorescent treponemal antibody-absorption (FTA-ABS) test or the *T. pallidum* passive particle agglutination (TP-PA) test (CDC, 2010c; Fischbach & Dunning, 2009). The sensitivity for FTA-ABS ranges from 84 to 100 percent and for TP-PA from 86 to 100 percent, depending on stage of syphilis at the time of diagnosis (Fischbach & Dunning, 2009) (see Chapter 14).

HEPATITIS TESTING

A serum sample can be used to test for hepatitis types A, B, C, D, E, and G. Hepatitis types tested for most often in women's health are hepatitis B and C. Hepatitis B is considered an STD, although it is also blood borne and can be transmitted by exposure to contaminated blood. It is discussed at length in Chapter 14. The tests for acute infection with hepatitis B are HBcAb IgM (hepatitis B core antibody immunoglobulin M) and HBsAg (hepatitis B surface antigen). A positive result for HBsAg may also indicate chronic infection. It is used as a screening test for presence of chronic infection. Those who have received the hepatitis B vaccine will have a positive HBsAb (hepatitis B surface antibody) test (Fischbach & Dunning, 2009). See Chapters 19 and 20 for prenatal testing recommendations for hepatitis B.

Hepatitis C was previously called hepatitis non-A, non-B. It is transmitted parenterally. This hepatitis type can be tested for by measurement of anti-hepatitis C virus (anti-HCV). This test should be confirmed with measurement of viral load: HCV RNA. As hepatitis C is transmitted parenterally, those who are IV drug abusers, those with tattoos, and those with body piercings are at increased risk (Fischbach & Dunning, 2009). See Chapter 23 for more information.

Hepatitis A is transmitted by fecal-oral contamination. Those with acute infection will have a positive HAV-Ab/IgM (hepatitis A virus antibody/immunoglobulin M).

There is a vaccine for hepatitis A, and those who have been vaccinated or have prior immunity from exposure can be assessed with a total anti-HAV (measurement of both HAV-Ab/IgM and HAV-Ab/IgG). See Chapter 23 for more information.

Hepatitis D can occur only in the presence of hepatitis B and, therefore, is tested for only in persons who are hepatitis B positive. Hepatitis E is present in contaminated waters and is transmitted by the fecal–oral route, but is very rare in the developed world. Hepatitis G is transmitted by contaminated blood and can be present only in those who are dually infected with hepatitis B and C (Fischbach & Dunning, 2009).

OVERVIEW OF COMMONLY USED PROCEDURES AND DIAGNOSTIC IMAGING

BREAST IMAGING

Mammography and other methods for breast imaging are fully discussed in Chapter 17.

COLPOSCOPY

Colposcopy is a procedure performed by a trained clinician. Training includes a didactic program as well as a mentorship and successfully completing an examination upon completion of the mentorship. Colposcopy is done to provide a magnified view of the cervix, vagina, and/or vulva to assess for invasive disease and is performed as indicated in cases of cervical cell abnormalities identified with the Pap smear. In some cases, the indication for colposcopy may be presence of suspicious vaginal or vulvar lesions. Biopsy specimens may be obtained during the colposcopy procedure (Apgar et al., 2008).

The colposcope is a "binocular microscope with a built-in light source and a converging objective lens attached to a support appliance" (Apgar et al., 2008, p. 104). For visualization of the cervix and vagina, the objective lens is placed externally in close enough proximity to the outlet of the vaginal speculum to allow for a magnified view of these structures while still allowing the clinician access to obtain tissue samples.

For the procedure, the patient is in the dorsal lithotomy position and draped. The vulva is inspected with the colposcope; if indicated, 3 to 5 percent acetic acid solution or vinegar may be applied to better visualize the epithelium. Either of these solutions is taken up by tissues with epithelial abnormalities differently than normal tissues and abnormalities present with an "acetowhite" response. A speculum is then inserted into the vagina to allow visualization of the cervix. Under magnification of the colposcope, the vascular pattern of the cervix is determined, and then a 3 to 5 percent acetic acid or vinegar solution is applied to the cervix twice to obtain an acetowhite response. Next, an iodine solution (Lugol's solution) may be applied to the cervix (unless the patient is allergic to iodine), endocervical curettage is performed, and suspicious lesions are then biopsied (Monsel's solution or silver nitrate may be used to control bleeding post biopsy). The speculum is then slowly removed to allow evaluation of the vagina. Specimens are sent to pathology, the procedure findings are documented by the clinician, and a follow-up plan is discussed with the patient (Apgar et al., 2008). See Chapter 16 for information on management of cervical, vaginal, or vulvar abnormalities.

ENDOMETRIAL BIOPSY

The endometrial biopsy is an in-office procedure that uses a pipelle device that, while a speculum is in the vagina, is passed through the cervix into the endometrial cavity in order to obtain a small amount of tissue for examination. Inform the client about the purpose and risks of the test. Most clinicians obtain a written informed consent, as there is a very small risk of uterine perforation and infection with any instrumentation to the uterus. Encourage relaxation breathing and convey the progression of each step to the client to alleviate her discomfort and anxiety. The biopsy usually takes no longer than 1 minute and is generally described as causing moderate menstrual-like cramps. The tissue sample is sent to pathology for analysis. Spotting and cramping may occur up to 48 hours following biopsy. Nonsteroidal anti-inflammatory drugs (NSAIDs) can be recommended if there are no contraindications. The client is generally able to proceed with her day as usual without any need for assistance with driving, returning to work, and so on.

HYSTEROSCOPY

Hysteroscopy allows transcervical visualization of the endometrial cavity. The procedure is done in the office or operating room under local anesthesia (such as a paracervical block), or minimal anesthetic control (MAC), or a combination of both. A vaginal speculum is inserted, the cervix is dilated, and then the telescope-like hysteroscope is passed into the cervical os and the uterine cavity. A camera at the proximal end of the scope transmits an image of the uterine cavity to a screen for the clinician to view. Minor surgical procedures such as removal of polyps can be performed. The hysteroscope is inserted when the cervix is dilated. The uterus is distended with Dextran 70, carbon dioxide, or another distention medium to facilitate visualization of the endometrial cavity (Petrozza & Rivlin, 2011) (see Chapter 11).

HYSTOSALPINGOGRAM

The hystosalpingogram is a radiological study that may be performed as part of an infertility workup. See Chapter 13 for more information.

ULTRASONOGRAPHY

Ultrasound has been used extensively in both obstetrical and gynecological settings. The high-frequency sound waves transmitted by the ultrasound transducer bounce off differently based on tissue density and character and are analyzed to provide a picture of internal organs and structures on a screen. There are abdominal, transvaginal, and transrectal probes. The abdominal and transvaginal probes are the most frequently used probes in women's imaging. The procedure has no known harmful effects. Sonogram is another name for ultrasonography (Fischbach & Dunning, 2009). See Chapters 20 and 21 for more discussion on use of this imaging in obstetrics.

Pelvic Ultrasound

Transvaginal pelvic ultrasound can be used to evaluate the ovaries and the uterus. It is also used in early pregnancy to evaluate location of gestational sac and/or fetal viability. The procedure needs to be performed by a clinician who is trained in ultrasonography. Measurement of the endometrial stripe is part of any uterine evaluation. An endometrial stripe less than 5 mm in width generally excludes significant endometrial pathology. More than 90 percent of symptomatic menopausal women with endometrial cancer or other endometrial pathology have a stripe greater than 5 mm in width (Greenspan, Cardillo, Davey, Heller, & Moriarty, 2006). However, further evaluation is recommended for all symptomatic menopausal women not on hormone replacement therapy whose endometrial stripe is greater than 4 mm in width.

Saline-Infusion Sonohystogram

Saline-infusion sonohystogram may be utilized prior to hysteroscopy to identify if abnormality exists within the uterine cavity. For this procedure, a catheter is passed through the cervical os and the endometrial cavity is distended with saline prior to insertion of the vaginal ultrasound probe (see Chapters 11 and 13).

CONCLUSION

The list of diagnostic tests, procedures, and imaging methods covered in this chapter is not meant to be exhaustive of all such methods utilized in assessing women's health. It is meant to serve as a broad overview. The reader will also find these and other tests, procedures, or imaging methods discussed in subsequent chapters.

REFERENCES

ACOG Practice Bulletin. (2004, reaffirmed 2010). *Gynecologic herpes simplex viral infections* (No. 57). Washington, DC: ACOG.

ACOG Practice Bulletin. (2006, reaffirmed 2011). *Vaginitis* (No. 72). Washington, DC: ACOG.

ACOG Practice Bulletin. (2009). *Cervical cytology screening* (No. 114). Washington, DC: ACOG.

American Academy of Orthopaedic Surgeons. (2009). *Position statement: Osteoporosis/bone health in adults as a national public health priority*. Retrieved from http://www.aaos.org/about/papers/position/1113.asp

Apgar, B.S., Brotzman, G.L., & Spitzer, M. (2008). *Colposcopy: Principles and practice* (2nd ed.). Philadelphia: Saunders Elsevier.

Apgar, B.S., Kittendorf, A.L., Bettcher, C.M., Wong, J., & Kaufman, A.M. (2009). Update on ASCCP consensus guidelines for abnormal cervical screening tests and cervical histology. *American Family Physician, 80*(2), 147–155.

Arbyn, M., Bergeron, C., Klinkhamer, P., Matin-Hirsch, P., Siebers, A.G., & Bulten, J. (2008). Liquid compared with conventional cervical cytology: A systematic review and meta-analysis. *Obstetrics and Gynecology, 111*, 167–177.

Arbyn, M., Herbert, A., Schenck, U., Nieminen, P., Jordan, J., McGougan, E., et al. (2007). European guidelines for quality assurance in cervical cancer screening: Recommendations for collecting samples for conventional and liquid-based cytology. *Cytology, 18*, 133–139.

ASCCP. (2007). *Cytology algorithms*. Retrieved August 13, 2011, from http://www.asccp.org/ConsensusGuidelines/tabid/7436/Default.aspx

Banerjee, D., Wong, E.C., Shin, J., Fortmann, S.P., & Palaniappan, L. (2011). Racial and ethnic variation in lipoprotein (a) levels among Asian Indian and Chinese patients. *Journal of Lipids*. doi:10.1155/2011/291954

Bernstein, A.S., Makuc, D.M., & Bilheimer, L.T. (2010). *Chartbook: Health, United States, 2010*. Hyattsville, MD: National Center for Health Statistics.

BD. (2011). *BD SurePath™ liquid-based Pap test*. Retrieved August 13, 2011, from http://www.bd.com/tripath/physicians/surepath.asp

Brown, D.L., & Frank, J.B. (2003). Diagnosis and management of syphilis. *American Family Physician, 63*(2), 283–290.

Centers for Disease Control and Prevention. (2008). *Cervical cancer*. Retrieved May 14, 2011, from http://www.cdc.gov/cancer/cervical/

Centers for Disease Control and Prevention. (2010a). *National chronic kidney disease fact sheet, 2010*. Atlanta, GA: U.S. Department of Health and Human Services. Retrieved from http://www.cdc.gov/diabetes/pubs/factsheets/kidney.htm

Centers for Disease Control and Prevention. (2010b). *Sexually transmitted diseases treatment guidelines, 2010: Chlamydial infections*. Retrieved August 13, 2011, from http://www.cdc.gov/std/treatment/2010/chlamydial-infections.htm

Centers for Disease Control and Prevention. (2010c). *2010 STD treatment guidelines*. Retrieved August 13, 2011, from http://www.cdc.gov/std/treatment/2010/

Centers for Disease Control and Prevention. (2011a). *Fatal injury data*. Atlanta, GA: U.S. Department of Health and Human Services. Retrieved from http://www.cdc.gov/injury/wisqars/fatal.html

Centers for Disease Control and Prevention. (2011b). *HIV surveillance in adolescents and young adults*. Atlanta, GA: U.S. Department of Health and Human Services. Retrieved from http://www.cdc.gov/hiv/topics/surveillance/resources/slides/adolescents/index.htm

Centers for Disease Control and Prevention. (2011c). *Revised recommendations for HIV testing in healthcare settings in the U.S.* Atlanta, GA: U.S. Department of Health and Human Services. Retrieved from http://www.cdc.gov/hiv/topics/testing/slidesets.htm

Centers for Disease Control and Prevention. (2011d). *Falls among older adults: An overview*. Atlanta, GA: U.S. Department of Health and Human Services. Retrieved from http://www.cdc.gov/homeandrecreationalsafety/falls/adultfalls.html

Centers for Disease Control and Prevention, Cancer Prevention and Control. (2011). *Cancer among women*. Atlanta, GA: U.S. Department of Health and Human Services. Retrieved from http://www.cdc.gov/cancer/dcpc/data/women.htm

Centers for Disease Control and Prevention, Office of Women's Health. (2010). *Leading causes of death in females: United States, 2007*. Atlanta, GA: U.S. Department of Health and Human Services. Retrieved from http://www.cdc.gov/women/lcod

Chapin, K. (1999). Probing the STDs. *American Journal of Nursing, 99*(7), 24–27.

Cheng, Y.J., Hootman, J.M., Murphy, L.B., Langmaid, G.A., & Helmick, C.G. (2010). Prevalence of doctor-diagnosed arthritis and arthritis-attributable activity limitation—United States, 2007–2009. *Morbidity and Mortality Weekly Report, 59*(39), 1261–1265.

Childtrends Data Bank. (2011). Retrieved from http://www.childtrendsdatabank.org/?q=node/

Chlebowski, R.T., Kuller, L.H., Prentice, R.L., Stefanick, M.L., Manson, J.E., Gass, M., et al. (2009). Breast cancer after use of estrogen plus progestin in postmenopausal women. *New England Journal of Medicine, 360*, 573–587.

Cong, X., Cox, D.D., & Cantor, S.B. (2007). Bayesian meta-analysis of Papanicolaou smear accuracy. *Gynecologic Oncology, 107*, S133–S137.

Davey, D.D., Austin, R.M., Birdson, G., Buck, H.W., Cox, J.T., Darragh, T.M., et al. (2002). ASCCP patient management guidelines: Pap test specimen adequacy and quality indicators. *Journal of Lower Genital Tract Disease, 6*(2), 195–199.

Fahey, M.T., Irwig, L., & Macaskill, P. (1995). Meta-analysis of Pap test accuracy. *American Journal of Epidemiology, 141*, 680–689.

Fairweather, D., & Rose, N.R. (2004). Women and autoimmune diseases. *Emergent Infectious Diseases*. Retrieved from http://wwwnc.cdc.gov/eid/article/10/11/04-0367.htm

Fischbach, F.T., & Dunning, M.B. (2009). *A manual of laboratory and diagnostic tests* (8th ed.). Philadelphia: Wolters Kluwer/Lippincott Williams & Wilkins.

Gravitt, P.E., Belinson, J.L., Salmeron, J., & Shah, K.V. (2011). Looking ahead: A case for human papillomavirus testing of self-sampled vaginal specimens as a cervical cancer screening strategy. *International Journal of Cancer, 129*, 517–527.

Greenspan, D.L., Cardillo, M., Davey, D.D., Heller, D.S., & Moriarty, A.T. (2006). Endometrial cells in cervical cytology: Review of cytological features and clinical assessment. *Journal of Lower Genital Tract Disease, 10*, 111–122.

Guendelman, S., Thornton, D., Gould, J., & Hosang, N. (2005). Social disparities in maternal morbidity during labor and delivery between Mexican-born and US-born white Californians, 1996–1998. *American Journal of Public Health, 95*, 2218–2224.

Guerra, R., Zhaoxia, Y., Marcovina, S., Peshock, R., Cohen, J.C., & Hobbs, H.H. (2005). Lipoprotein(a) and apolipoprotein(a) isoforms: No association with coronary artery calcification in the Dallas Heart Study. *Circulation, 111*, 1471–1479. Retrieved from http://circ.ahajournals.org/content/111/12/1471.full

Hathaway, J.K., Pathak, P.K., & Maney, R. (2006). Is liquid-based pap testing affected by water-based lubricant? *Obstetrics and Gynecology, 107*(1), 66–70.

Henley, S.J., Eheman, C., Richardson, L., Plescia, M., Asman, K.J., Dube, S.R., et al. (2011). State-specific trends in lung cancer incidence and smoking—United States, 1999–2008. *Morbidity and Mortality Weekly Report*. Retrieved from http://www.cdc.gov/mmwr/preview/mmwrhtml/mm6036a3.htm

Heron, M. (2010). Deaths: Leading causes for 2006. *National Vital Statistics Reports, 58*(14). Hyattsville, MD: National Center for Health Statistics.

Hologic. (2011). *ThinPrep Pap test specimen collection: Brush/spatula protocol and broom-like device protocol*. Retrieved August 13, 2011, from http://www.thinprep.com/hcp/specimen_collection.html

Howlader, N., Noone, A.M., Krapcho, M., Neyman, N., Aminou, R., Waldron, W., et al. (2010). *SEER cancer statistics review, 1975–2008*. Bethesda, MD: National Cancer Institute. Retrieved from http://seer.cancer.gov/csr/1975_2008/

Iglesias, E., Alderman, E., & Fox, A. (2000). Use of wet smears to screen for sexually transmitted diseases. *Infections in Medicine, 17*(3), 175–185.

Jemal, A., Siegel, R., Ward, E., Murray, T., Xu, J., & Thun, M.J. (2007). Cancer statistics. *A Cancer Journal for Clinicians, 57*, 43–66.

Jemal, A., Siegel, R., Ward, E., Hao, Y., Xu, J., Murray, T., & Thun, M.J. (2008). Cancer statistics. *A Cancer Journal for Clinicians, 58*, 71–96.

Juckett, G., & Hartman-Adams, H. (2010). Human papillomavirus: Clinical manifestations and prevention. *American Family Physician, 82*(10), 1209–1214.

Kaiser Women's Health Survey. (2005). *Women and health care: A national profile*. Retrieved from http://www.kff.org/womenshealth/upload/Women-and-Health-Care-A-National-Profile-Key-Findings-from-the-Kaiser-Women-s-Health-Survey-Report-Highlights.pdf

Koutsky, L. (2009). The epidemiology behind the HPV vaccine discovery. *Annals of Epidemiology, 19*, 239–244.

Leisure, M., Dudley, S., & Donowitz, L. (1993). Does a clean-catch urine sample reduce bacterial contamination? *New England Journal of Medicine, 328*(4), 289–290.

Levit, K., Stranges, E., Ryan, K., & Elixhauser, A. (2008). *HCUP facts and figures, 2006: Statistics on hospital-based care in the United States*. Rockville, MD: Agency for Healthcare Research and Quality. Retrieved from http://www.hcup-us.ahrq.gov/reports/factsandfigures/facts_figures_2006.jsp

Lu, C., Chang, C., Chang, M., Chen, S., Jan, Y., Fu, T., & Ho, E.S. (2010). Clinical parameters associated with unsatisfactory specimens of conventional cervical smears. *Diagnostic Cytopathology, 39*(2), 91.

Mandelblatt, J., Lawrence, W., Womack, S., Jacobson, D., Yi, B., Hwang, Y., et al. (2002). Benefits and costs of using HPV testing to screen for cervical cancer. *Journal of the American Medical Association, 287*(18), 2372–2381.

Mariotto, A.B., Yabroff, K.R., Shao, Y., Feuer, E.J., & Brown, M.L. (2011). Projections of the cost of cancer care in the U.S.: 2010–2020. *Journal of the National Cancer Institute, 103*(2), 117–128. Retrieved form http://www.ncbi.nlm.nih.gov/pubmed/21228314

Mata, J. (1998). Bacterial infections of the urinary tract in females. In R.E. Rakel (Ed.), *1998 Conn's current therapy* (pp. 668–670). Philadelphia: W. B. Saunders Co.

Mauck, K.F., & Clarke, B.L. (2006). Diagnosis, screening, prevention, and treatment of osteoporosis. *Mayo Clinic Proceedings, 81*(5), 662–672.

Meyers, D.S., Halvorson, H., & Luckhaupt, S. (2007). Screening for chlamydial infection: An evidence update for the U.S. Preventive Services Task Force. *Annals of Internal Medicine, 147*, 135–142.

Monif, G. (2002, April 15). Infectious vulvuvaginal disease: Obstacles to performing wet mount exams. *Consultant*, pp. 621–624.

Narayan, K.M.V., Aviles-Santa, L., Oza-Frank, R., Pandey, M., Curb, J.D., McNeely, M., et al. (2010). Report of a National Heart, Lung, and Blood Institute Workshop: Heterogeneity in cardiometabolic risk in Asian Americans in the U.S.: Opportunities for research. *Journal of the American College of Cardiology, 55*, 966–973.

National Adolescent Health Information Center. (2006). *Fact sheet on suicide: Adolescents & young adults*. San Francisco: Author. Retrieved from http://nahic.ucsf.edu/downloads/Suicide.pdf

National Cancer Institute (NCI). (2010a). *Cancer advances in focus, cervical cancer*. Retrieved October 15, 2011, from http://www.cancer.gov/cancertopics/factsheet/cancer-advances-in-focus/cervical

National Cancer Institute (NCI). (2010b). *Human papillomaviruses and cancer*. Retrieved May 14, 2011, from http://www.cancer.gov/cancertopics/factsheet/Risk/HPV

National Center for Health Statistics. (2010). *Health, United States, 2010: With special features on death and dying*. Hyattsville, MD: Author.

National Highway Traffic Safety Administration (NHTSA). (2009). *Fatal crashes involving young drivers*. Traffic Safety Facts: Research Note, DOT HS 811218. Retrieved from http://www-nrd.nhtsa.dot.gov/Pubs/811218.pdf

National Institute of Mental Health (NIMH). (2010). *Suicide in the U.S.: Statistics and prevention* (NIH Publication No. 06-4594). Washington, DC: U.S. Department of Health and Human Services. Retrieved February 9, 2012, from http://www.nimh.nih.gov/health/publications/suicide-in-the-us-statistics-and-prevention/index.shtml

National Osteoporosis Foundation. (2011). *Advocacy resources: Prevalence report*. Retrieved from http://www.nof.org/advocacy/resources/prevalencereport

National Transportation Safety Board, U.S. Department of Transportation. (2009). *Driver distraction fact sheet*. Retrieved from http://www.distraction.gov/content/get-the-facts/facts-and-statistics.html

Owens, P.L., & Mutter, R. (2010). *Emergency department visits for adults in community hospitals, 2008*. Retrieved from http://www.hcup-us.ahrq.gov/reports/statbriefs/sb100.pdf

Petrozza, J.C., & Rivlin, M.E. (2011). Hysteroscopy. *Medscape Reference: Drugs, Diseases & Procedures*. Retrieved from http://emedicine.medscape.com/article/267021-overview

Rose, D.P., Haffner, S.M., & Baillargeon, J. (2007). Adiposity, the metabolic syndrome, and breast cancer in African-American and white American women. *Endocrine Reviews, 28*(7), 763.

Sacks, J.J., Helmick, C.G., Langmaid, G., & Sniezek, J.E. (2002). Trends in deaths from systemic lupus erythematosus—United States, 1979–1998. *Morbidity and*

Mortality Weekly Report. Retrieved from http://www.cdc.gov/mmwr/preview/mmwrhtml/mm5117a3.htm

Saslow, D., Solomon, D., Lawson, H.W., Killackey, M., Kulasingam, S.L., Cain, J., et al. (2012). American Cancer Society, American Society for Colposcopy and Cervical Pathology, and American Society for Clinical Pathology screening guidelines for the prevention and early detection of cervical cancer. *Journal of Lower Genital Tract Disease, 16*(3). doi:10.1097/LGT.0b013e31824ca9d5

Smith, K., Harrington, K., Wingood, G., Oh, M.K., Hook, E.W., & DiClemente, R.J. (2001). Self-obtained vaginal swabs for diagnosis of treatable sexually transmitted diseases in adolescent girls. *Archives of Pediatric and Adolescent Medicine, 155*, 676–679.

Solomon, D., Davey, D., Kurman, R., Moriarty, A., O'Connor, D., Prey, M., et al. (2002). The 2001 Bethesda System: Terminology for reporting results of cervical cytology. *Journal of the American Medical Association, 287*, 2114–2119.

Solomon, D., Schiffman, M., Tarone, R., & ALTS Study Group. (2001). Comparison of three management strategies for patients with atypical squamous cells of undetermined significance: Baseline results from a randomized trial. *Journal of the National Institute of Cancer, 93*(4), 293–299.

Spigarelli, M.G. (2006). Urine gonococcal/chlamydia testing in adolescents. *Current Opinion on Obstetrics and Gynecology, 18*, 498–502.

Spigarelli, M.G., & Biro, F.M. (2005). An update on diagnosing STIs and HIV. *Contemporary OB/GYN, 50*(5), 76, 79–80.

Strander, B., Andersson-Ellström, A., Milsom, I., Rådberg, T., & Ryd, W. (2007). Liquid-based cytology versus conventional Papanicolaou smear in an organized screening program: A prospective randomized study. *Cancer, 111*(5), 285–291.

Substance Abuse and Mental Health Services Administration, Center for Behavioral Health Statistics and Quality (SAMHSA). (2011). *Drug abuse warning network (DAWN)*. Retrieved from http://oas.samhsa.gov/2k10/DAWN034/EDHighlights.htm

Table 22. Life expectancy at birth, at 65 years of age, and at 75 years of age, by race and sex: United States, selected years 1970–2007. (2010). Hyattsville, MD: National Center for Health Statistics.

Taylor, P., Jr., Andersen, W.A., Barber, S.R., Covell, J.L., Smith, E.B., & Underwood, P.B., Jr. (1987). The screening Papanicolaou smear: Contribution of the endocervical brush. *Obstetrics and Gynecology, 70*(5), 734–738.

Tierney, B., Westin, S.N., Schlumbrecht, M.P., & Ramirez, P.T. (2010). Early cervical neoplasia: Advances in screening and treatment modalities. *Clinical Advances in Hematology & Oncology, 8*(8), 547–555.

Toye, B., Woods, W., Bobrowska, M., & Ramotar, K. (1998). Inhibition of PCR in genital and urine specimens submitted for *Chlamydia trachomatis* testing. *Journal of Clinical Microbiology, 36*(8), 2356–2358.

Tripepi, G., Jager, K.J., Dekker, F.W., & Zoccali, C. (2009). Diagnostic methods 2: Receiver operating characteristic (ROC) curves. *Kidney International, 76*, 252–256.

Tucker, M.J., Berg, C.J., Callaghan, W.M., & Hsia, J. (2007). The black–white disparity in pregnancy-related mortality from 5 conditions: Differences in prevalence and case-fatality rates. *American Journal of Public Health, 97*, 247–251.

Turner, C., Rogers, S., Miller, H., Miller, W., Gribble, J., Chromy, J., et al. (2002). Untreated gonococcal and chlamydial infection in a probability sample of adults. *Journal of the American Medical Association, 287*(6), 726–733.

U.S. Cancer Statistics Working Group. (2010). *United States cancer statistics: 1999–2007 incidence and mortality web-based report*. Atlanta, GA: U.S. Department of Health and Human Services, Centers for Disease Control and Prevention, and National Cancer Institute.

U.S. Census Bureau. (2009). *Survey of income and program participation, 2004 panel, wave 5, June–September 2005*. Retrieved from http://www.cdc.gov/mmwr/preview/mmwrhtml/mm5816a2.htm#tab2

USDHHS. (2009). Summary health statistics for U.S. adults: National health interview survey, 2005. *Vital and Health Statistics, 10*(242), 7.

USDHHS, Office of Minority Health. (2010). *Obesity and African Americans*. Retrieved from http://minorityhealth.hhs.gov/templates/content.aspx?ID=6456

U.S. Preventive Services Task Force. (2007). Screening for chlamydial infection: Recommendations and rationale. *American Journal for Nurse Practitioners, 6*(13), 13, 19–20, 23–24.

van Stralen, K.J., Stel, V.S., Reitsma, J.B., Dekker, F.W., Zoccali, C., & Jager, K.J. (2009). Diagnostic methods I: Sensitivity, specificity, and other measures of accuracy. *Kidney International, 75*, 1257–1263.

Velásquez-Mieyer, P.A., Cowan, P.A., Pérez-Faustinelli, S., Nieto-Martínez, R., Villegas-Barreto, C., Tolley, E.A., et al. (2008). Racial disparity in glucagon-like peptide 1 and inflammation markers among severely obese adolescents. *Diabetes Care, 31*(4).

Véronique, R.L., Go, A.S., Lloyd-Jones, D.M., Adams, R.J., Greenlund, K.J., Hailpern, S., et al. (2011). AHA statistical update: Heart disease and stroke statistics—2011 update. *Circulation, 123*, e18–e209. Retrieved from http://circ.ahajournals.org/content/123/4/e18.full

World Health Organization. (2005). *Make every mother and child count: World Health Report 2005*. Retrieved from http://www.who.int/whr/2005/whr2005_en.pdf

World Health Organization. (2007). *Maternal mortality in 2005*. Retrieved from http://www.who.int/whosis/mme_2005.pdf

Wright, P.K., Marchall, J., & Desai, M. (2010). Comparison of SurePath and ThinPrep liquid-based cervical cytology using positive predictive value, atypical predictive value and total predictive as performance indicators. *Cytopathology, 21*(6), 374–378.

Wright, T.C., Jr., Massad, S., Twiggs, L., Dunton, C.J., Spitzer, M., Wlikinson, E.J., & Solomon, S. (2007a). 2006 consensus guidelines for the management of women with abnormal cervical cancer screening tests. *American Journal of Obstetrics & Gynecology*, 346–355.

Wright, T.C., Jr., Massad, S., Twiggs, L., Dunton, C.J., Spitzer, M., Wlikinson, E.J., & Solomon, S. (2007b). 2006 consensus guidelines for the management of women with cervical intraepithelial neoplasia or adenocarcinoma in situ. *American Journal of Obstetrics & Gynecology*, 340–345.

Xu, J.Q., Kochanek, K.D., Murphy, S.L., & Tejada-Vera, B. (2010). Deaths: Final data for 2007. *National Vital Statistics Reports, 58*(19). Hyattsville, MD: NCHS. Retrieved from http://www.cdc.gov/nchs/data/nvsr/nvsr58/nvsr58_19.pdf

CHAPTER ❖ 4

ASSESSING ADOLESCENT WOMEN'S HEALTH

Sarah A. Stoddard ◆ *Renee Sieving*

Adolescence offers unique opportunities for investment in the health and well-being of future generations.

Highlights

- Adolescent Growth and Development
- Selected Issues That Impact Adolescent Women's Health
- Adolescent Health Screening and Evaluation
- Recommendations for Gynecologic Examination With Adolescents

❖ INTRODUCTION

Adolescence is a critical period in human development. It is the period between childhood and adulthood, and a time of important changes and transition. It is a time characterized by rapid, dramatic physical, social, emotional, and intellectual change. Experimentation and exploration are hallmarks of adolescence as young people seek to find their place in society. Experimentation and exploration can manifest in high-risk behaviors that can affect young people's health. While adolescence can be a time of increased risk-taking behaviors, it also offers unique opportunities to invest in health and well-being. Healthy behaviors such as healthy sexual practices, exercise, and use of health care resources develop during the adolescent years. Both health and risk behaviors during adolescence have long-term implications later in life. Consequently, understanding this unique developmental period is important.

ADOLESCENT GROWTH AND DEVELOPMENT

Adolescence is characterized by distinct and dramatic developmental changes such as physical changes due to puberty; social changes related to social roles, expectations, and relationships with family and peers; as well as emotional and intellectual changes in a transition from concrete to abstract thought and reasoning. The rate of these developmental changes is second only to infancy. Three distinct phases are recognized: early (approximately ages 10 to 14), middle (approximately ages 15 to 17), and late (approximately ages 18 to 21) adolescence. Early adolescence involves the transition from childhood to adolescence, whereas late adolescence is a time of transition to adulthood. It is important to understand adolescence in the continuum of the life span. The experiences of childhood have a significant impact on adolescence, whereas adolescence lays a foundation for the experiences of adulthood. Table 4–1 provides an overview of the physical, social, emotional, and intellectual changes that occur during adolescence.

PUBERTAL GROWTH AND DEVELOPMENT

Physical development during adolescence is characterized by the onset of puberty, with changes in hormones, height, weight, body composition, and sexual development. The physical changes that take place during adolescence are linked to changes in peer relationships, adults' views of adolescents, and adolescents' views of themselves.

Hormonal Changes and Development

Pubertal changes are triggered by hormones during early adolescence, with changes in physical characteristics continuing into late adolescence. The developmental changes of puberty are attributable to the hypothalamic-pituitary-gonadal (HPG) axis and the presence of sex hormones. The HPG axis is a cyclic phenomenon involving activity of gonadotrophin-releasing hormone (GnRH) from the hypothalamus, pituitary secretion of gonadotropins (i.e., follicle-stimulating hormone [FSH] and luteinizing hormone [LH]), and estradiol positive feedback triggering a preovulatory surge in LH, follicular rupture, and corpus luteum formation (Fritz & Speroff, 2011). The HPG axis is established in utero, becomes dormant during childhood, and is reactivated during the second decade of life with a resurgence of GnRH, LH, FSH, and estrogen secretion (Neinstein & Kaufman, 1996).

It has been suggested that the timing of puberty is controlled by bloodborne substances that convey metabolic information related to carbohydrate or protein utilization as an indicator of growth and nutrition of the body and that these substances influence the body's hormonal biochemistry, thereby directing GnRH secretion. Although the exact mechanism for reactivating the HPG axis is unclear, sequential maturation of the central nervous system and decreased sensitivity of the hypothalamus and pituitary to circulating levels of estradiol are thought to play significant roles (Baram, 1996). Consequently, puberty is a brain-driven event controlled by maturation of the somatic component of the HPG axis.

Release of GnRH in a pulsatile fashion coincident with sleep initiates increased secretion of hormones. Eventually, the pulsatile pattern increases in frequency and magnitude, extending beyond sleep time to encompass the entire 24-hour period (Baram, 1996). Gonadotrophic secretion causes progressive changes in the morphology of ovarian follicles and an increase in estrogen secretion. In females, the final stage of HPG axis maturation involves development of a positive feedback

TABLE 4–1. Characteristics of Healthy Adolescent Development

	Developmental Milestones and Tasks		
	Early Adolescence (10–14 years)	Middle Adolescence (15–17 years)	Late Adolescence (18–21 years)
Physical growth[a]	Puberty; menstruation; Secondary sexual characteristics begin to develop	Secondary sexual characteristics advanced; 95% of adult height reached	Physical maturity and reproductive growth complete
Body image	Preoccupation with physical changes and critical of appearance; Peers viewed as standard for normal appearance	Less concern about physical changes but extremely concerned with appearance	Increased comfort with body
Brain maturation	Limbic system development—increased emotional arousal, sensation seeking, reward orientation	Period of heightened vulnerability to risk taking and problems in regulating affect and behavior	Maturation of frontal lobe facilitates reasoning, advanced thought, and impulse control
Cognitive development	Concrete thought dominates; Cause–effect relationships underdeveloped	Growth in abstract thought; Revert to concrete thought under stress; Cause–effect relationships better understood; Self-absorbed	Abstract thought established; Future oriented (understand, plan, and pursue long-range goals); Philosophical and idealistic
Emotional development	Stronger "self" than "social" awareness	Increased examination of inner experiences/feelings; Emotional regulation increases; Concern for others increases	Increased social awareness
Identity development	"Am I normal?" Imaginary audience; Daydreaming; Desire for privacy; Magnify own problems: "no one understands me" Begin to develop own value system; Emerging sexual feelings and sexual exploration; Vocational goals change frequently	Alternate between unrealistic high expectations and worries about future; Experimentation—friends, jobs, sex, drugs, and/or other risk-taking behaviors	Pursue realistic vocational goals through education or employment; Realization of own limitations and mortality; Establishment of sexual identity or sexual activity is common; Establishment of ethical and moral value systems
Autonomy	Challenge authority, family; Loneliness; Wide mood swings; At times, argumentative and disobedient	Conflict with family predominates due to ambivalence about emerging independence; May feel parents interfere with independence	Emancipation: continued education and/or work; More self-reliant and able to make independent decisions
Social relationships (peers/family)	Close friendships gain importance; Intense friendships with same-sex peers; Contact with opposite sex in groups; Increasing peer influences; Occasional rudeness to parents; Complaints that parents interfere with independence	Strong emphasis on peer group—strong peer allegiances; Increased tolerance of differences; Sexual drives emerge, begin to explore ability to date and attract a partner; Engagement with parents declines	Decisions/values less influenced by peer groups; Relates to individuals more than to peer group; Social networks expand; Selection of partner based on individual preference; More capable of intimate, complex relationships; Relate to family as adult

[a]See Table 4–2 for additional information on physical growth during adolescence

Sources: Adapted from McNeely and Blanchard, 2009; Neinstein, 1996

system in which critical levels of estrogen trigger a large release of GnRH, stimulating LH to initiate ovulation (Neinstein & Kaufman, 1996).

Reactivation of the HPG axis is responsible for the physical changes of puberty. However, after reproductive maturity is reached, the HPG axis is replaced as the mediator of hormone secretion. Mature ovaries, with positive and negative feedback loops based on the secretion of estrogen and progesterone, take over control of hormone levels. Thus, the gonadal component of the axis becomes the regulating force throughout women's reproductive years.

Physical Development

Physical changes during puberty are typified by the development of secondary sexual characteristics, a growth spurt, the maturation of genital organs, and the onset of menstruation. These physical changes occur in an orderly and sequential pattern. For females (as noted in Table 4–2), breast buds develop (thelarche), pubic hair appears (pubarche), a physical growth spurt starts, menstruation begins (menarche), and hips widen. While there is a typical sequence to pubertal changes, great variability exists in the timing of the onset of puberty, influenced by health status, genetics, and nutrition. For females, normal puberty can start as early as age 8 years, with pubertal growth and development spanning from ages 8 to 16 years. Pubertal changes have been categorized into sequential stages. See Figure 4–1 for images of pubertal stages (Tanner staging).

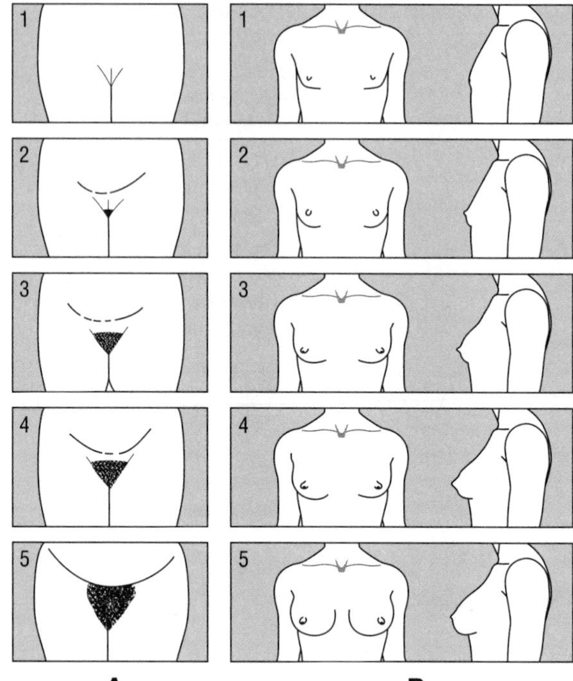

FIGURE 4–1. Sexual Maturity Rating in Females by Pubic Hair (A) and Breast (B) Development
Stage 1 is prepubertal. Breast stages (right panel): 2—a subareolar breast bud, 3—elevation of the breast contour and enlargement of the areolae, 4—the areolae form a secondary mound above the contour of the breast, and 5—mature female breast with recession of the secondary mound and a dependent breast contour. Pubic hair stages (left panel): 2—sparse, fine, straight pubic hair; 3—long, dark, curly hair; 4—pubic hair resembles adult pubic hair in quality but not distribution, having not yet spread to the thighs; 5—pubic hair has adult quality and distribution, with spread to the medial thighs.

BRAIN MATURATION

The brain begins its final stages of maturation during adolescence, growing and changing continually throughout this period. Two of the primary brain functions develop at different rates during the adolescent years. The limbic system, the part of the brain that perceives rewards from risk, begins rapid development in early adolescence. This reward orientation causes early adolescents to no longer be stimulated by activities that excited them as younger children. Thus, they often engage in activities of greater risk in efforts to achieve similar levels of excitement. In addition, because the frontal regions of their brains are not fully developed, early and middle adolescents rely heavily on the parts of the brain that house the emotional centers for making decisions, thus further increasing risk.

The largest part of the brain, the cortex, is divided into lobes that mature from front to back. The prefrontal cortex (frontal lobe), which governs the "executive functions" of reasoning, advanced thought, and impulse control, is the final area of the human brain to mature and does not fully mature until later adolescence and young adulthood.

TABLE 4–2. Normal Physical Development for Adolescent Females

- Appearance of breast buds (between 8 and 12 years of age), followed by breast development (between 13 and 18 years of age)
- Development of pubic hair (ages 11–14)
- Growth spurt begins (on average at age 10), adding inches to height and hip circumference
- Menses begins (on average at age 12, normal age range between 9 and 16 years)
- Enlargement of ovaries, uterus, labia, and clitoris; thickening of the endometrium and vaginal mucosa
- Appearance of underarm hair (ages 13–16)
- Dental changes including jaw growth and molar development
- Development of body odor and acne

Source: Adapted from McNeely and Blanchard, 2009

The time between the development of the limbic system and the maturation of the frontal lobe may create a period of increased vulnerability to problems in regulating emotions and behavior, which may increase the potential during middle adolescence for risk taking and the onset of emotional and behavioral problems (Spear, 2003). This difference in the timing of development of brain functions may explain why individuals take more risks during middle adolescence than during late adolescence. During late adolescence, as the frontal lobe becomes more developed, individuals develop better self-control and are better able to determine cause and effect. In addition, more areas of the brain become involved in processing emotions, so older adolescents are better at accurately interpreting other people's emotions. The brain continues this rapid development well into early adulthood, concluding around the age of 25.

Cognitive Development

Cognitive development is related to brain maturation during adolescence. It includes three major tasks. First, advanced reasoning skills expand during adolescence, including the ability to think about multiple options and possibilities, ponder things hypothetically, and follow a logical thought process. Second, abstract thinking skills emerge during these years (i.e., the ability to think about things that cannot be seen, heard, or touched). Abstract thought allows the ability to think about concepts such as faith, love, trust, beliefs, and spirituality. Third, the capacity to think about thinking, a process known as *metacognition*, develops during adolescence. Metacognition allows young people to consider how they feel and what they are thinking, and includes the ability to think about how they are perceived by others (Luna, 2009).

IDENTITY DEVELOPMENT

Adolescence is a time of discovering oneself and forms the basis of personal identity or sense of self. Due to changes with cognition and brain development, adolescents develop tools to start building a personal identity. Defining oneself focuses on clarification of personal values, attitudes, knowledge, and behaviors and involves defining a clear sense of identity, a positive sense of self-worth, and control over one's life. This includes developing a positive identity around gender, physical attributes, sexuality, and ethnicity. Two key aspects of defining oneself include self-concept and self-esteem. Self-concept, or what persons believe about themselves, is determined by their perception of their talents, qualities, goals, and life experiences. Self-esteem refers to feelings about self-concept, in other words, whether people feel good about themselves. Self-esteem is affected by the approval of others—parents, other adults, or peers—and by personal success. During adolescence, ups and downs in self-esteem are normal, particularly during early adolescence.

Identity development during adolescence includes identifying oneself sexually. Sexual identity is one's identification with a gender and a sexual orientation. Gender identity (masculine/feminine) may differ from biological sex (male/female). Sexual orientation is based on an awareness of being attracted to persons of the same and/or opposite sex. However, sexual identity is more than identifying one's sexual orientation; it is also how a young person identifies as a member of a social group. While the foundation of sexual identity begins during childhood, adolescence is the first time young people experience sexual feelings and are cognitively mature enough to think about their sexuality. Often, adolescents explore different sexual identities through experimentation. Through friendships, dating, and romantic relationships, adolescents come to know their sexual identities. By mid-to-late adolescence, young people become more comfortable with their changing bodies and sexual feelings.

In addition to defining oneself, identity formation includes two additional sets of tasks ("finding one's place in the world" and "achieving one's personal goals, hopes, and aspirations") that encompass other important facets of identity development: becoming independent (developing autonomy), achieving mastery or a sense of competence, and establishing social status. Finding one's place in the world focuses a person on finding or creating his or her place in the environment. It involves forming relationships with others, using available support systems, finding a valued place in the world, and finding ways to be useful to others. Achieving one's personal goals, hopes, and aspirations involves mastering social skills, developing advanced lifelong learning habits, continuing to develop a sense of curiosity and exploration, seeing a promising future with real opportunities, acquiring skills to participate in the economy, and establishing a respect for diversity.

EMOTIONAL AND SOCIAL DEVELOPMENT

Emotional competence is the ability to perceive, assess, and manage one's own emotions. Social competence is the capacity to be sensitive and effective in relating to others. Brain and cognitive development during adolescence increase adolescents' ability to manage their emotions and relate to others. Adolescents achieve emotional and social competence through the development of self-awareness, social awareness, self-management, friendships, and peer relationships. Self-awareness or "what do I feel?" focuses on recognizing one's own emotions. Learning to accurately identify one's feelings and the source of these feelings is important for figuring out constructive ways to manage feelings and solve problems. Social awareness centers on developing empathy and taking into account the feelings of others. In addition to understanding the thoughts and feelings of others, appreciating individual differences is an important aspect of social awareness. Immature brain and cognitive development makes social awareness more difficult for the younger adolescent. Until the prefrontal cortex fully develops in late adolescence and early adulthood, individuals may misinterpret body language and facial expressions. Self-management includes monitoring and regulating one's emotions, and establishing and working toward positive goals. During adolescence, self-management involves using emerging abstract thinking skills to examine emotions and to consider how those emotions impact goals. During this time, adolescents begin to learn how to manage their emotions rather than reacting to them, and they begin to realize that they can choose how to react in a situation. In addition, they learn that the way they react can change the way they experience that situation.

Healthy social and emotional development depends on establishing and maintaining healthy, rewarding relationships—based on cooperation and effective communication—and on the ability to resolve conflict and manage social influences. During adolescence, social skills are fostered by involvement in peer groups, which provide an opportunity to form social skills and an identity outside the family. Adolescents often prefer to spend more time with peers than with family. While peers take on a very influential role, parents and families remain a central influence throughout adolescence. Adolescents depend on their parents and families for affection, identification, values, and decision-making skills. They may also seek out other adults (teachers, other relatives, or neighbors) as role models and for guidance and support.

SELECTED ISSUES THAT IMPACT ADOLESCENT WOMEN'S HEALTH

As noted earlier, adolescence is a unique developmental period that presents distinct challenges and opportunities for improving health. Sexual and reproductive health issues create substantial challenges to the health of adolescents. Unsafe sexual behavior is a leading cause of morbidity among U.S. adolescents (Kirby, 2007; Mulye et al., 2009). Moreover, patterns of behavior related to sexual and reproductive health begun during adolescence set trajectories for adulthood (McIntyre, Williams, & Peattie, 2002). The following section describes prevalence and trends in various aspects of adolescent women's health including sexual behaviors; contraceptive use; sexually transmitted infections (STIs) including HIV; pregnancy, births, and abortions; menstrual disorders; depression; dating violence; sexual violence; and substance use and abuse.

SEXUAL AND REPRODUCTIVE ISSUES

Sexual Behaviors

The proportion of adolescents who are sexually experienced is of public health interest as it is this group of young people who are at risk for STIs and pregnancy. Just under half of all U.S. adolescents report ever having had sexual intercourse; this proportion increases steadily with age. About one quarter (27.7%) of 15- to 17-year-old females reported ever having had sex compared with 59.7 percent of females aged 18 to 19 years (Abma, Martinez, & Copen, 2010). Among 9th- to 12th-grade students in 2009, 46 percent reported ever having had sexual intercourse, ranging from 31.6 percent of 9th graders to 62.3 percent of 12th graders (Eaton et al., 2010). The proportion of sexually experienced adolescents also varies with race and ethnicity, although much of this variation disappears when studies take into account poverty and other indicators of disadvantage (Kirby, 2007). In 2009, 65 percent of African American, 49 percent of Hispanic, and 42 percent of white high school students had ever had sexual intercourse. However, the proportion of adolescents who have ever had sex has declined over the past two decades. For example, the prevalence of sexually experienced high school students decreased from 54.1 percent in 1991 to 46.0 percent in 2009 (Eaton et al., 2010).

Among sexually experienced adolescents, there is wide variation in how recently and how often teens have sex. These parameters are important to consider in understanding individuals' risk for STI and pregnancy. In a recent national survey of never-married 15- to 19-year-old females 28 percent had sex within a month of the survey, 30 percent within 3 months, and 38 percent within 12 months (Abma et al., 2010). Having had sex in the past 3 months is a commonly used indicator of current risk. In

2009, 34.2 percent of U.S. high school students had had sex within the past 3 months, ranging from 21.4 percent of 9th graders to 49.1 percent of 12th graders (Eaton et al., 2010).

Most sexually experienced adolescents do not have more than one partner during any given period of time; that is, they practice serial monogamy. In a recent national survey of 15- to 19-year-old females 25 percent reported having had sex with one partner while 3 percent reported having had sex with four or more partners during the year prior to the survey (Abma et al., 2010). Having a greater numbers of sexual partners increases the risk of STI exposure. In 2009, 13.8 percent of U.S. high school students reported having had sex with four or more partners during their life, ranging from 8.8 percent of 9th graders to 20.9 percent of 12th graders. A higher percentage of male (16.2%) than female (11.2%) students had had sex with four or more partners in their life (Eaton et al., 2010).

While most sexually active adolescents have partners close to their own age, some have partners who are much older. Among adolescent women, having a much older partner increases the odds that their first sexual experiences are involuntary and that they will become pregnant (Kirby, 2007). In a national survey, 22 percent of sexually experienced 15- to 19-year-old females first had sex with a male partner four or more years older than them (Gavin et al., 2009).

Contraceptive Use

Most sexually experienced adolescents report that they use contraception, at least some of the time. Among sexually experienced females aged 15 to 19 year old, 79 percent reported using a contraceptive method the first time they had sex and 84 percent noted using contraception the most recent time they had sex. The condom is the most common method used at both first and most recent sex, followed by birth control pills. The percentages of sexually active adolescent women who used contraception with first sex and with most recent sex increased substantially from the mid-1990s to the early 2000s, and remained stable through the late 2000s (Abma et al., 2010).

Data from nationwide surveys suggests that an increasing percentage of sexually active adolescents are protecting themselves from both STI and pregnancy. In 1995, about 8 percent of sexually active young women reported using condoms plus hormonal contraception with most recent sex. A decade later, 21 percent of sexually active young women reported using condoms plus hormonal contraception with most recent sex (Abma et al., 2010).

Contraceptive use with first sex or most recent sex does not necessarily mean consistent use. Many adolescents do not use contraception consistently, thereby increasing the risk of pregnancy and STI. For example, among sexually active 15- to 19-year-old females, about one half reported using condoms consistently in the past 4 weeks. Among 15- to 19-year-old females relying primarily on birth control pills, only 70 percent said that they took a pill every day (Abma, Chandra, Mosher, Peterson, & Piccinino, 1997). See Chapter 12 for information on specific contraceptive methods.

Sexually Transmitted Infections

Adolescents' patterns of sexual activity and contraceptive use, in combination with their biologic susceptibility and limited access to health care services, lead to high rates of STIs (Centers for Disease Control and Prevention [CDC], 2006). While young people ages 15 to 24 represent only 25 percent of the sexually active population, they account for about half of all new cases of STIs (Weinstock, Berman, & Cates, 2004). Recent data suggests that 26 percent of 14- to 19-year-old females have at least one of the most common STIs (human papillomavirus, chlamydia, herpes simplex virus, trichomoniasis) (CDC, 2008). Substantial disparities in STI rates exist among racial and ethnic populations, with African American adolescent women having the highest rates of gonorrhea and chlamydia of any age/gender group (CDC, 2009).

Because of the long and variable time between HIV infection and the onset of AIDS, HIV infection rates provide an accurate picture of current trends in the AIDS epidemic. Among 13- to 15-year-olds in the United States, the majority (77%) of HIV diagnoses occurred in female teens, whereas among 16- to 19-year-olds, slightly more than half (52%) of HIV diagnoses occurred in male teens. For adolescent women, the most common mode of transmission was heterosexual contact, while for adolescent men it was male-to-male sex (Rangel, Gavin, Reed, Fowler, & Lee, 2006).

Adolescents who have not yet received or completed the immunization series for hepatitis B and/or human papillomavirus should receive information about the benefits and risks of these vaccines and offered the vaccination series if desired.

Pregnancy, Births, and Abortions

Despite steady declines since the early 1990s, pregnancy and birth rates among U.S. teens remain high. Each year, more than 740,000 young women under the age of 20 become pregnant (Ventura, Abma, Mosher, & Henshaw,

2009). Before they reach the age of 20, more than 30 percent of U.S. adolescent women will have experienced a pregnancy (Kirby, 2007). Among 15- to 19-year-old females, about 57 percent of pregnancies end in a live birth, 27 percent in induced abortion, and 16 percent in fetal losses (Ventura et al., 2009). In 2009, women under the age of 20 had 415,000 live births and 203,000 abortions (Hamilton, Martin, & Ventura, 2010; Ventura et al., 2009). The United States continues to have the highest teen pregnancy and birth rates among industrialized nations (Bearinger, Sieving, Ferguson, & Sharma, 2007), with rates being disproportionately high among young women of color (Hamilton et al., 2010; Martin et al., 2010; Ventura et al., 2009).

Adolescent childbearing has adverse outcomes for teen mothers, their children, and society. When adolescents give birth, their prospects for the future decline. They become less likely to finish high school and attend college and more likely to be single parents and have large families. Being the child of an adolescent parent carries adverse social and health risks including delays in cognitive development, behavior problems, school failure, and increased likelihood of adolescent childbearing. In 2004, teen childbearing cost U.S. taxpayers at least $9.1 billion in lost tax revenues, public assistance, health care, child welfare, and criminal justice expenditures (Hoffman, 2006).

Menstrual Disorders

By the time they reach late adolescence, 75 percent of young women experience some problem associated with menstruation (Mitan & Slap, 2000). Many of the problems are minor, including minor dysmenorrhea and minor variations in cycle length or amount of flow. However, the dysfunction can become more severe when debilitating dysmenorrhea, severe dysfunctional uterine bleeding, or amenorrhea occurs (Neinstein, 1996). Clinical evaluation and management of menstrual disorders is addressed in Chapter 11.

In one of the only population-based studies of menstrual problems among U.S. adolescents aged 12 to 17 years, Klein and Litt (1981) found that 60 percent of adolescent women reported some level of pain during menses, with 9 percent reported severe dysmenorrhea. Dysmenorrhea is the leading reason for school absenteeism among adolescent women, with 14 percent of adolescents frequently missing school because of cramps. Those with severe cramps (50%) were more likely to miss school than those with mild cramps (17%).

It is not uncommon for adolescents to have irregular menstrual patterns during the first few years following menarche. While most abnormal bleeding is the result of anovulatory menstrual cycles, it must be differentiated clinically from organic lesions, although such lesions account for less than 10 percent of abnormal uterine bleeding among adolescents (Neinstein, 1996). Amenorrhea, the complete absence or cessation of menses, requires careful clinical evaluation and management. The distinction between primary and secondary amenorrhea, together with the presence or absence of secondary sex characteristics, will guide the differential diagnosis of amenorrhea (see Chapter 11).

MENTAL HEALTH AND SOCIAL ISSUES

Depression

Depressive symptoms, major depression, dysthymia (chronic depression), and other mood disorders are common in adolescents (Eaton et al., 2010; Lewinsohn, Hops, Roberts, Seeley, & Andrews, 1993; Saluja et al., 2004). According to the National Comorbidity Survey-Adolescent Supplement (NCS-A), about 11 percent of adolescents have a depressive disorder by age 18. Girls are more likely than boys to experience depression. During the past year, 34 percent of U.S. female high school students reported feeling so sad or hopeless almost every day for 2 or more weeks that they stopped some usual activities. In addition, 17.4 percent of female students reported seriously considering suicide attempt and 8.1 percent of female students had attempted suicide (Eaton et al., 2010). While emotional extremes are common during the adolescent years, prolonged, severe, and emotional distress is not part of normal adolescent development (Offer, Ostrov, Howard, & Atkinson, 1990; Rutter, Graham, Chadwick, & Yule, 1976). See Chapter 25 for more information.

Research suggests that depression increases adolescents' likelihood of engaging in sexual risk behaviors and acquisition of STIs (DiClemente et al., 2001; Lehrer, Buka, Gortmaker, & Shrier, 2006; Shrier, Harris, & Beardslee, 2002; Shrier, Harris, Sternberg, & Beardslee, 2001). Depressive symptoms have been linked with having multiple sex partners, inconsistent condom use, IV drug-using partners, and having partners with an STI (Mazzaferro et al., 2006; Orr, Celentano, Santelli, & Burwell, 1994).

Dating Violence

Dating violence among adolescents is an understated public health problem. Dating violence can be physical, emotional, or sexual. Estimates of dating violence vary as it is often underreported. One in four adolescents reports verbal, physical, emotional, or sexual abuse from a dating partner each year (Forshee & Matthews, 1996). One in 10 (10 percent) U.S. high school students reports having been the victim of physical violence from a dating partner (Eaton et al., 2010). Rates of lifetime dating violence victimization among adolescent and young adult women are as high as 36 percent (Erickson, Gittelman, & Dowd, 2010). While adolescent women can be victims of dating violence, they can also be aggressive toward their dating partners. Reciprocal relationship violence is common among adolescent and young adult women who report being victims of dating violence (Archer, 2000; Jain, Buka, Subramanian, & Molnar, 2010; Rothman, Johnson, Azrael, Hall, & Weinberg, 2010; Swahn, Alemdar, & Whitaker, 2010; Wolfe et al., 2009).

For young women, the consequences of dating violence include increased risk of STIs and pregnancy (Kreiter et al., 1999; Silverman, Raj, & Clements, 2004; Silverman, Raj, Mucci, & Hathaway, 2001). Teen victims of dating violence are at increased risk for depression, poor school performance, risky behaviors (e.g., drug and alcohol use), and eating disorders (see Chapter 25 for information on adolescence and eating disorders) (Ackard & Neumark-Sztainer, 2002; Banyard & Cross, 2008). In addition, adolescent victims of dating violence are at higher risk for victimization during college and adulthood (Smith, White, & Holland, 2003).

Sexual Violence

Adolescence is a time of greatest risk for sexual violence, and it is a time during which sexual violence can have the most devastating effects. Twenty to 25 percent of young women who attend college report experiencing an attempted or completed rape in college (Fisher, Cullen, & Turner, 2000). In a national survey, 60 percent of female victims were first sexually assaulted before the age of 18 (Basile, Chen, Black, & Saltzman, 2007). Almost 11 percent of female high school students report being forced to have sexual intercourse at some time in their lives (CDC, 2006). Sexual violence can negatively impact the social, emotional, and intellectual changes that occur during adolescence (Pharris & Nafstad, 2002). Health consequences for young women who have a history of sexual violence can include chronic pelvic pain, gastrointestinal disorders, premenstrual syndrome, gynecological and pregnancy complications, frequent headaches, back pain, and facial pain (Jewkes, Sen, & Garcia-Moreno, 2002). Immediate psychological consequences of sexual violence include shock, denial, fear, confusion, anxiety, withdrawal, guilt, distrust of others, and symptoms of post traumatic stress disorder (PTSD) (emotional detachment, sleep disturbances, flashbacks, and mental replay of assault) (Felitti et al., 1998; Yuan, Koss, & Stone, 2006). Chronic psychological consequences can include depression, suicide attempt or completion, alienation, and PTSD symptoms. Some young women also report increases in risky behaviors after experiencing sexual violence. These behaviors include engaging in high-risk sexual behaviors (unprotected sex; early sexual initiation; high-risk sexual partners; multiple sex partners; and trading sex for food, money, or drugs), substance use (alcohol and drug use), and unhealthy eating behaviors (Basile et al., 2006; Champion et al., 2004; Jewkes et al., 2002; Raj, Silverman, & Amaro, 2004).

Substance Use and Abuse

Experimenting with tobacco, alcohol, marijuana, and other drugs is common during adolescence. Alcohol is used by more young people in the United States than tobacco or illicit drugs (U.S. Department of Health and Human Services [USDHHS], 2007). In 2009, almost three quarters of U.S. high school students reported having consumed alcohol during their lifetime. Almost 25 percent of students reported binge drinking (i.e., five or more drinks of alcohol in a row) during the past 30 days. Approximately 36 percent of students reported using marijuana during their lifetime, with 21 percent of students having used marijuana during the past 30 days. In their lifetime, 6 percent of high school students reported cocaine use, 7 percent reported ecstasy use, and 4 percent reported methamphetamine use (Eaton et al., 2010; USDHHS, 2009).

Alcohol and the propensity for risk taking have been linked to motor vehicle accidents (MVAs) during adolescence. MVAs are the leading cause of death for adolescents and young adults, and alcohol plays a significant role in MVA mortality (Mulye et al., 2009). In 2007, alcohol involvement in fatal crashes was reported for 23 percent of drivers ages 16 to 20 and 41 percent of drivers ages 21 to 24. In 2009, 28 percent of high school students reported riding with a driver who had been drinking alcohol and 10 percent of students reported drinking and driving (Eaton et al., 2010). Adolescent males are more likely to be involved in MVAs than adolescent females (Allen & Brown, 2008; Eaton et al., 2010; Mulye et al., 2009). The use of alcohol, marijuana, and other substances affects decision making and may increase the likelihood of engaging in risky sexual behaviors. Adolescents' use of cigarettes, alcohol, marijuana, and other drugs has been associated with early initiation of sexual activity, more frequent sexual activity, multiple lifetime sex partners, nonuse of contraception, and sexual risk taking in general (Biglan et al., 1990; Donovan & Jessor, 1985; Duncan, Strycker, & Duncan, 1999; Epstein & Tamir, 1984; Flora & Thoresen, 1988; Lowry et al., 1994; Zabin, 1984; Zapata, Hillis, Marchbanks, Curtis, & Lowry, 2008). Sexual contact commonly occurs after drinking, and the use of alcohol reduces the likelihood of engaging in safer sexual practices (Hingson, Strunin, Berlin, & Heeren, 1990). These risky sexual behaviors may lead to STIs including HIV and unintended pregnancy.

TABLE 4–3. Building Trust: Key Interviewing Strategies

Active Listening
Suspend analysis and judgment
Attend to verbal and nonverbal messages
Listen to understand the teen's experience in a situation, rather than to "get the facts"
Responding to Emotions
Verbally acknowledge the adolescent's emotions
Legitimate the adolescent's feelings
Express support for the adolescent
Demonstrating Respect
Acknowledge teen's developmental stage, cultural and religious values and practices, and rights
Ensure privacy
Discuss confidentiality
Offer explanation for questions that are asked
Model honesty; reveal hidden agendas
Give the adolescent control over some things during a clinical encounter
Engage the adolescent in decisions affecting her health

ADOLESCENT HEALTH SCREENING AND EVALUATION

APPROACH TO THE ADOLESCENT

Health care providers can play a critical role in helping adolescents prevent negative health outcomes described earlier. One-on-one clinical interactions provide a particular opportune time for clinicians to offer preventive services to adolescent women. An important goal of such interactions is to establish trusting relationships in which adolescents are willing to disclose personal or sensitive information that allow clinicians to tailor preventive services to their particular situations (Street & Epstein, 2008). Interviewing strategies related to active listening, responding to emotions, and demonstrating respect, listed in Table 4–3, can be very useful in building trust. *Active listening* involves suspending judgment and seeking to understand what is being said. While listening to understand a teen's experience of a situation differs from a direct pursuit of "the facts" (e.g., who, what, where, when), this style is essential to encourage communication during one-on-one clinical interactions. *Responding to emotions* involves strategies such as verbally reflecting emotions that an adolescent conveys (verbally or nonverbally) as well as validating feelings that a young woman shares. To *demonstrate respect*, clinicians must use language appropriate to an adolescent woman's developmental level, sexual orientation, and cultural and religious values and practices. Clinicians can also demonstrate respect by offering a nonthreatening explanation for the questions asked during the interview, modeling honesty in the interview (e.g., "your mom called me before our visit today with some concerns that you might be pregnant"), giving the adolescent control over some things during the clinical visit ("would you like your aunt to be present during your exam?"), encouraging the adolescent to share her concerns and perspectives, and actively engaging the adolescent in making decisions that affect her health (strategies for engaging teens in decision making are described later in this chapter).

Legal Considerations

The notion that many adolescents have the right to make important decisions about their health care has been well established in federal and state policy. English (2007) notes laws offer several different kinds of protection related to adolescents' access to sexual and reproductive health care. First, federal and state laws allow minor adolescents to give their own consent for care; second, laws ensure that information about care will not be disclosed without a young person's agreement, except in uncommon circumstances. Finally, laws provide financial support for the provision of confidential services to minors.

The necessity for the law to provide for and protect confidential access to sexual and reproductive care is not inconsistent with the idea that parents play an important role in decisions related to their adolescent children's health care. Clinicians, parents, and adolescents interact to different degrees around health care decisions, depending on the nature of medical issues, family dynamics, developmental maturity, and legal status of the minor. Many adolescents voluntarily involve their parents in health care decisions, and many parents are aware of health care services that their adolescents receive. Some adolescents, however, cannot or will not involve their parents when seeking care. For these young people, legal protection of the ability to give consent and to receive confidential services is necessary.

Many states specifically authorize minors to consent to contraceptive services, testing and treatment for STIs including HIV, prenatal care and delivery services, treatment for alcohol and other drug abuse, and outpatient mental health care. The Center for Adolescent Health and the Law (2010) provides a state-by-state review of minor consent statutes for clinicians to familiarize themselves with existing laws and educate others about the effects of these laws on adolescent care (English, Bass, Boyle, & Eshragh, 2010).

PSYCHOSOCIAL HEALTH SCREENING AND INTERVENTION

Individuals face many risks to their health as they venture through the developmental stages of adolescence. However, as noted in Figure 4–2, individual assets and environmental supports act as important protective buffers against these risks. In the span of a brief office visit, the HEEADSSS mnemonic (Goldenring & Rosen, 2004) provides an optimal strategy for assessing risk and protective factors present in the life of an individual adolescent. A HEEADSSS assessment focuses on *h*ome environment; *e*ducation and employment; *e*ating and exercise; social *a*ctivities; *d*rug, alcohol, and tobacco use; *s*exuality and sexual behaviors; *s*afety, violence, and abuse; and *s*uicide, depression, and emotional distress. Assessment within these psychosocial domains provides information on important influences on adolescents' health.

An important quality of a HEEADSSS approach is that it proceeds from questions in less-threatening domains to questions in more personal and sensitive domains. Before beginning a HEEADSSS assessment, clinicians should offer a brief explanation for the questions they will ask (e.g., "Like I do with all young people I see in clinic, I'm going to ask you several questions to give me a better sense of things that

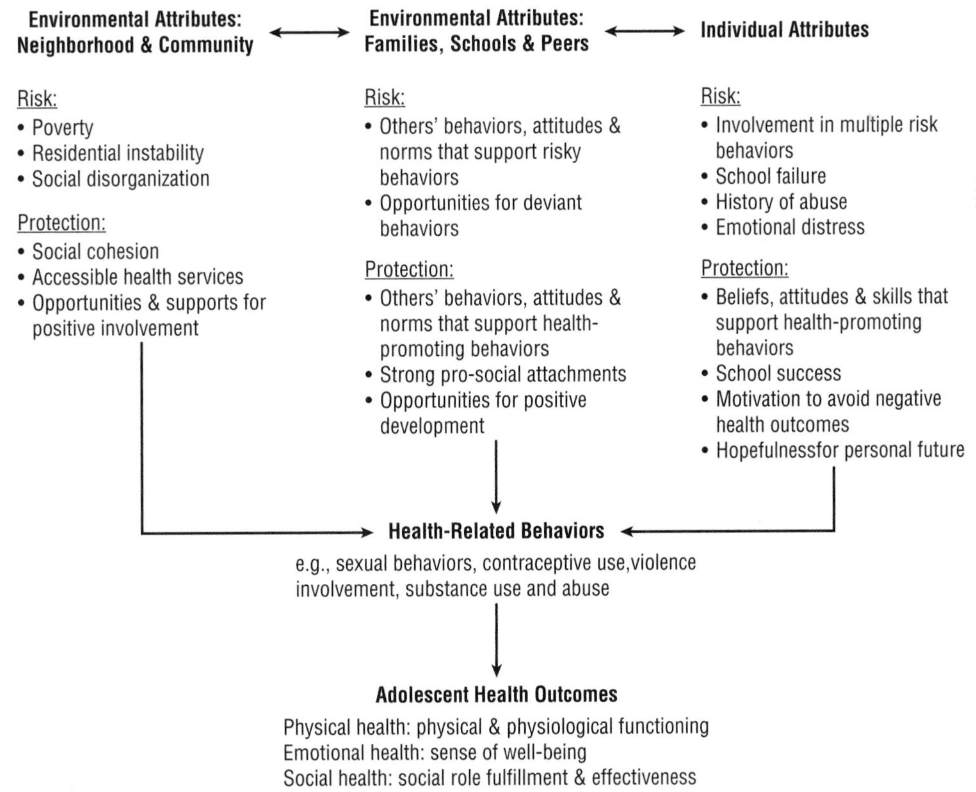

FIGURE 4–2. Risk and Protective Factors for Adolescent Health. Source: Adapted from Sieving, Oliphant, and Blum, 2002.

can affect your health"). This explanation may be especially important with new adolescent patients and with younger adolescents who may be acutely aware of the physical, emotional, and social changes they are experiencing.

Table 4–4 offers screening questions in each HEEADSSS domain. Within each domain, adolescents are most likely to respond honestly to open-ended, nonjudgmental versus close-ended, seemingly judgmental questions.

In the domain of sexuality, screening questions should be phrased in ways that allow adolescents to discuss same- and opposite-sex attractions and behaviors. For adolescents who note that they have been involved in sexual relationships, specific questions can be asked such as "Are you having sex with anyone now?" Asking questions that define sexual intercourse helps both the clinician and the adolescent clarify what types of sexual risk taking are occurring. For instance, the clinician might ask, "There are different kinds of sex—anal, oral, and penis in vagina sex. What kinds of sex are you having?" Discussing types of sexual activity is important because understanding and involvement vary greatly among adolescents. While surprising, some providing a range of choices will legitimize honest responses from others. Questions such as "What are you doing to protect yourself from pregnancy?" or "What are you doing to protect yourself from sexually transmitted infections?" work well for sexually active adolescents and allow sexually abstinent adolescents to answer truthfully. With adolescents who indicate using condoms or hormonal contraception, it is important to assess consistency of use, both over time and across sexual partners. Asking such questions allows tailoring of counseling and education to the specifics of an adolescent's situation.

Guidelines for Brief Office-Based Interventions

Among the "best bets" in brief office-based interventions are those that (1) include a dual focus on building

TABLE 4–4. HEEADSSS Psychosocial Screening Questions

Home
Where do you live? Who lives with you?
What are relationships like at home? To whom are you closest at home? To whom can you talk at home?
Have you moved recently?
Is there anyone new at your home? Has someone left recently?
Education and Employment
What are your favorite subjects at school? Your least favorite subjects?
How are your grades? Any recent changes? Any big changes in the past?
How often have you changed schools in the past few years?
Tell me about ideas, plans, or goals you have for school and work.
Are you working? (Where? How much?)
Eating and Exercise
What do you consider a healthy diet? How does that compare to your current eating patterns?
How much exercise do you get in an average week?
What do you like and do not like about your body?
Have you had any recent changes in your weight?
Have you dieted in the past year? (How? How often?)
Have you done anything else to try to manage your weight?
Activities
What do you and your friends do for fun? (With whom? Where? When?)
What do you and your family do for fun? With whom? Where? When?
Do you participate in sports or other activities?
Do you regularly attend an organized group (like a youth group at a church, synagogue, or mosque)?
Drugs
How many of your friends use tobacco? Alcohol? Other drugs?
Do any of your family members use tobacco? Alcohol? Other drugs?
Do you use tobacco? Alcohol? Other drugs?
Is there a history of problems with alcohol or drug problems in your family?
Sexuality
Have you ever been in a romantic relationship? Tell me about someone you've dated.
Is there someone in your life right now that you consider as your boyfriend or your girlfriend?
Have any of your relationships been sexual relationships?
What does the term *safe sex* mean to you?
Are you interested in boys? Girls? Both?
Safety, Violence, and Abuse
Have you ever been seriously injured? (How?) How about anyone else you know in real life?
How often do you wear a seat belt?
Do you use safety equipment for sports and other physical activities? (e.g., helmets for biking or skateboarding)
Have you ever ridden with a driver who was drunk or high? (When? How often?)
Do you feel safe in your home? Is there loud shouting and swearing in your home? Is there physical fighting or violence in your home?
Is there physical fighting or other violence among your friends?
Is there a lot of violence at your school? Do you feel safe at school?
Is there a lot of violence in your neighborhood? Do you feel safe in your neighborhood?
Have you ever worried about being physically or sexually abused?
Suicide, Depression, and Emotional Distress
Do you feel sad or down more than usual? Do you find yourself crying more than usual?
Are you "bored" all of the time?
Are you having trouble sleeping?
Have you thought a lot about hurting yourself or someone else?

Source: Adapted from Goldenring and Rosen, 2004

protective factors *and* reducing risk and (2) build motivation and/or skills needed for behavior change.

A Dual Approach: Building Protection While Reducing Risk. While some individual-level and environmental forces increase adolescents' risk, other factors within individual-level and environmental domains act as protective buffers. Jessor (1991), Resnick (2000), and others suggest that to promote the health and well-being of adolescents, the most effective clinical interventions simultaneously build protection *and* address risks that are amenable to change. As depicted in Figure 4–2, protective and risk factors are present within social contexts and environments in which adolescents live, as well as in the perceptions, beliefs, skills, and behaviors of individual adolescents.

Behavior Change: Understanding Motivation and Skills. Adopting healthy behaviors, or giving up risky behaviors, can be thought of as a process involving several distinct stages, noted in Table 4–5. From this perspective, change is a spiral process (Prochaska, Redding, & Evers, 2008). An important concept related to behavior change is that of motivation. Motivation has been defined as involving two core elements: *importance* or an individual's perceptions of the risks and benefits related to changing a behavior and *confidence* or self-efficacy in performing specific set of skills and/or behaviors (Rollnick, Mason, & Butler, 1999). Assessing an adolescent's level of perceived importance and confidence to engage in, or avoid, a particular behavior gives clinicians a reference for where to begin brief office-based counseling. For example, a clinician might ask an adolescent to respond to the following questions using a scale of 1 to 10, with 10 being high interest and confidence: "How *interested* are you in ____ (e.g., using birth control)?" and "how *confident* are you that you could start ____ (e.g., using birth control)?" A clinician can follow with probes such as "what would it take to move your interest/confidence from (current rating) to (higher rating)?"

Depending on where an adolescent is at in the process of change, different types of interviewing strategies are particularly useful in promoting healthy decision making and action. Rollnick and colleagues (Emmons & Rollnick, 2001; Rollnick et al., 1999) provide detail on office-based strategies to support healthy behavior change. Table 4–6 offers guidelines for clinicians to help adolescent women develop and practice decision-making skills.

TABLE 4–5. Stages of Behavior Change

Precontemplation—no intention to change behavior in the foreseeable future
Example: Sexually active adolescent who is not currently using condoms and has no intention to start doing so.
Contemplation—thinking about a change in behavior; considering the pros and cons of change
Example: Sexually active adolescent who is currently not using condoms, but is considering use because she is worried about getting an STI.
Preparation—intention to take action in the near future
Example: The adolescent who has decided to talk with her partner tomorrow about using condoms when they have sex.
Action—actively modifying behavior, experiences, or environment in order to make a change
Example: The teen who insists that her partner use a condom when they have sex.
Maintenance—work on continuing or reinforcing behaviors adopted during the action stage
Example: The teen who has used condoms every time she's had sex with this partner over the past 6 months.

Source: Prochaska et al., 2008

TABLE 4–6. Supporting Teens With Decision Making

- Don't rush the teen into a decision-making mode
- Present options for the future rather than a single course of action
- Describe what other teens faced with similar situations have done
- Emphasize "You are the best judge of what's best for you"
- Provide information in a neutral, nonpersonal manner
- Remember that failure to reach a decision is *not* a failed counseling session
- Resolutions to change often break down. Make sure the adolescent understands this and doesn't avoid future contact if things change
- Acknowledge that commitment to change is likely to fluctuate; empathize

Source: Adapted from Sieving, Oliphant, and Blum, 2002

RECOMMENDATIONS FOR GYNECOLOGIC EXAMINATION WITH ADOLESCENTS

Health care providers working with adolescents commonly encounter gynecologic issues including questions related to pubertal development, menstrual disorders, contraception, STIs, and non-STIs. The gynecologic examination is a key element in assessing pubertal status and documenting physical findings. However, most adolescents do not need an internal examination involving a speculum or a bimanual exam because of newer STI screening tests that can be performed with urine, vaginal, or cervical samples, as well as recent changes in recommendations for initiation of cervical cancer screening (Braverman, Breech, & Committee on Adolescence, 2010).

In the past, a history of sexual activity was an automatic indication for a full pelvic exam to perform STI and Papanicolaou (Pap) tests and a prerequisite for prescribing hormonal contraception. Certainly, the external genitalia of all adolescent female patients should be examined to confirm normal anatomy, assess pubertal development, and look for evidence of trauma or pathology (Braverman et al., 2010). However, with available urine-based and vaginal-swab STI tests, a speculum exam in an asymptomatic patient is not necessary for diagnosing asymptomatic STIs (Huppert et al., 2005; Johnson et al., 2002). Other nonsexually transmitted vaginal infections (e.g., bacterial vaginosis and yeast infection) can also be diagnosed with a vaginal swab obtained by the clinician or the patient (Blake, Duggan, Quinn, Zenilman, & Joffe, 1998; Sobel, 2005). A speculum or bimanual exam is considered unnecessary before prescribing most forms of contraception (American College of Obstetricians and Gynecologists [ACOG], 2007). Two exceptions would be the intrauterine device (IUD) and diaphragm, for which anatomic variation could affect insertion or appropriate sizing of the device (Braverman et al., 2010).

Previous recommendations to perform a Pap test at the onset of vaginal intercourse have changed. Current guidelines state that a first Pap test should be at age 21 years, except if an adolescent has immune suppression or HIV infection, in which cases annual Pap tests are started with the onset of vaginal intercourse. Adolescents who have been screened previously and have documented cervical intraepithelial neoplasia 2 or 3 or carcinoma require continued screening as outlined in the new guidelines (ACOG, 2010).

Table 4–7 lists indications for a pelvic exam. A complete exam (external exam, speculum exam, or bimanual exam) is always indicated in cases of suspected or reported rape or sexual abuse and as part of an evaluation for lower abdominal pain. A complete exam is also indicated with menstrual disorders (Braverman et al., 2010). A speculum exam is indicated in cases with persistent symptomatic vaginal discharge. Some nucleic acid amplification tests to detect chlamydia and gonorrhea infections are more sensitive with cervical or vaginal specimens than with urine samples (Johnson et al., 2002). Visualizing the cervix allows for assessment of mucopurulent discharge and friability, symptoms associated with chlamydia and gonorrhea. Finally, a speculum exam can rule out other causes of vaginal discharge (e.g., foreign body).

TABLE 4–7. Indications for a Pelvic Examination With Adolescents

Suspected/reported rape or sexual abuse
Dysmenorrhea unresponsive to nonsteroidal anti-inflammatory drugs
Amenorrhea
Abnormal vaginal bleeding
Lower abdominal pain
Pregnancy
Contraceptive counseling for IUD or diaphragm
Performing Pap test (as per current guidelines)
Persistent vaginal discharge
Urinary tract symptoms in a sexually active female

Source: Adapted from Braverman et al., 2010

The first pelvic examination should be approached with care and gentleness. The clinician should be aware of the adolescent's developmental level as the internal examination is a source of anxiety for most adolescents. Common concerns include the fear of pain, embarrassment, or discovery of an anomaly as well as inadequate knowledge of the vaginal anatomy and physiology. In nonsexually active younger adolescents, a rectovaginal examination and pelvic ultrasonography are alternatives to a pelvic exam that may provide information about possible abnormalities of the vaginal, uterine, and adenexal structures (Fritz & Speroff, 2011). Prior to a first pelvic exam, the adolescent should receive a thorough explanation and demonstration of what will be done and offered the opportunity to voice questions or concerns. Establishing a good rapport prior to the examination and maintaining eye contact and a professional, reassuring presence during the exam are essential (Raines, 2004).

CONCLUSION

Adolescence is a time of positive growth and development. It is a time of rapid physical, cognitive, and emotional changes, and new expectations, norms, and social roles. While this developmental period is often been viewed as a time of increased risk for negative health outcomes, it can also be an important time for developing healthy behaviors. By fostering protective individual assets and environmental supports, health care providers who work with adolescents have unique and important opportunities to invest in the health and well-being of future generations.

REFERENCES

Abma, J.C., Chandra, A., Mosher, W.D., Peterson, L.S., & Piccinino, L.J. (1997). Fertility, family planning, and women's health: New data from the 1995 National Survey of Family Growth. *Vital and Health Statistics, 23*(19), 1–114.

Abma, J.C., Martinez, G.M., & Copen, C.E. (2010). Teenagers in the United States: Sexual activity, contraceptive use, and childbearing, national survey of family growth 2006–2008. *Vital and Health Statistics, 23*(30), 1–47.

Ackard, D.M., & Neumark-Sztainer, D. (2002). Date violence and date rape among adolescents: Associations with disordered eating behaviors and psychological health. *Child Abuse and Neglect, 26*(5), 455–473.

Allen, J.P., & Brown, B.B. (2008). Adolescents, peers, and motor vehicles. The perfect storm? *American Journal of Preventive Medicine, 35*(3S), S289–S293.

American College of Obstetricians and Gynecologists. (2007). *Guidelines for women's health care: A resource manual* (3rd ed.). Washington, DC: American College of Obstetricians and Gynecologists.

American College of Obstetricians and Gynecologists. (2010). Committee opinion no. 463: Cervical cancer in adolescents: Screening, evaluation, and management. *Obstetrics & Gynecology, 116*(2), 469–472.

Archer, J. (2000). Sex differences in aggression between heterosexual partners: A meta-analytic review. *Psychological Bulletin, 126*(5), 651–680.

Banyard, V.L., & Cross, C. (2008). Consequences of teen dating violence: Understanding intervening variables in ecological context. *Violence Against Women, 14*(9), 998–1013.

Baram, D.A. (1996). Sexuality and sexual function. In J.S. Berek, E.Y. Adashi, & P.A. Hillard (Eds.), *Novak's gynecology* (12th ed.). Baltimore: Williams & Wilkins.

Basile, K.C., Black, M.C., Simon, T.R., Arias, I., Brener, N.D., & Saltzman, L.E. (2006). The association between self-reported lifetime history of forced sexual intercourse and recent health-risk behaviors: Findings from the 2003 National Youth Risk Behavior Survey. *Journal of Adolescent Health, 39*(5), 752.e1–752.e7.

Basile, K.C., Chen, J., Black, M.C., & Saltzman, L.E. (2007). Prevalence and characteristics of sexual violence victimization among U.S. adults, 2001–2003. *Violence and Victims, 22*(4), 437–448.

Bearinger, L.H., Sieving, R.E., Ferguson, J., & Sharma, V. (2007). Global perspectives on the sexual and reproductive health of adolescents: Patterns, prevention, and potential. *Lancet, 369*(9568), 1220–1231.

Biglan, A., Metzler, C.W., Wirt, R., Ary, D., Noell, J., Ochs, L., et al. (1990). Social and behavioral factors associated with high-risk sexual behavior among adolescents. *Journal of Behavioral Medicine, 13*(3), 245–261.

Blake, D.R., Duggan, A., Quinn, T., Zenilman, J., & Joffe, A. (1998). Evaluation of vaginal infections in adolescent women: Can it be done without a speculum? *Pediatrics, 102*(4, Pt. 1), 939–944.

Braverman, P.K., Breech, L., & Committee on Adolescence. (2010). Gynecologic examination for adolescents in the pediatric office setting. *Pediatrics, 126*(3), 583–590.

Center for Adolescent Health and the Law (2010). *Promoting the health of adolescents and their access to comprehensive health care.* Retrieved from www.cahl.org

Centers for Disease Control and Prevention. (2006). *HIV/AIDS surveillance report, 2005.* Atlanta, GA: Author.

Centers for Disease Control and Prevention. (2008). *Nationally representative CDC study finds 1 in 4 teenage girls has a sexually transmitted disease* [Press release]. Retrieved from http://www.cdc.gov/stdconference/2008/press/release-11march2008.htm

Centers for Disease Control and Prevention. (2009). *Trends in the prevalence of sexual behaviors: National YRBS 1991–2009.* Retrieved from http://www.cdc.gov/healthyyouth/yrbs/pdf/us_sexual_trend_yrbs.pdf

Champion, H.L., Foley, K.L., DuRant, R.H., Hensberry, R., Altman, D., & Wolfson, M. (2004). Adolescent sexual victimization, use of alcohol and other substances, and other health risk behaviors. *Journal of Adolescent Health, 35*(4), 321–328.

DiClemente, R.J., Wingood, G.M., Crosby, R.A., Sionean, C., Brown, L.K., Rothbaum, B., et al. (2001). A prospective study of psychological distress and sexual risk behavior among black adolescent females. *Pediatrics, 108*(5), E85.

Donovan, J.E., & Jessor, R. (1985). Structure of problem behavior in adolescence and young adulthood. *Journal of Consulting and Clinical Psychology, 53*(6), 890–904.

Duncan, S.C., Strycker, L.A., & Duncan, T.E. (1999). Exploring associations in developmental trends of adolescent substance use and risky sexual behavior in a high-risk population. *Journal of Behavioral Medicine, 22*(1), 21–34.

Eaton, D.K., Kann, L., Kinchen, S., Shanklin, S., Ross, J., Hawkins, J., et al. (2010). Youth risk behavior surveillance—United States, 2009. *MMWR Surveillance Summaries, 59*(5), 1–142.

Emmons, K.M., & Rollnick, S. (2001). Motivational interviewing in health care settings: Opportunities and limitations. *American Journal of Preventive Medicine, 20*(1), 68–74.

English, A. (2007). Sexual and reproductive health care for adolescents: Legal rights and policy challenges. *Adolescent Medicine: State of the Art Reviews, 18,* 371–381.

English, A., Bass, L., Boyle, A.D., & Eshragh, F. (2010). *State Minor Consent Laws: A summary* (3rd ed.). Chapel Hill, NC: Center for Adolescent Health & the Law.

Epstein, L., & Tamir, A. (1984). Health-related behavior of adolescents: Change over time. *Journal of Adolescent Health Care, 5*(2), 91–95.

Erickson, M.J., Gittelman, M.A., & Dowd, D. (2010). Risk factors for dating violence among adolescent females presenting to the pediatric emergency department.*Journal of Trauma, 69*(Suppl. 4), S227–S232.

Felitti, V.J., Anda, R.F., Nordenberg, D., Williamson, D.F., Spitz, A.M., Edwards, V., et al. (1998). Relationship of childhood abuse and household dysfunction to many of the leading causes of death in adults: The adverse childhood experiences (ACE) study. *American Journal of Preventive Medicine, 14*(4), 245–258.

Fisher, B.S., Cullen, F.T., & Turner, M.G. (2000). *The sexual victimization of college women* (Volume Publication No. NCJ 182369). Washington, DC: National Institute of Justice.

Flora, J.A., & Thoresen, C.E. (1988). Reducing the risk of AIDS in adolescents. *American Psychologist, 43*(11), 965–970.

Forshee, V.A., & Matthews, R.A. (1996). Adolescent dating abuse perpetration: A review of findings, methodological limitations and suggestions for future research. In D.J. Flannery, A.T. Vazsonyi, & I.D. Waldman (Eds.), *The Cambridge handbook of violent behavior and aggression* (pp. 431–449). New York: Cambridge University Press.

Fritz, M.A., & Speroff, L. (2011). *Clinical gynecological endocrinology and infertility* (8th ed.). Philadelphia: Wolters Kluwer/Lippincott Williams & Wilkins.

Gavin, L., MacKay, A.P., Brown, K., Harrier, S., Ventura, S.J., Kann, L., et al. (2009). Sexual and reproductive health of persons aged 10–24 years—United States, 2002–2007. *MMWR Surveillance Summaries, 58*(6), 1–58.

Goldenring, J.M., & Rosen, D.S. (2004). Getting into adolescent heads: An essential update. *Contemporary Pediatrics, 21*(1), 64–92.

Hamilton, B.E., Martin, J.A., & Ventura, S.J. (2010). Births: Preliminary data for 2009. *National Vital Statistics Reports, 59*(3), 1–19.

Hingson, R.W., Strunin, L., Berlin, B.M., & Heeren, T. (1990). Belief about AIDS, use of alcohol and drugs, and unprotected sex among Massachusetts adolescents. *American Journal of Public Health, 80*(3), 295–299.

Hoffman, S.D. (2006). *By the numbers: The public costs of teen childbearing*. Washington, DC: National Campaign to Prevent Teen Pregnancy.

Huppert, J.S., Batteiger, B.E., Braslins, P., Feldman, J.A., Hobbs, M.M., Sankey, H.Z., et al. (2005). Use of an immunochromatographic assay for rapid detection of Trichomonas vaginalis in vaginal specimens. *Journal of Clinical Microbiology, 43*(2), 684–687.

Jain, S., Buka, S.L., Subramanian, S.V., & Molnar, B.E. (2010). Neighborhood predictors of dating violence victimization and perpetration in young adulthood: A multilevel study. *American Journal of Public Health, 100*(9), 1737–1744.

Jessor, R. (1991). Risk behavior in adolescence: A psychosocial framework for understanding and action. *Journal of Adolescent Health, 12,* 597–605.

Jewkes, R., Sen, P., & Garcia-Moreno, C. (2002). Sexual violence. In E.G. Krug, L.L. Dahlberg, J.A. Mercy, A.B. Zwi, & A.B. Lozano (Eds.), *World report on violence and health* (pp. 213–239). Geneva, Switzerland: World Health Organization.

Johnson, R.E., Newhall, W.J., Papp, J.R., Knapp, J.S., Black, C.M., Gift, T.L., et al. (2002). Screening tests to detect Chlamydia trachomatis and Neisseria gonorrhoeae infections, 2002. *MMWR Recommendation Reports, 51*(RR-15), 1–38.

Kirby, D. (2007). *Emerging answers 2007: Research findings on programs to reduce teen pregnancy and sexually transmitted diseases*. Washington, DC: National Campaign to Prevent Teen Pregnancy.

Klein, J.R., & Litt, I.F. (1981). Epidemiology of adolescent dysmenorrhea. *Pediatrics, 68*(5), 661–664.

Kreiter, S.R., Krowchuk, D.P., Woods, C.R., Sinal, S.H., Lawless, M.R., & DuRant, R.H. (1999). Gender differences in risk behaviors among adolescents who experience date fighting. *Pediatrics, 104*(6), 1286–1292.

Lehrer, J.A., Buka, S., Gortmaker, S., & Shrier, L.A. (2006). Depressive symptomatology as a predictor of exposure to intimate partner violence among US female adolescents and young adults. *Archives of Pediatrics and Adolescent Medicine, 160*(3), 270–276.

Lewinsohn, P.M., Hops, H., Roberts, R.E., Seeley, J.R., & Andrews, J.A. (1993). Adolescent psychopathology: I. Prevalence and incidence of depression and other DSM-III-R disorders in high school students. *Journal of Abnormal Psychology, 102*(1), 133–144.

Lowry, R., Holtzman, D., Truman, B.I., Kann, L., Collins, J.L., & Kolbe, L.J. (1994). Substance use and HIV-related sexual behaviors among US high school students: Are they related? *American Journal of Public Health, 84*(7), 1116–1120.

Luna, B. (2009). Developmental changes in cognitive control through adolescence. *Advances in Child Development and Behavior, 37,* 233–278.

Martin, J.A., Hamilton, B.E., Sutton, P.D., Ventura, S.J., Mathews, T.J., & Osterman, M.J. (2010). Births: Final data for 2008. *National Vital Statistics Reports, 59*(1), 1–72.

Mazzaferro, K.E., Murray, P.J., Ness, R.B., Bass, D.C., Tyus, N., & Cook, R.L. (2006). Depression, stress, and social support as predictors of high-risk sexual behaviors and STIs in young women. *Journal of Adolescent Health, 39*(4), 601–603.

McIntyre, P., Williams, G., & Peattie, S. (2002). *Adolescent friendly health services: An agenda for change*. Geneva, Switzerland: World Health Organization.

McNeely, C., & Blanchard, J. (2009). *The teen years explained: A guide to healthy adolescent development*. Baltimore, MD: Center for Adolescent Health, Johns Hopkins Bloomberg School of Public Health.

Mitan, L.A., & Slap, G.B. (2000). Adolescent menstrual disorders: Update. *Medical Clinics of North America, 84*(4), 851–868.

Mulye, T.P., Park, M.J., Nelson, C.D., Adams, S.H., Irwin, C.E., Jr., & Brindis, C.D. (2009). Trends in adolescent and young adult health in the United States. *Journal of Adolescent Health, 45*(1), 8–24.

Neinstein, L.S. (1996). *Adolescent health care: A practical guide* (3rd ed.). Baltimore: Williams & Wilkins.

Neinstein, L.S., & Kaufman, F.R. (1996). Normal growth and development. In L.S. Neinstein (Ed.), *Adolescent health care:*

A practical guide (3rd ed., pp. 3–39). Baltimore: Williams & Wilkins.

Offer, D., Ostrov, E., Howard, K.I., & Atkinson, R. (1990). Normality and adolescence. *Psychiatric Clinics of North America, 13*(3), 377–388.

Orr, S.T., Celentano, D.D., Santelli, J., & Burwell, L. (1994). Depressive symptoms and risk factors for HIV acquisition among black women attending urban health centers in Baltimore. *AIDS Education and Prevention, 6*(3), 230–236.

Pharris, M.D., & Nafstad, S.S. (2002). Nursing care of adolescents who have been sexually assaulted. *Nursing Clinics of North America, 37,* 475–497.

Prochaska, J.O., Redding, C.A., & Evers, K.E. (2008). The transtheoretical model and stages of change. In K. Glanz, B.K. Rimer, & K. Viswanath (Eds.), *Health behavior and health education: Theory, research and practice* (4th ed., pp. 97–122). San Francisco: Jossey-Bass.

Raines, D.A. (2004). Assessing adolescent women's health. In E.Q. Youngkin & M.S. Davis (Eds.), *Women's health: A primary care clinical guide* (3rd ed., p. 50). Upper Saddle River, NJ: Pearson Prentice Hall.

Raj, A., Silverman, J.G., & Amaro, H. (2004). The relationship between sexual abuse and sexual risk among high school students: Findings from the 1997 Massachusetts Youth Risk Behavior Survey. *Maternal and Child Health Journal, 2,* 125–134.

Rangel, M.C., Gavin, L., Reed, C., Fowler, M.G., & Lee, L.M. (2006). Epidemiology of HIV and AIDS among adolescents and young adults in the United States. *Journal of Adolescent Health, 39*(2), 156–163.

Resnick, M.D. (2000). Protective factors, resiliency and healthy youth development. *Adolescent Medicine: State of the Art Reviews, 11*(1), 157–165.

Rollnick, S., Mason, P., & Butler, C. (1999). *Health behavior change: A guide for practitioners.* New York: Churchill Livingstone.

Rothman, E.F., Johnson, R.M., Azrael, D., Hall, D.M., & Weinberg, J. (2010). Perpetration of physical assault against dating partners, peers, and siblings among a locally representative sample of high school students in Boston, Massachusetts. *Archives of Pediatrics & Adolescent Medicine, 164*(12), 1118–1124.

Rutter, M., Graham, P., Chadwick, O.F., & Yule, W. (1976). Adolescent turmoil: Fact or fiction? *Journal of Child Psychology and Psychiatry, 17*(1), 35–56.

Saluja, G., Iachan, R., Scheidt, P.C., Overpeck, M.D., Sun, W., & Giedd, J.N. (2004). Prevalence of and risk factors for depressive symptoms among young adolescents. *Archives of Pediatrics & Adolescent Medicine, 158*(8), 760–765.

Shrier, L.A., Harris, S.K., & Beardslee, W.R. (2002). Temporal associations between depressive symptoms and self-reported sexually transmitted disease among adolescents. *Archives of Pediatrics & Adolescent Medicine, 156*(6), 599–606.

Shrier, L.A., Harris, S.K., Sternberg, M., & Beardslee, W.R. (2001). Associations of depression, self-esteem, and substance use with sexual risk among adolescents. *Preventive Medicine, 33*(3), 179–189.

Sieving, R.E., Oliphant, J.A., & Blum, R.W. (2002). Adolescent sexual behavior and sexual health. *Pediatrics in Review, 23*(12), 407–415.

Silverman, J.G., Raj, A., & Clements, K. (2004). Dating violence and associated sexual risk and pregnancy among adolescent girls in the United States. *Pediatrics, 114*(2), e220–e225.

Silverman, J.G., Raj, A., Mucci, L.A., & Hathaway, J.E. (2001). Dating violence against adolescent girls and associated substance use, unhealthy weight control, sexual risk behavior, pregnancy, and suicidality. *Journal of the American Medical Association, 286*(5), 572–579.

Smith, P.H., White, J.W., & Holland, L.J. (2003). A longitudinal perspective on dating violence among adolescent and college-age women. *American Journal of Public Health, 93*(7), 1104–1109.

Sobel, J.D. (2005). What's new in bacterial vaginosis and trichomoniasis? *Infectious Disease Clinics of North America, 19*(2), 387–406.

Spear, L.P. (2003). Neurodevelopment during adolescence. In D. Cicchetti & E. Walker (Eds.), *Neurodevelopmental mechanisms in psychopathology.* New York: Cambridge University Press.

Street, R.L., & Epstein, R.M. (2008). Key interpersonal functions and health outcomes: Lessons from theory and research on clinician-patient communications. In K. Glanz, B.K. Rimer, & K. Viswanath (Eds.), *Health behavior and health education: Theory, research, and practice* (4th ed., pp. 237–270). San Francisco: Jossey-Bass.

Swahn, M.H., Alemdar, M., & Whitaker, D.J. (2010). Nonreciprocal and reciprocal dating violence and injury occurrence among urban youth. *Western Journal of Emergency Medicine, 11*(3), 264–268.

U.S. Department of Health and Human Services. (2007). *Substance abuse.* Retrieved from http://www.hhs.gov/ash/oah/adolescent-health-topics/substance-abuse/home.html

U.S. Department of Health and Human Services. (2009). *National youth risk behavior survey overview.* Retrieved from http://www.cdc.gov/HealthyYouth/yrbs/pdf/us_overview_yrbs.pdf

Ventura, S.J., Abma, J.C., Mosher, W.D., & Henshaw, S.K. (2009). Estimated pregnancy rates for the United States, 1990–2005: An update. *National Vital Statistics Reports, 58*(4), 1–14.

Weinstock, H., Berman, S., & Cates, W., Jr. (2004). Sexually transmitted diseases among American youth: Incidence and prevalence estimates, 2000. *Perspectives on Sexual and Reproductive Health, 36*(1), 6–10.

Wolfe, D.A., Crooks, C., Jaffe, P., Chiodo, D., Hughes, R., Ellis, W., et al. (2009). A school-based program to prevent adolescent dating violence: A cluster randomized trial. *Archives of Pediatrics & Adolescent Medicine, 163*(8), 692–699.

Yuan, N.P., Koss, M.P., & Stone, M. (2006). *The psychological consequences of sexual trauma.* National Online Resource Center on Violence Against Women. Retrieved from http://new.vawnet.org/Assoc_Files_VAWnet/AR_PsychConsequences.pdf

Zabin, L.S. (1984). The association between smoking and sexual behavior among teens in US contraceptive clinics. *American Journal of Public Health, 74*(3), 261–263.

Zapata, L.B., Hillis, S.D., Marchbanks, P.A., Curtis, K.M., & Lowry, R. (2008). Methamphetamine use is independently associated with recent risky sexual behaviors and adolescent pregnancy. *Journal of School Health, 78*(12), 641–648.

CHAPTER ❖ 5

ASSESSING ADULT WOMEN'S HEALTH

Diane Schadewald ◆ Catherine Juve ◆
Ellis Quinn Youngkin ◆ Marcia Szmania Davis

Consider any interaction with a client (e.g., a therapeutic intervention by permitting the free expression of issues and concerns).

Highlights

- Leading Risk Factors for Women
- Screening Methods/Approaches to Health History
- Physical Examination

❖ INTRODUCTION

Women's life span, opportunities and risks, challenges, and stresses are ever increasing. As perhaps the only person a woman sees for health care, the woman's health care provider must approach assessment holistically. Indeed, all factors impinging on the woman's health and well-being must be considered if significant omissions in detecting problems and offering care are to be avoided. Pender (1996), in discussing health and wellness, refers to Dunn's suggestion that optimum health, or high-level wellness, emanates only from an environment that is favorable. Thus, the provider must help the woman become more attuned to her body and its cues and use the assessment period as an opportunity for teaching and counseling.

Healthy People 2020 has as its main goal helping Americans improve the quantity and quality of their lives using a public health prevention framework (U.S. Department of Health and Human Services [USDHHS], 2010). Maternal health, family planning, sexually transmitted infections, and lifestyle issues are all targeted for improvement. Providers of women's health care are responsible for holistically assessing a woman's physical, social, and psychological risk factors and working with her to change her behaviors and lifestyle to more healthful ones.

LEADING RISK FACTORS FOR WOMEN

An overall evaluation of risk factors should include assessment of the following behaviors.

UNSAFE LIFESTYLE BEHAVIORS

Unsafe lifestyle behaviors are related to personal choices and are amenable to change in most instances.

- *Cigarette smoking* continues to be the "single most preventable cause of disease and death" in this country. Smoking is associated with many diseases, including lung cancer and chronic respiratory diseases; heart diseases; cerebrovascular and peripheral vascular diseases; cancers of the cervix, larynx, oral cavity, pharynx and esophagus, bladder, kidney, and pancreas; peptic ulcer disease; increased cataracts; deaths by fire; lowered estrogen levels and early menopause; rapid skin aging and wrinkling; and secondhand smoke risk (Centers for Disease Control and Prevention [CDC], 2011). Nonsmokers exposed to secondhand smoke have a 25 to 30 percent increased risk for heart disease. Secondhand smoke causes about 3,000 cancer deaths annually and increases children's risk of serious respiratory and middle ear infections (National Cancer Institute, 2004). Recently, we have become aware of the dangers to children and others from third-hand smoke (Winickoff et al., 2009). Although women's rates of smoking have dropped significantly since they peaked in 1965, 18.1 percent of adult women smoked in 2009 (Bernstein et al., 2010, Table 58). Women ages 35 to 44 had the highest number of smokers, 22.9 percent, with 18- to 24-year-olds at only 16.7 percent. Black women 45 to 64 years old and white females 35 to 44 years old had the highest percentage of smokers, and those with a bachelor's degree or higher smoked the least (Bernstein et al., 2010, Table 59). Overall, it is estimated that nearly 28 percent of American Indian and Alaskan Native women, nearly 21 percent of non-Hispanic white women, 17 percent of non-Hispanic black women, nearly 10 percent of Hispanic women, and about 5 percent of Asian/Pacific Islander women smoke (Barnes, Adams, & Powell-Griner, 2010). Smoking is associated with premature births, mental retardation, miscarriage, and low birth weight in infants, yet 13 percent of pregnant women 15 to 54 years of age smoke. The number of low birth weight infants was nearly two times higher in smokers than nonsmokers in 2007 (Bernstein et al., 2010, Table 9). Factors associated with smoking in women include higher body mass index (BMI), longer prior attempts to stop smoking, greater dependence on nicotine, lower education, lower exercise patterns, stress, and depressive symptoms (Borrelli et al., 2002; Ludman et al., 2002; Tseng, Yeatts, Millikan, & Newman, 2001). Assessment should include what a woman smokes, the number smoked per day, the number of years she has smoked, ill effects, the number of attempts to quit, current level of desire to quit, and others in the household who smoke or are affected.

- *Substance use/abuse* includes alcohol, nicotine, caffeine, heroin, cocaine, marijuana, tranquilizers, inhalants, and most recently, a number of designer drugs. Twenty to 25 percent of patients seen in primary care settings have alcohol-abuse problems. Women, particularly older women, require less alcohol to become intoxicated than younger women or men because they have less body water. Accompanying diagnoses of sexual abuse (including history in childhood), mental health disorders such as phobias, eating disorders, and post-traumatic stress disorder are often seen in women with alcohol use issues (Becker & Walton-Moss, 2001; McCutcheon et al., 2009; National Institute on Alcohol Abuse and Alcoholism [NIAAA], 2008). A family history of alcoholism and onset of alcohol use in adolescence predispose to this disease. Women with disabilities have a higher risk of alcohol dependence (Brucker, 2007). Breast cancer risk is increased if a woman drinks on average as little as one alcohol-containing drink a day (NIAAA, 2008). An alcohol intake of four or more drinks at a time or eight or more drinks in a week increases the chance of developing alcoholism for women. It is estimated that 5.3 million women in the United States can be considered heavy users of alcohol. Heavy use of alcohol increases a woman's risk for a number of health problems including alcoholic liver disease, obesity, type 2 diabetes, brain disease, cancer, suppression of the immune system, hypertension, stroke, and heart disease, as well as deaths from homicide, suicide, high-risk sexual behavior, and motor vehicle accidents (MVAs) (NIAAA, 2008; USDA & USDHHS, 2010). It is imperative to screen for alcohol abuse, particularly in women who could bear children, because fetal alcohol syndrome is a leading cause of birth defects (Enoch & Goldman, 2002; NIAAA, 2008).

    Illicit or recreational drug use is not uncommon in adult women. The most commonly used illicit drug is marijuana. The most chronically abused drug is cocaine, and relapse into drug use for any chronic drug user is common (Arkangel, 2005). Sexually transmitted disease (STD) and HIV/AIDS, tuberculosis (TB), strokes, heart failure, heart arrhythmias, convulsions, mental health disorders, and memory defects are associated with illicit drug use. Adult women who are substance abusers have been found more likely to be successful with treatment if they have personal and social resources such as education, job abilities, and past employment histories (Kelly, Blacksin, & Mason, 2001). Women with disabilities have a higher risk of illicit drug use associated with lower self-esteem, peer pressure, and other factors that influence use (Li & Ford, 1998). In addition, risk for drug abuse by women is related to the fact that women are treated significantly more often than men with drugs that have abuse potential (Simoni-Wastila & Tompkins, 2001).

    All women should be assessed for alcohol use. This should include the number and frequency of drinks per day, per week, or per month. If a woman acknowledges alcohol intake, then further screening with an appropriate screening tool for alcohol abuse such as the CAGE assessment questions should be used. All women should also be assessed for abuse of illicit or recreational drugs and offered counseling regarding risks of drug use and referral for treatment as indicated (see Table 5–1).

- *Overuse of any medication or supplement* may occur when clients fail to read warnings or are not cautioned about the excessive use of legal drugs, such as gastric mucosal irritation with nonsteroidal anti-inflammatory drugs (NSAID) or nutritional supplements. Neurological abnormalities associated with excessive vitamin B_6 ingestion is an example of potential harm from overuse of a supplement. Assess the type of drug or supplement, amount used, years of use, and effects.
- *Sedentary lifestyle and lack of exercise and personal fitness* have been known for some time to be associated with a shorter life span, more dependence on others for activities of daily living (ADL), and poorer quality of life. Diseases/conditions associated with lack of physical activity include hypertension, diabetes, heart disease, colon cancer, lower back problems, breast cancer, osteoporosis, and arthritis. The highest percentages of less or no-leisure activity have been found in African American and Hispanic women, the older adult, those with less education and funds, those with disabilities, and people living in the northeastern and southern states. It was determined

TABLE 5–1. CAGE Alcohol Abuse Screening Tool

C	Have you ever thought you should CUT DOWN on your drinking?
A	Have you ever felt ANNOYED by others' criticism of your drinking?
G	Have you ever felt GUILTY about your drinking?
E	Do you ever have a morning EYE OPENER?

Source: www.AddictionsAndRecovery.org

in 1997 that only 30 percent of women in the United States spent 20 minutes in physical activity 3 or more days per week (USDHHS, 2000). Factors associated with being more physically active include earning four times the poverty level or more, being better educated, being married, and being white. In 2008, the USDHHS published its first ever recommendations for physical activity: *2008 Physical Activity Guidelines for Americans*. These guidelines provide information about recommended levels of physical activity for all. For example, adults who are inactive are recommended to start with a walking program of slow walking for 5 minutes several times a day for 5 to 6 days out of the week working up to 10 minutes three times a day for 5 to 6 days out of the week while also increasing their pace of walking (USDHHS, 2008). Since these guidelines have been released, the number of women age 18 and over meeting the highest level of physical activity recommendations increased from 12 to 16 percent (Bernstein et al., 2010). The guidelines with details on recommendations for exercise are available for download online at www.health.gov/PAGuidelines/. All women should be assessed for their level of physical activity during routine health maintenance exams.

- *Nutritional excesses and deficits* are associated with many serious and potentially lethal conditions such as obesity, coronary heart disease, some cancers, stroke, type 2 diabetes, and osteoporosis (USDA & USDHHS, 2010). Eating disorders, such as binging, purging, and anorexia, occur primarily in younger women. Those diagnosed with eating disorders in adolescence have better outcomes (Attia & Walsh, 2007). Underweight women report having had more stress during mealtime communications with their families, while overweight women report more effects from emphasis by their families on appearance and weight control (Worobey, 2002). Women who have an eating disorder tend to think that their appearance will help them develop and maintain romantic relationships more so than women who do not have an eating disorder (Sanchez & Kwang, 2007) (see Chapter 25).

  More Americans than ever are overweight or obese, and these conditions are associated with a greater risk of hypertension; abnormal lipid levels; type 2 diabetes; cardiovascular and cerebrovascular diseases; cancers of the endometrium, breast, prostate, and colon; gallbladder disease; breathing disorders and sleep disturbances; and arthritis (USDA & USDHHS, 2010). Between 1960 and 1994, the incidence of obesity in U.S. women rose from 15.7 percent of the population to 26.0 percent. As of 2008, it was 36.2 percent (Bernstein et al., 2010, Table 71) (see Chapter 3). When overweight women are also included with obese women, the percentage of American women increases to 64 percent. The daily environment Americans currently live in has been described as an "obesogenic" environment (USDA & USDHHS, 2010, p. 10).

  Health is associated with eating a balanced diet that provides adequate sources of vitamins and minerals with adequate protein, complex carbohydrates, vegetables, fruits, low fat (especially limiting saturated fat and cholesterol), moderate salt and sugar, adequate whole grains, and moderate alcohol if it is consumed (American Dietetic Association, 2010; USDA & USDHHS, 2010). A study that looked at diet quality using the health eating index (HEI), food consumption patterns, and BMI found that BMIs were lowest among women who ate vegetarian diets or high carbohydrate/low fat diets (Kennedy, Bowman, Spence, Freedman, & King, 2001). The highest quality diets were high complex carbohydrate. Eating out usually provides diets with higher fat and sodium and lower grains, vegetables, and fruits (USDA & USDHHS, 2010). The American Cancer Society guidelines for diet to decrease cancer morbidity and mortality parallel those of the American Heart Association to prevent heart disease (Byers et al., 2002). Childbearing-age women need folic acid and adequate iron, and all women, especially those past menopause, need adequate calcium and vitamin D. The American Dietetic Association emphasizes total diet, not one food or another, the importance of moderation, balance in the diet, getting all needed nutrients from food, and participation in physical activity (Kreider, Serra, Beavers, & Jonnalagadda, 2011). Because changing eating habits is tied to so many factors—sociocultural, psychological, environmental, physiological, and genetic—assessment must focus on all these parameters to offer assistance for change to individuals and families (USDA & USDHHS, 2010).

  Women should be assessed for usual caloric intake. This can be done by inquiring about usual daily intake from meals and snacks (see Special Assessment Guides, Nutritional Assessment).

- *Unsafe automobile driving*, inattention to precautions, and lapses in driving safety are associated with a high level of morbidity and mortality for women up to age 64, especially young women. Talking on cell phones and texting while driving are recent factors related to risk for MVAs, and such use has been outlawed in many states. The greatest numbers of deaths from MVAs are in the 15-to-24 and 65-and-over age groups (Bernstein et al., 2010, Table 37). Older women are more likely to die if injured in an MVA than younger women, due to increased vulnerability to serious complications. Nonuse of protective devices (seat belts) and reckless driving need to be assessed. Safety cautions should be integrated into the history routinely.

- *Exposure to intimate partner, family, or stranger violence* increases women's risk for substance abuse, psychological distress, and development of stress-related chronic illness (Carbone-López, Kruttschnitt, & MacMillan, 2006; Svavarsdottir & Orlygsdottir, 2009). The lifetime prevalence for women to be violently attacked is somewhere between one in three and one in four adult women in the United States (McColgan, Dempsey, Davis, & Giardino, 2010). Both heterosexual and lesbian women experience sexual assault. Alcohol abuse and/or other substance abuse is associated with episodes of IPV in both groups of women (Stevens, Korchmaros, & Miller, 2010). The National Violence Against Women Survey identified those at highest risk for experiencing IPV in descending order as American Indian/Alaskan Native women and men, African American women, and Hispanic women (Tjaden & Thoennes, 2000). However, others have found neither race nor economic status as significant variable in identifying risk (McColgan et al., 2010). More than one third of women seen in emergency rooms of hospitals for violence-related injuries were victims of their intimate partners. The husband, ex-husband, or boyfriend, in 1995 data, was the murderer in almost 50 percent of 5,000 cases of murdered women. Past data indicates that rape, attempted rape, and sexual assault are much higher than actually reported (USDHHS, 2000). According to a 2009 report by the Bureau of Justice Statistics, 8 out of 10,000 females age 12 and older experienced attempted or completed rape or other sexual assault. A national study of more than 3,000 women identified risk factors for rape and physical assault separately (Acierno, Resnick, Kilpatrick, Saunders, & Best, 1999). Findings showed that having been a past victim, being young, and current post-traumatic stress disorder were all factors associated with an increased risk of being raped. Increased risk of physical assault was associated with a past history of being a victim, minority status, current active depression, and drug use. A study of 2,109 North Carolina women found that perception of health as fair or poor, past history of ill health or mental health problems in the last month, and a history of poor mental health were associated with sexual assault (Cloutier, Martin, & Poole, 2002).

  Reports of abuse in pregnancy have varied over the years. An older study reported an incidence as high as 60 percent, with 25 percent being teens (Anderson, 2002). A more recent study of 1,500 postpartum women noted that 7.4 percent of these women interviewed at their 6-week postpartum visit reported IPV in the past 12 months (Certain, Mueller, Jagodzinski, & Fleming, 2008). Another study by Brown, McDonald, and Krastev (2008) noted that 18 percent of women had experienced fear of their partner during pregnancy. See Chapter 19 for more information.

  An adult woman who was a victim of rape as an adolescent may not have reported it; therefore, it is important when screening for abuse that inquiry is also made regarding a past history of abuse. Assessment should include asking about dangerous, conflictual relationships and living conditions such as violent families and neighborhoods. The authors urge screening for sexual assault and adverse childhood experiences (ACEs) in all settings.

- *Exposure to HIV, hepatitis, and STDs* may cause life-threatening, incurable, or disabling conditions (see Chapters 14 and 15). Many of the same characteristics that put women at risk for HIV, such as nonmonogamous relationships and substance abuse, also put them at risk for non-HIV STDs. A recent study by Witte, El-Bassel, Gilbert, Wu, and Chang (2010) found that 3 percent of women thought they were in a monogamous relationship when they were not; this is lower than the percentage found in other studies where up to 33 percent were unaware (Riehman, Wechsberg, Francis, Moore, & Morgan-Lopez, 2006). In addition, in the most recent study the percentage of women unaware of their partner's risk behaviors increased for older women (Witte et al., 2010). Women whose only sexual partners are women are still at risk for STDs and should be tested, but many are not aware that they are at risk (Bauer & Welles, 2001; Marrazzo, Coffey, & Bingham, 2005).

Previously nonoxynol-9 was thought to decrease risk for STD transmission and was considered a part of safer sex practice. However, with further study it was found to actually increase risk of transmission (Cone et al., 2006). Therefore, women who use barrier methods, such as a diaphragm with spermicide or condoms with spermicide, may be at higher risk. A number of older studies have identified various other risk factors for STDs in women. Characteristics such as less self-efficacy, less self-esteem, less knowledge about sexual issues, less ability to communicate, being poor, and being African American or Hispanic have all been associated with higher risk (Aral, 2001; Raphan, Cohen, & Boyer, 2001; USDHHS, 2000).

Women's complications of STDs—pelvic inflammatory disease (PID), human papillomavirus (HPV), cervical malignancy, ectopic pregnancy, infertility, chronic pelvic pain—are far more serious than those of men. Assessment should include questions about the frequency of sexual contacts, the number of partners currently and in the past, the risk status of partners, forms of sexual expression, type of contraception, and/or barrier/chemical methods of protection. Perception of risk should be assessed; it may be significantly different from real risk.

- *Low health literacy and/or poor health maintenance behavior*, lack of knowledge regarding health-directed behaviors, or poor personal care is associated with a substandard health status and inadequate detection and prevention behaviors, such as lack of use of vaccines, regular routine screening exams, and contraception. Those with low health literacy also have decreased ability to read and comprehend prescription labels and patient information pamphlets (Berkman, Sheridan, Donahue, Halpern, & Crotty, 2011). A woman's ability to maintain or improve her health and the health of her family is directly related to her health literacy (Shieh & Halstead, 2009). Assessment should include inquiry regarding understanding of and recommendations for frequency of breast self-exam, dental and eye exams, general screening physical and diagnostic exams (including pelvic and rectal exams), cervical cytology and indicated cultures/tests, occult fecal blood testing, mammography, and vulvar self-exam.
- *Inadequate, excessive, or unusual sleep* in women can be impacted by physiologic events and hormonal changes related to the menstrual cycle, pregnancy, and menopause is found in the National Sleep Foundation's (NSF) 2007 study (Lee, Baker, Newton, & Ancoli-Israel, 2007). The NSF's 2004–2005 study found that about 25 percent of Americans thought they had a sleep problem. Further analysis of the NSF's 2007 survey concluded that 25 percent of American women have high risk for experiencing obstructive sleep apnea (OSA) and that it is underdiagnosed in women (Kapsimalis & Kryger, 2009). Sleep durations of both less than 5 hours and more than 9 hours have been associated with cardiovascular disease (Sabanayagam & Shankar, 2010). Some medical and psychiatric comorbidities associated with insomnia are anxiety, depression, diabetes, obesity, hypertension, chronic obstructive pulmonary disease (COPD), and asthma (Li et al., 2010; Rosekind & Gregory, 2010). Women ages 30 to 60 are typically sleep deprived, averaging 1.5 hours less sleep on weeknights (NSF, 2011). Daytime sleepiness also increases risk for injury, either work related or motor vehicle related. Shift work, employment status, increased age, and female gender have been associated with increased risk for insomnia (Rosekind & Gregory, 2010). Therefore, a complaint of insomnia necessitates further assessment for modifiable risk factors and underlying medical and psychiatric disorders as well as sleep disorders. Assessment should include evaluation of duration and quality of sleep, breathing difficulties, snoring, smoking, neuroses, alcohol use, medication use, menstrual symptoms, estrogen decline, time zone or job shift changes, sleepwalking, stress and depression, heavy exercise near bedtime, environmental conditions for sleep, and dozing off during the day. See Chapter 25 for further discussion of sleep dysregulation.

EXPOSURE TO ENVIRONMENTAL HAZARDS

Unsafe conditions may be found in the home or work environment.

- *Unsafe home environment* encompasses exposure to chemical/toxic/radon hazards, fire, excessive heat or cold, unsanitary living conditions, unsafe drinking water, lack of running water, rodent or insect infestation, airborne pollutants, and infections among people living in crowded conditions. People spend 90 percent of their time indoors where higher levels of allergens and pollutants are found. Dust mites, cockroaches, pets, mold, and rodents contribute to indoor allergens and the development of respiratory diseases. Indoor air pollution may also contribute to headaches, dizziness, fatigue, heart disease, and, in the long term, cancer risk. Radon levels may be too high in 1 out of 15 homes in the United States; older homes may have materials containing lead or asbestos. Volatile organic compounds can be released from many new furnishings and household products used for remodeling or cleaning, respectively (USDHHS, 2009). See Chapter 19 for a discussion of exposure to toxins and pregnancy. Inquire as to household living conditions. Measures to help decrease exposure to indoor air pollution can be found at www.epa.gov/iaq/pubs/residair.html.

- *Unsafe occupational situations* are associated with life-threatening, damaging, or debilitating conditions (also see unsafe home environment information). In general, women experience fewer work-related injuries than men, but women who work in service-related industries such as health care or as typists are at higher risk for musculoskeletal injury such as sprains, strains, and tendonitis (Hoskins, 2005; Treaster & Burr, 2004). Risk of low birth weight, when a pregnant woman is exposed to pesticides in her job, as well as problems with fertility when exposed to phthalates, is suggested in the literature (Burdorf et al., 2011). Working in adverse conditions (whole-body vibrations, prolonged standing, sitting, reaching, bending, or squatting) or where one is exposed to hazardous substances (radiation, chemicals, solvents, gases, and antineoplastic drugs) is associated with an increase in one or more of the following: problems with fertility, spontaneous abortions, preterm births, and low birth weight infants, as well as cancers and musculoskeletal injuries (Croteau, Marcoux, & Brisson, 2007; Figà-Talamanca, 2006; Hoskins, 2005). Job strain—that is, work with high demands, either psychologically or physically, and low control without a good support network—and/or working more than 5 days in a row were also associated with preterm delivery (Croteau et al., 2007). Military women exposed to heavy metals, pesticides, petroleum products, and chemicals have a greater risk of abnormal pregnancy outcomes (Hourani & Hilton, 2000). Clinicians need to take a detailed workplace history. Assessment should include the individual's type of work, work hazards and conditions, and effects. Biological, chemical, environmental-mechanical, physical, and psychosocial hazards should be assessed (see Special Assessment Guides in this chapter and Chapter 19 on pregnancy). Clinicians should also be familiar with their local, state, and national resources such as the local poison control center hotline and Occupational Safety and Health Administration (OSHA) (toll-free at 1-800-321-6742 or online at www.osha.gov).
- *Access to firearms* in the household can increase risk for injury, especially if household members are not properly educated about their use and/or if the firearm is not locked in a gun safe away from the reach of children (Narang et al., 2010).

NEGATIVE INFLUENCES ON EMOTIONAL HEALTH

Such influences vary widely from family crises to unrealistic values of thinness.

- *Stress* is associated with a wide array of physical and emotional problems. Individual response to a stressor will vary from woman to woman. However, high levels of stress have been associated with physical function limitations in women ages 44 to 55 similar to those seen with older women (Pope, Sowers, Welch, & Albrecht, 2001).

  Lazarus (1981), a pioneer on research regarding stress, closely linked the effects of hassles (the little irritating or distressing occurrences that happen daily) rather than major life events to emotional health. Women living in a poor, urban city community described stressors as finances, work, family, safety, police, and municipal services; depression in this group of women was significantly associated with increased problems with finances, police, and safety stress and unfair treatment factors (Schulz et al., 2006). Stress can affect the person physically (reduced immune responses and increased risk of cardiovascular, reproductive, and gastrointestinal [GI] conditions) and mentally (post-traumatic stress syndrome, neuroses, and transient situational disturbances) (see Chapter 25). Assessment should include stressors related to work, home, family, and other relationships.
- *A poor or absent support system* is associated with feelings of loneliness, helplessness, hopelessness, and powerlessness. Pender's (1996) work has shown that social support appears to be related to better health and feelings of well-being. Social networks have long been known to decrease health risks

associated with occupational stress, cancer, and pregnancy (Auslander, 1988). In a study that examined social support as a predictor of health-related quality of life in chronic heart failure patients, changes in social support significantly predicted changes in health-related quality of life (Bennett et al., 2001). Loneliness has been confirmed as a risk factor for depression in a longitudinal study of women ages 50 to 67 (Cacioppo, Hughes, Waite, Hawkley, & Thisted, 2006). Loneliness has also been linked to risk for increased systolic blood pressure (Hawkley, Thisted, Masi, & Cacioppo, 2010). Assessment of supports should include determining distance from friends, relatives, cultural group, health resources; quality of relationships with friends; and access to support systems, such as church.

- *Family crises* mean increased physical and emotional risks for both the individual and the family. Assessment includes family health, values, health care beliefs, cultural influences, and coping abilities, as evidenced by past coping with crises, individual, and family. Such crises include a wide array of problems such as marriage, birth, death, serious illness, divorce, loss of a job, loss of a home, moving, or substance abuse of a member.
- *Depression and other mood disorders* are common psychiatric illnesses in women (see Chapter 25 on depression). One in four U.S. women will be clinically depressed at some time in her life and twice as many women as men become depressed (Kessler et al., 2005). Depression, the most common U.S. mental illness, causes more disability than any other illness and is a factor in most suicides (National Institute of Mental Health [NIMH], 2009). Eighteen to 44-year-olds are most affected. The childbearing years and the hormone-level fluctuations are often associated with more stress and mental illness than any other period in women's lives (Lee et al., 2007). Depression following childbirth affects between 6 and 13 percent of women (Gaynes et al., 2005). Women often experience depression during the menopause transition attributed to the interaction between vasomotor symptoms, changing hormone levels, and sleep problems (Lee et al., 2007). Assessment requires recognizing four or more signs and symptoms that cluster and persist for a 2-week period and are a change from usual patterns (American Psychiatric Association, 2000). These signs include changes in mood, sleep patterns, weight, appetite, and activity or energy level; decreased motivation, interest in life, concentration and memory, and self-esteem/self-worth; and suicidal ideation. A family history of mental disorders is also a warning sign.
- *Unrealistic values* of youth, beauty, and thinness lead to unhealthy, excessive concerns and behaviors related to appearance. Much of the emphasis on attractiveness and youth from the media is thought to be at the root of the increase in cosmetic surgery in those age 44 to 55 (Slevec & Tiggemann, 2010). These concerns may also indicate an inability to accept the aging process. Assessment includes appearance, age, weight, height, history of unusual or overuse of plastic/reparative surgery, diet and exercise history, any verbal and nonverbal cues, such as great concern with being overweight when in reality one is underweight (see nutritional excesses and deficits in this chapter and Chapter 25 on eating disorders).
- *Lack of recreational and relaxation activities* can contribute to unhealthy stress response, overwork, anxiety, and in some instances depression. Assessment includes financial, social, physical, and psychological conditions and barriers. Relaxation takes planning and considered time to break from life's usual pressures and competitions.

POVERTY, INSUFFICIENT INSURANCE, AND INADEQUATE MATERIAL RESOURCES

Poverty increased during the Great Recession that started in 2007. The rate of poverty in 2009 was 14.3 percent. Women and children (including adolescents) continue to be the fastest growing segment of those living in poverty (U.S. Census Bureau, 2011). In addition, all of the gains in alleviating poverty of the 1990s were eliminated, leading up to and during the Great Recession (KIDS COUNT, 2011). For the year 2011, the poverty line was $22,350 for a family of four. For a single person, it was $10,890 (USDHHS, 2011). There are more women ages 55 to 64 who live in poverty than men in the same age span. This may be related to the fact that, according to Jennifer Tucker from the Center for Women Policy Studies, women typically earn only 77 percent of what men earn for full-time work (Young, 2011). Also, the consistent decrease in the value of low-skilled labor over the last several decades is inversely related to the increasing number of children in working poor families, according to the executive director of KIDS COUNT 2011. Lower income is associated with greater risk of heart disease, diabetes, and obesity (CDC, 2011). Loss of insurance coverage with loss of employment has swelled the ranks of the uninsured.

In an examination of uterine cancer outcome, those with insurance, regardless of race, had better outcomes than those covered by Medicaid or those uninsured (Fedewa, Lerro, Chase, & Ward, 2011). Mammography usage, according to the 2005 National Health Interview Survey, was found to be lowest for low-income uninsured Asian and Hispanic women; however, previous lower use by American Indian/Alaskan Native women was no longer present (Sabatino et al., 2008). Poor people have often delayed seeking health care when ill, used fewer measures to prevent or alleviate illness, had less accurate information about health, and had fewer choices for access to health care. Gains in health that have occurred for those in higher-income brackets are not mirrored in lower-income groups.

Disparities in health for minorities are significantly determined by socioeconomic factors. Minorities in general have increased barriers to access to care and a higher incidence of chronic disease. Use of preventive services, such as mammography, and risk behaviors, such as smoking, are not uniform within any particular ethnic group across the United States. However, lack of use may be prevalent in a particular community and clinicians, in order to address health care disparities, need to be aware of practices of ethnic groups within the community in which they practice (CDC, 2011).

The Affordable Care Act (ACA), signed into law in March 2010, holds promise to improve access to affordable health insurance and decrease health disparities. It falls short of universal coverage, but is targeted to decrease the number of those uninsured. All provisions of the ACA will be fully in effect by 2014. In August 2011, the DHHS announced guidelines for preventive health services for women that will go into effect in August 2012. These services are to be provided with no cost sharing and include annual well woman visits; gestational diabetes screening; HPV DNA testing; STI counseling; HIV counseling and screening; contraception and contraceptive counseling (with the exception of abortifacient drugs); breastfeeding support, supplies, and counseling; and domestic violence screening. The decision to provide these services without cost sharing was based on the finding that more than 50 percent of women postpone these services because of cost if there is a required co-pay (HealthCare.gov, 2011). These provisions may alleviate many previous health disparities for women.

HEREDITARY, CULTURAL, AND ETHNIC INFLUENCES

Family history and culture impact health.

- *Familial diseases* may be detected by assessing family history. Diabetes, breast cancer, colorectal cancer, ovarian cancer, diabetes, heart disease, asthma, and allergies are examples of disease risks inherited from family members.
- *Race* is another consideration. Some diseases are more common among people of certain races; for example, osteoporosis is more prevalent in light- or yellow-skinned women; sickle cell disease is found in African Americans; and glucose-6-phosphate dehydrogenase (G-6-PD) deficiency occurs more often in people of Mediterranean descent. Also, African American women are excessively prone to chronic illness and disability, regardless of their socioeconomic status; Geronimus has proposed early health insults related to the stress of living in a race-conscious society as a potential cause of this increased risk (Geronimus, 2001; Geronimus, Hicken, Keene, & Bound, 2006).
- *Ethnic, cultural, and religious influences* may be associated with unhealthy practices: eating uncooked meat, prolonged fasting, refusing to see a health care provider, or lacking health-directed behaviors. These influences may also be protective. A study of women with fibromyalgia found that religiosity had a potential protective impact on stress response (Dedert et al., 2004). Religiosity has also been positively associated with mental health in women in a study of patients with cancer (Holt, Oster, Clay, Urmie, & Fouad, 2011) and reduced anxiety in a group of pregnant women (Mann, McKeown, Bacon, Vesselinov, & Bush, 2008). Sensitivity to a client's culture, religion, and ethnic influences is essential in trying to assist her with any health behavior changes, for these variables strongly affect her health beliefs.

CURRENT OR PAST MEDICAL PROBLEMS

Of particular concern are the risks of past and present problems and the potential or real effects of current or past illness on new disease conditions. For example, research indicates a past history of smoking, even if the person no longer smokes, increases the risk of multiple myeloma and colon cancer. Multiple drug interactions may cause increased risks and confusing presentations. Past PID increases the risk of ectopic pregnancy or infertility.

SCREENING METHODS/ APPROACHES TO HEALTH HISTORY

HEALTH HISTORY

Interview and Approach Considerations

Effective interviewing and interpersonal skills are required in order to gather accurate, useful data.

- Consider any interaction with a client (e.g., a therapeutic intervention by permitting the free expression of issues and concerns). Treat the client with dignity and respect; be nonjudgmental, accepting, supportive, concerned, and an appropriate role model.
- Use clear language and terminology matched to the client's level of understanding, culture, and background. Consider the client's age, education, response to the interview, and ethical, cultural, and religious taboos. Avoid medical jargon and clarify by restating confusing information. Use an interpreter if necessary.
- Appropriate questioning technique includes using open questions early in the interview to facilitate broad information gathering and to assist with mental status and general survey assessment. Ask the client about her concerns. Avoid interrupting, which may cause valuable data to be lost. Use pointed, directive questions to obtain specific data. Avoid leading questions and phrase-sensitive questions in a nonjudgmental manner.
- Be aware of nonverbal cues such as facial expressions, body movements, and signs of anxiety. The client may avoid making eye contact or answering questions. She may be reluctant to give information. Such cues may indicate fears or concerns.
- Help the woman understand the importance of telling you her concerns. If the client is able to talk freely, the interaction becomes healing, and there is the increased probability that something will be said that will help in understanding a problem or help in management. Recognize that the client's real concerns may not surface until she feels comfortable with you.

Physical and psychological factors affect interaction.

- Provide a quiet, private place for the interview.
- Maintain the client's comfort. Permit her to remain dressed during the interview and provide comfortable seating that will allow client and interviewer to be at the same eye level. Never obtain a history with the client in lithotomy position.
- Due to the limited time frames for most visits in primary care today, seek to find out early what problems at most concern her. Keep the interview focused to stay within a reasonable time limit, using more than one session if needed.

Components of Health History

- Demographic and biographical data, called identifying data (ID), must be accurate.
- Record the chief complaint (CC) or reason for visit (RFV). Use the client's own words in a brief statement and put into a time frame (e.g., "I've had chest pain for 2 days" or "I need a Pap test and checkup").
- Inquire about history of present illness (HPI) or current health status (CHS). An introductory statement is essential: gravidity (G); parity—full-term (T) or premature pregnancies (P); abortions (A)—spontaneous and induced, with reasons and length of gestation; number of living children (L); dates of last and previous normal menstrual periods based on first day of bleeding (LNMP, PNMP); and methods of contraception used by client and/or partner—for how long or when stopped. If appropriate, include date of menopause.

Write the remainder of the paragraph as a narrative, giving the following:

- Usual state of health
- Clear, chronological development/analysis of complaints: sequencing (starting with onset), causes or associated phenomena, factors worsening/lessening/relieving/aggravating, quality or character of complaint, quantity of problem, effect on activities, location, radiation, severity (on a scale of 1 to 10), timing, past occurrence, others with problem
- Relevant family history
- Degree of disability
- Significant negatives

If the visit is related to the menstrual cycle, a complete description of the menstrual cycles is needed, including characteristics before and after the use of hormonal or other contraception that may affect the cycles.

If the visit is for routine health maintenance, elicit information about the client's usual health, last exams or tests and their results, current medications, habits, and significant problems or negatives, such as diabetes mellitus or cardiac disease.

- Assess and record the past medical history (PMH) or past health status (PHS).
    - *Childhood Diseases.* Measles, mumps, frequent infections, and so on.

TABLE 5–2. Adult Immunizations

Vaccine	Schedule/Timing	Indications	Comments	Precaution/Contraindications
Adult tetanus/ diphtheria toxoid (Td)	Booster q 10 years through life; repeat dose with contaminated wounds if 5 years post booster. Substitute one-time dose of Tdap for next Td (this one-time booster of Tdap can be given regardless of when last Td given)	All previously immunized adults	1. If pregnant and update needed, give Td in second or third trimesters. If update not needed, give Tdap postpartum. (See Chapter 19 for more information about Tdap and pregnancy.)	Neurologic or immediate hypersensitivity after prior dose; severe local reaction after prior dose
Influenza (whole or split-virus) LAIV or TIV	One dose (whole or split-virus) annually; generally in November, but may be offered as early as September LAIV—intranasal TIV—intramuscular	1. LAIV or TIV to healthy nonpregnant adults age 19–49 2. Give TIV to persons with high-risk medical conditions, pregnant women, and persons age 50 and older	1. Provides protection against strains identified as high risk for the season (may include A, B, H1N1, etc.) 2. Does not cause the flu 3. May cause fever, malaise, myalgia 6–12 hours after given; lasts 1–2 days 4. Healthy adults benefit through less work time lost; less money spent on treatment	1. Acute febrile illness (wait until all symptoms abate) 2. Known hypersensitivity to eggs 3. Delay in pregnancy until after first trimester (give TIV then) 4. Moderately to severely ill persons
Measles, mumps, rubella (MMR) vaccine	One or two doses subcutaneous	1. Birthdate prior to 1957 generally gives immunity. Except health care personnel born prior to 1957 need proof of immunity 2. Childbearing age women and persons entering college, health care work, military, traveling internationally, or adults exposed in an outbreak are also candidates 3. No evidence of documented vaccination requires two doses 1 month apart	1. Is live virus vaccine 2. MMR is vaccine of choice 3. HIV persons may receive if CD4 + T lymphocyte count ≥ 200 c/μL 4. Breastfeeding is not contraindication	1. Pregnant women (give vaccine postpartum if not immune) 2. Immunocompromised persons, other than those with HIV 3. History of anaphylactic reaction after ingesting egg or after receiving neomycin 4. Moderately to severely ill persons 5. Recent receipt of antibody-containing blood products
Varicella zoster vaccine (VZV; Varivax)	Two doses 4–8 weeks apart; if > 8 weeks apart, may still give second dose	1. All adults without evidence of immunity	1. Live, attenuated vaccine 2. Herpes zoster risk ≤ natural disease 3. 25% have erythema/soreness at injection site; 5%—rash	1. Contraindicated in pregnancy. Avoid in immunocompromised, hypersensitive, or neomycin-allergic people 2. Avoid pregnancy for 1 month after vaccine 3. HIV persons may receive if CD4 + T lymphocyte count ≥ 200 c/μL. Avoid in moderately to severely ill persons 5. Do not give if recent receipt of antibody-containing blood products
Zostavax		1. All adults over age 60 regardless of history of a previous herpes zoster infection		1. Contraindicated in pregnancy. Avoid in immunocompromised, hypersensitive, or neomycin-allergic people
Hepatitis A vaccine	One dose IM; booster at 6–12 months	1. Adults at risk such as international travelers, those with hepatitis C or other chronic liver disease, HIV, persons who use street drugs, persons who receive clotting factor concentrates, persons in close contact to international adoptee from HAV endemic area	1. Inactivated virus 2. Side effects: soreness at site, malaise, headache	1. Use only in pregnancy if risk > without

(*continued*)

Vaccine	Schedule/Timing	Indications	Comments	Precaution/Contraindications
Hepatitis B vaccine	First dose at first visit Second dose in 4 weeks Third dose in 5 months after second dose	1. All health care workers 2. All who are at increased risk occupationally or socially (includes family exposure)	1. Recombinant vaccine	1. Not contraindicated in pregnancy (see Chapters 19 and 22 for pregnancy and postpartum recommendations)
Pneumococcal	One dose IM; another dose every 6 years may be considered	1. Immunocompetent adults with chronic disease 2. Immunocompromised adults 3. HIV-infected adults 4. Those living where increased risk of disease exists 5. All persons with asplenia	1. Vaccinate high-risk women before or after pregnancy 2. Half experience injection site pain, erythema; 1% have fever, myalgias, severe local reaction	1. Contraindicated in pregnant women
Meningoccocal vaccine (meningococcal conjugate vaccine [MCV], meningococcal polysaccharide vaccine [MPSV])	MCV—give a two-dose series at 0 and 2 months. MCV—give one dose for revaccinating those under age 54 every 5 years MPSV—alternative for those age 19–55 and for revaccination if over age 56	1. Immunocompromised adults (complement deficiency, HIV, asplenia) 2. Travelers to endemic regions, military personnel, lab personnel, college bound living in dorms		

HPV vaccination with Gardasil (HPV4) or Cervirex (HPV2) can be offered to women under the age of 27 who have not yet been immunized. Full immunization consists of a series of three IM injections at 0, 1 to 2, and 6 months. It is contraindicated in pregnancy.

For catch-up schedule for nonimmunized adults and for information about immunizations for travel, see CDC (2011).

Those over age 18, including foreign-born adults, no longer need polio vaccination unless they are traveling to an area where wild poliovirus exists.

Sources: Akinsanya-Beysolow and Wolfe, 2009; CDC, 2011; Marcy, 2007.

- *Immunizations and Screening Tests.* Dates of childhood immunizations: hepatitis B, diphtheria, pertussis, tetanus, Hemophilus influenza type B, measles, mumps, rubella, chickenpox, polio vaccines (types); dates of adult immunizations: tetanus (Td or Tdap), pneumococcus, influenza, hepatitis B, measles (those born after 1956), rubella (women without immunity), varicella; dates of other vaccinations: meningococcus, smallpox, typhoid, and other special vaccines (BCG) for at-risk populations; screening tests (HIV, rubella, TB, sickle cell, G-6-PD). (See Table 5–2 for recommended routine adult immunizations.)
- *Hospitalizations, Surgeries, and Serious Illnesses.* Dates, places, health care providers, reasons, courses of recovery, sequelae.
- *Accidents and Injuries.* Type of injury, how it occurred, severity, treatment, where, by whom, sequelae.
- *Obstetric History.* All pregnancies, regardless of outcome; dates and types of deliveries, sex and weights of infants, lengths of gestations; antepartum, intrapartum, and postpartum complications.
- *Contraceptive History.* Types of contraceptives used by client or partner, length of use, complications, side effects, satisfaction with method.
- *Sexual History.* Assess safer sex methods used and sexual satisfaction (see Chapter 7).
- *Allergies.* Specific allergens (food, environmental, medication), types of reactions, treatments, and results.
- *Medications.* Prescription, over-the-counter, herbs, supplements, dosages, administration routes, frequencies, reasons for use, side effects.
- *Transfusions/Transplants.* Dates, reasons, exposure to HIV, hepatitis B and C.

- Social history includes recreational or illicit substance use, tobacco, alcohol, type of substances, frequency, duration of use, effects, routes of administration, risk practices such as needle sharing.
- Violence history includes incidents of assault, incest, rape, other violence; injuries, treatment, counseling, sequelae. Assess for IPV and or ACEs. See Appendix B for assessment tools.
- Family history (FH) includes hereditary, communicable, and environmental family diseases; causes of death of maternal and paternal grandparents, parents, siblings, children, partners, aunts, uncles, and cousins (if indicated). A genogram can be visually helpful (see Special Assessment Guides, Family Assessment). Note if family history is unknown or the client

is adopted. Of particular importance is a family history of breast, colon, or ovarian cancer in mother or sister, congenital anomalies or retardation, multiple births, CVD, and anemia.

- Psychosocial history taking (PSH) and personal history taking and assessment require sensitivity.
  - *Nutrition.* See Special Assessment Guides, Nutritional Assessment.
  - *Family Relationships, Friendships, and Support Systems.* Significance and quality of relationships and interactions, areas of concern or conflict, verbal or physical abuse, living arrangements, availability of support systems, club and organization memberships, activities enjoyed with friends and relatives (see Special Assessment Guides, Family Assessment).
  - *Culture/Ethnicity.* Foods, religion, values, and beliefs affecting health.
  - *Occupation.* Full- or part-time employment, length of employment, type of work, hazards, stressors (see Special Assessment Guides, Occupational Assessment).
  - *Education.* Highest level obtained (formal and informal); client's feelings of satisfaction and how she learns best.
  - *Economic Status.* Adequacy of income for basic and recreational needs, monetary concerns, adequacy of insurance.
  - *Exercise and Activity.* Current levels and types of activity, length of time spent, frequency, tolerance, safety.
  - *Developmental Status.* Current level of task accomplishment according to developmental stage (see Chapters 2 and 4).
  - *Self-Concept.* Locus of control, positive and negative feelings about self, satisfaction with self, perceived strengths and weaknesses.
  - *Coping Mechanisms.* Stressors and usual methods of coping, perceived effectiveness (see Special Assessment Guides, Stress/Risk Assessment).
  - *Patterns and Maintenance of Health Care.* Types, sources, and frequency of health care visits; home/folk remedies; general experiences and attitudes about health and care.
  - *Sleep and Wakefulness.* Patterns, effects, problems, dreams, medication used to sleep or to stay awake (see Special Assessment Guides, Sleep Assessment).
  - *Recreation/Relaxation.* Hobbies and activities for fun or relaxation; associated patterns, roles, and relationships.
  - *Living Environment.* Hazards (real or potential), level of comfort, privacy, space.
  - *Religion.* Importance to client, source of strength or stress, level of involvement.
  - *Daily Profile.* Description of a typical day for the client.
- A review of systems (ROS) includes a thorough past and present history of each system.
  - *General.* General health, fatigue, exercise tolerance, episodes of unusual weight/height loss or gain, malaise, ability to carry out ADL.
  - *Skin, Hair, Nails.* Diseases; primary or secondary skin lesions, itching, flaking; changes in texture, moisture, color, skin temperature, amount of hair, care practices.
  - *Head and Neck.* Injuries and their treatments, sequelae; headaches (type); range-of-motion limitations, pain, or stiffness; enlarged nodes; swelling.
  - *Eyes.* Use of corrective lenses, reason for prescription, results of last exam and glaucoma test, diseases or infections, pain, itching, discharge, diplopia, cataracts, blurred vision, spots, halos, flashing lights, blind spots.
  - *Ears.* Hearing acuity, test results and dates, use of aids and their effectiveness, diseases, pain, ringing, vertigo, infection, discharge, care habits.
  - *Mouth, Teeth, and Throat.* Diseases; condition of teeth (loose, missing, caries), last exam and results, knowledge of routine care; sore throats, lesions, bleeding, hoarseness, voice changes; chewing, swallowing, or taste problems.
  - *Nose and Sinuses.* Diseases; problems with sense of smell; nosebleeds; allergies/seasonal problems, sneezing, congestion, drainage, pain; trauma; breathing difficulties; infections and their treatments.
  - *Chest and Lungs.* Diseases; dyspnea, cough, hemoptysis, exertion breathing difficulty, wheezing, asthma, pneumonia, bronchitis, TB, emphysema, orthopnea, night sweats, smoking; time of last chest x-ray, reason, and results; last TB test and results.
  - *Cardiovascular.* Diseases; pain, cyanosis, palpitations, murmurs, bruits, irregular heart rate, mitral valve prolapse, hypertension, edema, varicosities, rheumatic fever; coldness, tingling, color changes, hair loss on extremities; recent cholesterol and lipid screening results.
  - *Breasts and Axillae.* Diseases; pain, masses, changes related to menstrual cycle, discharge,

color, characteristics; skin, vascular, temperature changes; breast self-exam (when, how); last provider exam; last mammogram results; breastfeeding history.

- *Gastrointestinal.* Diseases; abdominal pain, distention, masses, indigestion, food intolerances, belching, nausea, vomiting (character), reflux, jaundice, ascites, diarrhea, constipation, character of stools; hemorrhoids; use of antacids or laxatives; last hemoccult test, results.
- *Genitourinary*

  Reproductive. Onset of puberty, menarche (when, character, regularity of menses), current menstrual pattern (frequency, duration, flow amount); premenstrual syndrome (PMS); dysmenorrhea; tampon or pad use, size, correct use, number per day of flow, saturation; problems related to menses; use of medications or hormones, reasons, problems; history of female genital cutting (female circumcision); genital piercings; last pelvic exam and Pap smear (if abnormal results, follow-up, sequelae); vaginitis, itching, discharge, lesions, diseases, abnormalities; STDs, including pain, fever, chills; diethylstilbestrol (DES) exposure; fertility problems; sexual satisfaction, discomfort, problems. (Obstetric, sexual, contraceptive, and menopause history data may go here, or in HPI or CHS if it relates to the RFV; see Chapter 19 for further information about obstetric history.)

  Urinary. Character and regularity of urination; diseases, infections (cystitis or pyelonephritis); dysuria, polyuria, oliguria, anuria, incontinence, hematuria, nocturia, urgency, stones, flank pain, fever, chills.
- *Musculoskeletal.* Diseases, fractures, or other injuries, cramping, pain, fasciculations, weakness/strength, range-of-motion/ADL limitations, gait problems, joint complaints (swelling, redness, pain, deformity, crepitus); back discomfort, ache, or deformity; loss of height.
- *Neurological.* Diseases; fainting, loss of consciousness, seizures (and medication for them), sensory problems (numbness, tingling, paresthesia), motor problems (balance, gait, spasm, paralysis), cognitive problems (mood changes, memory loss, disorientation, loss of judgment, hallucinations); sleep disturbances.
- *Blood and Immune.* Diseases; anemias, bleeding tendencies, easy bruising, transfusions, allergies, treatments; unexplained infections or node enlargement; blood type.
- *Endocrine.* Diseases; unusual changes in weight, height, glove, or shoe size; increased thirst, urination, appetite; heat/cold intolerance; weakness/fatigue; changes in skin and hair (loss, excessive growth, hirsute, texture).

SPECIAL ASSESSMENT GUIDES

Family Assessment

Determine who lives in the family, their relationships, cultural origins, religious preferences, health practices; the role of each member (education, occupation), communication among members, material management (home, money), goals of the family, relaxation and recreational family activities; and strengths, weaknesses, conflicts, problems, past resolution methods (Sawin & Harrigan, 1995; Seidel, Ball, Dains, & Benedict, 2011).

- The *Calgary Family Assessment Model* (CFAM) can be used for assessment of families and also as a structure for planning interventions for families. It assesses the family in three main areas: (1) structural, (2) developmental, and (3) functional. Each of these areas has subcategories that may be included in the assessment. The clinician may choose to assess in only one of the main areas and may also use discretion regarding which subcategories to include within each area. This will depend on whether the clinician needs assessment in a specific area or if a global assessment is necessary (see Figure 5–1). The clinician utilizing the CFAM may develop genograms and/or ecomaps when assessing family structure. It can be considered a snapshot of the family seen through the lens of the clinician providing the assessment (Wright & Leahey, 2009). Familiarity with the model is necessary in order to utilize accurately and fully.
- *"Family APGAR"* is a quick screening tool for identifying satisfaction with family function. It was introduced by Smilkstein in 1978. Chao, Zyzanski, and Flocke (1998) propose that obtaining the score on just the female head of household correlates well with the score that would be obtained if all family members were evaluated. One study found that it does not accurately identify families as functional or dysfunctional and concluded it shouldn't be used for this purpose as it was developed to measure level of satisfaction with family support that may or may not be reflective of function (Gardner et al., 2001). It uses five areas for scoring: *adaptation*, *partnership*, *growth*, *affection*, and *resolve*. Each category receives a score of 0 to 2 points. The provider asks the client to score 2 points

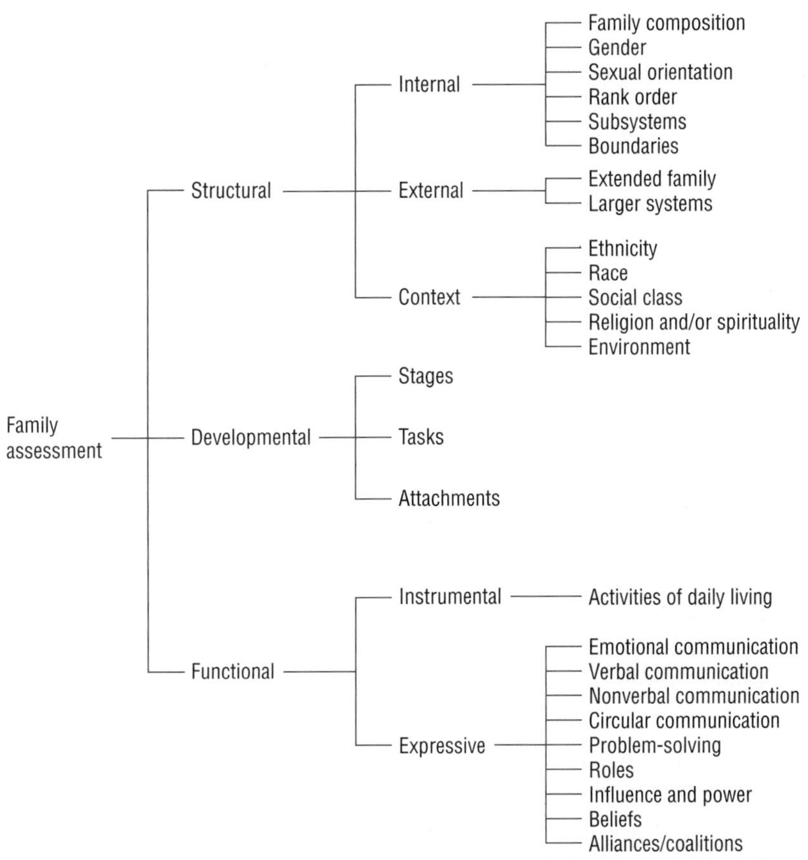

FIGURE 5–1. Calgary Family Assessment Model. *Source:* Adapted from Kaakinen, J.R., Padgett Coehlo, D. Gedaly-Duff, V., & Harmon Hanson, S.M. (2010). *Family Health Care Nursing: Theory, Practice and Research, 4th ed.* Philadelphia, PA: F.A. Davis Company; Wright, L.M. & Leahey, M. (2005). *Nurses and Families: A Guide to Family Assessment and Intervention, 4th ed.* Philadelphia, PA: F.A. Davis Company.

for "almost always," 1 point for "some of the time," and 0 point for "hardly ever." The following statements are given to the client for scoring:

- I am satisfied with the help that I receive from my family* when something is troubling me (adaptation).
- I am satisfied with the way my family* discusses items of common interest and shares problem solving with me (partnership).
- I find that my family* accepts my wishes to take on new activities or make changes in my lifestyle (growth).
- I am satisfied with the way my family* expresses affection and responds to my feelings, such as anger, sorrow, and love (affection).
- I am satisfied with the amount of time my family* and I spend together (resolve).

*Substitute spouse, partner, significant other, parent, or children if necessary.

A score of 0 to 3 is associated with a severely dysfunctional family; 4 to 6 with a moderately dysfunctional family; and 7 to 10 with a highly functional family. This tool is easy to use and focuses on perception of satisfaction (Sawin & Harrington, 1995).

- The *genogram* is a family tree picture that contains a family's relationships, structure, health, and other important data, such as ethnic heritage, over three generations (Sawin & Harrington, 1995). Standardization has not been accomplished yet. However, the genogram may be considered useful for helping a family understand genetic risks and make decisions regarding pursuit of genetic testing (Tavernier, 2009).
- The *ecomap* is a family picture of up-to-date family functioning and the relationship of the family members with each other and surrounding environments. It indicates whom the family is interacting with and the strength of these contacts. This tool can be of assistance in helping the family problem solve (Wright & Leahey, 2009).

Nutritional Assessment

Appropriate nutrition swith adequate exercise will ensure better health. Assess the client's 24-hour diet recall of food/drink intake for balance and adequacy of nutrients. For nonpregnant, nonlactating women, tables in *Dietary Guidelines for Americans, 2010* give daily intake recommendations (the amounts are listed both by age and by activity level) (USDA & USDHHS, 2010). See Table 5–3 for examples of servings and foods from the food groups appropriate for nonpregnant women 25 years of age and over who have average activity level.

Healthy, active women who are not dieting need between 1,800 and 2,000 calories daily. These calories should be distributed with carbohydrates comprising 45 to 65 percent, protein 10 to 35 percent, and fat no more than 20 to 35 percent. No more than 10 percent of fat should come from saturated fats such as animal fat or tropical oils such as coconut oil. Trans-fat-free foods are advised to decrease low-density lipoprotein cholesterol (LDL-C) levels also (USDA & USDHHS, 2010). Blood lipid levels should be maintained at healthful levels (see Chapter 23).

TABLE 5–3. Examples of Foods and Serving Sizes From Food Groups Appropriate for Nonpregnant Women 25 Years of Age and Above

Food Group	Foods and Serving Sizes	
Fruits/vegetables		
High in vitamin A	Cantaloupe	¼ medium
	Tomato	2 medium
	Papaya	½ medium
	Apricot	3 medium
	Carrot, spinach, greens, sweet potato, winter squash	½ cup cooked or 1 cup raw
	Chili peppers	2 tbsp. raw/cooked
High in vitamin C	Juices (orange, grapefruit)	6 oz (¾ cup)
	Cantaloupe, papaya	¼ medium
	Grapefruit	½ medium
	Orange, lemon, kiwi	1 medium
	Tomato	2 medium
	Broccoli, brussels sprouts, strawberries, cauliflower, green pepper, cabbage	½ cup cooked or 1 cup raw
Other	Raisin	¼ cup
	Grapes/watermelon	½ cup
	Apple, banana, peach	1 medium
	Asparagus, green beans, potato, peas, yellow squash, corn	½ cup cooked or 1 cup raw
	Lettuce	1 cup raw
Milk products	Milk, yogurt, custard	1 cup
	Cheese (cheddar)	1½ oz
	Cheese (American)	2 oz
	Frozen yogurt, ice milk, ice cream	1½ cups
	Cottage cheese	2 cups
Breads/cereals/ grains	Bread	1 slice
	Tortilla	1 small
	Cereal, cold	¾ cup
	Cereal, hot	½ cup
	Macaroni/noodles/spaghetti, cooked	½ cup
	Rice, cooked	½ cup
	Hot dog/hamburger bun	½
	Biscuit, roll, muffin	1 small
	Pancake	1 medium
	Crackers	8
Protein foods	Cooked dry beans/peas	½ cup
	Peanut butter	2 tbsp.
	Soyburger	2½ oz
	Nuts/seeds	⅓ cup
	Meat/poultry/fish (serving size 2–3 oz)	1 piece
	Eggs	1 substituted for 1 oz meat/poultry/fish
	Canned tuna/fish	¼ cup
Unsaturated fats	Avocado	⅛ medium
	Margarine, mayonnaise, vegetable oil	1 tsp
	Salad dressing—mayonnaise-based	2 tsp.
	oil-based	1 tsp.

Diet should contain less than 10 percent of calories from fat; less than 300 mg cholesterol; avoidance of trans fats if at all possible; limit caloric intake from solid fats and added sugars; choose whole grains over refined grains; sodium intake should be <2,300 mg prior to age 51 and <1,500 mg after age 51 or if have hypertension, diabetes, or chronic kidney disease or are African American. Make half your plate fruits and vegetables.

Source: USDA, 2011, ChooseMyPlate, www.choosemyplate.gov; USDA and USDHHS, 2010.

Sugar and salt should be used in moderation. The maximum amount of salt daily in foods and added in cooking or at the table should be no more than 2,300 mg until age 51, and from then on it decreases to no more than 1,500 mg. A variety of foods that provide the proper number of food group servings should be eaten daily. Moderate alcohol consumption is advised for a woman who uses alcohol. This equates to less than 1 to 1.5 oz of 80 proof distilled liquor daily or under 7 oz per week; 5 oz of wine or one 12-oz beer daily (USDA & USDHHS, 2010).

Eating adequate fruits and vegetables (optimum is nine servings a day) provides the body with antioxidants (five or more of vegetables and four or more of fruits). Six to eight servings of grains are needed daily. Fiber-rich foods—such as apples, carrots, whole grains, bran, and legumes—are important for reducing risks of bowel cancer, diabetes, obesity, and decreasing serum cholesterol (Tapper-Gardzina, Cotugna, & Vickery, 2002; USDA & USDHHS, 2010). Adequate fiber intake (25–30 g daily) is advised. Oat bran, kidney beans, and a pear are examples of 4 g of soluble fiber per serving. Raisins, prunes, and figs provide insoluble fiber that increases transit time and decreases constipation.

Megadoses of vitamins and minerals are not advised. To reduce the risk of neural tube defects in fetuses, women of childbearing age are advised to take folate 400 mcg daily or a daily women's multivitamin supplement (ACOG, 2003; Hilton, 2002). Fortification is added to most enriched breads, flours, and grain products. Women under age 60 in the Nurses' Health Study who had a daily consumption of 352 mg or more of vitamin C were 57 percent less likely to develop cataracts than if they had less than 140 mg per day (Vitamin C and Cataract Risk in Women, 2002). Calcium-rich foods daily are advised, or calcium supplements, if diet is not adequate or not tolerated. Women 24 to 50 years (premenopausal) need 1,000 mg of calcium daily. Women 50 to 64 years (postmenopausal) need 1,200 mg daily. Pregnant and nursing women need 1,000 to 1,300 mg daily. Foods high in calcium include dairy products, broccoli, kale, turnip greens, some legumes, canned fish, seeds, nuts, and fortified products. Not all calcium supplements are as bioavailable as others. Calcium citrate is one of the better sources providing more bioavailable elemental calcium. Best absorption of calcium supplements is in doses of 500 mg or less taken between meals. Calcium carbonate absorption is impaired without the presence of gastric acid, however, and so should be taken with foods promoting secretion of gastric acid. Calcium citrate is not dependent on gastric acid for absorption. Six to eight glasses of water in addition to other fluids are recommended daily for optimal body functioning.

Vegetarians can get all the nutrients needed from a diet comprised mainly of plant foods, such as vegetables, grains, legumes, fruits, seeds and nuts, small amounts (three servings per day) of low or nonfat dairy foods per day, and three to four egg yolks a week. Readers are referred to the *Dietary Guidelines for Americans, 2010* for complete coverage of vegetarian diets, including vegan and lacto-ovo vegetarian subtypes, and nutrients requiring special attention, such as folate, calcium, vitamins B_{12} and D, iron, and protein. Vegetarian diets are especially beneficial in providing fiber and antioxidants.

Correlate diet patterns with other history, physical examination, and diagnostic test findings; for example, high fat intake may be correlated with obesity and abnormal lipid levels. The BMI is the accepted measure for assessing weight most accurately. The normal BMI range is 18.5 to 24.9 (Gennaro, 2001). A BMI of 25.0 to 29.9 equates with being overweight; 30.0 to 34.9 with obesity; 35.0 and over with being extremely obese; and 40.0 and over with being morbidly obese. If a woman's BMI is under 18.5, she is considered underweight. As body fat increases and lean body mass decreases, the risk for cardiovascular disease increases. Waist/hip ratio is another helpful measure for assessing health status related to weight. This ratio is calculated by dividing the waist measurement in inches by the hip measurement in inches. The optimal ratio should be 0.80 or under for women (Gennaro, 2001; Gerchufsky, 1996). In general, the waist size is important alone as a measure (Gennaro, 2001). A waist size greater than 35 in in women is considered a high risk for health problems. If a woman has both a high BMI (25.0 or greater) and a waist size greater than 35 in, she is at high to extremely high risk (see Tables 5–4 and 5–5). Any ratio above this optimum indicates a tendency for central obesity, a significant risk factor for heart disease. (See Chapter 19 for nutritional recommendations during pregnancy.)

Stress/Risk Assessment

Stress with ineffective coping is associated with the development of illnesses, such as hypertension, coronary artery disease, headaches, back pain, and GI upsets; decreased immunity; mental health problems such as depression and substance abuse; and domestic violence, to name a few. Distress is stress overload; therefore, look at factors such as financial problems; changing situations or relationships with family or significant others; and employment, unemployment, or underemployment problems or concerns (such as lack of control or input into the job situation). In addition, assess personal information (age, hereditary factors such as family history of depression, lifestyle, living conditions, and habits), coping strategies, and social support.

Helpful assessment tools for evaluating stress or anxiety are the Holmes and Rahe Life-Change Index, which measures the degree of change from major life events in one's life to predict the chance of illness (Holmes & Rahe, 1967); the hassles and uplift scales (Kanner, Cyne, Schaefer, & Lazarus, 1980); and Speilberger's State-Trait Anxiety Inventory (Spielberger, 1983), which measures the amount of anxiety a person feels at the time of testing. The Perceived Stress Scale (PSS) is another measurement tool to consider for use (Cohen, Kamarck, & Mermelstein, 1983). The PSS has been translated into several different languages and used worldwide. It has been found to be valid across cultures (Leung, Lam, & Chan, 2010; Mimura & Griffiths, 2004; Örücü & Demir, 2009). The tool consists of 14 questions that are answered on a scale of 0 to 4 with 0 being never and 4 being very often. It provides for quantification of perceived stress for the individual (see Appendix B). Signs of excessive stress (mood swings, disposition changes, physical signs and symptoms) must be correlated

TABLE 5–4. Body Mass Index

BMI	19	20	21	22	23	24	25	26	27	28	29	30	31	32	33	34	35
Height (inches)								Body Weight (pounds)									
58	91	96	100	105	110	115	119	124	129	134	138	143	148	153	158	162	167
59	94	99	104	109	114	119	124	128	133	138	143	148	153	158	163	168	173
60	97	102	107	112	118	123	128	133	138	143	148	153	158	163	168	174	179
61	100	106	111	116	122	127	132	137	143	148	153	158	164	169	174	180	185
62	104	109	115	120	126	131	136	142	147	153	158	164	169	175	180	186	191
63	107	113	118	124	130	135	141	146	152	158	163	169	175	180	186	191	197
64	110	116	122	128	134	140	145	151	157	163	169	174	180	186	192	197	204
65	114	120	126	132	138	144	150	156	162	168	174	180	186	192	198	204	210
66	118	124	130	136	142	148	155	161	167	173	179	186	192	198	204	210	216
67	121	127	134	140	146	153	159	166	172	178	185	191	198	204	211	217	223
68	125	131	138	144	151	158	164	171	177	184	190	197	203	210	216	223	230
69	128	135	142	149	155	162	169	176	182	189	196	203	209	216	223	230	236
70	132	139	146	153	160	167	174	181	188	195	202	209	216	222	229	236	243
71	136	143	150	157	165	172	179	186	193	200	208	215	222	229	236	243	250
72	140	147	154	162	169	177	184	191	199	206	213	221	228	235	242	250	258
73	144	151	159	166	174	182	189	197	204	212	219	227	235	242	250	257	265
74	148	155	163	171	179	186	194	202	210	218	225	233	241	249	256	264	272
75	152	160	168	176	184	192	200	208	216	224	232	240	248	256	264	272	279
76	156	164	172	180	189	197	205	213	221	230	238	246	254	263	271	279	287

To use the table, find the appropriate height in the left-hand column labeled Height. Move across to a given weight. The number at the top of the column is the BMI at that height and weight. Pounds have been rounded off.

Source: http://www.nhlbi.nih.gov/guidelines/obesity/bmi_tbl.htm

with other assessment findings (sleep, appearance, nutrition, relaxation, recreation, self-concept, social supports, use of medications/substances, or unusual behaviors).

Offering ways for managing stress to decrease the potential adverse effects becomes important as a routine part of women's health care in our society today. Using relaxation techniques is one effective way to inhibit the stress effects on the body. Mindfulness-based stress reduction is one such technique with proven effectiveness (Grossman, Niemann, Schmidt, & Walach, 2004).

Fitness Assessment

Assess activities at work, home, or play for aerobic quality, stretching/flexibility movement, strength components, and sufficient intensity to meet therapeutic cardiovascular levels without compromising safety. Determine the duration of the exercise session, frequency per week, and the motivation of the client to exercise. To achieve a realistic assessment, evaluate fitness within a framework of lifestyle, diet, weight, stress, and substance use. *Healthy People 2010* objectives

TABLE 5–5. Classification of Overweight and Obesity by BMI, Waist Circumference, and Associated Disease Risks

			Disease Risk[a] Relative to Normal Weight and Waist Circumference[b]	
	BMI (kg/m^2)	Obesity Class	Men 102 cm (40 in) or Less Women 88 cm (35 in) or Less	Men >102 cm (40 in) Women >88 cm (35 in)
Underweight	<18.5		—	—
Normal	18.5–24.9		—	—
Overweight	25.0–29.9		Increased	High
Obesity	30.0–34.9	I	High	Very High
Extreme obesity	35.0–39.9	II	Very High	Very High
Morbid obesity	≥40.0	III	Extremely High	Extremely High

[a]Disease risk for type 2 diabetes, hypertension, and CVD.

[b]Increased waist circumference can also be a marker for increased risk even in persons of normal weight.

Source: http://www.nhlbi.nih.gov/health/public/heart/obesity/lose_wt/bmi/dis.htm

aimed to increase the proportion of U.S. adults who engage in moderate physical activity for a minimum of 30 minutes daily to 30 percent (USDHHS, 2000). This goal was not met. However, recommended activity levels were updated in 2008 with the release of *2008 Physical Activity Guidelines for Americans*. The current recommendations are for 150 minutes a week of moderate-intensity physical activity or 75 minutes of vigorous activity. It has been determined that benefit can still occur if physical activity is broken into increments of at least 10 minutes of continuous aerobic activity. Muscle-strengthening activity is also recommended in order to obtain optimal health benefit. Furthermore, activities ideally should be spread throughout the week (USDHHS, 2008).

Provide the woman with information on the benefits of exercise, such as the positive effects on blood pressure and cholesterol, the improved immunity effects, the decrease in body fat and improved glucose tolerance, the maintenance of bone density and increased lean muscle mass, and the improved self-concept. A study of the effect of a single walking bout on a treadmill on serum lipids and lipoproteins in groups of premenopausal and postmenopausal women found that in the immediate postexercise period, even a single exercise event lowered the total cholesterol and LDL-C in the premenopausal women and lowered the LDL-C in the postmenopausal group (Pronk, Crouse, O'Brien, & Rohack, 1995). Over 11 months, total cholesterol, LDL-C, and high-density lipoprotein cholesterol (HDL-C) all changed positively with the combined regimen. (Refer to Chapter 18 for current information related to hormone replacement therapy and risks.)

For any exercise regimen, teach the value of beginning slowly for short periods of time, then gradually building it, with emphasis on increasing tone, strengthening, reducing stress, enhancing flexibility and coordination, promoting relaxation, preventing injury, and improving self-concept. For a healthy woman who has no contraindications for exercise, advise building up to 20 to 40 minutes of aerobic activity, with a warm-up and cool down of 5 to 10 minutes.

The intensity of exercise is aimed at safely improving cardiovascular function. Referral to an exercise therapist may be necessary for full assessment and program management. A good guideline is that the client should be able to talk while in the safe target percentage range for the heartbeat, but probably not sing. Activities that the usually sedentary individual can integrate into her life to provide short opportunities for moderate exercise include brisk walking, stair climbing, yard work, play with children, and gardening (Pender, 1996). Suggestions include taking every opportunity to walk, such as changing channels by walking to the television, parking farther from the destination, and taking the stairs instead of the elevator (Brown, Bauman, & Owen, 2009). Researchers found that women in the Nurses' Health Study II who were underweight or overweight based on BMI had an increased risk of ovulatory infertility, that vigorous activity of 1 hour each week reduced the risk, and that each hour of increased activity decreased the risk by 7 percent (Rich-Edwards et al., 2002). Another study found that women at risk for type 2 diabetes who included exercise as part of lifestyle changes for management had a 58 percent reduction in incidence of diabetes as compared to a 38 percent reduction of incidence for those on medication alone (Knowler et al., 2009). Even light exercise has been shown to improve postprandial glucose levels (Healy et al., 2007). Culturally appropriate interventions are important in success of lifestyle modifications (Young & Stewart, 2006). Walking programs of exercise statistically decreased resting systolic and diastolic blood pressure in adults ≥18 years old (Kelley, Kelley, & Tran, 2001).

Occupational Assessment

Assess the type of work, amount, duration, physical labor involved, rest breaks, environmental risks, and stress overload. Problem areas include prolonged standing or sitting, heavy lifting, excessive noise, excessive heat or cold, exposure to toxins, exposure to chemicals or radiation, excessive hours on the job, boredom, low pay, low recognition, and little or no control over work. An area of increasing concern is environmental tobacco smoke exposure. An increased incidence of coronary heart disease and all-cause mortality was noted in the Nurses' Health Study related to exposure to particulate matter (Puett et al., 2008). A 39 percent excess risk of lung cancer was found with exposure in the workplace in a multicenter study that looked at lifetime lung cancer relative risk associated with environmental exposure (Fontham et al., 1994).

Be especially concerned about a pregnant woman (see Chapter 19); determine if she has been exposed to chemicals, anesthetic gases, radiation, or infections. Consider the influence of multiple variables, such as secondhand smoke, stress, nutrition, lack of sleep, and exposure to hazardous materials. Three questions have been found to be essential for a simple occupational history: (1) What is your job like? Describe it; (2) Have you ever worked with any health hazard, such as asbestos, chemicals, noise, or repetitive motion? and (3) Do you have any health problems that you believe may be related to your work or home? The CC should always be examined for a relationship with the person's work or home activities or exposures. A more in-depth occupational history as presented by Twinings (1995) is needed if the simple history indicates problems.

Sleep Assessment

Assess the sleep and rest patterns of the woman. Seven to 9 hours of sleep each night is recommended by the NSF (2011) for adults. Sleep is composed of five stages: Stage 1, non-rapid eye movement (NREM) sleep for a few minutes as the person moves in transitional sleep with dreamlike thoughts; Stage 2, NREM sleep that is deeper with fragmented thoughts for 15 to 20 minutes; Stages 3 and 4, deeper NREM sleep stages (delta sleep) lasting 40 to 70 minutes; REM Stage, follows the first four stages and is sleep (dream sleep) that can be considered as restorative, or as calisthenics, for the brain. The cycles of sleep stages are repeated through the sleep period with increasingly lengthening REM stages until the person awakens. Many activities can interrupt the normal circadian rhythms, disrupting sleep, and causing distress. Lack of sufficient REM sleep affects memory and learning.

If the woman complains of awakening to go to the bathroom, look further because sleep apnea may be the cause (Lowenstein et al., 2008). Sleep apnea affects 4 percent of women moderately and 2 percent of women severely enough to be categorized as OSA and cause physiologic change. Those with OSA are at increased risk for cardiovascular disease and diabetes (Al Lawati, Patel, & Ayas, 2009). Loud snoring, especially with gasping/choking episodes, indicates apnea. Because obstructive problems decrease oxygen to the brain, the body nearly awakes as a warning. If this pattern is repeated multiple times a night, serious repercussions can occur. The woman needs to be seen by a sleep specialist. A history of accidents on the job, sleeping on the job, and/or personality-cognitive changes should raise suspicions. A referral is also needed for women with narcolepsy (periods of sudden sleeping), which can lead to accidents.

Ask the following questions: Does it take you at least an hour to fall asleep? Do you wake up too early? Does your sleep partner complain that you are restless? Do you worry about getting enough sleep most nights? If you wake up in the night, can you go back to sleep? Do you use aids (pills or alcohol) to get to sleep? Do you feel exhausted from lack of sleep? Do you sleep in on days off or take daytime naps to make up for lack of sleep? Do you need caffeine to stay alert during the day? How much? Does your mind continue to work excessively during times when your body is resting? Any "yes" responses can indicate a problem.

PHYSICAL EXAMINATION

OVERVIEW

Accurate inspection, palpation, percussion, and auscultation are critical, as is the precise use of appropriate equipment. Understanding the findings is also essential.

- In preparation for the exam, explain all procedures to the client. Ensure privacy, draping, and comfort. Have all necessary equipment available and clean and use good lighting. Ask the client to void before the exam. Clean hands and the use of universal precautions are essential.
- During the exam, give anticipatory advice and information; for example, teach abdominal breathing to help the client relax. Use the exam as an opportunity to teach. Be gentle, systematic, and sensitive. Avoid facial expressions or utterances indicating disgust. Provide tissues for the client after the pelvic exam. When finished, wash hands and allow the client to dress before reviewing findings.
- An abbreviated physical examination of a well woman, as done in some family planning clinics or private offices, includes assessment of blood pressure, height and weight, lymph nodes (head/neck, axillae, groin), thyroid, heart, lungs, breasts, abdomen, extremities, and genitourinary tracts and rectum.
- A selective exam related to those systems indicated by the CC is required for episodic visits for problems such as vaginal itching or breast pain. Remember that more than one system may be involved.
- Refer to any current and complete physical assessment text for information on the correct considerations by system for the physical examination. The following information provides special hints for some select systems.

GENERAL SURVEY

Obtain an overall first impression of the client. Obvious and more subtle clues are obtained primarily by sensory observation and listening with a sixth sense. Be sure to measure height and weight with clothes on and shoes off. Consider age and gender effects: Women should have height measured yearly after menopause. Note body type and posture, whether the woman is obese, slender, average, or stocky; and her fat distribution and any deformities.

Skin, Hair, Nails. Teach the client to evaluate moles for changes. Check piercings and tattoos for infection, keloid scarring. Check for cosmetic surgery because clients often fail to provide this in the history. Observe for hair dye, permanent wave, cosmetic damage. Check nails for infection and damage from artificial nail applications.

Thyroid. Be vigilant in checking for nodules and enlargement and associated signs of disease.

Breasts, Areolae, Nipples, and Axillae. Note sexual maturity, size, symmetry, dimpling, retractions, color, edema, thickening, vascular pattern, lesions/rashes/scaling, discharge, masses/nodules, rash, unusual pigmentation, and abnormal lymph nodes. Discuss breast self-exam. The reproductive years (Tanner Stage V) involve potential cyclic changes, for example, changes in the size, nodularity, and tenderness of the breasts, related to hormonal changes in the menstrual cycle. These changes, along with an increase in total breast volume, occur maximally 3 to 4 days before the onset of menses and minimally in days 4 through 7 of the menstrual cycle. Structural changes also occur, unrelated to the cycle. As women age, breast density decreases. Especially after menopause fat become the predominant tissue in the breast (Fritz & Speroff, 2011).

Abdomen. Observe color of skin, lesions, contour, masses, distention, symmetry, vascularity, peristalsis, pulsations, and the umbilicus. Using percussion and/or palpation, assess pulsations, bowel sounds, bruits, ascites, organomegaly, and masses. Note inguinal node enlargement, tenderness/pain, rebound, and rigidity. Perform iliopsoas and obturator maneuvers with acute abdomen.

PELVIC EXAMINATION

Use gloves on both hands; maintain strict medical aseptic technique to prevent spread of organisms. Some clinicians recommend double gloves or special high-risk gloves if the HIV AIDS/hepatitis B status is known to be positive. For those with a history of female genital cutting, the following internal exam techniques may be difficult or impossible to perform. The World Health Organization (WHO) has a good description of various types of female genital cutting available at the following web address: www.who.int/reproductivehealth/topics/fgm/overview/en/index.html. The WHO (2010) has issued statements advocating for abandonment of this practice with the latest statement, along with a World Health Assembly resolution (WHA61.16), being made in 2008.

- *Inspect and palpate* femoral nodes, external genitalia, and Bartholin's, urethra, and Skene's (BUS) glands. This includes, in addition to the Bartholin's and urethra glands, the mons pubis, labia minora and majora, clitoris, urethral meatus, and vaginal opening. Assess sexual maturity and check pubic hair for pattern/parasite. Pubic hair may spread onto the inner aspect of the upper thighs. The female hair pattern is triangular, while the male is diamond-shaped, a possible clue that testosterone is too abundant if seen in the female. The labia majora increase in prominence; the labia minora and clitoris enlarge. Note any swelling, enlargement, inflammation, lesions (e.g., excoriations, leukoplakia, folliculitis from shaving), pigmentation, discharge, relaxation/celes, and tenderness. Teach self-examination of the vulva (Seidel et al., 2011). The 2 minutes it takes to provide the woman with a tour of her genital area may save her life. The self-exam should be done monthly.
- *The vagina and cervix* are examined with a warmed speculum; lubricate with water or may use a small amount of water-based lubricant on the outer surface of the posterior blade. Inspect the cervix and os: size, shape, color, lesions, discharge/bleeding, and position. Obtain the Pap smear and prepare cultures and wet prep specimens (see Chapter 3). Inspect the vagina for color, rugae, lesions (erosions, leukoplakia, masses, ulcerations), inflammation, and discharge. With a cotton-tipped applicator, gently remove any discharge that prevents adequate visualization of surfaces.
- *Assess the uterus and adnexa.* Lubricate index and middle gloved fingers; insert into vagina with other hand on abdomen above pubis. Premenopausal adult women should have increased elasticity of vaginal tissue along with attainment of a mature vagina and

ovarian size. Note vaginal nodules, masses, or tenderness; note cervical size, consistency, nodules or masses, tenderness, pain with movement of the cervix, and closure of the os. Assess the position, size, shape, consistency, mobility, and tenderness of the uterus, adnexal organs, and any masses.

- *The rectovaginal area* is evaluated after gloves are changed and fingers lubricated again. Inspect the external anal area and palpate the sphincter, rectal walls, septum, posterior surface of the uterus, and palpable adnexal areas for tumors and tenderness. Retroverted or retroflexed uteri are more accessible by rectal exam. Obese women may be evaluated more fully by the rectovaginal route. The reproductive organs of women who are virgins may be more easily assessed via the rectal exam.

Neurological/Psychological

- General mental status is observed. Assessment of reflexes may be appropriate depending on the patient history. In-depth neurological exam generally requires referral when working in a gynecological setting.
- Case-finding instruments are valuable adjuncts in gathering data to diagnose major depression in primary care settings (Mulrow et al., 1995). Several instruments such as the *Beck Depression Inventory* and the *Zung Self-Assessment Depression Scale* can be administered in 2 to 5 minutes, are easy in relation to literacy level, and are depression specific. However, the PHQ-2 is frequently used as an initial screen in many primary care settings, proceeding to the PHQ-9 as indicated (see Appendix B). About 20 percent of depressed clients can be identified with use of a case-finding instrument, a decided improvement over the 50 percent missed if usual history and physical methods are used without a full diagnostic interview. Depression instruments should not be used to the exclusion of other instruments for case-finding additional disorders, however, such as anxiety or drug/alcohol abuse. Some instruments are multidimensional, such as the *Primary Care Evaluation of Mental Disorders* and the *Symptom Driven Diagnostic System* and should be considered in gathering data. Additionally, specific examinations and tests are needed to rule out physical pathology of somatic complaints, such as chest pain in the woman with panic disorder or headache associated with depression. The reader is referred to Chapter 25, Psychosocial Health Concerns for Women, for more in-depth assessment information.

PLAN

Guidelines for Routine Examinations and Screening Tests

See Table 5–6 for guidelines for routine health maintenance exams for women ages 19 to 39, 40 to 49, and 50 to 65 adapted from ACOG Committee Opinion (2011) and U.S. Preventive Services Task Force (USPSTF, 2010). See Chapter 4 for exam and screening of adolescents and Chapter 6 for exam and screening of older women.

Guidelines for General Education and Anticipatory Guidance

Education and guidance should be targeted for certain age groups. Suggestions for targeting health information/guidance to all age groups include discussion of the following: sun exposure, smoking, alcohol use, prescription/over-the-counter drug and supplement use, nutrition, driving accidents/seat belt use, family/marital/other relationships, school and work safety/stressors, fitness, stress, sleep, breast cancer, dental care, sexuality, sexually transmitted infections/HIV/AIDS, immunizations, and violence/abuse.

After menarche until death, self-examination of the breasts, vulva, and skin is appropriate for all women. Signs and symptoms of cancer should be taught. Despite recent controversy regarding the value of mammography to prolong life, it offers the best breast screening test available at this date. Breast self-examination is no longer advised monthly; however, the American Cancer Society states that women should be encouraged to become familiar with how their breasts feel normally in order to be able to detect a change and also advises that women check their breasts occasionally while showering. The USPSTF (2010) recommends daily aspirin for women starting at age 55 for prevention of stroke in those whose risk of GI hemorrhage is less than their risk for stroke. Readers are encouraged to access the USPSTF website and ACOG for their latest recommendations.

TABLE 5–6. Guidelines for Selected Screening Examinations and Tests for Healthy Nonpregnant Adult Women

Exam/Test	19–39 Years	40–49 Years	50–65 Years
Physical examination[a]	q1y	q1y	q1y
Height/weight/BMI	q1y	q1y	q1y
Breast clinical examination	q1y ≥ age 20	q1y	q1y
Pelvic[c]	q1y[c]	q1y	q1y
Pap[d]	See Pap guidelines	See Pap guidelines	See Pap guidelines
Rectal exam	q1y if at risk	q1y	q1y
Mammography	[i]	q1–2y[i]	q1–2y
Hematocrit/hemoglobin	[e]	q10y or[e]	
Blood glucose (fasting)	[e]	q3y ≥ age 45 or q1y[e]	q3y or q1y[e]
Cholesterol, lipids (fasting)	[e]	q5y ≥ age 45	q5y or q1y[e]
Hepatitis C viral testing	[e]	[e]	[e]
STI testing[c]	q1y ≤ 25[c]	[c]	[c]
Stool for occult blood	[e]	q1y	q1y
Sigmoidoscopy/colonoscopy	[e]	[e]	q10y
Blood pressure	q1–2y[g]	q1–2y[g]	q1–2y[g]
Urinalysis	[e]	[e]	[e]
Skin exam	q1y	q1y	q1y
Dental exam	q1y	q1y	q1y
Eye exam	Baseline & q1–2y or[e]	1–2y or[e]	q1y
Glaucoma test		Start age 50 q1y	q1y
Hearing exam[h]	Baseline @ 40	Repeat @ 50[g]	
Endometrial sampling	[e]	[e]	[e]
Tuberculosis	[e]	[e]	[e]
Chest x-ray or CT lung scan	[e]	[e]	[e]
Thyroid testing (TSH)	[e]	[e]	q5y ≥ age 50
Bone density screening		[e]	[e] or q2y ≥ age 65

[a]After three consecutive normal physical examinations, clinical discretion advised for need for annual exam.

[b]Ultrasound and/or mammography indicated if clinical or risk factors present. Women on HRT with denser breasts may need to avoid HRT for a period prior to mammography.

[c]STD/HIV screen advised for any client < 25 and/or at risk. Otherwise as indicated. Also recommend HIV for preconceptual visit.

[d]See Pap guidelines in Chapter 3. Women with hysterectomies for noncancer reasons do not need annual Pap smears, unless they were exposed to DES in utero.

[e]Indicated if risk factors present. Recommend Hgb if excessive menstrual flow or Caribbean, Latin American, Asian, Mediterranean, or African ancestry. Recommend fasting glucose if BMI ≥ 25 or if BP > 135/80. Recommend fasting lipid panel if BMI ≥ 30.

[f]After age 50, should have two consecutive annual negative evaluations before extending years between tests.

[g]Every year if BP is 130–139/85–89 mm HG; if higher, repeat within 2 months and evaluate for hypertension.

[h]Audiogram may be needed as the woman ages.

[i]Researchers at the University of Toronto reported no increased survival with early screening (Miller, To, Baines, & Wall, 2002).

Sources: ACOG, 2011; Board of Trustees, 2002; Mammography Screening Revisited, 2002; Slanetz, 2002; USPSTF, 2010.

REFERENCES

Acierno, R., Resnick, H., Kilpatrick, D.G., Saunders, B., & Best, C.L. (1999). Risk factors for rape, physical assault, and post-traumatic stress disorder in women. *Journal of Anxiety Disorders, 13*(6), 541–563.

ACOG. (2003, reaffirmed 2011). Neural tube defects (Practice Bulletin No. 44). *Obstetrics & Gynecology, 102,* 203–213.

ACOG Committee Opinion. (2011). Primary and preventive care: Periodic assessments (No. 483). *Obstetrics & Gynecology, 117*(4), 1008–1015.

Akinsanya-Beysolow, I., & Wolfe, C. (2009). Update: Vaccines for women, adolescence through adulthood. *Journal of Women's Health, 18*(8), 1101–1108.

Al Lawati, N.N.A., Patel, S.R., & Ayas, N.T. (2009). Epidemiology, risk factors, and consequences of obstructive sleep apnea and short sleep duration. *Progress in Cardiovascular Diseases, 51*(4), 285–293.

American Dietetic Association. (2010). Whole-grain consumption is associated with diet quality and nutrient intake in adults: The national health and nutrition examination survey 1999–2004. *Journal of the American Dietetic Association, 110*(10), 1461–1463.

American Psychiatric Association. (2000). *Diagnostic and statistical manual of mental disorders* (4th ed., text revision). Washington, DC: Author.

Anderson, C. (2002). Battered and pregnant: A nursing challenge. *AWHONN Lifelines, 6*(2), 95–99.

Aral, S. (2001). Sexually transmitted diseases: Magnitude, determinants and consequences. *International Journal of STD AIDS, 12*(4), 211–215.

Arkangel, C. (2005). *Cocaine abuse*. Retrieved August 17, 2011, from http://www.emedicinehealth.com/cacaine-abuse/article-em.htm

Attia, E., & Walsh, T. (2007). Anorexia nervosa. *American Journal of Psychiatry, 164*(12), 1805–1810.

Auslander, G.K. (1988). Social networks and the functional health status of the poor: A secondary analysis of data from the national survey of personal health practices and consequences. *Journal of Community Health, 13,* 197–209.

Barnes, P.M., Adams, P.F., & Powell-Griner, E. (2010). Health characteristics of the American Indian or Alaska Native adult population: United States, 2004–2008. *National Health Statistics Reports, 20*. Hyattsville, MD: National Center for Health Statistics. Retrieved February 13, 2011, from http://www.cdc.gov/nchs/products/nhsr.htm

Bauer, G., & Welles, S. (2001). Beyond assumptions of negligible risk: Sexually transmitted diseases and women who have sex with women. *American Journal of Public Health, 91*(8), 1282–1286.

Becker, K., & Walton-Moss, B. (2001). Detecting and addressing alcohol abuse in women. *Nurse Practitioner, 26*(10), 13–16, 19–23.

Bennett, S., Perkins, S., Lane, K., Deer, M., Brater, D., & Murray, M. (2001). Social support and health-related quality of life in chronic heart failure patients. *Quality of Life Research, 10*(8), 671–682.

Berkman, N.D., Sheridan, S.L., Donahue, K.E., Halpern, D.J., & Crotty, K. (2011). Low health literacy and health outcomes: An updated systematic review. *Annals of Internal Medicine, 155,* 97–107.

Bernstein, A.S., Makuc, D.M., & Bilheimer, L.T. (2010). *Chartbook: Health United States, 2010*. Hyattsville, MD: National Center for Health Statistics.

Board of Trustees of the North American Menopause Society. (2002). Management of postmenopausal osteoporosis: Position statement of the North American Menopause Society. *Menopause, 9*(2), 84–101.

Borrelli, B., Hogan, J.W., Bock, B., Pinto, B., Roberts, M., & Marcus, B. (2002). Predictors of quitting and dropout among women in a clinic-based smoking cessation program. *Psychology of Addict Behavior, 16*(1), 22–27.

Brown, S.J., McDonald, E.A., & Krastev, A.H. (2008). Fear of an intimate partner and women's health in early pregnancy: Findings from the maternal health study. *Birth, 35*(4), 293–302.

Brown, W.J., Bauman, A.E., & Owen, N. (2009). Stand up, sit down, keep moving: Turning in circles in physical activity research? *British Journal of Sports Medicine, 43,* 86–88.

Brucker, D. (2007). Estimating the prevalence of substance use, abuse, and dependence among social security disability benefit recipients. *Journal of Disability Policy Studies, 18*(3), 148–159.

Burdorf, A., Brand, R., Jaddoe, V.W., Hofman, A., Mackenbach, J.P., & Steegers, E.A.P. (2011). The effects of work-related maternal risk factors on time to pregnancy, preterm birth and birth weight: The Generation R Study. *Occupational and Environmental Medicine, 68,* 197–204.

Bureau of Justice Statistics. (2009). *Rape and assault*. Retrieved August 17, 2011, from http://bjs.ofp.usdoj.gov/index.cfm?ty=tp&tid=317

Byers, T., Nestle, M., McTiernan, A., Doyle, C., Currie-Williams, A., Gansler, T., et al. (2002). American Cancer Society guidelines on nutrition and physical activity for cancer prevention: Reducing the risk of cancer with healthy food choices and physical activity. *CA: A Cancer Journal for Clinicians, 52*(20), 92–119.

Cacioppo, J.T., Hughes, M.E., Waite, L.J., Hawkley, L.C., & Thisted, R.A. (2006). Loneliness as a specific risk factor for depressive symptoms: Cross-sectional and longitudinal analyses. *Psychology and Aging, 21*(1), 140–151.

Carbone-López, K., Kruttschnitt, C., & MacMillan, R. (2006). Patterns of intimate partner violence and their associations with physical health, psychological distress, and substance use. *Public Health Reports, 121,* 382–392.

Centers for Disease Control and Prevention (CDC). (2011). *Vaccines*. Retrieved from http://www.cdc.gov/vaccines

Certain, H.E., Mueller, M. Jagodzinski, T. & Fleming M. (2008). Domestic abuse during the previous year in a sample of postpartum women. *Journal of Obstetric, Gynecologic & Neonatal Nursing, 37*(1), 35–41.

Chao, J., Zyzanski, S., & Flocke, S. (1998). Choosing a family level indicator of family function. *Families, Systems & Health, 16*(4), 367–374.

Cloutier, S., Martin, S.L., & Poole, C. (2002). Sexual assault among North Carolina women: Prevalence and health risk factors. *Journal of Epidemiology and Community Health, 56*(4), 242–243.

Cohen, S., Kamarck, T., & Mermelstein, R. (1983). A global measure of perceived stress. *Journal of Health and Social Behavior, 24,* 385–396.

Cone, R.A., Hoen, T., Wong, X., Abusuwwa, R., Anderson, D.J., & Moench, T.R. (2006). Vaginal microbicides: Detecting toxicities in vivo that paradoxically increase pathogen transmission. *BMC Infectious Diseases, 6,* 90. doi:10.1186/1471-2334-6.90

Croteau, A., Marcoux, A., & Brisson, C. (2007). Work activity in pregnancy, preventive measures, and the risk of preterm delivery. *American Journal of Epidemiology, 166,* 951–965.

Dedert, E.A., Studts, J.L., Weissbecker, I., Salmon, P.G., Banis, P.L., & Sephton, S.E. (2004). Religiosity may help preserve the cortisol rhythm in women with stress-related illness. *International Journal of Psychiatry in Medicine, 34*(1), 61–77.

Enoch, M., & Goldman, D. (2002). Problem drinking and alcoholism: Diagnosis and treatment. *American Family Physician, 65*(3), 449–450.

Fedewa, S.A., Lerro, C., Chase, D., & Ward, E.M. (2011). Insurance status and racial differences in uterine cancer survival: A study of patients in the National Cancer Database. *Gynecologic Oncology, 122*(1), 63–68.

Figà-Talamanca, I. (2006). Occupational risk factors and reproductive health of women. *Occupational Medicine, 56*, 521–531.

Fontham, E., Correa, P., Reynolds, P., Wu-Williams, A., Buffler, P.A., Greenberg, R.S., et al. (1994). Environmental tobacco smoke and lung cancer in nonsmoking women. *Journal of the American Medical Association, 27*(22), 1752–1759.

Fritz, M.A., & Speroff, L. (2011). *Clinical gynecologic endocrinology and infertility* (8th ed.). Philadelphia: Wolter Kluwer/Lippincott Williams & Wilkins.

Gardner, W., Nutting, P.A., Kelleher, K.J., Werner, J.J., Farley, T., Stewart, L., et al. (2001). Does the family APGAR effectively measure family functioning? *Journal of Family Practice, 50*(1), 19–25.

Gaynes, B.N., Gavin, N., Meltzer-Brody, S., Lohr, K.N., Swinson, T., Gartlehner, G., et al. (2005). *Perinatal depression: Prevalence, screening accuracy, and screening outcome* (Evidence Report/Technology Assessment No. 119 and AHRQ Publication No. 05-E006-2). Rockville, MD: Agency for Healthcare Research and Quality. (Prepared by the RTI-University of North Carolina Evidence-based Practice Center, under Contract No. 290-02-0016)

Gennaro, S. (2001). Weighty matters. In *Every woman: The essential guide for healthy living*. Washington, DC: AWHONN.

Gerchufsky, M. (1996). How much is too much? Weight questions. *Advance for Nurse Practitioners, 4*(1), 17–19, 60.

Geronimus, A. (2001). Understanding and eliminating racial inequalities in women's health in the United States: The role of the weathering conceptual framework. *Journal of the American Medical Women's Association, 56*(4), 133–136, 149–150.

Geronimus, A., Hicken, M., Keene, D., & Bound, J. (2006). "Weathering" and age patterns of allostatic load scores among black and whites in the United States. *American Journal of Public Health, 96*(5), 826–833.

Grossman, P., Niemann, L., Schmidt, S., & Walach, H. (2004). Mindfulness-based stress reduction and health benefits: A meta-analysis. *Journal of Psychosomatic Research, 57,* 35–43.

Hawkley, L.C., Thisted, R.A., Masi, C.M., & Cacioppo, J.T. (2010). Loneliness predicts increased blood pressure: 5-year cross-lagged analyses in middle-aged and older adults. *Psychology and Aging, 25*(1), 132–141.

HealthCare.gov. (2011). *Affordable care act rules on expanding access to preventive services for women.* Retrieved August 21, 2011, from http://www.healthcare.gov/news/factsheets/womensprevention08012011a.html

Healthy people 2020: National health promotion and disease prevention objectives. (2010). Washington, DC: U.S. Public Health Service.

Healy, G.N., Dunstan, D.W., Salmon, J., Cerin, E., Shaw, J.E., Zimmet, P.Z., et al. (2007). Objectively measured light-intensity physical activity is independently associated with 2-h plasma glucose. *Diabetes Care, 30,* 1384–1389.

Hilton, J. (2002). Folic acid intake of young women. *Journal of Obstetric, Gynecologic, and Neonatal Nursing, 31*(2), 172–177.

Holmes, T., & Rahe, R. (1967). The social readjustment rating scale. *Journal of Psychosomatic Research, 11,* 213.

Holt, C., Oster, R.A., Clay, K.S., Urmie, J., & Fouad, M. (2011). Religiosity and physical and emotional functioning among African American and White colorectal and lung cancer patients. *Journal of Psychosocial Oncology, 29*(4), 372–393.

Hoskins, A.B. (2005). Occupational injuries, illnesses, and fatalities among women. *Monthly Labor Review, 128*(10), 31–37.

Hourani, L., & Hilton, S. (2000). Occupational and environmental exposure correlates of adverse live-birth outcomes among 1032 U.S. Navy women. *Journal of Occupational Medicine, 42*(12), 1156–1165.

Kanner, A., Cyne, J., Schaefer, C., & Lazarus, R. (1980). Comparison of two modes of stress management: Daily hassles and uplifts versus major life events. *Journal of Behavioral Medicine, 4*(1), 1–35.

Kapsimalis, F., & Kryger, M. (2009). Sleep breathing disorders in the U.S. female population. *Journal of Women's Health, 18*(8), 1211–1219.

Kelley, G., Kelley, K., & Tran, Z. (2001). Walking and resting blood pressure in adults: A meta-analysis. *Preventive Medicine, 33*(2, Pt. 1), 120–127.

Kelly, P.J., Blacksin, B., & Mason, E. (2001). Factors affecting substance abuse treatment completion for women. *Issues in Mental Health Nursing, 22*(3), 287–304.

Kennedy, E., Bowman, S., Spence, J., Freedman, M., & King, J. (2001). Popular diets: Correlation to health, nutrition, and obesity. *Journal of the American Dietetic Association, 101*(4), 411–420.

Kessler, R.C., Berglund, P., Demler, O., Jin, R., Merikangas, K.R., & Walters, E.E. (2005). Lifetime prevalence and age-of-onset distributions of DSM-IV disorder in the National Comorbidity Survey Replication. *Archives of General Psychiatry, 62*(6), 593–602.

KIDS COUNT. (2011). *America's children, America's challenge: Promoting opportunity for the next generation.* Baltimore, MD: Annie E. Casey Foundation (KINETIK). Retrieved August 25, 2011, from http://datacenter.kidscount.org/DataBook/2011/Default.aspx

Knowler, W.C., Fowler, S.E., Hamman, R.F., Christophi, C.A., Hoffman, H.J., Brenneman, A.T., et al. (2009). 10-year follow-up of diabetes incidence and weight loss in the Diabetes Prevention Program Outcomes Study. *Lancet, 374*(9702), 1677–1686.

Kreider, R.B., Serra, M., Beavers, K.M., & Jonnalagadda, S.S. (2011). A structured diet and exercise program promotes favorable changes in weight loss, body composition, and weight maintenance. *Journal of the American Dietetic Association, 110*(10), 1461–1463.

Lazarus, R.S. (1981, July). Little hassles can be hazardous to health. *Psychology Today*, pp. 59–62.

Lee, K.A., Baker, F.C., Newton, K.M., & Ancoli-Israel, S. (2007). The influence of reproductive status and age on women's sleep. (National sleep foundation: Proceedings of the women and sleep workshop, Washington, DC, March 5–7, 2007). *Journal of Women's Health, 17*(7), 1209–1214.

Leung, D.Y.P., Lam, T., & Chan, S.S.C. (2010). Three versions of perceived stress scale: Validation in a sample of Chinese cardiac patients who smoke. *BMC Public Health, 10,* 513.

Li, C., Ford, E.S., Zhao, G., Croft, J.B., Balluz, L.S., & Mokdad, A.H. (2010). Prevalence of self-reported clinically diagnosed sleep apnea according to obesity status in men and women: National Health and Nutrition Examination Survey, 2005–2006. *Preventive Medicine, 51,* 18–23.

Li, L., & Ford, J. (1998). Illicit drug use by women with disabilities. *American Journal of Drug and Alcohol Abuse, 24*(3), 405–418.

Lowenstein, L., Kenton, K., Brubaker, L., Pillar, G., Undevia, N., Mueller, E.R., et al. (2008). The relationship between obstructive sleep apnea, nocturia, and daytime overactive bladder syndrome. *American Journal of Obstetrics & Gynecology, 198*(5), 598.e1–598.e5.

Ludman, E., Curry, S., Grothaus, L., Graham, E., Stout, J., & Lozano, P. (2002). Depressive symptoms, stress, and weight concerns among African American and European American low-income female smokers. *Psychology of Addiction Behavior, 16*(1), 68–71.

Mammography screening revisited. (2002). *Clinician Reviews, 12*(3), 41.

Mann, J.R., McKeown, R.E., Bacon, J., Vesselinov, R., & Bush, F. (2008). Religiosity, spirituality and antenatal anxiety in Southern U.S. women. *Archives of Women's Mental Health, 11*(1), 19–26.

Marcy, A.M. (2007). Recommendations and promising developments for vaccines in adolescents and adults. *Family Practice Recertification, 29*(4), 38–43.

Marrazzo, J.M., Coffey, P., & Bingham, A. (2005). Sexual practices, risk perception and knowledge of sexually transmitted disease risk among lesbian and bisexual women. *Perspectives on Sexual & Reproductive Health, 37*(1), 6–12.

McColgan, M.D., Dempsey, A., Davis, M., & Giardino, A.P. (2010). Overview of the problem. In A.P. Giardino & E.R. Giardino (Eds.), *Intimate partner violence: A resource for professional working with children and families* (pp. 1–29). St. Louis, MO: STM Learning.

McCutcheon, A.A., Heath, A.C., Edenberg, H.J., Grucza, R.A., Hesselbrock, V.M., Kramer, J.R., et al. (2009). Alcohol criteria endorsement and psychiatric and drug use disorders among DUI offenders: Greater severity among women and multiple offenders. *Addictives Behaviors, 34,* 432–439.

Miller, A., To, T., Baines, C., & Wall, J. (2002). Mammograms in women age 40 to 49: Results of the Canadian Breast Cancer Screening Study. *Annals of Internal Medicine, 137,* 305–312.

Mimura, C., & Griffiths, P. (2004). A Japanese version of the perceived stress scale: Translation and preliminary test. *International Journal of Nursing Studies, 41,* 379–385.

Mulrow, C., Williams, J., Jr., Gerety, M., Ramirez, G., Montiel, O.M., & Kerber, C. (1995). Case-finding instruments for depression in primary care settings. *Annals of Internal Medicine, 122,* 913–921.

Narang, P., Paladugu, A., Manda, S.R., Smock, W., Goshay, C., & Lippmann, S. (2010). Do guns provide safety? At what cost? *Southern Medical Journal, 103*(3), 151–153.

National Cancer Institute. (2004). *Cancer progress report 2003.* Washington, DC: U.S. Department of Health and Human Services, Public Health Service, National Institutes of Health.

National Institute on Alcohol Abuse and Alcoholism (NIAAA). (2008). *Alcohol: A women's health issue.* Retrieved August 16, 2011, from http://www.niaaa.nih.gov/Publications/Pamphlets BrochuresPosters/English/Documents/WomensBrochure

National Institute of Mental Health (NIMH). (2009). *Women and depression* (NIH Publication No 09 4779). Washington, DC: U.S. Department of Health and Human Services, National Institutes of Health.

National Sleep Foundation (NSF). (2011). *Women and sleep.* Retrieved August 31, 2011, from http://www.sleepfoundation.org/article/sleep-topics/women-and-sleep

Örücü, M., & Demir, A. (2009). Psychometric evaluation of perceived stress scale for Turkish university students. *Stress and Health, 25,* 103–109.

Pender, N.J. (1996). *Health promotion in nursing practice* (3rd ed.). Stamford, CT: Appleton & Lange.

Pope, S., Sowers, M., Welch, G., & Albrecht, G. (2001). Functional limitations in women at midlife: The role of health conditions, behavioral and environmental factors. *Women's Health Issues, 11*(6), 494–502.

Pronk, N., Crouse, S., O'Brien, B., & Rohack, J. (1995). Acute effects of walking on serum lipids and lipoproteins in women. *Journal of Sports Medicine and Physical Fitness, 35*(1), 50–57.

Puett, R.C., Schwarts, J., Hart, J.E., Yanosky, J.D., Speizer, F.E., Suh, H., et al. (2008). Chronic particulate exposure, mortality, and coronary heart disease in the Nurses' Health Study. *American Journal of Epidemiology, 168*(10), 1161–1168.

Raphan, G., Cohen, S., & Boyer, A. (2001). The female condom, a tool for empowering sexually active urban adolescent women. *Journal of Urban Health, 78*(4), 605–613.

Rich-Edwards, J., Spiegelman, D., Garland, M., Hertzmark, E., Hunter, D., Colditz, G., et al. (2002). Physical activity, body mass index, and ovulatory disorder infertility. *Epidemiology, 13*(2), 184–190.

Riehman, K.S., Wechsberg, W.M., Francis, S.A., Moore, M., & Morgan-Lopez, A. (2006). Discordance in monogamy beliefts, sexual concurrency, and condome use among your adult-substance-involved couples: implication for risk of sexually transmitted infections. *Sexually Transmitted Disease, 33*(11), 677–682.

Rosekind, M., & Gregory, K.B. (2010). Insomnia risks and costs: Health, safety, and quality of life. *American Journal of Managed Care, 16*(8), 617–626.

Sabanayagam, C., & Shankar, A. (2010). Sleep duration and cardiovascular disease: Results for the National Health Interview Survey. *Sleep, 33*(8), 1037–1042.

Sabatino, S.A., Coates, R.J., Uhler, R.J., Breen, N., Tangka, F., & Shaw, K.M. (2008). Disparities in mammography use among US women aged 40-60 years, by race, ethnicity, income, and health insurance status, 1993–2005. *Medical Care, 46*(7), 692–700.

Sanchez, D.T., & Kwang, T. (2007). When the relationship becomes her: Revisiting women's body concerns from a relationship contingency perspective. *Psychology of Women Quarterly, 31,* 301–414.

Sawin, K., & Harrington, M. (1995). *Measures of family functioning for research and practice.* New York: Springer Publishing.

Schulz, A., Israel, D., Zenk, S.N., Parker, E., Lichtenstein, R., Shellman-Weir, S., et al. (2006). Psychosocial stress and social support as mediators of relationships between income, length of residence and depressive symptoms among African American Women on Detroit's eastside. *Social Science & Medicine, 62,* 510–522.

Seidel, H., Ball, J., Dains, J., & Benedict, G. (2011). *Mosby's guide to physical examination* (7th ed.). St. Louis, MO: Mosby.

Shieh, C., & Halstead, J.A. (2009). Understanding the impact of health literacy on women's health. *Journal of Obstetric, Gynecologic, and Neonatal Nursing, 38,* 601–612.

Simoni-Wastila, L., & Tompkins, C. (2001). Balancing diversion control and medical necessity: The case of prescription drugs with abuse potential. *Substance Use and Misuse, 36,* 1275–1296.

Slanetz, P. (2002). Hormone replacement therapy and breast tissue density on mammography. *Menopause, 9*(2), 82–83.

Slevec, J., & Tiggemann, M. (2010). Attitudes toward cosmetic surgery in middle-aged women: Body image, aging, anxiety, and the media. *Psychology of Women Quarterly, 34,* 65–74.

Smilkstein, G. (1978). The family APGAR: A proposal for a family function test and its use by physicians. *Journal of Family Practice, 6,* 1231–1239.

Spielberger, C.D. (1983). *Manual for state-trait anxiety inventory.* Palo Alto, CA: Consulting Psychologists Press.

Stevens, S., Korchmaros, J.D., & Miller, D. (2010). A comparison of victimization and perpetration of intimate partner violence among drug abusing heterosexual and lesbian women. *Journal of Family Violence, 25,* 639–649.

Svavarsdottir, E.K., & Orlygsdottir, B. (2009). Intimate partner abuse factors associated with women's health: A general population study. *Journal of Advanced Nursing, 65*(7), 1452–1462.

Tapper-Gardzina, Y., Cotugna, N., & Vickery, C. (2002). Should you recommend a low-carb, high protein diet? *Nurse Practitioner, 27*(4), 52–59.

Tavernier, D.L. (2009). The genogram: Enhancing student appreciation of family genetics. *Journal of Nursing Education, 48*(4), 222–225.

Tjaden, P., & Thoennes, N. (2000). *Extent, nature, and consequences of intimate partner violence: Findings from the national violence against women survey* (NCJ Publication No. 181867). Washington, DC: National Institute of Justice and Centers for Disease Control and Prevention.

Treaster, D.E., & Burr, D. (2004). Gender differences in prevalence of upper extremity musculoskeletal disorders. *Ergonomics, 47,* 495–526.

Tseng, M., Yeatts, K., Millikan, R., & Newman, B. (2001). Area-level characteristics and smoking in women. *American Journal of Public Health, 91*(11), 1847–1850.

Twinings, S. (1995). The occupational and environmental health history: Guidelines for the primary care nurse practitioner. *Nurse Practitioner Forum, 6*(2), 64–71.

U.S. Census Bureau. (2011). *Poverty.* Retrieved August 21, 2011, from http://www.census.gov/hhes/www/poverty/index.html

U.S. Department of Agriculture and U.S. Department of Health and Human Services. (2010, December). *Dietary guidelines for Americans, 2010* (5th ed.). Washington, DC: U.S. Government Printing Office.

U.S. Department of Health and Human Services (USDHHS). (2000). *Healthy people 2010* (Conference Edition, in Two Volumes). Washington, DC: U.S. Government Printing Office.

U.S. Department of Health and Human Services (USDHHS). (2010). *Healthy people 2020.* Retrieved from www.healthypeople.gov/2020/default.aspx

U.S. Department of Health and Human Services (USDHHS). (2008). *2008 physical activity guidelines for Americans.* Retrieved August 17, 2011, from http://www.health.gov/PAGuidelines/

U.S. Department of Health and Human Services (USDHHS). (2009). *The environment and women's health, fact sheet.* Retrieved August 19, 2011, from http://www.womenshealth.gov/ppublications/our-publications/fact-sheet/environment-womens-health.cfm

U.S. Department of Health and Human Services (USDHHS). (2011). *The 2011 HHS poverty guidelines.* Retrieved August 21, 2011, from http://aspe.hhs.gov/poverty/11poverty.shtml

U.S. Preventive Services Task Force (USPSTF). (2010, December). *Recommendations.* Retrieved October 24, 2011, from http://www.uspreventiveservicestaskforce.org/recommendations.htm

Vitamin C and cataract risk in women. (2002). *Harvard Women's Health Watch, IX*(9), 1.

Winickoff, J.P., Friebely, J., Tanski, S.E., Sherrod, C., Matt, G.E., Howell, M.F., et al. (2009). Beliefs about the health effects of "thirdhand" smoke and home smoking bans. *Pediatrics, 123,* e74–e79.

Witte, S.S., El-Bassel, N., Gilbert, L., Wu, E., & Chang, M. (2010). Lack of awareness of partner STD risk among heterosexual couples. *Perspectives on Sexual and Reproductive Health, 42*(1), 49–55.

World Health Organization. (2010). *Female genital mutilation.* Retrieved October 23, 2011, from www.who.int/mediacentre/factsheets/fs241/en/

Worobey, J. (2002). Early family mealtime experiences and eating attitudes in normal weight, underweight and overweight females. *Eating and Weight Disorders, 7*(1), 39–44.

Wright, L.M., & Leahey, M. (2009). *Nurses and families: A guide to family assessment* (5th ed.). Philadelphia: F. A Davis Company.

Young, C. (2011). The pay bias between the sexes lingers on. *Madam Noire*. Retrieved February 25, 2012, from http://madamenoire.com/120639/the-pay-bias-between-the-sexes-lingers-on/

Young, D.R., & Stewart, K.J. (2006). A church-based physical activity intervention for African American women. *Family and Community Health, 29*(2), 103–117.

CHAPTER ❖ 6

ASSESSING OLDER WOMEN'S HEALTH

Debra Hain

Highlights

- Dimensions of Aging
- Leading Risk Factors
- Screening Methods
- Physical Examination
- General Survey

❖ INTRODUCTION

Many people define aging in terms of chronology along with physical features such as graying hair, wrinkles, and changes in posture and gait (Hooyman & Kiyak, 2011). However, it may be prudent to consider the various dimensions of aging, such as physical and psychological, as a more appropriate way to define aging (Morgan & Kunkel, 2011). In fact, one of the American Nurses Association's, *Gerontological Nursing: Scope and Standards of Practice* (2010), assumptions of aging that drive the approach and philosophy of care to older adults states, "aging encompasses physical, cognitive, emotional, psychological, sociological, and spiritual changes" (p. 2). For the purposes of clarification, this chapter will provide a chronological age (women ≥ 65). However, the chapter content will be guided by a framework that considers the physical and psychosocial dimensions of aging.

DIMENSIONS OF AGING

DEMOGRAPHICS AND EPIDEMIOLOGY

It would be impossible to live in the United States and not be aware that we are experiencing an aging society. In 1904, only 4 percent of the population were over the age of 65 as compared to 13 percent who are living today. As health care improves and people live longer, the number of older adults in the United States is expected to continue to grow. By 2030, the number of people over age 65 will nearly double, to 71 million. The fastest growing segments of older adults are those 85 and older (Figure 6–1). In 2000, the life expectancy was 76.9 years, and today, people who reach age 65 can expect to live to age 82.9. Older women outnumber older men by 2 to 1. In 2008, women ≥ 65 represented about 58 percent of the population cohort and 67 percent in those 85 and older (Federal Interagency Forum on Aging-Related Statistics, 2010). In the future, there will also be a considerable shift in racial and ethnic composition among older adults. The proportion of older adults who consider themselves non-Hispanic will decrease from 80 to 58.5 percent by 2050, while the proportion of other groups will increase. It is anticipated that the population of Hispanic older adults will increase from 7.0 to 19.8 percent and non-Hispanic African Americans from 8.2 to 11.2 percent (Administration on Aging, 2010). The aging population will place a significant burden on our health care system, making it critical for health care professionals, including advanced practice nurses, to discover effective and efficient ways to improve health outcomes of a diverse older population.

PSYCHOSOCIAL DIMENSIONS OF AGING

Social Aging

The process of aging is complex, and many social factors may affect people as they age. Aging people may face many losses, both personal and financial. Genetics play a role in the aging process; however, goals, values, preferences, and actions specific to a person are shaped by a lifetime of individual experiences and social circumstances (Morgan & Kunkel, 2011). As a person ages, the role of social support, which includes the network of people in their lives, can have a positive effect on health and well-being (Antonucci & Akiyama, 1987; Krause, 2001).

Many sociological theories of aging have been proposed; however, only a few will be briefly discussed. The Role Theory suggests that the role of individuals evolves as they age and that the ability to adapt predicts adjustment to personal aging (Cottrell, 1942). The Activity Theory supports the belief that activity level has a significant impact on the person's life satisfaction and positive self-concept (Maddox, 1963). The foundation of the Age-Stratification Theory is that elders exist in cohorts sharing similar life experiences with others (Marshall, 1996). For example, many women who were born prior to 1930 stayed home and raised their families. It was not until the feminist movement in the 1960s that this changed and women had more opportunities outside the home (see Chapter 2). It is important for the clinician to consider sociological aging and its impact on health. Cultural beliefs and expectations can be related to roles; current level of activity may influence life satisfaction and the fear of losing one's mobility may lead to resistance to recommended interventions; and the historical context of individual life experience may influence the person's perception and responses to care.

Number of Persons 65+, 1900–2030 (numbers in millions)

Year (as of July 1)	1900	1920	1940	1960	1980	1990	2000	2010	2020	2030
Number (millions)	3.1	4.9	9	16.6	25.5	31.2	35	40.2	54.8	72.1

FIGURE 6–1. Number of Persons Age 65 and Over in the United States: 1900 Projected to 2030

Increments in years are uneven.

The source of the data for 1900 to 2000 is Table 5. Population by Age and Sex for the United States: 1900 to 2000, p. A-9, by Hobbs, Frank, and Nicole Stoops, in *Demographic Trends in the 20th Century*, U.S. Census Bureau, Census 2000 Special Reports, Series CENSR-4. The figures for 2008 are from the U.S. Census Bureau 2008 population estimates. The projections for 2010 to 2030 are from Table 12. Projections of the Population by Age and Sex for the United States: 2010 to 2050 (NP2008-T12), Population Division, U.S. Census Bureau. *Source:* Administration on Aging, 2010.

Psychological Aging

According to Erikson's eight stages of development, as discussed in Chapter 2, specific tasks in life must be accomplished before the person is able to master the next task. The task of later life is ego integrity as opposed to ego despair (Erikson, 1950). This is a sense of wholeness and cohesion of self. This has also been described as the achievement of late-life wisdom; something that should be considered when developing strategies aimed at helping the older woman attain and/or maintain health.

Considering Maslow's Hierarchy of Needs (1954), the clinician should ensure that the basic needs are met before higher levels of health are achievable. Once these are met, the older woman may feel safe and secure and be able to move to the next level of belonging. Maslow views people as social beings needing to interact with others. As older women experience personal losses, such as the loss of a loved one or friends, it is important to identify ways to reduce the risk of social isolation and depression that may occur (Ebersole, Hess, Touhy, Jett, & Luggen, 2008). The Family APGAR (Smilkstein, 1978) is a valid and reliable tool that can be used to assess social support for the older woman (see Chapter 5). Social isolation and depression will be discussed later in this chapter.

LEADING RISK FACTORS

HEALTH ISSUES

Health behaviors begin early in life, are shaped by life experiences, and have a significant impact on health and functioning of older women. Although women cannot control genetic predisposition to certain diseases, they can engage in disease prevention and health promotion behaviors that can lead to optimal health. Ageism is prevalent in the United States and may prevent older women from receiving information regarding their best options for care (Kane, Ouslander, Abrass, & Resnick, 2009). It is essential that clinicians take an individual approach to education and provision of resources for older women as they make informed decisions about disease prevention and health promotion. Preventable problems specific to older adults warrant attention. The most preventable problem that clinicians can address is iatrogenic disease.

Pharmacotherapeutics, Polypharmacy, and Aging

As people age, their responses to therapeutic interventions decrease, which makes them more susceptible to toxic side effects of medications. These changes can be attributed to many factors, including metabolism of medications, changes in receptor behavior, and altered chemical environment from medications (Kane et al., 2009). Due to reduced capacity for metabolizing and excreting many medications, there is a narrower therapeutic window resulting in the need for less medication to achieve desired results. Changes in receptors may also make older women more sensitive to medications. Polypharmacy (a person taking multiple medications at the same time) increases the risk of drug–drug interactions and of the person experiencing adverse events (Gallagher, 2001). When a person is prescribed two medications, there is a 6 percent chance that an adverse event will occur. This substantially increases to 50 percent when five or more medications are used and to 100 percent when eight or more medications are taken (Shaughnessy, 1992). Therefore, it is crucial that a thorough medication review that includes having the woman bring in all her medications be conducted on a regular basis (at least annually). Another important issue related to iatrogenic problems is hospitalization.

Complications From Hospitalization

Older women are more likely to experience untoward events during a hospitalization. This can be related to preexisting physical and psychological problems. Functional decline during hospitalization also increases the risk of having poor outcomes. The risk factors for functional decline during hospitalization include 75 years and older, Mini-Mental State Examination (MMSE) score 24/30, dependence in two or more activities of daily living (ADL) prior to admission, pressure wounds, baseline functional dependency, and history of low social activities (Inouye & Charpentier, 1996; Sager et al., 1996). All efforts should be employed to keep older women out of the hospital, but in cases when this is necessary, strategies to reduce iatrogenesis should be implemented. This begins with a good assessment of who may be at risk, monitoring for adverse events, and appropriate discharge planning.

In a fragmented health care system, older adults are at a high risk for potentially avoidable 30-day rehospitalization after being discharged. This not only increases the chances of poor health outcomes for the older woman, but it also results in increased health care costs. Therefore, adequately identifying those needing additional help before discharge, assessing the individual's strengths and weaknesses, clarifying goals, and effectively communicating with the person/family and other health care professionals are essential.

Nutrition

Many factors impact nutritional status in older adults. Eating a well-balanced diet may present challenges for some older adults. If the person is unable to eat a well-balanced diet, malnutrition can occur, which leads to increased risk for disease and death. It may seem obvious that food has to be available in order to eat; however, social factors such as limited finances and transportation or mobility problems that decrease the ability to purchase food. Other factors to consider are physical activity level, disease burden, and advancing age.

There is a close association of physical activity and nutrition. Changes in body composition occur with advancing age. After age 60, a person's weight usually stabilizes, and then begins to decline making weight maintenance challenging as the person ages. Older adults experience a progressive loss of lean body mass, an increase in fat mass, and redistribution of fat from peripheral to central locations within the body (Halter et al., 2009). A change in appetite and energy intake regulation occurs with advancing age. The metabolic, neural, and humoral pathways that maintain the balance between appetite and hunger begin to lose their compensatory mechanisms to respond to changes in energy demand. As people age, they can experience a loss of taste and smell, which may lead to a decreased nutrient intake. The aroma of food is a powerful appetite stimulant, and without this, individuals may not have the desire to eat a meal.

Nutritional Needs. Nutritional needs may vary among older adults. The following focuses on general needs of the population. Dietary needs of special populations will be addressed later in this chapter under Special Assessments.

In 2005, the U.S. Department of Agriculture (USDA) changed the food pyramid that many of us followed throughout our lives. It supports an individual approach that considers sex, age, height, weight, and exercise patterns. In 2007, Tufts University modified its older adults' food pyramid to integrate the new recommendation from the USDA (Figure 6–2). It incorporated foods that could meet the unique needs of older adults along with an emphasis on the importance of regular activity. It continues to stress the value of foods with the best nutrients as well as the importance of fluid balance.

Older adults generally consume fewer calories, but there may be situations in which they will require more calories, such as acute illness and fever. Basically, they should consume a variety of foods and reduce fat intake by 20 to 30 percent of total calories (substitute unsaturated fats for saturate fats and limit cholesterol). Carbohydrate intake should make up about 50 to 60 percent of total caloric intake, with majority being from complex sugars such as fresh fruits and vegetables. If possible they should avoid junk foods and ensure adequate mineral and vitamin intake (Saxon, Etten, & Perkins, 2010). Protein is essential for maintenance of lean body mass, organ system performance, and optimal immune system function. The recommended daily allowance (RDA) for protein intake should be about 0.8 g/kg of body weight per day (Biggs, 2007), which is about 20 to 30 percent of total caloric intake. There is some controversy whether this is adequate for older women. The results of a subset of the Women's Health Initiative Observational Study of 24,417 women aged 65 to 79 indicated that higher protein intake was associated with lower risk of frailty (Beasley et al., 2010). Gaffney-Stomberg, Insogna, Rodriguez, and Kerstetter (2009) recommend RDA of 1.0 to 1.2 g/kg of body weight per day (for about 13–16% of total calories) to support muscle and bone health in older adults. More research is needed exploring protein needs in a diverse older population; however, until then clinicians should

Modified MyPyramid for Older Adults

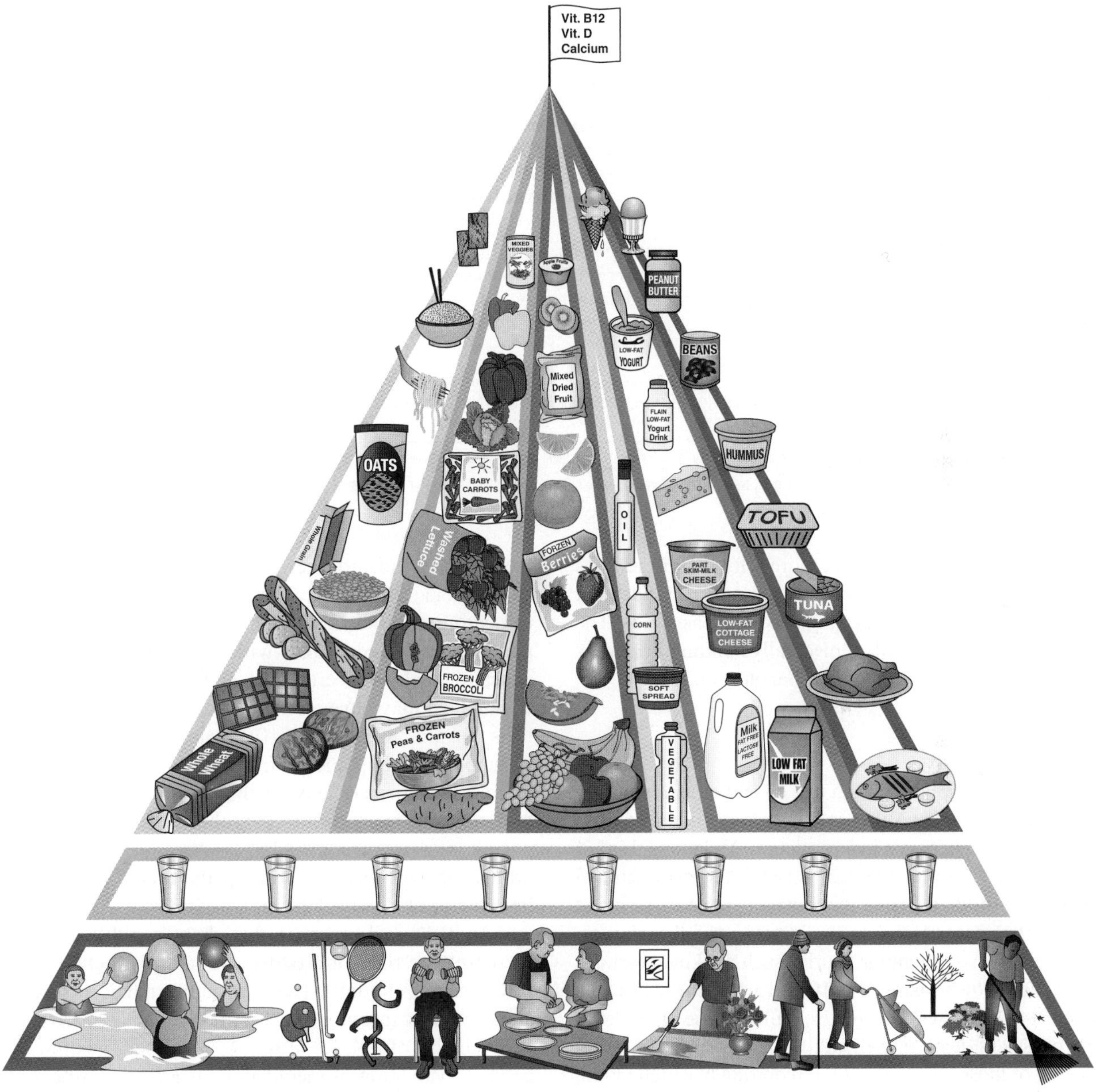

FIGURE 6–2. Modified MyPyramid for Older Adults

This pyramid represents the need for whole, enriched, and fortified grains and cereals such as brown rice and 100 percent whole-wheat bread; bright-colored vegetables such as carrots and broccoli; deep-colored fruits such as berries and melon; low- and nonfat dairy products such as yogurt and low-lactose milk; dry beans and nuts, fish, poultry, lean meat, and eggs; liquid vegetable oils and soft spreads low in saturated and trans fat; fluid intake; and physical activity such as walking, house work, and yard work. *Source:* © 2007 Tufts University, http://www.nutrition.tufts.edu/research/modified-mypyramid-older-adults.

base the decision on protein intake on an individual basis. Although vitamins are important, they are not without risk. Older women should seek the guidance of a health professional when making a decision to take vitamins (see Table 6–1).

DEHYDRATION RISKS

Many older adults experience dehydration caused by limited fluid intake. This is in part due to the fact that older adults have decreased thirst mechanism and may not

TABLE 6–1. Recommended Vitamins for Older Women and Assessment Pearls Related to Specific Vitamins

Vitamin	RDA[a]	Assessment Pearls
• Vitamin B_1 (thiamin) • Vitamin B_2 (riboflavin) • Niacin • Vitamin B_6 (pyridoxine) • Vitamin B_{12} • Folic acid (folate) • Vitamin C (ascorbic acid)	• 1.1 mg • 1.1 mg • 14 mg • 1.5 mg • 2.4 μg • 400 μg • 75 mg	• Deficiencies in B vitamins include skin flaking, dermatitis, mucous membranes may atrophy and become painful, anemia, seizures, constipation, diarrhea, anorexia, irritability, depression, and confusion • In particular, vitamin B_{12} deficiency is common on older women, and you may see smooth beefy red tongue, macrocytic anemia, peripheral neuropathy (including paresthesias and numbness), sensory ataxia, limb weakness. The signs and symptoms in older adults may be nonspecific and common in older women; thus, screening all older women for vitamin B_{12} deficiency should be considered and supplementation started • Assessment for reversible causes of dementia include screening for vitamin B_{12} deficiency
• Vitamin E • Vitamin A • Vitamin K	• 15 mg 22 IU (natural vitamin E) 33 IU (synthetic vitamin E) • 700 μg • 90 μg	• Major symptoms of vitamin E deficiency include anemia, reduced blood clotting times, neuromuscular degeneration, weakness, leg cramps, and difficulty ambulating. High doses of vitamin can interact with anticoagulant therapy as well as potentiate the antiplatelet effects of supplements such as ginko biloba, ginger, ginseng, and garlic (the tolerable upper limit is 1,000 mg/day)
• Calcium • Vitamin D	• 1,200 mg • 400 IU (age 51 to 70) • 600 IU (age > 70)	• Early signs of vitamin D deficiency include nonspecific musculoskeletal pain, particularly in bones and muscles of the back, hips, legs, and shoulders, and can see proximal weakness

[a]The recommended daily allowance (RDA) is the recommended average daily intake that will fulfill the nutritional needs of many healthy older adults.

Source: Halter et al., 2009; Office of Dietary Supplements, National Institutes of Health. (2011). *Dietary supplement fact sheet: Vitamin D.* Retrieved July 20, 2011, from http://ods.od.nih.gov/factsheets/VitaminD/; Tabloski, 2010.

realize that they need to drink more. Physical limitations may reduce access to fluids and persons with advance dementia may not recognize the need to drink fluids. The average fluid intake, unless medically contraindicated, is about 1,500 to 2,500 cc per day (Saxon et al., 2010).

FALLS

Falls among men and women age 65 and older are a public health problem. Aging is a risk factor for falls that may threaten a person's independence. About one third of community-residing older adults (≥ 65) fall on an annual basis; two thirds fall after experiencing the first fall; and about 50 percent of nursing home residents fall each year. Many falls result in minor injuries such as skin abrasions, lacerations, or bruising, but 10 to 15 percent result in a fracture or other serious injuries. Falls are one of the leading causes of death in men and women age 65 and older. In fact, of those who suffer a fall requiring hospitalization, 50 percent will die within the first year. Falls are associated with a decline in function, greater chance of nursing home admission, greater increase of medical services, and development of fear of falling (a risk factor for falling) (American Geriatrics Society [AGS], 2010). Considering the risk for falling and associated poor health outcome, it is critical that a fall assessment be performed on a regular basis and whenever a person has experienced a fall.

Older adults have many risk factors for falls, and these can be classified as intrinsic factors and extrinsic factors and divided further by modifiable and nonmodifiable factors (Table 6–2). There is inconclusive evidence indicating an associated risk of falls with sociodemographic status. Individuals with less than a high school education, below poverty level, and considered to be disadvantaged may have an increased risk for falls (Fabre, Ellis, Kosma, & Wood, 2010); more research is needed to support this hypothesis. Increased risk related to cardiovascular disease may be the result of arrhythmias, hypotension, heart failure, or other conditions predisposing them to syncope. Many older adults experience orthostatic hypotension requiring education regarding the importance of slowly changing positions.

As discussed earlier in this chapter, polypharmacy increases the risk for adverse events; this includes the increased risks for falls. There are certain medications that are potentially inappropriate for the older adult because of a higher risk of falls, delirium, or other poor health outcomes. Evaluation of medications is a crucial aspect of the health assessment. The Beers Criteria provides a list of medications that if possible should be avoided in older adults and at the very least modified (available at https://www.dcri.org/trial-participation/the-beers-list/).

Vitamin D insufficiency/deficiency has been linked to falls due to decreased muscle strength, and replacement therapy has shown some promising benefits. Zhu, Austin, Devine, Bruce, and Prince (2010) studied the effects of vitamin D replacement therapy (1,000 IU of vitamin D_2 per day and 1 g of calcium citrate per day) on muscle

TABLE 6–2. Risk Factors for Falls

	Intrinsic Factors	Extrinsic Factors	Environmental Factors
Nonmodifiable	• Age (≥65) • Gender (females have more risk for nonfatal injury) • Race/ethnicity (white, non-Hispanic and white women have higher rate of fall-related hip fractures than women of other races) • Chronic illness (Parkinson's disease, osteoarthritis, stroke, cardiovascular disease [hypertension, heart disease], respiratory, normal pressure hydrocephalus, and dementia) • Chronic psychological problems (stress, depression, and anxiety)		
Modifiable	• History of falls (one or more falls in past year have three times risk of falling again) • Fear of falling • Decreased physical activities • Functional decline/gait instability • Acute illness (influenza, infection, delirium stroke, transient ischemic attack, seizure) • Drop attacks (sudden leg weaknesses without loss of consciousness) • Somatosensory and vestibular dysfunction (dizziness and/or vertigo) • Orthostatic hypotension: hypovolemia, or low cardiac output, autonomic dysfunction, impaired venous return, prolonged bed rest, drug induced, postprandial hypotension • Vision problems (poor lens elasticity, lack of lens transparency, decreased peripheral field view, decreased contrast sensitivity, and decreased accommodation during lighting changes. Other includes cataracts, macular degeneration, and glaucoma) • Urinary: overactive bladder, urge incontinence, nocturia • Osteoporosis	• Prescribed/taking three or more medications (which include herbal and over-the-counter medications) • Classifications of medications: antidepressants, antipsychotics, long and short acting benzodiazepines, anticonvulsants, antihypertensive, cardiac medications, analgesics, antihistamines, and gastrointestinal-histamine receptors) • Environmental factors include hazards in the home and outside the home	• Beds and toilets at inappropriate height • Unavailability of grab bars • Slippery floors and bathtubs • Throw rugs, frayed carpets cords, wires • Inadequate lighting • Walking with improper footwear • Cracked and uneven sidewalks • Pets that get under foot • Poorly designed or unstable furniture • Changing positions incorrectly • Lack of access to bathroom • Untrained or lack of staff to assist person

Sources: Adapted from Fabre et al., 2010; Kane et al., 2009.

strength and mobility in older women with vitamin D insufficiency (25[OH]D concentration less than 24 ng/mL). The authors reported that women who showed the most promising effects of increased muscle strength and mobility were those who were the weakest and slowest at baseline. More research is needed, but in the meantime consideration of assessing vitamin D levels and initiating replacement therapy may help to reduce the risk of falls. It is believed that vitamin D alone will not reduce the risk of falls. This is complex issue requiring a multicomponent approach (Papas & Cluxton, 2011).

SENSORY CHANGES

Vision

As women age there are normal age-related changes in vision that over time can impact functional abilities. Visual impairment can result in loss of independence (Tabloski, 2010), something that many older women fear. Some visual changes include decreased rod and cone function; pigmentation accumulation; decreased speed of eye movements; ciliary muscle atrophy; increased lens size and yellowing of the lens that may result in decreased visual acuity, visual fields, and light/dark adaptation; increased sensitivity to glare; distorted depth perception with increased risk for falls; and less ability to differentiate blues, greens, and violets. Increased intraocular pressure increases the risk for glaucoma. Decreased tear secretion can cause increased eye dryness and irritation (Kane et al., 2009).

Hearing

Although hearing loss is more common among men than women, auditory problems and loss of hearing can have a significant impact on the quality of life of many women. Hearing loss is common as a person ages; over 30 percent of people age 65 to 74 have hearing loss, and the risk increases as the person ages, with about 66 percent of those over age 75 experiencing some hearing loss

(Demers, 2007). Hearing changes such as loss of auditory neurons and loss of hearing from high to low frequency cause decreased auditory acuity and decreased ability to hear consonants. Older adults have increased cerumen that can cause cerumen impaction, which should be considered when a woman presents with hearing loss. Older women have problems hearing in noisy places or when speech is rapid, so it is important to reduce noise and to speak slowly (Kane et al., 2009).

Olfactory

Olfactory dysfunction is common in older adults; it affects about 50 percent of people over age 60. A diminished sense of smell (hyosmia) may be due to age-related changes, but can also be related to olfactory nerve damage (Bickley, 2007). Upper respiratory, head trauma, inflammatory conditions, and neurodegenerative diseases (Alzheimer's disease and Parkinson's disease) are major causes of olfactory nerve damage (Tabloski, 2010). A decreased number of olfactory nerve fibers may lead to a decreased sense of smell, which may impact a woman's nutritional intake as described earlier in this chapter (Kane et al., 2009).

Taste

The sense of taste is essential for the appreciation of flavor and palatability of food, and it also is a way to recognize if food is spoiled or should not be eaten. The diminished sense of taste (hypogeusia) is common after age 70 (Tabloski, 2010) and increases the risk for consumption of spoiled food. Also, older people often use excessive sugar or salt to compensate for hypogeusia (Kane et al., 2009).

Tactile

Due to slower conduction of nerve impulses and reduced function of the peripheral nerves, tactile sensation diminishes as a woman ages. This may lead to a decreased perception of pain and extreme temperatures (Tabloski, 2010). The loss of this sensation increases the risk of injury for older adults and should be considered during the assessment.

LONELINESS

Four decades ago, Burnside (1971) described factors that contribute to loneliness in older adults as geographical and language barriers; cultural loneliness; lifestyle loneliness; loneliness due to illness and/or pain; loss loneliness, and loneliness caused by impending death. Despite having recognition of this as a problem, loneliness may be underrecognized as a factor contributing to functional decline and depression among older women. Loneliness in older women often is the result of the loss of a spouse. This involves the end of a shared past and future, companionship, social networks, and sometimes economic security (Hooyman & Kiyak, 2011). Other causes of loneliness are prolonged periods of separation from loved ones (i.e., friends and family), loss of social role functioning, and loss of social status (Berman & Furst, 2011). Loneliness is associated with cognitive decline, social isolation, hopelessness, and challenge performing ADL. Women may not present with reports of depression, but rather have vague aches and pains, sleep disturbances, problems with their memory, apathy, and withdrawn from others. A thorough assessment will help differentiate these symptoms from typical physical and functional health problems associated with aging (Hooyman & Kiyak, 2011). Women in long-term care facilities may experience different levels of loneliness (Hicks, 2000). Assessment should include evaluation for grieving, depression, financial situation, and social support (Ebersole et al., 2008). Some questions that may be asked include (1) what time of the day do you like to be with other people, (2) tell me what you like to do socially, and (3) what recent losses or changes have you experienced? (Hicks, 2000). Chapter 5 provides additional information about impact of loneliness on physical health.

COGNITIVE CHANGES

Crystallized intelligence (information and skills gained from experience) remains stable as a person ages, whereas fluid intelligence (flexible reasoning and problem solving) and speed of processing decline. Older adults are able to stay focused on one thing for a period of time; however, they may experience challenges with divided attention (ability to concentrate on more than one thing at a time). Executive function (ability to plan, organize, carry out tasks, and having appropriate judgment) generally remains intact. Memory change is one of the most common complaints of older adults, often causing the person to question what is normal and what is not. Remote memory (recall of events that occurred in distant past) and sensory memory remain intact. Procedural memory and semantic memory (vocabulary and general information) remain stable until very late in life. Even though older women can learn, it might take a little longer to achieve success. A deficit in recalling new information may be present as well. Language comprehension and vocabulary normally remain relatively stable throughout the life span. Aging is associated with psychomotor slowing and slowing of cognitive speed (Halter et al., 2009).

CHRONIC DISEASE

An essential aspect of keeping older adults healthy is preventing chronic disease(s) and health promotion in those who experience chronic disease(s). About 80 percent of older adults have one chronic condition and 50 percent have at least two (Centers for Disease Control and Prevention [CDC], 2011). More specific information on chronic disease(s) can be found in Chapters 23 and 24. Heart disease and malignant neoplasm are the most common causes of death in women 65 years and older. There is an emerging epidemic of diabetes in the United States, and older adults are among the many experiencing this disease. There are over 20 million people diagnosed with diabetes and another 5 million who remain undiagnosed, calling for prevention and early recognition (Gambert & Pinkstaff, 2006). In 2006, diabetes was the sixth leading cause of death. However, hypertension and arthritis are the most prevalent among older adults, and they do not make the list of leading causes of death. Stroke and lung disease are also very common and can be debilitating but are not the most common causes of death (Albert & Freedman, 2010). Even though hypertension, arthritis, stroke, and lung disease are not the main causes of death, they can have a significant impact on an older person's life, and ways to improve quality of life should be considered as part of health promotion (see Figure 6–3).

Osteoporosis is the most common metabolic disease in older women; about 50 percent of women will be affected in their lifetime. Over 20 million women in the United States have osteoporosis. Major risk factors include advancing age, female sex, white or Asian race, family history, and thin body habitus. In 2005, osteoporosis was responsible for more than 2 million fractures with almost 300,000 hip fractures and about 547,000 vertebral fractures. The number of fractures is expected to increase to more than 3 million by 2025. Women who have experienced a hip fracture are at a fourfold greater risk of having a second one. Quality of life is impacted when a woman has a hip fracture, and about 24 percent of those who sustain a hip fracture die within a year; in 2005, about 15,000 women age 65 and over died as the result of injuries sustained from an osteoporotic fracture that resulted in a fall. If women survive the fracture, they may experience limited mobility; within 6 months after the hip fracture, only about 15 percent of women can walk across the room (National Osteoporosis Foundation, 2011). This alarming statistics makes assessment for osteoporosis and treatment as indicated an essential aspect of caring for older women (assessment will be discussed later in this chapter).

COMMON GYNECOLOGICAL DISORDERS

Atrophic vaginitis or inflammation of the vagina due to the decreased estrogen levels is common among women age 55 and older. Pelvic organ prolapse (cystocele,

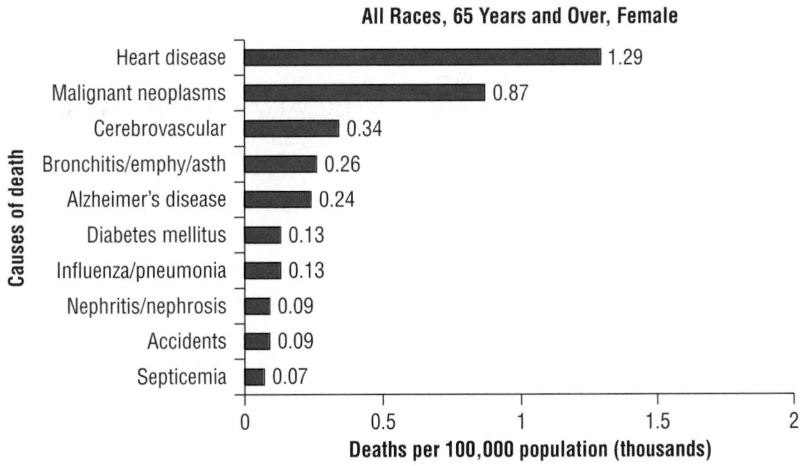

FIGURE 6–3. Causes of Death in Older Women

Data is not age adjusted.

Sources: Centers for Disease Control and Prevention, National Center for Health Statistics; National Vital Statistics System, 2006.

rectocele, and prolapsed uterus), which is influenced by estrogen depletion and/or having multiple children, also can occur among older women. Cancer of the vulva and vagina are not common diseases, but when they occur it is often in older women. Cancer of the uterus occurs most frequently after menopause as the result of hormone imbalances. In fact, cancer of the uterus or endometrium is the most common gynecological cancer in older women. Cancer of the ovary tends to occur primarily in women over age 50; 75 percent of ovarian cancer is in women over age 55 (Ries et al., 2002). Even though ovarian cancer has the highest mortality rate, there is only a 5 percent occurrence. Breast cancer remains the most common malignancy in the United States (Saxon et al., 2010). (See Chapter 16 for more information on common gynecologic pelvic disorders.)

SCREENING METHODS

HEALTH HISTORY

It is recommended that a comprehensive geriatric assessment be conducted on an annual basis, after hospitalization for acute illness, when considering nursing home placement, and/or with abrupt changes in cognitive function or physical function. Performing the health history in older women can be challenging. Clinicians must be sensitive to concerns of older women, be aware of atypical presentation of illness, and create an environment that supports disclosure. The health history must consider physical, psychological, socioeconomic factors, as well as functional abilities (Kane et al., 2009). The history should include the following:

- Review of acute and chronic health problems
- Comprehensive medication review that includes prescribed and over-the-counter medications; recommend having women bring in all medications for review
- Health promotion and disease prevention, immunizations, and cancer screening. A schedule of recommended vaccines can be found at http://www.cdc.gov/vaccines/recs/schedules/default.htm#adult.
- Functional status (ADL and instrumental ADL); using a valid and reliable instrument will help guide the questions. Tools for achieving best practice are available from the Hartford Institute for Geriatric Nursing's Try This Series at http://www.hartfordign.org/practice/try_this/
- Social support (caregiver issues, family/friends)
- Social (living arrangements, transportation, economic factors [i.e., ability to purchase food and medication])
- Home environment: stairs, emergency numbers, safety of neighborhood, grab bars, absence of scatter rugs, assistance in the home, ability to cook (accidents in the kitchen, such as leaving the stove on)
- Driving status and safety record: ask "if" questions that can help determine if a woman experiences geographical disorientation (i.e., has there been episodes in which you were in a familiar place and you were not sure what direction to go; have you ever made the wrong turn in a familiar place and experienced difficulties finding your way?)
- Geriatric-focused review of systems should include memory, nutrition, pain, intake senses, falls, bowel and bladder function, sleep

Interview and Approach

Impaired hearing and vision may interfere with effective communication so it is essential that clinicians develop techniques that can facilitate communication with the patient. Adequate lighting, elimination of extraneous noises, speaking slowly and in deep tones while facing the person may be helpful. Many times older women may underreport potentially essential information because they feel it is not important or they may forget. Women may be fearful about illness and loss of independence so they may minimize symptoms (Kane et al., 2009). It is important to ask specific questions, and with the woman's approval, you may consider having a family member present to assist with the history. Asking the person to write down questions/information for pending appointments may help. Most importantly, be patient and take the time needed to obtain a comprehensive history.

SPECIAL ASSESSMENTS

Nutritional Assessment

Under nutrition can impact older women's quality of life, and malnutrition can lead to poor health outcomes, such as poor wound healing, functional decline, altered immune system, alter pharmacokinetics, and increased risk for hospitalization or placement in other institutions. Overweight or obesity can also impact quality of life and lead to adverse outcomes such as chronic disease (Chapman, 2006). Therefore, it is important to routinely assess older women who are ≥65 for nutritional problems (Kane et al., 2009). A comprehensive assessment should include anthropometric measurements, laboratory values, and clinical findings from the history and physical examination. Laboratory studies should include albumin (≤3.5 mg/dL indicates mild malnutrition, but some studies use ≤3.0 mg/dL as an indication); prealbumin has a shorter half-life so it can be used to provide current information about protein status, complete blood count (CBC), serum folate, and vitamin B_{12} assays. Dehydration or overhydration will cause inaccurate albumin levels. Nephritic syndrome increases urinary excretion of albumin, and liver disease can result in decreased albumin synthesis (Tabloski, 2010).

The health history should include a 24-hour diet recall. If needed, a food frequency questionnaire could be used to fill in the gaps when there is poor recall. The Nutrition Screening Initiative (NSI) is a public health strategy that provides screening tools that clinicians can use to identify risk factors in community-residing older adults. The DETERMINE is a checklist that can be used to identify warning signs of poor nutrition and is available at http://www.cdaaa.org/images/Nutritional_Checklist.pdf. The Mini-Nutritional Assessment (MNA) is a valid and reliable tool that can be used for screening and assessment in older adults. The Try This Series from the Hartford Institute for Geriatric Nursing provides information on how to use this simple and quick method to identify those at risk; the instrument is available at http://consultgerirn.org/uploads/File/trythis/try_this_9.pdf as well as the Nestle Nutrition Institute at http://www.mna-elderly.com/.

A common nutritional concern is unintentional weight loss (about 25% of people have a known cause). Weight loss of ≥5 percent in 1 month, ≥7.5 percent in 3 months, and ≥10 percent over 6 months are risk factors for malnutrition. Some of the causes of unintentional weight loss include depression; medication side effects; social isolation; improper feeding assistance; pain; dehydration; sensory changes; cognitive impairment; personal, cultural, or religious food preferences; diarrhea; alcoholism; fever; wounds; bone factors; advanced chronic obstructive pulmonary disease; or polypharmacy (Tabloski, 2010). Assessment for dysphagia or difficulty swallowing should be considered, especially for long-term care residents; about 60 percent have dysphagia and are at risk for aspiration pneumonia (American Dietetic Association [ADA], 2005).

Fall Risk Assessment

Before strategies aimed at reducing the risk of falls can be implemented, it is essential that fall screening (Table 6–4) and assessment (Table 6–5) are completed. In 2010, the AGS and British Geriatrics Society (BGS) Clinical Practice Guideline, *Prevention of Falls in Older Persons*, published evidence-based guidelines for assessment and possible interventions aimed at reducing the risk of falls. These well-organized and easy-to-use guidelines are available at http://www.americangeriatrics.org/health_care_professionals/clinical_practice/clinical_guidelines_recommendations/2010/.

The get-up-and-go test can be used in any setting (Resnick, Corcoran, & Spellbring, 2001) to assist with the assessment of gait disorders. The woman should be asked to rise from a straight-back chair, turn around, and sit down. Performance is graded on a 5-point scale from 1 (normal) to 5 (severely abnormal). The quality of movement is assessed for impaired balance. A score of 3 or higher suggests a high risk of falling. Gait speed and agility are related to functional level. Marked gait disturbance is not a normal part of aging and is most likely indicative of an underlying disorder (Ebersole et al., 2008). The Hendrich II Fall Risk Model (Hendrich, Bender, & Nyhuis, 2003) is a valid and reliable tool that can be used in acute settings. A description and copy of the instrument are available through the Hartford Institute for Geriatric Nursing Try This assessment at http://consultgerirn.org/uploads/File/trythis/try_this_8.pdf.

Sleep Assessment

Sleep complaints are common among older adults and the risk of experiencing sleep disturbances increases as a person ages. Health history includes past and present health issues, medications, chronic pain or pruritus, psychological problems, change in living situations or sleep routines, current stressors or worries, nocturia, and need for sleep medications. Tylenol® PM is commonly used by older adults for sleep. The diphenhydramine component of the medication can affect cognitive function, so if possible this medication should be avoided and instead the clinician may prescribe acetaminophen without an antihistamine for pain that may be disrupting sleep. Women should be instructed to limit caffeine and alcohol before bedtime. It is important to assess for snoring, which may indicate the presence of sleep apnea. Sleep apnea is more prevalent among men than women (Phillips & Ancoli-Israel, 2001), but women should still be assessed. Risk factors for sleep apnea are obesity (body mass index >30), hypertension, cigarette smoking, and large neck size (see Chapter 5). The Epworth Sleepiness Scale (Ancoli-Israel & Ayalon, 2006) is a brief instrument used to screen for severity of daytime sleepiness and the Pittsburgh Sleep Quality Index is used to screen for sleep problems in the home environment and monitor changes in sleep

TABLE 6–3. Recommended Immunizations for Person Age 65 and Older

Vaccine	Indications	Dose	Precaution/Contraindications
Pneumococcal polysaccharide (PPSV)	1. Any unvaccinated person over age 65	1. Administer 0.5 mL PPSV either intramuscularly (22–25 g; needle length according to the patient's age/body mass [1–1½"]) or subcutaneously (23–25 g, 5/8" needle) 2. Can be given concurrently with other vaccines at different sites 3. A second dose should be given to any person ≥65 years who was previously vaccinated and 5 years or more have lapsed; this is not needed for persons vaccinated at age ≥65 4. One-time second dose after 5 years for persons with chronic kidney disease, nephritic syndrome, functional or anatomic asplenia	1. Don't give to someone who has history of serious reaction (e.g., anaphylaxis) after a previous dose of PPSV or a PPSV component 2. Minor illnesses with or without fever are not contraindications 3. Use caution in cases of moderate or severe acute illness 4. Pneumococcal conjugate vaccine (PCV) not approved for use in older adults
Influenza	1. All adults ≥65 years old, including those with high-risk health conditions 2. All nursing home residents and chronic care facilities 3. All household contacts of high-risk adults or ≥65 years	1. One dose annually 2. Use trivalent influenza vaccine (TIV) only: Afluria, FluLaval (5.0 mL multidose vial), or Fluarix (0.5 mL prefilled syringe) 3. Vaccinate in deltoid muscle using needle length ≥1" (>25 mm)	1. Any prior anaphylactic reaction to vaccine or components (e.g., eggs) 2. Do not give live attenuated influenza vaccine (LAIV) to persons ≥50 years 3. Guillain-Barré syndrome within 6 weeks of a previous dose
Herpes zoster	1. All adults ≥65 years old regardless of report of prior zoster infection 2. Neither taking varicella history nor serologic testing for varicella immunity is needed before administration of zoster vaccine	1. One-time single dose; no second dose needed 2. Subcutaneous administration in upper arm (0.65 mL dose) 3. Lyophilized zoster vaccine stored frozen, at 5°F (–15°C) 3. Should be given within 30 minutes of reconstitution to maintain potency	1. Contraindicated if previous anaphylactic reaction to any component of the zoster vaccine (e.g., gelatin, neomycin) 2. Contraindicated in immunocompromised condition; HIV infection with <200 CD4 cells/μL 3. Persons with chronic medical conditions may be vaccinated unless the condition is among contraindications listed above 4. Use caution in cases of moderate or severe acute illness 5. If patient is known to be varicella zoster virus (VZV) seronegative, then a two-dose series of varicella vaccine should be administered 6. Not indicated to treat herpes zoster or ongoing postherpetic neuralgia
Td	1. Complete vaccine series is indicated for older adults with uncertain vaccine history or with fewer than three recorded doses	1. Primary: three doses of tetanus and diphtheria toxoid; two doses at least 4 weeks apart; third dose 6–12 months later; boosters at 10-year intervals; more often with high-risk injuries (burns, puncture wounds, extensive soft tissue injury)	1. Prior anaphylaxis with Td vaccine; acute illness
Tdap (updated by CDC in 2010; available at www.cdc.org)	1. Older adults ≥65 years and older (e.g., grandparents, childcare providers, and health care practitioners) who have or who anticipate having close contact with an infant less than 12 months of age and who previously have not received Tdap should receive a single dose of Tdap to protect against pertussis and reduce the likelihood of transmission 2. For other adults aged 65 years and older, a single dose of Tdap vaccine may be given instead of Td vaccine, in persons who have not previously received Tdap	1. Tdap can be administered regardless of interval since the last tetanus- or diphtheria toxoid–containing vaccine. After receipt of Tdap, persons should continue to receive Td for routine booster immunization against tetanus and diphtheria, according to previously published guidelines. Either Tdap vaccine product may be used 2. Further recommendations on the use of both Tdap vaccines in adults aged 65 years and older will be forthcoming should one or more Tdap products be licensed for use in this age group	

Source: American Geriatrics Society, 2009, *A Pocket Guide to Common Immunizations for Older Adult (≥65 Years)*, http://www.americangeriatrics.org/files/documents/AGS_PocketGuide.pdf.

TABLE 6–4. Summary of Screening for Falls

- All individuals over the age of 65 should be asked about falls on an annual basis
- An older person who reports a fall should be asked about the frequency and circumstances
- Older individuals should be asked about gait and balance difficulties; if demonstrate a problem with gait or balance, the woman should be under a multifactorial fall risk assessment
- The person who has a single fall should be evaluated for gait and balance problems
- Older women who present for medical attention because of a fall, report recurrent falls in the past year, or report difficulties in walking or balance should have a multifactorial fall risk assessment
- Older women who can't perform or perform poorly on a standardized gait and balance test should be given a multifactorial fall risk assessment
- Older women reporting only a single fall and demonstrates no difficulty or unsteadiness during the evaluation of gait and balance assessment do not require a fall risk assessment
- The multifactorial fall risk assessment should be performed by a clinician (or clinicians) with appropriate skills and training

Source: Adapted to women from AGS/BGS Clinical Practice Guideline, *Prevention of Falls in Older Persons (2010)*, http://www.americangeriatrics.org/health_care_professionals/clinical_practice/clinical_guidelines_recommendations/2010/.

TABLE 6–5. Multifactorial Fall Risk Assessment

Focused history	1. Description of the circumstances of the fall(s): frequency, symptoms at time of fall, injuries, other circumstances 2. Medication review: all prescribed, over-the-counter, herbal and supplements; include dosages and times of administration; discuss how to self-manage medications (use of divided pill container, etc.); consider brown bag approach and have woman bring in all medications she is taking 3. History of relevant risk factors (see Table 6–4)
Physical examination	1. Detailed assessment gait, balance, and mobility levels and lower extremity joint function 2. Neurological function: cognitive evaluation, lower extremity peripheral nerves, proprioception reflexes, tests of cortical, extrapyramidal and cerebellar function 3. Muscle strength (lower extremities) 4. Cardiovascular status: heart rate and rhythm, postural pulse, blood pressure, and if appropriate, heart rate and blood pressure response to carotid sinus stimulation 5. Assessment of visual acuity, and if appropriate, have woman undergo ophthalmological examination 6. Examination of the feet and footwear
Functional assessment	1. Assessment of activities of daily living (ADL) skills including use of adaptive equipment and mobility aids, as appropriate 2. Assessment of the woman's perceived functional ability and fear related to falling (assessment of current activity levels with attention to the extent to which concerns about falling are protective [i.e., appropriate given abilities] or contributing to deconditioning and/or compromised quality of life [i.e., individual is curtailing involvement in activities she is safely able to perform due to fear of falling]) 3. Consider use of a valid and reliable instruments if needed to assist with functional assessment
Environmental factors	1. Home assessment (Table 6–4) 2. Institutions such as hospital, nursing home: untrained staff, faulty equipment, call light not within reach, inadequate supervision, unclear path to bathroom, and dim lighting

Source: Adapted to women from AGS/BGS Clinical Practice Guideline, *Prevention of Falls in Older Persons (2010)*, http://www.americangeriatrics.org/health_care_professionals/clinical_practice/clinical_guidelines_recommendations/2010/.

TABLE 6–6. Suggested Interventions for Community-Residing Older Women

- Treat orthostatic hypotension and cardiovascular conditions; teach women to slowly change positions
- Modify medications and reduce the number if possible, especially antihypertensive medication; withdrawal or minimization of psychoactive medications
- Assistive devices as needed
- Exercise, particularly balance, strength, and gait training. An exercise program that targets strength, gait and balance, such as Tai Chi or physical therapy, is recommended as an effective intervention to reduce falls
- Exercise programs should take into account the physical capabilities and health profile of the older person (i.e., be tailored) and be prescribed by qualified health professionals or fitness instructors
- All older adults who are at risk of falling should be offered an exercise program incorporating balance, gait, and strength training. Flexibility and endurance training should also be offered, but not as sole components of the program
- In older women in whom cataract surgery is indicated, surgery should be expedited as it reduces the risk of falling
- Multifactorial/multicomponent intervention should include an education component complementing and addressing issues specific to the intervention being provided, tailored to individual cognitive function and language.
- Vitamin D supplements of at least 800 IU per day should be provided to older persons with proven or suspected vitamin D deficiency or at risk for falls
- Management of foot problems and selection of appropriate footwear. Discussion of appropriate footwear; advise about walking with shoes of low heel height and high surface contact area may reduce the risk of falls
- Modify environmental hazards; if a home assessment is warranted, consult a professional who has the expertise to conduct a comprehensive home assessment (i.e., gerontological nurse practitioner, physical or occupational therapist)

Sources: AGS/BGS Clinical Practice Guideline, *Prevention of Falls in Older Persons (2010)*, http://www.americangeriatrics.org/health_care_professionals/clinical_practice/clinical_guidelines_recommendations/2010/; Kane et al., 2009.

quality index (Buysse, Reynolds, Monk, Berman, & Kupfer, 1989). They are available from the Hartford Institute for Geriatric Nursing at ConsultGeriRN.org.

Pain Assessment

One in five people age 65 and older experience chronic pain, especially pain related to musculoskeletal disorders (spinal stenosis, osteoporosis with compression fractures, osteoarthritis, degenerative disk disease), cancer, and neuropathic disorders. A subjective pain assessment should be included in the history. Pain assessment is an ongoing process (Hadjistavropoulos et al., 2007) that should be addressed at each encounter. Pain scales can be helpful to quantify pain for evaluation of interventions aimed at alleviating or reducing pain to a tolerable level. Pain assessment can be more complicated in person with dementia. Asking a family member may help, but other things to assess include change in facial expression, body movements, interaction with others, mental status, and activity level (Herr, 2010).

Cognitive Assessment

Impaired memory is frequently one of the first signs of Alzheimer's disease, but not all women who complain of memory problems have Alzheimer's disease. However, early evaluation has many benefits, such as early treatment to slow the progression of the disease, preparation of advanced directives, and addressing care issues as the disease progresses. An evaluation of cognitive function should be considered in women who present with complaints about their memory, family members who report a change in their loved ones' memory, or if the clinician identifies that there may be a problem based on conversations with the woman, missed appointments that the woman does not recall, or making medication errors. Evaluation should include laboratory studies to assess for reversible causes such a thyroid disease, metabolic disturbances, anemia, or vitamin B_{12} deficiency, evaluation of medications, and assessment for depression. It is also important to identify if acute mental status changes (delirium) may be contributing to the woman's presentation (Ebersole et al., 2008). Clinicians may be challenged with distinguishing between normal aging memory changes and a neurodegenerative disease. Many standardized screening tools are available at ConsultGeriRN.org for clinicians to screen for problems. When possible memory impairment is suspected, neuropsychological evaluation may prove beneficial to assist with diagnostic determination.

PHYSICAL EXAMINATION

OVERVIEW

Although components of a comprehensive geriatric assessment should include physical, psychological, and socioeconomic interrelated complex factors that can impact health and functional status of older women, this section will focus only on gynecological changes in older women. However, these other issues should be considered during the physical examination. The most obvious gynecological change that older women experience is menopause, which is covered at length in Chapter 18. Once menopause occurs, estrogen levels dramatically decrease and remain low for the rest of the women's life. A low estrogen level has many physical and physiological effects; however, these may be minimized if women take hormone replacement therapy.

- Vaginal tissues become thin and less elastic, and the vagina narrows and shortens and there is less lubrication; many women may experience atrophic vaginitis due to this change.
- Pubic hair becomes sparse and gray.
- Labia and clitoris become thin, pale, and dry (from the loss of lubrication), making sexual intercourse painful.
- Uterus decreases in size to about half the size of the woman's fist postmenopausally, making it challenging to palpate; the ligaments and connective tissue of the pelvis sometimes lose elasticity and tone leading to prolapse of the uterus; the ovaries and fallopian tubes atrophy; the cervix, urethra, and trigone of the bladder atrophy (Bellino, 2007). If there is significant vagina stenosis, then the clinician should consider using a one-finger bimanual examination.
- Breasts become less firm, and somewhat pendulous.
- Glandular tissue in the breast is gradually replaced by fat and Cooper's ligaments no longer support the lobular shape of the breast.
- The ducts near the areola become less elastic and palpation may reveal firm string-like structures.
- The level of circulating androgens is no longer opposed by estrogen causing the skin to become to become more coarse and hirsutism may develop on the face (lip and chin), chest, abdomen, and back.
- Older women may experience a change in sexual responses, taking longer to become aroused and to produce vaginal lubricant.
- The clitoris remains an important aspect of orgasm, but may become more irritated because clitoral blood is less protective (Duffy, 1998).

- Older women continue to need intimacy and may continue to engage in sexual activities. Dyspareunia (painful intercourse) due to deceased lubricant, extension of the labia, and lack of elevation of the uterus during sexual arousal may occur. During the exam, the clinician should discuss sexual activity, transmission of sexually transmitted diseases (if appropriate), and ways to reduce dyspareunia. In addition, discussing alternative expressions of intimacy can be suggested (Tabloski, 2010).

Although there are changes to the bladder and urethra that increase the risk for urinary tract infections and urinary incontinence (UI), UI is not a normal part of aging. The detrus or muscles become less contractile and somewhat unstable. This leads to difficulty completely emptying the bladder and involuntary contractions of the bladder (Ouslander & Johnson, 2003). Urethral changes are due to the low estrogen levels. In addition, the sphincter muscle becomes thinner and less able to resist the pressure of urine. Older women may not present with the same symptoms of a urinary tract infection as younger women; instead, they may experience a new onset of urinary frequency or incontinence, or altered mental status that warrants evaluation.

Urinary incontinence is the most prevalent symptom encountered by older women; women are twice as likely to experience UI as men (Mason, Newman, & Palmer, 2003). So it is important to assess for various forms of incontinence such as:

- Stress incontinence: loss of urine with increased intra-abdominal pressure, such as sneezing, laughing, or exercising
- Urge incontinence: overactive bladder ("got to go")
- Functional incontinence: unable to get to the bathroom (i.e., wheelchair bound, persons with dementia, and frail older persons)

GENERAL SURVEY

Guidelines for Routine Examination and Testing

Recommendations from the American College of Obstetricians and Gynecologists (2011) for periodic assessment in women over age 65 include the following:

- *Physical exam:* height, weight, body mass index, blood pressure, oral cavity, neck adenopathy, thyroid, breast (encourage breast self-examination), axillae, abdomen, pelvic exam (if a woman's age or other health issues may cause her to choose no interventions if something were to be detected, then the clinician may decide not to perform this evaluation), and skin
- *Laboratory testing:* bone mineral density (screen no more than every 2 years); cervical cytology (consider discontinuing at age 65 or 70 years if the woman has had three or more normal results in a row, or no abnormal results in 10 years, no history of cervical cancer or diethylstilbestrol exposure in utero, and is HIV negative); if discontinued, then the clinician should evaluate risk factors on an annual basis and reinstitute screening if necessary. Colorectal screening every 10 years, fasting glucose every 3 years, lipid profile every 5 years, mammography, TSH every 5 years, urinalysis. If high risk, then hemoglobin, hepatitis C, HIV, STD testing, TB skin test
- *Evaluation and counseling:* sexuality, fitness and evaluation, psychosocial evaluation, cardiovascular risk factors (diabetes mellitus, hypertension, dyslipidemia, obesity, sedentary lifestyle), health/risk behaviors, and immunizations (these were covered previously in this chapter)

Guidelines for General Education and Anticipatory Guidance

Although many older women may live long healthy lives, as a woman ages there are many risk factors that could lead to poor health outcomes. Therefore, it is critical that the clinician consider the risk factors that have been described in this chapter and proactively implement strategies aimed at reducing the risk. Consultation with other disciplines, such as gerontological experts, may assist the clinician in making evidence-based clinical decisions.

CONCLUSION

This chapter provides an overview of how to asses older women (≥65) and is not meant to be all inclusive of the many health problems older adults may face. What is important is that clinicians consider health promotion and preventative measures to improve health outcomes of older women. It is critical to consider physical, psychological, socioeconomic, and functional status when conducting a health history and physical examination. In addition, differentiating between what is normal and what is not, considering patient/family preferences and wishes, and what the outcome of the intervention may be are crucial aspects of the shared decision-making process (between clinicians and patient/family).

REFERENCES

Administration on Aging. (2010). *A profile of older Americans*. Retrieved June 16, 2011, from www.aoa.gov/aoaroot/aging-statistics/Profile/2010/docs/2010profile.pdf

Albert, S.M., & Freedman, V.A. (2010). *Public health and aging: Maximizing function and well-being* (2nd ed.). New York: Springer Publishing Company.

American College of Obstetricians and Gynecologists (ACOG) Committee Opinion. (2011). *Primary and preventive care: Periodic assessments* (No. 483). *Obstetrics & Gynecology, 117*(4), 1008–1015.

American Dietetic Association (ADA). (2005). Position statement of the American Dietetic Association: Liberalization of the diet prescription improves quality of life for older adults in long-term care. *Journal of the American Dietetic Association, 105,* 1955–1965.

American Geriatric Society (2010) AGS/BGS Clinical Practice Guideline: *Prevention of Falls in Older Persons* retrieved from: http://www.americangeriatrics.org/health_care_professionals/clinical_practice/clinical_guidelines_recommendations/2010/

American Nurses Association. (2010). *Gerontological Nursing: Scope and standards of practice*. Silver Spring, MD: Nursesbooks.org.

Ancoli-Israel, S., & Ayalon, L. (2006). Diagnosis and treatment of sleep disorders in older adults. *American Journal of Geriatric Psychiatry, 14*(2), 95–103.

Antonucci, T.C., & Akiyama, H. (1987). Social networks in adult life and a preliminary examination of the convoy model. *Journal of Gerontology, 42,* 519–527.

Beasley, J.M., LaCroix, A.Z., Neuhouser, M.L., Huang, Y., Tinker, L., Woods, N., et al. (2010). Protein intake and incident frailty in the Women's Health Initiative Observational Study. *Journal of the American Geriatrics Society, 58,* 1063–1071.

Bellino, E. (2007). Female reproductive aging and menopause. In P.S. Timiras (Ed.), *Physiological basis of aging and geriatrics* (4th ed., pp. 160–184). New York: Inform Healthcare.

Berman, J., & Furst, L.M. (2011). *Depressed older adults: Education and screening*. New York: Springer Publishing Company.

Bickley, L.S. (2007). *Bate's guide to physical examination and history taking* (9th ed.). Philadelphia: Lippincott Williams & Wilkins.

Biggs, A.J. (2007). Nutritional considerations. In A.D. Linton & H.W. Lach (Eds.), *Matteson & McConnell's gerontological nursing* (3rd ed., pp. 161–197). St. Louis, MO: Saunders.

Burnside, I.M. (1971). Loneliness in old age. *Mental Hygiene, 33*(3), 391–397.

Buysse, D.J., Reynolds, C.F., Monk, T.H., Berman, S.R., & Kupfer, D.J. (1989). The Pittsburgh Sleep Quality Index: A new instrument for psychiatric practice and research. *Psychiatry Research, 28*(2), 193–213.

Centers for Disease Control and Prevention (CDC). (2011). Healthy aging: Helping people to live long and productive lives and enjoy a good quality of life. *At a Glance 2011*. Retrieved from http://www.cdc.gove/chronicdisease/resources/publications/AG/aging.htm

Chapman, J.M. (2006). Nutritional disorders in the elderly. *Medical Clinics of North America, 90,* 887–907.

Cottrell, L. (1942). The adjustment of the individual to his age and sex roles. *American Sociological Review, 7,* 617–620.

Demers, K. (2007). Hearing screening in older adults: A brief hearing loss screener. Try this: Best practice in nursing care of older adults. *Hartford Institute for Geriatric Nursing*, p. 12.

Duffy, L.M. (1998). Lovers, loners, and lifers: Sexuality and the older adult. *Geriatrics, 53*(Suppl. 1), S66–S69.

Ebersole, P., Hess, P., Touhy, T., Jett, K., & Luggen, A.S. (2008). *Toward healthy aging: Human needs & nursing response* (7th ed.). St. Louis, MO: Mosby Elsevier.

Erikson, E.H. (1950). *Childhood and society*. New York: Norton.

Fabre, J.M., Ellis, R., Kosma, M., & Wood, R.H. (2010). Falls risk factors and a compendium of falls risk screening instruments. *Journal of Geriatric Physical Therapy, 33,* 184–197.

Federal Interagency Forum on Aging-Related Statistics. (2010, July). *Older Americans 2010: Key indicators of well-being*. Washington, DC: U.S. Government Printing Office. Retrieved June 2011 from http://www.agingstats.gov/Main_Site/Data/2010_Documents/docs/Introduction.pdf

Gaffney-Stomberg, E., Insogna, K.L., Rodriguez, N.R., & Kerstetter, J.E. (2009). Increasing dietary protein requirements in elderly people for optimal muscle and bone health. *Journal of American Geriatrics Society, 57,* 1073–1079.

Gallagher, L.P. (2001). The potential for adverse drug reactions in elderly patients. *Applied Nursing Research, 14*(4), 221–224.

Gambert, S.R., & Pinkstaff, S. (2006). Emerging epidemic: Diabetes in older adults: Demography, economic impact, and pathophysiology. *Diabetes Spectrum, 19*(4), 221–228.

Hadjistavropoulos, T., Herr, K., Turk, D., Fine, P., Dworkin, R.H., Helme, R., et al. (2007). An interdisciplinary expert consensus statement on assessment of pain in older persons. *Clinical Journal of Pain, 23*, S1–S43.

Halter, J.B., Ouslander, J.G., Tinetti, M.E., Studenski, S., High, K.P., & Asthana, S. (2009). *Hazzard's geriatric medicine and gerontology* (6th ed.). New York: McGraw Medical.

Hendrich, A.L., Bender, P.S., & Nyhuis, A. (2003). Validation of the Hendrich II Fall Risk Model: A large concurrent CASE/control study of hospitalized patients. *Applied Nursing Research, 16*(1), 9–21.

Herr, K. (2010). Pain in the older adult: All imperative across all health care settings. *Pain Management in Nursing, 11*(2), S1–S10.

Hicks, T.J. (2000). What is your life like now? Loneliness and elderly individuals residing in nursing home. *Journal of Gerontological Nursing, 26,* 15–19.

Hooyman, N.R., & Kiyak, A.H. (2011). *Social gerontology: A multidisciplinary perspective* (9th ed.). Boston: Allyn & Bacon.

Inouye, S.K., & Charpentier, P.A. (1996). Precipitating factors for decline in hospitalized patients. *Journal of American Medical Association, 275*(11), 852–857.

Kane, R.L., Ouslander, J.G., Abrass, H.B., & Resnick, B. (2009). *Essentials of clinical geriatrics* (6th ed.). New York: McGraw-Hill Medical.

Krause, N. (2001). Social support. In R.H. Binstock & L.K. George (Eds.), *Handbook of aging and the social sciences* (5th ed., pp. 272–294). San Diego: Academic Press.

Maddox, G. (1963). Activity and moral: A longitudinal study of selected elderly subjects. *Social Forces, 42,* 195.

Marshall, V.W. (1996). The state of theory in aging and the social sciences. In R.H. Binstock & L.K. George (Eds.), *Handbook of aging and the social sciences* (4th ed., pp. 11–26). San Diego, CA: Academic Press.

Maslow, A. (1954). *Motivation and personality*. New York: Harper & Row.

Mason, D.J., Newman, D.K., & Palmer, M.H. (2003). Changing UI practice. *American Journal of Nursing, 103*(3), 129.

Morgan, L.A., & Kunkel, S.R. (2011). *Aging, society, and the life course* (4th ed.). New York: Springer Publishing Company.

National Osteoporosis Foundation. (2011). *Fast facts*. Retrieved September 5, 2011, from http://www.nof.org/node/40

Office of Dietary Supplements, National Institutes of Health. (2011). *Dietary supplement fact sheet: Vitamin D*. Retrieved July 20, 2011, from http://ods.od.nih.gov/factsheets/VitaminD/

Ouslander, J.G., & Johnson, T.M. (2003). Incontinence. In W.R. Hazzard, J.P. Blass, J.B. Halter, J.G. Ouslander, & M.E. Tinetti (Eds.), *Principle of geriatric medicine and gerontology* (5th ed., pp. 1571–1586). New York: McGraw-Hill.

Papas, E., & Cluxton, R.J. (2011). Vitamin D: Beneficial for pain, fracture, and falls in long-term care residents? *Annals of Long Term Care, 19*(5), 33–36.

Phillips, B., & Ancoli-Israel, S. (2001). Sleep disorders in the elderly. *Sleep Medicine, 2*, 99–114.

Resnick, B., Corcoran, M., & Spellbring, A.M. (2001). Gait and balance disorders. In A.M. Adelman & M.P. Daly (Eds.), *Twenty common problems in geriatrics* (pp. 277–307). New York: McGraw-Hill.

Ries, L.A.G., Eisner, M.P., Kosary, C.L., Hankey, B.F., Miller, B.A., Clegg, L., et al. (Eds.). (2002). *SEER cancer statistics review, 1973–1999*. Bethesda, MD: National Cancer Institute. Retrieved September 12, 2011, from http://seer.cancer.gov/csr/1973_1999/

Sager, M.A., Rudberg, M.A., Jalaloddin, M., Franks, T., Inouye, S.K., Landfeld, C.S., et al. (1996). Hospital admission risk profile (HARP) identifying older patients at risk for functional decline following an acute hospitalization. *Journal of the American Geriatrics Society, 44,* 251–257.

Saxon, S.V., Etten, M.J., & Perkins, E.A. (2010). *Physical change & aging: A guide for helping professions* (5th ed.). New York: Springer Publishing Company.

Shaughnessy, A.F. (1992). Common drug interactions in the elderly. *Emergency Medicine, 24*(21), 21.

Smilkstein, G. (1978). The family APGAR: A proposal for a family function test and its use by physicians. *Journal of Family Practice, 6*(6), 1231–1239.

Tabloski, P.A. (2010). *Gerontological nursing* (2nd ed.). Upper Saddle River, NJ: Pearson.

Tufts University Health and Nutrition Newsletter. (2008). *26*(5), 1–4.

Zhu, K., Austin, N., Devine, A., Bruce, D., & Prince, R.L. (2010). A randomized controlled trial of the effects of vitamin D on muscle strength and mobility of older women with vitamin D insufficiency. *Journal of American Geriatric Society, 58,* 2063–2068.

II ❖ Promotion of Wellness for Women

CHAPTER ❖ 7

WOMEN AND SEXUALITY

Melissa A. Dahir

All women deserve to be able to feel safe in expression of their sexuality, have access to knowledge to dispel myths, treatments to address problems, and live free from sexual degradation and violence.

Highlights

- Working Definitions
- Evolution of Sexual Response Cycles: Linear to Circular
- Female Sexual Dysfunction Classification

❖ INTRODUCTION

Sexuality is an essential and important component of a woman's biological lifecycle. A woman's sexuality emerges from early sexual relationships, evolves, and continues to evolve past menopause. When this cycle has been interrupted, a woman's identity, health, and well-being are affected. According the World Health Organization's (WHO) International Classifications of Diseases-10 (ICD-10) (1992), sexual dysfunction occurs when a woman is not able to engage in a sexual relationship as she desires.

In 1998, the Food and Drug Administration (FDA) approved sildenafil (Viagra) as the first oral medication for the treatment of male erectile dysfunction (ED). After the approval, Pfizer launched an Erectile Dysfunction Awareness Campaign; television commercials featured former Senator Bob Dole encouraging men to discuss treatment options for ED with their physicians. As a result, primary care physicians and urologists were bombarded with men inquiring about Viagra—the magical "blue pill." The blockbuster success of Viagra for men propelled a strong medical interest in female sexual dysfunction (FSD) in hopes of discovering a magical "pink pill" for women.

Multiple factors can contribute to FSD such as psychogenic, physical, mixed, or unknown causes (Women's Sexual Health Foundation, 2005). Psychogenic factors include a woman's lack of knowledge about her own body, a lack of knowledge about the sexual response cycle, personal religious beliefs and religious upbringing, social pressures, a history of sexual abuse, negative sexual experiences, unrealistic expectations, resentment toward a partner, and relationship conflict. Physical factors include medications (birth control pills [BCPs], antidepressants, chemotherapy); chronic illness or disease (diabetes mellitus, coronary artery disease, cancer, hypothyroidism, depression, spinal cord injury); and other processes such as childbirth, menopause, and oophorectomy.

The International Society for the Study of Women's Sexual Health (ISSWSH) is the leading international organization committed to women's sexual health and advancing the field of female sexuality. It advocates a collaborative approach in the assessment, diagnosis, and treatment of women with sexual health problems. It composed the following Women's Initiative on Sexual Health (WISH) position statement on FSD:

> Female sexual disorders are valid conditions that warrant assessment, diagnosis and appropriate therapeutic intervention. The etiology of female sexual problems is often complex. It may include sexual medicine issues related to biologic etiologies including neurologic, hormonal, vascular and anatomic components as well as psychological issues relating to socio-cultural, emotional, cognitive and relationship concerns. We are aware that female sexual dysfunction research is still a relatively new field and continuing research is needed to further elucidate the etiological factors that contribute to female sexual disorders. We advocate the development of safe and effective treatments, both biological and psychosocial-cultural in nature, for women who are suffering from these conditions. Although not all treatments will work equally for everyone, women deserve to have a variety of treatment options and for their voices to be heard. In light of this, we call upon all the stakeholders, including government regulators, to move the bar of available therapies forward. (www.isswsh.org/resources/Positions/docs/Womens Initiative on Sexual Health.pdf).

WORKING DEFINITIONS

Many experts do not agree on what constitutes "normal" sexual health. In January 2002, a group of working definitions was developed after a WHO conference, and the definitions have been updated as experts throughout the world engaged in discussions about sexual health. (Although the following definitions are available on the WHO website [www.who.org], they do not represent an official WHO position.)

> **Sex**
>
> Sex refers to the biological characteristics that define humans as female or male. While these sets of biological characteristics are not mutually exclusive, as there are individuals who possess both, they tend to

differentiate humans as males and females. In general use in many languages, the term sex is often used to mean "sexual activity," but for technical purposes in the context of sexuality and sexual health discussions, the above definition is preferred.

Sexuality

Sexuality is a central aspect of being human throughout life and encompasses sex, gender identities and roles, sexual orientation, eroticism, pleasure, intimacy and reproduction. Sexuality is experienced and expressed in thoughts, fantasies, desires, beliefs, attitudes, values, behaviours, practices, roles and relationships. While sexuality can include all of these dimensions, not all of them are always experienced or expressed. Sexuality is influenced by the interaction of biological, psychological, social, economic, political, cultural, ethical, legal, historical, religious and spiritual factors.

Sexual health

Sexual health is a state of physical, emotional, mental and social well-being in relation to sexuality; it is not merely the absence of disease, dysfunction or infirmity. Sexual health requires a positive and respectful approach to sexuality and sexual relationships, as well as the possibility of having pleasurable and safe sexual experiences, free of coercion, discrimination and violence. For sexual health to be attained and maintained, the sexual rights of all persons must be respected, protected and fulfilled.

Sexual rights

Sexual rights embrace human rights that are already recognized in national laws, international human rights documents and other consensus statements. They include the right of all persons, free of coercion, discrimination and violence, to:

- the highest attainable standard of sexual health, including access to sexual and reproductive health care services;
- seek, receive and impart information related to sexuality;
- sexuality education;
- respect for bodily integrity;
- choose their partner;
- decide to be sexually active or not;
- consensual sexual relations;
- consensual marriage;
- decide whether or not, and when, to have children; and
- pursue a satisfying, safe and pleasurable sexual life.

EVOLUTION OF SEXUAL RESPONSE CYCLES: LINEAR TO CIRCULAR

ALFRED KINSEY

One of the earliest sexologists in American history was Alfred Kinsey. In the early 1900s, Kinsey was a biology and zoology instructor at Harvard University, where he became interested in the taxonomy of gall wasps. In the 1920s, Kinsey continued to study gall wasps and was an assistant professor at Indiana University. In 1938, Kinsey's interest in gall wasps shifted and transitioned to human sexuality when he taught a course on marriage. The marital class quickly gained popularity because it was a place for students to inquire about their sexuality. It was believed that Kinsey's taxonomic technique used to classify gall wasps crossed over into how he studied human sexuality. Kinsey objectively categorized human sexual behavior without making value judgments—the same way a biologist would study the sexual behavior in animals (Rosen & Rosen, 2006).

In 1953, Kinsey, Pomeroy, Martin, and Gebhard published *Sexual Behavior in the Human Female*. The book was controversial because it removed the moral element of female sexuality and analyzed it scientifically. The public and scientific communities were offended by Kinsey's strong views. For example, Kinsey rejected the Victorian view that women who engage in masturbation are unhealthy and dangerous. He noticed a consistent correlation in which women who masturbated before getting married were more likely to reach orgasm during intercourse after being married. Kinsey concluded that sexual behavior and the physiology of orgasm were essentially the same in men and women. *Sexual Behavior in the Human Female* and the Kinsey project containing almost 5,000 female sexual histories remain some of the most reliable accounts of sexual behavior in America today.

LINEAR MODELS OF SEXUAL RESPONSE

In the 1950s, William Masters and Virginia Johnson studied the sexual response cycle of men and women through direct laboratory observation. Masters was trained in obstetrics and gynecology, and Johnson was trained in psychology and sociology. In 1966, Masters and Johnson were the first sexologists to publish a summary of the female sexual response cycle in their groundbreaking book *Human Sexual Response*. The book comprised more than 10 years of data, including more than 14,000 sexual encounters and 10,000 human orgasms. Through direct observation, Masters and Johnson discovered similarities in sexual physiology among both sexes. They also explained the role of vaginal lubrication and the physiology of multiple orgasms. As a result, a linear sexual response cycle known as the "four-stage model" was proposed in which each phase occurs in a progressively orderly fashion: excitement, plateau, orgasm, and resolution.

Sex therapist Helen Singer Kaplan founded the first clinic for sexual disorders located within a medical school in the United States. In 1970, she founded the Human Sexuality Program at the Payne Whitney Clinic (Saxon, 1995). In 1974, Kaplan published *The New Sex Therapy* and began work on a new linear model. Kaplan modified Masters and Johnson's four-stage model because it was based on physical stimulation. Masters and Johnson had excluded sexual desire from their model; they felt it was subjective, and therefore, not measurable. In 1979, Kaplan published *Disorders of Sexual Desire* and proposed the idea that the psychological component of sexual desire influences the overall sexual response cycle and a woman's sexual drive is the motivation for engaging in sexual activity. Kaplan dichotomized Masters and Johnson's first stage of excitement into desire and arousal and eliminated the plateau and resolution stages. The result was a three-stage linear model comprised of desire, arousal, and orgasm.

In summary, the models proposed by Masters and Johnson and Kaplan were the first depictions of female sexual response. Both models were linear with sequential stages in which one stage preceded the next under normal circumstances. However, as sexual health experts attained a deeper understanding of female sexual response, Kaplan's model seemed too simplistic because it did not include the emotional desire for intimacy and other motivations. In 1991, Beck, Bozman, and Qualtrough evaluated the role of sexual desire in a woman's sexual experience. They discovered initial desire was absent in 66 percent of women less than 25 years of age and absent in 97 percent of women greater than or equal to 25 years of age.

CIRCULAR MODEL OF SEXUAL RESPONSE: AN UPDATED MODEL

In the new millennium, Rosemary Basson (2000, 2001a, 2001b, 2004) redefined the female model of sexual response based on a deeper understanding of sexuality and advances in research (Beck et al., 1991; Tiefer, 1991; Tiefer, Hall, & Tavris, 2002). Basson (2001b) proposed a "circular" model in which female sexual response is affected by emotional intimacy, sexual stimuli, and relationship satisfaction. In the circular model, all women begin in sexually neutral position until motivated to engage in sexual activity; the combination of psychological and physiological functioning allows for the phases to overlap and occur more than once during a single sexual experience.

Unlike Kaplan's 1979 linear model where sexual desire is present initially, Basson's (2001b) model is more complex and suggests that women have many reasons for engaging in sexual activity. This includes physical, emotional, and cognitive feedback as possible triggers for sexual desire. Sexual desire may or may not be initially present, and the motivation for future sexual activity is affected by sexual and nonsexual outcomes. Past sexual experiences with positive rewards such as emotional closeness or increased commitment can also stimulate sexual desire and motivation to initiate sexual activity in the future.

Research validates that women engage in sexual activity for a variety of personal reasons and incentives, especially in long-term relationships (Basson, Wierman, van Lankveld, & Brotto, 2010; Cain, Johannes, & Avis, 2003). In 2003, a community-based study by Cain and colleagues discovered the most common reasons for engaging in sexual activity included expressing love, relieving tension, because their partner initiated, and for pleasure. In 2007, Meston and Buss surveyed 1,287 undergraduate students and community volunteers on reasons for engaging in sexual activity. They identified 237 reasons including desire, spirituality, altruism, and revenge. They also reported the following primary factors for motivation: physical, goal attainment, emotional, and insecurity.

Responsive sexual desire is described as a longing for sexual activity to continue or become more intensified (Basson, 2000). Therefore, sexual activity may precipitate a woman's physical and subjective arousal, and in turn, trigger "responsive" desire (Basson, 2004). Finally, receptivity is affected by a combination of biological and psychological influences. When these factors affect the mind's ability to process sexual information, subjective arousal is inhibited. Examples of biological factors include fatigue, depression, or medication side effects. Examples of psychological factors include a fear of intercourse causing pain, the fear of an unwanted pregnancy, past negative sexual experiences, or feelings of shame (Basson, 2001a; Graham, Sanders, Milhausen, & McBride, 2004). See Figure 7–1 for a graphic depiction of Basson's model.

FEMALE SEXUAL DYSFUNCTION CLASSIFICATION

The two most commonly used classification systems for FSD are the WHO's ICD-10 (1992) and the American Psychiatric Association's (APA) *Diagnostic and*

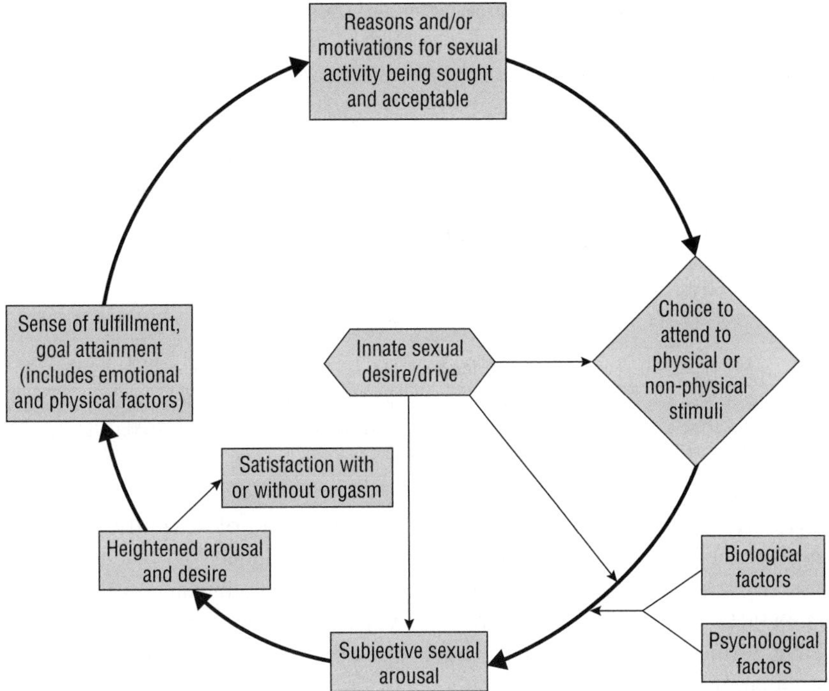

FIGURE 7–1. Basson's Model of Female Sexual Response. *Adapted from:* Association of Reproductive Health Professionals, 2008; Basson et al., 2001; Parish, 2009.

Statistical Manual of Mental Disorders, text revision (*DSM-IV-TR*) (2000). Both classification systems use four categories: sexual desire disorder, sexual arousal disorder, sexual pain disorders, and orgasmic disorder. The ICD-10 focuses on physical factors that affect sexual response. The *DSM-IV-TR* involves the emotional and psychological factors that affect sexual response and classifies sexual disorders by onset (lifelong or acquired), context (generalized or situational), and etiology (psychological or combined).

A major criticism to the ICD-10 and *DSM-IV-TR* sexual disorder classifications is that they both reflect a linear model of sexual response, which is thought to be more representative of men than women (Basson et al., 2003; Bean, 2002). In addition, many sexual health experts believe the ICD-10 and *DSM-IV-TR* definitions of FSD are unacceptable because they do not encompass women's authentic sexual encounters and do not reflect current trends in research.

In 2000, the American Foundation for Urologic Diseases (AFUD) sponsored the International Consensus Panel on women's sexual dysfunction to redefine the categories of desire, orgasm, and sexual pain. The categories (as previously used in the ICD-10 and *DSM-IV-TR*) were expanded to include biological (organic) factors in addition to psychological causes. The AFUD omitted the criterion for interpersonal distress and added personal distress as a diagnostic criterion. The AFUD classification system for FSD is also based on the traditional linear model (see Table 7–1).

New recommendations for the 2012 publication of *DSM-V* have been proposed for the categories of hypoactive sexual desire disorder (HSDD) and female sexual arousal disorder (FSAD). The current definition of HSDD views an absence of sexual fantasies as an indicator of sexual dysfunction, but sexual fantasies have not been shown to influence a woman's sexual desire (Brotto, Heiman, & Tolman, 2009). Research suggests that spontaneous sexual thoughts of sexual fantasies may occur in a new relationship, but is less common in long-term relationships (Meston & Buss, 2007). It has been recommended that the new definition include other sexual motivational incentives for sexual desire such as the need to feel tenderness and appreciation for her partner is derived from a sexually motivated incentive in which subjective desire is only one of many different components (Basson et al., 2010; Meston & Buss, 2007). Also, because a lack of sexual desire can occur in any phase of Basson's sexual response cycle, experts have recommended that the definition of HSDD included the recurrent, or consistent, inability to experience sexual arousal or desire (Basson & Schultz, 2007).

TABLE 7–1. American Foundation for Urologic Diseases Female Sexual Dysfunction Classification and Definitions

Sexual desire disorders	
Hypoactive sexual desire disorder	Absence of sexual fantasies, thoughts, and/or desire for, or receptivity to, sexual activity, which causes personal distress
Sexual aversion disorder	Phobic aversion to and avoidance of sexual contact with a sexual partner, which causes personal distress
Sexual arousal disorders	
Female sexual arousal disorder	Inability to attain or maintain sufficient sexual excitement, causing personal distress, which may be expressed as a lack of subjective excitement, or genital (lubrication/swelling) or other somatic responses
Orgasmic disorders	
Female orgasmic disorder	Delay in or absence of attaining orgasm following sufficient sexual stimulation and arousal, which causes personal distress
Sexual pain disorders	
Dyspareunia	Genital pain associated with sexual intercourse
Vaginismus	Involuntary spasm of the musculature of the outer third of the vagina that interferes with vaginal penetration, which causes personal distress
Noncoital pain	Genital pain induced by noncoital sexual stimulation

Source: Basson et al., (2000) Report of the international consensus development conference on female sexual dysfunction: Definitions and classifications. *Journal of Urology, 163*(3), 888–893.; Berman, J.R. (2005). Physiology of female sexual function and dysfunction. *International Journal of Impotence Research* 17, S44–S51. doi:10.1038/sj.ijir.3901428; Mimoun, S. & Wylie, K. (2009) Female sexual dysfunctions: Definitions and classification. *Maturitas*, "http://www.maturitas.org/issues?issue_key=S0378-5122%2809%29X0008-3" *63*(2), 116–118.

The current definition of FSAD focuses on "lubrication/swelling response" of the vaginal tissues, but women do not typically seek medical treatment for inadequate lubrication. In fact, healthy women diagnosed with FSAD usually have normal vasocongestion of the genitals with sexual stimulation. Therefore, the woman's perception of impaired arousal becomes the cause of her distress and not a result of impaired genital congestion. In addition, subjective and genital sexual arousal appears to be poorly correlated. Therefore, it is recommended that the four subtypes of FSAD (genital sexual arousal disorder, subjective arousal disorder, combined genital and subjective arousal disorder, and persistent genital arousal disorder) become distinguishable and the diagnostic foundation is based upon the woman's self-report of genital arousal and lubrication in addition to the identification of possible underlying pathology (e.g., atrophy of the vaginal tissues or vaginal infection) (Basson et al., 2010).

EPIDEMIOLOGY

In early reports, it has been suggested that up to 60 percent of women under the age of 60 experience some type of sexual dysfunction (Frank, Anderson, & Rubinstein, 1978). Limited data is available on the epidemiology of FSD. However, a few community studies have been published, and the results suggest that sexual dysfunction is more prevalent in women (25 to 63%) than men (10 to 52%) (Frank et al., 1978; Rosen, Taylor, Leiblum, & Bachmann, 1993; Spector & Carey, 1990). These findings have been supported by results from the 1992 National Health and Social Life Survey (NHSLS). The survey used a national probability sample that was demographically characteristic of sexually active adults in the United States. It included 1,410 men and 1,749 women ages 19 to 59. In 1999, Laumann, Paik, and Rosen analyzed the survey results and reported that sexual dysfunction is more prevalent in women (43%) than in men (31%). Analysis of the survey also offered insight into the prevalence of sexual dysfunction based on demographics such as marital status, education, and ethnicity. Women who were divorced, widowed, separated, or never married were at an increased risk of developing sexual dysfunction. Women who were not married were also 1.5 times more likely to have sexual anxiety and difficulty with orgasm functioning. Women with lower levels of education are more likely to experience problems with sexual functioning. In fact, female college graduates are less likely (about 50%) to experience HSDD, difficulty achieving climax, sexual anxiety, and dyspareunia. The correlation between FSD and race/ethnicity varied. Caucasian women were more likely to experience dyspareunia than African American women. In contrast, African American women reported lower sexual desire than Caucasian women. Hispanic women consistently reported lower rates of sexual issues in all categories when compared to other ethnic groups.

Laumann et al. (1999) identified the following lifestyle and health factors that increase the risk of sexual dysfunction: stress, urinary tract symptoms, lower socioeconomic status, and history of sexual abuse. Women who are emotionally stressed are more likely to experience problems with desire, arousal, and pain. Sexual pain and arousal disorders were commonly reported in women with irritative urinary tract symptoms, and women in poor health were more likely to report sexual pain. A decline in economic status and household income was associated with an increased risk for all categories of sexual dysfunction. Women with a history of sexual exploitation, such as childhood abuse by an adult perpetrator or coercion, are much more likely to experience problems with sexual arousal. Laumann et al. found that women in same-sex relationships did not have an increased risk for sexual dysfunction.

BARRIERS TO TREATMENT

The epidemiology results from Laumann et al. (1999) give strong evidence that there is a need to treat FSD. Many experts agree FSD is a prevalent problem with multifactorial causes that remain undiagnosed by health care providers (Bachmann, 2006). Women want to know that other women have similar issues to validate their concerns and be reassured they are not alone, but many are not comfortable approaching the subject with their health care provider (Feldhaus-Dahir, 2009a). A survey by Berman and colleagues (2003) found that up to 40 percent of women did not seek treatment for sexual dysfunction because they were too embarrassed, they thought their physician could not help, or they had never thought about seeking medical treatment for their sexual complaint. In women who did seek treatment for their sexual complaint, more than half of the women felt they were not thoroughly examined. In addition, less than a quarter of these women thought their health care provider performed appropriate medical tests, made a diagnosis, developed a treatment plan, and followed up with the patient.

Health care providers may not be comfortable or competent to appropriately manage women with sexual dysfunction. This may be due to inadequate clinical habits developed as students if their education did not include sexual health as an important component of the patient's medical history and examination (Feldhaus-Dahir, 2009a). Unfortunately, these poor habits often continue throughout one's medical career, which contributes to a cycle of misunderstanding and poor communication patterns with the patient and health care provider. When health care providers choose not to address sexual concerns among their patients, it contributes to the perception of sexual health as being unimportant. Therefore, many women have low expectations regarding their providers' ability to treat their sexual complaint (McGarvey, Peterson, Pinkerton, Keller, & Clayton, 2003). Marwick (1999) reported that women did not seek medical treatment because 75 percent believed their doctor would dismiss their complaint, and 68 percent were concerned about embarrassing their doctor. Marwick also found that primary health care physicians did not initiate discussions regarding sexual functioning due to time constraints, a lack of knowledge, inadequate training, and limited ability for referrals. Rosenqvist and Sarkadi (2001) validated Marwick's finding and found that primary health care providers did not initiate discussion about sexual functioning due to a lack of time, limited ability for secondary referrals, patient embarrassment, lack of knowledge, and inadequate training and skills due to lack of education.

In 2003, Solursh et al. conducted a survey of medical schools to evaluate how well physicians were prepared to address sexual dysfunction. It was found that more than half of the schools offered less than 10 hours of human sexuality, with the main focus on reproduction and sexually transmitted diseases. In 2005, Pauls et al. conducted a study to evaluate practice patterns regarding sexuality among members of the American Urogynecologic Society. In regard to training in FSD, it was reported that 50 percent of the respondents rated their training as unsatisfactory, and only 8 percent of the respondents were very satisfied with their training.

Ageism is another barrier to addressing sexual dysfunction. It is important to understand that sexual health is important throughout a woman's life span and not just during her reproductive years. Older adults are often labeled "asexual" based on societal beliefs. This stereotypical view provokes feelings of shame, embarrassment, and fear and hinders them from seeking medical treatment (Berman et al., 2003). Some health care professionals view aging and sexual problems as normal and irreversible, while others believe sexuality is a "life pleasure" and problems with sexuality are not serious or damaging to one's health.

Laumann et al. (2007) conducted a more recent survey of sexual activity, behaviors, and problems of men and women 57 to 85 years of age. They found the following prevalence rates among older women: 43 percent experienced low libido (HSDD), 39 percent had difficulty with vaginal lubrication (sexual arousal disorder), and 34 percent were unable to achieve orgasm (orgasmic disorder). In the highest age category of sexually active men and women (ages 75 to 85), 54 percent were sexually active two to three times per month, and 23 percent were sexually active at least once a week. Overall, 22 percent of the older women reported they had attempted discussing sexual issues with their physician since the age of 50. Laumann et al. concluded that contrary to beliefs, older adults are sexually active. Many older adults experience sexual problems, but they are infrequently discussed with their health care providers.

SEXUAL HEALTH ASSESSMENT

Health care professionals may find it challenging to discuss sexual issues with patients due to time constraints and a lack of formalized training. Most health care providers do not have difficulty discussing bowel movements with their patients, but many avoid discussing topics of a sexual nature based on their own cultural biases (Shell, 2007). Nurse practitioners, physician assistants, and physicians, regardless of their specialty, must proactively screen female patients for problems with sexual functioning through a comprehensive evaluation (Feldhaus-Dahir, 2009a). The discussion should take place in a private, comfortable setting while the patient is fully clothed. The evaluation should include a complete medical history to identify potential underlying medical conditions (see Table 7–2). Clinicians can practice role-playing with a colleague, a partner, or an existing patient to increase their comfort level in using sexual terminology and initiating a conversation regarding sexual functioning (Kingsberg & Janata, 2007).

Kingsberg and Janata (2007) proposed a brief model for FSD screening and suggest legitimizing the sexual issue so that patients feel comfortable in future discussion and normalize the screening by explaining that it is a normal part of the history and physical examination. They also suggest starting with asking the patient:

"Do you have any questions or concerns about your sexual health?"

If the patient responds:

- "None," the health care provider can respond, "Please feel free to ask me questions in the future."
- "Yes," the health care provider can ask more detailed questions:
  1. "Are you in a current sexual relationship?" If yes, "Do you have any problems in your relationship?" "Does your partner have any issues with sexual functioning?"
  2. "Do you have a history of physical, sexual, or emotional abuse?"
  3. "What major stressors do you have?"
  4. "Do you have difficulty with sexual interest (desire), lubrication (arousal), pain, or the ability to climax (orgasm)?" You can ask the patient to rate their sexual problem on a scale of 1 to 10.
  5. "How long have you been aware of the problem? Did it occur suddenly or gradually or has it always occurred?"
  6. "Is the sexual problem associated with a particular event or circumstance? Does it occur in certain situations or with certain partners?"

In addition, the algorithm proposed by Basson, Althof, et al. (2004) may be helpful in making a diagnosis (see Figure 7–2).

SCREENING TOOLS

The Female Sexual Function Index

The Female Sexual Function Index (FSFI) is a 19-item multidimensional self-report questionnaire and takes 10 to 15 minutes to complete. The FSFI uses a 5-point ordinal scale to assess six dimensions of sexual functioning: desire, arousal (physical and mental), lubrication, orgasm,

TABLE 7–2. Medical Conditions and Female Sexual Dysfunction

Medical Condition	Decreased Desire	Impaired Arousal	Impaired Orgasm	Pain
Depression	X			
Thyroid disease	X			
Diabetes		X	X	
Cardiovascular disease		X		
• Coronary artery disease				
• Myocardial infarction				
Neurological disease		X	X	
• Multiple sclerosis				
• Spinal cord injuries				
Androgen insufficiency	X			X
• Natural, surgical, or chemical menopause				
• Hormonal contraceptives				
Estrogen deficiency		X		X
• Natural, surgical, or chemical menopause				
• Hormonal contraceptives				

Source: Basson & Schultz, 2007; Kingsberg & Janata, 2007.

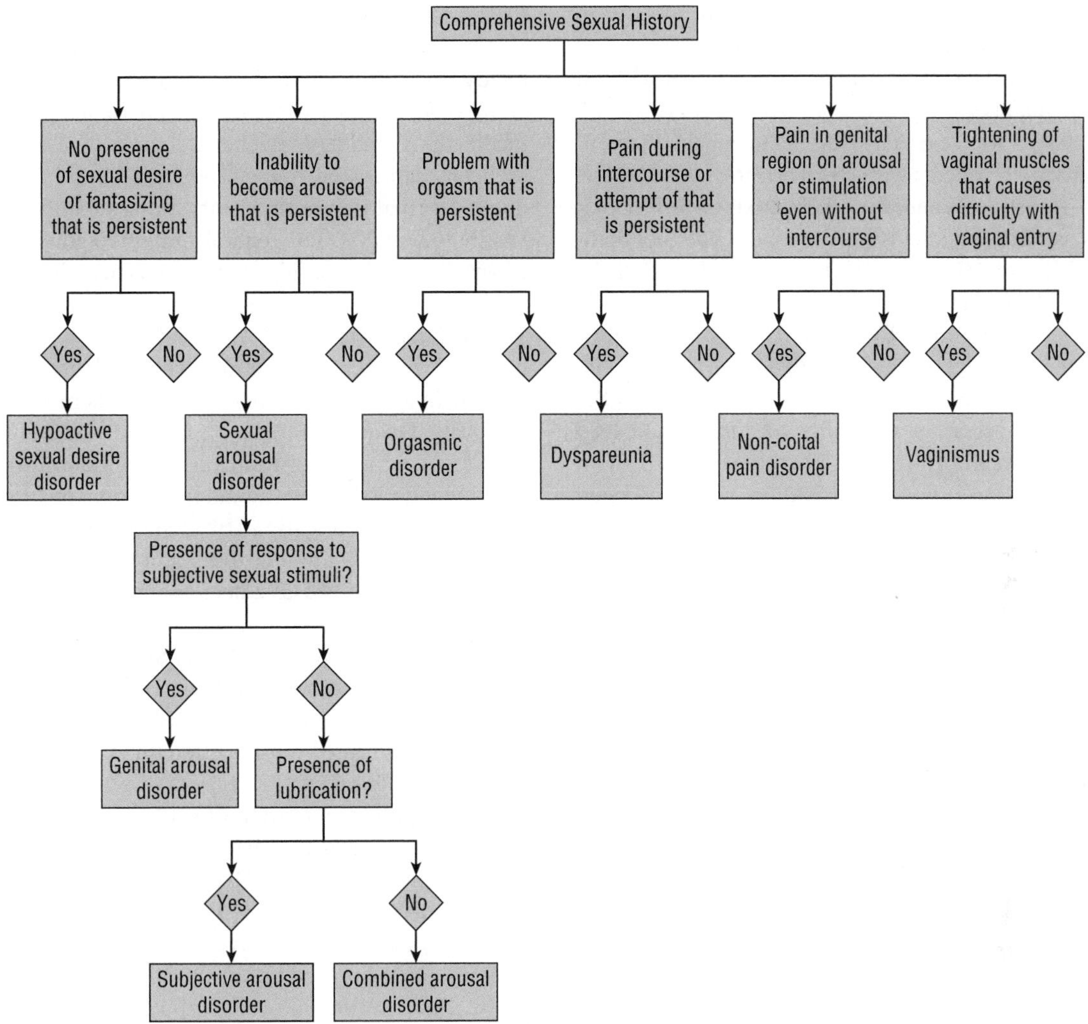

FIGURE 7–2. Algorithm for Diagnosing Female Sexual Dysfunction *Adapted from:* ACOG, 2010; Basson et al., 2004; Graziottin, Serafini & Palacios, 2009.

satisfaction, and pain over a 4-week period (Rosen et al., 2000). A score less than 26.5 indicates FSD. The FSFI tool has been used in clinical trials and community populations including multinational, heterosexual, and lesbian women. Reliability of the tool has been established through internal consistency (Cronbach's alpha ≥ 0.82) and test–retest reliability (r = 0.79–0.86). Discriminant and divergent validity of the tool has also been established. One criticism to the FSFI is that the tool is based on the modified linear sexual response cycle. Based on this model, a lack of initial desire is a determinant of sexual dysfunction and will result in a lower score (Hayes, 2011).

The FSFI questionnaire is free to use and can be accessed at http://www.fsfiquestionnaire.com (FSFI, 2000).

The Female Sexual Distress Scale

According to the AFUD, *DSM-IV-TR*, and ICD-10 criteria, personal distress must occur to diagnose a woman with FSD. The ability to measure female sexual distress has been increasingly important because the FDA has required the presence of personal distress as inclusion criteria in recent clinical drug trials for FSD (Sills et al., 2005). The Female Sexual Distress Scale (FSDS) is a 12-item self-report questionnaire and takes 10 to 15 minutes to complete (Derogatis, Rosen, Leiblum, Burnett, & Heiman, 2002). The FSDS uses a 4-point ordinal scale to assess a woman's distress in relation to her sexual functioning through quantitative measurement and is able to distinguish from healthy sexually functioning women. The validity has been established through clinical trials and population studies. Discriminant validity has been established in naturally and surgically postmenopausal women with HSDD when compared to women without sexual complaints.

The FSDS was revised (FSDS-R) to enhance screening sensitivity in patients with HSDD (Derogatis, Clayton, Lewis-D'Agostino, Wunderlich, & Fu, 2008). The FSDS-R includes an additional item: How often did you feel bothered by low sexual desire? Derogatis et al. tested the FSDS, FSDS-R, and FSDS-R item 13; both instruments demonstrated discriminant validity. There was a significantly higher recall period at 7 and 30 days in women with FSD or HSDD when compared to women without FSD ($p < 0.0001$). Test–retest reliability was also established in both instruments (intraclass correlation coefficient [ICC] > 0.74) and internal consistency was confirmed using Cronbach's alpha (> 0.86).

SEXUAL DESIRE DISORDER

Low sexual desire is also known as low libido and HSDD. HSDD is the most common type of FSD, and HSDD is more common in men than women. Laumann et al. (1999) reported a prevalence rate of 22 percent among women, compared to 5 percent among men. This was further supported by a large-scale international survey, the Global Study of Sexual Attitudes and Behaviors (GSSAB), in which 26 to 43 percent of women experienced HSDD compared to 13 to 28 percent of men (Gingell et al., 2005).

HSDD negatively impacts a woman's quality of life, physical and emotional satisfaction, and overall happiness (Laumann et al., 1999). In 2006, the Women's International Study of Health and Sexuality (WISHes) evaluated the effects of HSDD on the quality of life in women based on reproductive status and age. The WISHes study reported 24 to 36 percent of women ranging in age from 20 to 70 years experienced HSDD. In regard to reproductive status, younger surgically menopausal women (20 to 49 years of age) had significantly higher rates of HSDD compared to premenopausal women in the same age category (26% and 14%, respectively) (Barton, Koochaki, Leiblum, Rodenberg, & Rosen, 2006). Results from the WISHes study concluded that HSDD is prevalent among women of all ages, particularly among younger oophorectomized women.

It is difficult to assess the exact cause of HSDD because it is often complicated and multifactorial. The causes may be related to a number of physiological, psychological, environmental, and social factors (Nappi, Rosella, Schmitt, & Wawra, 2006). Other causes of HSDD include hormone imbalances related to pregnancy, the postpartum phase, and lactation; the use of certain medications such as antidepressants, psychiatrics medications, and beta blockers; chronic illnesses such as diabetes, depression, and cancer; and painful intercourse due to vaginal/pelvic floor conditions such as provoked vestibulodynia (PVD), generalized vulvodynia, endometriosis, interstitial cystitis, and urinary incontinence (Warnock, 2002). When interpersonal and sociological factors such as relationship conflict, sexual abuse, strict religious upbringing, and stress are involved, collaborative treatment with a mental health/sex therapist is recommended (Feldhaus-Dahir, 2009b).

Testosterone contributes to the initiation of sexual activity and modulates vaginal and clitoral engorgement, sensation, and lubrication (Brundu et al., 2003). A lack of testosterone is thought to be a contributing factor to HSDD because it causes a decrease in sexual receptivity, fatigue, lack of motivation, and overall reduced sense of well-being (Davis & Tran, 2001; Simon, 2002). Testosterone deficiency can also result in dysphoric mood (sadness, depression, anxiety, and irritability), hot flashes, bone loss, decreased muscle strength, and cognitive and memory changes (Lobo, 2001).

Androgens are a group of C19 steroids and include testosterone, androstenedione, dehydroepiandrosterone (DHEA), DHEA-sulfate (DHEA-S), and 5a-dihydrotestosterone (DHT) (Garcia-Banigan & Guay, 2005). Testosterone and DHT have the strongest androgenic activity. Women produce about 300 μg of testosterone daily. Testosterone is produced by the ovaries, by the adrenal glands, and through the peripheral conversion of androstenedione. Testosterone levels begin to decline for women in their late 20s and continue to decline at a steady rate (Bjornson, Sunley, Zussman, & Zussman, 1981). A bilaterateral oophorectomy (surgical removal of the ovaries) decreases testosterone production immediately by 50 percent and testosterone levels further decline even if a woman has an oophorectomy after menopause (Bjornson et al., 1981; Basaria & Dobs, 2006).

Women transitioning through menopause may experience HSDD due to a hormonal deficiency from the natural aging process and the use of hormone replacement therapy. During menopause, oral estrogen replacement is often prescribed to relieve hot flashes, mood changes, and sleep disturbances. However, oral estrogen replacement lowers testosterone levels and may contribute to HSDD (Abdallah & Simon, 2007). Oral estrogen increases circulating levels of sex hormone binding globulin (SHBG). SHBG is a protein that binds to testosterone and lowers the level of free testosterone. Therefore, the higher the level of SHBG, the lower the level of free testosterone. Oral estrogen also suppresses follicle-stimulating hormone (FSH) and luteinizing hormone (LH), which reduces ovarian synthesis and lowers total testosterone levels (Bowen, Klaiber, Simon, Wiita, & Yang, 1999; Buster et al., 1997). BCPs are also known to have the same lowering effect on testosterone levels. The exogenous estrogen also found in BCPs suppresses LH to prevent ovulation. As a result, ovarian production of testosterone is inhibited (Biggs, Clayton, Croft, Segraves, & Warnock, 2006). Therefore, the use of oral estrogen or hormonal contraceptives may be a contributing factor in HSDD.

The History of Testosterone

Testosterone has been used off-label in women since the turn of the century. In the early 1900s, clinicians prescribed testosterone based on clinical observation without controlled clinical trials, safety data, or the capability of measuring testosterone levels. Testosterone is not excreted in breast milk and has been used to treat fatigue, depression, and mastitis in lactating women (Glaser, Newman, Parsons, Zava, & Glaser-Garbrick, 2009). It has also been used to treat abnormal uterine bleeding, dysmenorrhea, benign and malignant tumors, and sexual dysfunction (Abel, 1945; Carter, Cohen, & Shorr, 1947; Kennedy & Nathanson, 1953; Salmon & Geist, 1943; Salmon, Geist, Gaines, & Walter, 1941; Sarrel, Dobay, & Wiita, 1998).

The off-label use of testosterone-only for the treatment of menopausal symptoms has been reported to be more efficacious than combination estrogen/testosterone and estrogen-only hormone replacement (Traish & Gooren, 2010).

Testosterone replacement does not require endometrial protection with subsequent progesterone replacement unless it is used with systemic estrogen (Perrone et al., 2009; Zang, Sahlin, Masironi, Eriksson, & Linden Hirschberg, 2007). Some view this as a benefit because it potentially avoids the slightly increased risk of breast cancer as previously reported in women who received synthetic progestin therapy (Campagnoli, Clavel-Chapelon, Kaaks, Peris, & Berrino, 2005).

Methyltestosterone is an anabolic steroid and a synthetic derivative of testosterone. In June 1974, the FDA approved methyltestosterone for the treatment of male androgen deficiency and female metastatic breast cancer. Methyltestosterone has also used off-label to treat dysmenorrhea, abnormal uterine bleeding, chronic mastitis, and female sexual dysfunction (Traish, Feeley, & Guay, 2009). There is limited research on the use of methyltestosterone for FSD. Penteado et al. (2008) published a study ($N = 60$) on the sexual effects of adding methyltestosterone to combined hormone replacement therapy (estrogen and progestogen). A significant improvement in sexual energy was reported with the addition of methyltestosterone ($p = 0.021$), but there was no effect on orgasm functioning.

Intrinsa is transdermal testosterone patch manufactured by Proctor & Gamble for the treatment of HSDD in postmenopausal women (Basaria & Dobs, 2006). Intrinsa has been approved for use in Europe, but it is not FDA approved in the United States. In December 2004, the FDA Advisory Committee reviewed clinical trial data and voted in favor of Intrinsa (14 to 3) based on its effectiveness. However, the FDA did not approve Intrinsa because they felt the 18-month clinical trial lacked safety data. The FDA recommended a large cardiovascular and breast safety study. The FDA has mandated a high standard for approving the use of testosterone in women for HSDD after adverse events occurred in patients taking Vioxx (Shames, Monroe, Davis, & Soule, 2007). Some medical professionals felt the FDA was apprehensive due to Women's Health Initiative (WHI). In regard to this statement, WHI published frightening results that triggered women and health care providers to discontinue the use of estrogen/progestin for fear that it would cause breast cancer. Unfortunately, WHI did not fully publicize the study's limitations such as a misrepresented sample of women ranging in age from 50 to 79. It also did not publicize that there was no increased risk of breast cancer when estradiol/progestin was used for 5 years or less, or that the absolute risk of breast cancer was an extra 4 to 6 additional invasive breast cancers per 10,000 women after 5 to 10 years of use. Also, WHI did not report that the estrogen-only arm actually had decreased risk of breast cancer when compared to the placebo-arm (Rossouw et al., 2002).

LibiGel (BioSante Pharmaceuticals, 2011) is a testosterone gel that is currently in the developmental stages for the treatment of HSDD in oophorectomized women. The LibiGel trials have been designed to show that the medication can increase women's sexual desire safely, increase the number of satisfying sexual encounters, and decrease personal distress from HSDD. The Phase II clinical trials revealed that LibiGel significantly increased the number of satisfying sexual events by 238 percent when compared to baseline results ($p < 0.0001$). BioSante has also completed two double-blinded, placebo-controlled Phase III safety and efficacy trials including more than 500 surgically menopausal women. A Phase III trial related to cardiovascular events and breast cancer safety in 3,656 women is currently in progress. BioSante plans to submit a new drug application to the FDA for LibiGel by the end of 2012.

Subcutaneous Testosterone Therapy

Testosterone replacement therapy in the form of a subcutaneous pellet has been used in women since the late 1930s. Research on the use of subcutaneous testosterone with doses ranging from 75 to 225 mg has demonstrated safety and efficacy in women (Burger et al., 1984; Dimitrakakis, Jones, Liu, & Bondy, 2004; Gambrell & Natrajan, 2006; Garnett, Studd, Watson, & Savvas, 1991; Thom, Collins, & Studd, 1981). Higher doses of subcutaneous testosterone ranging from 500 to 1,800 mg have also been used to safely treat breast cancer patients (Segaloff, 1975).

Subcutaneous testosterone has also been reported to have no effect on the menstrual cycle when administered to premenopausal women (Dewis, Newman, Ratcliffe, & Anderson, 1986; Glaser, Wurtzbacher, & Dimitrakakis, 2009). The subcutaneous route of administration does not increase the risk of thrombosis because it bypasses the liver and hepatic circulation (Sands et al., 1997; Seed, Sands, McLaren, Kirk, & Darko, 2000).

Glaser, York, and Dimitrakakis (2010) noted beneficial effects (somatic, psychological, and urogential symptoms) of subcutaneous testosterone therapy in pre- and postmenopausal women ($N = 300$). The study included a total of 300 women: 108 were premenopausal, 106 were naturally menopausal, 57 were surgically menopausal, and 29 had a hysterectomy with one or both ovaries remaining. The mean dose of implanted testosterone was 121 mg; the initial dose was partially based on weight (the patient's weight in kg × 2) and repeated doses were adjusted based on side effects and clinical response. The Menopause Rating Scale (MRS) was administered to compare the means score values before and after testosterone replacement. The MRS is a self-administered validated tool that measures 11 symptom categories using a severity scale ranging from 0 (none) to 4 (extremely severe). The symptom categories include hot flashes, heart discomfort, sleep problems, depressive mood, irritability, anxiety, physical/mental exhaustion, sexual problems, bladder problems, vaginal dryness, and joint/muscular discomfort. There was a statistically significant improvement in all 11 symptom categories after testosterone implantation ($p < 0.0001$). When higher doses of testosterone were administered, women reported a greater improvement in all symptom categories except vaginal dryness and anxiety ($p < 0.05$). More than 90 percent of the patients reported less irritability and less than 5 percent reported a mild increase in irritability. Some women in the study reported a slight increase in hirsutism, but none of them discontinued treatment as a result and only six women discontinued treatment due to a lack of effect or for nonmedical reasons. There were no adverse events reported; in addition, laboratory testing revealed no adverse effects on blood glucose or lipid profiles.

SEXUAL AROUSAL DISORDER

According to Laumann et al. (1999), the prevalence rate of FSAD is 14 percent, with an estimated lifetime prevalence of 20 percent. Women often require increased stimulation to achieve lubrication with aging. When lubrication is not adequate, women report that sensitive touching that was once pleasurable is now annoying, painful, or irritating. A survey by Gamble, Heiman, Nusbaum, and Skinner (2000) estimated that up to 75 percent of women have problems with sexual arousal, but may not seek treatment. The incidence of FSAD is higher in peri- and postmenopausal women. A study by Bachmann, Leiblum, Rosen, and Taylor (1993) reported that 44 percent of postmenopausal women experienced persistent or recurrent problems with lubrication.

During arousal, vasocongestion occurs due to increased blood flow to the genitals. As the vaginal walls engorge, pressure inside the capillaries creates transudation of plasma through the vaginal epithelium. This process forms a lubricative film that covers the vaginal wall, heightens sensation, and facilitates penetration (Levin, 1980). Then, the upper vagina expands due to smooth muscle relaxation and vaginal blood flow increases. Meanwhile, the lower portion of the vagina engorges and narrowing of the structures further increases sensation.

At this time, there in no definitive model that depicts an endocrinological response to arousal. However, studies in animals suggest a hormonal role in the modulation of sexual response (Bindert et al., 1999). In these studies, it is apparent that neuropeptides, neurotransmitters, and hormones play an important role in sexual arousal and inhibition.

Experts agree that sexual arousal stimulates a cardiovascular response, but the exact effect on the central nervous system is not fully understood (Carmichael, Davidson, Dixen, & Warburton, 1994). In 1999, Bindert et al. evaluated the neuroendocrine response to sexual arousal in men and women. They revealed increased subjective and

TABLE 7–3. Proposed Biological Causes of Persistent Genital Arousal Disorder

Vascular	Neurologic	Pharmacologic	Hormonal
• Pelvic arteriovenous malformations with unregulated arterial communications to the genitalia • Secondary to pelvic congestion syndrome with ovarian venous incompetence and large varices draining the genitalia	Occurs secondary to: • Tourette's syndrome • Epilepsy • Post-blunt central nervous system (CNS) trauma • Surgical intervention of central arteriovenous malformation or cervical/lumbosacral region • Pudendal nerve entrapment • Hypersensitivity	Occurs secondary to: • Trazodone (serotonin receptor antagonist) • Sudden withdrawal of selective serotonin reuptake inhibitors (SSRIs)	Occurs secondary to: • Initiation or discontinuation of hormone replacement therapy (HRT) • Excessive use of herbal estrogens

Sources: Goldmeier & Leiblum, 2008; Goldstein, De, & Johnson, 2006; Leiblum, Brown, Wan, & Rawlinson, 2005; Leiblum & Goldmeier, 2008; Leiblum, Seehuus, Goldmeier, & Brown, 2007.

physiological arousal with masturbation-induced orgasm. In addition, heightened sexual arousal increased heart rate, blood pressure, and serum adrenaline and noradrenaline concentrations. Orgasm induced a significant increase in serum prolactin and remained elevated for 60 minutes after arousal. There was also a slight increase in serum LH and testosterone levels; there were no changes reported in beta-endorphin, FSD, progesterone, or estradiol levels. In 2000, Exton et al. studied the effects of norepinephrine on sexual arousal. They discovered increased levels of norepinephrine when women were exposed to sexually arousing films compared to prefilm levels.

A decrease in blood flow to the genitals reduces vaginal, labial, and clitoral engorgement. When estrogen levels decrease due to menopause, ovarian removal, or the use of hormonal contraceptives, women often report overlapping symptoms of sexual dysfunction. A decline in estrogen level can interrupt nerve transmission and disrupt arousal due to thinning and atrophy of the vaginal tissues. This can result in vaginal dryness, impaired arousal, and dyspareunia (Berman & Goldstein, 1998).

Persistent Genital Arousal Disorder

Another disorder of sexual arousal is persistent genital arousal disorder (PGAD). PGAD is a rare condition that causes extreme frustration in women and often leads to suicidal thoughts and attempts (Korda, Pfaus, Kellner, & Goldstein, 2009). PGAD causes unwanted, excessive genital arousal and engorgement; it is unrelated to sexual interest and usually does not resolve with orgasm (Basson, Leiblum, et al., 2004; Goldstein, De, & Johnson, 2006; Hatzimouratidis & Hatzichristou, 2007). There is very little known about the pathophysiology of PGAD. The exact cause remains unknown, but it may be associated with psychological conditions such as anxiety or depression; biological causes such as vascular, neurologic, pharmacologic, and hormonal factors; or idiopathic (Goldmeier & Leiblum, 2008; Goldstein, De, et al., 2006; Leiblum, Brown, Wan, & Rawlinson, 2005; Leiblum & Goldmeier, 2008; Leiblum, Seehuus, Goldmeier, & Brown, 2007) (see Table 7–3).

Treatments

Topical Lubricants. Women experiencing vaginal dryness or a lack of lubrication often purchase an over-the-counter lubricant. A supplementary lubricant temporarily increases moisture to the vaginal tissues, which can decrease vaginal discomfort and improve the overall sexual experience (Herbenick et al., 2009).

Petroleum-based lubricants such as Vaseline and mineral oil are commonly used because they are easily accessible. However, women should be advised against using petroleum-based products because they can cause vaginal irritation and increase the risk of infection (Krychman, 2007). In addition, the use of oil-based lubricants (such as petroleum jelly, vitamin E, olive oil, clear mineral oil, and coconut butter) with condoms should be discouraged because they can cause the condom to break down. The use of glycerin-based lubricants has been thought to increase the risk of yeast infections. There is no data to support this, but if a woman is susceptible to vaginal yeast, a glycerin-free lubricant (such as Slippery Stuff or FemGlide) should be recommended. Silicone lubricants are a good option for women with sensitive skin because they are usually hypoallergenic. Lubricants containing silicone are not absorbed by the skin and stay fluid longer. The lubricant must be cleaned off with soap and water, and silicone lubricants must be used with caution around bathroom floors or other wet surfaces as they can increase the risk of falling or injury (Katz, 2009).

Adriaens and Remon (2008) examined mucosal irritation caused by different lubricants. They discovered not all water-based lubricants are created equal and reported that lubricant osmolality was an important determinant of mucosal tolerability. The results were Pre-Seed (an isoosmotic lubricant) was tolerated the best and caused no changes in mucosal irritation; FemGlide, also known as Slippery Stuff (a hypoosmotic lubricant), decreased the natural response and caused negative mucus production; Replens and K-Y jelly (moderately hyperosmotic lubricants) caused mild to moderate irritation; and Astroglide (a highly hyperosmotic lubricant) caused severe irritation and tissue damage.

Vaginal Moisturizers. Replens contains polycarbophil, which has the capability of retaining up to 60 times its weight in water. It delivers continuous moisture for up to 3 days and helps restore the vaginal pH. The gel produces a moist film over the vaginal tissues and attaches to the epithelial surface. As the epithelial cells regain moisture, elasticity is restored and the vaginal tissues are rejuvenated. The hydration of the epithelium has been shown to reduce the incidence of vaginal itching, irritation, and dyspareunia (de Bie, de Leeuw, de Wilde, Hanselaar, & van der Laak, 2002). During this process, the dead cells slough away and a discharge commonly occurs. It also claims to replenish natural vaginal moisture when used regularly. Although Replens should make intercourse more comfortable, a lubricant is often needed.

A study by Gelfand and Wendman (1994) evaluated the use of a polycarbophil moisturizing gel in women with a history of breast cancer. They found a statistically significant reduction in the vaginal pH, improvement in vaginal moisture and elasticity, and overall improvement in vaginal tissues. Eighty percent of the subjects rated the polycarbophil gel as a good to excellent vaginal moisturizer. In addition, two other studies found that Replens was just as effective as conjugated vaginal estrogen cream in treating vaginal atrophy (Abu-Ghazaleh et al., 1997; Bygdeman & Swahn, 1996). This suggests that a polycarbophil moisturizing gel such as Replens is helpful in relieving vaginal dryness in breast cancer patients and may be a good alternative in women who cannot or prefer not to use vaginal estrogen.

Estrogen. Estrogen plays an important role in female sexual functioning. Estrogen is required for the development of female reproductive organs and estrogen maintains the integrity of female genital tissues. It has vasoprotective and vasodilatory effects that increase vaginal, clitoral, and urethral blood flow. Estrogen also helps maintain female sexual response and prevents atherosclerotic compromise of the pelvic arteries (Sherwin, Gelfand, & Brender, 1985). It has been suggested that estrogen protects the vaginal tissues because it facilitates nitric oxide synthase (NOS), an enzyme that controls vaginal and clitoral arterial blood flow. Nitric oxide (NO) is a potent relaxer of vascular and nonvascular smooth muscle and has been isolated in human tissues and is thought to be the primary facilitator of clitoral and labial engorgement (Gendrano, Phillips, & Rosen, 1999). In fact, some studies suggest vasoactive intestinal polypeptide (VIP) and NO are responsible for vaginal lubrication due to increased blood flow and smooth muscle relaxation (Berman, 2005).

An estradiol level below 35 pg/mL can cause thinning of the vaginal mucosa, atrophy of vaginal walls. When genital response is inhibited due to estrogen deficiency, it can be replaced using a vaginal tablet, ring, or topical cream. The use of topical vaginal estrogen in women with breast cancer has been controversial. When initiating local estrogen therapy, it is common for the circulating serum levels of estrogen to rise initially due to atrophied vaginal tissues that are more absorbent than normal vaginal mucosa (Dizon & Wiggins, 2008). In 2003, a group of researchers evaluated the effects of topical vaginal estrogen on women with a history of breast cancer. They concluded that topical estrogen did not appear to place them at an increased risk for recurrence (Dew, Eden, & Wren, 2003).

Prostaglandin E1 (Alprostadil). During arousal, dilation of the vessels along the vaginal epithelium occurs. Therefore, the use of a locally applied vasodilator may be a good approach to treating FSAD. Prostaglandin E1 is a potent vasodilator that naturally regulates blood flow throughout the reproductive tract (Coleman, Narumiya, & Smith, 1994). It increases intracellular levels of cyclic adenosine monophosphate (cAMP) through the stimulation of adenylate cyclase and leads to a decrease in free calcium concentration. As a result, smooth muscle relaxation and vasodilatation occurs (McVary, Pelham, Polepalle, & Riggi, 1999). Prostaglandins also enhance the activity of sensory afferent nerves, which improves sensation and facilitates the central nerve stimulation that occurs during arousal. Alprostadil is a prostaglandin and is not FDA approved for use in women, but it can be compounded into a topical cream.

In 2006, a study by Costabile et al. evaluated the effects of topical alprostadil on naturally or surgically postmenopausal women with FSAD. The women were treated with 100 mcg alprostadil, 400 mcg alprostadil, or placebo. They found that genital vasocongestion was significantly improved in both treatment groups in comparison to placebo. The group of women using 400 mcg of alprostadil also reported increased physical and emotional sexual arousal and sexual satisfaction. The only adverse event noted was mild genital burning that typically lasted less than a minute.

Sildenafil Citrate (Viagra). It has been proposed that FSAD may occur due to vasculogenic factors. For this reason, it has been thought that vasodilators and smooth muscle relaxants used for ED may also help treat FSAD (Berman & Goldstein, 1998). Sildenafil citrate (Viagra) is the only phosphodiesterase type 5 (PDE5) inhibitor that has been studied in clinical trials for the treatment of FSD. In 2004, Pfizer announced that it would no longer conduct research on the use of Viagra in women with FSAD due to inconclusive results. Pfizer had conducted several large-scale, placebo-controlled studies in about 3,000 women. It discovered that Viagra was generally well tolerated in women, but offered little or no benefit to most women with sexual dysfunction.

L-Arginine Glutamate. ArginMax is a nutritional supplement for women that contains L-arginine, Panax ginseng, Ginkgo biloba, damiana leaf, multivitamins, and minerals. L-arginine is thought to enhance NO pathways that cause smooth muscle relaxation and vascular dilatation (Ito, Polan, Trant, & Whipple, 2006). In 2006, a study by Ito et al. evaluated the sexual effects of ArginMax on women ranging from 22 to 73 years of age. After 4 weeks of treatment, the premenopausal group reported a significant increase in sexual desire (72%) in comparison to the placebo group. In the perimenopausal group, 86 percent reported an increase in frequency of intercourse, 79 percent reported satisfaction with their sexual relationship, and 64 percent noted a decrease in vaginal dryness. In the postmenopausal group, 51 percent of women had an increase in sexual desire compared to only 8 percent in the placebo group. From these results, it is apparent that nutritional supplementation may have a positive effect on female sexual functioning. Because ArginMax does not affect estrogen activity, it may be an appropriate alternative to patients with breast cancer or for those who are reluctant to use hormone replacement therapy.

Eros-Clitoral Therapy Device. The Eros-Clitoral Therapy Device (Eros-CTD) was approved by the FDA on April 28, 2000. It was designed to increase blood flow to the clitoris in order to maintain clitoral engorgement while facilitating arousal and orgasm in women. The battery-operated device provides three levels of gentle vacuum suction when applied to the glans clitoris. The nonpharmacologic device has been shown to improve genital sensation, vaginal lubrication, orgasm, and overall sexual satisfaction.

A study by Wilson, Delk, and Billups (2001) evaluated the effects of the Eros-CTD on sexual functioning in women with and without FSAD. The subjects were instructed to use the device at least three times per week for 6 weeks. The subjects applied the vacuum device to the clitoris for 3 to 5 minutes per session. A significant improvement in sensation was reported by both groups: 80 percent in the FSAD group and 89 percent in the non-FSAD group. Also, 70 percent of the FSAD subjects and 67 percent of the non-FSAD subjects reported an increase in lubrication.

Treatment of PGAD. There is limited data on the treatment of PGAD. Psychologically based treatments such as couples therapy or cognitive-behavioral therapy (CBT) may be helpful. Interventions such as distraction or hypnosis may help manage anxiety and/or depression and facilitate relaxation (Goldstein, De, et al., 2006; Hiller & Hekster, 2007). Other treatments such as ice or the use of topical anesthetics may also offer relief (Wylie, Levin, Hallman-Jones, & Goddard, 2006). If the suspected cause is due to medications such as trazodone, venlafaxine, or herbal estrogen products, discontinuation is recommended (Amsterdam, Abu-Rustum, Carter, & Krychman, 2005; Mahoney & Zarate, 2007). The patient should be evaluated for a surgical or radiological intervention if the symptoms are due to a known vascular cause (Thorne & Stuckey, 2008). The use of off-label medications has also been recommended. This includes drugs from the following categories: tricyclic or selective serotonin reuptake inhibitor (SSRI) antidepressants, prolactin-elevating agents, or antiseizure medications (Goldstein, De, et al., 2006; Leiblum & Goldmeier, 2008; Wylie et al., 2006).

In 2009, a case report was published on a woman with primary lifelong PGAD who was prescribed Chantix (varenicline) for smoking cessation (Korda, Pfaus, & Goldstein, 2009). Varenicline is a partial agonist at the alpha-4 beta-2 nicotinic receptor in which the ability to stimulate mesolimbic dopamine is decreased (Rollema, Chambers, et al., 2007; Rollema, Coe, et al., 2007). After a few weeks on Chantix, the woman reported a significant reduction in PGAD symptom. Interestingly, when she discontinued Chantix, her symptoms returned, and when she restarted the medication, her symptoms of PGAD improved again. Korda, Pfaus, and Goldstein proposed that Chantix is a good treatment option for women with hyperactive dopamine release because it reduces dopamine concentrations at the extracellular level, thereby restoring normal dopamine functioning.

Korda, Pfaus, Kellner, et al. (2009) also published a case report on the use of electroconvulsive therapy (ECT) for symptomatic management of PGAD. A woman with bipolar disorder developed symptoms of PGAD upon abrupt discontinuation of paroxetine. As the genital symptoms worsened, she became severely depressed and had suicidal ideation. ECT treatments were started to manage her psychiatric symptoms. After the fourth ECT treatment, her PGAD symptoms resolved and she continued to receive ECT when her PGAD symptoms returned. The side effects of ECT were cited as "minimal" and included temporary short-term memory loss, headache, and muscle aches.

SEXUAL PAIN DISORDER (DYSPAREUNIA)

Sexual pain, or painful intercourse, is also known as dyspareunia. Laumann et al. (1999) reported a prevalence rate of 7 percent. Vulvodynia is the most common cause of dyspareunia. It is a chronic pain disorder that affects the vulva and often occurs without an identifiable cause or visible pathology. The National Institutes of Health estimates that 13 million women suffer from vulvodynia at some point during their lifetime (Harlow & Stewart, 2003). Vulvodynia was once thought to affect only white, nulliparous women, but has been found to affect Caucasian, African American, and Hispanic women ranging in age from 16 to 80 years (Hengge & Runnebaum, 2005). Comorbid conditions associated with vulvodynia include interstitial cystitis, fibromyalgia, irritable bowel syndrome, chronic fatigue syndrome, depression, chronic yeast infections, and chronic urinary tract infections (Arnold, Bachmann, Rosen, Kelly, & Rhoads, 2006). Arnold et al. mailed questionnaires regarding the comorbidities of vulvodynia. Of the 208 eligible responses, fibromyalgia and irritable bowel syndrome were significantly related to vulvodynia. According to a study by Munday, Buchan, Ravenhill, Wiggs, and Brooks (2007), many women reported a lack of sexual desire because intercourse was associated with pain rather than pleasure. It was found that more than half of the women developed sexually avoidant behaviors for fear that closeness with their partner would lead to vaginal penetration.

Weinstein (1987) proposed an adapted pain cycle in women with vulvar pain. The cycle included the following related sets of symptoms: (1) pain often leads to anxiety, stress, depression; (2) a loss of control and self-esteem; (3) dyspareunia and sexual dysfunction; (4) deteriorating relationships and ineffective communication; and (5) hopelessness due to decreased support and social isolation. At any point during the cycle, the patient may seek treatment from another health care professional due to the patient's perception of failure or rejection (Shepphard, Hallam-Jones, & Wylie, 2008).

Vulvodynia Subtypes: PVD and Generalized Vulvodynia

There are two subtypes of vulvodynia: (1) PVD (formerly known as vulvar vestibulitis syndrome) and (2) generalized vulvodynia. These subtypes are classified according to the site of pain as generalized or localized and whether the pain is provoked, unprovoked, or mixed (Collins et al., 2005). In 2003, a population-based study in the United States by Harlow and Stewart estimated the lifetime prevalence of vulvodynia and PVD was 16 and 12 percent, respectively. Of the women surveyed, 10 percent experienced dyspareunia. However, the aforementioned prevalence rates were underreported because up to 30 percent of women surveyed did not seek medical treatment.

Provoked Vestibulodynia. PVD is the most common subtype of vulvodynia (Moyal-Barracco & Lynch, 2004). PVD interferes with a woman's sexual functioning and psychological well-being (Pukall, Smith, & Chamberlain, 2007). Education about this condition is lacking among women and health care professionals. PVD was originally believed to occur as a result of an unusual psychosomatic gynecologic dysfunction (Binik & Meana, 1994). The exact etiology remains unknown, but the pathogenesis is thought to be multifactorial, including physical and psychosexual causes (Ayers et al., 2006; Graziottin & Brotto, 2004). In more recent years, experts have isolated possible causes for vestibulodynia such as a neuroproliferation, hormone imbalance, hypertonic pelvic floor muscle dysfunction, vaginitis (desquamative inflammatory vaginitis, allergic vaginitis, and recurrent vaginal yeast), vulvar dermatologic conditions (lichen sclerosus or lichen planus) (Babula, Bongiovanni, Ledger, & Witkin, 2004; Bornstein, Goldschmid, & Sabo, 2004; Glazer, Jantos, Hartmann, & Swencionis, 1998; Goldstein & Burrows, 2008; Harlow, He, & Nguyen, 2009; Witkin, Gerber, & Ledger, 2002).

Congenital neuroproliferative PVD occurs due to the increased density of C-afferent nociceptors in the vestibular mucosa. Burrows, Goldstein, Klingman, and Pukall (2008) suggested that primary PVD is congenital due to a defect in the urogenital sinus during embryologic development. Acquired neuroproliferative PVD may cause chronic vestibular inflammation due to inhibited production of interferon alpha. Acquired neuroproliferation often occurs after an allergic reaction or severe/recurrent candidiasis infection (Harlow et al., 2009). Acquired neuroproliferation may also occur due to the activation of mast cells. Bornstein et al. (2004) reported that women with PVD have increased mast cells in the vestibular tissues. They believe the increased mast cells release nerve growth factor, thereby causing proliferation of nociceptors.

It is likely that some women have an altered peripheral and central neuropathic response to pain. Research has demonstrated hyperplasia of C-afferent nociceptors in the vestibular tissue. Neurotransmitters such as glutamate and substance P have also been isolated in the vestibular mucosa, which has been thought to alter sensory perception (Bohm-Starke, Hilliges, Falconer, & Rylander, 1999; Westrom & Willen, 1998). Abbott, Amsel, Binik, Khalife, and Pukall (2002) supported the theory of vulvar pain being a manifestation of central neuropathic pain processing. They reported that patients with PVD had an overall hypersensitivity to touch and pain throughout their body.

There is strong evidence that a hormonal imbalance (such as hormonal contraceptives, breastfeeding, menopause, or surgical removal of the ovaries) increases the risk for developing PVD. This is known as hormonally mediated PVD. A lack of estrogen to the vaginal tissues also causes pain and hypersensitivity due to hyperplasia of nociceptive nerve fibers (Bradshaw & Berkley, 2002). As a result, the vaginal walls shorten and lose elasticity (Bachmann & Leiblum, 2004). This often leads to vaginal dryness, unpleasant hypersensitivity of the vestibular glands, vulvar pain, and dyspareunia (de Freitas et al., 2009).

Low-dose estrogen hormonal contraceptives are thought to be a contributing factor in vestibulodynia; it increases inflammatory cytokines in the vestibular epithelium (Foster & Hasday, 1997). Goldstein, Pukall, and Goldstein (2009) suggest this is due to an increase in SHBG and a decrease in free testosterone. In 1994, Bazin et al. reported that women who use oral contraceptive pills (OCPs) before the age of 17 have relative risk of 9.2 (920% increased risk) for developing vestibulodynia and women who start OCPs after the age of 17 still have a relative risk of 4.6 (460% increased risk). Another study in 1997 by Nylander Lundqvist and Sjoberg supported the OC theory. They observed that women who used OCPs for a longer period of time were more likely to have PVD when compared to the control groups.

Women with PVD usually report the onset of pain to be acute or gradual with symptoms ranging from moderate to severe such as vulvar burning, stinging, irritation; knife-like pain; or the feeling of acid being poured on the vulva (National Vulvodynia Association, 2010). The pain occurs at the vaginal opening (vestibule) and often inhibits vaginal penetration with sexual activity, gynecologic examination/Pap smear, or tampon insertion. The pain can also be provoked when pressure is exerted on the vestibule, such as riding a bicycle, wearing tight clothing, or sitting for an extended period of time. In 2003, a web-based survey found that yeast infections and stress were the two most common factors that contributed to the development of PVD and 55 percent reported that stress made their symptoms of vulvar pain worse (Gordon, Panahian-Jand, McComb, Melegari, & Sharp, 2003).

Currently, there is no data available on the morbidity, mortality, or economic impact of PVD (Goldstein et al., 2009). An online study of 428 women with vulvar pain reported that more than half of the women sought treatment from four to nine physicians and the estimated medical expenses ranged from $500 to $75,000 per patient (Gordon et al., 2003). In addition, chronic pain conditions have been associated with higher health care costs, lower work production, and other debts to society (Turk & Burwinkle, 2005). Therefore, health care costs related to PVD and dyspareunia are assumed to be high because PVD is highly comorbid with other costly medical conditions such as interstitial cystitis, pelvic inflammatory disease, chronic pelvic pain, and endometriosis (Mathias et al., 1996; Mirkin, Murphy-Barron, & Iwasaki, 2007; Nyrop et al., 2007; Wu et al., 2006).

Generalized Vulvodynia. Generalized vulvodynia is the second subtype of vulvodynia and it can occur in conjunction with the first subtype, PVD. Generalized vulvodynia is thought of as a complex regional pain syndrome (CRPS) as seen in fibromyalgia and interstitial cystitis (Edwards, 2003). Women with CRPS appear to have an enhanced systemic pain perception, which is also known as central nervous system sensitization. Also, women with generalized vulvodynia are more likely to have other CRPS conditions such as endometriosis or fibromyalgia (Gordon et al., 2003). This may be due to a phenomenon known as "wind up" in which there is increased activity in dorsal horn cells of the spinal cord after repetitive activation of primary C-afferent fibers (Burrows & Goldstein, 2008).

In generalized vulvodynia, pain occurs spontaneously and is usually constant. On occasion, there are periods of relief from pain. Women with generalized unprovoked vulvodynia typically have no abnormal physical signs on examination. The pain is usually exacerbated when pressure is applied to the vulva such as wearing pants or sitting for a prolonged period of time. Women experience pain in a generalized area such as the labia majora, the perineum, or the entire vulva.

Vaginismus. In 1547, Trotula of Salerno, a female physician from Salerno, Italy, provided the earliest known definition of vaginismus in the book *The Diseases of Women* (1940). Trotula of Salerno described a condition in which a woman may appear virginal because the vulva tightens despite seduction. Vaginismus occurs due to an involuntary spasm of the muscles that surround the vagina making penetration painful or impossible. Women with vaginismus report a heightened fear of pain and emotional distress due to vaginal penetration (tampon insertion, penile penetration, or gynecologic exam) (Reissing, Binik, Khalife, Cohen, & Amsel, 2004).

The prevalence of vaginismus among the population is unknown because many women avoid gynecological exams, but prevalence in the clinical setting has been reported to range from 5 to 17 percent (Spector & Carey, 1990). A study by Reissing et al. (2004) reported that two independent gynecologists agreed on the diagnosis of vaginismus only 4 percent of the time. Coincidentally, the background literature on vaginismus has been described as "virginal" due to a lack of consensus on the definition and diagnostic criteria. Weijmar Schultz and van de Wiel (2005) proposed the following criteria to help identify symptoms:

- Vaginal penetration is impossible in all/the majority of attempts because of vaginal and/or pelvic muscle hypertonicity and/or muscle guarding at the entrance to the vagina
- Vaginal penetration is avoided for all/the majority of opportunities because of recurrent or chronic vulvar, vaginal, or pelvic pain
- Vaginal penetration is avoided for all/the majority of opportunities because of associated, significant anxiety and/or panic, and may be accompanied by feelings of disgust, dread, and/or fear

Psychological factors are believed to cause vaginismus, but few psychological theories have been supported by empirical research. Proposed psychological factors include a lack of sexual knowledge, sexual guilt, and negative attitudes about sexuality/sex before marriage; a dysfunctional relationship between the couple; and history of abuse (Biswas & Ratnam, 1995; Ellison, 1968, 1972; Van de Wiel, 1990). However, in a review of studies, the prevalence of vaginismus in women with a history of physical or sexual abuse was unsupportive. Five out of six studies did not reveal a higher incidence of vaginismus in this population (Barnes, 1986; Hawton & Catalan, 1990; O'Sullivan, 1979; van Lankveld, Brewaeys, ter Kuile, & Weijenborg, 1995; van Lankveld et al., 2006).

Biological factors such as hymenal abnormalities, vaginal infections, genital trauma, radiation, vaginal atrophy, exposure to irritants, pelvic floor muscle dysfunction (hypertonicity and reduced muscle control), and vestibulodynia are thought to play a role in vaginismus as well (Abramov, Wolman, & Higgins, 1994; American College of Obstetricians and Gynecologists, 1995; Crowley, Richardson, & Goldmeier, 2006; Leiblum, 2000; Reissing et al., 2004). However, there is limited evidence regarding organic pathologies at this time. Interestingly, women with vaginismus and PVD have similar descriptions of their pain and it is possible that acquired vaginismus occurs secondary to PVD (de Kruiff, ter Kuile, Weijenborg, & van Lankveld, 2000; Fordney, 1978; Lamont, 1978; Reissing et al., 2004; Steege, 1984; ter Kuile, van Lankveld, Vlieland, Wilekes, & Weijenborg, 2005). Vaginismus and dyspareunia due to PVD demonstrate overlapping symptoms such as vulvar pain and tightness of the pelvic floor muscles (Reissing et al., 2004). Studies have also shown that 42 to 100 percent of women with vaginismus also meet the criteria for PVD (de Kruiff et al., 2000; Engman, Lindehammar, & Wijma, 2004; Reissing et al., 2004). This may be due to the fact that health care providers often have a difficult time distinguishing between these pain disorders, but it is helpful to remember that the key characteristic of PVD is superficial pain (Reissing et al., 2004).

Physical Examination

Vestibulodynia is diagnosed by signs and symptoms because a defined pathophysiology does not exist (Goldstein et al., 2009). In 1987, Edward Friedrich proposed the following diagnostic criteria: (1) severe pain upon touch of the vulvar vestibule (vaginal opening) or attempted vaginal entry; (2) discomfort localized to the vulvar vestibule with the application of pressure; and (3) varying degrees of vulvar erythema.

A thorough examination is necessary to rule out other causes of vulvar pain. The vulva should be examined for evidence of infection such as yeast or HPV; dermatologic condition, such as an allergic reaction, contact dermatitis, or lichen sclerosus; and trauma or injury. An examination using vulvoscopy may be helpful during the examination to identify microfissure tears, excoriation, induration, ulceration, pigmentation changes, lichenification, fusing of the vulvar tissues or clitoral hood, and loss of labial architecture. Any suspicious lesions should be biopsied and sent to a dermatopathologist for diagnosis. Biopsy of nonspecific findings such as erythema is not recommended because the results are often uninformative (Burrows & Goldstein, 2008). If the tissues are atrophic, the patient can be prescribed topical estrogen cream such as Estrace. The topical vaginal estrogen can be applied to the vaginal opening one to two times daily for at least 1 week to decrease discomfort during the biopsy and facilitate healing (Feldhaus-Dahir, 2011). It is also important to treat any underlying yeast or bacterial infection as this can interfere with the biopsy results.

During the examination, a moistened cotton swab should be used to gently palpate the area along the labia majora and minora, intersulcus, clitoral hood, posterior fourchette, and Hart's line. On the labia minora, if the tissue lateral to Hart's line elicits normal sensation on Q-tip touch and the tissue medial to Hart's line causes severe allodynia, a diagnosis of PVD can be made. Next, a Q-tip test should be performed along the vestibule and vestibular glands. Place the Q-tip anterior, inferior, and laterally along the urethra and posteriorly at the 4, 6, and 8 o'clock positions. A single-digit examination of the pelvic floor should also be performed to assess for pelvic muscle tightness (e.g., hypertonus of the levator ani muscles).

In addition, the health care provider should evaluate pain using the visual analog scale (VAS) to record baseline measurements and monitor treatment effectiveness. The VAS is a scale from 0 to 10 in which the patients rates their pain (0 = absence of pain and 10 = the worst pain imaginable) (Carlsson, 1983).

Treatments

Topical Lidocaine. Topical lidocaine is a safe and fairly inexpensive treatment for vestibulodynia. Lidocaine may help relieve chronic vulvar pain because it blocks the transmission of C-fibers and inhibits the irritable nociceptors that are responsible for pain. Zolnoun, Hartmann, and Steege (2003) prospectively evaluated the effectiveness of 5 percent lidocaine ointment for symptoms of vulvar pain. The patients were instructed to apply a copious amount of lidocaine ointment to the vestibule at bedtime. A cotton ball saturated with lidocaine was placed inside the vestibule to ensure direct contact for at least 8 hours. Prior to the study, only 36 percent of the patients were able to have intercourse. After a mean of 7 weeks, 76 percent of the patients were able to engage in intercourse and more than half of the women had a reduction of dyspareunia by at least 50 percent.

Vaginal Estrogen and Testosterone. Diminished levels of testosterone (as seen with the use of hormonal BCPs or menopause) have been associated with sexual pain disorders such as PVD. Androgen receptors have been isolated in the vagina and the vestibule; adequate levels of testosterone are required to maintain healthy vaginal tissues (Giraldi et al., 2004; Hodgins, Spike, Mackie, & MacLean, 1998; Taylor, Guzail, & Al-Azzawi, 2008). The effects of testosterone have been studied in the vaginal tissues of rabbits and rats. The administration of testosterone in these animals has shown structural improvements in the vaginal tissues such as enhanced NOS activity, increased blood flow, smooth muscle relaxation, and maintenance of the vaginal muscularis layer (Giraldi et al., 2004; Traish et al., 2003, 2004).

Topical vaginal estrogen has been used as a treatment for vestibulodynia. Estrogen has an immunomodulatory effect because it can stimulate antibody response while inhibiting T-cell-mediated inflammation (Josefsson, Tarkowski, & Carlsten, 1992).

Capsaicin. Capsaicin has been used to treat neurologic and inflammatory pain disorders such as arthritis, diabetic neuropathy, postherpetic neuralgia, and overactive bladder. Capsaicin is vanillyl amide that activates A-delta sensory neurons and unmyelinated C fibers. It allows depolarization of afferent nerve fibers and causes desensitization due to the activation of substance P, thereby inducing a burning sensation at the application site (Clapham, 1997).

In 2005, Kellogg-Spadt, Oyama, Rejba, Steinberg, and Whitmore retrospectively evaluated the use of 0.025 percent of capsaicin in acid mantle cream for vestibulodynia. The patients applied 2 percent of lidocaine gel to the vaginal opening for at least 10 minutes prior to the application of capsaicin. The lidocaine was wiped off and capsaicin was applied to the vaginal opening at 1, 4, 6, 8, and 11 o'clock for 20 minutes. The patients continued to use the compounded capsaicin cream for 20 minutes daily over the next 12 weeks. They were allowed to use the lidocaine gel as needed for the first 2 weeks and then ice packs only for the remaining 10 weeks. Prior to treatment, 62 percent of the patients were able to have vaginal intercourse, and this number increased to 95 percent following capsaicin treatment. All patients reported a significant increase in frequency; however, one criticism is that the pretreatment of lidocaine gel made it difficult to isolate the effects of capsaicin alone.

Injectable Steroids. Bianco, Murina, Roberti, and Tassan (2001) suggested using injectable methylprednisolone and lidocaine as an alternative approach for the treatment of vestibulodynia. The mixture contained 40 mg of methylprednisolone acetate and 10 mg of lidocaine in a saline medium for a total volume of 1 mL. The patients were given 1 mL on day 1, 0.5 mL on day 8, and 0.3 mL on day 15. Each dose was divided into three equal parts and was injected into the vestibule using a 26-gauge needle at 4 and 8 o'clock, and along the posterior fourchette. More than half of the patients had a favorable response: 32 percent had complete resolution of pain and 36 percent reported significant improvement in dyspareunia and vulvar burning while 32 percent of the patients had no improvement in symptoms. None of the patients reported negative side effects. Segal, Tifheret, and Lazer (2003) published a case study on a 24-year-old woman with persistent vestibulodynia. The patient received weekly injections containing 6 mg of betamethasone diluted in 1 percent lidocaine to three points along the vestibule. The patient reported complete resolution of vulvar pain and improved quality of sexual relations.

Botulinum Toxin Type A. Over the past few years, botulinum toxin type A (Botox) has been used to treat facial wrinkles, hyperhydrosis, and pain disorders without causing significant side effects. Therapeutic Botox has been shown to be effective in the treatment of PVD, vaginismus, and pelvic floor spasms (Bohm-Starke et al., 1999; van Lankveld et al., 1995). However, research findings have been mixed and many of the published studies contain small sample sizes. Botox is thought to relieve vulvar pain due to its paralytic effect on muscle fibers that become painful due to pelvic floor hypertonicity and because it blocks the neurotransmission of nociceptive pain receptors throughout the vestibule (Bohm-Starke et al., 1999; Chung, Shim, & Yoon, 2007).

In 2007, Chung et al. published promising results on the use of Botox for vulvodynia. They had a small sample of seven women with intractable vulvar pain. The patients received 20 to 40 units of Botox per injection along the vestibule, levator ani muscle, or perineum. Five of the patients were reinjected with Botox 2 weeks after the first series of injections. All patients had resolution of pain and no adverse outcomes were identified. The patients had a mean follow-up of 11.6 months and none of them had a recurrence of vulvar pain.

In 2009, Petersen, Giraldi, Lundvall, and Kristensen published less-promising results from a randomized, placebo-controlled, double-blinded study in Denmark. Sixty-four women were randomized to receive Botox ($N = 32$) and saline placebo ($N = 32$). A total of 60 women completed the 6-month study. The following tools were used to measure outcomes: the VAS, the FSFI, the FSDS, and the 36-item short form (SF-36) quality of life. Both treatment groups reported a significant reduction in pain ($p < 0.001$), and at the 6-month follow-up, there was no significant difference in VAS scores between the two groups ($p > 0.984$). There was no significant difference between both groups' FSFI scores from baseline to 6 months ($p = 0.635$). Interesting, the placebo group had a close to significant decrease in sexual distress at the 6-month follow-up ($p = 0.444$). There was no significant difference in SF-36 quality of life scores between the groups.

Vulvar Vestibulectomy. If conservative therapy for vestibulodynia has failed, the patient should be evaluated for a vestibulectomy. Surgical intervention for vestibulodynia has evolved over the last 25 years. In 1981, Genadry, Poliakoff, and Woodruff were the first to use perineoplasty for the treatment of vaginal outlet distortion. Two years later, the same technique was used to treat patients with vestibulodynia. The hymen and areas of vestibular sensitivity were excised and the vagina was advanced to cover the defect. The area anterior to the urethra was also excised, but was left to heal by secondary intention. More than half of the patients reported cure or significant improvement after surgical intervention (Friedrich, 1987).

A review of 32 published case studies containing 1,275 patients from 1981 to 2006 demonstrated promising results. Even though the case studies used several different surgical approaches, 28 of the 32 publications had at least an 80 percent success rate (Goldstein, Klingman, Christopher, Johnson, & Marinoff, 2006).

Multidisciplinary Treatment Options for PVD

Providing quality health care to patients with sexual pain disorders often requires a multidisciplinary approach because the causes of PVD are multifactorial (Ehrstrom, Kornfeld, Rylander, & Bohm-Starke, 2009). The organization of interdependent health care teams provides the patient with better long-term outcomes in regard to functional status and pain (Goldstein et al., 2009). In the past, a surgical vestibulectomy was thought to be the best treatment option for PVD with a partial or complete success rate of 50 to 100 percent (Haefner, 2000). Recently, a multidisciplinary approach involving medical, physical, and sexual therapy has been proposed because it helps patients increase coping skills, reduce stress, and decrease pain (Bachman, Widenbrant, Bohm-Starke, & Dahlof, 2008).

Bachman et al. (2008) published a study on the effects of combined physical and psychosexual therapy for PVD. Physical therapy included desensitization of the vestibular mucosa and techniques to relax the pelvic floor. Psychosexual therapy included patient education of the pain response cycle and the use of a cognitive model to address the patient's coping skills. Bachman et al. reported a significant increase in the frequency of intercourse, positive attitudes regarding sexuality, and an overall increase in sexual functioning. In addition, patients reported a decrease in dyspareunia and general life stressors.

Another study by Hartmann, Strauhal, and Nelson (2007) found that the use of visceral manipulation by a physical therapist in women with generalized vulvodynia and PVD significantly reduced pain. Seventy-one percent of the women had an overall improvement in vulvar pain and 62 percent of the women had an improvement in sexual functioning.

Vaginismus. Throughout the early 1900s, psychotherapy was the preferred treatment because vaginismus was thought to be a symptom of hysteria or a phobia of pain (Fenichel, 1945; Musaph & Haspels, 1976; Walthard, 1909). In the 1970s, Masters and Johnson reported great success in vaginismus treatment with behaviorally oriented sex therapy and vaginal dilatation.

Current treatments for vaginismus include pelvic floor physical therapy to improve mobility, decrease pain and anxiety, and gain control of the pelvic muscles. Physical therapists who treat vaginismus have specialized training in techniques such as breathing/relaxation, tissue desensitization, vaginal dilators varying in size, manual stretching, and biofeedback therapy (Binik, 2010; Rosenbaum, 2005, 2008). Medication management has also been used to treat vaginismus. This included the use of local/topical anesthetics such as lidocaine ointment, muscle relaxants such as botulinum toxin, and anxiolytics (Bertolasi et al., 2009; Brin & Vapnek, 1997; Ghazizdeh & Nikzad, 2004; Hassel, 1997; Plaut & RachBeisel, 1997; Shafik & El-Sibai, 2000). Unfortunately, studies using pharmacologic interventions are inconclusive due to small sample sizes, lack of control groups, nonrandomized, and use of nonstandardized outcome instruments (Lahaie, Boyer, Amsel, Khalife, & Binik, 2010). Psychological treatments such as relationship enhancement and hypnosis have been used based on the belief that vaginismus originates from past negative sexual experiences, a lack of sexual education, and relationship/marital conflict (Gottesfeld, 1978; Harman, Waldo, & Johnson, 1994). CBT is another treatment option. In 2006, van Lankveld et al. published the first randomized, controlled trial using CBT for the treatment of vaginismus. Women received sexual education and they were instructed on the use of vaginal dilators, relaxation, and sensate focus techniques.

ORGASMIC DISORDER

The female orgasm inspires interest because it is often absent and it does seem to play a role in the reproductive process (Symons, 1979). About 90 percent of women experience orgasm from sexual stimulation (Lloyd, 2005). Less than 25 percent of women experience orgasm through vaginal penetration only, which may be even lower in reality because many women experience indirect stimulation of the clitoris with vaginal penetration. According to the National Social and Health Life Survey, 24 percent of women reported a lack of ability to achieve orgasm within the last year and occurring for several months or longer (Laumann, Gagnon, Michael, & Michaels, 1994). The etiology of female orgasmic disorder is multifactorial due to causes such as genetics, other health conditions, alcohol, drug use (prescription or illicit), stress, and relationship conflict (Rellini & Clifton, 2011).

Women are variable in the type and/or intensity of stimulation needed to facilitate orgasm. Sexual stimulation and orgasm often arise from the clitoris and vagina (Levin, 1992, 2001; Masters & Johnson, 1966). Anatomically, the clitoris consists of external structures—the shaft and clitoral glans—and internal structures—two clitoral bulbs and two clitoral bodies that form a vaulted structure superior to the anterior vaginal wall. Stimulation of the periurethral glands, breasts, and mons has also been shown to induce orgasm. The exact mechanism for inducing orgasm is not fully understood. However, studies using brain imaging have shown increased activity of the hippocampus, cerebellum, hypothalamus (paraventricular nucleus), and midbrain (periaqueductal gray area). It is difficult to define the meaning of orgasm due to its subjective nature. Meston, Levin, Sipski, Hull, and Heiman

(2004) proposed the following operational definition of female orgasm:

> An orgasm in the human female is a variable, transient peak sensation of intense pleasure, creating an altered state of consciousness, usually with an invitation accompanied by involuntary, rhythmic contractions of the pelvic striated circumvaginal musculature, often with concomitant uterine and anal contractions, and myotonia that resolves the sexually induced vasocongestion (sometimes only partially) and myotonia, general with an induction of well-being and contentment.

Different types of orgasms have been identified in women through self-report (Fisher, 1973, pp. 72–73). Orgasm achieved through clitoral stimulation has been described as warm, ticklish, electric, and sharp; vaginal stimulation has been described as throbbing, deep, soothing, and comfortable. Singer (1973, pp. 72–73), a philosopher, analyzed nonscientific findings and suggested the following three categories of orgasm: (1) "vulval," rhythmic contractions of the vagina through clitoral or coital stimulation; (2) "uterine," apnoea and gasping due to penile-cervix contact without vaginal contractions; and (3) "blended," which contains elements of vulval and uterine orgasms due to coitus and accompanied by apnoea.

Treatment

The treatment of anorgasmia (the inability to achieve orgasm) involves a psychoanalytic, cognitive-behavioral, and/or pharmacological approach (Heiman, 2000). CBT increases the ability to achieve orgasm and decreases anxiety by changing attitudes and thoughts about sexuality. To facilitate change, behavioral techniques such as sensate focus, systematic desensitization, and direct masturbation are used. CBT also includes the use of sexual education, interpersonal training, and Kegel exercises.

When a woman is not able to achieve orgasm with her partner, treatment modalities include reducing anxiety, improving communication and building trust with her partner, and maximizing clitoral stimulation manually or by changing sexual positions (Meston, Hull, Levin, & Sipski, 2004).

CONCLUSION

Sexual functioning is a healthy part of the human life cycle. Addressing issues with sexual functioning is important for both sexes, but the absence of FDA-approved medications has resulted in a lack of screening and treatment for women. It is also important to remember that there is no "magical cure" for FSD. For example, if a woman loses interest in her sexual relationship because her partner is verbally abusive or there is underlying conflict in their relationship, the use of testosterone will not restore her desire for intimacy (Feldhaus-Dahir, 2009c). There are several complicated causes (e.g., medical, psychological, or interpersonal) that can disrupt a woman's sexual functioning and it is important to remember that FSD can occur at any time during the female life cycle. Oftentimes, FSD does not occur as a single diagnosis. Rather, it seems to have a domino effect in which multiple problems with sexual functioning coexist. For example, a woman diagnosed with breast cancer is at an increased risk for FSD due to the following factors. She must deal with emotional issues as she adapts to the new diagnosis, and stress as she selects a treatment plan. If she is premenopausal, she will likely experience premature ovarian failure due to chemotherapy (chemical menopause), radiation, or oophorectomy (surgical menopause). As a result, she will probably experience vaginal atrophy and vaginal dryness, which may lead to painful intercourse. She may also experience fatigue as a side effect from chemotherapy and body image disturbance following a mastectomy. Next, she may report symptoms of depression or hot flashes to her health care provider and be prescribed venlafaxine (Effexor). This may result in delayed or absent orgasm, or further decline in libido. The final outcome is a vicious cycle with the added stress of relationship conflict and a poor prognosis for sexual functioning (Feldhaus-Dahir, 2009b).

Because FSD is multidimensional in nature, it requires a multispecialty approach. This includes collaboration with physical therapists trained in pelvic floor dysfunctions, sex therapists, and other health care providers. As FSD becomes more recognized as a medical condition that negatively impacts a woman's quality of life, increased knowledge to appropriately screen, diagnose, and treat these women is warranted. However, sexuality remains a taboo subject, causing many women to experience physical and emotional distress, decreased quality of life, divorce, and problems with future relationships (Aslan & Fynes, 2008). It is not professional or compassionate to ignore or dismiss women's complaints and doing so prohibits total disease management (Mick, 2007). When sexual issues are not addressed, it may leave patients feeling anxious, self-doubting, and resistant to treatment. It can also lead to low self-esteem, poor quality of life, and deterioration of interpersonal relationships (Basson et al., 2000). Therefore, it is imperative for health care professionals to be educated in disorders related to sexual functioning so that women can be diagnosed in a timely manner with appropriate treatments, or referred to a specialist who is qualified to manage their care. For a list of experts in sexual medicine, or "ISSWSH Fellows," refer to the International Society for the Study of Women's Sexual Health website at www.isswsh.org.

REFERENCES

Abbott, F., Amsel, R., Binik, Y., Khalife, S., & Pukall, C. (2002). Vestibular tactile and pain thresholds in women with vulvar vestibulitis syndrome. *Pain, 96*(1–2), 163–175.

Abdallah, R., & Simon, J. (2007). Testosterone therapy in women: Its role in the management of hypoactive sexual desire disorder. *International Journal of Impotence Research, 19*(5), 458–463.

Abel, S. (1945). Androgenic therapy in malignant disease of the female genitalia. *American Journal of Obstetrics and Gynecology, 49,* 327–342.

Abramov, L., Wolman, I., & Higgins, M.P. (1994). Vaginismus: An important factor in the evaluation and management of vulvar vestibulitis syndrome. *Gynecologic and Obstetric Investigation, 38*(3), 194–197.

Abu-Ghazaleh, S., Ellison, N., Hammer, A., Kaur, J., Law, M., Loprinzi, C., et al. (1997). Phase III randomized double-blind study to evaluate the efficacy of a polycarbophil-based vaginal moisturizer in women with breast cancer. *Journal of Clinical Oncology, 15*(3), 969–973.

Adriaens, E., & Remon, J. (2008). Mucosal irritation potential of personal lubricants relates to product osmolality as detected by the slug mucosal irritation assay. *Sexually Transmitted Diseases, 35*(5), 512–516.

American College of Obstetricians and Gynecologists. (1995). Sexual dysfunction. *International Journal of Gynecology and Obstetrics, 51,* 265–277.

American Psychiatric Association. (2000). *Diagnostic and statistical manual of mental disorder* (4th ed., text revision). Washington, DC: Author.

Amsterdam, A., Abu-Rustum, N., Carter, J., & Krychman, M. (2005). Persistent sexual arousal syndrome associated with increased soy intake. *Journal of Sexual Medicine, 3,* 338–340.

Arnold, L.D., Bachmann, G.A., Rosen, R., Kelly, S., & Rhoads, G.G. (2006). Vulvodynia: Characteristics and associations with comorbidities and quality of life. *Obstetrics and Gynecology, 107*(3), 617–624.

Aslan, E., & Fynes, M. (2008). Female sexual dysfunction. *International Urogynecology Journal, 19*(2), 293–305.

Ayers, C., Bachmann, G., Basson, R., Binik, Y., Brown, C., Foster, D., et al. (2006). Vulvodynia: A state-of-the-art consensus on definitions, diagnosis, and management. *Journal of Reproductive Medicine, 51*(6), 447–456.

Babula, O., Bongiovanni, A.M., Ledger, W.J., & Witkin, S.S. (2004). Immunoglobulin E antibodies to seminal fluid in women with vulvar vestibulitis syndrome: Relation to onset and timing of symptoms. *American Journal of Obstetrics and Gynecology, 190,* 663–667.

Bachmann, G. (2006). Female sexuality and sexual dysfunction: Are we stuck on the learning curve? *Journal of Sexual Medicine, 3*(4), 639–645.

Bachmann, G., & Leiblum, S. (2004). The impact of hormones on menopausal sexuality: A literature review. *Menopause, 11,* 120–130.

Bachmann, G., Leiblum, S., Rosen, R., & Taylor, J. (1993). Prevalence of sexual dysfunction in women: Results of a survey of 329 women in an outpatient gynecological clinic. *Journal of Sex and Marital Therapy, 19*(3), 171–188.

Bachman, H., Widenbrant, M., Bohm-Starke, N., & Dahlof, L. (2008). Combined physical and psychosexual therapy for provoked vestibulodynia: An evaluation of a multidisciplinary treatment model. *Journal of Sex Research, 45*(4), 378–385.

Barnes, J. (1986). Lifelong vaginismus: Social and clinical features. *Irish Medical Journal, 79,* 59–62.

Barton, I., Koochaki, P., Leiblum, S., Rodenberg, C., & Rosen, R. (2006). Hypoactive sexual desire disorder in postmenopausal women: U.S. results from the Women's International Study of Health and Sexuality (WISHeS). *Menopause, 13*(1), 46–56.

Basaria, S., & Dobs, A.S. (2006). Clinical review: Controversies regarding transdermal androgen therapy in postmenopausal women. *Journal of Clinical Endocrinology and Metabolism, 91*(12), 4743–4752.

Basson, R. (2000). The female sexual response: A different model. *Journal of Sex and Marital Therapy, 26,* 51–65.

Basson, R. (2001a). Using a different model for female sexual response to address women's problematic low sexual desire. *Journal of Sex and Marital Therapy, 27,* 395–402.

Basson, R. (2001b). Female sexual response: The role of drugs in the management of sexual dysfunction. *American College of Obstetrics and Gynecology, 98*(2), 350–352.

Basson, R. (2004). Recent advances in women's sexual function and dysfunction. *Menopause, 11,* 714–725.

Basson, R., Althof, S., Davis, S., Fugl-Meyer, K., Goldstein, I., Leiblum, S., et al. (2004). Summary of the recommendations on sexual dysfunctions in women. *Journal of Sexual Medicine, 1,* 24–34.

Basson, R., Berman, J., Burnett, A., Derogatis, L., Ferguson, D., Fourcroy, J., et al. (2000). Report of the international consensus development conference on female sexual dysfunction: Definitions and classifications. *Journal of Urology, 163*(3), 888–893.

Basson, R., Brotto, L., Derogatis, L., Fourcroy, J., Fugl-Meyer, K., Graziottin, A., et al. (2003). Definitions of women's sexual dysfunction reconsidered: Advocating expansion and revision. *Journal of Psychosomatic Obstetrics and Gynecology, 24*(4), 221–229.

Basson, R., Leiblum, S., Brotto, L., Derogatis, L., Fourcroy, J., Fugl-Meyer, K., et al. (2004). Revised definitions of women's sexual dysfunction. *Journal of Sexual Medicine, 1,* 40–48.

Basson, R., & Schultz, W.W. (2007). Sexual sequelae of general medical disorders. *Lancet, 369*(9559), 409–424.

Basson, R., Wierman, M.E., van Lankveld, J., & Brotto, L. (2010). Summary of the recommendations on sexual dysfunctions in women. *Journal of Sexual Medicine, 7,* 314–326.

Bazin, S., Blanchette, C., Bouchard, C., Brisson, J., Fortier, M., Meisels, A., et al. (1994). Vulvar vestibulitis syndrome: An exploratory case-control study. *Obstetrics and Gynecology, 83*(1), 47–50.

Bean, J.L. (2002). Expressions of female sexuality. *Journal of Sex and Marital Therapy, 28*(1), 29–38.

Beck, J.G., Bozman, A.W., & Qualtrough, T. (1991). The experience of sexual desire: Psychological correlates in a college sample. *Journal of Sex Research, 28,* 443–456.

Berman, J. (2005). Physiology of female sexual function and dysfunction. International *Journal of Impotence Research, 17* (Suppl. 1), S44-S51.

Berman, J., & Goldstein, I. (1998). Vasculogenic female sexual dysfunctions: Vaginal engorgement and clitoral erectile insufficiency syndromes.*International Journal of Impotence Research, 10*(Suppl. 2), S84–S90.

Berman, L., Berman, J., Chhabra, S., Felder, S., Miles, M., Pollets, D., et al. (2003). Seeking help for sexual function complaints: What gynecologists need to know about the female patient's experience. *Fertility and Sterility, 79*(3), 572–576.

Bertolasi, L., Frasson, E., Cappelletti, J.Y., Vicentini, S., Bordignon, M., & Graziottin, A. (2009). Botulinum neurotoxin type A injections for vaginismus secondary to vulvar vestibulitis syndrome. *Obstetrics and Gynecology, 114*(5), 1008–1016.

Bianco, V., Murina, F., Roberti, P., & Tassan, P. (2001). Treatment of vulvar vestibulitis with submucous infiltrations of methylprednisolone and lidocaine: An alternative approach. *Journal of Reproductive Medicine, 46*(8), 713–716.

Biggs, F., Clayton, A., Croft, H., Segraves, R., & Warnock, J. (2006). Comparison of androgens in women with hypoactive sexual desire disorder: Those on combined oral contraceptives vs. those not on combined oral contraceptives. *Journal of Sexual Medicine, 3*(5), 878–882.

Bindert, A., Exton, M., Hartmann, U., Kruger, T., Schedlowski, M., & Scheller, F. (1999). Cardiovascular and endocrine alterations after masturbation-induced orgasm in women. *Psychosomatic Medicine, 61*(3), 280–289.

Binik, Y.M. (2010). The DSM diagnostic criteria for vaginismus. *Archives of Sexual Behavior, 39*(2), 278–291.

Binik, Y., & Meana, M. (1994). Painful coitus: A review of female dyspareunia. *Journal of Nervous Mental Disease, 182*(5), 264–272.

BioSante Pharmaceuticals. (2011). *LibiGel.* Retrieved December 7, 2011, from http://www.biosantepharma.com/LibiGel.php

Biswas, A., & Ratnam, S.S. (1955). Vaginismus and outcome of treatment. *Annals of the Academy of Medicine, 24,* 755–758.

Bjornson, E., Sunley, R., Zussman, L., & Zussman, S. (1981). Sexual response after hysterectomy-oophorectomy: Recent studies and reconsideration of psychogenesis. *American Journal of Obstetrics and Gynecology, 140*(7), 725–729.

Bohm-Starke, N., Hilliges, M., Falconer, C., & Rylander, E. (1999). Neurochemical characterization of the vestibular nerves in women with vulvar vestibulitis syndrome. *Gynecologic and Obstetrical Investigation, 48*(4), 270–275.

Bornstein, J., Goldschmid, N., & Sabo, E. (2004). Hyperinnervation and mast cell activation may be used as a histopathologic diagnostic criteria for vulvar vestibulitis. *Obstetrics and Gynecology, 58*(3), 171–178.

Bowen, A., Klaiber, E., Simon, J., Wiita, B., & Yang, H. (1999). Differential effects of estrogen-androgen and estrogen-only therapy on vasomotor symptoms, gonadotropin secretion, and endogenous androgen bioavailability in postmenopausal women. *Menopause, 6*(2), 138–146.

Bradshaw, H.B., & Berkley, K.J. (2002). Estrogen replacement reverses ovariectomy-induced vaginal hyperalgesia in the rat. *Maturitas, 41,* 157–165.

Brin, M.F., & Vapnek, M.V. (1997). Treatment of vaginismus with botulinum toxin injections. *Lancet, 349,* 252–253.

Brotto, L.A., Heiman, J.R., & Tolman, D.L. (2009). Narratives of desire in mid-age women with and without arousal difficulties. *Journal of Sex Research, 46,* 387–398.

Brundu, B., Detaddei, S., Ferdeghini, F., Nappi, R., Polatti, F., & Sommacal, A. (2003). Role of testosterone in female sexuality. *Journal of Endocrinological Investigation, 26*(Suppl. 3), 97–101.

Burger, H.G., Hailes, J., Menelaus, M., Nelson, J., Hudson, B., & Balazs, N. (1984). The management of persistent menopausal symptoms with oestradiol-testosterone implants: Clinical, lipid and hormonal results. *Maturitas, 6*(4), 351.

Burrows, L., & Goldstein, A. (2008). Vulvodynia. *Journal of Sexual Medicine, 5*(1), 5–15.

Burrows, L., Goldstein, A., Klingman, D., & Pukall, C. (2008). Umbilical hypersensitivity in women with primary vestibulodynia. *Journal of Reproductive Medicine, 53*(6), 413–416.

Buster, J., Carson, S., Casson, P., Elkind-Hirsch, K., Hornsby, P., & Snabes, M. (1997). Effect of postmenopausal estrogen replacement on circulating androgens. *Obstetrics and Gynecology, 90*(6), 995–998.

Bygdeman, M., & Swahn, M. (1996). Replens versus Dienoestrol cream in the symptomatic treatment of vaginal atrophy in postmenopausal women. *Maturitas, 23*(3), 259–263.

Cain, V.S., Johannes, C.B., & Avis, N.E. (2003). Sexual functioning and practices in a multi-ethnic study of mid-life women: Baseline results from SWAN. *Journal of Sex Research, 40,* 266–276.

Campagnoli, C., Clavel-Chapelon, F., Kaaks, R., Peris, C., & Berrino, F. (2005). Progestins and progesterone in hormone replacement therapy and the risk of breast cancer. *Journal of Steroid Biochemistry and Molecular Biology, 96*(2), 95–108.

Carlsson, A.M. (1983). Assessment of chronic pain. I. Aspects of the reliability and validity of the visual analogue scale. *Pain, 16,* 87–101.

Carmichael, M., Davidson, J., Dixen, J., & Warburton, V. (1994). Relationships among cardiovascular, muscular, and oxytocin responses during human sexual activity. *Archives of Sexual Behavior, 23*(1), 59–79.

Carter, A.C., Cohen, C.J., & Shorr, E. (1947). The use of androgens in women. *Vitamins and Hormones, 5,* 317–391.

Chung, W., Shim, B., & Yoon, H. (2007). Botulinum toxin A for the management of vulvodynia. *International Journal of Impotence Research, 19,* 84–87.

Clapham, D. (1997). Some like it hot: Spicing up ion channels. *Nature, 389,* 783–784.

Coleman, R., Narumiya, S., & Smith, W. (1994). International Union of Pharmacology classification of prostanoid receptors: Properties, distribution, and structure of the receptors and their subtypes. *Pharmacological Reviews, 46*(2), 205–229.

Collins, M., Davis, G., Edwards, L., Foster, D., Gordon, D., Hartmann, E., et al. (2005). The vulvodynia guideline. *Journal of Lower Genital Tract Disease, 9*(1), 40–51.

Costabile, R., Dietrich, J., Friedman, A., Gittelman, M., Guay, A., Heard-Davison, A., et al. (2006). Topical alprostadil (PGE1) for the treatment of female sexual arousal disorder: In-clinic evaluation of safety and efficacy. *Journal of Psychosomatic Obstetrics and Gynecology, 27*(1), 31–41.

Crowley, T., Richardson, D., & Goldmeier, D. (2006). Recommendations for the management of vaginismus: BASHH special interest group for sexual dysfunction. *International Journal of STD and AIDS, 17,* 14–18.

Davis, S., & Tran, J. (2001). Testosterone influences libido and well-being in women. *Trends in Endocrinology and Metabolism, 12*(1), 33–37.

de Bie, L., de Leeuw, H., de Wilde, P., Hanselaar, A., & van der Laak, J. (2002). The effect of Replens on vaginal cytology in the treatment of postmenopausal atrophy: Cytomorphology versus computerised cytometry. *Journal of Clinical Pathology, 55*(6), 446–451.

de Freitas, M., de Sa, M., Ferriani, R., Lara, L., Reis, R., Rosa e Silva, A., et al. (2009). The effects of hypestrogenism on the vaginal wall: Interference with the normal sexual response. *Journal of Sexual Medicine, 6*(1), 30–39.

de Kruiff, M.E., ter Kuile, M.M., Weijenborg, P.T., & van Lankveld, J.J. (2000). Vaginismus and dyspareunia: Is there a difference in clinical presentation? *Journal of Psychosomatic Obstetrics and Gynaecology, 21*(3), 149–155.

Derogatis, L.R., Clayton, A., Lewis-D'Agostino, D., Wunderlich, G., & Fu, Y. (2008). Validation of the female sexual distress scale-revised for assessing distress in women with hypoactive sexual desire disorder. *Journal of Sexual Medicine, 5,* 357–364.

Derogatis, L.R., Rosen, R., Leiblum, S., Burnett, A., & Heiman, J. (2002). The Female Sexual Distress Scale (FSDS): Initial validation of a standardized scale for assessment of sexually related personal distress in women. *Journal of Sex and Marital Therapy, 28,* 317–330.

Dew, J., Eden, A., & Wren, B. (2003). A cohort study of topical vaginal estrogen therapy in women previously treated for breast cancer. *Climacteric, 6*(1), 45–52.

Dewis, P., Newman, M., Ratcliffe, W.A., & Anderson, D.C. (1986). Does testosterone affect the normal menstrual cycle. *Clinical Endocrinology (Oxford), 24*(5), 515–521.

Dimitrakakis, C., Jones, R.A., Liu, A., & Bondy, C.A. (2004). Breast cancer incidence in postmenopausal women using testosterone in addition to usual hormone therapy. *Menopause, 11*(5), 531.

Dizon, D., & Wiggins, D. (2008). Dyspareunia and vaginal dryness after breast cancer treatment. *Sexuality, Reproduction, and Menopause, 6*(3), 18–22.

Edwards, L. (2003). New concepts in vulvodynia. *American Journal of Obstetrics and Gynecology, 189*(Suppl. 3), S24–S30.

Ehrstrom, S., Kornfeld, D., Rylander, E., & Bohm-Starke, N. (2009). Chronic stress in women with localized provoked vestibulodynia. *Journal of Psychosomatic Obstetrics and Gynecology, 30*(1), 73–79.

Ellison, C. (1968). Psychosomatic factors in the unconsummated marriage. *Journal of Psychosomatic Research, 21,* 61–65.

Ellison, C. (1972). Vaginismus. *Medical Aspects of Human Sexuality, 6,* 34–54.

Engman, M., Lindehammar, H., & Wijma, B. (2004). Surface electromyography diagnostics in women with partial vaginismus with or without vulvar vestibulitis and in asymptomatic women. *Journal of Psychosomatic Obstetrics and Gynecology, 25*(3–4), 281–294.

Exton, M., Exton, N., Hartmann, U., Leygraf, N., Saller, B., Schedlowski, M., et al. (2000). Neuroendocrine responses to film-induced sexual arousal in men and women. *Psychoneuroendocrinology, 25*(2), 187–199.

Feldhaus-Dahir, M. (2009a). Female sexual dysfunction: Barriers to treatment. *Urologic Nursing, 29*(2), 81–85.

Feldhaus-Dahir, M. (2009b). The causes and prevalence of hypoactive sexual desire disorder: Part I. *Urologic Nursing, 29*(4), 259–260.

Feldhaus-Dahir, M. (2009c). Testosterone for the treatment of hypoactive sexual desire disorder: Part II. *Urologic Nursing, 29*(5), 386–389.

Feldhaus-Dahir, M. (2011). The causes and prevalence of vestibulodynia: A vulvar pain disorder. *Urologic Nursing, 31*(1), 51–54.

Female Sexual Function Index (FSFI). (2000). *FSFI.* Retrieved November 27, 2011, from http://www.fsfiquestionnaire.com

Fenichel, L. (1945). *The psychoanalytic theory of neurosis.* New York: Norton.

Fisher, S. (1973). *The female orgasm.* New York: Basic Books.

Fordney, D.S. (1978). Dyspareunia and vaginismus. *Clinical Obstetrics and Gynecology, 21,* 205–221.

Foster, D.C., & Hasday, J.D. (1997). Elevated tissue levels of interleukin-1 beta and tumor necrosis factor-alpha in vulvar vestibulitis. *Obstetrics and Gynecology, 89*(2), 291–296.

Frank, E., Anderson, C., & Rubinstein, D. (1978). Frequency of sexual dysfunction in "normal" couples. *New England Journal of Medicine, 299*(3), 111–115.

Friedrich, E.G. (1987). Vulvar vestibulitis syndrome. *Journal of Reproductive Medicine, 32*(2), 110–114.

Gamble, G., Heiman, J., Nusbaum, M., & Skinner, B. (2000). The high prevalence of sexual concerns among women seeking routine gynecological care. *Journal of Family Practice, 49*(3), 229–232.

Gambrell, R.D., Jr., & Natrajan, P.K. (2006). Moderate dosage estrogen-androgen therapy improves continuation rates in postmenopausal women: Impact of the WHI reports. *Climacteric, 9*(3), 224–233.

Garcia-Banigan, D.C., & Guay, A.T. (2005). Testosterone treatment in women. *Contemporary Sexuality, 39*(7), i–vii.

Garnett, T., Studd, J., Watson, N., & Savvas, M. (1991). A cross-sectional study of the effects of long-term percutaneous hormone replacement therapy on bone density. *Obstetrics and Gynecology, 78*(6), 1002.

Gelfand, M., & Wendman, E. (1994). Treating vaginal dryness in breast cancer patients: Results of applying a polycarbophil moisturizing gel. *Journal of Women's Health, 3*(6), 427–434.

Genadry, R., Poliakoff, S., & Woodruff, J. (1981). Treatment of dyspareunia and vaginal outlet distortions by perineoplasty. *Obstetrics and Gynecology, 62,* 750–753.

Gendrano, N., Phillips, N., & Rosen, R. (1999). Oral phentolamine and female sexual arousal disorder: A pilot study. *Journal of Sex and Marital Therapy, 25*(2), 137–144.

Ghazizdeh, S., & Nikzad, M. (2004). Botulinum toxin in the treatment of refractory vaginismus. *Obstetrics and Gynecology, 104,* 922–925.

Gingell, C., Glasser, D., Laumann, E., Moreira, E., Nicolosi, A., & Wang, T. (2005). Sexual problems among women and men aged 40-80y: Prevalence and correlates identified in the global study of sexual attitudes and behaviors. *International Journal of Impotence Research, 17*(1), 39–57.

Giraldi, A., Marson, L., Nappi, R., Pfaus, J., Traish, A.M., Vardi, Y., et al. (2004). Physiology of female sexual function: Animal models. *Journal of Sexual Medicine, 1,* 237–253. doi:10.1111/j.1743-6109.04037

Glaser, R., Newman, M., Parsons, M., Zava, D., & Glaser-Garbrick, D. (2009). Safety of maternal testosterone therapy during breast feeding. *International Journal of Pharmaceutical Compounding, 13,* 314–317.

Glaser, R., Wurtzbacher, D., & Dimitrakakis, C. (2009). Efficacy of testosterone therapy delivered by pellet implant. *Maturitas, 63*(Suppl. 1), 283.

Glaser, R., York, A.E., & Dimitrakakis, C. (2010). Beneficial effects of testosterone therapy in women measured by the validated menopause rating scale (MRS). *Maturitas, 68,* 355–361.

Glazer, H.I., Jantos, M., Hartmann, E.H., & Swencionis, C. (1998). Electromyographic comparisons of the pelvic floor in women with dysesthetic vulvodynia and asymptomatic women. *Journal of Reproductive Medicine, 43,* 959–962.

Goldmeier, D., & Leiblum, S. (2008). Interaction of organic and psychological factors in persistent genital arousal disorder in women: A report of six cases. *International Journal of STD and AIDS, 19,* 488–490.

Goldstein, A.T., & Burrows, L. (2008). Vulvodynia. *Journal of Sexual Medicine, 5,* 5–15.

Goldstein, A.T., Klingman, D., Christopher, K., Johnson, C., & Marinoff, S.C. (2006). Surgical treatment of vulvar vestibulitis syndrome: Outcome assessment derived from a postoperative questionnaire. *Journal of Sexual Medicine, 3*(5), 923–931.

Goldstein, A.T., Pukall, C.F., & Goldstein, I. (2009). *Female sexual pain disorders: Evaluation and management.* Hoboken, NJ: Wiley-Blackwell.

Goldstein, I., De, E.J.B., & Johnson, J. (2006). Persistent sexual arousal syndrome and clitoral priapism. In I. Goldstein, C.M. Meston, S.R. Davis, & A.M. Traish (Eds.), *Women's sexual function and dysfunction: Study, diagnosis, and treatment* (pp. 674–685). Boca Raton, FL: Taylor Francis.

Gordon, A.S., Panahian-Jand, M., McComb, F., Melegari, C., & Sharp, S. (2003). Characteristics of women with vulvar pain disorders: Responses to a web-based survey. *Journal of Sex and Marital Therapy, 29*(Suppl. 1), 45–58.

Gottesfeld, M.L. (1978). Treatment of vaginismus by psychotherapy with adjunctive hypnosis. *American Journal of Clinical Hypnosis, 4,* 272–277.

Graham, C.A., Sanders, S.A., Milhausen, R.R., & McBride, K.R. (2004). Turning on and turning off: A focus group study of the factors that affect women's sexual arousal. *Archives of Sexual Behavior, 33,* 527–538.

Graziottin, A., & Brotto, L.A. (2004). Vulvar vestibulitis syndrome: A clinical approach. *Journal of Sex and Marital Therapy, 30*(3), 125–139.

Haefner, H.K. (2000). Critique of new gynecologic surgical procedures: Surgery for vulvar vestibulitis. *Clinical Obstetrics Gynecology, 43,* 689–700.

Harlow, B.L., He, W., & Nguyen, R.H. (2009). Allergic reactions and risk of vulvodynia. *Annals of Epidemiology, 19*(11), 771–777.

Harlow, B.L., & Stewart, E. (2003). A population-based assessment of chronic unexplained vulvar pain: Have we underestimated the prevalence of vulvodynia? *Journal of American Medical Women's Association, 58*(2), 82–88.

Harman, M.J., Waldo, M., & Johnson, J.A. (1994). Relationship enhancement therapy: A case study for treating vaginismus. *Family Journal, 2*(2), 122–128.

Hartmann, D., Strauhal, M.J., & Nelson, C.A. (2007). Treatment of women in the United States with localized, provoked vulvodynia: Practice survey of women's health physical therapists. *Journal of Reproductive Medicine, 52*(1), 48–52.

Hatzimouratidis, K., & Hatzichristou, D. (2007). Sexual dysfunctions: Classifications and definitions. *Journal of Sexual Medicine, 4,* 241–250.

Hassel, B. (1997). Resolution of primary vaginismus and introital hyperesthesia by topical anesthesia. *Anesthesia and Analgesia, 85,* 1415–1416.

Hawton, K., & Catalan, J. (1990). Sex therapy for vaginismus: Characteristics of couples and treatment outcome. *Journal of Sex and Marital Therapy, 5,* 39–48.

Hayes, R.D. (2011). Circular and linear modeling of female sexual desire and arousal. *Journal of Sex Research, 78*(2–3), 130–141.

Heiman, J.R. (2000). Orgasmic disorders in women. In S.R. Leiblum & S.C. Rosen (Eds.), *Principles and practice of sex therapy* (3rd ed., pp. 118–153). New York: Guildford Press.

Hengge, U.R., & Runnebaum, I.B. (2005). Vulvodynia. *Hautarzt, 56*(6), 556–559.

Herbenick, D., Reece, M., Hensel, D., Sanders, S., Jozkowski, K., & Fortenberry, J.D. (2009). Association of lubricant use with women's sexual pleasure, sexual satisfaction and genital symptoms: A prospective daily diary study. *Journal of Sexual Medicine, 6,* 1867–1874.

Hiller, J., & Hekster, B. (2007). Couple therapy and cognitive behavioural techniques for persistent sexual arousal syndrome. *Sex Relationship Therapy, 22,* 91–96.

Hodgins, M.B., Spike, R.C., Mackie, R.M., & MacLean, A.B. (1998). An immunohistochemical study of androgen, oestrogen and progesterone receptors in the vulva and vagina. *British Journal of Obstetrics and Gynaecology, 105*(2), 216–222.

Ito, T., Polan, M., Trant, A., & Whipple, B. (2006). The enhancement of female sexual function with ArginMax, a nutritional supplement, among women differing in menopausal status. *Journal of Sex and Marital Therapy, 32*(5), 369–378.

Josefsson, E., Tarkowski, A., & Carlsten, H. (1992). Anti-inflammatory properties of estrogen. I. In vivo suppression of leukocyte production in bone marrow and redistribution of peripheral blood neutrophils. *Cell Immunology, 142*(1), 67–78.

Kaplan, H.S. (1974). *The new sex therapy.* New York: Brunner/Mazel.

Kaplan, H.S. (1979). *Disorders of sexual desire.* New York: Brunner/Mazel.

Katz, A. (2009). *Women cancer sex.* Pittsburgh, PA: Oncology Nursing Society.

Kellogg-Spadt, S., Oyama, I., Rejba, A., Steinberg, A., & Whitmore, K. (2005). Capsaicin for the treatment of vulvar vestibulitis. *American Journal of Obstetrics and Gynecology, 192*(5), 1549–1553.

Kennedy, B.J., & Nathanson, I.T. (1953). Effects of intensive sex steroid hormone therapy in advanced breast cancer. *Journal of the American Medical Association, 152,* 1 135–1141.

Kingsberg, S.A., & Janata, J.W. (2007). Female sexual disorders: Assessment, diagnosis, and treatment. *Urologic Clinics of North America, 34*(4), 497–506.

Kinsey, A.C., Pomeroy, W.B., Martin, C.E., & Gebhard, P.H. (1953). *Sexual behavior in the human female.* Philadelphia: W.B. Saunders.

Korda, J.B., Pfaus, J.G., & Goldstein, I. (2009). Persistent genital arousal disorder: A case report in a woman with lifelong PGAD where serendipitous administration of varenicline tartrate resulted in symptomatic improvement. *Journal of Sexual Medicine, 6,* 1479–1486.

Korda, J.B., Pfaus, J.G., Kellner, C.H., & Goldstein, I. (2009). Persistent genital arousal disorder (PGAD): Case report of long-term symptomatic management with electroconvulsive therapy. *Journal of Sexual Medicine, 6*(10), 2901–2909.

Krychman, M.L. (2007). *Vaginal atrophy: The 21st century health issue affecting quality of life.* Retrieved from http://www.medscape.org/viewarticle/561934

Lahaie, M.A., Boyer, S.C., Amsel, R., Khalife, S., & Binik, Y.M. (2010). Vaginismus: A review of the literature on the classification/diagnosis, etiology and treatment. *Women's Health, 6*(5), 705–719.

Lamont, J.A. (1978). Vaginismus. *American Journal of Obstetrics and Gynecology, 131,* 633–636.

Laumann, E.O., Gagnon, J.H., Michael, R.T., & Michaels, S. (1994). *The social organization of sexuality: Sexual practices in the United States.* Chicago: University of Chicago Press.

Laumann, E.O., Paik, A., & Rosen, R.C. (1999). Sexual dysfunction in the United States: Prevalence and predictors. *Journal of the American Medical Association, 281*(6), 537–544.

Laumann, E.O., Levinson, W., Lindau, S.T., O'Muircheartaigh, C.A., Schumm, L.P., & Waite, L.J. (2007). A study of sexuality and health among older adults in the United States. *New England Journal of Medicine, 357*(8), 762–774.

Leiblum, S., Brown, C., Wan, J., & Rawlinson, L. (2005). Persistent sexual arousal syndrome: A descriptive study. *Journal of Sexual Medicine, 2,* 331–337.

Leiblum, S., & Goldmeier, D. (2008). Persistent genital arousal disorder in women: Case reports of association with anti-depressant usage and withdrawal. *Journal of Sexual Medicine, 34,* 150–159.

Leiblum, S., Seehuus, M., Goldmeier, D., & Brown, C. (2007). Psychological, medical and pharmacological correlates of persistent genital arousal disorder. *Journal of Sexual Medicine, 4,* 1358–1366.

Leiblum, S.R. (2000). Vaginismus: A most perplexing problem. In S.R. Leiblum & R.C. Rosen (Eds.), *Principles and practice of sex therapy* (pp. 181–202). New York: Guilford Press.

Levin, R.J. (1980). The physiology of sexual function in women. *Clinical Obstetrics and Gynecology, 7*(2), 213.

Levin, R.J. (1992). The mechanisms of human female sexual arousal. *Annual Review of Sex Research, 3,* 1–48.

Levin, R.J. (2001). Sexual desire and the deconstruction and reconstruction of the human female sexual response model of Masters & Johnson. In W. Everaerd, E. Waan, & S. Both (Eds.), *Sexual appetite, desire and motivation: Energetics of the sexual* (pp. 63–93). Amsterdam: Royal Netherlands Academy of Arts and Sciences.

Lobo, R.A. (2001). Androgens in postmenopausal women: Production, possible role, and replacement options. *Obstetrical and Gynecological Survey, 56*(6), 361.

Lloyd, E. (2005). *The Case of the Female Orgasm.* Boston, MA: Harvard university Press.

Mahoney, S., & Zarate, C. (2007). Persistent sexual arousal syndrome: A case report and review of the literature. *Journal of Sex and Marital Therapy, 33,* 65–72.

Marwick, C. (1999). Survey says patients expect little physician help on sex. *Journal of the American Medical Association, 281*(23), 2173–2174.

Masters, W.H., & Johnson, V.E. (1966). *Human sexual response.* Boston: Little Brown.

Masters, W.H., & Johnson, V.E. (1970). *Human sexual inadequacy.* Boston: Little Brown.

Mathias, S.D., Kuppermann, M., Liberman, R.F., Lipschutz, R.C., & Steege, J.F. (1996). Chronic pelvic pain: Prevalence, health-related quality of life, and economic correlates. *Obstetrics and Gynecology, 87,* 321–327.

McGarvey, E., Peterson, C., Pinkerton, R., Keller, A., & Clayton, A. (2003). Medical students' perceptions of sexual health issues prior to a curriculum enhancement. *International Journal of Impotence Research, 15*(Suppl. 5), S58–S66.

McVary, K., Pelham, R., Polepalle, S., & Riggi, S. (1999). Topical prostaglandin E1 SEPA gel for the treatment of erectile dysfunction. *Journal of Urology, 162*(Suppl. 3, Pt. 1), 726–730.

Meston, C.M., & Buss, D.M. (2007). Why humans have sex. *Archives of Sexual Behavior, 36,* 477–507.

Meston, C.M., Hull, E., Levin, R.J., & Sipski, M. (2004). Disorders of orgasm in women. *Journal of Sexual Medicine, 1*(1), 66–68.

Meston, C.M., Levin, R.J., Sipski, M.L., Hull, E.M., & Heiman, J.R. (2004). Women's orgasm. *Annual Review of Sex Research, 15,* 173–257.

Mick, J.M. (2007). Sexuality assessment: 10 strategies for improvement. *Clinical Journal of Oncology Nursing, 11*(5), 671–675.

Mirkin, D., Murphy-Barron, C., & Iwasaki, K. (2007). Actuarial analysis of private payer administrative claims data for women with endometriosis. *Journal of Managed Care Pharmacy, 13,* 262–272.

Moyal-Barracco, M., & Lynch, P.J. (2004). 2003 ISSVD terminology and classification of vulvodynia: A historical perspective. *Journal of Reproductive Medicine, 49,* 772–777.

Munday, P., Buchan, A., Ravenhill, B., Wiggs, A., & Brooks, F. (2007). A qualitative study of women with vulvodynia: II. Response to a multidisciplinary approach to management. *Journal of Reproductive Medicine, 52*(1), 15–18.

Musaph, H., & Haspels, A.A. (1976). Vagisime. *Ned Tijdschr Geneekunde, 120,* 1589–1592.

Nappi, R., Rosella, E., Schmitt, S., & Wawra, K. (2006). Hypoactive sexual desire disorder in postmenopausal women. *Gynecological Endocrinology, 22*(6), 318–323.

National Vulvodynia Association. (2010). *NVA history.* Retrieved from https://www.nva.org

Nylander Lundqvist, E., & Sjoberg, I. (1997). Vulvar vestibulitis in the north of Sweden: An epidemiologic case-control study. *Journal of Reproductive Medicine, 42*(3), 166–168.

Nyrop, K.A., Palsson, O.S., Levy, R.L., Korff, M.V., Feld, A.D., Turner, M.J., et al. (2007). Costs of health care for irritable bowel syndrome, chronic constipation, functional diarrhea and functional abdominal pain. *Alimentary Pharmacology and Therapeutics, 26,* 237–248.

O'Sullivan, K. (1979). Observations of vaginismus in Irish women. *Archives of General Psychiatry, 36,* 824–826.

Pauls, R.N., Kleeman, S.D., Segal, J.L., Silva, W.A., Goldenhar, G.M., & Karram, M.M. (2005). Practice patterns of physician members of the American Urogynecologic Society regarding female sexual dysfunction: Results of a national survey. *International Urogynecology Journal, 16*(6), 460–467.

Penteado, S.R.L., Fonseca, A.M., Bagnoli, V.R., Abdo, C.H.N., Junior, J.M.S., & Baracat, E.C. (2008). Effects of the addition of methyltestosterone to combined hormone therapy with estrogens and progestogens on sexual energy and on orgasm in postmenopausal women. *Climacteric, 11,* 17–25.

Perrone, A.M., Cerpolini, S., Salfi, N.C.M., Ceccarelli, C., De Giorgi, L.B., Formelli, G., et al. (2009). Effect of long-term testosterone administration on the endometrium of female-to-male (FtM) transsexuals. *Journal of Sexual Medicine, 6*(11), 3193–3200.

Petersen, C.D., Giraldi, A., Lundvall, L., & Kristensen, E. (2009). Botulinum toxin type: A novel treatment for provoked vestibulodynia? Results from a randomized, placebo controlled, double blinded study. *Journal of Sexual Medicine, 6*(9), 2523–2537.

Plaut, A.M., & RachBeisel, J. (1997). Use of anxiolytic medication in the treatment of vaginismus and severe aversion to penetration: Case report. *Journal of Sex Education and Therapy, 22,* 43–45.

Pukall, C.F., Smith, K.B., & Chamberlain, S.M. (2007). Provoked vestibulodynia. *Women's Health, 3*(5), 583–592.

Reissing, E.D., Binik, Y.M., Khalife, S., Cohen, D., & Amsel, R. (2004). Vaginal spasm, pain, and behavior: An empirical investigation of the diagnosis of vaginismus. *Archives of Sexual Behavior, 33,* 5–17.

Rellini, A.H., & Clifton, J. (2011). Female orgasmic disorder. *Advances in Psychosomatic Medicine, 31,* 35–56.

Rollema, H., Chambers, L.K., Coe, J.W., Glowa, J., Hurst, R.S., Lebel, L.A., et al. (2007). Pharmacological profile of the alpha-4-beta-2 nicotinic acetylcholine receptor partial agonist varenicline, an effective smoking cessation aid. *Neuropharmacology, 52,* 985–994.

Rollema, H., Coe, J.W., Chambers, L.K., Hurst, R.S., Stahl, S.M., & Williams, K.E. (2007). Rationale, pharmacology and clinical efficacy of partial agonists of the alpha-4-beta-2 nicotinic acetylcholine receptors for smoking cessation. *Trends in Pharmacological Sciences, 28,* 316–325.

Rosen, L.J., & Rosen, R.C. (2006). Fifty years of female sexual dysfunction research and concepts: From Kinsey to present. In I. Goldstein, C.M. Meston, S.R. Davis, & A.M. Traish (Eds.), *Women's sexual function and dysfunction: Study, diagnosis, and treatment* (pp. 3–10). Boca Raton, FL: Taylor & Francis.

Rosen, R.C., Brown, C., Heiman, J., Leiblum, S., Meston, C., Shabsigh, R., et al. (2000). The female sexual function index (FSFI): A multidimensional self-report instrument for the assessment of female sexual dysfunction. *Journal of Sex and Marital Therapy, 26,* 191–208.

Rosen, R.C., Taylor, J.F., Leiblum, S.R., & Bachmann, G.A. (1993). Prevalence of sexual dysfunction in women: Results of a survey study of 329 women in an outpatient gynecologic clinic. *Journal of Sex and Marital Therapy, 19,* 171–188.

Rosenbaum, T.Y. (2005). Physiotherapy treatment of sexual pain disorders. *Journal of Sex and Marital Therapy, 31,* 329–340.

Rosenbaum, T.Y. (2008). The role of physiotherapy in female sexual dysfunction. *Current Sexual Health Reports, 5,* 97–101.

Rosenqvist, U., & Sarkadi, A. (2001). Contradiction in the medical encounter: Female sexual dysfunction in primary care contacts. *Family Practice, 18*(2), 161–166.

Rossouw, J.E., Anderson, G.L., Prentice, R.L., La Croix, A.Z., Kooperberg, C., Stefanick, M.L., et al. (2002). Risks and benefits of estrogen plus progestin in healthy postmenopausal women: Principal results from the women's health initiative randomized controlled trial. *Journal of the American Medical Association, 288,* 321–333.

Salmon, U.J., & Geist, S.H. (1943). Effect of androgens upon libido in women. *Journal of Clinical Endocrinology, 3,* 235–238.

Salmon, U.J., Geist, S.H., Gaines, J.A., & Walter, R.I. (1941). The treatment of abnormal uterine bleeding with androgens. *American Journal of Obstetrics and Gynecology, 41,* 991–1009.

Sands, R., Studd, J., Seed, M., Doherty, E., Kelman, D., Andrews, G., et al. (1997). The effects of exogenous testosterone on lipid metabolism & insulin resistance in postmenopausal women. *Maturitas, 27*(Suppl. 1), 50.

Sarrel, P., Dobay, B., & Wiita, B. (1998). Estrogen and estrogen-androgen replacement in postmenopausal women dissatisfied with estrogen-only therapy. Sexual behavior and neuroendocrine responses. *Journal of Reproductive Medicine, 43,* 847–856.

Saxon, W. (1995). Dr. Helen Kaplan, 66, dies; pioneer in sex therapy field. *New York Times*. Retrieved from http://www.nytimes.com

Seed, M., Sands, R.H., McLaren, M., Kirk, G., & Darko, D. (2000). The effect of hormone replacement therapy and route of administration on selected cardiovascular risk factors in post-menopausal women. *Family Practice, 17*(6), 497.

Segal, D., Tifheret, H., & Lazer, S. (2003). Submucous infiltration of betamethasone and lidocaine in the treatment of vulvar vestibulitis. *European Journal of Obstetrics, Gynecology, and Reproductive Biology, 107*(1), 105–106.

Segaloff, A. (1975). Hormone therapy of breast cancer. *Cancer Treatment Reviews, 2,* 129–135.

Shafik, A., & El-Sibai, O. (2000). Vaginismus: Results of treatment with botulinum toxin. *Journal of Obstetrics and Gynecology, 20,* 300–302.

Shames, D., Monroe, S.E., Davis, D., & Soule, L. (2007). Regulatory perspective on clinical trials and end points for female sexual dysfunction, in particular, hypoactive sexual desire disorder: Formulating recommendations in an environment of evolving clinical science. *International Journal of Impotence Research, 19,* 30–36.

Shell, J. (2007). Including sexuality in your nursing practice. *Nursing Clinics of North America, 42*(4), 685–696.

Shepphard, C., Hallam-Jones, R., & Wylie, K. (2008). Why have you both come? Emotional, relationship and social issued raised by heterosexual couples seeking sexual therapy (in women referred to a sexual difficulties clinic with a history of vulvar pain). *Sexual and Relationship Therapy, 23*(3), 217–226.

Sherwin, B., Gelfand, M., & Brender, W. (1985). Androgen enhances sexual motivation in females: A prospective, cross-over study of sex steroid administration in the surgical post-menopausal. *Psychometric Medicine, 47*(4), 339–345.

Sills, T., Wunderlich, G., Pyke, R., Segraves, R.T., Leiblum, S., Clayton, A., et al. (2005). The Sexual Interest and Desire Inventory-Female (SIDI-F): Item response analysis of data from women diagnosed with hypoactive sexual desire disorder. *Journal of Sexual Medicine, 2*(6), 801–818.

Simon, J. (2002). Estrogen replacement therapy: Effects on the endogenous androgen milieu. *Fertility and Sterility, 77*(Suppl. 4), S77–S82.

Singer, I. (1973). *The goal of human sexuality*. New York: W.W. Norton.

Solursh, D.S., Ernst, J.L., Lewis, R.W., Prisant, L.M., Mills, T.M., Solursh, L.P., et al. (2003). The human sexuality education of physicians in North American medical schools. *International Journal of Impotence Research, 15*(Suppl. 5), S41–S45.

Spector, I.P., & Carey, M.P. (1990). Incidence and prevalence of the sexual dysfunctions: A critical review of the empirical literature. *Archives of Sexual Behavior, 19,* 389–408.

Steege, J.F. (1984). Dyspareunia and vaginismus. *Clinical Obstetrics and Gynecology, 27,* 750–759.

Symons, D. (1979). *The evolution of human sexuality*. New York: Oxford University Press.

Taylor, A.H., Guzail, M., & Al-Azzawi, F. (2008). Differential expression of oestrogen receptor isoforms and androgen receptor in the normal vulva and vagina compared with vulval lichen sclerosus and chronic vaginitis. *British Journal of Dermatology, 158*(2), 319–328.

ter Kuile, M., van Lankveld, J., Vlieland, C.V., Wilekes, C., & Weijenborg, P.T.M. (2005). Vulvar vestibulitis syndrome: An important factor in the evolution of lifelong vaginismus? *Journal of Psychosomatic Obstetrics and Gynaecology, 26,* 245–249.

Thom, M.H., Collins, W.P., & Studd, J.W.W. (1981). Hormonal profiles in postmenopausal women after therapy with subcutaneous implants. *British Journal of Obstetrics and Gynaecology, 88,* 426–433.

Thorne, C., & Stuckey, B. (2008). Pelvic congestion syndrome presenting as persistent genital arousal: A case report. *Journal of Sexual Medicine, 5,* 504–508.

Tiefer, L. (1991). Historical, scientific and feminist criticisms of "the Human Sexual Response Cycle" model. *Annual Review of Sex Research, 7,* 252–282.

Tiefer, L., Hall, M., & Tavris, C. (2002). Beyond dysfunction: A new view of women's sexual problems. *Journal of Sex and Marital Therapy, 28,* 225–232.

Traish, A.M., Feeley, R.J., & Guay, A.T. (2009). Testosterone therapy in women with gynecological and sexual disorders: A triumph of clinical endocrinology from 1938 to 2009. *Journal of Sexual Medicine, 6,* 334–351.

Traish, A.M., & Gooren, L.J. (2010). Safety of physiological testosterone therapy in women: Lessons from female to male transsexuals (FMT) treated with pharmacological testosterone therapy. *Journal of Sexual Medicine, 7*(11), 3758–3764.

Traish, A.M., Huang, Y.H., Min, K., Kim, N.N., Munarriz, R., & Goldstein, I. (2004). Binding characteristics of [3H] delta(5)-androstene-3beta,17beta-diol to a nuclear protein in the rabbit vagina. *Steroids, 69*(1), 71–78.

Traish, A.M., Kim, N.N., Huang, Y.H., Min, K., Munarriz, R., & Goldstein, I. (2003). Sex steroid hormones differentially regulate nitric oxide synthase and arginase activities in the proximal and distal rabbit vagina. *International Journal of Impotence Research, 15*(6), 397–404.

Trotula of Salerno. (1940). *The diseases of women*. W. Mason-Hohl Trans (Ed.). Los Angeles, CA: The Ward Ritchie Press.

Turk, D.C., & Burwinkle, T.M. (2005). Clinical outcomes, cost-effectiveness and the role of psychology in treatments for chronic pain sufferers. *Professional Psychology: Research and Practice, 36,* 602–610.

Van de Wiel, H.B. (1990). Treatment of vaginismus: A review of concepts and treatment modalities. *Journal of Psychosomatic Obstetrics and Gynecology, 11,* 1–18.

van Lankveld, J.J., Brewaeys, A.M., ter Kuile, M.M., & Weijenborg, P.T. (1995). Difficulties in the differential diagnosis of vaginismus, dyspareunia and mixed sexual pain disorder. *Psychosomatic Obstetrics and Gynaecology, 16,* 201–209.

van Lankveld, J.J., ter Kulie, M.M., de Groot, H.E., Melles, R., Nefs, J., & Zandbergen, M. (2006). Cognitive-behavioral therapy for women with lifelong vaginismus: A randomized waiting-list controlled trial of efficacy. *Journal of Consulting and Clinical Psychology, 74*(1), 168–178.

Walthard, M. (1909). Die psychogene aetiologie und die psychotherapie des vaginismus. *Munch Med Wochenschr, 56,* 1997–2000.

Warnock, J. (2002). Female hyperactive sexual desire disorder: Epidemiology, diagnosis, and treatment. *CNS Drugs, 16*(11), 745–753.

Weijmar Schultz, W.C.M., & van de Wiel, H.B.M. (2005). Vaginismus. In R. Balon & R.T. Segraves (Eds.), *Handbook of sexual dysfunction* (pp. 301–316). New York: Taylor & Francis.

Weinstein, K. (1987). *Living with endometriosis*. New York: Addison Wesley.

Westrom, L., & Willen, R. (1998). Vestibular nerve fiber proliferation in vulvar vestibulitis syndrome. *Obstetrics and Gynecology, 91*(4), 572–576.

Wilson, S.K., Delk, J.R., & Billups, K.L. (2001). Treating symptoms of female sexual arousal disorder with the Eros-Clitoral Therapy Device. *Journal of Gender-Specific Medicine, 4*(2), 54–58.

Witkin, S.S., Gerber, S., & Ledger, W.J. (2002). Differential characterization of women with vulvar vestibulitis syndrome. *American Journal of Obstetrics and Gynecology, 187*(3), 589–594.

Women's Sexual Health Foundation. (2005). *Educational materials: Are you a woman experiencing sexual difficulties?* Retrieved December 2, 2011, from http://www.twshf.org/pamphlets.html

World Health Organization (WHO). (1992). *ICD-10: International statistical classification of diseases and related health problems*. Geneva: Author.

World Health Organization (WHO). (n.d.). *Sexual and reproductive health: Working definitions*. Retrieved November 19, 2011, from http://www.who.int/reproductivehealth/topics/gender_rights/sexual_health/en/

Wu, E.Q., Birnbaum, H., Mareva, M., Parece, A., Huang, Z., Mallett, D., et al. (2006). Interstitial cystitis: Cost, treatment and co-morbidities in an employed population. *Pharmacoeconomics, 24,* 55–65.

Wylie, K., Levin, R., Hallman-Jones, R., & Goddard, A. (2006). Sleep exacerbation of persistent sexual arousal syndrome in a postmenopausal woman. *Journal of Sexual Medicine, 3,* 296–302.

Zang, H., Sahlin, L., Masironi, B., Eriksson, E., & Linden Hirschberg, A. (2007). Effects of testosterone treatment on endometrial proliferation in postmenopausal women. *Journal of Clinical Endocrinology and Metabolism, 92*(6), 2169–2175.

Zolnoun, D.A., Hartmann, K.E., & Steege, J.F. (2003). Overnight 5% lidocaine ointment for treatment of vulvar vestibulitis. *Obstetrics and Gynecology, 102*(1), 84–87.

CHAPTER ❖ 8

HEALTH NEEDS OF LESBIANS AND OTHER SEXUAL MINORITY WOMEN

Debera Jane Thomas

Although the health care needs of lesbians are the same as those of all women in most instances, lesbians and other sexual minority women face additional unique health problems to which health care providers must attend.

Highlights

- Care Barriers for Lesbians
- An Inclusive Approach and Environment for Acceptance
- Assessing the Woman's Coping Status
- Special Groups at Greater Risk
- Health Problems of Lesbians
- Desire to Parent
- Health Resources and Organizations

❖ INTRODUCTION

There is no standard definition for the term *lesbian*; it generally describes a woman's sexual identity, but is not necessarily an indication of sexual behavior (Ben-Natan & Adir, 2009). Women who form sexual and affectional relationships with other women are considered lesbian; however, they may or may not self-identify as lesbian. Several factors influence a woman's decision to identify or not to identify herself as lesbian, such as race, ethnicity, socioeconomic class, cultural values, age, religion, or personal history. Women may identify themselves as lesbian at any time during their lives, from youth to old age, and sexual orientation may be fluid across a woman's life with periods of heterosexuality and same-sex relationships. Sexual preference is only one aspect of why a person considers herself or himself same-sex identified.

Sexuality, sexual orientation, and gender expression exist on a continuum from exclusively heterosexual to exclusively homosexual, with bisexuality somewhere in the middle. Likewise, gender expression occurs along a similar continuum from extremely male to extremely female. Gender dysphoria occurs when individuals are discontented with their biological sex. Transgender refers to those individuals who live or wish to live as individuals opposite of their biologic sex. When an individual transitions from one gender to the other, it is called *sex* or *gender reassignment* (American Psychiatric Association [APA], 2011).

Lesbians, bisexual women, and transgendered individuals are as diverse as the population at large, crossing all age, occupation, ethnic/racial, religious, economic, and geographic boundaries. The number of lesbians in the United States by any definition is not known, but is estimated to be between 8 and 20 percent of U.S. women (Marrazzo, 2004); because of the fear of social stigma, this may be an underestimation. Updated demographics may be gleaned from the 2010 U.S. census when data is analyzed. One goal of Healthy People 2020 is to "Improve the health, safety, and well-being of lesbian, gay, bisexual, and transgender (LGBT) individuals" (2011). Although the health care needs of lesbians are the same as those of all women in most instances, lesbians can experience some health problems with greater frequency than the average. Further, it is imperative that nurses caring for women be attuned to and respectful of this population and their health care needs and problems.

The decrease in the number of articles appearing in the nursing literature since 2005 relating to the special needs and concerns of this population and an increase in the number of lesbians, bisexual women, and transgendered individuals appearing in popular media would seem to indicate a tolerant attitude, but prejudice and ignorance remain. The existence of prejudice prevents many women in this group from seeking health care until the condition becomes more emergent, resulting in more debilitating, costlier medical problems. Providers can help to decrease barriers by acknowledging any internalized homophobia of their own and attempting to be as impartial as humanly possible to all their women clients.

Health care providers need to understand that, regardless of age, social status, education, and so on, every woman who becomes woman identified and eventually self-identifies as a lesbian has generally gone through a period of coming-out—realizing that her sexual and affectional preference is not the societal norm and, in fact, may be condemned by major religious and political groups. Health care in the United States is generally delivered on the assumption that everyone is heterosexual (Spidsberg, 2007). This, often unconscious, assumption can lead to uncomfortable encounters within the health care system because of homophobic and heterosexist attitudes among health care providers (Irwin, 2007). The fear of a negative encounter may lead a patient to not disclose her sexual orientation. A newly identified lesbian, bisexual, or transgendered (LBT) woman may have had to make a shift in core identity and had to process the pros and cons of disclosure. Therefore, she may require positive support and counseling. In fact, 87 percent of sexual minority people report being discriminated against (McCabe, Bostwick, Hughes, West, & Boyd, 2010). For the adolescent coping with developmental tasks as well as for the woman who finally begins to acknowledge that the heterosexual way of life is not fulfilling, it can be a time of great emotional distress, with greater risks of depression or suicide. Both families and health care providers need to consider questions about sexual identity as a reason for significant behavioral changes. Until the individual becomes comfortable with her choice, *every* coming-out is a mine field: Will I be rejected, shunned, mocked? Can I live with that? Eventually, lesbians, bisexual women, or transgendered individuals begin to understand that homophobia is the other person's problem. The hard part is knowing that the other's homophobia—internalized or externalized—can indeed affect the LBT's life in very real and tangible ways.

Providing a safe, comfortable atmosphere, where truth can be told without repercussion, is the ideal. A client who allows a provider to know she is an LBT has imparted a gift of self. That information should be handled gently and professionally.

CARE BARRIERS FOR LESBIANS

Little current information has been published on barriers to health care for lesbians, bisexual women, and transgendered individuals. Most of the literature published in this area dates from the 1990s to the early 2000s. It is reasonable to assume that little has changed; however, this lack of knowledge serves to keep this group invisible. Nursing as a profession has been particularly silent on the issues of health care for sexual minorities (Eliason, Dibble, & DeJoseph, 2010). Lesbians, bisexual women, and transgendered individuals experience the same barriers to care that other women do, such as having no transportation, childcare, or leave time from work; inconvenient times and location of clinics/practices; inability to communicate due to language barriers or reading ability; physical or cultural barriers; "ism" barriers (race, sex, class, age, ability); putting others ahead of self for care; avoiding health screening as a way to deny problems or viewing it as a nonnecessity; seeking care for serious problems only; history of abuse causing distancing from body; fear of procedures causing pain, embarrassment, or fear of the unknown; fear of findings of tests; inability to pay; and/or lack of recommendation for a procedure by a health care provider (Bernhard, 2001; Institute of Medicine [IOM], 2011). In addition, lesbians and bisexual women may also face barriers that are particular to a gay identity/behavior (see Table 8–1).

TABLE 8–1. Special Barriers to Health Care Experienced by Lesbians

- Homophobia from the health care provider
- Internalized homophobia
- Heterosexist assumptions
- Lack of knowledge about special risks and screening needs of lesbians by lesbians themselves
- Incorrect knowledge about health care needs of lesbians by health care providers
- Belief (false) by lesbians and health care providers that lesbians are immune to STDs, cervical cancer, and HIV
- Preventive care sought less because lesbians need routine contraceptive and prenatal care less often
- Lack of insurance and/or of access under partner's coverage
- Excluded or believe they are excluded from health promotion campaigns

Source: Bernhard, 2001; IOM, 1999; Marrazzo et al., 2001.

Most LBT women do have regular primary care providers, but the majority seek care only if they are experiencing a problem. Of concern is the fact that care is often delayed. In a groundbreaking narrative study of 45 lesbians in the San Francisco area, Stevens (1994a, 1994b) found that "noncare" was common. Noncare was negative care, such as feeling a lack of respect, feeling not safe enough to continue with a particular provider, feeling generally poorly cared for. These results confirm the findings of the prior studies in which providers' negative behaviors included actions such as clipped voice tones; constricted affect; roughness in handling; a hurried pace that frightened, humiliated, or hurt; and use of false endearments. There is little information to indicate that this has changed since 1994. One small study conducted in the Midwest found nursing students and faculty to be neutral in their homophobia attitudes. The researchers hypothesize, however, that the scores reflect heterosexism, continuing the invisibility of sexual minorities in nursing (Dinkel, Patzel, McGuire, Rolfs, & Purcell, 2007).

Other reasons and examples of why lesbians may not seek health care, may delay health care, or may not disclose their sexual orientation to health care providers include the following (Claes & Moore, 2000; Deevey, 1995; IOM, 1999; Stevens, 1994b):

- *Prejudicial language:* For example, when taking a history, do not ask any woman if she is married, but ask who her support person is. Do not use the term *homosexual*; rather, use *lesbian*, which is thought to have a more positive connotation. Do not ask if she is "having intercourse"; rather, ask if she is "sexually active." Better questions are "Are you single, partnered, or married?" "Who is in your immediate family?" If your client uses the term *lesbian* about herself and her family, she is probably relatively at ease with herself. The term *homosexual* generally refers to males in the gay culture.

- Negative behavior changes by the provider upon learning that the patient is lesbian. These can be avoiding touching her, superficial or condescending interaction with her, or outright hostility.
- Isolation from those they love—friends and relatives of choice—when in or visiting the hospital. The "traditional family" may be the only people allowed by the hospital staff to visit and support the client.
- Fear that coming-out or disclosure will lead to loss of confidentiality. If the client is labeled in the charts or records, it may become public knowledge, leading to personal, social, and work losses.
- Fear of substandard care or perhaps hurtful care.
- Fear after prior negative experiences.
- Lack of female provider (MD, NP, PA, CNM).

AN INCLUSIVE APPROACH AND ENVIRONMENT FOR ACCEPTANCE

Interview techniques and written materials that do not make the assumption that the woman is heterosexual and that use inclusive language will give the lesbian the message that disclosing her sexual orientation to the health care provider is safe, thus promoting disclosure of more useful information. It is imperative to establish an open, sensitive, and nonjudgmental climate from the onset, reassuring the woman that everything she discloses will be kept confidential. Beginning the conversation with something like the following may be helpful: "In order for me to provide you with care that is specific for your needs, I need to ask some sensitive questions about your sexual history and your support network." In addition, a safe environment can be created that facilitates disclosure by using open body language, inviting the woman's partner or friend to participate if she wishes, assuring the confidentiality of medical documentation, and having a posted nondiscrimination policy as well as diversified reading materials prominently displayed in the waiting room.

Because heterosexuality is the accepted societal norm, too often providers assume that the client is heterosexual. A provider who asks a woman if she is sexually active, learns that she is, and then immediately asks what form of contraception is being used is insensitive, judgmental, and exhibiting heterosexism.

Questions that give a woman an opportunity to disclose her sexual and affectional relationships should be used. By asking if a woman is in a committed relationship or partnership rather than asking if she is married opens the door for disclosure. An open question about who she relies on for support and who are the most important people in her world also gives the woman an invitation to disclose. Follow-up questions should include inquiry about the people the woman considers to be in her family circle by birth and by choice. After establishing a relationship with the patient, the provider should ask about the person the woman lives with and what the relationship is. This may be considered prying until a relationship is established between the provider and the patient.

Asking "Are you sexually active?" and receiving a "Yes" response should then lead to asking "Are you sexually active with men, women, or both?" "Have your partners been men, women, or both?" Asking these questions in a matter-of-fact way allows the client to feel free to be truthful because the provider expects any of the answers. However, questions about sexual relationships need to go further than the sex of partner(s) and the number of partners. The provider needs to determine if the patient's sexual relationship is a committed one—where the partner is the most important support person for the woman. This data is important for future reference in case of illness and hospitalization. Because of possible stigma attached to lesbian sexual orientation and the possibility that this information could negatively influence care, permission to place this information in the medical record should be obtained from the patient.

Though the woman may identify herself as lesbian, she may be reluctant to disclose that she is bisexual, and the provider may need to ask if there is a need to discuss contraception. If the woman is in a committed, long-term monogamous relationship, there may be no need to discuss issues of safer sex, but if she is in a new relationship, a non-monogamous relationship, or a bisexual relationship, then the provider is compelled to discuss the possibility of sexually transmitted diseases (STDs). Additionally, the provider should ask the woman if she has any concerns she would like to discuss, thereby opening the door to discussions about domestic violence, stress, and any other health concerns.

ASSESSING THE WOMAN'S COPING STATUS

Heterosexism and sexism are pervasive in our society and can be stressful for LBT women and can impact health (Szymanski & Owens, 2009). It is essential for health care providers to assess the coping skills of patients in order to best meet their needs. After a trusting relationship is established, the health care provider can ask questions that may help identify how the patient is dealing with her sexuality. How does she feel about being a lesbian, bisexual, or transgender? Does she share information about her sexual orientation with others and, if so, does she feel comfortable about this? How has she been and how is she now treated by health care professionals? Has she been treated before by or know of health care providers who are open to caring for LBT women? What health needs and risks does she feel she has? Is she aware of support networks? The answers to these questions will allow the provider to give the client more information to help herself and to uncover areas for care.

Lesbians, bisexual women, and transgendered individuals may, in fact, share little or nothing about their self-identification. By controlling this information, the patient may believe her environment is safer (Stevens, 1995). She feels less likely to be mistreated, ignored, or misdiagnosed. This is seen as a survival method. Some women may increase their feelings of safety by bringing a friend who will be a witness if they are mistreated or be an advocate if needed. The provider needs to allow this type of support unless there is concern that the friend is abusive or coercive.

Our society assumes everyone is heterosexual. This heterosexism is most often unintentional but may be associated with the belief that heterosexuality is the only acceptable form of sexuality (Irwin, 2007). Homophobia is the fear of same-gendered sexual identity and can result in hatred of a group of people that one has never met. Although heterosexism is unintentional, homophobia is strong antihomosexual feelings associated with some form of behavior and is most often intentional. An unrealistic fear of anyone who has a different sexual identity from the socially acceptable "norm" is the basis of homophobia, and in the U.S. culture, a person is raised with the unconscious fear of anyone different. Lesbians, bisexual women, and transgendered individuals are no exception. This may lead to issues of low self-esteem, self-hatred, and internalized homophobia leading to depression, substance abuse, or negative behaviors.

SPECIAL GROUPS AT GREATER RISK

CHILDREN AND ADOLESCENTS

Little is known about the specific developmental issues that may exist for lesbian children or adolescents. Very little current research exists, and much of the older research may not be relevant in the context of society today because of a more tolerant attitude toward homosexuality and a move away from considering it as a pathologic condition. Current contextual changes in society have brought homosexuality to a position of increased visibility and less stigma, as witnessed by the popularity of several gay/lesbian television sitcoms in recent years. However, unless the young LBT child or adolescent is lucky enough to be part of a family who is able to accept and support her in her development regardless of sexual orientation, she may be vulnerable to psychological trauma in her growth and development. Young girls battling inwardly with their same-sex feelings and are in a situation where they are being told outwardly that same-sex feelings are wrong may be prone to poor self-identity development, perhaps becoming runaways, homeless, isolated, depressed, or suicidal; furthermore, they may abuse substances, experience domestic violence, and fail in school or work (National Institute on Drug Abuse, 2006; Padilla, Crisp, & Rew, 2010). These girls need positive role models and support in developing self-respect to help decrease the risks of these consequences. A number of larger cities have gay and lesbian adolescent social services organizations to which such clients can be referred. (See addresses for several such organizations at the end of this chapter.)

OLDER LESBIANS, BISEXUAL WOMEN, AND TRANSGENDERED INDIVIDUALS

As the population ages in general, the number of LBT women also increases. This presents a unique situation for older LBT women because more health care events occur later in life. As previously stated, the health care system operates on a heterosexual assumption. This impacts caregiving situations as well as end-of-life care. Nursing home personnel should be educated to understand the special needs of all patients, including LBT women. The National Resource Center on LGBT aging is a valuable resource for older LBT women as well as a resource for health care providers. Older heterosexual women are at a greater risk for unmet health needs. Add the status of also being LBT and the risk is even greater. Additionally, older women may have been too afraid of negative consequences of affirming publicly their sexual orientation and thus may never have come out. Consequently, health care providers may not pick up on clues so that effective assistance can be offered to the older person, especially through support from the significant other (Stevens, 1995). Poverty and increasing health problems of aging add to the significant risks for LBT elders. Health care providers will need to be particularly aware and sensitive to offer needed assistance.

LESBIANS, BISEXUAL WOMEN, AND TRANSGENDERED INDIVIDUALS WITH DISABILITIES

Disabilities can be physical, mental, or intellectual. To some degree, a disability is evident, whereas being LBT is not. This can render sexual identity invisible. Another common misconception about disabled individuals is that they are asexual (Hunt, Matthews, Milsom, & Lammel, 2006). Homosexuality and disability (particularly mental disability) are often stigmatized conditions causing LBT women with disabilities to avoid or delay seeking health care. Because of a fear of negative consequences, these women may put off seeking care until their condition is very acute. Health care providers can ease this problem by being sensitive to the situation and approaching the women with respect and compassion.

RACIAL AND ETHNIC MINORITY LBT WOMEN

Not only do LBT women face unique challenges because of their sexual orientation, but if they are members of a minority race/ethnic group or have religious beliefs that are outside of the mainstream beliefs in the United States, they face even greater risks of rejection based on racial, ethnic, or religious prejudices. If a woman is lesbian, African American, and Muslim, she must overcome many "isms" (racism, sexism, heterosexism, and religious discrimination).

HEALTH PROBLEMS OF LESBIANS

Some lesbians and bisexual woman seek health care for menstrual problems (painful or irregular periods), vaginal infections and STDs (primarily vaginal infections and herpes), reproductive problems (pelvic pain, uterine infections, infertility problems, painful coitus, or orgasms), urinary tract infections, musculoskeletal problems, and breast problems (IOM, 1999). Many women never seek health care for these problems, except for musculoskeletal problems. Unique health concerns of lesbians and bisexual women that may go unaddressed if the provider assumes heterosexuality include appropriate screening for cancer, domestic violence, depression, substance abuse, STDs, HIV, as well as relationship issues, pregnancy, and parenting (Hutchinson, Thompson, & Cederbaum, 2006; IOM, 2011; Weber, 2010).

An early study by Buenting (1992) that compares lesbian and heterosexual women's lifestyles found no difference between the groups on items of regular exercise, cigarettes smoking, social activities, community service, monthly self-breast exams, spiritual-religious activities, abstinence from alcohol, and alcohol consumption. Heterosexual women had significantly higher mean scores on regular Papanicolaou (Pap) smears, use of prescribed medications, and fulfilling family obligations. Lesbians had significantly higher mean scores on use of recreational drugs, alternative diets, and meditation/relaxation techniques. A recent study supported the finding that lesbian-identified women had a higher chance of using complementary and alternative medicine (Smith et al., 2010). Other research has found that lesbian and bisexual women between the ages of 20 and 34 were at higher risk for cigarette smoking and alcohol use than heterosexual women (Gruskin, Hart, Gordon, & Ackerson, 2001). This reflects the 1999 IOM findings that, in general, a greater percentage of lesbians describe themselves as being in recovery from alcohol than do heterosexual women, and that limited research on lesbians and drug use seems to point to a greater use of illegal drugs for lesbians than other women.

PHYSICAL HEALTH PROBLEMS

Menstrual Problems and Pelvic Pain

Dysmenorrhea is a common complaint of lesbians and is often severe. Because lesbians are hesitant to seek care for a number of reasons previously discussed, they may never seek treatment for this problem. Endometriosis is presumed to be high, based on the severe dysmenorrhea rate and the high rate of nulliparity. However, no data exist that support this assumption.

STDs and Vaginal Infections

The prevalence of STDs among lesbians is reported as low. The problem with the data is that there are no current large-scale contemporary studies and no delineation of women who have never had sex with men, who have sex with men and women, or who have sex with multiple female partners who may also have sex with men (IOM, 1999). Complicating the issue is the fact that there is little data on the actual sexual practices of lesbians and bisexual women. The data is limited with respect to the prevalence of STDs in women who have had sex only with other women, but classical infections such as syphilis, gonorrhea, and chlamydia are rare because of anatomical transmission inefficiency. However, it is possible to transmit these infections by the use of shared sex toys. Also, many women who identify as lesbian have had sex with men at some point and may transmit a previously acquired STD to a current female partner (Addis, Davies, Greene, MacBride-Stewart, & Shepherd, 2009). Lesbians should be reminded that oral sex can transmit some infections, such as herpes and HIV.

Evidence suggests that the incidence of bacterial vaginosis (BV) is higher in lesbians than in heterosexual women. The Centers for Disease Control and Prevention (CDC) considers BV an extremely common vaginal infection and not necessarily sexually transmitted. Women who have never had sexual intercourse can still get BV. The CDC (2011) identifies two behaviors that increase the risk: (1) having new or multiple-sex partners and (2) douching. Because BV is not well understood and can result from a bacterial imbalance in the vagina, information from small studies with lesbians is not conclusive.

Several types of human papillomavirus (HPV) cause genital warts and cervical neoplasia but are often asymptomatic and go undetected, increasing the risk of transmission and delaying effective treatment. The epidemiology of HPV among lesbians has only recently been explored. In a study of 149 lesbians, the prevalence of HPV was 19 percent in women who had never had sex with men and 30 percent in the entire sample (Marrazzo, 2000). Marrazzo, Koutsky, Kiviat, Kuypers, and Stine (2001) reviewed data for the previous two decades on the occurrence of HPV in lesbians and validated the possibility of transmission in this population. Health care providers need to educate lesbians about the possibility of HPV infection and stress the importance of routine Pap smears.

Although early studies of HIV in lesbians indicated that HIV infection was rare and many lesbian and bisexual women believed themselves to be at low risk, this is not true today. The research is limited (and somewhat outdated), but some unexpected findings regarding women having sex with women are the following:

- Higher HIV seroprevalence rates among women who have sex with both women and men (i.e., behaviorally bisexual women) compared to their exclusively homosexual or heterosexual counterparts.
- High levels of risk for HIV infection through unprotected sex with men and through injection drug use.
- Risk for HIV infection of unknown magnitude owing to unprotected sex with women and artificial insemination with unscreened semen (IOM, 1999, p. 76).

Screening for HIV is more common in lesbians and bisexual women than in the general heterosexual population. In a study conducted by Conron, Mimiaga, and Landers (2010), lesbians and bisexual women were 1.8 and 2.7 times, respectively, more likely to have HIV screening than heterosexual women. Use of dental dams and latex gloves offer some protection against the spread of the virus but more accurate information about increasing sexual safety and appropriate prevention rests in knowing the sexual preference of the client. It shows lack of awareness and insensitivity to ask every woman who walks in what kind of contraception she uses and to advise that her partner use condoms without knowing her sexual preference. Women who have male and female partners need to use condoms and spermicide with male partners and other barriers with female partners. Avoidance of contact with blood and secretions/discharges of any partner is important protection from HIV infection.

Obesity

Obesity rates in the United States have escalated in the last 50 years, increasing from 13.4 percent of the population in 1960 to more than 33.8 percent by the late 2000s (Flegal, Carroll, Ogden, & Curtin, 2010; Gaziano, 2010). Some data from population-based studies indicates that lesbians may be at a greater risk for obesity than their heterosexual counterparts, but that data is less clear on other sexual minority women (Boehmer, Bowen, & Bauer, 2007). Overweight and obesity are determined by BMI (body mass index). Normal weight is considered a BMI less than 25 kg/m^2, overweight between 27 and 27.5 kg/m^2, and obesity more than 27.5 kg/m^2. Morbid obesity is a BMI over 40 kg/m^2 (Golden, Thomas, & Porter, 2011). A recent study found that lesbians were more likely to be obese than heterosexual women and that bisexual women were more likely to be at a normal weight than lesbians (Conron et al., 2010). Whether lesbians have a higher incidence of diseases attributable to obesity is unknown. Conron and colleagues (2010) found that even though sexual minority women did have more risk factors for chronic disease, there was no difference in the reporting of diabetes or heart disease diagnoses between them and heterosexuals. Health care providers need to consider these general risks, however, in providing preventive care.

Cancer Risks

Many factors have been identified that put women at greater risk for certain types of cancer. Many of the identified risk factors are nonmodifiable, such as advancing age and family history of cancer; however, many behavioral factors may increase the risk of cancer. Cigarette smoking, secondhand smoke exposure, alcohol use, and a history of HPV infection are some commonly identified risk factors for the development of several types of cancer. Lesbians and bisexual women are more likely to smoke, use drugs, and drink alcohol than their heterosexual counterparts (Conron et al., 2010). Certain behaviors decrease the risk of certain cancers. For example, women who have been pregnant and who have taken oral contraceptives are at a lower risk for developing breast cancer. It has been assumed that lesbians would be at a greater risk because of less use of oral contraceptives and less likelihood of childbearing.

The risk for cervical cancer is strongly associated with HPV infection, which is, in turn, associated with certain sexual behaviors including multiple (male) sexual partners or partners who have had multiple male sexual partners, early age at first intercourse, and unprotected sex (Kaloczi, Latendresse, & Morgan, 2010). Considering the high-risk behaviors for HPV, it has been assumed that lesbians are at a lower risk for developing cervical cancer than their heterosexual counterparts. HPV can also be transmitted by oral sex and shared sex toys. Therefore, there is no difference in the screening recommendations for lesbians or bisexual women, and health care providers need to inform their patients of the risk.

In general, the incidence of breast cancer among lesbians and bisexual women is not known because data is not collected with sexual orientation as a descriptor. Although there have been reports of lesbians performing self-breast exams and obtaining screening mammograms less often than their heterosexual counterparts, recent studies indicate that sexual minority women were no different in screening mammography than heterosexual women (Conron et al., 2010). More research needs to be conducted to determine if lesbians are at an increased risk for breast cancer because of a lack of or delayed childbearing, lack of oral contraceptive use, or higher alcohol consumption.

The cause of ovarian cancer is not yet known. Evidence suggests that any condition that suppresses ovulation (multiple pregnancies, prolonged lactation, oral contraceptives) decreases the risk for ovarian cancer (Latendresse, McCance, & Morgan, 2010). Conversely, factors that increase lifetime ovulation (early menarche, late menopause, and nulliparity) increase the risk for ovarian cancer. So the health care provider should assess each of the areas in order to determine each individual's risk for ovarian cancer.

Heart Disease and Stroke

Those factors that may increase the risk of colon, breast, and endometrial cancer also may increase the lesbian's risk for heart disease and stroke. It is not known what the actual incidence among this group is for these diseases, but a recent study found no difference in the reported incidence in diabetes or heart disease (Conron et al., 2010).

The glaring truth is that for all the cancer and cardiovascular risk factors, routine screening is one safeguard leading to early detection as well as to health promotion efforts that lesbians are less likely to have due to delayed care and irregular care. Both increase the risk of more serious disease.

MENTAL HEALTH ISSUES

In a recent study, depression among sexual minority women was reported at 38 percent (Lehavot & Simoni, 2011). The researchers postulate that this high rate of depression is related to stigmatization and stress related to being a member of a minority group. Several studies have illustrated a risk for suicide in lesbians, bisexual women, and transgendered individuals (Lehavot & Simoni, 2011; Meyer, Dietrich, & Schwartz, 2008; Mustanski, Garofalo, & Emerson, 2010). These studies purport that suicide attempts are more prevalent in youth and could possibly be related to coming-out. Suicide is an issue for all youth in the United States.

If the provider assesses that depression is a health factor, it is appropriate to ask the client, in the course of narrowing down cause, if she has any problems relating to sexual orientation. Once disclosure has been made, the provider—who can comfortably do so—may then ask some or all of the following questions:

- How do you feel about your sexual orientation?
- When did you first come out to yourself?
- Have you been able to talk about this with your friends or family of origin? How did they respond?
- Have you been discriminated against or been victimized because of your orientation? By whom?
- Do you have a support system who you can turn to?
- Do you need information on how to find gay organizations in the area?

Providing the client with information about mental health professionals who routinely deal with these issues and/or support groups can be immensely helpful and affirming. Even in these so-called tolerant times, the client experiencing emotions toward someone of the same sex for the first time—or acknowledging it for the first time—may still think she is the only one on earth this has happened to. Being gay is a statement of selfhood and identity. Coming to terms with it can involve depression when too many forget that sexual identity is a spectrum and in fact seems to have a genetic basis.

Drinking alcohol has been reported as higher in lesbians and bisexual women (Conron et al., 2010; Lehavot & Simoni, 2011). Some older studies have been criticized because they recruited subjects in bars, but the two most recent studies are methodologically sound. A more recent study found that in sexual minority adults who reported discrimination, substance abuse disorders were four times greater (McCabe et al., 2010). A referral resource for practitioners to be aware of are Alcoholics Anonymous meetings specifically conducted for women or lesbians.

Lesbian relationships are much the same as heterosexual relationships. Issues that cause conflict center around money, sex, and roles much the same as heterosexual relationships. One difference is that in heterosexual relationships, there are societal role expectations. In a lesbian relationship, roles must be negotiated and renegotiated. This is often a source of conflict. Other relational conflicts may exist when one partner in the relationship wishes to keep her sexuality private and the other wishes to be more public or out.

Little is reported about the frequency of intimate partner violence in LBT women's relationships. Old estimates of intimate partner violence in the LBT community are between 12 and 50 percent, and in a recent study, researchers found that lesbians and bisexual women were more likely than heterosexual women to experience intimate partner violence (Conron et al., 2010). One big difference for LBT women is that same-sex domestic violence remains virtually invisible, whereas heterosexual domestic violence is very visible in the media and legislation. Heterosexism and homophobia successfully keep same-sex domestic violence invisible. Another factor contributing to the invisibility of this type of domestic violence is the fact that women in general are not seen as violent persons and, therefore, are not seen as perpetrators of domestic violence. Most states do not offer protection for the victims of same-sex intimate partner violence.

Although domestic violence in general includes physical, sexual, and emotional abuse as well as property damage and economic control, same-sex domestic violence can also include the use of an individual's internalized homophobia and the homophobia of other significant people in the victim's life to exercise control (Gruskin, 1999). For example, the perpetrator may threaten to out her partner or expose her sexual identity to family, friends, coworkers, or boss. This could threaten her employment or affect her relationship with her family and friends, possibly losing their love and support. The perpetrator can effectively maintain control, especially if the woman is considering leaving the relationship.

The implications for health care professionals include the creation of an environment where a woman feels comfortable talking about her sexual identity and the abuse she suffers. The health care provider also must be aware of internal and external homophobia and the ways that a perpetrator can use this to control her partner. As with reports of any domestic violence, the health care provider needs to understand the ramifications of the patient's reporting of the violence. Ramifications can include retaliation from the perpetrator, negative reactions from the police when learning of the woman's sexual orientation, and loss of support from the lesbian community. Support groups are available for assistance.

Of course, other forms of violence are experienced by lesbians, bisexual women, and transgendered individuals just as by heterosexual women. However, the special acts of violence born of hate, often unreported in years past, are being reported more often today. The National Gay and Lesbian Task Force prepares reports and offers support. Its hotline in Washington, DC, is 202-393-5177.

DESIRE TO PARENT

Having children is highly valued by U.S. society, and many lesbians and bisexual women are no different. However, one study found that childless lesbian couples had less desire to become parents than their childless heterosexual counterparts (Riskind & Patterson, 2010). In an analysis of the National Survey of Family Growth (NSFG), 41 percent of lesbian respondents had the desire for children, whereas 53 percent of heterosexual women had the desire for children (Gates, Badgett, Macomber, & Chambers, 2007). Health care providers must be aware of and open to the idea that many lesbians and same-sex couples have the desire to be parents and they should address this area in the history.

Artificial insemination is the usual choice of reproductive technology for lesbians and lesbian couples who wish to become pregnant. Information about this process is often requested from the health care provider. It is advisable that the sperm comes from a screened donor bank to decrease the possible risk of HIV and other STDs. Seeking a male to have intercourse with for insemination purposes is another option for pregnancy but may be distasteful for some lesbians. Adoption poses problems legally, especially if the legal parent dies or the couple separates. It is advisable for lesbians who wish to become pregnant to consult a legal practitioner who is knowledgeable about issues of same-sex parenting.

Practitioners also need to be aware that, because of LBT sexual orientation, increased support may be needed when from a previous heterosexual relationship or from the lesbian relationship are involved in custody battles. Other common fears for LBT parents relate to telling their children about their orientation and interacting with the straight community—people in the schools, churches, and health care system.

CONCLUSION

Lesbians, bisexual women, and transgendered individuals represent a large group of clients with unique medical, psychological, and social needs. Often, providers remain unaware of a woman's sexual orientation and, therefore, unique and diverse needs may go unrecognized. The opportunity to provide sensitive and optimal care is missed. More research in the area of sexual minority women's health would benefit both the women and the practitioners. Although there are studies that examine these areas, most of them are small. Data collected by governmental agencies on health and health care often does not identify sexual orientation and so data is missing for sexual minority women.

HEALTH RESOURCES AND ORGANIZATIONS

Gay & Lesbian Medical Association
1326 18th Street NW, Suite 22
Washington, DC 20036
202-600-8037
http://www.glma.org/

World Professional Association for Transgender Health (WPATH)
1300 South Second Street, Suite 180
Minneapolis, MN 55454
http://www.wpath.org/

Center of Excellence for Transgender Health
http://transhealth.ucsf.edu

Sexual Violence Prevention
http://www.cdc.gov/ViolencePrevention/sexualviolence/index.html

Intimate Partner Violence Prevention
http://www.cdc.gov/ViolencePrevention/intimatepartnerviolence/index.html

Lesbian Health
http://womenshealth.gov/faq/lesbian-health.cfm (National Women's Health Information Center)

Cancer Facts for Lesbians and Bisexual Women
http://www.cancer.org/Healthy/FindCancerEarly/WomensHealth/cancer-facts-for-lesbians-and-bisexual-women (American Cancer Society)

COMMUNITY SERVICES CENTERS

The Community of LGBT Centers
CenterLink
http://www.lgbtcenters.org/Centers/find-a-center.aspx

The Lesbian, Gay, Bisexual & Transgender Community Center
208 West 13th Street
New York, NY 10011
212-620-7310
http://www.gaycenter.org

Gay & Lesbian Center
McDonald/Wright Building
1625 N. Schrader Blvd.
Los Angeles, CA 90028-6213
323-993-7400
http://www.laglc.org

The Lesbian, Gay, Bisexual & Transgender Community Center of Greater Cleveland
6600 Detroit Avenue
Cleveland, Ohio 44102
216-651-5428
http://www.lgbtcleveland.org

The Gay & Lesbian Community Center of Southern Nevada
953 E. Sahara Ave, B-31
Las Vegas, NV 89104
702-733-9800
http://www.thecenterlv.com

YOUTH

The Gay Student Center Web Community
http://gaystudentcenter.student.com

Long Island Gay and Lesbian Youth
34 Park Ave
Bay Shore, NY 11706-7309
631-665-2300
http://www.ligaly.org

Boston Alliance of Gay, Lesbian, Bisexual and Transgender Youth (BAGLY)
14 Beacon St. #620
Boston, MA 02108-3738
http://www.bagly.org/

Boston Gay and Lesbian Social Services (GLASS) Community Center
http://www.jri.org/glass/

Indiana Youth Group (IYG)
2943 East 46th Street
Indianapolis, IN 46205-2408
317-541-8726
http://www.indianayouthgroup.org/

Out Youth Austin
909 E. 49 1/2 Street
Austin, TX 78751
512-419-1233
http://www.outyouth.org/

National Runaway Switchboard
(800) runaway
http://www.nrscrisisline.org/

ELDERS

National Resource Center on LGBT Aging
c/o Services & Advocacy for GLBT
Elders (SAGE)
305 Seventh Avenue
6th Floor
New York, NY 10001
212-741-2247
http://www.lgbtagingcenter.org/

Old Lesbians Organizing for Change (OLOC)
P.O. Box 5853
Athens, OH 45701
1-888-706-7506 or email: info@oloc.org
http://www.oloc.org/

Services & Advocacy for GLBT Elders (SAGE)
305 7th Ave
15th Floor
New York, NY 10001
212-741-2247
http://www.sageusa.org/index.cfm

LGBT Aging Project
555 Amory Street
Jamaica Plain, MA 02130
617-522-1292
http://www.lgbtagingproject.org/

FAMILIES AND FRIENDS

Parents, Families and Friends of Lesbians and Gays (PFLAG)
http://community.pflag.org/

Gay Family Support
http://www.gayfamilysupport.com/

Family Equality Council
http://www.familyequality.org/

Violence
http://www.rainbowdomesticviolence.itgo.com/
http://www.lagaycenter.org/site/PageServer?pagename=YH_DV_Family_Violence_Partner_Abuse

New York City Gay and Lesbian Anti-Violence Project
240 West 35th Street, Suite 200
New York, NY 10001-2515
212-714-1141 (24-hour bilingual hotline)
http://www.avp.org/

Tucson United Against Domestic Violence/Brewster Center
1535 West St. Mary's Road
Tucson, AZ 85719
Tucson-Pima Shelter
520-622-6347

LEGAL SERVICES

The WilmerHale Legal Services Center
Harvard Law School
122 Boylston Street

Jamaica Plain, MA 02130
617-522-3003
http://www.law.harvard.edu/academics/clinical/lsc/clinics/gay.htm

Transgender Law Center
870 Market Street, Room 400
San Francisco, CA 94102
415-865-0176
http://www.transgenderlawcenter.org/

OTHER

Sexuality Information and Education Council of the United States (SIECUS)
90 John St. Suite 402
New York, NY 10038
212-819-9770

SIECUS Washington, DC, Office
1012 14th Street, NW, Suite 107
Washington, DC 20005
202-265-2405
http://www.siecus.org

National Women's Health Network
1413 K Street NW, 4th Floor
Washington, DC 20005
202-682-2640
http://nwhn.org/

REFERENCES

Addis, S., Davies, M., Greene, G., MacBride-Stewart, S., & Shepherd, M. (2009). The health, social care and housing needs of lesbian, gay, bisexual and transgender older people: A review of the literature. *Health and Social Care in the Community, 17*(6), 647–658.

American Psychiatric Association (APA). (2011). *Healthy minds. Healthy lives. Sexual orientation.* Retrieved February 17, 2011, from http://healthminds.org/More-Info-For/Gay-LesbianBisexuals.aspx

Ben-Natan, M., & Adir, O. (2009). Screening for cervical cancer among Israeli lesbian women. *International Nursing Review, 56*, 433–441.

Bernhard, L.A. (2001). Lesbian health and health care. *Annual Review of Nursing Research, 19*, 145–177.

Boehmer, U., Bowen, D.J., & Bauer, G.R. (2007). Overweight and obesity in sexual-minority women: Evidence from population-based data. *American Journal of Public Health, 97*, 1134–1140.

Buenting, J.A. (1992). Health life-styles of lesbian and heterosexual women. *Health Care for Women International, 13*, 165–171.

Centers for Disease Control and Prevention (CDC). (2011). *Sexually transmitted diseases (STDs): Bacterial vaginosis—CDC fact sheet.* Retrieved March 15, 2011, from http://www.cdc.gov/std/bv/STDFact-Bacterial-Vaginosis.htm

Claes, J.A., & Moore, W. (2000). Issues confronting lesbian and gay elders: The challenge for health and human services providers. *Journal of Health and Human Services Administration, 23*(2), 181–202.

Conron, K.J., Mimiaga, M.J., & Landers, S.J. (2010). A population-based study of sexual orientation identity and gender differences in adult health. *American Journal of Public Health, 100*(10), 1953–1960.

Deevey, S. (1995). Lesbian health care. In C.I. Fogel & N.F. Woods (Eds.), *Women's health care: A comprehensive handbook.* Thousand Oaks, CA: Sage Publications.

Dinkel, S., Patzel, B., McGuire, M.J., Rolfs, E., & Purcell, K. (2007). Measures of homophobia among nursing students and faculty: A Midwestern perspective. *International Journal of Nursing Education Scholarship, 4*(1), Article 24. Retrieved from http://www.bepress.com/ijnes/vol4/iss1/art24

Eliason, M.J., Dibble, S., & DeJoseph, J. (2010). Nursing's silence on lesbian, gay, bisexual, and transgender issues: The need for emancipatory efforts. *Advances in Nursing Science, 33*(3), 206–218.

Flegal, K.M., Carroll, M.D., Ogden, C.L., & Curtin, L.R. (2010). Prevalence and trends in obesity among U.S. adults, 1999–2008. *Journal of the American Medical Association, 303*, 235–241.

Gates, G.J., Badgett, M.V., Macomber, J.E., & Chambers, K. (2007). *Adoption and foster care by gay and lesbian parents in the United States.* Los Angeles: The Williams Institute, University of California at Los Angeles.

Gaziano, J.M. (2010). Fifth phase of the epidemiologic transition: The age of obesity and inactivity. *Journal of the American Medical Association, 303*, 275–276.

Golden, A., Thomas, D., & Porter, B. (2011). Endocrine and metabolic problems. In L. Dunphy, J. Winland-Brown, B. Porter, & D. Thomas (Eds.), *Primary care: The art and science of advanced practice nursing* (3rd ed., pp. 830–906). Philadelphia: F.A. Davis Company.

Gruskin, E.P. (1999). *Treating lesbians and bisexual women: Challenges and strategies for health professionals.* Thousand Oaks, CA: Sage Publications.

Gruskin, E.P., Hart, S., Gordon, N., & Ackerson, L. (2001). Patterns of cigarette smoking and alcohol use among lesbians and bisexual women enrolled in a large health maintenance organization. *American Journal of Public Health, 91*(6), 976–979.

Healthy People 2020. (2011). *Lesbian, gay, bisexual, and transgender health.* Retrieved February 17, 2011, from http://healthypeople.gov/2020/topicsobjectives2020/overview.aspx?topicid=25

Hunt, B., Matthews, C., Milsom, A., & Lammel, J.A. (2006). Lesbians with physical disabilities: A qualitative study of experiences with counseling. *Journal of Counseling and Development, 84*, 163–173.

Hutchinson, M.K., Thompson, A.C., & Cederbaum, J.A. (2006). Multisystem factors contributing to disparities in preventive health care among lesbian women. *Journal of Obstetric, Gynecologic, and Neonatal Nursing, 35*(3), 393–402.

Institute of Medicine (IOM). (1999). *Lesbian health: Current assessment and directions for the future*. Washington, DC: National Academies Press.

Institute of Medicine (IOM). (2011). *The health of lesbian, gay, bisexual, and transgender people: Building a foundation of better understanding*. Washington, DC: National Academies Press.

Irwin, L. (2007). Homophobia and heterosexism: Implications for nursing and nursing practice. *Australian Journal of Advanced Nursing, 25*(1), 70–76.

Kaloczi, L., Latendresse, G., & Morgan, K. (2010). Sexually transmitted infections. In K. McCance & S. Huether (Eds.), *Pathophysiology: The biologic basis of disease in adults and children* (6th ed., pp. 923–951). Maryland Heights, MO: Mosby Elsevier.

Latendresse, G., McCance, K., & Morgan, K. (2010). Alteration of the reproductive systems. In K. McCance & S. Huether (Eds.), *Pathophysiology: The biologic basis of disease in adults and children* (6th ed., pp. 816–922). Maryland Heights, MO: Mosby Elsevier.

Lehavot, K., & Simoni, J. (2011). The impact of minority stress on mental health and substance use among sexual minority women. *Journal of Consulting and Clinical Psychology, 79*(2), 159–170.

Marrazzo, J.M. (2000). Genital human papillomavirus infection in women who have sex with women: A concern for patients and providers. *AIDS Patient Care and STDs, 14*(8), 447–451.

Marrazzo, J.M. (2004). Barriers to infectious disease care among lesbians. *Emerging Infectious Diseases, 10*(11), 1974–1978. Retrieved from www.cdc.gov/eid

Marrazzo, J.M., Koutsky, L.A., Kiviat, N.B., Kuypers, J.M., & Stine, K. (2001). Papanicolaou test screening and prevalence of genital human papillomavirus among women who have sex with women. *American Journal of Public Health, 91*(6), 947–952.

McCabe, S.E., Bostwick, W.B., Hughes, T.L., West, B.T., & Boyd, C.J. (2010). The relationship between discrimination and substance use disorders among lesbian, gay, and bisexual adults in the United States. *American Journal of Public Health, 100*(10), 1946–1952.

Meyer, I.H., Dietrich, J., & Schwartz, S. (2008). Lifetime prevalence of mental disorders and suicide attempts in diverse lesbian, gay, and bisexual populations. *American Journal of Public Health, 98*(6), 1004–1006.

Mustanski, B.S., Garofalo, R., & Emerson, E.M. (2010). Mental health disorders, psychological distress, and suicidality in a diverse sample of lesbian, gay, bisexual, and transgender youths. *American Journal of Public Health, 100*(12), 2426–2432.

National Institute on Drug Abuse. (2006, February). *NIDA community drug alert bulletin—stress & substance abuse*. Retrieved February 3, 2011, from http://archives.drugabuse.gov/stressalert/StressAlert.html

Padilla, Y.C., Crisp, C., & Rew, D.L. (2010). Parental acceptance and illegal drug use among gay, lesbian, and bisexual adolescents: Results from a national survey. *Social Work, 55*(3), 265–275.

Riskind, R.G., & Patterson, C.J. (2010). Parenting intentions and desires among childless lesbian, gay, and heterosexual individuals. *Journal of Family Psychology, 24*(1), 78–81.

Smith, H.A., Matthews, A., Markovic, N., Youk, A., Danielson, M.E., & Talbott, E.O. (2010). A comparative study of complementary and alternative medicine use among heterosexually and lesbian identified women: Data from the ESTHER project (Pittsburg, PA, 2003–2006). *Journal of Alternative and Complementary Medicine, 16*(11), 1161–1170.

Spidsberg, B.D. (2007). Vulnerable and strong—lesbian women encountering maternity care. *Journal of Advanced Nursing, 60*(5), 478–486.

Stevens, P.E. (1994a). Lesbians' health-related experiences of care and noncare. *Western Journal of Nursing Research, 16*(6), 639–659.

Stevens, P.E. (1994b). Protective strategies of lesbian clients in health care environments. *Research in Nursing and Health, 17*, 217–229.

Stevens, P.E. (1995). Structural and interpersonal impact of heterosexual assumptions on lesbian health care clients. *Nursing Research, 44*(1), 25–30.

Szymanski, D.M., & Owens, G.P. (2009). Group-level coping as a moderator between heterosexism and sexism and psychological distress in sexual minority women. *Psychology of Women Quarterly, 33*, 197–205.

Weber, S. (2010). A stigma identification framework for family nurses working with parents who are lesbian, gay, bisexual, or transgendered and their families. *Journal of Family Nursing, 16*(4), 378–393.

CHAPTER ❖ 9

HEALTH NEEDS OF WOMEN WITH DISABILITIES

Michele R. Davidson

Being disabled does not contradict responsible, effective parenting, yet judgmental attitudes continue.

Highlights

- Overview
- Lifestyle, Developmental, and Cultural Issues
- Health Promotion for Women With Disabilities
- Risk for Abuse for Women With Disabilities
- Fostering Accessibility to Clinic Services
- Pregnancy
- Parenting
- Resources for Women, Their Families, and Professionals

❖ INTRODUCTION

Wellness is the lens of self-perception. Many women with conditions such as cerebral palsy, spinal cord injury, lupus, multiple sclerosis, and rheumatoid arthritis do not view themselves as disabled in spite of immense physical limitations. However, women with disabilities frequently face discrimination and economic vulnerability. Nearly half of them live alone (Davidson, Ladewig, & London, 2012). For those who are married, rates of divorce reach as high as 75 percent (Rowe, 2009). Women with physical disabilities may also have unmet needs such as accessibility to gynecologic care and accessibility to professionals with knowledge of how disability impacts primary care. In addition, the discrimination that women with disabilities face is twofold: First, they are women, and second, they are individuals with disabilities. Sexual minority women with disabilities face a threefold level of discrimination as they are also discriminated against for their sexual preference.

Narrow negative social attitudes set unnecessary barriers to the optimal growth and development of women with disabilities and the health care they obtain (Groce, 1999). An example is the stereotypic image of American women having two major functions—caretaker and object of beauty. The ideal woman is physically perfect; women with disabilities are seen as dependent and nonproductive and may be judged incompetent to perform women's work or seen as invisible (Banks, 2010). Also women with disabilities are often not viewed as sexual beings by members of society (Ostrander, 2009). Globally, women with disabilities are seen as unequal to women without physical disabilities. In some cultures, these women are shunned and are hidden by their families and become isolated (Kim, 2009). They receive less education, face unemployment, are often prohibited from marrying and having children, are less likely to be included in social services programs, and are often barred from social and religious activities within the community (Bergoffen, Gilbert, Harvey, & McNeeley, 2011).

The Americans with Disabilities Act (ADA) became law in 1990. Employment discrimination against persons with disabilities who are qualified for the job is illegal. The ADA is enforced by the U.S. Equal Employment Opportunity Commission and other related agencies. As of July 26, 1994, this law applied to all employers with 15 or more employees. In 2008, the ADA was further amended to include broader coverage of individuals with a disability.

Nevertheless, women with disabilities have the lowest employment rankings falling behind men with disabilities (Parent et al., 2008). They earn less, work less, and studied less. Their employment rate is 26.8 percent compared to 65 percent for nondisabled women (Davidson et al., 2012). Multiple factors, including the narrowing of available jobs women with disabilities can accomplish, competitiveness in the job market, and decreased educational attainment, are thought to contribute to these low rates (Kruse, Schur, & Ali, 2010).

All in all, women around the world are more limited by prevailing social, cultural, and economic factors than by physical, psychosocial, sensory, or cognitive impairments.

OVERVIEW

DEFINING DISABILITY

The term *disability* can have multiple definitions that vary accordingly to whose writing the definition. Under the ADA, the statutory definition of a disability is that an individual with disabilities has "a physical or mental impairment that substantially limits one or more of the major life activities of such individual; a record of such an impairment; or being regarded as having such an impairment" (U.S. Equal Employment Commission, 2008, Section 902.1).

PREFERRED TERMINOLOGY

The preferred term for people not affected by a disability is *nondisabled* or *persons without disabilities*. The term *normal* should be avoided as it equates to a woman with any disability being categorized as not normal. Language is a powerful communicator of negative attitudes; therefore, communication needs to be inclusive and limiting, stereotypic terms must be avoided (see Table 9–1).

There are multiple terms that have been used in the past to describe a woman with a disability that are no longer considered politically appropriate. *Crippled*,

TABLE 9–1. Language Guidelines for Use When Interacting With Women Who Have a Disability

1. Where possible, emphasize an individual, not a disability. Say "people or persons with disabilities" or "person who is blind" rather than "disabled persons" or "blind person." (Many individuals prefer to use the words *physically challenged* to describe this population.)
2. When speaking of people with disabilities, always choose words that accurately describe the disability. Avoid using emotional descriptors such as unfortunate and pitiful. Do not refer to or focus on a disability unless crucial for the purpose of communication.
3. Talk directly to the person with a disability. If using an interpreter, speak facing the person with hearing impairment.
4. Avoid labeling persons into groups, as in "the disabled," "the deaf," "retardate," and "the arthritic"; instead, say "people who are deaf," "person with arthritis," and "persons with disabilities."
5. Do not sensationalize a disability by saying "afflicted with," "victim of," and so on. Instead, say "person who has multiple sclerosis" or "person who has polio."
6. Avoid portraying persons with disabilities who succeed as superhuman. This implies that persons who are disabled have no talents or unusual gifts.
7. Avoid use of "confined to wheelchair." Instead, consider "wheelchair user." Indeed, many individuals are liberated by a wheelchair rather than limited by the chair.
8. Emphasize abilities, such as "walks with a cane (braces)," rather than "is crippled"; "is partially sighted" rather than "partially blind." Never use the term *normal* in contrast.
9. After an initial greeting, sit down so that a person using a wheelchair won't have to crane her neck to make eye contact.
10. Shake whatever a person offers in greeting—a hand, prosthesis, or elbow.
11. When speaking with a person with a hearing loss, try to keep your face out of the shadows and your hands away from your mouth as you speak.
12. If someone's ability to read, write, or handle documents is limited, be prepared to provide assistance in completing paperwork.
13. When someone with a disability enters your clinic, don't assume she needs your help. Greet the person and tell her you're available for assistance.
14. Always speak directly to a person with a disability. Don't assume a companion is a conversational go-between.
15. When you offer to assist someone who is visually impaired, allow the person to take your arm so you can guide, rather than propel her.
16. Act naturally. Do not be afraid to use expressions such as "Would you like to see that?" or "Let me run over there." On the other hand, don't ask personal questions you wouldn't ask someone without a disability.
17. When speaking with a person with speech difficulty, talk normally. Don't pretend to understand when you don't. If necessary, ask the person to repeat. She has experienced this before and knows problems can arise.

Specific Language Guidelines

Disability (disabled, physically disabled). General term used for a (semi)permanent condition that interferes with a person's ability to do something independently—walk, see, hear, learn, lift. It may refer to a physical, mental, or sensory condition. Preferred usage is as a descriptive noun or adjective, as in persons who are disabled, people with disabilities, or disabled persons. Terms such as the disabled, crippled, deformed, and invalid are inappropriate.

Handicap. Often used as a synonym for disability. Usage, however, has become less acceptable (one origin is from "cap in hand," as in begging). Except when citing laws or regulations, *handicap* should not be used to describe a disability. This word can be used to describe the society or environment that limits accessibility.

Mute or Person Who Cannot Speak. Preferred terms to describe persons who cannot speak. Terms such as *deaf-mute* and *deaf* and *dumb* are inappropriate. They imply that persons without speech are always *deaf.*

Nondisabled. In a media portrayal of persons with and without disabilities, *nondisabled* is the appropriate term for persons without disabilities. Able-bodied should not be used, as it implies that persons with disabilities are less able. *Normal* is appropriate only in reference to statistical norms.

Seizure. Describes an involuntary muscular contraction symptomatic of the brain disorder epilepsy. Rather than saying "epileptic," say a "person with epilepsy" or "person with a seizure condition." The term *convulsion* should be reserved for seizures involving contractions of the entire body. The term *fit* is used by the medical profession in England, but it has strong negative connotations.

Spastic. Describes a muscle with sudden, abnormal involuntary spasms. It is not appropriate for describing a person with cerebral palsy. *Muscles* are spastic; people are not.

Speech Impaired. Describes persons with limited or difficult speech patterns.

Cesarean Birth. Should be used to describe a surgical birth. Avoid "section," it depersonalizes. Grapefruits get sectioned; women give birth.

Sources: Adapted from *Guidelines for reporting and writing about people with disabilities.* (1987). Media Project, Research and Training Center on Independent Living (348 Haworth Hall, University of Kansas, Lawrence, KS 66045); Sawin, K.J. (1986). *Physical disability in contemporary women's health.* Menlo Park, CA: Addison-Wesley; and *Disability etiquette.* Virginia Commonwealth University: Office of EEO/Affirmative Action Services; Dajani, K.F. (2001). What's in a name? Terms used to refer to people with disabilities. *Disability Studies Quarterly, 21*(3), 196–209.

handicapped, *mentally retarded*, and *insane* are examples of terms that are considered no longer acceptable when describing a person with a disability. The American Psychological Association (2011) and other groups advise phrases such as "people or a person with a disability" to describe the person first and disability second. For example, women with schizophrenia should be described as such and not as schizophrenics.

The term *disability* can also refer to an intellectual disability previously referred to as mentally disabled, cognitively disabled, mentally challenged, mongoloid, or mentally retarded. These traditionally describe women with a lower intelligence score, typically less than 70 on an IQ test.

Mental disabilities, women with psychological disabilities, and women with mental illness describe women who have a psychological diagnosis. Mental illness is a common source for disability in women, with depression being the leading cause. This chapter will focus on physical disability.

LIFESTYLE, DEVELOPMENTAL, AND CULTURAL ISSUES

COMMUNITY VERSUS INSTITUTIONAL DWELLING

Community-based care models focus on keeping persons with disabilities in a home-like setting and providing subsidies to the family or to the individual with disabilities to augment care services. Many women with disabilities utilize this funding to hire a personal care attendant. Personal care attendants provide individualized care services that may include bathing, feeding, dressing, and driving to medical appointments. Some care attendants are paid through state-funded Medicaid waivers, whereas others are paid directly by family members or the woman's personal finances. The political issues surrounding reimbursement, regulation, and licensing of personal care attendants may dramatically affect the quality of life for women with disabilities.

The number of adults living in institutional settings has changed over the past 20 years. In that the number of older adults in institutional settings has risen while the number of individuals in psychiatric facilities has dramatically decreased. The majority of people in institutions within the United States are older adults. Mental illness and physical disability are factors associated with being institutionalized. The cost of institutionalization represents the highest cost of providing care. Many states prefer this mode of care to independent living community-based programs despite the cost-savings involved. Although home care can offer a higher quality of care, it is not always feasible or available to all women who need this level of care.

SPECIAL PROBLEMS

Sight and Hearing Impairment

Clients who are deaf or blind are limited in their ability to communicate with providers if interpreters are not available. If a woman is provided an interpreter, she loses the option of having private interaction with the provider. If sign language is used in relating issues of sexuality and sexual intercourse, it should be remembered that sign communication is easily interpreted across the room; therefore, attention must be given to the interview area (Davidson et al., 2012). Few clinics and providers have readily available interpreters and many women rely on community-based services to meet their needs, which adds another level of complexity in scheduling appointments.

Severe Disability

Women institutionalized with severe multiple disabilities, including intellectual impairment, may have clinical problems such as vaginal discharge, menstrual cycle dysfunction, and oligomenorrhea, menorrhagia, and dysmenorrhea. Sensitive on-site management is essential. The severity of physical impairment, however, is not a good predictor of the impact of a disability on a woman (Davidson et al., 2012). Many women with severe physical and intellectual impairments are now making choices to become sexually active or opting to become mothers. Care providers must be familiar with choices available for women with severe disabilities and their own unique needs in evaluating the potential for new roles.

Service Animals

Some women with disabilities utilize service animals to provide assistance with activities of daily living (ADLs) and other care activities. Service dogs have been utilized for individuals with visual disabilities, hearing deficits, mobility issues, and psychological disorders. The federal law was changed in 2011, tightening requirements on the use of service animals, limiting it to dogs and, in some cases, miniature horses (Alifanz, 2011). The new law does not allow for emotional support or comfort alone as an indication for use; however, individuals with a psychiatric impairment can utilize a service dog.

Increased Risk for Latex Allergy

Women with multiple congenital malformations, especially multiple urinary anomalies, have a higher incidence of latex allergy. Those with spina bifida are at highest risk and should be tested for latex allergy with radioallergosorbent test (RAST) (Blumchen et al., 2010). Latex gloves are the most common source of reaction; however, condoms, dental dams, and urinary catheters have also created allergic response. The Spina Bifida Association of America has a comprehensive list of nonlatex options, which is updated regularly, and a short well-done video useful to both families and professionals (see Resources list).

CHANGES IN MENARCHE/ MENSTRUATION

It appears that some variations in menarche occur among women with disabilities. Individuals with blindness experience menarche earlier than usual occurrence. Head injury is also associated with precocious puberty (Flynn-Evans, Stevens, Tabandeh, Schernhammer, & Lockley, 2009). Bedridden young women who are intellectually impaired also have been noted to have an earlier onset of menses (Davidson et al., 2012). For some women with mobility impairments, lack of manual dexterity, and difficulty transferring can impair independence and may lead a woman to seek a means to reduce or eliminate the menstrual cycle. The practice is widespread in well-meaning parents of women with intellectual impairment and severe physical disabilities (Zacharin, Savasi, & Grover, 2010). Depo-Provera®, for example, has been associated with osteoporosis with long-term use and is generally not recommended for long-term use in adolescence (Davidson et al., 2012). Combination contraceptives can be used to decrease menstrual frequency and are associated with a reduction in absenteeism in school, fewer menstrual-related difficulties, and greater satisfaction; however, they carry the risk of thrombophlebitis and pulmonary embolism (Hicks & Rome, 2010). Women and their families must carefully weigh the risks and benefits of interventions to manage menstrual hygiene with potential long-term effects. The following are some condition-specific potential menstrual-related changes.

Cystic Fibrosis

Many adolescents with cystic fibrosis have delayed menarche, averaging approximately 2 years later than their unaffected peers (Umławska, Sands, & Zielińska, 2010).

Spinal Cord Injury

Temporary cessation of menses is normal for up to 1 year following injury. Cessation of menses may persist for up to 2 years, with the average duration being 6 months. Resumption of ovulation is unpredictable. It may occur before menstruation. Artificial induction of menses may be required to reestablish menstruation (Saulino & Vaccaro, 2009). In addition, menstrual discomfort may remain, even if altered.

Multiple Sclerosis

Multiple sclerosis (MS) is the most common neurologic disease among young adults. Women are affected twice as often as men. Female sex hormones, estrogen and progesterone, may be involved. Clinical symptoms often appear during changes in hormonal balance during the menstrual cycle, after pregnancy, and during the climacteric. No change, however, occurs in fertility or menstruation.

Epilepsy

Epilepsy does not substantially alter puberty in adolescents. Approximately 70 percent will have no change in seizure frequency, 15 percent experience increase, and 15 percent experience a decrease in seizure frequency, with more seizures at ovulation and immediately before and after the menstrual flow (Emory University Health Sciences Center, 2004). Some women with epilepsy experience variations in seizure frequency with hormonal changes, a condition known as catamenial epilepsy (Emory University Health Sciences Center, 2004). Women should chart their seizures in relation to their menstrual cycle and/or ovulation to see if a pattern emerges. If a pattern is present, women may benefit from supplemental hormonal therapy.

AGING/MENOPAUSE

People with disabilities are now living into old age. Post-polio syndrome is a reality for many women in their 60s and 70s. It is characterized by increased joint weakness and joint stiffness. We do know that the major causes of death to persons with spinal cord injuries are respiratory infections, urinary tract infections, and external causes such as suicide. There is little data, however, explaining why most other people with lifelong disabilities die. Individuals with disabilities are asking questions such as the following: What are the implications of aging to 70 if you have had osteoarthritis since 20? What is menopause like for women with disabilities or what are the implications on joint health of walking for many years with altered gait or of the early transition to wheelchair as primary source of mobility? As women with disabilities age, they have less access to health care services, less support, less needed equipment to preserve functioning, and inadequate assistance (Rosso, Wisdom, Horner-Johnson, McGee, & Yvonne, 2011).

Women with disabilities may experience unique changes in addition to or independently from the customary aging processes. Women with physical disabilities are less likely to ambulate, participate in physical exercise, and are more likely to have a history of phlebitis. They enter menopause with fewer years of weight bearing and little or no participation in aerobic activity (Rosso et al., 2011). Thus, they are at risk for obesity, cardiovascular deconditioning, and cardiovascular illnesses. Women with disabilities also have an increased risk of osteoporosis, with some already diagnosed in their 20s or 30s. In addition, menopause can bring decreased skin turgor and strength, loss of elasticity, and decreased blood supply. This can put a woman with disabilities at increased risk for skin breakdown (Davidson et al., 2012).

It is also clear that menopause may occur earlier in women with Down syndrome and women with epilepsy. Women with Down syndrome may also experience sensory, adaptive, or cognitive losses earlier than other women (Antonia et al., 2010).

In the last decade, use of estrogen replacement has often been eliminated from consideration due to concerns over thrombotic events. The transdermal route for estrogen therapy, however, may be a safer option and can be considered (Canonico, Plu-Bureau, Lowe, & Scarabin, 2008). Nevertheless, with recent research findings related to hormone replacement therapy and stroke, myocardial infarction, and deep vein thrombosis, management of menopausal symptoms by nurse practitioners in collaboration with gynecologist, geriatrician, and/or physiatrist consultation is advised to optimize care for older women with disabilities (see Chapter 18 for more information).

We need further research to know how the aging trajectory differs for people with disabilities since childhood or young adulthood. In addition, we know little about the impact of lifelong disability or chronic illness on menopause or about sexuality issues in those aging with disability.

CULTURE AND DISABILITY

Activists and scholars writing about the civil rights movement of individuals with disabilities reject the traditional view of disability as being physically defective and needing to be fixed. Instead, these activists are asserting that individuals with disabilities are a legitimate cultural minority. This philosophy is based on the belief that most of the problems faced by individuals with disabilities are not caused by the body but by a society that refuses to accommodate their differences. This culture proposes that medical needs are only a small part of the disability experience, with the larger, more pressing problems being social and political (Balcazar, Suarez-Balcazar, Taylor-Ritzler, & Keys, 2010).

Nevertheless, culture shapes women's experience with disabilities. The prevalence of disability is higher among minority women, yet little is written about the experience of disability for women in diverse cultures. The more the disability experience is divergent from the societal norm of the referent culture group, the more issues women will face. For women who are immigrants, the experience is more difficult as the woman must deal with her marginality, social isolation, and alienation in a foreign culture (Balcazar et al., 2010). The devaluation of self is not only rooted in the disability experience but also from the definition of self that is constructed in dealing with the migration experience.

For African American women with disabilities, there may be issues of identity, role conflict, employment, and sexuality. African American women may experience greater difficulty with multiple role conflict. They tend to have more roles, more children, and greater environmental stress and may be more likely to be single parents. The kinship network of the African American woman, however, is usually a positive protective factor. If the disability causes collapse of that network, health care providers need to aggressively assist the woman to repair or renew her support network. Employment is a challenge for African American women. Women of color with disabilities have lower employment income levels than all other men and women with and without disabilities. Women with disabilities earn 65 percent of what men with disabilities earn; women of color earn even less (Balcazar et al., 2010).

CONFRONTING NEGATIVE ATTITUDES AND BARRIERS

Attitudes Among Health Care Providers

Women with disabilities face multiple barriers to quality reproductive health care services and receive fewer services. Health care providers often have negative attitudes toward women with disabilities expect less of them and overestimate the negative impact of disability on family life (Balcazar et al., 2010). Often, health care providers speak without sensitivity. They are frequently unaware of how many adults with disabilities live independently in the community, use adaptive equipment, modify homes, and use attendant care (Davidson et al., 2012). Health care providers' perception of issues such as appearance, ease of communication, and autonomy can influence their response to women. Moreover, professionals are more aware of predominately male disabilities and underestimate the frequency of disabilities among women (Neal & Guillet, 2004).

Health care providers should look at their own attitudes and expectations to determine potential problems before eliciting a history from women with disabilities. Do not vary the history protocol to omit potential issues. If you usually ask about first sexual experiences, birth control, episodes of unwanted intercourse, or satisfaction with intimate relationships, then ask the same questions to women with disabilities. In doing so, it is important to watch your "handicapism" terms and use inclusive and sensitive language (see Table 9–1). Providers need to assess the assumptions they hold. They may be surprised to learn that the severity of physical impairment is not a good predictor of impact of the disability on women (Davidson et al., 2012). In fact, fatigue and pain have been found to be better predictors of health outcomes even after the impact of functional ability has been taken into consideration.

Invisible Asexual Misperception

As noted in the introduction of this chapter, women with disabilities, especially those growing up with a disability, are often seen as asexual and not in need of discussions regarding sexuality. To the contrary, these women have numerous needs. Even though opportunities for sexual experiences may be more limited, many women with physical disabilities do engage in sexual activities and report stronger relationships and better satisfaction rates than nondisabled women (Ostrander, 2009). Denying the sexuality of a woman with disabilities limits the services that are provided for her and may put the woman at risk for adverse health conditions and disease.

Lowered Expectations

Health care providers are among those who often send the message that a woman's body is unacceptable and somehow broken. Expectations are that women with disabilities are less likely to marry or have children; they may be seen as more dependent, weak, and less able to care for themselves or a child (Balcazar et al., 2010). In fact, a significant factor in whether young women with disabilities have active social lives was their parent's expectations (Howland & Rintala, 2001; Nelson, 1995). Unfortunately, although these parents had educational goals for their daughters, only a small percentage expected their daughters to be socially active (Nelson, 1995). Furthermore, career counseling for women with disabilities is often limited because they may be viewed as unemployable in the workforce (Neal & Guillet, 2004).

Surmised Intellectual Impairment

Often women with disabilities are treated as if physical disability means intellectual impairment, especially if their speech is impaired. Characteristically, clinic and hospital personnel talk to the person who is accompanying the individual with a disability, not to the individual herself. In addition, they frequently talk down or use language patterns appropriate for a child (Neal & Guillet, 2004). Frequently, inebriation is assumed in addition to low IQ. Talking more loudly or more simply is a frequent reaction to speech disability.

Perceived Parenthood Conflict

Conflict is perceived between carrying out the responsibilities of parenthood and complying with a medical regimen. Mothers report that health care providers seem unable to recognize the profound interrelationship between their mothering responsibilities and disabilities.

HEALTH PROMOTION FOR WOMEN WITH DISABILITIES

Healthy People 2020's priority goal is to reduce health disparities among Americans. A major goal of the Healthy People 2020 initiatives is to decrease health disparities among people with disabilities. Women with disabilities often lack preventative care services such as annual dental screenings, regular mammograms, and recommended Pap testing (Healthy People 2020, 2011). However, women with mobility problems were likely to get immunizations such as pneumonia and influenza (Davidson et al., 2012). Many women with disabilities have unhealthy lifestyles that include tobacco use, lack of physical activity, and lack of routine medical care for conditions associated with obesity, such as hypertension (Healthy People 2020, 2011). Identifying interventions to support health-promoting behaviors in persons with disabilities is the top priority of researchers in rehabilitation nursing. Additionally, there is a growing emphasis both from clinicians/researchers and from the National Institutes of Health (NIH) to generate knowledge about an area ignored until recently—health promotion or wellness needs of women with disabilities. The Center for the Study of Women with Disabilities has been created at Baylor University; NIH has held a consensus conference on the health of women with disabilities; and organizations, such as the Spina Bifida Association and the American Epilepsy Society, have created either an organizational committee or a task force to address the unique needs of this population.

Public health initiatives also aim to improve the life of women with disabilities by encouraging access for women with disabilities within their environment. The need for inclusion within the general community is imperative. Access can be improved by facilitating more health promotion programs for women with disabilities and providing appropriate services, enhancing work and educational opportunities, increasing social engagement, and improving access to assistive technology and assistive supports (Healthy People 2020, 2011).

NUTRITION RELATED TO WOMEN WITH DISABILITIES

Optimal health promotion includes adequate nutrition and certain disabilities require higher calorie or nutrient needs. For example, women with spastic quadriplegia cerebral palsy utilize a great deal of calorie consumption due to spasticity and need more nutrient-dense foods. Women with osteoporosis-related disabilities should have diets enriched with calcium and vitamin D. Women who are non–weight bearing are at an increased risk for lowered bone mineral density and also need these additional minerals and nutrients. Some women are at risk for osteoporosis based on their medication regimens. Vitamin D and calcium supplementation is important in women with epilepsy as well because they are at increased risk for osteoporosis with long-term antiepileptic drug (AED) treatment. All well women with epilepsy (WWE), including adolescents, capable of becoming pregnant should be taking 0.4 mg of folic acid. Select AEDs have been shown to lower folic acid levels, which increases the risk for neural tube conditions (Caughley, 2011).

PHYSICAL ACTIVITY/SPORTS

Individuals with disabilities have demonstrated physiological responses to exercise similar to women without disabilities. In addition, exercise has been shown to yield positive overall fitness and psychological outcomes (Healthy People 2020, 2011; Motl & Gosney, 2008). Normal wheelchair propulsion is not sufficient to maintain physical condition, and training programs yield positive changes in physical conditioning. A steady exercise program should be customized based on a woman's specific interests, abilities, and available activities within the community. Research is needed that explores the responses of women with disabilities to a variety of recreational and sports programs and the interaction of women's health status with these programs. Opportunities for physical activity for women with disabilities need to be expanded. This is particularly important for girls in physical education classes who are experiencing segregation inclusion and social isolation (Hutzler & Levi, 2008).

BREAST SELF-EXAMINATION/ MAMMOGRAPHY

In some rehabilitation and primary care settings, breast self-examination is not discussed with women with disabilities, even when they present for gynecologic examinations. Clinical breast exam is especially important for older women with arthritis or neuropathies (Cristian, 2009). Women with intact manual dexterity and sensation can be taught breast self-examination. Moreover, some women with impaired sensation can perform a modified examination, or an attendant or partner can perform it. If neither of these plans is acceptable, more frequent examination by a health care provider should be considered (Davidson et al., 2012).

CONTRACEPTION

Information on contraception is often not offered to women with disabilities (Davidson et al., 2012). It is important for health care providers to examine the options with clients. The choice may be a balance of risk factors: for example, the risk of pregnancy versus the risk of the contraceptive method. If oral contraception or an intrauterine device (IUD) is considered and the method carries risk, consultation with or referral to a gynecologic specialist needs to be initiated.

Discussion of alternatives needs to take place with the woman who is allergic or whose partner is allergic to latex. Contraceptive options may be significantly restricted for women with mobility impairment or with a latex allergy. Joint management with a physician colleague is indicated.

Barrier Methods

Barrier methods are often an optimal choice. If a client has manual limitations and, consequently, difficulty manipulating a barrier device, it is important to determine the availability of a partner or personal care attendant and their roles. A client may need to explore ways to ask her partner to assist with a barrier method. Many women have not considered asking a personal care attendant to assist with placement of a contraceptive device before sexual activity, but could be open to asking for this kind of assistance when made aware of the possibility.

- *Condoms.* Condoms, which also provide protection against AIDS and other sexually transmitted infections (STIs), are an option. Water-soluble lubricants can ease vaginal dryness. Caution should be taken to identify women who have, or whose partners have, latex allergies. A nonlatex condom (LifeStyles® Skyn) is available. This is the only nonlatex condom that has been FDA approved to prevent the transmission of HIV and other STIs.
- *Cervical Cap.* For some women, a cervical cap is attractive, as it can be inserted in the morning by a personal care attendant and removed 24 hours later, eliminating the need for assistance during lovemaking.
- *Diaphragm.* An increase in urinary infections is associated with the arch diaphragm. It may present particular problems and not be appropriate for women with urinary stasis. Caution should be taken to identify women who have, or whose partners have, latex allergies.

Hormonal Contraceptives

Depo-Provera® was once widely used as a means of menstrual suppression for women with intellectual impairment and women with other disabilities; however, recent studies have shown its long-term use can cause osteoporosis. This risk warranted a black-box warning by the FDA in 2004. Current recommendations advise its use for no longer than 2 years as a protective means to protect bone mineral density in women (Pascall & Kaunitz, 2008).

Hormonal contraceptives offer a means of menstrual suppression that can be administered by care providers for women with severe disability. Oral contraceptive pills can be given consecutively without interruption to suppress monthly menses and provide contraceptive benefits as well. The Mirena® IUD can be used in nulliparous and parous women to suppress menses and provide contraception, but insertion is not well tolerated in some nulliparous women and may not be a viable option for most women with severe disability. The vaginal ring can be placed by a care provider and replaced on a regular basis to suppress a woman's menstrual cycle (Hicks & Rome, 2010). Contraceptive patches can also be used and may be preferred for some women, although there is a higher incidence of thrombolytic events that warrant careful assessment prior to their use (Davidson et al., 2012).

An additional benefit of hormonal contraceptives is derived by women with severe mobility restrictions. If these women are dependent on others for menstrual hygiene care, the possible lack or decreased frequency of menstrual periods may increase their functional status.

Women with disabilities who are active in the political arena warn that we do not have enough data on any of these methods to be clear about their long-term impact for women with disabilities and recommend cautious use until more data is available.

Specific Conditions and Contraceptive Needs

Although research is limited, the data that is available regarding contraceptive needs for the most frequent disabilities is reported here and may be presented in discussions with clients. Because women with disabilities are considered high risk medically, joint management with a physician colleague or referral for a form of contraception other than a barrier method is recommended.

Spinal Cord Injury

The fertility of women with spinal cord injury is unaffected. Their decreased mobility and the increased incidence of deep vein thrombosis place them at high risk with respect to hormonal contraceptives, especially those containing estrogen. Hormonal contraceptives containing estrogen are absolutely contraindicated if a woman has uncontrolled hypertension or if she is known to have circulatory problems (Davidson et al., 2012).

Use of IUDs poses a risk because of the woman's decreased sensation and ability to determine warning signs of infection. Some women, however, indicate that dysreflexia is triggered by the pain that they are unable to perceive. They may thus be able to identify infection with the occurrence of dysreflexia. In addition, they propose that checking the IUD string placement could be carried out by their partners. IUDs may be a preferred method because they do not pose risks associated with thrombolytic events.

Most women with paraplegia can usually manage barrier methods with no or minimal assistance in positioning legs for effective insertion. Women with higher spinal cord lesions require assistance from a partner or an attendant.

Multiple Sclerosis

The menstrual and fertility patterns of women with MS rarely change. Oral contraceptive use has no effect on the risk of developing MS. Smoking has been associated with early conversion of the disease and should be avoided in childbearing women whenever possible (Di Pauli et al., 2008).

Women with MS do not have contraindications in contraceptive choices. They should discuss contraceptive options with care providers to determine the best choice for their specific personal needs. Although some studies have indicated that conceptive use is protective against MS, none have been conclusive. Contraceptives do not cause or precipitate MS (Alonso et al., 2005).

Cystic Fibrosis

Data on hormonal contraception is limited. It is estimated that two thirds of women with cystic fibrosis use a means of contraception, with oral contraceptive pills being the most commonly used (Plant et al., 2008). The use of hormonal contraceptives has not been found to increase the need for antibiotics or interfere with pulmonary functioning (Kernan, Cullinan, Alton, Bilton, & Griesenbach, 2010). There is no contraindication to the use of barrier methods among women with cystic fibrosis.

Rheumatoid Arthritis

There appears to be no change in disease patterns when hormonal contraceptives are used (Farr, Folger, Paulen, & Curtis, 2010). Barrier methods may be difficult for some women to use if they experience weakness and decreased manual dexterity (Davidson et al., 2012). An IUD may also be a viable option.

Cerebral Palsy

The effect of cerebral palsy on contraception varies greatly. If the client is paralyzed or has decreased mobility, hormonal contraception is risky because of the risk for deep vein thrombosis. Independent use of barrier methods, especially the diaphragm or cervical cap, may be troublesome for women with spasticity; however, these methods are viable with partner participation.

Epilepsy

Estrogen levels are related to seizure threshold in WWE. Seizures vary during the menstrual cycle: Incidence is highest during the estradiol spike before ovulation and the rapid drop in progesterone immediately before and during menstruation. The relationship between oral hormonal therapy and seizures is less evident; however, drug interaction has been associated with the use of combined oral contraceptives (COCs) and implantable devices such as Norplant. There has been no negative association with progestin-only contraceptives, which may represent a good choice of birth control for WWE (Gaffield, Culwell, & Lee, 2011). WWE metabolize drugs differently, and when COCs are used, higher doses are generally indicated. COCs can actually cause an increase in seizure activity as well (Reddy, 2010). Depo-Provera® may be a viable choice because it is progesterone-only contraceptive with high effectiveness rates; however, as previously mentioned, long-term use, greater than 2 years, has been associated with a reduction of bone mineral density and a risk factor for osteoporosis (Bonnema, McNamara, & Spencer, 2010).

Intrauterine devices are a very good option and do not interfere in metabolism of drugs or increase seizure activity (Bonnema et al., 2010).

Down Syndrome

Fertility is unaffected. For many women with Down syndrome, the choice of contraception is affected by mobility, chronic illness, and intellectual factors. In the use of contraception, informed consent is a critical aspect.

- Oral hormonal contraception requires that a woman's memory skills be adequate for the regimen.
- Implants may be attractive to some.
- Women who have multiple disabilities (motor and intellectual) may not be able to manage a diaphragm.
- Adolescents and young women need comprehensive ongoing sex education and accessible adults to assist with problem solving and skill development.

Some women with Down syndrome are now making the decision to pursue pregnancy and parenting options. Women with intellectual impairment need ongoing education and skills training when considering pregnancy. Most of these women who do conceive have a strong social support network. Also, most have a social service intervention that assesses their ability to care for themselves and children independently (Davidson et al., 2012).

Women With Sickle Cell Disease

Contraception for women with sickle cell disease (SCD) is important for two reasons: (1) Women with this condition can get pregnant and (2) their pregnancies are high risk and need careful planning. All barrier methods, most low-dose pills, Implanon®, and Depo-Provera® are options to consider for women with this condition. Depo-Provera®, although associated with low bone mineral density, is known to decrease the incidence of sickle cell crisis and is widely used in women with SCD.

Women With Lupus

Oral contraceptives increase risk of hypertension, thrombosis, and disease exacerbation. The use of IUDs has been associated with infection. Barrier method in combination with spermicide is safest. Permanent sterilization may be an option chosen by some women.

SEXUALITY

It is not clear what impact the timing of disability onset has on a woman's satisfaction with contraception and sexuality information. Women whose onset of disability is after menarche are identified by some as having special needs for contraception and sexuality. Other data suggests that women who grow up with their disability and those with developmental disabilities do not have adequate sexuality and contraception counseling (Tice & Hall, 2008). The need for sexuality and contraception counseling must be assessed regardless of the time of onset. Women report that professionals rarely initiate discussion of sexuality issues. Some authors propose that the primary barriers to full expression of sexuality are the negative attitudes of others, especially family members and medical and rehabilitation professionals. The attitude that the disability has somehow neutered a woman interferes with her belief in her right to sexual feelings and expression (Higgins, 2010).

From in-depth qualitative interviews conducted two decades ago, Nosek et al. (1994) identified tasks important to developing a wellness perspective of sexuality among women with physical disabilities (see Table 9–2). In the quantitative portion of this study, 475 women with disabilities were compared with a population of 425 women without disabilities. There was no difference between groups in sexual desire. Further, there was no impact of the severity of disability on sexual activity. Women with disabilities did report lower amounts of sexual activity, sexual response, and sexual satisfaction. Women with disabilities since childhood had more sexual thoughts and higher desire. No differences were found in sexual frequency, arousal, or satisfaction. The psychological factors predicted the greatest amount of sexual variance: 35 percent of variance in sexual satisfaction and 40 percent of variance in sexual activity. Since then other researchers agree, reporting decreased function without changes in interest or importance of sexual activity (Higgins, 2010).

Patterns of sexual activity for women with a disability may be decreased. Many women report the lack of a partner. Women also report a need to avoid spontaneity and instead plan for sexual activity. This need, however, can be seen as a benefit: Because many persons with disability must communicate with their partners about sexual possibilities and restrictions, this opens up avenues for communication in other areas of the relationship. Unfortunately, many people who are totally physically independent may never experience such communication.

Many women with mobility or sensory limitations employ a personal care attendant. She may address some unique sexuality issues; for example, she may place the cervical cap or diaphragm and carry out the bowel or bladder program before sexual activity. Spouses and significant others often function as personal care attendants, but it can be difficult to be both care provider and lover. Each couple needs to address this issue. If both the woman and her partner are disabled, the attendant may assist in positioning the couple.

A number of drugs may have a negative impact on sexual function. A full assessment of both prescription and over-the-counter drugs is critical when addressing issues of sexuality with women who have a disability. Certain medications may also be contraindicated for pregnancy so it is essential that women have contraceptive counseling with each office visit.

Sexuality and Adolescents With Disability

To prove that they are normal, adolescents with disability may sometimes increase their sexual behavior (Maart & Jelsma, 2010). Consequently, they are at increased risk of pregnancy, STIs, and abuse. Primary care of all adolescent women with disabilities must include assessment of the potential for sexual activity or actual sexual activity and the need for contraception.

Multiple myths related to sexuality and disability in adolescents exist and health care providers often fail to realize their needs and aspirations most frequently mirror those of their nondisabled peers (Maart & Jelsma, 2010). In addition, parents of children with disabilities are often

TABLE 9–2. Wellness Perspective of Sexuality Among Women With Physical Disabilities

Having a Positive Sexual Self-Concept
She appreciates her own value.
She asserts her right to make a choice.
She feels ownership of her body.
She is able to restrict the limitations resulting from her disability to physical functioning only and does not impose those limitations to her sexual self.
She is accepting, not ashamed, of her body.
Having Sexual Information
She has general information about sexuality and is able to apply to herself.
She actively seeks information about how her disability affects her sexuality.
Having Positive, Productive Relationships
She feels generally satisfied with her relationships.
She is able to communicate effectively with others.
She feels stability in her relationships.
She is able to control the amount and nature of contact with others.
Managing Barriers
She is able to recognize psychological, physical, and sexual abuse and its exploitation and take action to reduce or eliminate it or neutralize its impact.
She has learned to reduce her vulnerability.
She understands her disability-related environmental needs and seeks information on how to meet these needs.
She recognizes her right to live in a barrier-free environment and takes action to achieve it.
She confronts societal barriers by using good communication skills to educate her partner, friends, and family.
Maintaining Optimal Health and Physical Sexual Functioning
She participates in health maintenance activities and engages in health-promoting behaviors.
She feels congruity between her values/desires and her sexual behaviors.
She manages her environment to optimize privacy for intimate activities.
She is satisfied with the frequency and quality of sexual activity.
She is able to communicate freely with her partner about limitations and devices and about what pleases her sexually.

Source: Adapted from Nosek et al., 1994.

overprotective and may not educate these children in terms of sexuality, contraception, STIs, and exploitation and abuse. Recommendations for adolescents with disabilities include a comprehensive sex education program that should be tailored to fit their specific needs.

DISABILITY CONDITIONS THAT IMPACT SEXUALITY

Spasticity

Spasticity can be elicited by a variety of tactile stimulations. Each woman needs to determine the ability of a variety of sexual activities to produce this response. Slow-building stimulation may produce less spasticity than more-intense stimulation. Women with spasticity might experience spasticity with sexual activity and orgasm (Stevenson, 2010). The knee-chest position during sexual activities may facilitate decrease in spasticity.

Spinal Cord Injury

Because a women's fertility is not affected in spinal cord injury, many providers and researchers have assumed no sexuality problems exist. Women with complete lesions experience neither traditional orgasm nor clitoral or vaginal sensation; however, women with spinal cord injury do report satisfying pleasurable orgasm-like sensations from stimulation of the breasts, ears, or other sensitive areas. Even women with complete lesions report psychological and even physical sensations of orgasm or intense pleasure during sex. Vaginal lubrication may occur via reflex for women with lesions at T9–T11 or above and has also been reported in relation to masturbation unrelated to level of lesion. In addition, some women report cervical and vaginal pressure (Kreuter, Siösteen, & Biering-Sørensen, 2008). Arousal was present in women regardless of level of lesion and not correlated with type of stimulation (vaginal, cervical, or hypersensitive area). Clearly, the mechanism of sexual response in women with spinal cord injuries does not totally follow the traditional physiological model. Alternative areas of sexual stimulation and strategies for sexual expression need to be identified, including alternative positions, such as side-lying, knee-chest positions, and chair sitting, for paraplegics and quadriplegics and the stuffing technique (of flaccid penis) for women whose partner is paraplegic. If graphic depiction of positions for sexual intercourse would be helpful, the health care provider needs to communicate the appropriate resources (Kreuter et al., 2008). The normal sexual responses that may occur are opening of the labia, contraction of the outer third of the vagina, expansion of the inner two thirds of the vagina, and uterine contraction. Many women are satisfied with postinjury sexual experience.

Joint Inflexibility and Pain

Arthrogryposis congenita, sickle cell anemia with joint involvement, arthritis, severe scoliosis, amputation, cerebral palsy, and dwarfism may result in joint inflexibility and pain. With respect to sexual activity, careful assessment of physical parameters, such as range of motion, is helpful. Discussion about alternative positioning may follow. The importance of extended foreplay, possible gentle warming up and stretching, warm showers, and use of vibration, massage, or masturbation to achieve orgasm may also be considered. Prolonged rest should be avoided in order to decrease likelihood of joint stiffness. Sexual activity may augment an overall sense of comfort, as orgasm releases endorphins. The client may profit from some helpful suggestions.

- Choose the time of day for sexual activity relative to pain history.
- Consider a warm shower or compress in foreplay if effective in pain relief.
- Consider medicine for pain relief before intercourse if pain is limiting.
- Consider referral to a physical therapist for comprehensive muscle assessment in complex cases.

Multiple Sclerosis

The symptoms of MS may vary greatly and may include spasticity, dry vagina, fatigue, muscle weakness, pain, bladder and bowel incontinence, and difficulty achieving orgasm. Balance and fatigue may necessitate energy-sparing sexual activities and positions for intercourse. A water-soluble lubricant may be used if the vagina is dry. Vibrators have been found to be helpful to those who tried them, as a way to increase stimulation and achieve orgasm. Data indicates that about half of women who have MS report changes in their sexual life (Fletcher et al., 2009). The duration of MS, degree of disability, number of exacerbations in the last year, disability score, and presence of bowel problems or fatigue have little impact on the presence of sexual dysfunction, although the amount of sexual activity may decrease. Corticosteriods are most often used to reduce the duration of the attacks and severity of symptoms and can help reduce sexual dysfunction.

Sexual difficulties for women with MS can be divided into three categories. Primary symptoms are directly related to neurological changes that can impact the sexual response cycle, such as decreased desire, unpleasant sensations, and decreased ability to reach orgasm. Secondary sexual dysfunction occurs from symptoms not directly related to neurological functioning such as bowel and bladder issues, tremors, spasticity, and muscle weakness. Tertiary dysfunction refers to cultural and psychological issues associated with having MS and the associated feelings that can interfere with sexual functioning (Multiple Sclerosis International Foundation, 2011).

Epilepsy

Several concerns exist for WWE, however, including the effect of their hormones and menstrual cycle on seizures, contraception, fertility, and sexuality issues (Davidson et al., 2012). A healthy development of sexuality has been affected for some. Some sexuality issues may be related to AEDs.

Presence of Urinary and Bowel Appliances

Apparatus may discourage sexual activity. The following steps can be taken to ease discomforts:

- Foley catheters can be taped out of the way or removed, but may need to be reinserted soon after sexual activity; individuals using intermittent catheterizations should catheterize before sexual activity to prevent urine leakage.
- Stomal appliances can be ignored, changed, covered, or removed before sexual activity, based on what has been ordered and individual preference.
- Clients should be told that masturbation and coitus may stimulate bladder or bowel incontinence.
- Discussing how to tell potential partners about bladder and bowel issues may be critical. Role-playing may be helpful.

Intellectual Impairment

It is difficult for women with intellectual impairment or developmental delays to achieve sexual options available to other women with disabilities. Women with severe intellectual impairments are often seen as nonadults and as unequal to their peers without disabilities. Issues of sexual education, effective birth control, sexual expression, and pregnancy are complex. Even when parents verbalize the opinion that young adults with intellectual impairment should have sexual options, it is difficult for the same parents to prepare their own children to make sexual decisions, consider teaching their teen the appropriate use of masturbation, or teach abuse prevention skills. Better understanding of the needs of young women who grow up with intellectual delay or developmental disabilities is crucial to provision of effective care (Davidson et al., 2012).

Visual/Hearing Impairment

Many women who are deaf/blind enter adulthood sexually unaware but with normal sexual drives and desires. They often lack basic sexual information such as physical differences between the sexes, information related to reproduction and contraceptive options, and knowledge of STIs. This deficit in sexual and reproductive education created by parents' and health care providers' lack of alternate methods of communication is compounded by the youth's inability to learn about sexuality by observing others model appropriate and inappropriate sexual behaviors. Sexuality education for women who are deaf/blind should be taught throughout their life span. The better informed the women are, the less likely they will be sexually maladjusted or abused (Davidson et al., 2012).

SEXUALLY TRANSMITTED INFECTIONS

Little is written about how women with disabilities experience STIs. If sensation is impaired, women may have special issues with STIs. For example, if women with disabilities have HSV (herpes simplex virus), they may have limited ability to promptly respond to a prodrome if it is tingling or itching in the affected area. Inability to identify developing painful lesions may have severe consequences to these women. These women will need to learn to identify and monitor more subtle cues. Many of these women may be in the habit of frequent visual skin inspection and should be advised to include the genital area in this visual inspection.

RISK FOR ABUSE FOR WOMEN WITH DISABILITIES

Women with physical and intellectual disabilities are at higher risk for abuse (Davidson et al., 2012). Abuse is a serious problem for women with disabilities because they have even fewer options for escaping or resolving the abuse than women in general.

There is combined cultural devaluation of women with disabilities, devaluation based on age, and devaluation of disability. A woman with disabilities often has experienced overprotection and has internalized social expectations. Combine this with a lack of knowledge, overcompliance, an unrealistic view that everyone is a friend, limited social opportunity, constant negative feedback (women with disabilities are ugly, worthless, etc.), low self-esteem, and limited or no assertiveness or refusal skills, and it is understandable that this population has a high incidence of abuse. Women may not report abuse because of fear of not being believed due to their devalued status or the abuse may have been perpetrated by a valued friend, family member, or caretaker. If a teenager or adult who is disabled feels undesirable, she may become vulnerable to exploitation, particularly in sexual relations (Davidson et al., 2012). Women with intellectual disabilities are also at the greatest risk for abuse (Hope, 2011). Lesbian women who are disabled are more likely to be targets of violence and to face relationship-based intimate partner violence (Higgins, 2010). Of women with disabilities, 65 to 90 percent have been sexually abused at some time in their lives (Hope, 2011).

Women with disabilities are frequently not educated on the risks of sexual exploitation, abuse, and violence (Davidson et al., 2012). Health care providers need to provide information on how to lessen risk of violence and safe practices. Educational programs need to be developed to address skill building in coping with potential or real abuse and orientation to sexuality rights and responsibilities. If abuse has occurred, a woman should be reassured that it was not her fault and reporting options should be examined. Practitioners are required by law to report cases of abuse against minors and, in some states, against vulnerable individuals. It is important that the health care provider acknowledge the sexuality of women with disabilities, teach healthy sexuality in the context of family, reinforce a positive sense of self, learn to recognize signs of abuse, listen to the patient, and act on reports of abuse. Assessment of abuse and treatment interventions for women with disabilities will be the same as their peers without disabilities. In order to increase services, considerably more needs to be known about interventions that are most effective for this population. Prevention of exploitation, abuse, and violence, however, is the major key.

In addition, health care providers need to advocate for inclusion of sexual assertiveness skills in sex education or family life education curricula. The optimal time for this education is in childhood or adolescence. Professionals need to seek out opportunities to act as a consultant to schools and community groups that serve this population (YWCA, local school districts, and schools). These women may need a myriad of specialized services for treatment. Agencies such as independent living centers may be useful partners in these endeavors.

FOSTERING ACCESSIBILITY TO CLINIC SERVICES

ADA REQUIREMENTS

The ADA, enacted in 1990, mandates that all new buildings meet minimal accessibility standards; section 504 of the Persons with Disabilities Act of 1978 applies to all facilities receiving any federal funds. The regulations do not require that a facility have special programs or services. The regulations do, however, require that the same services offered to women without disabilities must be offered to women with disabilities (Federal Register, 1990). For example, if women without disabilities are weighed, accurate mechanisms are needed to weigh women with disabilities. Wheelchair-accessible scales can be used to weigh ambulating women as well. If the clinic offers Pap smears and pelvic examinations, it needs to offer women with disabilities the same services and to make necessary accommodations.

PSYCHOLOGICAL ACCESSIBILITY

It has been suggested that the client may find it more difficult to gain psychological accessibility to the health care provider than physical accessibility to the clinic. Providers must limit stereotypes, actively pursue optimal communication procedures, value mutual problem solving and goal setting, and use every opportunity to reaffirm normalcy. In a clinical setting, guidelines are needed to enhance accessibility, beginning with the first telephone contact. When the first appointment is made, clients should be asked the following:

- Do you have a physical disability? If so, ask the client to specify if it is difficult getting around, hearing, or seeing, and so on.
- What accommodations will be necessary for your visit to the clinic? Arrangements may need to be made that will allow for a longer visit.

PHYSICAL ACCESSIBILITY OF CLINIC

Physical Layout

In assessing the physical layout of a clinic, determine wheelchair accessibility: for example, ramp dimensions, bathrooms, and doorways. Using a wheelchair may be helpful in assessing the environment. Lack of accessibility promotes the dependence of clients.

Accessible Supportive Examination Table

A table at wheelchair height facilitates transfer of women with motor disabilities. One such table adjusts to wheelchair height to facilitate transfer to the table; it provides armrests to support women with cerebral palsy and spasticity who may fear falling off the table when severe or unexpected spasms occur. The absence of leg support, however, may be a major drawback for women with leg weakness or paralysis. Examination tables that have leg support but are not at wheelchair height may be preferred in some settings. Each setting needs to assess its target population for services and provide the most accessible examination table.

Client's Equipment

The health care provider must realize that the wheelchair, crutches, and/or other equipment are part of the client's personal space. Ask permission from the client before sitting or leaning on the equipment or moving it, particularly when the client is in it or on the examination table, where she may want her equipment close by. The use of service animals needs the same sensitivity. Do not approach, speak to, or pet these animals without their owners' permission. Such activities only detract the animals from their jobs—caring for the person with a disability.

Special Considerations

Women with disabilities may need assistance in gaining accessibility to examination tables, scales, and other office equipment. They may need assistance with urine collection and other procedures. Equipment such as nonlatex gloves, plastic catheters, and nonlatex pads need to be available.

Considerations in Obtaining Health History

The practitioner should inquire about current functioning levels and if any intermittent decreases in functioning. How does function level impact her physically, socially, economically, and psychologically? What was her family life while in school? Does she understand what implications her disability has for sexuality, contraception, birth control, and routine health needs? Ask if sexual information given either in adolescence or during rehabilitation was sufficient. From discussions with the client, determine knowledge deficits. In addition, identify unmet sexual and health needs. Include review of condition-specific issues such as dysreflexia for women with spinal cord injury, latex allergy for women with spina bifida, or spasticity issues for women with cerebral palsy. Ask the client what problems the disability has presented and how she has overcome these barriers.

Altered Pelvic Examination/Mutual Problem Solving

A health care provider must be aware that a client with disabilities may need an altered pelvic examination (Cristian, 2009). Discussion with the client should attempt to solve problems she might have had during previous pelvic exams. Ask what positions caused problems and what worked best for her. Even though autonomic dysreflexia is more common in males than females, women with SCI are at risk for this to occur with pelvic examination, labor, or intercourse positions (Campagnolo, 2009). Additional personnel may be needed to assist in supporting the client (e.g., holding legs) during the exam. The client should collaborate in deciding the need. She may prefer to bring a family member or friend with her to the exam. All movements in the examination should be gradual to allow patient accommodation. Schedule appointments for times of the day when joint stiffness is at a minimum. Also, medications can be appropriately utilized to decrease pain during the examination process. Assistance with getting onto the examination table and extended time for the actual appointment should be prearranged by the medical office. The woman should be asked for direction in how staff can best support her while providing minimum discomfort with movements.

- *Altered Range of Motion.* A side-lying position or speculum exam with "handle up" may be necessary because of alterations in range of motion. This handle-up technique may also make viewing a midposition or anteverted cervix easier.
- *Spasticity.* Women with cerebral palsy report spasms, especially adductor spasms, which may be controlled if the woman takes the knee-chest position, with an assistant "hugging" her, or the side-lying position, with the bottom leg flexed and upper leg on the examiner's shoulder (similar to left lateral delivery position) (Cristian, 2009). Keeping the woman's extremities close to the body decreases movement that may stimulate additional spasms.
- *Amputation and Decreased Range of Motion.* The client may be examined in a semisitting position. She may choose to hold the stump herself and place the other leg on the examiner's shoulder or she may choose to have assistance with holding her stump so she can hold a mirror and participate in the examination.
- *Insertion of Speculum.* In patients who have a history of autonomic dysreflexia or spasticity, pain on insertion of the speculum may be decreased and the exam made more effective and comfortable, if xylocaine gel is applied generously to the perineal area, as long as the gel will not interfere with any specimens needed.
- *Specific Examination.* Examination of the genitalia must include inspection of the vaginal walls for atrophic changes, determination of intravaginal tone, and assessment of hair distribution in the genital region to help rule out possible endocrinopathies (Cristian, 2009).

Some authors suggest select use of the Q-Tip Pap smear for the rare woman with disabilities who is unable to tolerate a speculum examination. A Q-Tip Pap is collected by inserting a dacron swab into the vaginal vault and blindly sweeping the cervical region to obtain a sample of cervical cells. The sample is then either transferred on to a slide or into a liquid Pap collection container. This technique is much less accurate, however, and every effort should be made to assist the client and her family to understand the implications of its use (Cristian, 2009). During the pelvic examination, reaffirm the client's identified normalcy and healthy status. This makes a strong positive impact on her perception of self.

PREGNANCY

CONFRONTING NEGATIVE ATTITUDES AND BARRIERS

Disability is not a contraindication to responsible, effective parenting, yet judgmental attitudes continue. Moreover, few agencies exist to assist the increasing number of pregnant women and mothers with disabilities. The majority of registered nurses, nurse practitioners, and occupational and physical therapists indicate that their experience, education, and training have not prepared them adequately for this high-risk population. Many fail to correlate the interaction of specific health problems directly impacting pregnancy. Health care providers who are involved in coordinating care and have no disability-related experience must consult with others. For example, consideration should be given to speaking with a colleague in rehabilitation or an experienced, active consumer with disabilities. Resources for perinatal educators need to provide specific information on pregnancy for women and families affected by disability.

Education of Health Care Providers

Programs must be developed to address health care providers' lack of information about the needs of mothers with disabilities. Information that is modified to answer questions about the unique situation of women with disabilities is needed. What are the emotional and physical changes of pregnancy? What are the special demands of labor and delivery? What are the adaptive parenting skills and equipment necessary for responsible parenting?

Case Management

During pregnancy, case management may be indicated for a woman with disabilities. The case manager is responsible for assuring that the client's unique health care needs are being met, especially if numerous agencies are involved.

Partner Preparation

It is important for the health care provider to assess whether a woman's partner needs preparation. The partner may require information from the provider about the woman's special needs in order to give realistic support and avoid unnecessary restrictions. A typical concern of any couple experiencing pregnancy—hesitancy to have sexual relations for fear of hurting the baby—may be expanded for couples in which the woman has a disability; they may be afraid of hurting the woman.

Although it is especially important for health care providers to interact with partners, data indicates that women with disabilities feel their partners are unwanted by health care providers during labor and delivery. A prenatal care provider or case manager may need to initiate educational sessions to discuss attitudinal barriers. These activities should be organized well before delivery. If the partner also has a disability, special considerations may be needed to facilitate his involvement.

ACCESSIBILITY TO LABOR AND DELIVERY FACILITIES

Several questions should be asked about the structure of health care facilities and their accessibility to women with mobility and sensory impairment. Are labor and delivery rooms and bathrooms large enough to transfer women from a wheelchair? Are large showers available without a raised lip, which would prevent a woman from rolling her wheelchair into the shower? Are select rooms large enough to accommodate wheelchairs, consumer-owned specially padded commode chairs, leg braces, crutches, and other equipment? Can a woman in a wheelchair be weighed in labor and delivery settings? Are exam tables available that can be adjusted for a woman with mobility impairment?

Specific Adaptive Needs of Client

Determine what the client needs with respect to her condition. Is a pressure relief mattress or raised toilet seat needed? Does she want to bring equipment from home? Plan a tour of the hospital during the fifth or sixth month of pregnancy so that the need for special equipment can be identified and the equipment ordered.

Accessibility to Equipment

Having necessary equipment within reach is critical to the well-being and comfort of the client. Previous arrangements should be made prior to the onset of labor to ensure all needed equipment is accessible for both labor and birth and unexpected antenatal admissions.

Education for All Staff

Housekeeping personnel may need to know that a wheelchair positioned in a particular way next to a bed allows a woman to be independent. To move the chair makes the woman essentially a prisoner, as it removes her independence. Nursing staff may need to review prevention of skin shearing, management of dysreflexia, and implications of contraction monitoring.

PRENATAL AND PERINATAL PERIODS

Generally, in perinatal management, a health care provider needs to determine if a woman with a disability has access to a role model who has the same disability as she or if the client needs case management services. Specialized groups may offer support persons and role models from women with similar conditions.

Self-Assessment

The client should be able to identify the stressors and fears, both general and specific, that are related to her disability.

Staff Assessment

A woman's muscle strength, ADLs, and childcare skills must be assessed. Determinations may be made by direct observation, by reports of activities, and by a self-assessment from the woman and her family. A referral may be made to a physical or occupational therapist, depending on resources and the severity of the woman's limitations. Assessment needs to be made early in pregnancy in order to design adaptive equipment. For example, one woman with minimal distal muscle strength who wished to breast-feed was able to place the child at the breast and initiate nursing but did not have the strength to hold the child throughout nursing. Believing that she could not breast-feed, she switched to formula. If she had been assessed early in pregnancy, her strength deficiency might have been identified and referral made to a rehabilitation engineer to design or modify a fabric infant carrier that would support the child during nursing. Most women with a disability are able to nurse their newborns. Indeed, the convenience of breastfeeding can be an advantage for women with mobility limitations.

Dependency Increase

If a woman's dependency increases during pregnancy, there is a need to assess her specific level of function. Similarly, assess the body image issues generated by pregnancy.

Normal Emotional Changes

Reassure the client of the normalcy of emotional fluctuations during pregnancy.

Cesarean Birth

If cesarean birth is a possibility, discuss the options available, including father participation, positioning and precautions during the surgical procedure, and strategies to prevent complications in the postpartum period.

Breastfeeding

Breastfeeding is generally not contraindicated for women with spinal cord injury, MS, arthritis, or epilepsy but is contraindicated for women with SCD who are on certain medications. Women with lupus taking immunosuppressive medications should not breast-feed. Women with lupus not on these medications need to have close monitoring of their child's growth while breastfeeding as well as the fatigue level in the mother. Some women may need adaptive equipment or counseling about specific strategies to make breastfeeding successful. Consultation with a lactation consultant knowledgeable in caring for women with disabilities is warranted.

SELECTED DISABILITIES AND PREGNANCY

Impaired Vision and Hearing

The changing body of a woman with impaired vision may dramatically affect her ability to function as her center of gravity changes and alters her relation to objects. Use tactile models and assist to palpate abdomen. Lack of materials in Braille or on audiotape may necessitate increased need for individual teaching. A birth rehearsal in a labor room may be helpful to orient to the room, bed, and bathroom. For a woman with impaired hearing, it is important to talk to the woman even if an interpreter is used. Always get her attention before proceeding with any exam. Visual interaction is critical. For delivery, assess if she would prefer to be in a room where the nurses station can be seen and arrange for this as part of any birth plan (Sawin & Horton, 2004).

Cystic Fibrosis

Some women with cystic fibrosis may have impaired fertility. Although pregnancy can be tolerated in women with mild disease, those with poor lung function, severe disease, and diabetes had increased risk of prematurity and decline after delivery (March of Dimes, 2011). Pregnancy can be a significant risk for both mother and infant.

Rheumatoid Arthritis

Rheumatoid arthritis is known to improve during pregnancy. Recently, lactation and prolactin have been shown to reduce the onset of rheumatoid arthritis and decrease flare or relapse of arthritis (Ostensen, 2009). Among some women who may be genetically susceptible, breastfeeding is associated with an increased risk of rheumatoid arthritis, particularly after the first pregnancy and some of the medications used in treating rheumatoid arthritis are contraindicated in lactation (Temprano, Florea, & Scarbroough, 2009). Consultation with the rheumatologist is essential for women considering pregnancy and in the prenatal and postpartum period. The main concerns continue to be pharmacological management of symptoms.

Spinal Cord Injury

Fertility rates are unknown; however, when women with SCI do conceive, they should be managed by a perinatologist. They have increased risk for skin breakdown and urinary tract infections. Premature birth occurs in 33 percent. Autonomic dysreflexia commonly occurs during pregnancy and in second stage of labor and delivery (Ghidini & Simsonian, 2011). Women with spinal cord injury may be at risk for an unattended birth because they cannot sense uterine contractions.

Multiple Sclerosis

It is estimated that 20 percent of women with MS will bear children after being diagnosed with MS (Franklin & Tremlett, 2009). Pregnancies complicated with MS have a higher incidence of intrauterine growth restriction and antenatal hospitalizations (Kelly, Nelson, & Chakravarty, 2010). Many women with MS experience a reduction of flare-ups during the second and third trimesters of the prenatal period and an increase in the first 3 months of the postpartum period. Breastfeeding appears to reduce the number of flare-ups in the postpartum period and should be encouraged. There are no differences in long-term prognosis or maternal functioning in women with MS who have had a pregnancy and those who have not (Franklin & Tremlett, 2009).

Epilepsy

Women with epilepsy have normal fertility. Genetic counseling may be helpful to determine patterns of birth defects in the family. There are approximately 1 million women of childbearing age with epilepsy in the United States, and each year 20,000 of them give birth. Many of the AEDs taken to control seizures have teratogenic potential, especially if the young woman is on more than one medication. Infant malformations occur more in women using polytherapy rather than monotherapy. Safer sex becomes critical as the best outcomes of pregnancy are when the pregnancy is planned. The greatest risk for seizure recurrence when women attempt to withdraw from AEDs occurs in the first 6 months. Thus, if women have been seizure-free for 2 to 5 years and wish to consider withdrawal in collaboration with their neurologist, it is desirable that a slow taper be used and withdrawal be completed at least 6 months before any planned conception. After the pregnancy, it is too late to change medications or try to reduce the number as the risk of prolonged convulsions is also a risk for the fetus (Caughley, 2011).

PARENTING

Health care providers unfamiliar with the adaptive skills of women with disabilities may question the ability of these women to care for their babies. In fact, there are over 8 million families with children in which one or both parents have a disability (Parents with Disabilities Online, 2011). Many social institutions, however, such as family court, social services, and health care providers, continue to have discriminatory attitudes. Availability of a role model with a disability similar to a woman's can be very helpful to both the health care provider and the client. The roles of the parents and other caregivers must be assessed. Moreover, for the provider without expertise in infant care issues, consultation with a pediatric nurse practitioner, pediatrician, occupational therapist, rehabilitation consultant, or rehabilitation engineer may be helpful. In addition, an independent living center or a program that focuses on promoting positive parenting for women with disabilities is imperative. Frequently, support services in both the health and the social service arena are uninformed about resources that would make parenting and caretaking more effective for women with disabilities. Consultation with agencies that are knowledgeable in this area is critical to success. There are multiple online resources for both education and support for parents with disabilities.

ADAPTATION OF THE FAMILY

Equipment as Part of the Environment

It is common for children to consider a parent's equipment, such as wheelchairs and reachers, as ordinary parts of their environment without negative connotations. A toddler was overheard talking with her mom during a basketball tournament in which there was a wheelchair division. While observing a game played by nondisabled college students, she said, "Mom, what are they doing?" "Playing basketball, Honey." "But Mom, where are their wheelchairs?"

Service Animals

If a woman with a disability uses a guide dog or other animal to assist with impaired mobility, close assessment must be made of its impact on childcare. Planning to incorporate the child into the family with the service animal is similar to other families with pets.

Equipment Adaptation for Childcare

A woman with impaired mobility can alter equipment or procedures to assist with childcare.

- Women with mobility impairment may face special adaptation needs as parents. Women who previously used a manual wheelchair may choose to use an electric wheelchair to free hands for childcare. A specialized bracing system may be constructed to carry the baby while in the wheelchair.
- Furniture may need to be altered so that the woman can wheel up to the crib, changing table, or reclined stroller and be able to change the baby without moving him or her. Furniture may also be altered to create firm raised edges for infant safety and to assist the woman with decreased hand or arm strength.
- Velcro can be sewn on the clothes of both mother and baby for necessary alterations. For example, breastfeeding may be made easier if the mother's bra and blouse have Velcro fasteners. Also, Velcro fasteners on the infant's clothes assist the mother in dressing her baby. Women should practice prior to the birth to see what type of clothing works best for them.
- Bottle holders and bottle devices, such as a tactile calibrated bottle, may be helpful, as may adapting a breastfeeding position in the wheelchair.

Impaired Vision and Hearing

A woman with impaired vision or hearing can adapt procedures for childcare. The provider may need to facilitate the mother's interaction with her infant. The Brazelton (1973) tool is used to teach a mother about the states of the infant. For a woman with impaired vision, the focus is on her hearing and touching and how she increases interaction with the infant. On the other hand, for women with hearing impairment, a visual role model, tactile stimulation, and musical toys are used. If both parents have sensory impairment, referral to an infant stimulation program should be considered. Monitoring devices in a room or on a child can be helpful. Audiovisual resources may be useful.

Epilepsy

Infant care is often more of a concern of the family and friends than of the woman with epilepsy. The health professional needs to evaluate the real risks with the woman based on the type of seizure she experiences. Women with seizures at night may not need to adjust their daytime activities dramatically. Developing a reality-based concrete safety plan is recommended. Women can change the baby on a mat on the floor; use plastic bottles and containers; have two adults when giving an infant or child a bath; use sponge baths with tepid water in a separate bowl when alone; always feed the child in an infant seat, highchair, or appropriate chair; use a playpen for a safe play area; keep extra clothes on each level of the house to avoid stair climbing; move the child by stroller instead of being hand carried; and use microwave rather than conventional stove. Avoid holding the baby while cooking or performing other dangerous activities such as ironing (Epilepsy Foundation, 2011). Most women with active epilepsy cannot drive and should be counseled to always bring a car seat when traveling with other people.

FUTURE RESEARCH NEEDED

Several major official and voluntary organizations now have initiatives to explore the experiences of women with disabilities. This work, however, is early in its development. Many organizations now have policy statements on the need to accommodate women with disabilities in their health care choices. Research is needed that examines the use of contraception, preconception counseling, pregnancy, labor, birth, postpartum, and lactation issues for women with various disabilities. Women with disabilities are now effectively joining the workforce, engaging in social networks, marrying, having children, and engaging in parenting. Support services need to be in place to offer assistance for these needs and basic rights.

CONCLUSION

Women with disabilities are women first. Their similarities with other women are more common than their differences. One woman writes the following:

> We want to know that you value us as people and not just as examples of cultural diversity. We want you to know that life with a disability can be just fine. Sure, there are attitudinal and environmental barriers that make life difficult for us sometimes, but those obstacles are out there, not inside of us. Just imagine for a moment a woman in a wheelchair carrying a tiny baby. This woman is not being discharged from a maternity hospital where every woman must ride in a wheelchair. She is at the grocery store with her baby in an infant carrier and a cart full of groceries. Imagine her getting herself, her baby, her wheelchair,

and her groceries into the car alone and driving away. Imagine her independent, sexual, competent, mature, busy, happy, and, like all new parents, exhausted! To you she may be an amazement, but to me, I just feel like myself. (Craig, 1990)

If approached with

- a willingness to listen and hear the issues and concerns of these women,
- a willingness to see the woman as a true participant/partner in planning and one who may have more medical information about her disability than the provider does,
- an awareness of one's own comfort level with uncertainty and individuals with disability,
- a nonjudgmental approach,

the sensitive clinician can create a quality experience for the individual and build a new reality for women with disabilities.

RESOURCES FOR WOMEN, THEIR FAMILIES, AND PROFESSIONALS

INTERNET RESOURCES/ ORGANIZATIONS

Multiple Internet resources have been developed, and one study found that using websites aimed at women with disabilities was effective in increasing knowledge.

Antiepileptic Drug and Pregnancy Register
888-233-2334
http://www.epilepsyfoundation.org/livingwithepilepsy/gendertopics/womenshealthtopics/pregnancyandepilepsymedications/antiepileptic-drug-pregnancy-registry.cfm

Coalition on Sexuality and Disability
212-242-3900

CROWD, Center for Research on Women with Disabilities (Fact Sheet, Research Summary, and Bibliography)
http://www.bcm.edu/crowd/

Easter Seals
http://www.easter-seals.org

Epilepsy Foundation
http://www.epilepsyfoundation.org/

Multiple Sclerosis Foundation
http://www.msfacts.org

National Information Center for Children with Youth and Disabilities
800-999-5599
http://www.nichy.org

National Organization on Disability (NOD)
800-248-2253
http://www.nod.org

Parents With Disabilities Online
http://www.disabledparents.net

Spina Bifida Association of America
800-621-3141
http://www.spinabifidaassociation.org

UCP (United Cerebral Palsy)
http://www.ucpa.org

There are national groups for many disability conditions. Contact your local library for current addresses or toll-free numbers.

REFERENCES

Alifanz, M. (2011). *Service dogs limited to dogs and some miniature horses under new ADA laws.* Retrieved from http://www.stoelrivesworldofemployment.com/2011/03/articles/statutes/ada-1/service-animals-limited-to-dogs-and-some-miniature-horses-under-new-ada-rules/

Alonso, A., Jick, S.S., Olek, M.J., Ascherio, A., Jick, H., & Hernán, M.A. (2005). Recent use of oral contraceptives and the risk of multiple sclerosis. *Archives of Neurology, 62*(9), 1362–1365.

American Psychological Association. (2011). *Removing bias in language.* Retrieved from http://www.colby.edu/psychology/APA/Bias.pdf

Antonia, M.W., Coppus, H.M., Heleen, M.E., Evenhuis, G., Gert-Jan Verberne, F., Visser, E., et al. (2010). Early age at menopause is associated with increased risk of dementia and mortality in women with Down syndrome. *Journal of Alzheimer's Disease, 19*(2), 545–550. doi:10.3233/JAD-2010-1247

Balcazar, F.E., Suarez-Balcazar, Y., Taylor-Ritzler, T., & Keys, C.B. (2010). *Race, culture, and disability.* Sudbury, MA: Jones & Bartlett.

Banks, M.E. (2010). Feminist psychology and women with disabilities. *Psychology of Women Quarterly, 34*(4), 431–442. doi:10.1111/j.1471-6402.2010.01593.x

Bergoffen, D., Gilbert, P.R., Harvey, T., & McNeeley, C.L. (2011). *Confronting global gender justice.* Abingdon, Oxon: Routledge.

Blumchen, K., Bayer, P., Buck, D., Cremer, C.T., Fricke, H., Henne, H.P., et al. (2010). Effects of latex avoidance on latex sensitization, atopy and allergic diseases in patients with spina bifida. *Allergy, 65*(12), 1585–1583. doi:10.1111/j.1398-9995.2010.02447.x

Bonnema, R.A., McNamara, M.C., & Spencer, A.L. (2010). Contraception choices in women with underlying medical conditions. *American Family Physician, 82*(6), 621–628.

Brazelton, T.B. (1973). *Neonatal behavioral assessment scale.* Philadelphia: J. B. Lippincott.

Campagnolo, D.I. (2009). *Autonomic dysreflexia in spinal cord injury.* Retrieved from http://emedicine.medscape.com/article/322809-overview

Canonico, M., Plu-Bureau, G., Lowe, G.D., & Scarabin, P.Y. (2008). Hormone replacement therapy and risk of venous thromboembolism in postmenopausal women: Systematic review and meta-analysis. *British Medical Journal, 336*, 1227–1231. doi:10.1136/bmj.39555.441944.BE

Caughley, A.B. (2011). *Seizure disorders in pregnancy.* Retrieved from http://emedicine.medscape.com/article/272050-overview

Craig, D.I. (1990). The adaptation to pregnancy of spinal cord injured women. *Rehabilitation Nursing, 15*(1), 6–9.

Cristian, A. (2009). *Medical management of adults with neurological disabilities.* New York: Demos Medical Publishing.

Davidson, M.R., Ladewig, P.A.W., & London, M.L. (2012). *Olds' maternal-newborn nursing across the lifespan* (9th ed.). Upper Saddle River, NJ: Pearson Education.

Di Pauli, F., Reindl, M., Ehling, R., Schautzer, F., Gneiss, C., Lutterotti, A., et al. (2008). Smoking is a risk factor for early conversion to clinically definite multiple sclerosis. *Multiple Sclerosis, 14*(8), 1026–1030. doi:10.1177/1352458508093679

Emory University Health Sciences Center. (2004, May 3). *Monthly hormonal changes can exacerbate seizures in women with epilepsy.* Retrieved February 23, 2012, from http://www.sciencedaily.com/releases/2004/05/040503055734.htm

Epilepsy Foundation. (2011). *Pregnancy and parenting.* Retrieved from http://www.epilepsyfoundation.org/living/women/pregnancy/weiparenting.cfm

Farr, S.L., Folger, S.G., Paulen, M.E., & Curtis, K.M. (2010). Safety of contraceptive methods for women with rheumatoid arthritis: A systematic review. *Contraception, 82*(1), 64–71. (Epub March 29, 2010)

Federal Register (2010) ADA Standards for Accessible Design, Retrieved from: http://www.ada.gov/2010ADAstandards_index.htm

Fletcher, S.G., Castro-Borrero, W., Remington, G., Treadaway, K., Lemack, G.E., & Frohman, E.M. (2009). Sexual dysfunction in patients with multiple sclerosis: A multidisciplinary approach to evaluation and management. *Nature Reviews Urology, 6*, 96–107. doi:10.1038/ncpuro1298

Flynn-Evans, E.A., Stevens, R.G., Tabandeh, H., Schernhammer, E.S., & Lockley, S.W. (2009). Effect of light perception on menarche in blind women. *Ophthalmic Epidemiology, 16*(4), 243–248.

Franklin, G.M., & Tremlett, H. (2009). Multiple sclerosis and pregnancy: What should we be telling our patients? *Neurology, 73*(22), 1820–1822.

Gaffield, M.E., Culwell, K.R., & Lee, C.R. (2011). The use of hormonal contraception among women taking anticonvulsant therapy. *Contraception, 83*(1), 16–29. (Epub September 15, 2010)

Ghidini, A., & Simsonian, M.R. (2011). Pregnancy after spinal cord injury: A review of the literature. *Topics in Spinal Cord Injury Rehabilitation, 16*(3), 93–103. doi:10.1310/sci1603-93

Groce, N.E. (1999). Disability in cross-cultural perspective: Rethinking disability. *Lancet, 354*(9180), 756–757.

Healthy People 2020. (2011). *Disability and health.* Retrieved from http://www.healthypeople.gov/2020/topicsobjectives2020/overview.aspx?topicid=9

Hicks, C.W., & Rome, E.S. (2010, July). Menstrual manipulation: Options for suppressing the menstrual cycle. *Cleveland Clinic Journal of Medicine, 77*(7), 445–453. doi:10.3949/ccjm.77a.09128

Higgins, D. (2010). Sexuality, human rights and safety for people with disabilities: The challenge of intersecting identities. *Sexual and Relationship Therapy, 25*(3), 245–257. doi:10.1080/14681994.2010.489545

Hope, L.N. (2011). *Women against violence and exploitation.* Retrieved from http://www.nasuad.org/documentation/hcbs2010/PowerPoints/Monday/Women%20Against%20Violence%20and%20Exploitation.pdf

Howland, C., & Rintala, D.H. (2001). Dating behaviors of women with physical disabilities. *Sexuality and Disability, 19*(1), 41–70.

Hutzler, Y., & Levi, I. (2008). Including children with disability into physical education: General and specific attitudes of high school children. *European Journal of Adapted Physical Activity, 1*(2), 21–30.

Kelly, V.M., Nelson, L.M., & Chakravarty, E.F. (2010). Obstetric outcomes in women with multiple sclerosis and epilepsy. *Obstetrical and Gynecological Survey, 65*(3), 156–158. doi:10.1097/01.ogx.0000369670.88660.4c

Kernan, N.G., Cullinan, P., Alton, E.W., Bilton, D., & Griesenbach, U. (2010). Oral contraceptive use does not affect CF disease severity. *Thorax, 65*, A121. doi:10.1136/thx.2010.150987.4

Kim, M. (2009). Disability issues are women's issues. *Development, 52*(2), 230–232. doi:10.1057/dev.2009.10

Kreuter, M., Siösteen, A., & Biering-Sørensen, F. (2008). Sexuality and sexual life in women with spinal cord injury: A controlled study. *Journal of Rehabilitation Medicine, 40*(1), 61–69. doi:10.2340/16501977-0128

Kruse, D., Schur, L., & Ali, M. (2010). Disability and occupational projections. *Monthly Labor Review Online, 133*(10). Retrieved from http://www.bls.gov/opub/mlr/2010/10/art3exc.htm

Maart, S., & Jelsma, J. (2010). The sexual behaviour of physically disabled adolescents. *Disability Rehabilitation, 32*(6), 438–443.

March of Dimes. (2011). *Cystic fibrosis*. Retrieved from http://www.marchofdimes.com/birthdefects_cysticfibrosis.html

Motl, R.W., & Gosney, J.L. (2008). Effect of exercise training on quality of life in multiple sclerosis: A meta-analysis. *Multiple Sclerosis, 14*(1), 129–135.

Multiple Sclerosis International Foundation. (2011). *Sexual changes in MS*. Retrieved from http://www.msif.org/en/about_ms/ms_by_topic/relationships_intimacy_sexuality/sexual_changes/index.html

Neal, L.J., & Guillet, S.E. (2004). *Care of the adult with a chronic illness or disability: A team approach*. St. Louis, MO: Elsevier Mosby.

Nelson, M.R. (1995). Sexuality in childhood disability. *Physical Medicine and Rehabilitation: State of the Art Reviews, 9*(2), 451–462.

Nosek, M.A., Howland, C.A., Young, M.E., Georgiou, D., Rintala, D.H., Foley, C.C., et al. (1994). Wellness models and sexuality among women with physical disabilities. *Journal of Applied Rehabilitation Counseling, 25*(1), 50–58.

Ostensen, M. (2009). Management of early aggressive rheumatoid arthritis during pregnancy and lactation. *Expert Opinions in Pharmacotherapy, 10*(9), 1469–1479.

Ostrander, N. (2009). Sexual pursuits of pleasure among men and women with spinal cord injuries. *Sexuality and Disability, 27*(1), 11–19. doi:10.1007/s11195-008-9103-y

Parent, W., Foley, S., Balcazar, F., Ely, C., Bremer, C., & Gaylord, V. (Eds.). (2008, Summer/Fall). *Impact: Feature Issue on Employment and Women with Disabilities, 21*(1). Retrieved from http://ici.umn.edu/products/impact/211/

Parents with Disabilities Online. (2011). *Parents with disabilities: Did you know?* Retrieved from http://www.disabledparents.net/

Pascall, S., & Kaunitz, A.M. (2008). Depo-Provera and skeletal health: A survey of Florida obstetrics and gynecologist physicians. *Contraception, 76*(8), 370–376. doi:10.1016/j.contraception.2008.07.022

Plant, B.J., Goss, C.H., Tonelli, G., McDonald, G., Black, R.A., & Aitken, M.L. (2008). Contraceptive practices in women with cystic fibrosis. *Journal of Cystic Fibrosis, 7*(5), 412–414. doi:10.1016/j.jcf.2008.03.001

Reddy, D.S. (2010). Clinical pharmacokinetic interactions between antiepileptic drugs and hormonal contraceptives. *Expert Reviews in Clinical Pharmacology, 13*(2), 183–192.

Rosso, A.L., Wisdom, J.P., Horner-Johnson, W., McGee, M.G., & Yvonne, M.L. (2011). Aging with a disability: A systematic review of cardiovascular disease and osteoporosis among women aging with a physical disability. *Maturitas, 68*(1), 65–72.

Rowe, A. (2009). *Divorce rate among the chronically ill is over 75%*. Retrieved from http://www.associatedcontent.com/article/2333450/divorce_rate_among_the_chronically.html

Saulino, M.F., & Vaccaro, A.R. (2009). *Rehabilitation of persons with spinal cord injuries*. Retrieved from http://emedicine.medscape.com/article/1265209-overview

Sawin, K.J., & Horton, J.C. (2004). Health care concerns for women with physical disability and chronic illness. In E.Q. Youngkin & M.S. Davis (Eds.), *Women's health: A primary care clinical guide* (3rd ed., pp. 861–898). Upper Saddle River, NJ: Pearson.

Stevenson, V.L. (2010). Rehabilitation in practice: Spasticity management. *Clinical Rehabilitation, 24*(4), 293–304. doi:10.1177/0269215509353254

Temprano, K., Florea, S.C., & Scarbroough, E. (2009). *Rheumatoid arthritis and pregnancy*. Retrieved from http://emedicine.medscape.com/article/335186-overview

Tice, C.J., & Hall, D.M.K. (2008). Sexuality education and adolescents with developmental disabilities: Assessment, policy, and advocacy. *Journal of Social Work in Disability and Rehabilitation, 7*(1), 47–62. doi:10.1080/15367100802009749

Umławska, W., Sands, D., & Zielińska, A. (2010). Age of menarche in girls with cystic fibrosis. *Folia Histochemistry Cytobiology, 48*(2), 185–190.

U.S. Equal Employment Commission. (2008). *Section 902 definition of the term disability: Notice concerning the Americans with disabilities act amendments act of 2008*. Retrieved from http://www.eeoc.gov/policy/docs/902cm.html#902.2b

Zacharin, M., Savasi, I., & Grover, S. (2010). The impact of menstruation in adolescents with disabilities related to cerebral palsy. *Archives of Disease in Children, 95*, 526–530. doi:10.1136/adc.2009.174680

CHAPTER ❖ 10

INTEGRATING WELLNESS: COMPLEMENTARY THERAPIES AND WOMEN'S HEALTH

Jo Lynne W. Robins

Highlights

- Background
- Whole Medical Systems
- Natural Products
- Mind-Body Medicine
- Manipulative and Body-Based Practices
- Energy Therapies

❖ INTRODUCTION

This chapter presents an overview of complementary and alternative medicine (CAM) for women's health, including therapies during pregnancy and menopause. Although a comprehensive review of all CAM therapies with known or potential benefits in women's health is beyond the scope of this chapter, an organized, detailed overview is provided based on the categories of CAM set forth by the National Center for Complementary and Alternative Medicine (NCCAM). This, combined with the resources provided at the end of this chapter, will guide the exploration and integration of CAM into the practice of women's health. Particular therapies were chosen for inclusion based on one or a combination of the following criteria: safety, a substantial evidence base, and ease of incorporation into practice.

BACKGROUND

CAM is defined as a group of therapies that are not considered part of Western allopathic medicine. Experts in the field have stated that providers need to be informed and feel comfortable discussing CAM with patients and colleagues in order to improve safety and efficacy, quality of life, management of chronic conditions, and ultimately health outcomes (Adams et al., 2011; Hall, Griffiths, & McKenna, 2011; Peck, 2008).

According to the 2007 National Health Interview Survey, 38 percent of Americans use some form of CAM, an increase of 14.2 percent since 2002 (Su & Li, 2011), particularly in provider-based CAM such as massage and acupuncture. The highest use was in non-Hispanic whites. Having unmet medical needs or a cost-related delay in care also increased CAM use.

Research indicates that CAM is cost-effective compared to traditional therapies in the following areas: (1) acupuncture for migraine, (2) manual therapy for neck pain, (3) self-administered stress management in cancer patients undergoing chemotherapy, (4) biofeedback for "functional disorders" such as irritable bowel syndrome, and (5) guided imagery (GI) and relaxation therapy for cardiac patients (Herman, Craig, & Caspi, 2005). Another study found that individuals who self-administered two or more CAM therapies were significantly less likely to be hospitalized for any cause when compared to those who did not self-administer (Smith, Smith, & Ryan, 2008).

The National Institutes of Health's NCCAM is an evidence-based resource for information about CAM therapies. The center's mission is to rigorously explore CAM therapies in order to establish an evidence base of the safe and effective use of these therapies, including funding clinical trials and training CAM researchers. It also provides reliable information to practitioners and the public including descriptions, resources, and research on an extensive list of CAM therapies. Another valuable resource is "Time to Talk," a new initiative to facilitate open discussion of CAM between providers and patients (Koithan, 2009). For organizational clarity, it has grouped CAM therapies into the following categories:

- *Whole Medical Systems:* examples include traditional Chinese medicine (TCM), Ayurvedic medicine, and homeopathy
- *Natural Products:* examples include dietary supplements, herbal or botanical medicine, and probiotics
- *Mind-Body Medicine:* examples include deep breathing, meditation, GI, aromatherapy, yoga, tai chi (TC), and hypnotherapy
- *Manipulative and Body-Based Practices:* examples include chiropractic and osteopathic manipulation and massage
- *Other CAM Practices:* examples include movement therapies such as Rolfing, Trager, the Alexander Technique, and Feldenkrais; energy therapies such as Healing Touch, Therapeutic Touch, Reiki; magnet therapy; as well as traditional healers such as Shaman or Curanderas

The examples in these categories are not exhaustive. Additionally, some therapies fit into more than one category. For example, acupuncture is an integral component of TCM and is also an energy-based therapy. Because these categories provide a legitimate way of organizing, understanding, and applying CAM, they will be used to present a variety of ideas and therapies that may be useful in women's health.

WHOLE MEDICAL SYSTEMS

TRADITIONAL CHINESE MEDICINE

TCM comprises acupuncture, Chinese herbal medicine, and qigong and is based on the idea that disease results from disruption in the flow of energy ("chi," "qi") in the body. TCM has shown to be a promising treatment and possibly more effective than nonsteroidal anti-inflammatory drugs, oral contraceptive pills, acupuncture, and heat therapy for dysmenorrhea (Manheimer, Wieland, Kimbrough, Cheng, & Berman, 2009). The most commonly used and investigated TCM component is acupuncture. It is an effective therapy for the treatment of migraines, neck disorders, tension-type headaches, and osteoarthritis (Lee & Ernst, 2011). Also, it has been shown to be an effective treatment for polycystic ovary syndrome–related infertility and male idiopathic infertility, and to have beneficial effects on live birth rates when used on the day of embryo transfer (Franconi et al., 2011; Stone, Yoder, & Case, 2009). Additionally, a substantial amount of evidence is mounting to support the use of TCM in treating other common women's health disorders including dysmenorrhea, endometriosis, and vaginal discharge (Zhou & Qu, 2009). Darby (2009) has provided a comprehensive overview of integrating TCM into practice.

AYURVEDIC MEDICINE (AYURVEDA)

Ayurveda, often called the mother of TCM, is the oldest formal system of medicine. It is, in part, based on treating individuals according to their "dosha" or mind-body constitution. There are three dosha types: kapha (water), vata (air), and pitta (fire). Awareness of one's dosha helps to improve health even in the absence of disease by providing guidance for optimal diet and mind-body and physical exercise that is tailored for the individual. For example, those with a predominantly kapha dosha tend to be overweight and do not like to move fast so even fast walking may not be an ideal exercise to maintain. Those who are vata tend to have constipation and dry skin and like to be busy and moving quickly so maintaining hydration and helping them to sit still and train the mind with approaches like GI can help them maintain balanced health. Women with pitta dosha may be more troubled with hot flashes. Two books on applying Ayurveda by David Simon, a board certified neurologist and Ayurvedic practitioner, are provided in the Resources list at the end of this chapter. Although research on Ayurveda is limited, with most of it focusing on particular Ayurvedic herbs, a general understanding and application of the principles of this ancient healing system may be helpful in achieving optimal health.

HOMEOPATHY

Homeopathy is based on the theory of "like treats like." Homeopathy helps to restore the body's natural state of balance. Homeopathic preparations are created through a process of repeated dilutions and succussions (shaking the remedy). When completed, there is often no measurable trace of the active ingredient in the remedy. It is believed that through the series of dilutions and succussions, the active ingredient imprints itself on the water molecules and the effect of the remedy is energetic, not pharmacological. Generally, this makes homeopathic remedies safer than herbs. The advantage of homeopathy over herbs is the wrong remedy will cause no harm, whereas the right remedy will assist the body in healing. Therefore, it is the much-preferred treatment during pregnancy and breastfeeding. There have been many European studies documenting the effectiveness of homeopathy (Fontaine, 2005). Homeopathic prescribing is often complex, focusing on individual characteristics and symptomatology in choosing a remedy. However, some remedies are symptom focused such as arnica for muscle trauma and bruising, apis for bee stings, and calc phos for bone healing. Additionally, remedies are often marketed with their indication on the label making it easier to choose a remedy for a particular condition. Gregg (2010) has written multiple articles on the use of particular homeopathic remedies in pregnancy, labor, and birth.

NATURAL PRODUCTS

Almost 20 percent of individuals in the United States use herbal medicine for a condition or prevention, with a higher prevalence of use in individuals with cancer or chronic illness (Miller et al., 2008). Factors associated with use of herbal medicine include individuals who are female, non-Hispanic, ages 45 to 64, uninsured, more highly educated, living in the western United States, and using prescription or over-the-counter medications. The most commonly used herbs are echinacea, ginseng, gingko, and garlic for treating colds, musculoskeletal, and gastrointestinal conditions (Gardiner et al., 2007).

Herbal medicine is likely the most widespread complementary therapy with at least two types: traditional and pharmaceutical. Traditional herbalism has been practiced for thousands of years using single herbs in whole form such as the whole flower or leaf or formulas containing several herbs. Because these formulas do not extract and concentrate a particular active ingredient, they are pharmacologically weaker, work more gradually, and generally cause fewer adverse reactions than pharmacological preparations. Pharmacological herbalism is the more modern, Western approach. Extracts of the active constituent(s) in a plant are concentrated for maximal effect. These preparations tend to work faster, but potentially elicit more adverse reactions, including interactions with other pharmaceutical preparations. No legally imposed standards exist for manufacturing herbal products, and many reactions occur not because of the herb, but because of contaminants in the manufacturing process. Many herbal manufacturers have voluntarily adopted quality-control standards such as those imposed in European countries. To maintain safety, it is important to research manufacturers before recommending products. Additionally, looking for GMP (good manufacturing processes) on the label ensures safer products. Starting with herbal teas is generally safe because they are less potent and unlikely to cause serious adverse reactions. Teas can be taken internally or used topically in baths or poultices.

Lloyd and Hornsby (2009) reviewed the use of natural products for the treatment of common disorders in women's health. There was insufficient data to recommend thiamine, magnesium, vitamin E, or essential fatty acids for dysmenorrhea. Calcium (1,000–1,200 mg) and vitamin B_6 (50–100 mg) are beneficial for premenstrual syndrome ($\geq$100 IU dietary vitamin D may decrease symptom severity as well per Bertone-Johnson, Chocano-Bedoya, Zagarins, Micka, & Ronnenberg, 2010). Vitamin C (500–750 mg daily) and vitex agnus-castus or chasteberry may be useful in infertility. Vitamin B_6 as well as ginger is effective in treating nausea and vomiting in pregnancy. Dietary soy and black cohosh can be helpful in menopause but should be used with caution in women with a history of breast cancer. Dosing ranges were variable in this review for some natural products. The dosing range for black cohosh is 40 to 200 mg daily, with the typical dose being 40 to 80 mg (Ulbricht, 2011) (www.umm.edu). The typical therapeutic dose of vitex fruit extract is 420 mg daily, in divided doses (Ulbricht, 2011).

SOY

Soy has been the subject of great controversy for several years. It has been characterized both as a phytoestrogen and as a selective estrogen receptor modulator. It binds weakly to estrogen receptor sites, blocking the effects of excessive endogenous estrogens as well as augmenting insufficient endogenous estrogens. Research indicates soy may help reduce hot flashes, attenuate bone loss, and improve lipid profiles by lowering total and low-density lipoprotein (Borrelli & Ernst, 2010).

Soy is considered safe for most people when used as a food or when taken for short periods as a dietary supplement. Whole food sources of soy include soy beans and nuts, tofu, and tempeh. The safety of long-term use of soy isoflavone supplements has not been established and may increase the risk of endometrial hyperplasia. On the other hand, studies have not demonstrated an effect of dietary soy on risk for endometrial hyperplasia. It remains unclear if soy isoflavone supplement increases breast cancer risk, but in a recent study of 3,088 breast cancer survivors, soy food consumption was determined to cause no adverse effects (Caan et al., 2011). For now, women who are at increased risk should be cautioned about the use of soy, particularly in supplement form. The website of Soy Nutrition (www.soynutrition.com), sponsored by Silk, a major producer of soy products, contains factual, up-to-date information on soy for health care practitioners and consumers.

A soy isoflavone metabolite, S-equol has been discovered and heavily researched in Japan. It is now being introduced to clinicians and will likely soon be marketed in the United States. It has demonstrated significant improvement in menopausal symptoms as well as bone health without any stimulation of breast or uterine tissues (Aso, 2010; Jackson, Greiwe, Desai, & Schwen, 2011; Setchell & Clerici, 2010; Tousen et al., 2011).

HERBS IN PREGNANCY

In an extensive search of the literature, no studies were found on the prevalence of herbal use in pregnancy in the United States. Studies have been done in Germany. The most recent study indicated that half of the patients surveyed used CAM during pregnancy or delivery, with herbal use being one of the most popular (Kalder, Knoblauch, Hrgovic, & Münstedt, 2011). Historically, reviews have shown many herbs to be safe but studies are limited. Herbs that are unsafe in pregnancy are listed in Table 10–1. There are many herbs that can be incorporated into the diet or as supplements that are supportive and therapeutic during pregnancy. Most culinary herbs are safe; herbs that we eat

TABLE 10–1. Common Herbs to Avoid During Pregnancy

Aloe vera (oral)—cathartic	Goldenseal—uterine stimulant
Angelica—emmenagogue[a]	Gotu kola—CNS stimulant
Birthroot—uterine astringent	Juniper berries—possibly teratogenic
Black and blue cohosh—emmenagogue	Mugwort—emmenagogue
Cascara sagrada—laxative	Pennyroyal—emmenagogue
Coltsfoot—possibly teratogenic	Sage—emmenagogue (safe in cooking)
Damiana—CNS/hormonal activity	Sarsaparilla—hormonal activity
Dong quai—hormonal, carcinogenic properties	Senna—laxative
Ephedra (ma huang)—cardiac stimulant	Shepherd's purse—hemostatic
False unicorn root—uterine/hormonal effect	Tansy—emmenagogue
Feverfew—emmenagogue	Wormwood—emmenagogue

[a]Induces menstrual bleeding.

in food are more like soup than medicine. Herbal supplements should be used cautiously in the first trimester. For example, red raspberry, which provides calcium, magnesium, iron, and potassium as well as vitamins A, C, and E, is safe during pregnancy but should not be used in the first trimester in women with a history of early miscarriage. It is often recommended to take herbs individually rather than in combination to better assess their effects on the body. However, pregnancy tea is a common tonic that can gently support the body's adaptation to pregnancy. The benefits of teas may come from their high nutrient content. Pregnancy tea traditionally contains red raspberry leaf, oat straw, alfalfa, and stinging nettle. Red raspberry leaf is nourishing to the uterus. It is the safest, most widely used uterine/pregnancy tonic herb (American Pregnancy Association, 2011; Braun & Cohen, 2010; Weed, 2002). It is believed to have a normalizing effect on the uterus, increasing tone in lax muscle or relaxing a taut or irritable uterus, but studies of the exact mechanism are lacking (American Pregnancy Association, 2011; Weed, 2002). Nettle leaves contain chlorophyll as well as many vitamins and minerals (American Pregnancy Association, 2011; Weed, 2002). Nettles are a kidney tonic, enhancing the elimination of waste products (Belew, 1999). Oat straw is nourishing and strengthens capillaries. Alfalfa contains proteins, vitamins C and K, calcium, iron, phosphorus, and chlorophyll to help prevent anemia as well as hemorrhage during delivery (www.vitamins-supplements.org). Though there is no definitive agreement on dosing, it is usually recommended to mix 1 tablespoon of loose tea per cup, steep at least 10 minutes, covered to keep the nutrients in, and drink at least four cups per day. If women choose to solely take red raspberry leaf tea, the recommendations are the same. Or, she can take 4 to 8 g per day in tablet form.

Ginger (*Zingiber officinale*) has anti-emetic and anti-inflammatory properties. It is effective in the treatment of pregnancy-related nausea and vomiting (Braun & Cohen, 2010; www.nccam.nih.gov). It is available in a variety of forms such as tea, capsules, ginger chews, candied ginger root, and some types of ginger ale.

General guidelines for safe and effective integration of natural products include the following: identify reputable, updated resources such as NCCAM's "Herbs at a Glance"; locate experts in your community with expertise; and document use. Also, remember that growing and cooking with culinary herbs is a healthy and rewarding experience in self-care.

BIOIDENTICAL HORMONES

Bioidentical hormones (BH) are "hormone preparations that have a chemical structure identical to endogenous hormones" (Weil, 2009, p. 37). Weil and others have provided eloquent reviews of the literature on BH. This information is summarized here. Although BH are natural, they are synthesized in a laboratory from soy and wild yam. Other hormones such as conjugated equine estrogens (CEE) and esterified estrogens, while made from natural products, are not considered bioidentical. BH and synthetic hormones elicit very different physiological effects.

BH are manufactured by pharmaceutical companies (estradiol and progesterone) as well as licensed and regulated compounding pharmacists (estradiol, estriol, estrone, and progesterone). Extensive animal studies have been done as well as many small studies in humans. Holtorf (2009) completed a meta-analysis of 200 studies revealing a better safety profile for BH compared to synthetic hormones in healthy individuals as well as those at risk for breast cancer and cardiovascular disease. Progesterone, as well as certain synthetic progestins, may have anticarcinogenic effects on breast cancer cells and counters the proliferative effects of estradiol in health breast cells (Chen, Chien, Chen, & Ng, 2011; Foidart et al., 1998; Formby & Wiley, 1999). Although more well-designed research is needed, a significant amount of research exists on the physiological and clinical effects of BH, making them a viable option for women with menopausal symptoms.

MIND-BODY MEDICINE

Mind-body medicine therapies are among the safest, most valuable, and easy to incorporate. These therapies share the use of breathing to elicit the relaxation response, a state characterized by decreases in blood pressure and heart and respiratory rates and an increase in alpha wave activity in the brain (Benson, 1975). A conscious focus on breathing underlies many of these therapies. Learning breathing techniques and teaching them to clients or simply taking a few deep breaths is an inexpensive, efficient way to enhance well-being.

A systematic review of mind-body therapies for menopause found that while many studies were methodologically flawed and more well-designed research is needed, yoga and other mind-body therapies such as TC have been shown to significantly decrease vasomotor and musculoskeletal symptoms as well as improve sleep quality and enhance concentration and memory (Innes, Selfe, & Vishnu, 2010). Another systematic review of CAM and insomnia found yoga and TC (as well as acupressure) to be effective in the treatment of chronic insomnia (Sarris & Byrne, 2011).

GUIDED IMAGERY

GI is an accessible mind-body relaxation therapy that can reduce distress and improve immune function. It stimulates certain thoughts, which in turn produce physiological outcomes that have an effect on the immune system. GI has been shown to decrease anxiety and stress in pregnant women as well as enhance immunity, mood, and well-being (Gruzelier, 2002; Jallo, Bourguignon, Taylor, Ruiz, & Goehler, 2009–2010). There are many resources for GI. Belleruth Naparstek has developed a series of GI recordings for general health and wellness as well as a variety of health issues. These and others can be found at www.healthjourneys.com.

TAI CHI

In the west, TC is thought of as a moving meditation, a technique to promote relaxation and increase awareness of the mind-body connection by enhancing awareness of one's body as a means for expression of inner feelings and ideas (Chen & Snyder, 1999) and as a moderate intensity exercise (Lan, Chen, & Lai, 2008). The body of research on TC is extensive, consisting of hundreds of published studies and reviews. It has been shown to improve (1) blood pressure and glycemic control, (2) quality of life, (3) psychological well-being, (4) pain management, (5) sleep, (6) kinesthetic sense, (7) balance, (8) flexibility, (9) strength, (10) activity tolerance, (11) immune function, (12) cardiovascular and pulmonary function, (13) fall and fracture risk, (14) cardiorespiratory and musculoskeletal function, (15) state and trait anxiety, and (16) lipids (Klein & Adams, 2004; Kuramoto, 2006; Li and Chan 2001; Mansky et al., 2006; Yeh, Wang, Wayne, & Phillips, 2008). Many communities now have teachers of TC and related therapies such as qigong. Beginning level TC and qigong can be learned by DVD. Resources can be found at the end of this chapter.

AROMATHERAPY

Aromatherapy is the use of essential oils to stimulate the sense of smell for balancing mind, body, and spirit. Essential oils are derived from plants, flowers, trees, herbs, and shrubs. Essential oils are highly concentrated and are usually diluted before use. They can improve many discomforts of pregnancy including emotional changes (bergamot, ylang ylang), morning sickness (peppermint), constipation (rose), and backaches (lavender, clary sage) (Tillett & Ames 2010; Tisserand, 1988). Tillett and Ames provide a thorough overview of research and use of aromatherapy in women's health.

In 2002, Hawkins, Chestnut, and Gibbs reported that excessive stress-related catecholamines can adversely affect the developing fetus. Currently, the field of epigenetics is beginning to shed light on the effects of various stressors on fetal development and long-term health outcomes (Nelissen, van Montfoort, Dumoulin, & Evers, 2010; Paul, 2010). Enhancing maternal-infant well-being seems a wise approach. Using bergamot and lavender oils prenatally can decrease stress and aid in relaxation. Bringing these oils into the birthing room can help create a sense of safety and security, which is essential to birthing well. There are particular oils that should be avoided during pregnancy. Even during postpartum, oils can help with emotional well-being and healing (Table 10–2 and Table 10–3). Oils can be used singularly or blended. One useful blend for stretch marks combines 15 gtt lavender, 5 gtt neroli, 2 gtt rose, and 800 IU vitamin E in 4 oz carrier oil.

TABLE 10–2. Therapeutic Essential Oils to Use in Pregnancy

Chamomile (Roman)—calming	Mandarin—rejuvenating
Clary sage—morale booster, balancing	Peppermint—morning sickness
Geranium—uplifting, calming	Rosemary—energizing
Grapefruit—astringent, energizing	Rose bulgar—relaxing
Jasmine—emotional balance	Sandalwood—decreases heartburn
Lavender—calming, healing	Ylang ylang—uplifting, balancing

TABLE 10–3. Essential Oils to Avoid During Pregnancy

Aniseed	Clove[a]	Myrrh	Savoury[a]
Basil[a]	Fennel[a]	Nutmeg[a]	Spikenard
Bay[a]	Hops	Oregano[a]	Tarragon[a]
Black pepper[a]	Hyssop	Pennyroyal	Thyme[a]
Cedarwood	Juniper	Rosemary[a]	Valerian
Cinnamonbark	Marjoram[a]	Sage[a]	

[a]Safe for culinary use.

MANIPULATIVE AND BODY-BASED PRACTICES

In addition to chiropractic therapy, which is largely considered mainstream, massage therapy is likely the most popular and available body-based practice. It has been shown to modestly improve symptoms associated with fibromyalgia including anxiety, sleep quality, pain, and quality of life in women with fibromyalgia; decrease anxiety and blood pressure in African American women; and be a useful adjunct in women with chronic pelvic pain and female veterans with post-traumatic stress disorder (Castro-Sánchez, Matarán-Peñarrocha, Aguilera-Manrique, Quesada-Rubio, & Moreno-Lorenzo, 2011; Herbert, 2010; Jefferson, 2010; Kalichman, 2010; Price, McBride, Hyerle, & Kivlahan, 2007).

INTEGRATING WELLNESS WITH DIET AND EXERCISE

Diet and exercise are the cornerstones of achieving and maintaining health and wellness. Hippocrates stated "let thy food be thy medicine." A healthy diet improves overall health regardless of the health issue. Focusing on including whole foods in dietary intake such as grains and fresh vegetables and fruits has been shown to decrease risk of heart disease and cancer (Eilat-Adar & Goldbourt, 2010; Higdon, Delage, Williams, & Dashwood, 2007). Additionally, maintaining a healthy body weight, maintaining daily physical activity, eating a low saturated fat diet, limiting energy-dense foods and sugary drinks, limiting red meat and avoiding processed meats, and limiting consumption of alcohol and salt were all shown to decrease cancer risk (Bós et al., 2011; World Cancer Research Fund International/American Institute for Cancer Research, 2007; Yard, 2008). Also, be aware of potential adverse or allergic reactions to food and food additives, particularly in women with migraines (Alpay et al., 2010).

The human body is designed for motion. Exercise is good for prevention as well as treatment across the lifespan and it benefits physical and mental health. It improves antenatal depression as well as maternal perception of health (Barakat, Pelaez, Montejo, Luaces, & Zakynthinaki, 2011; Shivakumar et al., 2011). Exercise improves physical performance and decreases pain in osteoarthritis and fibromyalgia (Sañudo et al., 2010; Schlenk, Lias, Sereika, Dunbar-Jacob, & Kwoh, 2011). In addition to helping maintain healthy bone in women with and without osteopenia, exercise decreases fall and fracture risk and increases mobility and quality of life in women with osteoporosis (Bergland, Thorsen, & Kåresen, 2010; Korpelainen et al., 2010; Tolomio, Ermolao, Lalli, & Zaccaria, 2010). Walking may be the most efficient and economical form of exercise. Begin with a pedometer and visit "10,000 Steps a Day" at www.thewalkingsite.com.

ISSUES OF SAFETY AND EFFICACY

When considering these therapies, safety and efficacy are important. Begin with safety issues. Is there any empirical, theoretical, or intuitive information to suggest the therapy is harmful? If not, look for information regarding efficacy. Finding good CAM-related research can be challenging. Pilkington (2007) found that while systematic reviews of CAM are the same, if not better than, the quality of conventional medicine reviews, only 30 to 80 percent of all known published studies can be located using MEDLINE alone. Cochrane CENTRAL listed the highest proportion of studies across therapies. Additionally, because of variations in terminology for therapies, using a variety of search terms increases the likelihood of finding good research. While a substantial amount of CAM research exists, methodological flaws such as small sample size and lack of control groups are common. Fortunately, this is already improving, which will contribute to the integration of evidence-based CAM into practice. If the research is inadequate, convey this to your client but do not automatically dismiss the potential benefit of the therapy.

ENERGY THERAPIES

Energy medicine encompasses a variety of therapies based on the conceptualization of the body as an energetic system and includes healing touch, therapeutic touch, reflexology, acupuncture, and flower essences, among others. This conceptualization of the body as an energetic system stretches our view of the human body, but is not entirely foreign considering electrocardiograms and electroencephalograms are based on energy. The mechanism of action is believed to be the channeling of healing energy through the practitioner to the client (www.nccam.nih.gov).

ENERGY HEALING

Energy healing encompasses healing touch, Reiki, and therapeutic touch. The therapies share a common framework and each can be done with or without physical contact with the recipient. Consistently, these therapies have been shown to improve recipient and practitioner well-being. A recent systematic review indicated that these therapies decrease anxiety and pain in a variety of populations (Fazzino, Quinn Griffin, McNulty, & Fitzpatrick, 2010). Healing Touch International maintains a research and health care database citing the effects of healing touch in a variety of conditions and disease states (www.healingtouchinternational.org).

FLOWER ESSENCES

Perhaps the least known therapy in this category is the use of flower essences such as the Bach flower essences. Edward Bach, a physician, studied the effects of plants and flowers on mental and emotional states. Typically, the plant is placed in distilled water and exposed to sunlight and then the liquid is used to treat various psychological states. One of the most popular is "Rescue Remedy," which is a combination of five flowers and is safe for adults and children experiencing disorders such as anxiety and insomnia (Bach & Wheeler, 1997). The dosage is four drops in 4 to 6 oz of water.

CONCLUSION

Integrating wellness in the care of women through the use of CAM enhances awareness of the mind-body-spirit connection, fostering health and well-being. Given the minimal increases in self-administered CAM over the last several years and evidence that these therapies may enhance health and reduce hospitalizations, guidance and support is needed for self-care activities. Integrating complementary therapies will enable us to provide the best potential for treating, curing, and healing the women entrusted to our care.

ADDITIONAL RESOURCES

BOOKS

Buckle, J. (2003). *Clinical aromatherapy* (2nd ed.). Philadelphia: Churchill Livingstone.

Dossey, B., Keegan, L., Guzzetta, C., & Kolkmeier, L. (2008). *Holistic nursing: A handbook for practice*. Sudbury, MA: Jones and Bartlett.

Northrup, C. (2006). *The wisdom of menopause: Creating physical and emotional health and healing during the change*. New York: Bantam Books.

Northrup, C. (2010). *Women's bodies, women's wisdom: Creating physical and emotional health and healing*. New York: Bantam Books.

Simon, D. (1998). *The wisdom of healing: A natural mind-body program for optimal wellness*. New York: Three Rivers Press.

Simon, D. (1999). *Return to wholeness: Embracing body, mind, spirit in the face of cancer*. San Francisco: Wiley.

DVD

Element: Tai Chi for Beginners by Samuel Barnes (2009)

Scott Cole: Discover Tai Chi for Beginners (2009)

Getting Started With Qigong With Chris Pei (2009)

RELIABLE INFORMATION ON HERBS

Herbs at a Glance: www.nccam.nih.gov

Agricultural Research Service (Dr. James Duke): www.ars-grin.gov/duke

American Botanical Council: www.herbalgram.org

HOMEOPATHY

National Center for Homeopathy: www.homeopathic.org

ORGANIZATIONS

NCCAM: www.nccam.nih.gov

American Holistic Nurses Association: www.ahna.org

American Holistic Medical Association: www.ahma.org

American Association of Integrative Medicine: www.aaim.com

PEER-REVIEWED JOURNALS

Journal of Holistic Nursing

Holistic Nursing Practice

Journal of Complementary and Integrative Medicine

Evidence-Based Complementary and Alternative Medicine

Alternative Therapies in Health and Medicine

Journal of Alternative and Complementary Medicine

REFERENCES

Adams, J., Lui, C.W., Sibbritt, D., Broom, A., Wardle, J., & Homer, C. (2011). Attitudes and referral practices of maternity care professionals with regard to complementary and alternative medicine: An integrative review. *Journal of Advanced Nursing, 67*, 472–483.

Alpay, K., Ertas, M., Orhan, E.K., Ustay, D.K., Lieners, C., & Baykan, B. (2010). Diet restriction in migraine, based on IgG against foods: A clinical double-blind, randomised, cross-over trial. *Cephalalgia, 30*, 829–837.

American Pregnancy Association. (2011). Retrieved March 28, 2011, from http://www.americanpregnancy.org

Aso, T. (2010). Equol improves menopausal symptoms in Japanese women. *Journal of Nutrition, 140*, 1386S–1389S.

Bach, E., & Wheeler, F.J. (1997). *The Bach flower remedies*. New Canaan, CT: Keats Publishing.

Barakat, R., Pelaez, M., Montejo, R., Luaces, M., & Zakynthinaki, M. (2011). Exercise during pregnancy improves maternal health perceptions: A randomized clinical trial. *American Journal of Obstetrics and Gynecology, 204*(5), 402.e1–402.e7. Retrieved March 14, 2011, from http://www.ncbi.nlm.nig.giv/pubmed/21354547

Belew, C. (1999). Herbs and the childbearing woman: Guidelines for Midwives. *Journal of Nurse Midwifery, 44*(3), 231–251.

Benson, H. (1975). *The relaxation response*. New York: Morrow.

Bergland, A., Thorsen, H., & Kåresen, R. (2010). Effect of exercise on mobility, balance, and health-related quality of life in osteoporotic women with a history of vertebral fracture: A randomized, controlled trial. *Osteoporosis, 22*(6), 1863–1871. Retrieved March 14, 2011, from http://www.ncbi.nlm.nih.giv/pubmed/21060992

Bertone-Johnson, E.R., Chocano-Bedoya, P.O., Zagarins, S.E., Micka, A.E., & Ronnenberg, A.G. (2010). Dietary vitamin D intake, 25-hydroxyvitamin D3 levels and premenstrual syndrome in a college-aged population. *Journal of Steroid Biochemistry and Molecular Biology, 121*, 434–437.

Borrelli, F., & Ernst, E. (2010). Alternative and complementary therapies for the menopause. *Maturitas, 66*, 333–343.

Bós, A.M., Howard, B.V., Beresford, S.A., Urban, N., Tinker, L.F., Waters, H., et al. (2011). Cost-effectiveness analysis of a low-fat diet in the prevention of breast and ovarian cancer. *Journal of the American Dietetic Association, 111*, 56–66.

Braun, L., & Cohen, M. (2010). *Herbs & natural supplements: An evidence-based guide* (3rd ed.). Philadelphia: Churchill Livingstone.

Caan, B.J., Natarajan, L., Parker, B.A., Gold, E.B., Thomson, C.A., Newman, V.A., et al. (2011). Soy food consumption and breast cancer prognosis. *Cancer Epidemiology, Biomarkers, and Prevention, 20*(5), 854–858.

Castro-Sánchez, A.M., Matarán-Peñarrocha, G.A., Aguilera-Manrique, G., Quesada-Rubio, J.M., & Moreno-Lorenzo, C. (2011). Benefits of massage-myofascial release therapy on pain, anxiety, quality of sleep, depression, and quality of life in patients with fibromyalgia. *Evidence Based Complementary and Alternative Medicine, 2011*, 1–9.

Chen, F.P., Chien, M.H., Chen, H.Y., & Ng, Y.T. (2011). Effects of different progestogens on human breast tumor cell growth.*Climacteric, 14*, 345–351. Retrieved March 28, 2011, from http://www.ncbi.nlm.nih.gov/pubmed/21375453

Chen, K.M., & Snyder, M. (1999). A research-based use of Tai Chi/movement therapy as a nursing intervention. *Journal of Holistic Nursing, 17*, 267–279.

Darby, S.B. (2009). Traditional Chinese medicine: A complement to conventional. *Nursing for Women's Health, 13*, 198–206.

Eilat-Adar, S., & Goldbourt, U. (2010). Nutritional recommendations for preventing coronary heart disease in women: Evidence concerning whole foods and supplements. *Nutrition, Metabolism and Cardiovascular Diseases, 20*, 459–466.

Fazzino, D.L., Quinn Griffin, M.T., McNulty, R., & Fitzpatrick, J.J. (2010). Energy healing and pain: A review of the literature.*Holistic Nursing Practice, 24*, 79–88.

Foidart, J.-M., Colin, C., Denoo, X., Desreux, J., Béliard, J., Foumier, S., et al. (1998). Estradiol and progesterone regulate the proliferation of human breast epithelial cells. *Fertility and Sterility, 69*, 963–969.

Fontaine, K.L. (2005). *Complementary and alternative therapies for nursing practice*. Upper Saddle River, NJ: Pearson Prentice Hall.

Formby, B., & Wiley, T.S. (1999). Bcl-2, surviving and variant CD44 v7-v10 are downregulated and p53 is upregulated in breast cancer cells by progesterone: Inhibition of cell growth and induction of apoptosis. *Molecular and Cellular Biochemistry, 202*, 53–61.

Franconi, G., Manni, L., Aloe, L., Mazzilli, F., Giamvalvo, D.B.G., Lenzi, A., et al. (2011). Acupuncture in clinical and experimental reproductive medicine: A review. *Journal of Endocrinological Investigation, 34*(4), 307–311. Retrieved March 7, 2011, from http://www.ncbi.nlm.nih.gov/pubmed21297382

Gardiner, P., Graham, R., Legedza, A.T.R., Ahn, A.C., Eisenberg, D.M., & Phillips, R.S. (2007). Factors associated with herbal therapy use by adults in the United States. *Alternative Therapies in Health and Medicine, 13*, 22–29.

Gregg, D. (2010, Autumn). Like cures like: Homeopathy for labor and birth. *Midwifery Today, 16*, 13–64.

Gruzelier, J.H. (2002). A review of the impact of hypnosis, relaxation, guided imagery and individual differences on aspects of immunity and health. *Stress, 5*, 147–163.

Hall, H.G., Griffiths, D.L., & McKenna, L.G. (2011). The use of complementary and alternative medicine by pregnant women: A literature review. *Midwifery, 283*, 475–482.

Hawkins, J.L., Chestnut, C.P., & Gibbs, C.P. (2002). Obstetric anesthesia. In S.G. Gabbe, J.R. Niebyl, & J.L. Simpson

(Eds.),*Obstetrics: Normal and problem pregnancies* (p. 433). New York: Churchill Livingstone.

Herbert, B. (2010). Chronic pelvic pain. *Alternative Therapies in Health and Medicine, 16*, 28–33.

Herman, P.M., Craig, B.M., & Caspi, O. (2005). Is complementary and alternative medicine (CAM) cost effective? A systematic review. *BMC Complementary and Alternative Medicine, 5*, 11–25.

Higdon, J.V., Delage, B., Williams, D.E., & Dashwood, R.H. (2007). Cruciferous vegetables and human cancer risk: Epidemiologic evidence and mechanistic basis. *Pharmacological Research, 55*, 224–236.

Holtorf, K. (2009). The bioidentical hormone debate: Are bioidentical hormones (estradiol, estriol, and progesterone) safer or more efficacious than commonly used synthetic versions in hormone replacement therapy? *Postgraduate Medicine, 121*, 73–85.

Innes, K.E., Selfe, T.K., & Vishnu, A. (2010). Mind-body therapies for menopausal symptoms: A systematic review. *Maturitas, 66*, 135–149.

Jackson, R.L., Greiwe, J.S., Desai, P.B., & Schwen, R.J. (2011). Single-dose and steady-state pharmacokinetic studies of S-equol, a potent nonhormonal, estrogen receptor β-agonist being developed for the treatment of menopausal symptoms. *Menopause, 18*, 185–193.

Jallo, N., Bourguignon, C., Taylor, A.G., Ruiz, J., & Goehler, L. (2009-2010). The biobehavioral effects of relaxation guided imagery on maternal stress. *Advance, 24*, 12–22.

Jefferson, L.L. (2010). Exploring effects of therapeutic massage and patient teaching in the practice of diaphragmatic breathing on blood pressure, stress and anxiety in hypertensive African-American women: An interventional study. *Journal of the National Black Nurses Association, 21*, 17–24.

Kalder, M., Knoblauch, K., Hrgovic, I., & Münstedt, K. (2011). Use of complementary and alternative medicine during pregnancy and delivery. *Archives of Gynecology and Obstetrics, 283*, 475–482.

Kalichman, L. (2010). Massage therapy for fibromyalgia symptoms. *Rheumatology International, 30*, 1151–1157.

Klein, P.J., & Adams, W.D. (2004). Comprehensive therapeutic benefits of Taiji: A critical review. *American Journal of Physical Medicine and Rehabilitation, 83*, 735–745.

Koithan, M. (2009, March). Let's talk about complementary and alternative therapies. *Journal for Nurse Practitioners, 5*(3), 214–215.

Korpelainen, R., Keinänen-Kiukaanniemi, S., Nieminen, P., Heikkinen, J., Väänänen, K., & Korpelainen, J. (2010). Long-term outcomes of exercise: Follow-up of a randomized trial in older women with osteopenia. *Archives of Internal Medicine, 170*, 1548–1556.

Kuramoto, A.M. (2006). Therapeutic benefits of tai chi exercise: Research review. *Wisconsin Medical Journal, 105*, 42–46.

Lan, C., Chen, S.Y., & Lai, J.S. (2008). The exercise intensity of tai chi Chuan. *Medicine and Sport Science, 52*, 12–19.

Lee, M.S., & Ernst, E. (2011). Acupuncture for pain: An overview of Cochrane reviews. *Chinese Journal of Integrative Medicine, 17*, 187–189.

Li, J.X., & Chan, K.M. (2001). Tai chi: Physiological characteristics and beneficial effects on health. *British Journal of Sports Medicine, 35*, 148–160.

Lloyd, K.B., & Hornsby, L.B. (2009). Complementary and alternative medications for women's health issues. *Nutrition in Clinical Practice, 24*, 589–608.

Manheimer, E., Wieland, S., Kimbrough, E., Cheng, K., & Berman, B.M. (2009). Evidence from the Cochrane collaboration for traditional Chinese medicine therapies. *Journal of Alternative and Complementary Medicine, 15*(9), 1001–1014.

Mansky, P., Sannes, T., Wallerstedt, D., Ge, A., Ryan, M., Johnson, L.L., et al. (2006). Tai chi Chuan: Mind-body practice or exercise intervention? Studying the benefit for cancer survivors. *Integrative Cancer Therapies, 5*, 192–201.

Miller, M.F., Bellizzi, K.M., Sufian, M., Ambs, A.H., Goldstein, M.S., & Barbash, R. (2008). Dietary supplement use in individuals living with cancer and other chronic conditions: A population based study. *Journal of the American Dietetic Association, 108*, 483–494.

Nelissen, E.C., van Montfoort, A.P., Dumoulin, J.C., & Evers, J.L. (2010). Epigenetics and the placenta. *Human Reproduction Update, 17*(3), 397–417. Retrieved March 28, 2011, from http://www.ncbi.nlm.nih.gov/pubmed/20959349

Paul, A.M. (2010). *Origins*. New York: Free Press Simon & Schuster.

Peck. (2008). Integrating CAM into NP practice. *American Journal of Nurse Practitioners, 12*(5), 10–18.

Pilkington, K. (2007). Searching for CAM evidence: An evaluation of therapy-specific search strategies. *Journal of Alternative and Complementary Medicine, 13*, 451–459.

Price, C.J., McBride, B., Hyerle, L., & Kivlahan, D.R. (2007). Mindful awareness in body oriented therapy for female veterans with post-traumatic stress disorder taking prescription analgesics for chronic pain: A feasibility study. *Alternative Therapies in Health and Medicine, 13*, 32–40.

Sañudo, B., Baliano, D., Carrasco, L., Blagojevic, M., de Hoyo, M., & Saxton, J. (2010). Aerobic exercise versus combined exercise therapy in women with fibromyalgia syndrome: A randomized controlled trial. *Archives of Physical Medicine and Rehabilitation, 91*, 1838–1843.

Sarris, J., & Byrne, G.J. (2011). A systematic review of insomnia and complementary medicine. *Sleep Medicine Reviews, 15*, 99–106.

Schlenk, E.A., Lias, H.L., Sereika, S.M., Dunbar-Jacob, J., & Kwoh, C.K. (2011). Improving physical activity and function in overweight and obese older adults with osteoarthritis of the knee: A feasibility study. *Rehabilitation Nursing, 36*, 32–42.

Setchell, K.D., & Clerici, C. (2010). Equol: History, chemistry, and formation. *Journal of Nutrition, 140*, 1355S–1362S.

Shivakumar, G., Brandon, A.R., Snell, P.G., Santiago-Muñoz, P., Johnson, N.L., Trivedi, M.H., et al. (2011). Antenatal depression: A rationale for studying exercise. *Depression and Anxiety, 28*, 234–242.

Smith, T.C., Smith, B., & Ryan, M.A. (2008). Prospective investigation of complementary and alternative medicine use and subsequent hospitalizations. *BMC Complementary and Alternative Medicine, 8*, 19–28.

Stone, J.A., Yoder, K.K., & Case, E.A. (2009). Delivery of a full-term pregnancy after TCM treatment in a previously infertile patient diagnosed with polycystic ovary syndrome. *Alternative Therapies in Health and Medicine, 15*, 50–52.

Su, D., & Li, L. (2011). Trends in the use of complementary and alternative medicine in the United States: 2002–2007. *Journal of Health Care for the Poor and Underserved, 22*, 296–310.

Tillett, J., & Ames, D. (2010). The uses of aromatherapy in women's health. *Journal of Perinatal and Neonatal Nursing, 24*, 238–245.

Tisserand, M. (1988). *Aromatherapy for women*. Rochester, VT: Healing Arts Press.

Tolomio, S., Ermolao, A., Lalli, A., & Zaccaria, M. (2010). The effect of a multicomponent dual-modality exercise program targeting osteoporosis on bone health status and physical function capacity of postmenopausal women. *Journal of Women and Aging, 22*, 241–254.

Tousen, Y., Ezaki, J., Fujii, Y., Ueno, T., Nishimuta, M., & Ishimi, Y. (2011). Natural S-equol decreases bone resorption in postmenopausal non-equol-producing Japanese women: A pilot randomized, placebo-controlled trial. *Menopause, 18*(5), 563–574. Retrieved March 25, 2011, from http://www.ncbi.nlm.nih.gov/pubmed/21252728

Ulbricht, C. (2011). *Davis's pocket guide to herbs and supplements*. Philadelphia: F.A. Davis Company.

Weed, S. (2002). *The new menopausal years: Wise woman way*. Woodstock, NY: Ash Tree Publishing.

Weil, E. (2009, September). Bioidentical hormones: Examining the debate. *Advance for Nurse Practitioners*, pp. 37–41.

World Cancer Research Fund International/American Institute for Cancer Research. (2007). *Food, nutrition, physical activity, and the prevention of cancer: A global perspective*. Retrieved March 10, 2011, from http://www.dietandcancerreport.org

Yard, D.H. (2008, March). Dietary strategies for preventing cancer. *Clinical Advisor*, pp. 23–30.

Yeh, G.Y., Wang, C., Wayne, P.M., & Phillips, R.S. (2008). The effect of tai chi exercise on blood pressure: A systematic review. *Preventive Cardiology, 11*, 82–89.

Zhou, J., & Qu, F. (2009). Treating gynaecological disorders with traditional Chinese medicine: A review. *African Journal of Traditional, Complementary, and Alternative Medicine, 6*, 494–517.

III  Promotion of Gynecologic Health Care

CHAPTER ❖ 11

MENSTRUATION AND RELATED PROBLEMS AND CONCERNS

Kristine Alswager ◆ Christine Durler

Most women experience numerous changes in their menstrual cycle patterns during their reproductive life.

Highlights

- Normal Onset and Occurrence of Menses
- Abnormalities Related to the Menstrual Cycle

❖ INTRODUCTION

Menstruation is a normal, cyclically recurring event for women between the approximate ages of 12 and 50. Like childbirth, it usually occurs without major difficulties and is a universal event for most women. Historically, a menstruating woman has been viewed from unclean to possessing supernatural power. Some of these powers were regarded as good, while others instilled fear. In some cultures, women are to this day isolated during menstruation and allowed to be in the company of only other menstruating women. One theory is that women themselves started the practice of isolation during menstruation to have a time for quiet reflection and perhaps to provide a time for older women to impart their knowledge to younger women (Rome, Reame, & Stanford, 1998).

Throughout most of modern history, menstruation has been viewed as a disease rather than a normal condition. Medical treatment during the second half of the 19th century rested on an explicit view of women as fragile and vulnerable, totally dominated by the cyclicity and disability of their reproductive system. This heritage has objectively and subjectively colored society's perceptions of a menstruating woman as weak, suffering, unstable, or physically unable to execute her normal duties. There has been much argument in the literature about the effect of this on women's perceptions of menstrual symptoms and events. Feminist literature challenges much of medical and psychiatric literature on menstrual cycle research as being biased and sexist. Tools, such as the Menstrual Attitude Questionnaire and the Menstrual Distress Questionnaire, have revealed marked differences in women's perceptions and knowledge of menstruation and how these factors significantly influence one's personal and cultural experience of menstruation (Hoerster, Chrisler, & Gorman, 2003; Marvan, Espinosa-Hernandez, & Vacio, 2002).

In the past couple of decades, best sellers on menstrual changes associated with menopause opened the way for greater social awareness and knowledge of menstrual norms, made the topic more acceptable for discussion, and altered the attitudes of society toward menstruation. This is important because women can experience numerous changes in their menstrual cycle patterns during their reproductive life. Prevalence rates of primary dysmenorrhea are as high as 90 percent. Menstrual pain is a common cause of absenteeism and decreased quality of life for many females (Mannix, 2008). Adequate information about norms, increased comfort in discussing this bodily function, and access to reliable health care providers may decrease unnecessary office visits, reduce embarrassment and anxiety about common problems, and encourage further studies on women's menstrual experiences.

NORMAL ONSET AND OCCURRENCE OF MENSES

Menarche typically occurs within 2 to 3 years after thelarche (breast budding) (AAP&ACOG, 2006). See Chapter 4 for more information on these developmental milestones. The average age of menarche in the United States is 12 to 13 years old. Less than 10 percent of U.S. girls start to menstruate before 11 years of age; 90 percent of U.S. girls are menstruating by 13.75 years of age, and 98 percent by age 16. Popular perception is that menstruation is starting earlier and earlier. In reality, these percentages are not much different (0.34 years earlier) than those reported for U.S. girls in 1973.

Racial and/or ethnic differences have been found to exist regarding onset of menstruation. Compared to Caucasian females, non-Hispanic African American females experience menarche significantly earlier by approximately 1 year, whereas Mexican American females experience menarche only slightly earlier. Those who care for a large number of immigrant patients should be aware that age of menarche varies internationally, especially in less-developed countries. In Haiti, for example, the mean age of menarche is 15.37 years (AAP&ACOG, 2006). Possible explanations for these variations are differences in body mass index (BMI) and environmental factors including nutrition, socioeconomic conditions, and access to preventative health care (Chumlea, Schubert, & Roche, 2003).

THE NORMAL MENSTRUAL CYCLE

During the normal menstrual cycle, a series of events occur that lead to ovulation and the preparation of the endometrium for pregnancy. Under complex regulation by the hypothalamus, the pituitary gland, and the ovaries, cyclic changes induce development of a dominant follicle that results in ovulation and corpus luteum formation.

The endometrium responds to the cyclic changes in ovarian steroids by preparing for implantation and fertilization should occur. If pregnancy does not occur, the endometrium sloughs, resulting in menstruation. Most women have cycles lasting from 21 to 35 days, with 2 to 6 days of flow and an average blood loss of 20 to 60 mL.

The menstrual cycle involves cyclic changes in both the ovary and the uterus that are hormonally mediated (see Figure 11–1). The ovarian cycle is further divided into follicular and luteal phases. During the follicular phase, pulsatile gonadotropin-releasing hormone (GnRH) is released by the hypothalamus and results in pulses of follicle-stimulating

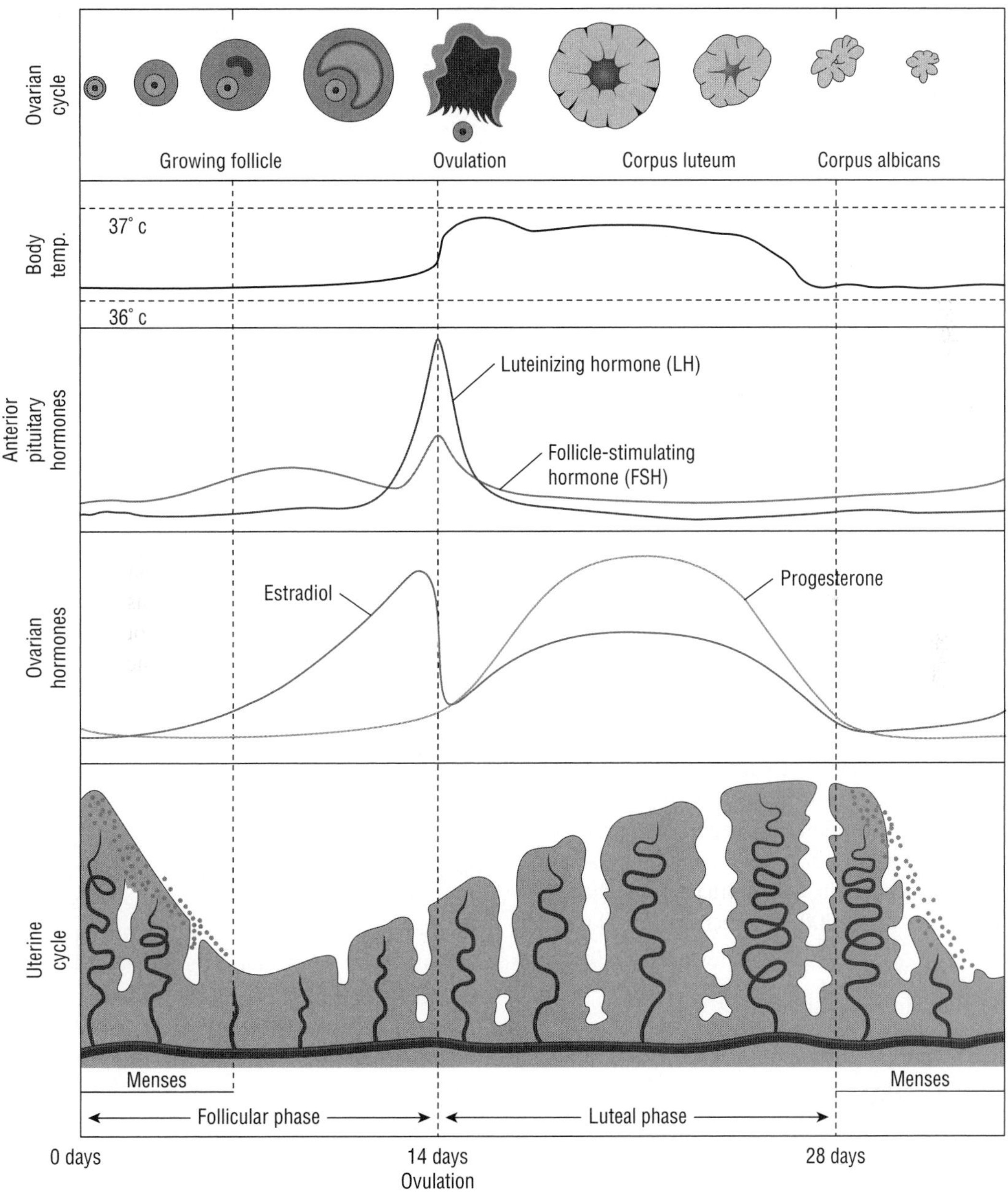

FIGURE 11–1. The Menstrual Cycle. *Sources:* Marieb, E.N. (2012). *Essentials of human anatomy and physiology* (10th ed., p. 555, Figure 16.12). Benjamin Cummings/Pearson; *The menstrual cycle*. Retrieved April 1, 2011, from http://www.uptodate.com/contents/physiology-of-the-normal-menstrual-cycle?source=search_result&selectedTitle=1~150; Boston Women's Health Collective. (1992). *The new our bodies, ourselves: A book by and for women updated and expanded for the 90s* (p. 256). New York: A Touchstone Book, Simon & Schuster Inc.

hormone (FSH) and luteinizing hormone (LH) from the anterior pituitary. This pulsatile stimulus recruits a number of follicles to begin developing, which increases estrogen levels. One follicle becomes the dominant follicle producing the most estrogen and the rest of the follicles stimulated in that cycle undergo atresia. Estrogen level reaches peak, about 24 hours before ovulation; LH level surges; and ovulation occurs 24 to 36 hours later.

Ovulation indicates transition to the luteal phase. During the luteal phase, there is a shift from estrogen dominance to progesterone dominance. Following the rupture of the follicle, the corpus luteum develops and produces large amounts of progesterone. Progesterone suppresses further follicular growth and causes secretory changes in the endometrium. The length of the luteal phase tends to be more constant than the follicular phase, approximately 14 days. Progesterone causes an elevation in basal body temperature; therefore, daily measurement of basal body temperature usually can determine whether ovulation has occurred. If a woman does not become pregnant, the corpus luteum rapidly deteriorates approximately 9 to 11 days after ovulation. This results in a sharp decline in serum levels of progesterone and estrogen and triggers menstruation.

The endometrium responds to the cyclic changes in ovarian steroids. The first phase of the uterine cycle, the proliferative phase, corresponds to the follicular phase of the ovarian cycle. Estrogen stimulates the endometrium to thicken and form progesterone receptors to increase blood flow to the endometrium. The second phase of the uterine cycle is called the secretory phase, which correlates with the luteal phase of the ovarian cycle. During this phase, progesterone causes the endometrium to differentiate and secrete proteins that are important in supporting implantation of an early embryo if fertilization of the egg occurs. As noted earlier, decrease of estrogen and progesterone results in the sloughing of the endometrium, or menstruation, and the cycle continues (Berek & Novak, 2007; Hatcher et al., 2011).

ABNORMALITIES RELATED TO THE MENSTRUAL CYCLE

DESCRIPTIVE TERMS

- Amenorrhea—absence of menses for at least three usual cycle lengths
- Oligomenorrhea—infrequently occurring menses at intervals greater than 35 days
- Polymenorrhea—menses at intervals of 21 to 24 days or fewer
- Hypomenorrhea—regular bleeding in less than normal amount
- Menorrhagia—regularly occurring bleeding excessive in duration and flow (greater than 80 mL/cycle or lasting longer than 7 days)
- Metrorrhagia—light bleeding occurring irregularly
- Menometrorrhagia—irregular, heavy bleeding
- Intermenstrual bleeding—bleeding at any time between otherwise normal menses (Fraser, Critchley, Munro, & Broder, 2007)

AMENORRHEA

Amenorrhea is a symptom, not a diagnosis, and is categorized as either primary or secondary. Primary amenorrhea is classically defined as the absence of menses by age 16. However, recent guidelines suggest a diagnosis of primary amenorrhea should be considered if a patient has not reached menarche by 14 to 15 years of age or has not done so within 3 years of thelarche (American Academy of Pediatrics, Committee on Adolescence, American College of Obstetricians and Gynecologists, 2006). Secondary amenorrhea is the absence of menses for more than three cycles or 6 months in women who previously had menses (Practice Committee of the American Society for Reproductive Medicine, 2006).

Epidemiology

Etiology. Primary amenorrhea has a number of origins such as obstructed flow, müllerian agenesis, androgen insensitivity syndrome, or a number of chromosomal abnormalities (Fritz & Speroff, 2011). Among women of reproductive age, secondary amenorrhea that is unrelated to pregnancy, lactation, or age-appropriate menopause may signal stress or a life-threatening disease. The three most common causes for secondary amenorrhea are hyperandrogenism, hypothyroidism, and pituitary adenoma (Hernandez, Cervera-Aguilar, Vergara, & Ayala, 1999). Other causative factors include other tumors, eating disorders, excessive exercise, medications, gynecological surgery injuries, a systemic illness, autoimmune diseases, chemotherapy, radiation therapy, defective enzyme systems, or anatomic deviations (Fritz & Speroff, 2011).

Incidence. Ninety-eight percent of girls are menstruating by age 15. In a study of 1,099 subjects between the ages of 15 and 50 years, Hernandez et al. (1999) found the prevalence of secondary amenorrhea was

4.9 percent between 26 and 35 years of age. Incidences of amenorrhea in subgroups such as college students and athletes are higher (Warren & Goodman, 2003). Polycystic ovary syndrome (PCOS) occurs in approximately 3 to 5 percent of the female population (Hoyt & Schmidt, 2004). Premature ovarian failure (POF) occurs in 1 out of 10,000 women below the age of 20, 1 out of 1,000 women below the age of 30, and 1 percent of women below the age of 40 (Christin-Maitre, Pasquire, Donadille, & Bouchard, 2006).

Subjective Data

The etiology of amenorrhea is revealed in a client's history most of the time. Questions should be asked in each of the following areas:

- Past medical and surgical history such as past illnesses, hospitalizations, and surgeries, particularly chronic diseases such as childhood leukemia, thyroid or adrenal dysfunction, and renal or hepatic diseases. Specifically ask about history of radiation therapy, chemotherapy, or gynecological surgery
- Obstetric history including history of infertility and the date(s) and course of any pregnancy; intrauterine or ectopic pregnancy; abortion; type of delivery; and occurrence of postpartum events such as hemorrhage requiring surgical intervention or infection
- A menstrual history including the following information: age of development of secondary sex characteristics and current status, absence of menarche or age it occurred, date of last menstrual period, symptoms associated with menses (such as pain), interval between menses, duration and characteristics of flow
- Review of systems for any other bodily changes or abnormalities, such as insomnia, headaches, visual field defects, weight loss or gain, nipple discharge, hot flashes, vaginal dryness, virilization (hirsutism, alopecia, acne, or voice changes)
- Lifestyle evaluation including disordered eating patterns, anorexia, bulimia, intense athleticism, life stressors, illicit drug use, smoking, and alcohol intake
- Prescription and over-the-counter drug use

Objective Data

Physical Examination

Vital signs: Include age, height, weight, and blood pressure.

General appearance and skin: Observe carefully and note general body habitus, stage of development of secondary sex characteristics (see Tanner developmental stages in Chapter 4), presence of signs of virilization such as acne, male pattern hair growth and fat distribution, and presence of striae. Observe skin for acanthosis nigricans.

Neck: Examine thyroid for nodules or enlargement.

Breasts: Observe breasts for spontaneous nipple discharge, palpate for masses. Gently manipulate nipple if nipple discharge is reported.

Abdomen: Palpate abdomen for masses or hernias.

Genitalia/reproductive: Examine genitalia for clitoromegaly, obstructive problems such as imperforate hymen. Note color and moisture of vaginal mucous membranes, presence of vaginal discharge and rugae. Check for presence of cervical mucus, cervical stenosis, vaginal agenesis, transverse vaginal septum. Cervical mucus should be clear and fern on microscopy if estrogen is present. Vaginal cells may be collected for a maturation index. With bimanual exam, note absent, enlarged, tender, or irregularly shaped uterus and/or ovaries.

Commonly Recommended Diagnostic Tests and Methods

Pregnancy Test. A pregnancy test should always be done first to rule out pregnancy or related complications. Urine pregnancy test (UPT) results are available within 3 to 5 minutes and at a lesser cost than quantitative human chorionic gonadotropin (HCG) blood tests.

Thyroid, Prolactin. Thyroid-stimulating hormone (TSH) and prolactin hormone levels are recommended because hypothyroidism (elevated TSH) and hyperprolactinemia (>50 ng/mL) can cause amenorrhea (Grubb, Chakeres, & Malarkey, 1987). Due to prolactin levels being influenced by breast stimulation, eating, and stress, it is recommended to reevaluate an initially elevated prolactin level while the patient is fasting and without any breast stimulation (Holt, 2008).

Hypothalamic-Pituitary-Ovarian (HPO) Axis. Evaluation of the hypothalamus, pituitary, ovary, and uterus.

- Measure serum levels of the gonadotropins: FSH and LH.
- An estradiol level is checked to evaluate how well the ovaries are producing estrogen.
- An elevated FSH and LH with a low estradiol level indicates ovarian failure.

- Low FSH, LH, and estradiol indicates hypogonadotropic hypogonadism.
- Low to normal FSH, LH, and estradiol indicates hypothalamic amenorrhea.

Progesterone Challenge Test or Evaluation of Endometrial Stripe. A progesterone challenge test or evaluation of the endometrial stripe may be performed if tests for pregnancy, thyroid disease, and prolactinoma are negative prior to proceeding with other hormonal testing unless other tests are indicated by patient history or exam. The progesterone challenge test confirms the presence of estrogen and the intactness of the outflow tract (uterus and vagina).

- Most commonly, 5 to 10 mg oral medroxyprogesterone is given for 7 to 10 days (Staggers, 2010a).
- An alternative regimen is 300 mg oral micronized progesterone for 7 to 10 days or 100 to 200 mg of progesterone in oil IM for one dose.
- If bleeding occurs in 2 to 7 days after completing the medication regimen, then it is clear that the cervix is patent, estrogen is being produced, and the endometrium is functional.
- If no bleeding occurs with the progesterone challenge test, consider administering oral-conjugated estrogen 0.625 mg/day or its equivalent (oral estradiol 1 mg/day or transdermal estradiol 0.05 mg/day) for 35 days to prime the endometrium. A progestin, such as 10 mg of oral medroxyprogesterone from days 26 to 35, is also added. If no bleeding occurs upon the cessation of this therapy, endometrial scarring is likely (Berman, 2008). Consultation with or referral to a medical provider prior to instituting this step would be appropriate.
- An alternative to the progesterone challenge test is to perform a pelvic ultrasound to measure the endometrial stripe. A thickness of ≥6.0 mm indicates adequate production of estrogen (Fritz & Speroff, 2011).

Ovarian/Adrenal Function Tests. These labs are checked and are particularly important if suspicion for PCOS exists or if any virilization is found on exam. Serum free and total testosterone, dehydroepiandrosterone sulfate (DHEA-S), 17-hydroxyprogesterone (17-OHP), cortisol, and fasting blood glucose are suggested for suspected abnormal androgenic and insulin states, such as with PCOS or androgen-secreting tumors.

- 17-OHP to rule out nonclassic 21-hydroxylase deficiency that accounts for more than 90 percent of congenital adrenal hyperplasia (Speiser & White, 2003).
- DHEA-S to assess for an adrenal tumor (suspected when DHEA-S is >700 mcg/dL).
- Testosterone to assess for an adrenal or ovarian androgen-secreting tumor (when >150 ng/mL).
- Cortisol may also be tested to rule out adrenal tumors and help rule out Cushing's syndrome, in which case salivary testing is ideal (Nieman et al., 2008).
- Fasting glucose elevation (indicating impaired glucose metabolism) as well as elevations of testosterone and DHEA-S can be (but not always) seen with PCOS (Devane, Czekala, Judd, & Yen, 1975).

Differential Medical Diagnoses

Pregnancy Related. Pregnancy, lactation, or pregnancy complications such as ectopic pregnancy, missed abortion, or trophoblastic neoplasm should be considered.

Thyroid Dysfunction. Amenorrhea can be seen when a patient is both hypo- and hyperthyroid states, with hypothyroid being the more commonly associated with amenorrhea (Krassass et al., 1999).

Pituitary Dysfunction. Hyperprolactinemia can cause amenorrhea. It is the most common endocrine disorder of the hypothalamic-pituitary axis and can lead to both short-term sexual dysfunction and galactorrhea, and long-term loss of bone mineral density. An elevated prolactin level can occur with a brain tumor (prolactinoma), necrosis, or injury of the brain. Hypothyroidism and certain medications can also cause hyperprolactinemia (Holt, 2008).

Drug Related. A number of medications and illegal drugs are associated with amenorrhea.

- Known medications that can cause hyperprolactinemia include some antipsychotics, antidepressants, and opiates as well as some gastrointestinal drugs and antihypertensive agents (Jerrell, Bacon, Burgis, & Menon, 2009).
- Cocaine may cause irregular menses. Chronic cannabis use may cause irregularity as well (it can increase prolactin levels, and therefore, galactorrhea) (Carey, 2006; Palha & Esteves, 2008).
- Combined or progestin-only contraceptives and other hormonally active medications, such as danazol and leuprolide, are frequently the source of diminished or absent menses. Upon discontinuing hormonal contraception, menses typically return to a woman's baseline in approximately 1 to 3 months (Davis et al., 2008). A notable exception to this is depot-medroxyprogesterone acetate (DMPA) where it is not unusual for menstruation to be delayed 6 to 12 months post discontinuation (see Chapter 12).

Hypothalamic Amenorrhea. Low FSH, LH, and estradiol will be found in women with increased exercise, intense athleticism, eating disorder, or weight loss more than 10 percent below the expected BMI. The hormone pattern seen in amenorrheic athletes includes a decrease in GnRH pulses from the hypothalamus, which results in decreased pulsatile secretion of LH and FSH and shut down of the ovary. The cause of menstrual irregularities is not due to the exercise alone, but to chronic inadequate or restrictive caloric intake that does not compensate for the energy expenditure. Complications associated with amenorrhea include compromised bone density, failure to attain peak bone mass in adolescence, and increased risk of stress fractures. The diagnosis of exercise-associated menstrual dysfunctions is one of exclusion (Warren & Goodman, 2003).

Chronic Disease and Stress-Related Amenorrhea. Similarly, conditions such as celiac disease, if left untreated, can lead to malnutrition and menstrual irregularity. Approximately 40 percent of women with celiac disease have menstrual cycle disorders (Moltini, Bardella, & Bianchi, 1990).

Mood disturbances including depression, anxiety, and psychological stress have been found to influence the hypothalamus, and therefore, the menstrual cycle (Barron, Flick, Cook, Homan, & Campbell, 2008; Sheinfeld, Gal, Bunzel, & Vishne, 2007).

Low FSH, LH, and estradiol can also be seen with chronic health conditions such as poorly controlled insulin-dependent diabetes mellitus (IDDM). Irregular menstrual cycles were diagnosed in 27.9 percent of IDDM girls, polymenorrhea in 50 percent, and oligomenorrhea in the remainder. Over follow-up, one third of the girls with oligomenorrhea had long-term noncompliance with glycemic control (HgbA1c 13.5%) and developed secondary amenorrhea (Snajderova et al., 1999).

Congenital Syndromes. Low FSH, LH, and estradiol may also be seen with rare congenital syndromes such as idiopathic hypogonadotropic hypogonadism, Prader-Willi syndrome, Laurence-Moon-Biedl syndrome, and Kallmann syndrome (Staggers, 2010a).

POF. An increase in FSH and LH and low estradiol is seen with physiologic menopause (onset approximately age 52 in the United States) or with POF (also called primary ovarian insufficiency). POF is defined by at least 4 months of amenorrhea with elevated gonadotropins (usually above 40 UI/L) detected on two occasions a few weeks apart in a woman before the age of 40. In 80 percent of POF cases, the etiology is unknown. The etiologies identified are (1) iatrogenic following chemotherapy and/or radiotherapy, (2) autoimmune, (3) viral, and (4) genetic (such as a17-hydroxylase deficiency–causing adrenal hyperplasia or Turner's syndrome). Infertility is common, as only 3 to 10 percent of the patients will have natural conception (Christin-Maitre, Pasquire, Donadille, & Bouchard, 2006).

Adrenal Function Related. Hyperandrogenism, insulin resistance, and hyperinsulinemia may be seen with androgen-secreting tumors, but are most commonly seen due to PCOS and in some cases of obesity (Pandey & Bhattacharya, 2010). There are elevations of DHEA-S, testosterone, cortisol, and fasting glucose levels.

PCOS occurs in approximately 3 to 5 percent of the female population and may be the leading cause of infertility in those of reproductive age (see Chapter 13). PCOS presents clinically with a variety of signs and symptoms; the most common being menstrual irregularities, hyperandrogenism, infertility, and obesity. The true pathophysiology has not been clearly elucidated; however, there is growing agreement that gonadotropin dynamic dysfunction, hyperandrogenism, and insulin resistance are key features. PCOS is not a benign condition. It may lead to complications involving glucose metabolism, dyslipidemias, cardiovascular disease, and cancer (Hoyt & Schmidt, 2004). Because of the continuing controversy regarding the definition of PCOS, the Androgen Excess Society (AES) proposed that PCOS should be diagnosed by the presence of three features: androgen excess (clinical and/or biochemical hyperandrogenism); ovarian dysfunction (oligoanovulation and/or polycystic ovarian morphology); and exclusion of other androgen excess or ovulatory disorders (Azziz et al., 2009).

Due to other possible, although rare, etiologies of virilization, the clinician should consider the following factors to best identify those women whose androgenic state is not related to PCOS: abrupt onset, short duration (typically less than 1 year), or sudden progressive worsening of hirsutism; onset of clinical symptoms in the third decade of life or later, rather than near puberty; and symptoms or signs of virilization, including frontal balding, severe pustular acne, clitoromegaly, increased muscle mass, or deepening of voice (Hatch & Rosenfield, 1981).

Anatomic Abnormalities. The following anatomic changes may also be the cause of amenorrhea.

- Congenital abnormalities such as imperforate hymen or a transverse vaginal septum can impede menstrual flow. Gross anatomical defects such as an absent uterus or ovaries can also occur.

- Asherman's syndrome is an anatomic variation that is in most cases associated with trauma to the endometrium from surgical procedures, primarily from curettage. Increasingly, cases have been associated with myomectomy (both abdominal and hysteroscopic), removal of septa, and any other intrauterine surgery. Pathology shows fibrous connective tissue bands ranging from filmy to dense with or without glandular tissue. The syndrome is characterized by a spectrum from amenorrhea to menstrual disturbance to normal menses. It is frequently associated with infertility. The true incidence is unknown. Most cases occur within close proximity to a pregnancy, usually within 4 months and usually while a woman is in a hypoestrogenized state (Berman, 2008).

Plan

The health care provider must address the diverse causes of amenorrhea, its relationship to sexual identity, perception of normal menstrual function, possible infertility, unplanned pregnancy, tumor, or life-threatening disease. Sensitive listening, interviewing, and individualized evaluation are essential. Educate a client about normal menstrual cycles and possible reasons for her abnormal pattern. Menstrual calendars are helpful with instruction about documenting any bleeding or spotting, days and dosages of medications, pad or tampon count, and associated menstrual symptoms such as dysmenorrhea. Choosing a management plan with the client (after morbidities are ruled out) will vary depending on the etiology and severity of the bleeding, associated symptoms, contraceptive needs, medical comorbidities and contraindications to hormonal or other medications. Appropriate referrals are made as needed.

Primary Amenorrhea. Refer all clients with primary amenorrhea for specialist evaluation as this situation generally warrants a genetic evaluation including karyotyping. Reassure young amenorrheic teens and their parents. Recommend watchful waiting if results of exam and tests are normal.

Secondary Amenorrhea. Refer all clients with secondary amenorrhea caused by central lesions, autoimmune diseases, or complex endocrine or metabolic diseases to a specialist for evaluation and management. Causes may be treated as suggested next.

Medication-Induced Amenorrhea. In the case of medications that may be influencing the client's menstrual pattern, it may be appropriate for the provider to reassure the patient, discontinue the medications, or have her medications reevaluated by the original prescriber.

Lifestyle Coaching and Education. Education on healthful diet and exercise regimens is often needed. The most effective treatment is to decrease the intensity of exercise and increase nutritional intake (Goodman & Warren, 2005). Inform the client of appropriate BMI range as well as appropriate rate of weight loss. Consider a referral to a nutritionist. Also provide emotional support as well as a referral to a psychologist and/or specialist if an eating disorder or unmanageable psychological stress or mood disorder is present (Sheinfeld et al., 2007).

Condition-Specific Treatment Plans

PCOS: The goals of treatment for PCOS should focus on restoring menstrual regularity, decreasing androgen excesses, and decreasing insulin resistance (Hoyt & Schmidt, 2004). The AES also suggests the following: Patients with normal glucose tolerance should be rescreened at least once every 2 years or more frequently if additional risk factors are identified. Patients with impaired glucose tolerance should be screened annually for development of type II diabetes (Salley et al., 2007).

Thyroid: Appropriate treatment and monitoring of hypothyroidism is often managed by either primary care or endocrinology. Hyperthyroidism requires a referral to endocrinology for either medical or surgical management depending on the etiology of the thyroid problem.

Hyperprolactinemia: Appropriate referral to an endocrinologist for diagnostic imaging with magnetic resonance imaging (MRI) is essential when the prolactin level is high. Prolactin-secreting tumors (prolactinomas) are benign neoplasms constituting about 40 percent of all pituitary tumors. Medical therapy with dopamine agonists is considered the treatment of choice. Transsphenoidal surgery is an option when medical therapy is neither effective nor well tolerated (Chanson & Salenave, 2004).

POF: All patients diagnosed with ovarian failure prior to age 30 require a specialist referral for karyotype determination. Screening tests for autoimmune disorders or systemic illness may also be indicated. Management of these patients includes hormone replacement therapy (HRT) in order to decrease risk for cardiovascular disease and osteoporosis related to hypoestrogenism. When fertility is desired, women with POF should be referred to reproductive endocrinology (see Chapter 13) (Christin-Maitre et al., 2006).

Asherman's syndrome: Refer to a gynecologist. The diagnosis is primarily by history and a high index of suspicion. Confirmatory tests are increasingly saline infusion sonohysterography (SIS) or hysterosalpingogram (HSG), although MRI has also been used. Ultimately, hysteroscopy is used for final diagnosis and treatment. Hysteroscopic lysis of adhesions is the main method of treatment. Treatment outcomes are difficult to assess as there is no universally agreed-upon classification system. However, intrauterine pregnancies rates range from 22 to 45 percent and live births range from 28 to 32 percent. The risk of complications for those who achieve pregnancy is significant with risk for placenta accreta and subsequent blood loss, transfusion, and hysterectomy (Berman, 2008).

Pharmacological Therapy. Once the underlying etiology of the amenorrhea is discovered, medications such as hormonal contraceptives are commonly prescribed as appropriately dictated by the diagnosis. The main indication for pharmacological treatment is to prevent amenorrhea-induced endometrial hyperplasia, which, if left untreated, can lead to endometrial cancer.

Low-Dose Combination Contraceptives

- Oral contraceptive pills are especially useful in those clients with PCOS, an immature/adolescent, suppressed/intense athleticism, or aging/perimenopausal HPO axis.
- Combined oral contraceptives (COCs) are superior to progesterone-only treatment in a sexually active, nonsmoking client who is younger than 35 as they prevent endometrial hyperplasia, provide contraception, and supplement estrogen for the protection of bone health.
- Note that the contraceptive patch and ring are other estrogen–progestin preparations that could be tried in place of regular monthly oral contraceptive use depending on the woman's personal preference. However, there are no data describing if control of uterine bleeding is indeed the same, superior, or less than with standard oral contraceptive use (ACOG, 2010). See Chapter 12 for further information on these methods.
- Contraindications include pregnancy, thromboembolic disorders, liver dysfunction, known or suspected malignancy of breast or reproductive organs, undiagnosed vaginal bleeding, or missed abortion.

Progesterone Therapy

- Medroxyprogesterone can be used to prevent endometrial hyperplasia in anovulatory clients who do not need contraception. Administer 5 to 10 mg orally for 12 days every 1 to 3 months of each month or during cycle days 16 to 26.
- Micronized progesterone (100 to 200 mg) daily orally or in a vaginal cream is an alternative to MPA. It resulted in regression of endometrial hyperplasia without atypia to normal endometrium in 91 percent of women treated from the 10th to the 25th day of the menstrual cycle for 3 to 6 months, with a relapse rate of 6 percent 6 months post treatment (Affinito, Di Carlo, Di Mauro, Napolitano, & Nappi, 1994).
- The levonorgestrel intrauterine system (LNG-IUS): Endometrial proliferation is suppressed, which results in prevention of endometrial hyperplasia in anovulatory clients who have contraindications to estrogen and desire contraception. It will not regulate cycles for most women as the endometrium is typically thinned to the point of scant menses to amenorrhea (Monteiro, Bahamondes, & Diaz, 2002). See Chapter 12 for more information.
- Contraindications include pregnancy, liver dysfunction, known or suspected malignancy of breast or reproductive organs, undiagnosed vaginal bleeding, or missed abortion. Some consider thromboembolic disorders as a contraindication to progesterone-only therapies.
- Anticipated outcome is that the client begins cyclic withdrawal spotting or bleeding 2 to 7 days after completing medication.
- Client teaching should include information about the possibility of heavy bleeding when medication is completed. Emphasize the importance of taking the medication to prevent endometrial hyperplasia or cancer. Inform the client of side effects and adverse reactions. Those most commonly reported are spotting, weight gain, fatigue, depression, or acne. Tell her to report any abnormal bleeding or the absence of withdrawal bleeding. Stress the necessity of consistently using reliable birth control measures as indicated.

HRT. HRT is indicated for hypoestrogenic states secondary to premature or physiological menopause, or in serious exercisers. See Chapter 18 for discussion of the most recent findings related to risks and benefits of HRT. Careful consideration of the individual characteristics of the woman must be considered before use. Only use HRT for women who do not need contraception.

Other. Other medication regimens are often times managed by or with a specialist because of the complex etiology of amenorrhea.

Follow-Up. Once workup is completed, follow-up is done annually. Prior to refilling medications, evaluate the client's menstrual charts, the client's adherence to the medication schedule, the presence of any new updates in her medical history that would be a contraindication to refilling her medication, as well as asking about and reviewing the side effects and danger signs of the medications.

DYSFUNCTIONAL UTERINE BLEEDING

Dysfunctional uterine bleeding (DUB) is traditionally described as noncyclic (metrorrhagia or menometrorrhagia) or excessive endometrial sloughing (menorrhagia) in the absence of a pelvic structural lesion or a systemic disease. The primary cause of abnormal uterine bleeding is anovulatory cycles. Some consider the terms *DUB* and *anovulatory cycles* synonymous. Clinically, anovulation frequently presents itself as stretches of amenorrhea (see section Amenorrhea) followed by irregular spotting and episodes of profuse and usually painless bleeding result (APGO, 2002). Women with DUB, especially when seen in those over 35 years, and/or those with exposure to unopposed estrogen either via medications or intrinsically, as with obesity or PCOS, are at risk for endometrial hyperplasia and carcinoma (Oriel & Schrager, 1999).

DUB can range from mild to severe where anemia and hypovolemic shock can occur. Irregular and excessive bleeding can impact a patient's quality of life including needing to stay home from work or school as well as interfering with sexual activity.

Menorrhagia, metrorrhagia, and menometrorrhagia are abnormal bleeding patterns that can also occur in ovulatory cycles, presenting as cyclic bleeding with superimposed abnormal bleeding. Menstrual flow requiring changes of menstrual products every 1 to 2 hours is considered excessive particularly when associated with flow that lasts more than 7 days at a time (AAP & ACOG, 2006; Staggers, 2010b).

Epidemiology

Etiology. The etiology of anovulatory-related DUB is some form of hormonal disturbance resulting in failure of ovarian follicular maturation. Progesterone is not properly produced causing a lack of control on endometrial growth as well as loss of control of synchronous shedding of the endometrium. The hormonal disturbance can originate from a variety of sources such as variations or derangements in the HPO axis, PCOS, endocrine disorders, or chronic illness as well as psychosocial issues.

The etiology of irregular bleeding in an ovulatory patient (generally regular cycles with superimposed abnormal bleeding) is likely related to an anatomic lesion (such as a fibroid), foreign body (such as an intrauterine device [IUD]), congenital malformation with partial obstruction, or endometriosis.

For abnormal cyclic bleeding, blood dyscrasias and uterine pathology are most likely. Other serious problems such as hepatic failure and malignancy are also possibilities in cyclic menorrhagia (AAP & ACOG, 2006; Staggers, 2010b).

Incidence. Approximately 25 percent of women report having menorrhagia (Shapely, Jordan, & Croft, 2004). DUB related to anovulation is most commonly seen in adolescence, obesity, PCOS, and perimenopause. In adolescents, the HPO axis is naturally immature. It can take 3 years from menarche for the majority of cycles to be ovulatory (AAP & ACOG, 2006). In perimenopausal women, anovulation is related to fluctuations in HPO functioning that accompany the natural decline in follicular number. Women between the ages of 40 and menopause commonly experience intermittent anovulatory cycles; that is, skipped periods. Heavy or prolonged periods are also typical of the menopause transition (Philipp et al., 2005).

Subjective Data

A complete history (see section Amenorrhea) is obtained, paying particular attention to the possibility of pregnancy. Is the bleeding related to any activities, such as intercourse? Is it interfering with daily activities? Are symptoms of ovulation (such as ovulatory mucus or breast tenderness) noted? Inquire if there are any associated symptoms such as systemic endocrine changes (virilization, hot flashes, breast discharge) or abdominal or genitourinary pain (infection, mass). Signs of anemia—including excessive fatigue, headaches, and dizziness—should also be assessed. Also, assessment of any family history of a bleeding disorder is important to help focus the diagnosis (Staggers, 2010b).

Note a history of the following, which may cause lack of ovulation and abnormal uterine bleeding: ovarian cysts (follicular, corpus-luteal), eating disorders, weight changes, increased exercise, stress, medication use, drug abuse, recent illnesses, infections, or a chronic illness.

Objective Data

- Check vital signs including height, weight (BMI), blood pressure, and age.
- Check hemoglobin for anemia.
- DUB is a diagnosis of exclusion; therefore, a complete physical examination is needed to rule out other

pathologies. The pelvic exam (speculum and bimanual) is a must. Note the site of bleeding, if it can be determined, and appearance of the cervix. If there is passage of tissue, send a specimen for pathology. Assess the size, contour, and tenderness of the uterus and ovaries.

Diagnostic Tests and Methods. A pregnancy test should be done for all women of reproductive age who are experiencing abnormal bleeding. Other common diagnostic tests include complete blood count (CBC), sexually transmitted infection (STI) screening, Papanicolaou (Pap), and endometrial biopsy. Additional tests to consider based on results of the physical exam include TSH, prolactin, partial thromboplastin time (PTT), prothrombin time (PT), factor VIII, von Willebrand factor (antigen and activity), DHEA-S, testosterone, ultrasound, saline sonohysterogram, and/or hysteroscopy.

- *CBC with platelets:* Obtained to rule out anemia, thrombocytopenia, and rarely, other systemic illnesses. Iron-deficiency anemia develops in 21 to 67 percent of cases (Milman, Clausen, & Byg, 1998).
- *STI screening:* Gonorrhea and chlamydia testing should be performed as indicated.
- *Cervical cancer screening:* Obtain a Pap smear if the client is not up-to-date. Changes to the cervix by HPV can lead to a more friable, or easy-to-bleed, cervix.
- *Endometrial biopsy:* After pregnancy is ruled out, an endometrial biopsy is recommended in all women over age 35 with DUB to rule out endometrial cancer or a premalignant lesion (endometrial hyperplasia). Consider an endometrial biopsy in women ages 18 to 35 who have risk factors for endometrial cancer: a family or personal history of ovarian, breast, colon, or endometrial cancer; tamoxifen use; chronic anovulation; obesity; estrogen therapy; prior endometrial hyperplasia; or diabetes (Santoro, Brown, Adel, & Skurnick, 1996). (See Chapter 3 for description of the endometrial biopsy procedure, risks of the procedure, and patient counseling recommendations.)
- *Thyroid:* Thyroid function tests, especially TSH, are indicated for women who may or may not have signs or symptoms of thyroid dysfunction because menorrhagia has been associated with hypothyroid disease (Krassass et al., 1999).
- *Prolactin:* A serum prolactin test may be indicated if the client reports periods of oligomenorrhea or galactorrhea.
- *Androgens:* Obtain serum for DHEA-S, cortisol, and testosterone if virilization reported or noted on exam.
- *Coagulation studies:* Further coagulation testing is recommended for those with a family history of bleeding disorder, excessive bleeding starting at menarche, or those with easy bruising (>5 cm) or excessive bleeding with dental or surgical procedures. A basic workup includes PTT, PT, factor VIII, and von Willebrand factor antigen and activity (Kouides, Conrad, Peyvandi, Lukes, & Kadir, 2005). Referral for this evaluation could be considered.
- *Ultrasound:* Transvaginal and/or transabdominal ultrasound can be helpful to confirm the abdominal or pelvic exam or to look for structural abnormalities such as a cyst or fibroid. An ultrasound may also be ordered to measure endometrial thickness, which is best assessed days 4 to 6 of the menstrual cycle. In reproductive-age women, normal proliferative phase endometrial thickness is 4 to 8 mm and secretory endometrium is 8 to 14 mm (APGO, 2002).
- *Sonohysterogram:* Saline-infused sonography (sonohysterogram) can better visualize the uterine cavity for small lesions such as polyps or submucosal fibroids. The procedure is performed by infusing sterile saline into the endometrial cavity and then evaluating by transvaginal ultrasound.
- *Hysteroscopy:* Hysteroscopy is visualization of the endometrium through a scope to search for uterine abnormalities. (See Chapter 3 for description of the procedure.) Minor treatments, such as polyp or septal removal, also can be done through hysteroscopy. Observation and directed tissue sampling is replacing dilation of the cervix and curettage (D&C) as the diagnostic procedure of choice. Inform the client that some cramps and bleeding may occur after the procedure. Also leakage of Dextran 70 through the cervix and vagina can be messy. Carbon dioxide distention may also cause shoulder pain. Pain medications should be provided. Advise the client to report signs of infection, excessive bleeding, or pain.

Finally, D&C may also be done for diagnostic evaluation. Endometrial D&C is recommended when medical regimens are ineffective or if polyps, incomplete abortion, or neoplasia is suspected. It may also be done if a more complete biopsy sampling of the endometrium is desired and hysteroscopy is unavailable. The procedure requires that the client be given local or general anesthesia. Specimens are sent to pathology. Provide the client with explanation of the procedure, anesthesia, cost, and risks. Postoperative instructions are given, advising the client to report signs of infection, excessive bleeding, and/or pain. Pain medication is also provided.

Differential Medical Diagnoses

- Pregnancy or pregnancy-related complications
- Cervical abnormalities: infection, polyp, carcinoma
- Uterine abnormalities: fibroids, infection, polyps, endometriosis, endometrial hyperplasia, endometrial intraepithelial neoplasia, carcinoma
- Medication use, including hormonal contraception
- Other diseases: thyroid or adrenal disorders, PCOS, liver or kidney failure, coagulopathies
- Other: foreign body such as an IUD

Plan

Educate the client about normal menstrual cycles and possible reasons for her abnormal pattern. Menstrual calendars are helpful with instruction given about documenting any bleeding or spotting, days and dosages of medications, pad or tampon count, and associated symptoms of dysmenorrhea. The results of the history, physical exam, laboratory evaluation, and diagnostic imaging or procedure are used to establish a diagnosis and guide treatment.

Choosing a management plan with the client (after pregnancy and malignancy have been ruled out) will vary depending on the etiology and severity of the bleeding, associated symptoms, contraceptive needs, medical comorbidities and contraindications to hormonal or other medications. Patients should be referred to a gynecologist if large structural lesions are noted on ultrasound or physical exam or if patients are not responding to treatment. Appropriate referrals are also made as needed for comorbidities, such as a clotting disorder.

Pharmacological Treatment. Once the underlying etiology of DUB is discovered, hormonal contraceptives are commonly prescribed as appropriately dictated by the diagnosis. The main indication for pharmacological treatment is to stop irregular and heavy bleeding and to increase the patient's quality of life as well as prevent anemia and endometrial hyperplasia, which can lead to endometrial cancer.

COCs. Low-dose COCs are known to control excessive or irregular bleeding and decrease menstrual flow. They cycle and suppress the endometrium. Oral contraceptives regulate bleeding patterns significantly more than placebo and result in a reduction of blood flow by 43 to 68 percent (Farquhar & Brown, 2009). The oral contraceptive regimen will depend on if the DUB is currently mild, moderate, heavy, or severe DUB. Note that the contraceptive patch and ring are other estrogen–progestin preparations that could be tried in place of oral contraceptives depending on the woman's personal preference. However, there are no data if control of uterine bleeding is indeed the same, superior, or less than the standard oral contraceptive (ACOG, 2010). See Chapter 12 for further information on these methods.

In cases of severe DUB, the main goal is to prevent anemia and hypovolemia. Ferrous sulfate 300 mg may be taken by mouth with orange juice 30 minutes after meals in addition to the following therapies if the hemoglobin level is below 12 g.

NSAIDs. NSAIDs inhibit the synthesis of prostaglandins that leads to vasoconstriction, reducing menstrual blood loss by 20 to 50 percent. Prescribe the following at the onset of menses. The client is to use NSAIDs for a minimum of 3 to 5 days and may use through the end of her menses. Treatment options are as follows:

- Mefenamic acid (Ponstel®) 500 mg po tid (41,47) *or* naproxen (Naprosyn®) 500 mg po at onset of menses and 3 to 5 hours later, then 250 to 500 mg twice a day (28,48,49) *or* ibuprofen (Motrin®) 600 mg every 6 hours with food.
- Side effects and adverse reactions include gastrointestinal upset (take with food to lessen), rash, and edema.
- Contraindications include pregnancy, peptic ulcers, asthma, sensitivity to aspirin, cardiovascular disease, coagulopathy, and inflammatory bowel disease.

Treatment Protocols for Varying Levels of Severity of DUB

- *Mild DUB:* If menses are longer than normal or cycles shortened for more than 2 months and Hgb is normal and contraception is not needed.
  - Reassurance and observation with a menstrual calendar, NSAIDs, and a multivitamin.
- *Moderate DUB:* Menses somewhat prolonged, heavier, cycle shortened with menses every 1 to 3 weeks, moderate to heavy flow with a mild anemia (Hgb greater than 10).
  - Start an oral contraceptive pill with a minimum of 30 μg estradiol to stabilize as well as start supplemental iron and high iron foods.
  - Alternatively, if currently bleeding, may take COCs twice a day until the bleeding stops and then continue on to once per day.
- *Heavy DUB:* Prolonged heavy bleeding with Hgb greater than 10.
  - Discuss plan with acute care provider.
  - The following regimen with a 35 μg oral contraceptive pill is recommended, in those without

contraindications to estrogen (keep in mind use of an antiemetic such as promethazine or ondansetron may be needed):
  - One pill four times a day for 4 days, one pill three times a day for 3 days, one pill twice a day for 2 weeks, then withdraw, slough 4 to 7 days. Then cycle one pill per day 3 to 6 months.
- *Severe DUB:* Prolonged heavy bleeding with Hgb less than 10.
  - Contact an acute care provider immediately.
  - Patients with severe anemia or life-threatening bleeding require immediate management for intravenous fluids, blood transfusion, and conjugated estrogen and/or a dilation and curettage may be necessary (Staggers, 2010b).

Progesterone. Progesterone is indicated for clients with anovulatory bleeding in whom estrogen is contraindicated and contraception is not needed.

Medroxyprogesterone or Micronized Progesterone

- If the client is currently bleeding, treatment with 200 mg of micronized progesterone can help stop bleeding. The client should take one pill every 4 hours until the bleeding stops. Once the bleeding stops, take one pill four times a day for 4 days, then three times a day for 3 days, then twice a day for 2 weeks.
- If the client is not currently bleeding, a cyclic oral regimen is used to induce regular withdrawal bleeding to prevent endometrial hyperplasia. This should be done monthly for a minimum of 3 months (Fraser, 1990). Ten milligrams of medroxyprogesterone or 200 mg of micronized progesterone is given once per day for 10 days each month.
- Contraindications (see *Progesterone* in Amenorrhea section of this chapter).
- Anticipated outcome on evaluation is that the first episode of bleeding after progesterone therapy will be heavy.
- Client teaching should include information about the possibility of bleeding being heavy when medication is completed. Emphasize the importance of taking medication to prevent endometrial hyperplasia or cancer. Inform the client of side effects (spotting, weight gain, fatigue, depression, or acne) as well as for her to report any abnormal bleeding or the absence of a withdrawal bleed (Fraser, 1990).

DMPA. More commonly known by its trade name Depo-Provera®, DMPA may be given to suppress the endometrium and provide contraception.

- It is given following the same guidelines and schedule as when it is being used for contraception.
- Anticipated outcome is reduced vaginal bleeding, perhaps cessation of menses. However, it is not unusual to experience unscheduled bleeding after the first injection(s).
- See Chapter 12 for more information.

LNG-IUS. Mirena® is a T-shaped contraceptive device placed within the uterine cavity that releases 20 μg per day of levonorgestrel. Menorrhagia generally improves on average by approximately 85 percent after 1 year of use. After 6 months, the majority of clients have amenorrhea or oligomenorrhea. It has been approved for the treatment of heavy menstrual bleeding (U.S. Food and Drug Administration [FDA], 2009). The LNG-IUS appears to be more effective than other hormonal treatments (Kaunitz et al., 2010). Like DMPA, for the first 3 to 6 months, unscheduled bleeding is quite common. Potential contraindications include pregnancy or suspicion of pregnancy, current cervical or endometrial infection, or uterine anomaly. See Chapter 12 for more information.

Other Medical Treatments

- Antifibrinolytic agents such as tranexamic acid—1,300 mg three times per day during menses for a maximum of 5 days—reduce menstrual flow by 30 to 50 percent. Tranexamic acid was approved by the FDA in 2009 for treatment of menorrhagia. However, the risk of thrombotic events with this group of medications is controversial (Roy & Bhattacharya, 2004).
- GnRH agonist, goserelin, causes amenorrhea by inducing a menopausal-like state. Cost and undesirable side effects limit its use (Irvine & Cameron, 1999).
- Danazol is an androgenic hormone that blocks gonadotropins and suppresses ovarian estrogen production. The endometrium thins and amenorrhea occurs. At 200 to 400 mg a day, it does reduce heavy menstrual bleeding. Side effects (possible virilization and thromboembolism) and the cost of Danazol limit its use (Stabinsky, Einstien, & Breen, 1999).

Surgical Interventions. Ablation or endometrial destruction techniques vary. Consultation and referral to a gynecologist is appropriate. Ablation of the endometrium reduces menstrual blood loss by approximately

85 percent, similarly as effective as the LNG-IUS. An advantage is it needs to be performed only once. However, a woman must be certain she has completed childbearing before undergoing ablation. Contraception is still required post procedure (Lethaby & Hickey, 2009). Hysterectomy is a last choice if medical treatment fails. Any surgical procedure and the expected course must be explained fully and follow-up planned.

Follow-Up. Anovulatory patterns tend to recur; therefore, clients should have a regular follow-up schedule and keep a menstrual and medication calendar. If more than a year elapses without a health care visit, notify the client. Cancer prevention should be a priority with this population. Ideally, the client is being seen every 3 to 6 months. Refer any patient who is not responding to treatments to appropriate specialist.

DYSMENORRHEA

Dysmenorrhea is the most common gynecologic condition experienced by menstruating women. The term *dysmenorrhea* is derived from the Greek words *dys* (difficult, painful, or abnormal), *meno* (month), and *rrhea* (flow). Dysmenorrhea is described as cramping pain in the lower abdomen that can range widely in severity and associated symptoms. Yet, its overall impact has significant medical and psychosocial implications (Morrow & Naumburg, 2009). Dysmenorrhea is divided into two categories: primary and secondary. Primary dysmenorrhea refers to the presence of crampy, lower abdominal pain that occurs just before and/or during menses in the absence of pelvic disease. Secondary dysmenorrhea refers to painful menstruation in the presence of a pelvic pathology, such as endometriosis, adenomyosis, uterine leiomyomas, or pelvic inflammatory disease (Proctor & Farquhar, 2006).

Epidemiology

Etiology. Primary dysmenorrhea is thought to occur in ovulatory cycles; therefore, symptoms typically do not begin with the first menstrual cycles after menarche, because they are likely to be anovulatory. Ovulation is thought to be associated with menstrual cycles 2 to 4 years after menarche in most women, but for some it may start earlier (Morrow & Naumburg, 2009). The most common explanation for dysmenorrhea is an overproduction of prostaglandins within the endometrium. Progesterone is the dominant hormone in the luteal phase and it stimulates the production of prostaglandins in endometrial cells. As menstruation begins, the production of prostaglandins with endometrium sloughing causes the uterus to contract. The contractions reduce blood flow and cause ischemia, and therefore, pain (Proctor & Farquhar, 2006). Vasopressin may also play a role by increasing uterine contractility, leading to vasoconstriction and ischemia. Elevated levels of prostaglandins and vasopressin have been observed in women with primary dysmenorrhea (French, 2008). Associated symptoms that are common with dysmenorrhea are nausea, vomiting, diarrhea, headache, malaise, or fatigue. It is thought that these symptoms may be related to prostaglandin release into the circulation (Morrow & Naumburg, 2009).

Secondary dysmenorrhea is painful menstruation due to pelvic or uterine pathology. These women may have other complaints such as nonmenstrual-related pelvic pain or pain with intercourse (Proctor & Farquhar, 2006).

Incidence. Most women experience some degree of dysmenorrhea. It is estimated that between 45 and 95 percent of women suffer from dysmenorrhea. It is the most common gynecological condition in women regardless of age, though it seems to be more common in adolescent females. Absenteeism from work and school as a result of dysmenorrhea is common, and if severe, it can be associated with restriction of activity and negative impact on quality of life (Proctor & Farquhar, 2006; Smith, 2008).

A number of factors have been associated with increased risk for primary dysmenorrhea, though the literature contains limited consensus. Some of the risk factors that have been identified are adolescence, anxiety or stress, BMI < 20 or > 30 kg/m^2, depression, eating disorder, disrupted social networks, family history, menarche at a young age, menorrhagia, metrorrhagia, nulliparity, and smoking (Morrow & Naumburg, 2009).

Subjective Data

Typically, the onset of primary dysmenorrhea is described as crampy, achy, or dull and located in the midline suprapubic region. Radiation of pain to the back, legs, and abdomen can be associated as well. This pain may begin hours to a few days before menses begins and often persists for 24 to 48 hours (Morrow & Naumburg, 2009). Some women experience related premenstrual symptoms that may include nausea, vomiting, fatigue, dizziness, diarrhea, nervousness, and headache (Proctor & Farquhar, 2006).

Secondary dysmenorrhea can occur at any time after menarche, but may arise as a new symptom later in a woman's life, after the onset of the underlying condition. The timing and intensity of the pain may change. Other symptoms may also be present such as dyspareunia, menorrhagia, metrorrhagia, postcoital bleeding, irregular cycles, urinary complaints, diarrhea, and vaginal discharge (Proctor & Farquhar, 2006; Reddish, 2006). A key defining factor in secondary dysmenorrhea is the presence of symptoms of pain and bleeding that persist beyond the normal menstrual cycle (Morrow & Naumburg, 2009).

A thorough history should be performed including assessment of the pain, associated symptoms, medications, family history, sexual history, gynecological history, social assessment and significance of the pain on the patient's life and daily activities, and cultural assessment of attitude toward menstruation (Reddish, 2006).

Objective Data

Physical Examination. It may be appropriate to perform only an abdominal examination in young adolescents with a typical history who have never been sexually active. For the sexually active female, a thorough pelvic exam is mandatory to establish diagnosis (French, 2005). Screening for STIs is indicated by the patient's history or symptoms. With primary dysmenorrhea, pelvic findings will be completely within normal limits except a mildly tender uterus on examination. Secondary dysmenorrhea, however, may reveal an assortment of pelvic pathologies, depending on the etiology of the problem. Endometriosis may present with a normal pelvic exam or the exam may reveal nodularity, thickening or focal tenderness of the uterosacral ligament, cervical stenosis, fixed ovaries or uterus due to adhesions, and possible adnexal fullness from endometrioma. An enlarged uterus that is soft and tender with normal mobility may be present in a woman with adenomyosis. Leiomyomas are to be suspected if the uterus is enlarged, firm, and/or of irregular shape. Infection is suspected with presence of discharge, cervical motion tenderness, adnexal tenderness, and/or uterine tenderness. Fever may also be present (Morrow & Naumburg, 2009).

Diagnostic Tests and Methods

Laboratory Tests

- Swabs as appropriate for gonorrhea, chlamydia, wet mount. Urinalysis and/or culture may be indicated based on symptoms. Pregnancy testing if suspicion for miscarriage is present.

Diagnostic Imaging

- Pelvic ultrasound may be indicated for a woman with an abnormal finding on physical exam that causes suspicion for secondary dysmenorrhea or structural abnormality such as leiomyoma, ovarian cyst, endometrioma, or congenital abnormality. It may also be indicated for women with severe dysmenorrhea that is unresponsive to initial treatment.
- Sonohysterogram may be useful in diagnosing endometriosis, although laparoscopy is the gold standard for this.
- MRI has been shown to be rather limited in its ability to diagnose endometriosis, but may be useful for detection of obstructive abnormalities.

Laparoscopy. Referral for laparoscopy is indicated if initial measures have not improved symptoms, if secondary dysmenorrhea is present, or if the patient has pain management problems that are impacting daily activities. Laparoscopy is useful for diagnosing and staging endometriosis. It may also be considered a treatment as removing endometrial implants may reduce pain (French, 2008; Morrow & Naumburg, 2009; Proctor & Farquhar, 2006).

Differential Medical Diagnoses

Although the clinical picture of dysmenorrhea is often clear cut, several differential diagnoses need to be considered. Secondary dysmenorrhea must be excluded before a diagnosis of primary dysmenorrhea can be assumed. Other etiologies to consider include pelvic infections, adenomyosis, leiomyomas, menorrhagia, endometrial/ovarian carcinoma, miscarriage, cervical stenosis, pelvic adhesions, ectopic pregnancy, retained tampon, IUD, polyps, congenital abnormalities, ovarian cysts, or dermoid tumors. A few other differentials to keep in mind are disorders of the urinary tract, renal calculi, irritable bowel syndrome, chronic constipation, inflammatory bowel disease, diverticulitis, psychosomatic disorders, depression, or musculoskeletal disorder (Harel, 2006; Reddish, 2006).

Plan

Psychosocial Interventions. Helping the client to understand the normal events surrounding the menstrual cycle and the etiology of the dysmenorrhea is an important part of intervention. It provides the client with the vocabulary to communicate more accurately about symptoms, and helps to dispel myths. In addition, intervention is directed toward pain relief and coping strategies that will promote a productive lifestyle. Give the client charts to record menses, onset of pain, timing of medication, relief afforded by the medication, and relationship of pain to basal body temperature. Charts can be used as a teaching tool as they provide the client with a realistic picture of her pain and an objective record for modifying future therapy.

Carefully explain the nature and severity of the pathology associated with secondary dysmenorrhea. Discuss in detail the rationales for selecting particular tests, treatments, medications, or surgery; this will enhance client understanding and compliance. Be sure to address the impact that the disease and treatment will have on fertility. Women may need social, financial, and emotional support related to the effects of missing school and work and should be referred as needed (Reddish, 2006).

Lifestyle Changes. Share information about lifestyle factors that can be initiated to restore some sense of control and alleviate the sense of frustration and victimization. For example, exercise increases endorphins, suppresses prostaglandin release, decreases endometrial proliferation, and shunts blood away from the uterus; pelvic congestion and pain are thereby decreased. Menus can be planned to limit salty foods, increase fiber with fresh fruits and vegetables, and increase water to serve as a natural diuretic. Heating pads or warm baths decrease muscle spasms and may increase comfort. Relaxation techniques, massage, physical exercise, and yoga may minimize dysmenorrhea, can supplement medication regimens, and enhance the client's ability to deal with pain (Reddish, 2006).

Medications

Prostaglandin Inhibitors. The most established initial therapy for dysmenorrhea is NSAIDs. They have direct analgesic effect through inhibition of prostaglandin synthesis, and they also decrease the volume of menstrual flow. Approximately 70 percent of women experience moderate to complete relief of painful cramping with the use of NSAIDs (Morrow & Naumburg, 2009). An extensive Cochrane review recommends ibuprofen, mefenamic acid, and naproxen as first-line treatment based on effectiveness and tolerability. Dosing ranges for NSAIDs vary considerably and women should be counseled to use the lowest effective dose that improves symptoms, but minimizes common side effects of nausea, gastrointestinal distress or dyspepsia, drowsiness, fluid retention, and diarrhea. Recommend that women take these medications with food to reduce the risk of gastrointestinal upset. There has been some research suggesting that beginning the medication before the onset of symptoms may be more effective than waiting for symptoms to occur; this may be difficult for women with irregular cycles. It is typically recommended that continuous use for the 2 to 5 days when symptoms persist is more effective than episodic use. The cyclooxygenase-2 (COX-2) inhibitors are effective in treating dysmenorrhea with less gastrointestinal side effects, but concerns about cardiovascular risks have prompted withdrawal of most of these agents from the market (Mannix, 2008; Proctor & Farquhar, 2006).

COCs. COCs are an appropriate second-line therapeutic option for dysmenorrhea if NSAIDs are inadequate or if a woman desires the added benefit of contraception. COCs suppress ovulation and reduce the amount of prostaglandin produced by the endometrial lining, which then reduces both uterine blood flow and cramps. Low-dose COCs containing less than 35 mcg of ethinyl estradiol have been shown to be effective and are the recommended preparation (Wong, Farquhar, Roberts, & Proctor, 2009). Nonsystematic reviews claim that COCs are up to 90 percent effective in the treatment of dysmenorrhea. A recent Cochrane review, however, concluded that there was insufficient evidence to support the statement that COCs were effective in treating primary dysmenorrhea (Morrow & Naumburg, 2009).

The vaginal contraceptive ring has also exhibited a reduction in dysmenorrhea, though the data is limited (Morrow & Naumburg, 2009). A small study using the transdermal contraceptive patch for at least 6 months found that 39 percent reported a decrease in dysmenorrhea, although 11 percent reported an increase in pain. The patch appeared to be less effective than oral contraceptives in another study (French, 2008).

Extended cycle or continuous use of low-dose monophasic COCs has become an increasingly popular option for treating a number of hormonal-related symptoms, including pelvic pain, premenstrual symptoms, menorrhagia, and the inconvenience of monthly menstrual cycles. Continuous use or extended cycles with COCs inducing a withdrawal bleed only every 3 months may offer additional benefit by elimination of menstruation and the associated symptoms. Although it seems reasonable that decreasing the frequency of menstrual periods would lead to diminished dysmenorrhea, there are no strong data to support this method as an effective treatment (Morrow & Naumburg, 2009). The data is also limited on the use of COCs for reducing severity of dysmenorrhea in women with endometriosis (ACOG, 2010).

Progesterone Contraceptives. Studies have established the usefulness of DMPA for secondary dysmenorrhea, but have not evaluated the efficacy in patients with primary dysmenorrhea. The single-rod contraceptive progestin implant, Implanon®, also appears to reduce dysmenorrhea symptoms in most users. Both DMPA and the progestin contraceptive implant have been proven to reduce pain with endometriosis (ACOG,

2010). The data on the effects of the LNG-IUS is limited, though the device decreases the amount of menstrual flow and suppresses endometrial thickening; therefore, it would seem to produce a positive benefit. It has been shown to decrease dysmenorrhea by as much as 50 percent (Morrow & Naumburg, 2009). The LNG-IUS has also been shown to reduce dysmenorrhea and chronic pelvic pain associated with endometriosis in several trials (ACOG, 2010).

Complementary and Alternative Therapies. Those women who do not respond to traditional treatment or women with contraindications for their use may seek alternative treatment options for dysmenorrhea. There is some evidence that behavioral therapy such as relaxation may be effective for dysmenorrhea. Progressive muscle relaxation with or without imagery and relaxation may help with spasmodic symptoms of menstrual pain (Proctor, Murphy, Pattison, Suckling, & Farquhar, 2011). Acupuncture also shows promising evidence for the treatment of primary dysmenorrhea when compared with pharmacological treatment of herbal medicine. Methodological flaws have limited results of recent studies and effectiveness is not evident when compared with sham acupuncture; therefore, further trials are needed (Cho & Hwang, 2010). Spinal manipulation has not been shown to be an effective therapy for dysmenorrhea (Proctor, Hing, Johnson, Murphy, & Brown, 2010).

Some women may desire to try herbal supplements or dietary treatments for dysmenorrhea. Vitamin B_1, or thiamine, is a water-soluble vitamin found in most diets. It has been suggested to be helpful with pain, muscle cramping, and fatigue. Recent studies have not proven that vitamin B_1 is any more beneficial than placebo. Additional studies are recommended. However, counseling on ensuring that women are receiving appropriate dietary intake would be reasonable. Magnesium is thought to help decrease prostaglandin synthesis and has been hypothesized to be helpful in the treatment of dysmenorrhea. Studies have not shown significant differences between taking magnesium or placebo in regard to pain scores; therefore, no recommendation can be made until further research is carried out (Braxton Loyd & Hornsby, 2009; Proctor & Murphy, 2010).

Follow-Up. Follow-up of clients with primary dysmenorrhea can be done on a regular gynecologic exam schedule once a medical regimen has been found that relieves pain adequately and is well tolerated. Follow clients with secondary dysmenorrhea according to the diagnosis, the type of medication prescribed, and the need for investigative or therapeutic surgery.

TOXIC SHOCK SYNDROME

Toxic shock syndrome (TSS) is a systemic disease marked by acute onset of fever, hypotension, myalgia, rash, multiple-organ failure, and late desquamation of hands and feet. It is associated with the colonization of toxin-producing *Staphylococcus aureus* in the vagina during menstruation, at other sites due to complications of a staphylococcal infection, or as a complication of a surgical procedure or other medical condition (Parsonnet et al., 2005). These bacteria have the ability to secrete toxins, called *superantigens*, which can trigger a widespread immune response. One *S. aureus* exotoxin has been identified in causing virtually all cases of menstrual TSS or TSST-1 (TSS toxin-1). It has the ability to absorb through the mucosa, such as the kind inside the vagina. When it enters the blood stream, it causes an exaggerated immune response (Lesher, DeCries, Danila, & Lynfield, 2009). The criteria established by the Centers for Disease Control and Prevention (CDC, 1997) to diagnose TSS include fever > 38.9°C, hypotension, diffuse erythroderma, desquamation of the palms and soles, and the involvement of three or more major organ systems.

Epidemiology

Etiology. The clinical manifestations of TSS result from the immune system's reaction to exotoxins produced by bacteria. Most TSS-susceptible patients are lacking specific antibodies that block the superantigens. A cause may never be identified (Lillitos, Harford, & Michie, 2007).

Incidence. The national incidence of TSS sharply declined after the removal of high-absorbency tampons from the market and public awareness campaigns during the years 1980 to 1996. However, the ability to recognize this condition remains important.

Subjective Data

Menstrual-related TSS presents with an abrupt onset of symptoms including high fever, chills, vomiting, diarrhea, myalgia, headaches, rash, or abdominal pain in a previously healthy young woman during or shortly after menstruation (Nikkanen, Sisson, & Blok, 2007).

Objective Data

Physical Examination Findings

- Fever ≥38.9°C (102.0°F)
- Hypotension has systolic blood pressure < 90 mm Hg for adults or <5th percentile by age for children

<16 years of age; orthostatic decrease in diastolic blood pressure >5 mm Hg from lying to sitting

- Diffuse macular erythroderma, sunburn-like rash develops 24 to 48 hours after onset of symptoms and progressed to desquamation
- Desquamation occurs 1 to 2 weeks after onset of illness, usually on the palms and soles
- Multisystem involvement is typical; hemodynamic instability is prominent
  - Gastrointestinal—vomiting or diarrhea at onset of illness, abdominal tenderness
  - Musculoskeletal—creatine phosphokinase level at least twice the upper limit of normal
  - Mucous membranes—vaginal, oropharyngeal, or conjunctival hyperemia
  - Renal—blood urea nitrogen or creatinine level at least twice the upper limit of normal, urinary sediment with pyuria (≥ 5 WBCs) in the absence of urinary tract infection
  - Hepatic—total bilirubin, alanine aminotransferase, or aspartate aminotransferase levels at least twice the upper limit of normal
  - Hematologic—platelet counts $\leq 100 \times 10^9$/L
  - Respiratory—acute respiratory distress syndrome, pneumonia, reactive airways
  - Central nervous system—disorientation or alterations in consciousness without focal neurologic signs when fever and hypotension are absent
- Negative laboratory results on blood, throat, or cerebrospinal fluid cultures (may be positive for *S. aureus*). No increase in titer for Rocky Mountain spotted fever, leptospirosis, or measles.

Differential Medical Diagnoses

Sepsis caused by other bacteria, staphylococcal scalded skin syndrome, typhoid fever, Rocky Mountain spotted fever, meningococcemia, exanthematous viral syndromes, necrotizing fasciitis, and leptospirosis needs to be considered and ruled out. Severe hyperthermia, heat stroke drug reactions, and insect-related allergic reactions are noninfectious causes on the differential list (Cosgrove, 2006; Lillitos et al., 2007).

Plan

TSS requires immediate physician referral and hospitalization. Early and aggressive hospital-based treatment is vital. Initial management should include cleaning of any obvious wounds, removal of foreign bodies, and drainage of affected tissues. TSS has a high mortality rate, although if treated quickly, most patients recover without long-term problems. Antibiotic therapy is necessary to remove the bacteria making the toxin. Clindamycin and anti-staphylococcal penicillin are used initially. Patients with TSS due to methicillin-resistant *Staphylococcus aureus* (MRSA) receive clindamycin plus either vancomycin or linezolid (Lillitos et al., 2007).

Follow-Up. Inform the client that subsequent milder attacks of TSS may develop within 2 to 3 months, encourage compliance with antibiotics, and discourage tampon use. If tampons are continued, only the lowest absorbency should be used. Advise good handwashing with soap prior to insertion or removal of tampons and recommend intermittent use with pads. Advise the woman to use barrier contraceptive methods carefully and to adhere to the manufacturer's directions. Also advise to seek medical care promptly if develops any reoccurrence of symptoms of TSS, such as fever or rash (Nikkanen et al., 2007).

PREMENSTRUAL SYNDROME AND PREMENSTRUAL DYSPHORIC DISORDER

Premenstrual syndrome (PMS) is a common cyclic disorder that is characterized by emotional and physical symptoms that consistently occur during the luteal phase of the menstrual cycle. Women with more severe affective symptoms may be classified as having premenstrual dysphoric disorder (PMDD) (Steiner et al., 2006). PMS and PMDD can negatively impact a woman's daily activities at home and work and negatively impact quality of life (Bahamondes, Cordova-Eguez, Pons, & Shulman, 2007).

Epidemiology

Etiology. The exact cause of PMS is not known, but research suggests that it involves the altered regulation of neurohormones and neurotransmitters. The rising and falling levels of hormones may influence chemicals in the brain, including serotonin, which affects mood. A number of studies have explored the role of a genetic predisposition to PMS and PMDD and find a strong correlation. In one of the largest twin studies, premenstrual symptoms were found to be highly heritable, although there was also noted contribution from individual environmental factors (Bahamondes et al., 2007). Androgens have also been considered to play a role due to the prominence of irritability in PMDD, but there has not been conclusive research. However, some success has been reported in treating PMDD with androgen antagonists (Vigod, Ross, & Steiner, 2009). Additionally, a history of depressive disorder appears to increase a woman's vulnerability to premenstrual symptoms, especially in regard to the severity and duration of the mood changes (Winer & Rapkin, 2006).

Incidence. It is estimated that up to 90 percent of women of reproductive age experience premenstrual symptoms or molimina. An estimated 20 to 40 percent of reproductive-age women have symptoms bothersome enough to meet ACOG criteria for PMS. A smaller subset of an estimated 3 to 8 percent of reproductive-age women meets the specific diagnostic criteria for PMDD (Winer & Rapkin, 2006).

Subjective Data

More than 300 symptoms have been associated with PMS (Freeman, 2007). The most common physical complaint is abdominal bloating, which occurs in 90 percent of women. Breast tenderness, headaches, fluid retention, increased appetite, weight gain, cravings, acne, fatigue, heart palpitations, dizziness, gastrointestinal symptoms, mood swings, irritability, anxiety, depression, libido changes, crying easily, poor concentration, and hot flashes are other common subjective findings (Steiner et al., 2006). The symptoms must be present in the luteal phase, approximately 2 weeks before menstruation begins to qualify as PMS symptoms.

Diagnostic Criteria for PMS. ACOG has identified guidelines for the diagnosis of PMS. These criteria require that one or more affective or somatic symptoms must be present in the 5 days before menstruation for at least three menstrual cycles in a row. The symptoms must end within 4 days after menstruation starts and cause significant impairment or distress on normal activities that cannot be accounted for by another diagnosis (Bahamondes et al., 2007).

Diagnostic Criteria for PMDD. The American Psychiatric Association's *Diagnostic and Statistical Manual of Mental Disorders* (*DSM-IV*) has outlined criteria for the diagnosis of PMDD, which is listed next. The primary difference between the ACOG guidelines for PMS and PMDD is the number of symptoms required for the diagnosis (Freeman, 2007).

- One-year duration of at least five or more of the following symptoms must have been present during the week prior to menses and resolving within a few days after menses starts. At least one symptom must be one of the first four listed.
    - Depressed mood, feelings of hopelessness, or self-deprecating thoughts
    - Feeling tense, anxious
    - Marked lability of mood with intermittent periods of tearfulness
    - Persistent irritability, anger, and increased interpersonal conflicts
    - Decreased interest in usual activities
    - Difficulty concentrating
    - Feeling fatigued, lethargic, or lacking of energy
    - Changes in appetite, cravings, binge eating
    - Hypersomnia or insomnia
    - Feeling of being overwhelmed or out of control
    - Physical symptoms such as breast tenderness, headache, join and muscle pains, bloating, or weight gain
- Symptoms must start or resolve within a few days of onset of menses and be absent during the week after menstruation stops.
- Symptoms must markedly impair the patient's ability to work, attend school, or conduct usual daily activities.
- The diagnosis must be confirmed by prospective daily ratings for at least two consecutive symptomatic menstrual cycles (Steiner et al., 2006).

Objective Data

There are no characteristic physical findings or laboratory testing associated with PMS and PMDD, but a complete medical history and physical examination should be performed to rule out any other illnesses. Some tests that are recommended to rule out other disorders with similar symptoms include pregnancy testing if indicated, and hormonal assays to rule out menopause, hypothyroidism, and hyperprolactinemia may be of some benefit. A CBC and other assays to assess for hyperandrogynism or hypoglycemia may be indicated as well as routine preventative health care screening based on guidelines (Freeman, 2007; Rapkin, 2006).

Differential Medical Diagnoses

To diagnose PMS and PMDD, it is important to rule out premenstrual exacerbation of an existing psychiatric disorder or underlying medical condition. Differential diagnoses include underlying major psychiatric disorders, such as depression, anxiety, dysthymia, personality- or panic-related disorders, eating disorders, anemia, drug or alcohol abuse, physical/sexual/emotional abuse, chronic medical conditions, endocrine disorders, autoimmune disorders, dysmenorrhea, endometriosis, and perimenopause (Dickerson, Mazyck, & Hunter, 2003; Freeman, 2007).

Plan

When PMS or PMDD is suspected, patients should be instructed to keep a premenstrual daily symptom diary for several consecutive months to confirm luteal-phase symptoms. The Calendar of Premenstrual Experiences is an example of a standardized calendar that is reliable and convenient (Dickerson et al., 2003) See Appendix B. The treatment for PMS and PMDD should involve an integrated approach tailored to each patient's individual circumstances. In all cases, it is critical to first address any underlying psychiatric disorders, medical conditions, life stressors, or any past or current physical or sexual abuse (Vigod et al., 2009).

Lifestyle Modifications. For women with mild symptoms, education about the condition and providing supportive counseling on healthy lifestyle measures, such as regular exercise, good amount of sleep, and healthy diet, may be sufficient to result in improvement of symptoms. Women should be encouraged to reduce or eliminate the intake of salty foods, sugar, caffeine, red meat, and alcohol (Vigod et al., 2009). It is recommended that women try to eat more frequent, small meals with consumption of complex carbohydrates, whole grains, fruits, vegetables, and legumes and reduced consumption of refined sugar and artificial sweeteners (Pearlstein & Steiner, 2008). Research supporting the benefit of exercise on limiting premenstrual symptoms is limited due to the difficulty of employing a double-blind study. However, regular exercise is recommended for all and may be helpful in decreasing fluid retention and the release of endorphins may help moods. Aerobic exercise should be recommended for 30 minutes, most days of the week (Kroll & Rapkin, 2006). It is also recommended that these women adhere to consistent bedtimes and waking times, especially during the premenstrual period, but also throughout the cycle (Vigod et al., 2009).

Psychosocial Treatments. Group psychoeducation can be effective in managing PMS and PMDD. Several studies noted efficacy of group support for managing symptoms of PMS. Relaxation therapy has also been shown to be effective in treating PMS. Cognitive-behavioral therapy (CBT) may be an effective treatment although there are limited quality studies and the effects do not approach those of pharmacotherapy or even behavioral treatments, such as relaxation (Kroll & Rapkin, 2006; Pearlstein & Steiner, 2008; Vigod et al., 2009).

Nonprescription Medications. Several nonprescription medications are available over the counter that contain mild diuretics, analgesics, prostaglandin inhibitors, and antihistamines. Women should be cautioned that these products may provide inadequate doses of some ingredients and excessive doses of others. NSAIDs can be effective in alleviating various physical symptoms, such as dysmenorrhea and headache (Dickerson et al., 2003).

Serotonergic Drugs. For women who do not respond to conservative therapies or who have severe symptoms requiring immediate treatment, selective serotonin reuptake inhibitors (SSRIs) are the first line of treatment (Vigod et al., 2009). Studies have shown that 50 to 60 percent of women with severe PMS or PMDD respond to SSRIs. One of the leading theories behind these disorders is related to an abnormal serotonergic response in vulnerable women (Freeman, 2007). Over the past several years, SSRIs were found to be highly effective in treating physical, functional, and behavioral symptoms. Luteal phase–only and continuous administration have both been found to be effective (Brown, O'Brien, Marjoribanks, & Wyatt, 2009). Continuous SSRI therapy may be a rational choice for patients with comorbid depressive or anxiety disorders, those not fully adherent to the dosing schedule, or those who experience adverse symptoms after abruptly discontinuing therapy postmenstrually. Intermittent SSRI therapy is the logical option for patients whose mood symptoms are limited to the luteal phase, those who do not want to take the medication for the entire month, or those who experience adverse effects, such as sexual dysfunction (Steiner et al., 2006). The FDA has approved fluoxetine, sertraline, and paroxetine for the treatment of PMDD (Vigod et al., 2009). A Cochrane database meta-analysis also suggests good evidence of effectiveness for fluvoxamine, citalopram, and tricyclic antidepressant clomipramine (Brown et al., 2009). Common side effects of SSRIs include insomnia, drowsiness, fatigue, nausea, nervousness, headache, mild tremor, and sexual dysfunction. Side effects are typically mild. Counsel patients that beneficial effects are not immediate and it may take 2 to 4 weeks (Dickerson et al., 2003).

Hormonal Manipulation of Menstruation. The goal with using hormonal treatments is to manipulate the usual hormonal fluctuations associated with the menstrual cycle. Although many hormonal regimens have been suggested for this purpose, few have demonstrated efficacy and their use can be limited by significant adverse effects and treatment costs (Dickerson et al., 2003; Vigod et al., 2009).

COCs. COCs have commonly been prescribed by clinicians for the treatment of PMS even though there were few studies demonstrating their efficacy until recently. COCs are a reasonably safe means of inhibiting ovulation.

Benefits from COCs are probably due to the estrogenic component; therefore, monophasic pills may be the most appropriate. COCs may improve physical symptoms such as bloating, headaches, abdominal pain, and breast tenderness (Dickerson et al., 2003). The FDA has approved a combination of 20 mcg of ethinyl estradiol with drospirenone for the treatment of PMDD. The efficacy of this particular COC may be due to its administration in a 24/4 regimen, which provides more stable hormone levels and reduces adverse symptoms that occur during withdrawal bleeding. Drospirenone may also be more efficacious due to its unique antimineralocorticoid and antiandrogenic properties (Pearlstein & Steiner, 2008). The potential for adverse effects with oral contraceptives, such as thromboembolic events, exceeds that of SSRIs; therefore, the FDA indication for this treatment has been limited to women who also wish to use the medication for contraceptive purposes (Vigod et al., 2009). A direct comparison of drospirenone-containing COC and the intravaginal contraceptive ring reported equivalent improvement in PMS. COCs containing 30 mcg of ethinyl estradiol with drospirenone have also been shown to decrease premenstrual mood deterioration in women receiving treatment for depression. Another approach that appears to be helpful for PMS is to suppress menstruation and further stabilize hormones with extended cycle or continuous COC regimens (ACOG, 2010).

Progesterone. There is limited evidence for treating premenstrual disorders with progesterone. It has been suggested that PMS might be caused by too little progesterone or falling levels after ovulation, though abnormal hormone levels have not been demonstrated in women with PMS or PMDD (Pearlstein & Steiner, 2008). Trials have not proven progesterone to be effective. The studies had flaws in methods or in handling outcome data; therefore, more research is needed to test claims for effectiveness of progesterone. Adverse effects were thought to be generally mild (Ford, Lethaby, Roberts, & Mol, 2009).

Other Ovulation Suppression Treatments. GnRH agonists, such as leuprolide acetate, have been clearly demonstrated to alleviate symptoms of PMS and PMDD. These drugs work by inhibiting the release of pituitary gonadotropins (Dickerson et al., 2003). However, GnRH agonists appear to be less effective in treating affective symptoms of PMDD than physical symptoms. Long-term use of these medications has been associated with a number of adverse side effects, including risk for hypoestrogenism and osteoporosis, especially when use is longer than 6 months. If treatment for more than 6 months is necessary, add-back estrogen therapy with estrogen and/or progesterone should be considered, but this may lead to a recurrence of premenstrual symptoms (Pearlstein & Steiner, 2008; Vigod et al., 2009).

Danazol is a synthetic steroid that can alleviate premenstrual symptoms when administered at dosages that suppress ovulation. However, it is limited by side effects, such as masculinization, as well as adverse effects on liver function tests and serum lipid profiles (Pearlstein & Steiner, 2008). It is also limited by the need for a concurrent contraceptive method due to possible virilization of the fetus if a woman became pregnant during treatment (Vigod et al., 2009).

The final treatment option for women with severe PMDD symptoms and no response to other therapies is permanent suppression of ovulation through oophorectomy. Because of the extremeness of this treatment and possibility of triggering mood problems associated with surgical menopause, it is not recommended (Vigod et al., 2009).

Dietary Supplements. Several dietary supplements are recommended in the lay press for treatment of premenstrual disorders, but unfortunately little scientific evidence is available to support these recommendations. Calcium supplementation has shown some promise at decreasing premenstrual symptoms. Because increased calcium intake is recommended for prevention of osteoporosis and there are no known adverse effects so long as doses do not exceed 1,500 mg/day, supplementing may be of benefit for women with PMS or PMDD (Kroll & Rapkin, 2006; Vigod et al., 2009). There is also some evidence for the efficacy of vitamin B_6 (pyridoxine) in the treatment of premenstrual symptoms, although reviews have been mixed. One study showed a greater decrease in psychiatric symptoms with 80 mg of vitamin B_6 compared with placebo. It should be noted that vitamin B_6 supplementation at higher doses has been associated with peripheral neuropathy, so patients should be cautioned (Vigod et al., 2009). There have been some small studies looking at the effect of magnesium, vitamin E, tryptophan, fish oil, and soy isoflavones on premenstrual symptoms, but results have been mixed; therefore, more research is needed (Pearlstein & Steiner, 2008).

Complementary and Alternative Therapies. Reviews of complementary treatments have reported that chasteberry or vitex agnus-castus have shown evidence for the treatment of premenstrual symptoms. It has been hypothesized that the benefit of chasteberry for premenstrual symptoms could be due to its effects as a dopamine agonist that possibly reduces FSH or prolactin levels. It has proven some benefit for physical more so than psychological symptoms (Pearlstein & Steiner, 2008; Vigod et al., 2009). Research has not suggested consistent benefit for Ginkgo biloba, evening primrose oil, and homeopathic treatments. Some studies have reported that saffron and Qi therapy were superior to placebo in women with confirmed PMS (Pearlstein & Steiner, 2008). There have been reports of initial positive trials of massage, reflexology, chiropractic manipulation, and biofeedback. Open trials also suggest support for yoga, guided imagery, photic stimulation, and acupuncture. Bright light therapy has been thought to be an effective treatment for PMDD with the rationale that it may induce rapid increase in serotonin (Vigod et al., 2009).

Follow-Up. Follow-up involves rescheduling the client in 1 or 2 months to evaluate her charts and progress and to arrive at a workable diagnosis and plan of care. The first few months involve intense examination of lifestyle, menstrual patterns, and coping strategies. Frequent visits provide time to review and provide more information, reinforce desired changes, give encouragement, assign reading, and discuss referrals. Results of initial lab work can be shared at this time, and continuation of symptom charting is stressed. As the client accrues knowledge and coping techniques and begins to see progress, her visits can be less frequent and shorter.

REFERENCES

Affinito, P., Di Carlo, C., Di Mauro, P., Napolitano, V., & Nappi, C. (1994). Endometrial hyperplasia: Efficacy of a new treatment with a vaginal cream containing natural micronized progesterone. *Maturitas, 20,* 191–198.

American Academy of Pediatrics, Committee on Adolescence, American College of Obstetricians and Gynecologists (AAP & ACOG). (2006). Menstruation in girls and adolescents: Using the menstrual cycle as a vital sign. *Pediatrics, 118,* 2245–2250.

American College of Obstetricians and Gynecologists (ACOG). (2010). Practice bulletin no. 110: Noncontraceptive uses of hormonal contraceptives. *Obstetrics and Gynecology, 115*(1), 206–212.

Association of Professors of Gynecology and Obstetrics. (APGO). (2002). Clinical management of abnormal uterine bleeding. *APGO Educational Series on Women's Health Issues*. Retrieved from http://www.apgo.org/bookstore/index.cfm?docid=0226D691-3FFF-6373-CF289B04C6D568D0

Azziz, R., Carmina, E., Dewailly, D., Diamante-Kandarakis, E., Escobar-Morreale, H.F., Futterweit, W., et al. (2009). The Androgen Excess and PCOS Society criteria for the polycystic ovary syndrome: The complete task force report. *Fertility and Sterility, 91,* 456–488.

Bahamondes, L., Cordova-Eguez, S., Pons, J., & Shulman, L. (2007). Perspectives on premenstrual syndrome/premenstrual dysphoric disorder. *Disease Management and Health Outcomes, 15*(5), 263–277.

Barron, M.L., Flick, L.H., Cook, C.A., Homan, S.M., & Campbell, C. (2008). Associations between psychiatric disorders and menstrual cycle characteristics. *Archives of Psychiatric Nursing, 22,* 254–265.

Berek, J.S., & Novak, E. (2007). *Berek and Novak's gynecology* (14th ed.). Philadelphia: Lippincott Williams & Wilkins.

Berman, J.M. (2008). Intrauterine adhesions. *Seminars in Reproductive Medicine, 26,* 349–355.

Braxton Lloyd, K., & Hornsby, L.B. (2009). Complementary and alternative medication for women's health issues. *Nutrition in Clinical Practice, 24*(5), 590–608.

Brown, J., O'Brien, P.M.S., Marjoribanks, J., & Wyatt, K. (2009). Selective serotonin reuptake inhibitors for premenstrual syndrome. *Cochrane Database of Systematic Reviews, 2,* CD001396.

Carey, J.C. (2006). Pharmacological effects on sexual function. *Obstetrics and Gynecology Clinic of North America, 33,* 599–620.

Centers for Disease Control (CDC). (1997). Case definitions for infectious conditions under public health surveillance. *Morbidity and Mortality Weekly Report, 46,* 39.

Chanson, P., & Salenave, S. (2004). Diagnosis and treatment of pituitary adenomas. *Minerva Endocrinology, 29*(4), 241–275.

Cho, S.H., & Hwang, E.W. (2010). Acupuncture for primary dysmenorrhoea: A systematic review. *BJOG: An International Journal of Obstetrics and Gynaecology, 117,* 509–521.

Christin-Maitre, S., Pasquire, M., Donadille, B., & Bouchard, P. (2006). Premature ovarian failure. *Annales d Endocrinologie, 67,* 557–566.

Chumlea, W.C., Schubert, C.M., & Roche, A.F. (2003). Age at menarche and racial comparisons in US girls. *Pediatrics, 111,* 110–113.

Cosgrove, S. (2006). *Staphylococcal toxic shock syndrome.* Retrieved March 20, 2011, from http://www.uptodate.com/contents/staphylococcal-toxic-shock-syndrome?source=search_result&selectedTitle=1~72#H18

Davis, A.R., Kroll, R., Soltes, B., Zhang, N., Grubb, G.S., & Constantine, G.D. (2008). Occurrence of menses or pregnancy after cessation of a continuous oral contraceptive. *Fertility and Sterility, 89,* 1059–1063.

DeVane, G.W., Czekala, N.M., Judd, H.L., & Yen, S.S. (1975). Circulating gonadotropins, estrogens, and androgens in polycystic ovarian disease. *American Journal of Obstetrics and Gynecology, 121,* 496–500.

Dickerson, L., Mazyck, P., & Hunter, M. (2003). Premenstrual syndrome. *American Family Physician, 67*(8), 1743–1752.

Farquhar, C., & Brown, J. (2009, October). Oral contraceptive pill for heavy menstrual bleeding. *Cochrane Database System Review,* CD000154.

Ford, O., Lethaby, A., Roberts, H., & Mol, B. (2009). Progesterone for premenstrual syndrome. *Cochrane Database of Systematic Reviews, 2,* CD003415.

Fraser, I.S. (1990). Treatment of ovulatory and anovulatory dysfunctional uterine bleeding with oral progestogens. *Australia and New Zealand Journal of Obstetrics and Gynaecology, 30,* 353–356.

Fraser, I.S., Critchley, H.O., Munro, M.G., Broder, M., & Writing group for this menstrual agreement process (2007). A process designed to lead to international agreement on terminologies and definitions used to describe abnormalities of menstrual bleeding. *Fertility and Sterility, 87,* 466–476.

Freeman, E. (2007). Distinguishing and treating PMS and PMDD. *Contemporary OB/GGYN, 2,* 60–66.

French, L. (2005). Dysmenorrhea. *American Family Physician, 71*(2), 285–291.

French, L. (2008). Dysmenorrhea in adolescents: Diagnosis and treatment. *Pediatric Drugs, 10*(1), 1–7.

Fritz, M.A., & Speroff, L. (2011). *Clinical gynecologic endocrinology and infertility* (8th ed.). Philadelphia: Wolters Kluwer/Lippincott Williams & Wilkins.

Goodman, L.R., & Warren, M.P. (2005). The female athlete and menstrual function. *Current Opinion in Obstetrics & Gynecology, 17*(5), 466–470.

Grubb, M.R., Chakeres, D., & Malarkey, W.B. (1987). Patients with primary hypothyroidism presenting as prolactinomas. *American Journal of Medicine, 83,* 765–769.

Harel, Z. (2006). Dysmenorrhea in adolescents and young adults: Etiology and management. *Journal of Pediatric Adolescent Gynecology, 19,* 363–371.

Hatch, R., & Rosenfield, R.L. (1981). Hirsutism: Implications, etiology, and management. *American Journal of Obstetrics and Gynecology, 140,* 815–830.

Hatcher, R.A., Trussell, J., Nelson, A.L., Cates, W., Jr., Kowal, D., & Policar, M.S. (2011). *Contraceptive technology* (20th rev ed.). New York: Ardent Media, Inc.

Hernandez, I., Cervera-Aguilar, R., Vergara, M.D., & Ayala, A.R. (1999). Prevalence and etiology of secondary amenorrhea in a selected Mexican population. *Ginecología y Obstetricia de México, 67,* 374–376.

Hoerster, K.D., Chrisler, J.C., & Gorman, J. (2003). Attitudes toward and experience with menstruation in the US and India. *Women and Health, 38,* 77–79.

Holt, R.I. (2008). Medical causes and consequences of hyperprolactinaemia: A context for psychiatrists. *Journal of Psychopharmacology, 22,* 28–37.

Hoyt, K.L., & Schmidt, M.C. (2004). Polycystic ovary (Stein-Leventhal) syndrome: Etiology, complications, and treatment. *Clinical Laboratory Science,* 155–163.

Irvine, G.A., & Cameron, I.T. (1999). Medical management of dysfunctional uterine bleeding. *Clinical Obstetrics and Gynaecology,* 189–194.

Jerrell, J.M., Bacon, J., Burgis, J.T., & Menon, S. (2009). Hyperprolactinemia-related adverse events associated with antipsychotic treatment in children and adolescents. *Journal of Adolescent Health, 45,* 70–76.

Kaunitz, A.M., Bissonnette, F., Monteiro, I., Lukkari-Lax, E., Muysers, C., & Jensen, J.T. (2010). Levonorgestrel-releasing intrauterine system or medroxyprogesterone for heavy menstrual bleeding: A randomized controlled trial. *Obstetrics and Gynecology,* 625–632.

Kouides, P.A., Conrad, J., Peyvandi, F., Lukes, A., & Kadir, R. (2005). Hemostasis and menstruation: Appropriate investigation for underlying disorders of hemostasis in women with excessive menstrual bleeding. *Fertility and Sterility, 84,* 1345–1351.

Krassass, G.E., Pontikides, N., Kaltsas, T., Papadopoulou, P., Paunkovic, J., Paunkovic, N., et al. (1999). Disturbances of menstruation in hypothyroidism. *Clinical Endocrinology, 50,* 655–659.

Kroll, R., & Rapkin, A. (2006). Treatment of premenstrual disorders. *Journal of Reproductive Medicine, 51*(4 Suppl.), 359–370.

Lesher, L., DeVries, A., Danila, R., & Lynfield, R. (2009). Evaluation of surveillance methods for staphylococcal toxic shock syndrome. *Emerging Infectious Diseases, 15*(5), 770–773.

Lethaby, A., & Hickey, M. (2009). Endometrial destruction techniques for heavy menstrual bleeding. *Cochrane Database System Review, 19,* CD001501.

Lillitos, P., Harford, D., & Michie, C. (2007). Toxic shock syndrome. *Emergency Nurse, 15*(6), 28–33.

Mannix, L. (2008). Menstrual-related pain conditions: Dysmenorrhea and migraine. *Journal of Women's Health, 17*(5), 879–891.

Marvan, M.L., Espinosa-Hernandez, G., & Vacio, A. (2002). Premenarcheal Mexican girls' expectations concerning perimenstrual changes and menstrual attitudes. *Journal of Psychosomatic Obstetrics and Gynecology, 23,* 89–96.

Milman, N., Clausen, J., & Byg, K.E. (1998). Iron status in 268 Danish women aged 18-30 years: Influence of menstruation, contraceptive method, and iron supplementation. *Annals of Hematology, 77,* 13–19.

Moltini, N., Bardella, M.T., & Bianchi, P.A. (1990). Obstetric and gynecological problems in women with untreated celiac sprue. *Journal of Clinical Gastroenterology, 12,* 37.

Monteiro, I., Bahamondes, L., & Diaz, J. (2002). Therapeutic use of levonorgestrel-releasing intrauterine system in women with menorrhagia: A pilot study. *Contraception, 65,* 325–328.

Morrow, C., & Naumburg, E. (2009). Dysmenorrhea. *Primary Care: Clinics in Office Practice, 36,* 19–32.

Nieman, L.K., Biller, B.M., Findling, J.W., Newell-Price, J., Savage, M.O., Stewart, P.M., et al. (2008). The diagnosis of

Cushing's syndrome: An endocrine society clinical practice guideline. *Journal of Clinical Endocrinology and Metabolism, 93*(5), 1526–1540.

Nikkanen, H., Sisson, S., & Blok, B. (2007). *Toxic shock syndrome. MD Consult.* Retrieved March 20, 2011, from http://www.mdconsult.com.floyd.lib.umn.edu/das/pdxmd/body/237615804-6/0?type=med&eid=9-u1.0-_1_mt_1014604

Oriel, K.A., & Schrager, S. (1999). Abnormal uterine bleeding. *American Family Physician, 60*(5), 1371–1380.

Palha, A.P., & Esteves, M. (2008). Drugs of abuse and sexual functioning. *Advanced Psychosomatic Medicine, 29,* 131–149.

Pandey, S., & Bhattacharya, S. (2010). Impact of obesity on gynecology. *Women's Health, 6,* 107–117.

Parsonnet, J., Hansmann, M.A., Seymour, J.L., Delaney, M.L., DuBois, A.M., Modern, P.A., et al. (2005). Persistence survey of toxic shock syndrome toxin-1 producing staphylococcus aureus and serum antibodies to this superantigen in five groups of menstruating women. *BMC Infectious Diseases, 10,* 249.

Pearlstein, T., & Steiner, M. (2008). Premenstrual dysphoric disorder: Burden of illness and treatment update. *Journal of Psychiatry and Neuroscience, 33*(4), 291–301.

Philipp, C.S., Faiz, A., Dowling, N., Dilley, A., Michaels, L.A., Ayers, C., et al. (2005). Age and the prevalence of bleeding disorders in women with menorrhagia. *Obstetrics and Gynecology, 105,* 61–66.

Practice Committee of the American Society for Reproductive Medicine. (2006). Current evaluation of amenorrhea. *Fertility and Sterility, 82,* 266–272.

Proctor, M., & Farquhar, C. (2006). Diagnosis and management of dysmenorrhoea. *British Medical Journal, 332(7550),* 1134–1138.

Proctor, M., Hing, W., Johnson, R.C., Murphy, P.A., & Brown, J. (2010). Spinal manipulation for dysmenorrhoea. *Cochrane Database of Systematic Reviews, 3,* CD002119.

Proctor, M., & Murphy, P.A. (2009). Herbal and dietary therapies for primary and secondary dysmenorrhoea. *Cochrane Database of Systematic Reviews, 2,* CD002124.

Proctor, M., Murphy, P.A., Pattison, H.M., Suckling, J.A., & Farquhar, C. (2011). Behavioural interventions for dysmennorhea. *Cochrane Database of Systematic Reviews, 2007*(3), CD002248.

Rapkin, A. (2006). Premenstrual symptoms: Current concepts in diagnosis and treatment. *Journal of Reproductive Medicine, 51,* 337–338.

Reddish, S. (2006). Dysmenorrhoea. *Australian Family Physician, 35*(11), 842–848.

Rome, E., Reame, N., & Stanford, W. (1998). *Our bodies, ourselves.* New York: Simon & Schuster.

Roy, S.N., & Bhattacharya, S. (2004). Benefits and risks of pharmacological agents used for the treatment of menorrhagia. *Drug Safety, 27,* 75–90.

Salley, K.E., Wickman, E.P., Cheang, K.I., Essah, P.A., Karjane, N.W., & Nestler, J.E. (2007). Glucose intolerance in polycystic ovary syndrome—A position statement of the Androgen Excess Society. *Journal of Clinical Endocrinology and Metabolism, 92,* 4546–4556.

Santoro, N., Brown, J.R., Adel, T., & Skurnick, J.H. (1996). Characterization of reproductive hormonal dynamics in the perimenopause. *Journal of Clinical Endocrinology and Metabolism, 81,* 1495–1501.

Shapely, M., Jordan, K., & Croft, P.R. (2004). An epidemiological survey of symptoms of menstrual loss in the community. *British Journal of General Practice, 54,* 359–363.

Sheinfeld, H., Gal, M., Bunzel, M.E., & Vishne, T. (2007). The etiology of some menstrual disorders: A gynecological and psychiatric issue. *Health Care for Women International, 28,* 817–827.

Smith, D.R. (2008). Menstrual disorders and their adverse symptoms at work: An emerging occupational health issue in the nursing profession. *Nursing & Health Sciences, 10*(3), 222–228.

Snajderova, M., Martinek, J., Horejsi, J., Novakova, D., Lebl, J., & Kolouskova, S. (1999). Premenarchal and postmenarchal girls with insulin-dependent diabetes mellitus: Ovarian and other organ-specific autoantibodies, menstrual cycle. *Journal of Pediatric and Adolescent Gynecology, 12,* 209–214.

Speiser, P.W., & White, P.C. (2003). Congenital adrenal hyperplasia. *New England Journal of Medicine, 349,* 776–788.

Stabinsky, S.A., Einstien, M., & Breen, J.L. (1999). Modern treatments of menorrhagia attributable to dysfunctional uterine bleeding. *Obstetrics and Gynecologic Survey, 54,* 61–72.

Staggers, B. (2010a). *Ways to think about amenorrhea. Adolescent health care.* Seattle, WA: Contemporary Forums.

Staggers, B. (2010b). *DUB: Dysfunctional uterine bleeding. Adolescent health care.* Seattle, WA: Contemporary Forums.

Steiner, M., Pearlstein, T., Cohen, L., Endicott, J., Kornstein, S., Roberts, C., et al. (2006). Expert guidelines for the treatment of severe PMS and PMDD, and comorbidities: The role of SSRIs. *Journal of Women's Health, 15*(1), 57–68.

U.S. Food and Drug Administration (FDA). (2009). *FDA approves additional use for IUD Mirena to treat heavy menstrual bleeding in IUD users.* Retrieved from www.fda.gov/newsevents/newsroom/pressannouncements/2009/ucm184747.htm

Vigod, S., Ross, L., & Steiner, M. (2009). Understanding and treating premenstrual dysphoric disorder: An update for the women's health practitioner. *Obstetrics and Gynecology Clinics of North America, 36,* 907–924.

Warren, M.P., & Goodman, L.R. (2003). Exercise induced endocrine pathologies. *Journal of Endocrinological Investigation, 26,* 873–878.

Winer, S., & Rapkin, A. (2006). Premenstrual disorders: Prevalence, etiology and impact. *The Journal of Reproductive Medicine, 51*(4), 339–347.

Wong, C.L., Farquhar, C., Roberts, H., & Proctor, M. (2009). Oral contraceptive pill for primary dysmenorrhoea. *Cochrane Database of Systematic Reviews, 4,* CD002120.

CHAPTER ❖ **12**

MANAGING CONTRACEPTION AND FAMILY PLANNING

Beth Walcker ◆ *Coralie Pederson*

More contraceptive methods that provide women safe, convenient, and effective options are available to women in the United States than in many other countries. However, many pregnancies in the United States remain unplanned.

Highlights

- Historical and Political Perspectives on Contraception
- Fundamentals
- Selecting a Method of Contraception
- Guidelines for Client Education and Informed Consent
- Induced Abortion
- Web Resources

❖ INTRODUCTION

Many options for contraception are currently available to women and men in the United States. These methods provide safe, effective, and convenient choices for people who wish to prevent or postpone pregnancy. Overall, 62 percent of women of reproductive age are currently using a contraceptive method. However, nearly half of all pregnancies among American women are unintended, and 4 in 10 of these pregnancies are terminated by abortion (Alan Guttmacher Institute, 2011). This chapter will address contraceptive methods available for use in the United States across the reproductive life span.

HISTORICAL AND POLITICAL PERSPECTIVES ON CONTRACEPTION

The desire of women and men to control reproduction has been evident since ancient times. Use of primitive barriers, spermicides, condoms, and withdrawal is documented in the writings of many ancient cultures. Until the mid-19th century, however, few reliable methods to prevent or delay pregnancy were available. Herbal and chemical spermicides, condoms, and coitus interruptus (withdrawal) carried relatively high risks of pregnancy; the latter two also depended on the cooperation of men (Wright, 2010).

Since the mid-19th century, major developments, feminist movements, and technological advances have fueled the movement in contraception across the reproductive life span. One of the earliest members of this movement was Margaret Sanger (1883–1966), a nurse and feminist and early leader of the U.S. family planning movement, who introduced the diaphragm into the United States and fought for women's rights. She founded the American Birth Control League, which later became the Planned Parenthood Federation of America (Lynaugh, 1991).

In the early 1960s, oral contraceptives and intrauterine devices (IUD) became available, beginning the "contraceptive revolution." A 1965 U.S. Supreme Court decision in the case of *Estelle T. Griswold and C. Lee Buxton v. State of Connecticut* declared birth control to be a basic right under the Bill of Rights. In the late 1960s, New York, California, and other states rewrote their abortion laws, culminating in the 1973 U.S. Supreme Court decision of *Roe v. Wade*, which limited the circumstances under which "the right to privacy" could be restricted by local abortion laws. Abortion was thus legalized. The ability to control the timing and circumstances under which they would conceive and give birth bestowed on women a higher degree of personal control and more freedom of choice in many dimensions of their lives (Boston Women's Health Book Collective, 2011; Hatcher et al., 2011). In 2005, the U.S. infant mortality rate was 6.86 infant deaths per 1,000 live births. The availability of modern birth control methods has dramatically reduced maternal and infant mortality (U.S. National Center for Health Statistics, 2009).

FUNDAMENTALS

DEFINITION AND PURPOSE

Contraception is defined as pregnancy prevention methods effective prior to implantation (Association of Reproductive Health Professionals [ARHP], 2011). Related terms often used interchangeably with contraception include *fertility control*, *birth control*, *family planning*, and *pregnancy prevention*. The reasons for contraception include personal convenience, economics, social values, health promotion, and lifestyle. Primary care clinicians are often the main source of information and advice on responsible family planning practices for clients. Family planning services/programs should offer clients a variety of safe, effective, acceptable, affordable contraceptive methods to help them prevent unwanted pregnancy.

GENERAL PRINCIPLES OF FERTILITY CONTROL

- When the goal is to prevent pregnancy, any contraceptive method is better than none.
- All sexually active women of every age must have access to effective, confidential, and nonpunitive contraceptive services.
- Women need to know their options, the risks and benefits, and which methods may be contraindicated for them and why.

- Health professionals are obligated to educate clients, without bias, about the range of possible methods so that fully informed choices can be made.
- No birth control method is 100 percent effective in preventing pregnancy.
- Information and counseling about sexually transmitted infections (STIs) is important because most contraceptive options do not provide protection against STIs.
- Responsibility for pregnancy prevention should be addressed during consultation with both men and women.
- Every woman needs to have knowledge about emergency contraception (EC) and how to obtain it.

ISSUES OF CONTROL AND SAFETY

A "perfect" contraceptive would be 100 percent effective in preventing pregnancy, highly acceptable, free from health hazards and side effects, not coitus related, low maintenance, and easily reversible. In addition, it would be inexpensive and offer noncontraceptive benefits such as protection against STIs. All methods of contraception carry some risks to users; therefore, advantages and disadvantages must be discussed. In assisting clients with contraceptive choices, it is often helpful to compare method risks with the risks of pregnancy. In most cases, the risks associated with pregnancy are much greater than those associated with contraceptive use (Hatcher et al., 2011; Zieman et al., 2010). Contraceptive safety concerns as well as apprehension about side effects appear to be more prevalent in minority communities (Dehlendorf, Rodriguez, Levy, Borrero, & Steinauer, 2010).

CONTRACEPTION AND SAFER SEX

When seeking to prevent pregnancy, both men and women bear responsibility. The question of whether a method offers any protection against STIs must be part of the decision-making process on contraceptive choice. For example, male condoms offer contraception with some protection against STIs, whereas combined hormonal methods provide no protection against STIs.

Safer Sex

There is no such entity as safe sex—hence the term *safer sex*. Though condoms are not 100 percent effective in preventing infections, male and/or female condoms are the best protection available at this time. Principal problems with male and/or female condom use are improper use, difficulty integrating use into sexual activity, and less often, condom breakage and slippage.

Sexual practices considered *safe* involve no exchange of body fluids of any kind and could include sexual fantasies; nongenital physical touch; mutual masturbation; and erotic books, movies, and conversations. *Possibly safe* activities include wet kissing when there are no breaks in the skin, lips, or mouth tissues, and use of latex or plastic barriers during all other oral, anal, and genital contact. *Unsafe sexual practices* include any direct contact with blood, semen, and vaginal secretions; any vaginal or anal intercourse without a condom; or sharing of sex toys.

SELECTING A METHOD OF CONTRACEPTION

A woman's reproductive life span is almost 40 years, and throughout those years, a variety of contraceptive methods may be used. Women need guidance in evaluating contraceptive choices as their needs change. Many individual factors may enhance or impair contraceptive behavior and impact the selection of birth control methods (Hatcher et al., 2011).

For example, new immigrants may anchor strongly to traditional religious and cultural expectations regarding family, sexuality, and fertility. Although health care providers must be cautious not to attribute stereotypical religious, social, and cultural characteristics to women seeking advice about contraception, they do need to recognize that different value systems may influence contraception decision making in couples of different cultures and faiths. This increased cultural awareness needs to be tempered by the understanding that each patient encounter is unique. The values that an individual woman holds may not be in keeping with the official teachings of her religion or the cultural norms reported by other members of the same culture (Srikanthan & Reid, 2008).

Emotional side effects were found to be of particular concern to Latina women, whereas for black women, menstrual irregularities caused by hormonal contraceptive methods were of particular concern, with menstruation seen as important for physical health and fertility as well as an important indicator regarding pregnancy. Studies have found minority women trust and rely more often on information from peers and family than from health care professionals (Dehlendorf, Rodriguez, Levy, Borrero, & Steinauer, 2010).

Guidelines to inform clinicians are available through the World Health Organization (WHO, 2009). There are

TABLE 12–1. Characteristics of Contraceptive Methods

Contraceptive Method	Cost	Ease of Use	Coitus Linked	Level of Convenience	Systemic Effects	Partner Involvement Required	Health Care System Contact Required	Time to Return of Fertility	Can Be Used While Lactating
CHCs	Mod to high	Great	No	High	Yes	None	Yes	Delay—possibly 2–3 months	Not recommended
POPs	Mod	Great	No	High	Yes	None	Yes	Rapid	Yes
Implants	High	Great	No	High	Yes	None	Yes	Delayed—possibly 2–3 months	Yes
Injections	Mod	Great	No	High	Yes	None	Yes	Delayed, 6–12 months	Yes
Diaphragms	Mod to high	Mod	Yes	Mod	No	None	Yes	Immediate	Yes
Sponge	Mod	Mod	Yes	Mod	No	No	No	Immediate	Yes
Cervical caps	Mod to high	Mod	Yes	Mod	No	None	Yes	Immediate	Yes
Postcoital emergency methods	High	Difficult	No	Low	Yes	None	Yes	Rapid	Not recommended
Male condoms	Low to mod	Mod	Yes	Mod to low	No	Yes	No	Immediate	Yes
Female condoms	Mod	Mod	Yes	Low	No	Some	No	Immediate	Yes
Vaginal spermicides	Low to mod	Mod	Yes	Low	No	None	No	Immediate	Yes
Intrauterine devices	High	Great	No	High	Some	None	Yes	Rapid	Yes
Fertility awareness methods	Low	Difficult	Yes	Low	No	Yes	Yes for teaching	Immediate	Not reliable
Lactational amenorrhea method	Low	Mod	No	High	No	None	No	Rapid	—
Withdrawal	None	Mod	Yes	Mod	No	Yes	No	Immediate	Yes
Female sterilization	High	Great	No	High	No		Yes	Not applicable	Yes
Male sterilization	Mod	Great	No	High	No		Yes	Not applicable	Yes

Source: Dickey, 2010; Hatcher et al., 2011; Rawlins & Smith, 2002.

four categories of medical eligibility recommendations identified by WHO for contraception:

Category	With Clinical Judgment	With Limited Clinical Judgment
1	Use method in any circumstances	Yes (use the method)
2	Generally use the method	Yes (use the method)
3	Use of method not usually recommended unless other more appropriate methods are not available or not acceptable	No (do not use the method)
4	Method not to be used	No (do not use the method)

Factors clinicians should consider during the contraceptive consult include the following:

- Desire for future fertility.
- Cultural and religious beliefs.
- Health/medical history.
- Presence of physical or mental limitations.
- Motivation of the woman.
- Degree of cooperation of the partner.
- Degree of comfort with one's body and one's sexuality.
- Lactation status.
- Short-term versus long-term contraceptive needs.
- Previous experience with birth control.
- Frequency of intercourse.
- Effectiveness of methods.
- Safety of methods.
- Access to health care.
- Noncontraceptive benefits.
- Cost of methods.
- Perceived convenience of methods.
- Confidence in methods.

Characteristics that may impact the selection and use of specific contraceptive methods are summarized in Table 12–1.

EVALUATION OF CLIENTS REQUESTING CONTRACEPTION

Women seeking care or advice about contraception are usually in a state of physical wellness. In addition, health care professionals must be aware that certain clients have limited or no access to contraceptive services. Clients with limited access may include teenagers, low-income women, and women in underserved areas. These women need services low in cost with convenient hours and accessible

TABLE 12–2. Contraceptive Selection in Special Populations

Special Populations or Medical Conditions	Contraceptive Options and/or Guidelines
Adolescence	• Methods not recommended include LAM, NFP, sterilization • Most other methods may be successfully used, STI protection is important • Strongly consider LARC methods • Hormonal methods • FP services for teens need to stress sex education at an early age, contraceptive use, prevention of STIs, affordability, teen-friendly approach, visual aids, and close supervision with follow-up to encourage continuation • Adolescents need skills and self-confidence to abstain or reduce risks
Perimenopause	• Long-term contraception is often preferred • Any IUD, combined hormonal methods (if no contraindications) are good choices • Progestin-only methods are good choices for women with contraindications to estrogen • Noncontraceptive benefits, such as cycle control and relief of vasomotor symptoms, may affect decision making • Sterilization is a good option • All methods may be used until menopause unless contraindicated
Physically disabled	• Progestin-only methods—good choices • Any IUD—good choice • Combined hormonal methods—generally good choices (though not recommended when client is immobile or has impaired circulation; caregiver or partner assistance may be needed) • Sterilization
Mental disability and psychiatric illnesses	• Long-acting progestins—DMPA, implants—good choices • Combination hormonal methods—generally good choices, review medication history carefully for drug–drug interactions • Any IUD—good choice

Sources: Adolescent Facts: Pregnancy, Birth and STDs, 2009; Best, 2000a, 2000b; Dickerson, 2001; Grimes, 1999.

locations. Other groups with special family planning concerns include women with chronic illnesses, women with cultural considerations, women with physical or mental disabilities, and perimenopausal women. For some women in these groups, unintended pregnancy could pose significant health risks. The contraceptive needs of special populations groups are briefly addressed in Table 12–2. Consider also that some women have more than one chronic condition.

Initial Evaluation

A thorough initial assessment seeks data to identify risk factors and other influences on method selection (as discussed previously) and contraindications to certain methods.

Necessary *subjective data* include the following:

- *Medical history:* cardiovascular disease (CVD), thromboembolic disorder, reproductive tract cancer, breast cancer, diabetes mellitus (DM), frequent urinary tract infections (UTIs), migraines, seizures, and so on.
- *Obstetric and gynecologic history:* menstrual, premenstrual syndrome (PMS), contraceptive, STIs, pelvic inflammatory disease (PID), vaginitis, and sexual.
- *Family history:* especially cancer, CVD, DM, stroke, and other significant problems.
- *Review of systems*
- *Personal and social data:* smoking status, comfort with touching oneself, use of tampons and female hygiene products, desire or plans for childbearing, and partner involvement.

Objective data are obtained from a screening physical examination including height, weight, and blood pressure (BP). Other components of physical examination may also require emphasis, depending on birth control methods being considered. Clinical breast exam, pelvic exam, and Pap smear, though customarily required, *are not essential* for prescribing hormonal contraceptives and could hinder some women's access to much-needed birth control. A thorough medical history and BP are essential because they reveal most of the medical conditions known to contraindicate hormonal contraceptive use. A woman should have the option to defer a breast exam, pelvic exam, and Pap smear to a later time and still receive hormonal contraception (New Approach, 2001).

Subsequent Evaluations

All women who are sexually active or using a method of contraception that requires a prescription should be seen annually to evaluate new risk factors, contraindications, side effects, concerns, or new problems associated with the present birth control method and to identify any other reproductive problems.

Subjective data needed in subsequent evaluations include a review of the client's history, any significant changes in her health status, and her method of birth control (including satisfaction with the method and any problems). Objective data may or may not include the client's weight and BP, screening physical, breast exam, pelvic exam, and Pap smear. Other lab tests are performed as indicated.

GUIDELINES FOR CLIENT EDUCATION AND INFORMED CONSENT

- A client must participate in choosing the birth control method; she must be an informed user.
- Always obtain informed consent. Consent should be written for a client choosing an IUD, implant, abortion, or sterilization. *Informed consent* implies that client makes a knowledgeable, voluntary choice; receives complete counseling about the procedure and its consequences; and is free to change her mind prior to the procedure.
- For a client planning to use any birth control method, carefully screen for contraindications.
- For certain methods (diaphragms, cervical caps, IUDs, implants, vaginal rings, sterilization), the health provider must receive formal education, training, and practice in fitting, insertion, and other technical aspects.
- During the visit, the health professional is responsible for providing client education and the opportunity for practice and validation of skills pertaining to selected methods (as applicable).
- Make all presentations, counseling, and educational materials compatible with the language, culture, and education of the client.
- Be aware of local myths and misperceptions about particular methods. Address misconceptions sensitively but directly.
- To prevent the omission of important information, use a standard teaching checklist outlining key information that the user should know.
- Instruct about female and male anatomy, using models and illustrations.
- Provide the client with method-specific teaching and counseling, using models, illustrations, and handouts to describe key information:
  - How the methods work.
  - Effectiveness of methods.
  - Advantages and disadvantages of methods.
  - Noncontraceptive benefits.
  - What to expect during the visit.
  - Recommendations concerning follow-up.
  - Descriptions of short- and long-term side effects that can occur and how to deal with them.
  - Danger signs associated with the method selected.
- Explore factors that could place the client at risk for method failure; counsel the client regarding these factors.
- If it is determined that the client is at risk for failure with her chosen method, recommend its use in combination with another method.
- Clients who choose a coitus-associated method need accurate understanding of the timing of ovulation and awareness of days with high risk for conception. An additional method and/or EC may be employed during high-risk times.
- Provide both oral and written instructions. Instruct the client to read specific package literature and follow the instructions carefully.
- Inform the client that regardless of the method chosen, she must always keep a second birth control method available and be familiar with its use.
- Advise the client to keep sufficient quantities of contraceptive products/supplies available at all times in a convenient location. Counsel her about the importance of budgeting for the purchase of products and supplies and for annual exams.
- Teach the proper care and storage of contraceptive devices and supplies.
- Ask the client to repeat important information.
- Inform all clients about the availability of EC in the event of method failure.

EFFECTIVENESS

The determination of contraceptive efficacy is, indeed, an inexact science; some statistics and trends are more measurable than others. Table 12–3 presents the best information available on the percentage of women in the United States experiencing contraceptive failure during the first year of typical use and the first year of perfect use, and the percentage of women continuing use of the method at the end of the first year. Typical use reflects how effective methods are for the average person who may not always use the methods correctly or consistently. Perfect use is when the method is used consistently, that is, correct use with every act of intercourse. Use of two contraceptive methods simultaneously dramatically lowers the risk of unintended pregnancy (Hatcher et al., 2011).

Because most women use a contraceptive method with adherence requirements, the majority of pregnancies result from incorrect or inconsistent method use rather than from method failure. Despite their proven safety, effectiveness, and cost-effectiveness, less than 3 percent of women in the United States use a long-acting reversible contraception (LARC), which includes intrauterine contraception (IUC) and subdermal implants (Secura, Allsworth, Madden, Mullersman, & Peipert, 2010).

TABLE 12–3. Percentage of Women Experiencing an Unintended Pregnancy During the First Year of Typical Use and the First Year of Perfect Use of Contraception and the Percentage Continuing Use at the End of the First Year: United States

Method	Typical Use	Perfect Use	% of Continuation at 1 year
No method	85	85	
Spermicides	29	18	42
Withdrawal	27	4	43
Fertility awareness methods	25	51	
Standard Days Method		5	
Ovulation Method		3	
TwoDay Method		4	
Sponge			
Parous women	32	20	46
Nulliparous women	16	9	57
Diaphragm	16	6	57
Condom			
Female	21	5	49
Male	15	2	53
COCs	8.7	0.3	68
POPs	3	0.5	68
Transdermal contraceptive patch	8	0.3	68
Vaginal contraceptive ring	8	0.3	68
Progestin-only injection	3	0.3	56
Copper-T IUD	0.8	0.6	78
LNG-IUS	0.2	0.2	80
Progestin-only implant	0.05	0.05	84
Female sterilization	0.5	0.5	100
Male sterilization	0.15	0.10	100
Emergency contraceptive pills	Treatment initiated within 120 hours reduces pregnancy by between 59 and 94%		
Lactational amenorrhea method (LAM)	LAM is a highly effective, temporary method of contraception		

Source: Trussell, 2007.

The American College of Obstetricians and Gynecologists (ACOG, 2009) recommends that LARC be offered as first-line contraceptive methods and encouraged as options for most women.

COMBINED HORMONAL CONTRACEPTION

Combined hormonal contraception (CHC) includes methods that contain combined estrogen and progestin formulations, with different delivery systems. The current available CHCs include combined oral contraceptives (COCs), a transdermal patch, or a vaginal ring.

The three estrogen compounds currently used in CHCs in the United States are ethinyl estradiol (EE), estradiol valerate, and mestranol. There are eight different progestins currently used in the United States. Progestins are categorized into "generations," which were introduced over time. First-generation progestins currently in use include norethindrone, norethindrone acetate, and ethynodiol diacetate; second-generation progestins are norgestrel and levonorgestrel; third-generation progestins are desogestrel and norgestimate; and fourth-generation progestin is drospirenone (Dickey, 2010; Hatcher et al., 2011).

These newer progestins are very potent in their ability to inhibit ovulation and to transform estrogen primed endometrium into secretory endometrium. The three newer agents—desogestrel, norgestimate, and drospirenone—have more specific progestational activity, have little estrogenic effect, have a longer half-life, and are weak antiestrogens. They have far less androgenic activity in animal studies in vivo than older progestins (Dickey, 2010; Hatcher et al., 2011). Drospirenone has antimineralocorticoid activity, including a risk of hyperkalemia comparable to that of a 25 mg dose of spironolactone. Drospirenone also has a unique property that mimics the antiandrogenic effect of spironolactone. It also has potential drug interactions (see Table 12–6) (Hatcher et al., 2011; Kupecz & Berandinelli, 2002). Third- and fourth-generation progestins may have a slightly higher risk than second-generation progestins of thrombolytic event, venous thromboembolism (VTE), because they allow for increased expression of estrogen (see Table 12–4).

Mechanism of Action

Pregnancy is prevented by several effects of estrogen and progestin.

- Gonadotropin-releasing hormone (GnRH) is suppressed, which in turn suppresses follicle-stimulating hormone (FSH) and luteinizing hormone (LH), inhibiting ovulation.
- Ovum/tubal transport is altered.
- Cervical mucus thickens, inhibiting sperm transport.

TABLE 12–4. Risk Factors for Venous Thromboembolism

1. Genetic predisposition, factor V Lieden mutation[a]
2. Acquired predisposition (e.g., lupus, anticoagulant, malignancy)
3. Increasing age
4. Physiologic factors (e.g., dehydration)[b]
5. Mechanical factors (e.g., immobility or trauma)
6. Obesity (defined here as BMI of 30 or over)
7. Varicose veins (the data on the magnitude of risk attributable to varicose veins is conflicting. Extensive varicosities are likely to be a risk factor)
8. Pregnancy

[a] Women with a family history of hereditary thrombophilia in a first-degree relative should not be prescribed combined oral contraceptives unless thrombophilia has been ruled out.
[b] May be acute and/or temporary risk factors.

Source: Dickey, 2010; Hatcher et al., 2011; Vandenbroucke et al., 2001.

- Implantation is inhibited by suppression of the endometrium and alteration of uterine secretions.
- Degeneration of the corpus luteum may occur (Bergett-Hanson, 2001; Dickey, 2010; Hatcher et al., 2011).

Effectiveness

CHCs are considered highly effective in preventing pregnancy (see Table 12–3). Failures are attributed to the following.

- Method failure, improper use, user error.
- Discontinuing method without immediate use of another method.
- Drug interactions.

Contraindications

See Table 12–5.

Advantages

- High rate of effectiveness.
- Use not associated with the act of intercourse.
- Use controlled by the woman.
- Easy to use, convenient.
- Rapid reversal of effects after discontinuing use.
- Considered safe for most women throughout their reproductive life span when there are no contraindications.
- Multiple noncontraceptive benefits.
- Continuous use: Continuous use of CHCs means that the user would skip the hormone-free interval and start a new cycle immediately. Continuous use eliminates a withdrawal bleed. Reduction in menstrual cycles also reduces symptoms such as headache, dysmenorrhea, breast tenderness, bloating, and/or swelling that occur during the hormone-free interval. Continuous dosing can be achieved with COCs, contraceptive vaginal ring (CVR), or transdermal contraceptive system (TCS) (Edelman, Gallo, Jensen, Nichols, & Grimes, 2005; Hatcher et al., 2011; Speroff & Darney, 2011).

Noncontraceptive Benefits

- *Improved menstrual characteristics:* CHCs minimize dysmenorrhea and usually decrease the amount and duration of bleeding so that periods are regular and predictable. CHCs relieve PMS in some women, and they lower the incidence of iron-deficiency anemia. They can be used to ameliorate amenorrhea and dysfunctional uterine bleeding. CHCs can also relieve symptoms related to perimenopause and early menopause.
- *Reduction in menstrual bleeding:* CHCs can be used continuously, skipping the hormone-free intervals, and eventually eliminating menstrual bleeding.
- *Protection against ovarian and endometrial cancer:* Compared with women who never used CHCs, users have half the risk of developing these cancers. Protection is noted after a minimum of 12 months of use and persists long after pills are discontinued.
- *Lower incidence of ovarian cysts:* Incidence is reduced by 90 percent, due to the suppression of ovulation.
- *Prevention of ectopic pregnancy:* Prevention occurs through the suppression of ovulation.
- *Lower incidence of endometriosis:* Incidence is reduced due to the suppression of endometrial growth.
- *Treatment for polycystic ovary syndrome:* Used in treatment once a diagnosis is established. Excessive androgen production of ovarian origin may be suppressed with CHCs that have high progestational and low androgenic activities.
- *Protection against loss of bone mineral density:* Because CHCs provide a consistent potent estrogen, higher peak bone mass is achieved. Women who have used CHCs enter menopause with stronger bones.
- *Some protection against PID:* Incidence of PID is 20 to 50 percent lower among users of CHCs than among those who use no contraceptive method. The greatest protection is against PID caused by gonorrhea.
- *Lower incidence of benign breast cysts and fibroadenomas:* As a result, breast biopsy procedures are decreased.
- *Reduction in vasomotor symptoms in perimenopausal women*
- *Other benefits:* CHCs may reduce acne in some women; may reduce the incidence of rheumatoid arthritis; are used in treatment of hirsutism. Risk of colon cancer may be reduced (Dickey, 2010; Hatcher et al., 2011; Pymar & Creinin, 2001).

Disadvantages

- Affect all body systems.
- Some forms require daily maintenance.
- Some users experience undesirable side effects that cause discontinuance.

TABLE 12–5. Summary Chart of U.S. Medical Eligibility Criteria for Contraceptive Use 2010 (Adapted From WHO Guidelines)

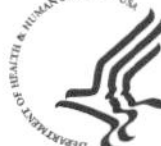

Summary Chart of U.S. Medical Eligibility Criteria for Contraceptive Use, 2010

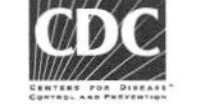

Key:
1 No restriction (method can be used)
2 Advantages generally outweigh theoretical or proven risks
3 Theoretical or proven risks usually outweigh the advantages
4 Unacceptable health risk (method not to be used)

This summary sheet only contains a subset of the recommendations from the US MEC. For complete guidance, see: www.cdc.gov/reproductivehealth/usmec

Most contraceptive methods do not protect against sexually transmitted infections (STIs). Consistent and correct use of the male latex condom reduces the risk of STIs and HIV.

(I = initiation, C = continuation; where a single value is shown it applies to both I and C.)

Condition	Sub-condition	Combined pill, patch, ring	Progestin-only pill	Injection	Implant	LNG–IUD	Copper-IUD
		I / C	I / C	I / C	I / C	I / C	I / C
Age		Menarche to <40=1; ≥40=2	Menarche to <18=1; 18-45=1; >45=1	Menarche to <18=2; 18-45=1; >45=2	Menarche to <18=1; 18-45=1; >45=1	Menarche to <20=2; ≥20=1	Menarche to <20=2; ≥20=1
Anatomic abnormalities	a) Distorted uterine cavity					4	4
	b) Other abnormalities					2	2
Anemias	a) Thalassemia	1	1	1	1	1	2
	b) Sickle cell disease‡	2	1	1	1	1	2
	c) Iron-deficiency anemia	1	1	1	1	1	2
Benign ovarian tumors	(including cysts)	1	1	1	1	1	1
Breast disease	a) Undiagnosed mass	2*	2*	2*	2*	2	1
	b) Benign breast disease	1	1	1	1	1	1
	c) Family history of cancer	1	1	1	1	1	1
	d) Breast cancer‡						
	i) current	4	4	4	4	4	1
	ii) past and no evidence of current disease for 5 years	3	3	3	3	3	1
Breastfeeding	a) < 1 month postpartum	3*	2*	2*	2*		
	b) 1 month or more postpartum	2*	1*	1*	1*		
Cervical cancer	Awaiting treatment	2	1	2	2	I: 4 / C: 2	I: 4 / C: 2
Cervical ectropion		1	1	1	1	1	1
Cervical intraepithelial neoplasia (CIN)		2	1	2	2	2	1
Cirrhosis	a) Mild (compensated)	1	1	1	1	1	1
	b) Severe‡ (decompensated)	4	3	3	3	3	1
Deep venous thrombosis (DVT) /Pulmonary embolism (PE)	a) History of DVT/PE, not on anticoagulant therapy						
	i) higher risk for recurrent DVT/PE	4	2	2	2	2	1
	ii) lower risk for recurrent DVT/PE	3	2	2	2	2	1
	b) Acute DVT/PE	4	2	2	2	2	2
	c) DVT/PE and established on anticoagulant therapy for at least 3 months						
	i) higher risk for recurrent DVT/PE	4*	2	2	2	2	2
	ii) lower risk for recurrent DVT/PE	3*	2	2	2	2	2
	d) Family history (first-degree relatives)	2	1	1	1	1	1
	e) Major surgery						
	(i) with prolonged immobilization	4	2	2	2	2	1
	(ii) without prolonged immobilization	2	1	1	1	1	1
	f) Minor surgery without immobilization	1	1	1	1	1	1
Depressive disorders		1*	1*	1*	1*	1*	1*
Diabetes mellitus (DM)	a) History of gestational DM only	1	1	1	1	1	1
DM (cont.)	b) Non-vascular disease						
	(i) non-insulin dependent	2	2	2	2	2	1
	(ii) insulin dependent‡	2	2	2	2	2	1
	c) Nephropathy/retinopathy/ neuropathy‡	3/4*	2	3	2	2	1
	d) Other vascular disease or diabetes of >20 years' duration‡	3/4*	2	3	2	2	1
Endometrial cancer‡		1	1	1	1	I: 4 / C: 2	I: 4 / C: 2
Endometrial hyperplasia		1	1	1	1	1	1
Endometriosis		1	1	1	1	1	2
Epilepsy‡§	See drug interactions	1*	1*	1*	1*	1	1
Gall-bladder disease	a) Symptomatic						
	(i) treated by cholecystectomy	2	2	2	2	2	1
	(ii) medically treated	3	2	2	2	2	1
	(iii) current	3	2	2	2	2	1
	b) Asymptomatic	2	2	2	2	2	1
Gestational trophoblastic disease	a) Decreasing or undetectable ß-hCG levels	1	1	1	1	3	3
	b) Persistently elevated ß-hCG levels or malignant disease‡	1	1	1	1	4	4
Headaches	a) Non-migrainous	I: 1* / C: 2*	I: 1* / C: 1*	I: 1* / C: 1*	I: 1* / C: 1*	I: 1* / C: 1*	1*
	b) Migraine						
	i) without aura, age <35	I: 2* / C: 3*	I: 1* / C: 2*	I: 2* / C: 2*	I: 2* / C: 2*	I: 2* / C: 2*	1*
	ii) without aura, age ≥35	I: 3* / C: 4*	I: 1* / C: 2*	I: 2* / C: 2*	I: 2* / C: 2*	I: 2* / C: 2*	1*
	iii) with aura, any age	I: 4* / C: 4*	I: 2* / C: 3*	I: 2* / C: 3*	I: 2* / C: 3*	I: 2* / C: 3*	1*
History of bariatric surgery‡	a) Restrictive procedures	1	1	1	1	1	1
	b) Malabsorptive procedures	COCs: 3; P/R: 1	3	1	1	1	1
History of cholestasis	a) Pregnancy-related	2	1	1	1	1	1
	b) Past COC-related	3	2	2	2	2	1
History of high blood pressure during pregnancy		2	1	1	1	1	1
History of pelvic surgery		1	1	1	1	1	1
HIV	High risk or HIV infected‡	1	1	1	1	I: 2 / C: 2	I: 2 / C: 2
	AIDS (see drug interactions)‡§	1*	1*	1*	1*	I: 3 / C: 2*	I: 3 / C: 2*
	Clinically well on ARV therapy§	If on treatment see drug interactions				I: 2 / C: 2	I: 2 / C: 2
Hyperlipidemias		2/3*	2*	2*	2*	2*	1*
Hypertension	a) Adequately controlled hypertension	3*	1*	2*	1*	1	1
	b) Elevated blood pressure levels (properly taken measurements)						
	(i) systolic 140-159 or diastolic 90-99	3	1	2	1	1	1

TABLE 12–5. (Continued)

Condition	Sub-condition	Combined pill, patch, ring	Progestin-only pill	Injection	Implant	LNG-IUD	Copper-IUD
	(ii) systolic ≥160 or diastolic ≥100‡	4	2	3	2	2	1
	c) Vascular disease	4	2	3	2	2	1
Inflammatory bowel disease	(Ulcerative colitis, Crohn's disease)	2/3*	2	2	1	1	1
Ischemic heart disease‡	Current and history of	4	I: 2; C: 3	3	I: 2; C: 3	I: 2; C: 3	1
Liver tumors	a) Benign						
	i) Focal nodular hyperplasia	2	2	2	2	2	1
	ii) Hepatocellular adenoma‡	4	3	3	3	3	1
	b) Malignant‡	4	3	3	3	3	1
Malaria		1	1	1	1	1	1
Multiple risk factors for arterial cardiovascular disease	(such as older age, smoking, diabetes and hypertension)	3/4*	2*	3*	2*	2	1
Obesity	a) ≥30 kg/m² body mass index (BMI)	2	1	1	1	1	1
	b) Menarche to < 18 years and ≥30 kg/m2BMI	2	1	2	1	1	1
Ovarian cancer‡		1	1	1	1	1	1
Parity	a) Nulliparous	1	1	1	1	2	2
	b) Parous	1	1	1	1	1	1
Past ectopic pregnancy		1	2	1	1	1	1
Pelvic inflammatory disease	a) Past, (assuming no current risk factors of STIs)						
	(i) with subsequent pregnancy	1	1	1	1	I: 1; C: 1	I: 1; C: 1
	(ii) without subsequent pregnancy	1	1	1	1	I: 2; C: 2	I: 2; C: 2
	b) Current	1	1	1	1	I: 4; C: 2*	I: 4; C: 2*
Peripartum cardiomyopathy ‡	a) Normal or mildly impaired cardiac function						
	(i) < 6 months	4	1	1	1	2	2
	(ii) ≥ 6 months	3	1	1	1	2	2
	b) Moderately or severely impaired cardiac function	4	2	2	2	2	2
Post-abortion	a) First trimester	1*	1*	1*	1*	1*	1*
	b) Second trimester	1*	1*	1*	1*	2	2
	c) Immediately post-septic abortion	1*	1*	1*	1*	4	4
Postpartum (in non-breastfeeding women)	a) < 21 days	3	1	1	1		
	b) ≥ 21 days	1	1	1	1		
Postpartum (in breastfeeding or non-breastfeeding women, including post-caesarean section)	a) < 10 minutes after delivery of the placenta					2	1
	b) 10 minutes after delivery of the placenta to < 4 weeks					2	2
	c) ≥ 4 weeks					1	1
	d) Puerperal sepsis					4	4
Pregnancy		NA*	NA*	NA*	NA*	4*	4*
Rheumatoid arthritis	a) On immunosuppressive therapy	2	1	2/3*	1	I: 2; C: 1	I: 2; C: 1
	b) Not on immunosuppressive therapy	2	1	2	1	1	1
Schistosomiasis	a) Uncomplicated	1	1	1	1	1	1
	b) Fibrosis of the liver‡	1	1	1	1	1	1
Severe dysmenorrhea		1	1	1	1	1	2

Condition	Sub-condition	Combined pill, patch, ring	Progestin-only pill	Injection	Implant	LNG-IUD	Copper-IUD
Sexually transmitted infections	a) Current purulent cervicitis or chlamydial infection or gonorrhea	1	1	1	1	I: 4; C: 2*	I: 4; C: 2*
	b) Other STIs (excluding HIV and hepatitis)	1	1	1	1	I: 2; C: 2	I: 2; C: 2
	c) Vaginitis (including trichomonas vaginalis and bacterial vaginosis)	1	1	1	1	I: 2; C: 2	I: 2; C: 2
	d) Increased risk of STIs	1	1	1	1	I: 2/3*; C: 2	I: 2/3*; C: 2
Smoking	a) Age < 35	2	1	1	1	1	1
	b) Age ≥35, < 15 cigarettes/day	3	1	1	1	1	1
	c) Age ≥35, ≥ 15 cigarettes/day	4	1	1	1	1	1
Solid organ transplantation‡	a) Complicated	4	2	2	2	I: 3; C: 2	I: 3; C: 2
	b) Uncomplicated	2*	2	2	2	2	2
Stroke‡	History of cerebrovascular accident	4	I: 2; C: 3	3	I: 2; C: 3	2	1
Superficial venous thrombosis	a) Varicose veins	1	1	1	1	1	1
	b) Superficial thrombophlebitis	2	1	1	1	1	1
Systemic lupus erythematosus‡	a) Positive (or unknown) antiphospholipid antibodies	4	3	I: 3; C: 3	3	3	I: 1; C: 1
	b) Severe thrombocytopenia	2	2	I: 3; C: 2	2	2*	I: 3*; C: 2*
	c) Immunosuppressive treatment	2	2	I: 2; C: 2	2	2	I: 2; C: 1
	d) None of the above	2	2	I: 2; C: 2	2	2	I: 1; C: 1
Thrombogenic mutations‡		4*	2*	2*	2*	2*	1*
Thyroid disorders	a) Simple goiter/hyperthyroid/hypothyroid	1	1	1	1	1	1
Tuberculosis‡	a) Non-Pelvic	1*	1*	1*	1*	1	1
	b) Pelvic	1*	1*	1*	1*	I: 4; C: 3	I: 4; C: 3
Unexplained vaginal bleeding	(suspicious for serious condition) before evaluation	2*	2*	3*	3*	I: 4*; C: 2*	I: 4*; C: 2*
Uterine fibroids		1	1	1	1	2	2
Valvular heart disease	a) Uncomplicated	2	1	1	1	1	1
	b) Complicated‡	4	1	1	1	1	1
Vaginal bleeding patterns	a) Irregular pattern without heavy bleeding	1	2	2	2	I: 1; C: 1	1
	b) Heavy or prolonged bleeding	1*	2*	2*	2*	I: 1*; C: 2*	2*
Viral hepatitis	a) Acute or flare	I: 3/4*; C: 2	1	1	1	1	1
	b) Carrier/Chronic	I: 1; C: 1	1	1	1	1	1
Drug Interactions							
Antiretroviral therapy (ARV)	a) Nucleoside reverse transcriptase inhibitors	1*	1	1	1	I: 2/3*; C: 2*	I: 2/3*; C: 2*
	b) Non-nucleoside reverse transcriptase inhibitors	2*	2*	1	2*	I: 2/3*; C: 2*	I: 2/3*; C: 2*
	c) Ritonavir-boosted protease inhibitors	3*	3*	1	2*	I: 2/3*; C: 2*	I: 2/3*; C: 2*
Anticonvulsant therapy	a) Certain anticonvulsants (phenytoin, carbamazepine, barbiturates, primidone, topiramate, oxcarbazepine)	3*	3*	1	2*	1	1
	b) Lamotrigine	3*	1	1	1	1	1
Antimicrobial therapy	a) Broad spectrum antibiotics	1	1	1	1	1	1
	b) Antifungals	1	1	1	1	1	1
	c) Antiparasitics	1	1	1	1	1	1
	d) Rifampicin or rifabutin therapy	3*	3*	1	2*	1	1

I = Initiation of contraceptive method; C = continuation of contraceptive method

* Please see the complete guidance for a clarification to this classification. www.cdc.gov/reproductivehealth/usmec

‡ Condition that exposes woman to increased risk as a result of unintended pregnancy.

§ Please refer to the US MEC guidance related to drug interactions at the end of this chart

TABLE 12–6. Oral Contraceptive Interactions With Other Drugs

Effect	Substances	Comments
Drugs whose effects may be enhanced in combination with oral contraceptives	Tricyclic antidepressants,[a] some benzodiazepines (alprozolam, chlordiazepoxide, clorazepate, diazepam, flurazepam), beta blockers, corticosteroids, theophylline, Troleandomycin (Tao)[b]	Monitor blood levels when available and monitor affected body systems. Use these drugs with caution
Drugs whose effects may be diminished in combination with oral contraceptives	Acetaminophen,[b] oral anticoagulants, some benzodiazepines (lorazepam, oxazepam, temazepam), guanethidine,[a] oral hypoglycemic agents (chlorpropamide, glipizide, glyburide, tolazamide, tolbutamide), methyldopa	Monitor physiological effect of drug, or use alternative drug, or use alternative contraceptive method
Drugs that may diminish the effectiveness of oral contraceptives	Anticonvulsants (carbamazepine, ethosuximide, phenobarbital, phenytoin, primidone, valproic acid, valproate), barbiturates, griseofulvin, rifampin, clofibrate, benzodiazepines, St. John's Wort, Orlistat	Could result in breakthrough bleeding or pregnancy. Use additional birth control method during drug use and for one cycle after drug discontinuation, or use alternative contraceptive method
Drugs that will interact with drospirenone-containing contraceptives to increase risk for hyperkalemia	ACE-Inhibitors, Angiotensin-II Receptor Antagonists, Potassium Sparing Diruetics, Heparin, Aldosterone Angatonists, Daily NSAIDS	Should have serum potassium checked during the first cycle of drospirenone use

[a] Clinical significance of this interaction is unknown.
[b] Increased risk of hepatotoxicity with simultaneous use.
Sources: Dickey, 2010; Hatcher et al., 2011.

- Should not be used while lactating.
- Provide no protection against STIs.
- High cost for some women.
- Prescription needed.
- May interact with other drugs (see Table 12–6).
- Many possible side effects.

Side Effects and Complications

Side effects and complications are caused by systemic effects of CHCs, and may be due to estrogenic, progestational, and/or androgenic activities, or their effects on one or more body systems. The lowest feasible biologic activity in each of these three areas should be chosen, because of potential long-term adverse effects on some body systems, particularly the cardiovascular system. Table 12–7 summarizes most common side effects of CHCs based on their relation to excess or deficient hormone activity.

Effects on Blood Lipids

Estrogen alone is known to beneficially affect blood lipids by lowering total cholesterol and low-density lipoprotein (LDL) cholesterol and elevating high-density lipoprotein (HDL) cholesterol. Estrogen can also elevate triglycerides.

High doses of progestins (19-nortestosterone derivatives) decrease triglyceride levels and HDL cholesterol levels, and elevate LDL cholesterol levels. Low doses, as used in progestin-only pills (POPs), show no significant effects, and depot formulations lower only HDL cholesterol levels. When synthetic estrogens and progestins are combined in CHCs, their effects on serum lipids seem to depend on the androgenicity of the progestin. Progestins that are more androgenic show the most unfavorable effects—that is, increasing LDLs, increasing triglycerides, and decreasing HDLs.

Formulations containing the third-generation progestins (desogestrel) show favorable effects on LDLs and HDLs, but they also raise triglycerides. No causal link between CHC use and cardiovascular morbidity resulting from blood lipid changes has been noted. Interest, however, has focused on lipoprotein changes that occur, because they are known indicators of increased risk for CVD.

Studies show no increased risk of atherosclerosis in women who use or have used CHCs. Data from the Nurses Health Study indicates no increased risk of coronary heart disease, stroke, or other heart disease among former CHC users. Lipid values may indeed vary somewhat in CHC users, but these variations tend to remain within the normal range. Women with known hyperlipidemia should be monitored while on CHCs, especially if they are hypertensive or diabetic (Bergett-Hanson, 2001; Mantel-Teeuwisse, Kloosterman, & Maitland-Van der Zee, 2001; Pymar & Creinin, 2001).

Cardiovascular Disease

A dose-response relationship between the risk of arterial and venous thrombosis and the amount of estrogen in CHCs has been well established. Therefore, the least amount of estrogen should be used when appropriate. Smoking and CHC use increase the risk of serious cardiovascular side effects, including myocardial infarction (MI) and stroke; this

TABLE 12–7. Hormone Content of Oral Contraceptives and Related Side Effects

Estrogen Excess			Estrogen Deficiency
Reproductive system	*PMS-type symptoms*	*Cardiovascular system*	Absence of withdrawal bleeding
Hypermenorrhea, menorrhagia, and clotting	Nausea	Vascular headaches	Spotting and bleeding (day 1 to day 9, or continuously)
Cervical extrophy	Edema, leg cramps	Hypertension	Hypomenorrhea
Dysmenorrhea	Nonvascular headaches	Cerebrovascular accident	Nervousness
Breast enlargement and tenderness	Irritability	Deep vein thrombosis	Atrophic vaginitis
Mucorrhea	Bloating	Thromboembolic disorders	Vasomotor symptoms
Uterine fibroid growth	Dizziness, syncope	Telangiectasias	Pelvic relaxation
Enlargement of uterus	Cyclic weight gain		
Cystic breast changes	*Miscellaneous symptoms*		
	Chloasma		
	Hayfever & allergic rhinitis		
	Urinary tract infection		
	Upper respiratory disorders		
	Epigastric distress		
Progestin Excess			**Progestin Deficiency**
Progestational	*Androgenic/anabolic*	*Cardiovascular system*	Breakthrough bleeding and spotting during late cycle (days 10 to 21)
Reproduction symptoms:	Increased libido	Hypertension	Delayed withdrawal bleeding
Post-pill amenorrhea	Acne	Dilation of leg veins	Dysmenorrhea
Libido decrease	Hirsutism	Lowered protective forms of high-density lipoproteins	Menorrhagia and clotting
Light menses	Oil skin and scalp		
Cervicitis	Cholestatic jaundice		
Monilial vaginitis	Rash		
Miscellaneous symptoms:	Pruritis		
Increased appetite	Edema		
Fatigue/weakness			
Depression, mood changes			
Noncyclic weight gain			

Sources: Dickey, 2010; Hatcher et al., 2011.

risk is greatly increasing after age 35 and/or in the presence of hypertension. Smokers over age 35 should not use CHCs. Formulations with the lowest amount of estrogen should be considered for all smokers, for women over age 35, and for women with other CVD risk factors such as DM and extreme obesity. A few studies have suggested a small increase in risk of VTE with desogestrel-containing CHCs as compared to the risk with other progestins (Bergett-Hanson, 2001; Mantel-Teeuwisse et al., 2001; Pymar & Creinin, 2001; WHO, 2009).

Stroke

A dose-response relationship has also been established between CHC estrogen dose and the risk of both hemorrhagic and ischemic (also called thrombotic) stroke. Studies over the last 10 years on women using CHCs containing less than 50 mcg of estrogen show the incidence of either type of stroke to be low, but not zero.

One study showed a higher risk of thrombotic stroke in women who used CHCs with second-generation progestins versus third-generation progestins, even after correcting for differences in estrogen dose. The 2009 WHO guidelines also characterized migraine with aura as a category 4 contraindication due to increased risk of cerebrovascular accident (CVA). CVAs are often preceded by persistent headache for weeks or months and/or transient hemiparesis, worsening migraine headaches, or uncontrolled hypertension (Bergett-Hanson, 2001; Lidegaard & Kreiner, 2002; Pymar & Creinin, 2001; Schwartz et al., 1998).

Factors that increase risk of CVA are the following:

- Increasing estrogen dosage, that is, lowest risk for POPs, slightly higher for 20 mcg estrogen pills, higher still for 30 to 40 mcg estrogen pills, and so on
- Smoking
- Moderate to severe hypertension
- Diabetes
- Obesity (linked to greater risk of ischemic stroke)
- African American descent

Carbohydrate Metabolism

Older high-dose CHCs were shown to increase glucose levels, increase plasma insulin levels, and slightly decrease glucose tolerance. These changes rapidly returned to normal after CHCs were discontinued. Some studies have also found that progestins and progesterone increase tissue resistance to insulin by decreasing the number of insulin receptors. Use of a low-dose pill with low progestin and low androgenicity is advised to decrease resistance to insulin and cardiovascular risks (Hatcher et al., 2011). WHO delineates guidelines specific to clients with endocrine conditions, including diabetes.

Risk of Breast Cancer

Long-term studies found that current and past CHC users aged 35 to 64 were at no higher risk for developing breast cancer than nonusers (Marchbanks et al., 2002). Even if there were a slight increased risk of breast cancer under 35, breast cancer is so rare in women in that age group that these are very reassuring findings about the safety of low-dose CHCs (Speroff & Darney, 2011). Several studies of high-risk women—BRCA-1/2 mutations or a strong family history of breast cancer—showed no increased risk of breast cancer if they used CHCs (Milne et al., 2005).

COMBINED ORAL CONTRACEPTIVES

COCs have been available in the United States for over 40 years. It is estimated that about 60 million women worldwide and almost 20 million U.S. women use COCs (Alan Guttmacher Institute, 2011). Pill use, its effectiveness, risks, benefits, and side effects have been well researched over the past since the 1950s. Low dosages of estrogen and progestin in today's pills make them very safe and effective for most women. Estrogen and progestin are combined in fixed dose pills (monophasic) or in variable amounts in relation to one another throughout the pill cycle, as in biphasic or triphasic preparations. The reason behind biphasic and triphasic cycles is to mimic the natural hormonal fluctuations.

Managing Side Effects

- Allow the client time to adjust to the pills (two or three cycles).
- Determine that she is taking the pills correctly.
- Determine whether any symptom indicates the possible development of a serious health problem or COC-related complication (especially MI, stroke, pulmonary embolism, thrombophlebitis, gallbladder or liver problems). Ask specific questions regarding early pill danger signs, remembering the acronym *ACHES*—severe *a*bdominal pain, severe *c*hest pain, severe *h*eadaches, *e*ye-visual changes, *s*evere leg pain. Other danger signs are shortness of breath, loss of coordination, speech problems, and depression.
- Determine whether the side effect may be due to an excess or deficiency of a hormonal component (see Table 12–7). If it is determined that the side effect is due to a deficiency or excess of a particular hormonal component, switch the client to a different COC product that has greater or lesser activity of the offending hormone.

Table 12-8 lists common side effects, suggested hormone adjustments, and other management considerations.

Client Counseling

COCs are available in 21-, 24-, or 28-day packs. Active pills are taken the first 21 or 24 days. The 24-day preparations contain 24 active and 4 hormone-free pills. The 28-day preparations contain 7 hormone-free tablets that are inert. Additionally, there are pill packs that contain 84 active pills and 7 hormone-free pills. The 84/7 packs are designed for menstrual suppression. Some preparations add estrogen during the hormone-free interval in order to decrease side effects from drop in estrogen levels. Although unnecessary to the mechanism of action, some preparations contain ferrous sulfate during the hormone-free interval. Another preparation now adds folic acid to the active and hormone-free interval. WHO recommends providing up to 1 year supply of COCs to women initiating the pill in order to reduce women's barriers to access to contraception (Faculty of Family Planning, 2005).

- Instruct that COCs do not protect against STIs, condom use should be encouraged.
- Initial pill selection is based on individual client characteristics. New COC users should generally be started on the lowest dose that is still effective: a 35 μg (or less) pill. Specific client characteristics that may influence initial COC selection include age, personal and family health history, contraindications, menstrual patterns, and hormone sensitivity (Dickey, 2010).
- Instruct the client to contact the provider if concerns arise. Early intervention and support when a client experiences bothersome side effects may prevent her from discontinuing the pill for nonmedical reasons.
- Instruct the client about how to take COCs. When first initiating pill use, one of the following methods is recommended (CDC, 2011; Hatcher et al., 2011; WHO, 2009):
  - *Quick start:* Start pack the day of clinical visit. Use backup method for 7 days (preferred method).
  - *Sunday start*: Start pack on first Sunday during menses.

TABLE 12–8. Management of Side Effects of Oral Contraceptives

Sign, Symptom, Side Effect	Estrogen Adjustment	Progestin Adjustment	Comments and Other Considerations
Acne	Increase	*or* Decrease—less androgenic	Hygiene, diet, topical, antibiotic therapy; choose a pill approved for acne treatment
Amenorrhea or light menses	Increase	Decrease	Rule out pregnancy; pill change not necessary; reassure
Anemia	No change	No change or increase	Diet, iron supplements, evaluate anemia
Bloating, fluid retention	Decrease	Decrease	Consider progestin-only method or drospirenone-containing COC
Breakthrough bleeding, spotting	Early cycle (days 1 to 14) increase estrogen	No change	Review history for misuse; check for infection, cervical changes, pregnancy
	Late cycle (days 15 to 21) No change	Increase or more biologically active	Change to pill with higher endometrial activity
Breast tenderness, fullness	Decrease	No change or decrease	Consider progestin-only method; decrease sodium, caffeine intake; vitamin E 400 IU bid
Breast or uterine cancer	Stop	Stop	Refer
Cervical ectopy and increased mucus	Decrease	No change or decrease	Examine for infection, annual Pap
Chloasma	Decrease or stop	Lower progestational and/or less estrogenic	Consider progestin-only method; avoid excessive sunlight
Contact lens discomfort, refractive changes	Decrease or stop	No change	Consider progestin-only method; have vision correction reevaluated
Cyclic weight gain	Decrease	No change or decrease	Consider drospirenone-containing COC
Decreased breast milk in nursing mothers	Stop	No change or decrease	COCs not recommended—consider progestin-only method
Depression	Decrease or stop	Decrease or stop	Try vitamin B_6 20–25 mg per day; monitor closely; treat depression and reevaluate frequently
Diplopia, any loss of vision, papilledema	Stop	Stop	Evaluate
Diabetes, worsening of	Decrease or stop	Decrease or stop; or try OC with desogestrel	Monitor closely
Dizziness	Decrease or stop	No change; or if hypoglycemia present, decrease	If hypoglycemia, eat regularly, and avoid simple carbohydrates
Dysmenorrhea	Decrease	Increase—higher progestational and androgenic	Rule out infection, other pathology
Gallbladder disease	Decrease or stop	Decrease or stop	Evaluate and monitor
Increased facial hair, hair changes, thinning scalp hair	Increase	Decrease—less androgenic	Rule out thyroid dysfunction
High-density lipoprotein (HDL) cholesterol, decrease	Decrease or stop	Decrease or stop	Triphasic pill or try pill with third generation progestin
Headache (nonmigraine)	Decrease or stop	Decrease or stop	Evaluate headaches, consult physician, see Table 12–2
Migraine with focal-neuro symptoms	Stop	Stop	Consider progestin-only method, or nonhormonal
Hypermenorrhea	Decrease	Increase—higher progestational and androgenic	Rule out pathology first; can combine decreasing estrogen with progestin/androgen change
Hypertension	Decrease or stop	Decrease or stop	Consider progestin-only method, stop smoking, increase exercise, lose weight, reduce stress, see Table 12–2
Hypoglycemia	Same or increase	Decrease—lower progestational and androgenic	Eat regularly, low CHO/high protein diet
Increased appetite	No change or decrease	Decrease—less androgenic	Dietary counseling
Increased growth of benign fibroid tumors	Decrease or stop	No change or decrease	Rule out malignancy
Libido decreased	Decrease	Decrease or higher androgenic	Sexual counseling
Liver disease, jaundice, or benign liver tumor	Stop	Stop	Evaluate

(*continued*)

TABLE 12–8. Management of Side Effects of Oral Contraceptives (CONTINUED)

Sign, Symptom, Side Effect	Estrogen Adjustment	Progestin Adjustment	Comments and Other Considerations
Myocardial infarction or stroke	Stop	Stop	Refer
Noncyclic weight gain	No change or decrease	Decrease—less androgenic	Avoid norgestrel and levonorgestrel
Nausea or vomiting	Decrease or change type	No change	Take after full meal; consider progestin-only method or another combined hormonal delivery system
Nervousness	No change	Decrease or stop	Rule out hypoglycemia; try monophasic pill
Ovarian cysts	No change or increase	Increase—moderate to high progestational activity	If on minipill, triphasic or very low dose OC, then switch to 35 µg dose monophasic or higher
Pulmonary embolism, thromboembolism, thrombophlebitis (or symptoms of)	Stop	Stop	Refer
Vaginal dryness	Increase	Decrease	Use additional lubrication
Varicose veins	Decrease	No change	Consider minipill or other progestin-only method
Yeast infections	No change	Decrease	Hygiene measures, treat infection

Sources: Dickey, 2010; Hatcher et al., 2011.

    - *First-day start:* Start pack first day of menstrual bleeding.
    - Postpartum women (not lactating) may begin COCs at day 21 postpartum, if they have no increased risk for VTE. Those with increased risk should wait until day 42 postpartum (see Chapter 22).
    - Postabortion or miscarriage may begin immediately (day 1 or 2).
- Periods may be very light while on pills. Even slight spotting or bleeding should be considered a period (as long as no pills were missed).
- Another method is always kept on hand to use in case of missed pills, when taking another medication that might interfere with pill effectiveness (see Table 12–3), or when vomiting or diarrhea occurs.
- Missed pills are a common problem. Studies have shown that the most risky time to miss pills is at the beginning of the pack, right after the hormone-free interval or during the third week of active pills, immediately prior to the start of the hormone-free interval. Preovulatory follicles may be present after 7 days without active pills. If the woman misses one or more pills close to the time of the hormone-free interval, thus extending the number of days without active pills to more than seven, she could ovulate and conceive. Missed pills during week 2 of the pack do not present a major concern. The following instructions apply if one or more pills are missed.
- If one pill is missed, take the missed pill as soon as remembered and the next pill at the usual time. If the missed pill is taken more than 12 hours late, a backup method must be used for the next 7 days.
- If two or more pills are missed, take two as soon as remembered and discard the remainder of the missed pills. The next day's pill will be the one normally taken for that day, had no pills been forgotten. Spotting is very likely to occur. Again, use a backup method for the next 7 days.
- If one or more pills are missed during week 3 of the pill pack, follow directions previously given, but skip the pill-free interval (spacer pills) and go directly to the first pill in the new pack. Advise the woman that she may not have a period.
- If a period is missed and pills were taken correctly, the client should begin a new pack as usual. Pregnancy is unlikely. If two consecutive periods are missed and pills were taken correctly, a pregnancy test is done. Emergency contraception should be provided.
- If a period is missed and the client missed one or more pills, pills are stopped; pregnancy test is done.
- If a decision is made to stop COCs and pregnancy is not desired, begin using another birth control method immediately. If pregnancy is desired, it is safe to become pregnant immediately; however, some providers recommend timing cycles for at least 1 month in order to better date the pregnancy. Encourage the client to take prenatal vitamins.
- The client who seems to consistently miss pills should consider other methods of contraception (Dickey, 2010; Hatcher et al., 2011).

TRANSDERMAL CONTRACEPTIVE SYSTEM

The TCS became available in 2002. The TCS consists of a three-layer patch with an area of 20 cm^2. When applied to one of four primary sites (lower abdomen, upper outer arm, buttocks, or upper torso, excluding the breast), it provides continuous, constant circulating levels of two hormones: 150 mcg of norelgestromin and 20 mcg of EE are delivered to the serum each day. Users may maintain all usual activities including sports, bathing, and swimming. One patch per week is applied for 3 consecutive weeks, followed by 1 week without use of a patch to allow scheduled withdrawal bleeding. The patch is changed the same day of each week. Serum hormone levels are maintained in a therapeutic range for up to 9 days, providing contraceptive effectiveness if patch replacement were delayed for up to 2 days. Studies showed a significantly higher rate of breakthrough bleeding and/or spotting only in the first two cycles of use when compared to a COC. After that, the breakthrough bleeding rates were comparable. A withdrawal bleed is usually experienced during the patch-free week. Side effects include a low incidence of application site reactions, breast discomfort, and dysmenorrhea. These decreased after the second cycle of use. Women with a body weight of 198 lb (90 kg) or greater had a significantly higher pregnancy rate than women with lower body weights (Rawlins & Smith, 2002; Speroff & Darney, 2011).

The U.S. Food and Drug Administration (FDA) released a press release (black-box warning) in November 2005, calling attention to the fact that women using the patch are exposed over time, to a greater amount of estrogen. Subsequently, the patch labeling has been updated to describe the higher estrogen exposure. However, follow-up studies showed no increased risk in venous thrombosis, stroke, or MI (Jick & Jick, 2007; Jick, Kaye, Li, & Jick, 2007; Jick, Kaye, Russman, & Jick, 2006).

The TCS can be used in several ways:

- *Quick start:* Apply TCS the day of clinical visit. Use backup method for 7 days (preferred method).
- *Sunday start*: Apply TCS on first Sunday during menses.
- *First-day start:* Apply TCS first day of menstrual bleeding.
- Postpartum women (not lactating) may begin at day 21 postpartum.
- Postabortion or miscarriage may begin immediately (day 1 or 2).

Advantages

- Hormone levels remain therapeutic for 9 days after the application of the second patch, suggesting that ovulation inhibition would be maintained even if a scheduled patch change was missed for as long as 2 days
- Weekly regimen
- Adheres well under a variety of conditions
- Verifiable, user can easily verify the presence of the patch
- Safe for women with latex allergy
- Delivery system avoids “first-pass” effect on the liver

Disadvantages

- Decreased effectiveness of Ortho Evra® patch for women weighing over 198 lb (90 kg)
- Women using the patch must remember to change it weekly
- Skin reactions
- Breast tenderness

Client Counseling

- Should be applied to clean, dry skin.
- Avoid areas of friction, such as under bra straps or thong underwear.
- If any stickiness or adhesive remains on the skin after removal, remove with oil.
- If the patch is partially detached, it should be firmly pressed in place for 10 seconds. If it sticks well, it can be used for the full 7 days; if not, apply a replacement patch.
- If it is completely detached, the client should try to reapply the same patch if it is clean and usable. If not, apply a new patch immediately.
- If the patch has been off for more than 24 hours, instruct her to use a backup method for 7 days and consider EC.
- Missed patches:
    - *First-week patch:* offer EC, place patch immediately, use a backup method for 7 days.
    - *Second- to third-week patch:* If late by 1 or 2 days, remove old patch and place a new one immediately, no backup or EC is needed. If late by more than 2 days, remove the old patch and place a new one immediately, offer EC, use a backup method for 7 days.
    - *Fourth-week patch:* remove the patch, she should place a new one on the usual day, no backup method or EC is needed.

CONTRACEPTIVE VAGINAL RING

A CVR was approved by the FDA in 2001 and became available in 2002. It consists of a flexible, soft, transparent ring made of ethylene vinyl acetate copolymer, with an outer diameter of 54 mm, which releases 120 mcg of etonogestrel (a metabolite of desogestrel) and 15 mcg of EE per day. Each ring is to be used for one cycle, which consists of a 3-week period of continuous ring use followed by a ring-free week to allow withdrawal bleeding. The CVR is inserted by the user: no fitting is necessary. The woman compresses the ring and inserts it into the vagina, as far back as possible. Precise placement is not critical. Although if the ring is bothersome, it could indicate that the ring should be inserted deeper into the vagina. The hormones are absorbed through the vaginal mucosa.

The CVR can be used in several ways:

- *Quick start:* Insert CVR the day of clinical visit. Use backup method for 7 days (preferred method).
- *Sunday start*: Insert CVR on first Sunday during menses.
- *First-day start:* Insert CVR first day of menstrual bleeding.
- Postpartum women (not lactating) may begin at day 21 postpartum.
- Postabortion or miscarriage may begin immediately (day 1 or 2).

The CVR can be left in place for 3 weeks, removed, and discarded. After 7 days without the ring, a new one is inserted, even if bleeding continues. During the 3-week wear period, if the ring is removed or expelled for 3 hours or more, backup contraception is needed for 7 days after it is reinserted. The CVR can also be inserted on the 1st of every month and removed on the 25th. It may easier for the patient to remember these insertion and removal dates. Using the CVR in this way could have economic benefit, as the patient would use 12 cycles in one year instead of 13. The CVR can also be used continuously, for menstrual suppression.

Advantages

- Elimination of the need for daily pill taking, so consistent use is improved
- Delivery systems avoid first-pass effect on the liver
- Low incidence of breakthrough bleeding
- Hormone levels remain therapeutic for at least 35 days, suggesting that ovulation inhibition would be maintained even if a woman forgets to remove the ring up to 2 weeks late (Hatcher et al., 2011)
- Safe for women with latex allergy

Disadvantages

- Vaginal ring not recommended for women with uterine prolapse, lack of vaginal muscle tone, or chronic constipation.
- Women must be comfortable with insertion and removal of the CVR.
- With CVR, women may experience a foreign body sensation in the vagina, problems with coitus, expulsion, or vaginal discomfort. These are the most common reasons for discontinuation.
- Side effects specific to CVR include a low incidence of headache, leukorrhea, and vaginitis (Rawlins & Smith, 2002; Speroff & Darney, 2011).
- Backup contraception needed for 7 days if the ring is removed for 3 or more hours.

Client Counseling

- Instruct the client to leave the CVR in the vagina for intercourse. If it is uncomfortable for either partner, it may be removed for up to 3 hours, cleansed with cool water, and replaced in the vagina.
- If the CVR has been out of the vagina for longer than 3 hours, a backup method should be used for 7 days. If the woman had unprotected intercourse, offer EC.
- Some women may experience an increase in normal vaginal secretions due to the localized estrogenic effect of CVR. Counsel patients on signs and symptoms of abnormal discharge.
- If the client is having trouble placing the CVR, she may find it helpful to use an empty tampon applicator to insert the CVR.

PROGESTIN-ONLY PILLS

Referred to as *minipills*, POPs were introduced 10 years after COCs. POPs are taken daily with no pill-free interval. Although much less popular than COCs, POPs are well suited to women who want to take contraceptive pills but have contraindications to COCs. Available POPs contain norethindrone or norgestrel; they contain a fixed dose of progestin in 28-day pack.

Mechanism of Action

There are four mechanisms by which POPs may prevent pregnancy.

- Ovulation is inhibited in a variable proportion of cycles.
- Cervical mucus maintains a thick consistency, inhibiting sperm penetration.

- The endometrium becomes thin and atrophic.
- Tubal changes occur, including altered tubal transport, contractility, and histology (Bergett-Hanson, 2001; Dickey, 2010; Hatcher et al., 2011, Speroff & Darney, 2011).

Effectiveness

See Table 12–3.

Advantages

- No estrogen-related side effects.
- Overall safer than CHCs (fewer and less serious complications).
- May be used by lactating women.
- May be used by clients with prior history of thrombophlebitis (no effect on blood clotting) or with history of other estrogen-related contraindications to CHC use.
- Minimal effect on carbohydrate metabolism; therefore, may be used (with caution) by diabetic women.
- Rapid reversal of effects after stopping.
- Several noncontraceptive benefits.

Noncontraceptive Benefits

Most health benefits are similar to those of CHCs. Menstrual cycle benefits include decreased cramping, lighter bleeding, shorter periods, decreased PMS-type symptoms, and lessened breast tenderness.

Disadvantages

- Must be taken with meticulous accuracy; no more than 27 hours between pills.
- Slightly less effective than CHCs.
- May cause irregular bleeding with unpredictable patterns (may include spotting, breakthrough bleeding, amenorrhea, prolonged bleeding).
- No protection against STIs.
- Interaction with other drugs can decrease effectiveness (see Table 12–6).
- Higher incidence of functional ovarian cysts.
- Higher incidence of ectopic pregnancy.
- Progestins may theoretically cause adverse effects on blood lipids by decreasing HDLs and increasing LDLs and triglycerides.
- Also refer to the section on CHCs and to Tables 12–7 and 12–8 to evaluate and manage side effects.

Contraindications/Precautions

According to the FDA, POPs are required to carry the same contraindications as CHCs, even though many of these contraindications are related to estrogen content (see Table 12–3). Several *relative* contraindications to POPs should be emphasized.

- History of functional ovarian cysts.
- History of ectopic pregnancy.
- Inability to take pills consistently.
- Undiagnosed abnormal vaginal bleeding during the preceding 3 months.
- Hyperlipidemia.

Client Counseling

- POPs may be used by women over 35 who smoke.
- Instruct that POPs do not protect against STIs.
- If decision is made to stop POPs and pregnancy is not desired, begin using another birth control method immediately.
- Spotting or bleeding between periods is not unusual for a woman on the minipill, especially during the first few months of use.
- Initiating use.
  - *Quick start:* Take the first pill the day of clinical visit. Use backup method for 7 days (preferred method).
  - *Sunday start*: Take the first pill on first Sunday during menses.
  - *First-day start:* Take the first pill the first day of menstrual bleeding.
  - Postpartum women may start immediately following delivery (6-week delay is recommended for breastfeeding).
  - Postabortion or miscarriage may begin immediately (day 1 or 2).
- One pill is swallowed daily until pack is finished; new pack is started the very next day—a day is never skipped. In addition, minipills must be taken at *exactly* the same time every day.
- When minipills are missed or forgotten, instruct the client as follows:
  - If pill is taken more than 3 hours late, use a backup birth control method for the next 48 hours.
  - If one pill is missed, take it as soon as remembered. Take the next pill at the regular time, even if this means taking two pills in one day. Use a backup method for the next 48 hours.
  - If two pills or more are missed in a row, there is a good chance of pregnancy occurring. Take two pills as soon as remembered and two the next day. Start using a second method of birth control right

away. If no period occurs in 4 to 6 weeks, a pregnancy test is needed.
- Emergency contraception may be used if pills were missed and client has had intercourse without adequate protection.

OTHER PROGESTIN-ONLY CONTRACEPTIVES: IMPLANT AND INJECTION

The newer long-acting progestin-only methods are ideal for women who desire long-term, continuous contraception and who may desire future pregnancies. Norplant and Implanon implants and depot-medroxyprogesterone acetate (DMPA) injections are discussed here.

Norplant

Norplant was marketed in the United States until 2002, when the U.S. distributor stopped selling it, citing limitations in product component supplies. Some women may still have Norplant in situ, and would need removal. This should be done by a provider who was trained in insertion and removal of Norplant.

Norplant is a timed-release implant of levonorgestrel. The system consists of six Silastic capsules, each measuring 2.4 × 34 mm and containing 36 mg of levonorgestrel. Capsules are implanted in a fanlike pattern through a 3 to 5 mm incision, usually in the medial aspect of the upper arm (Darney, 2001; Hatcher et al., 2011; Norplant Effective, 2000).

Implanon

Implanon is a 4 cm long and 2 mm diameter implant; it contains 68 mg of etonogestrel. Implanon is intended to provide contraception for 3 years after insertion.

Mechanism of Action

Implanon suppresses ovulation in almost all users throughout the first 3 years after insertion. It also alters endometrial structure and changes cervical mucus in a way that may impede sperm penetration. These mechanisms may contribute to the method's protective effect if ovulation does occur (Schering-Plough, 2009).

Effectiveness

See Table 12–3.

Advantages

- Ease of use
- No attention is required on the part of the user until time of removal
- Discreteness
- No adverse effect on acne
- Relief of dysmenorrhea
- Relief of endometriosis symptoms
- Few known clinically significant metabolic effects
- Reduces risk of ectopic pregnancy
- No estrogen
- Reversibility

Disadvantages

- Abnormal uterine bleeding
- 1/10 women discontinue the method due to unacceptable bleeding patterns
- Rare insertion complications
- Ovarian cysts
- Clinician dependency, must be inserted and removed by a trained clinician
- Does not protect against STIs
- Drug interactions
- Possible increased risk of thromboembolic conditions
- Infection can occur at the implant insertion site in rare instances
- No protection against STIs

Contraindications

- Breastfeeding women < 6 weeks postpartum
- Current deep vein thrombosis or pulmonary embolism
- Active, viral hepatitis, or severe cirrhosis
- Benign or malignant liver tumors
- Unexplained, unevaluated, abnormal vaginal bleeding
- Current breast cancer
- Past breast cancer without evidence of current disease within 5 years

Client Counseling

- Informed consent is obtained.
- Educate client regarding insertion and removal procedures.
- The insertion and removal of implant systems must be done by a professional specifically trained in the proper techniques.
- Be sure that both patient and clinician palpate the implant after insertion.
- Careful counseling regarding bleeding patterns is essential to user satisfaction; the user must be ready for unpredictable bleeding patterns.
- Initiation:
  - Insert any time during the first 5 days of the menstrual cycle if hormonal contraception is not being used.

- If hormonal contraception is being used, insert any time during the hormone-free interval.
- If on continuous-use CHCs, insert any time.
- If progestin-only contraception is being used, insert on the same day the next progestin injection is due, or implant, or IUD is removed.
- With progestin-only oral contraception, insertion can be performed any time.
- Insert any time within the first 5 days after an abortion or before the 4th-week postpartum in non-breastfeeding women.
- Insert before the 4th-month postpartum in breastfeeding women. However, if access to contraception is limited, it is appropriate to insert an implant immediately postpartum.
- No backup method is necessary if timing of insertion follows the above.
- If insertion occurs at other times, backup method is necessary for 7 days (Schering-Plough, 2009; Speroff & Darney, 2011).

Depot-Medroxyprogesterone Acetate

DMPA is an intramuscular (IM) injection that provides 12 weeks of protection. It was approved by the FDA for use as a contraceptive in the United States in 1992. The standard dosage is DMPA 150 mg IM every 12 weeks.

Mechanism of Action

- Ovulation is suppressed by inhibition of LH release from the anterior pituitary. Ovulation is inhibited in about 40 percent of cycles.
- Cervical mucus maintains a thick consistency, inhibiting sperm penetration.
- The endometrium becomes thin and atrophic.
- Tubal changes occur, including altered tubal transport, contractility, and histology.
- There is diminished functioning of corpus luteum.
- Progesterone receptor synthesis is inhibited (Dickey, 2010; Hatcher et al., 2011).

Effectiveness

See Table 12–3.

Advantages

- Long duration of action.
- Highly effective.
- Relative low doses of hormone.
- Few systemic complications.
- Reversible.
- Low ectopic pregnancy rates.
- Major complications are rare.
- Effects on blood lipids appear to be minimal (DMPA may lower HDL cholesterol).
- Estrogen free.
- Use not associated with coitus.
- Very light menses or amenorrhea.
- May be used while lactating.
- May be used by smokers over 35.
- Receiving the DMPA injection early by up to a week is not harmful. There is a grace period of 1 week if late receiving DMPA.
- Some noncontraceptive benefits.
- Culturally acceptable.
- Improvement of menstrual symptoms.
- Minimal drug interactions.
- Fewer seizures.
- Fewer sickle cell crises.
- Less pain from endometriosis.
- Benefit women with myomas.
- Decreased risk of PID.

Disadvantages

- Most women experience some side effects; most are usually minor and related to menstrual irregularities. If bleeding is heavy, anemia may occur.
- Return visit needed every 12 weeks for DMPA.
- If the woman is already depressed, signs and symptoms may increase on DMPA.
- No protection against STIs.
- Possible weight gain, nausea, headaches.
- Return to fertility may be delayed 6 to 12 months after injection of DMPA.
- Temporary, reversible decrease in bone density in long-term users.
- Not possible to discontinue immediately.
- Return visit to clinic every 3 months.

Contraindications

Progestin-only methods must carry the same contraindications as CHCs, even though many are related to estrogen content (see Table 12–3). Several relative contraindications to DMPA should be emphasized.

- Known or suspected pregnancy.
- History of undiagnosed abnormal vaginal bleeding during the 3 months prior to use of one of these methods.
- History of functional ovarian cysts.
- Acute liver disease.

- Jaundice.
- Significant concern about weight gain.
- When rapid return to fertility is desired.
- Hypercholesterolemia.
- Current significant depression.
- Women with existing or risk for bone density loss.

Client Counseling

- It takes 7 days to become effective.
- For nonbreastfeeding women, Depo-Provera may be initiated at 1-week postpartum or immediately postabortion (first trimester).
- Lactating women should wait until 6 weeks after delivery.
- Danger signs that indicate possible serious problems associated with use of the methods must be taught.
  - Severe abdominal pain.
  - Heavy vaginal bleeding.
  - Depression.
  - Severe headache.
  - Excessive weight gain.
- For spotting/bleeding with DMPA, provide reassurance that by second or third injection she may be amenorrheic.
- For amenorrhea, provide reassurance. Obtain pregnancy test if client is worried or if injection not done at the recommended time. No need to induce menses.

Management of Bleeding on Progestin-Only Methods

For prolonged and/or frequent bleeding, obtain the following information: history of bleeding pattern, sexual activity pattern, concurrent illness, unusual stressful events, medications, substance use/abuse. Examine for other causes of bleeding such as infection or genital lesions. Perform a pregnancy test, gonorrhea and chlamydia tests, saline and KOH preps. If no cause for bleeding can be determined from this evaluation, then may try one of the following methods. Each of these methods can help reduce bleeding in the short term; however, when these interventions are discontinued, irregular bleeding patterns may resume. Inform women the likelihood of amenorrhea will increase over time. Treatment options include the following:

- Ibuprofen 800 mg tid for 5 to 7 days.
- Doxycycline 100 mg bid for 5 days.
- Any currently available low-dose CHC for one or more cycles.
- Medroxyprogesterone acetate (Provera) 10 mg daily for 10 days.
- EE 20 or 50 mcg for 10 days. If bleeding persists, continue for 20 days *or* Premarin 0.625 mg daily for 25 days.
- If a low-dose estrogen supplement (oral, transdermal, or cream) is added to a progestin-only method to reduce a possible risk of lowered bone density, there may be a risk of thinned cervical mucus and unplanned pregnancy. Condoms are advised as long as the client is taking exogenous estrogen in this circumstance, or advise changing to another method of contraception (Advisor Forum, 2002). Serum estradiol levels below 20 pg/mL warrant evaluation for use of exogenous estrogen in some women (Hatcher et al., 2011; Speroff & Darney, 2011).

THE MALE CONDOM

The male condom, also referred to as a rubber, prophylactic, or skin, is a sheath that is worn over the erect penis to contain fluid from ejaculation. Most U.S. condoms are made from latex rubber. Other types include polyurethane or silicone rubber. Lambskin or lamb intestine condoms (natural skin condoms) are also still available. Organisms that cause STIs can penetrate natural skin condoms. Condoms are available in many colors, textures, sizes, shapes, and thicknesses. They are available lubricated with spermicide or without, and nonlubricated. Clients must be sure to purchase condoms that are labeled for use as contraceptives. Novelty condoms exist on the market, and may or may not prevent pregnancy or STIs. The user should be cautious of novelty products for this reason.

Mechanism of Action

A *condom* is a mechanical barrier to prevent sperm from entering the vagina and cervix. Condoms prevent direct contact with semen, penile lesions, discharges, and infected secretions. Condoms (except natural skin) prevent transmission of most STIs. Spermicidal condoms have the additional action of nonoxynol-9 to immobilize and kill sperm after ejaculation (see Spermicides, later in this chapter).

Effectiveness

Condoms are considered effective at preventing accidental pregnancy. Of 100 couples using condoms, 2 percent are estimated to become pregnant during *consistent and correct* use during the first 12 months of use (see Table 12–3). Couples vary in their ability to use male condoms consistently and correctly. Among those using condoms for contraception, about 15 of every 100 will become pregnant with *typical* use. Failure to prevent pregnancy is most frequently attributed to inconsistent use. Condom breakage can occur, but this is not a major cause of accidental pregnancy. Effectiveness increases significantly, approaching the effectiveness of oral contraceptives or an IUD, when used concurrently with a vaginal spermicide (Hatcher et al., 2011).

Advantages

- Available without a prescription or examination.
- Relatively inexpensive.
- Widely available.
- Physiologically safe.
- No adverse effect on fertility.
- Easily reversible contraception.
- Few side effects.
- Significant protection against most STIs.
- Possible protection against cancer of the cervix.
- Male participation in contraception is encouraged.
- Only reversible contraceptive available for use by men.
- May delay premature ejaculation in men for whom this is a concern.
- May be used during lactation.
- Lubricated condoms may reduce friction, preventing irritation to either partner.
- Postcoital drainage of semen from the vagina, which some women find objectionable, is eliminated.
- Polyurethane condoms are stronger than latex and thinner. It may improve sensation and pleasure.
- Polyurethane condom can be safely used with oil-based lubricants.

Disadvantages

- Fairly expensive for frequent use.
- Possible decreased sensation for man.
- Interferes with sexual spontaneity (requires forethought and preparedness).
- Necessity to interrupt foreplay to put condom on.
- Lambskin condoms made from animal membranes may not protect against STIs.
- Some women and men experience irritation with the use of particular lubricants or spermicides on condoms.
- Male partner may be unwilling to cooperate with condom use.
- Latex allergy (nonlatex condoms are an equally effective option).

Client Counseling

The following instructions will be helpful to couples using condoms:

- Store condoms in a cool, dry place. Heat, even body heat, may weaken the condom. Always keep the condom in its original package until use. Condoms should keep 5 years when properly stored. Check expiration date.
- Discuss condom use with partner before intercourse.
- The condom is placed on the erect penis (either partner can do this) *before* the penis comes in contact with the woman's genital area.
- Roll the condom all the way down to the base of the penis.
- Be careful not to tear the condom with sharp objects such as rings or long fingernails.
- If the condom does not have a built-in reservoir, leave one-half inch of empty space at the end of it to collect ejaculate. This is accomplished by pinching the tip of the condom as it is rolled on. Leave no air in the tip; this could contribute to tearing.
- Be sure that the vagina and/or condom are well lubricated to prevent condom tearing. If additional lubrication is needed, use only water, saliva, water-based jelly, or contraceptive foam, gel, or cream on latex condoms. Oil-based products, such as cold cream, mineral oil, cooking oil, petroleum jelly, body lotions, massage oil, and baby oil, will cause deterioration and weakening of latex. Other vaginal products that cause latex condom weakening include miconazole nitrate (Monistat), butoconazole nitrate (Femstat), estradiol (Estrace), and conjugated estrogen (Premarin) creams, Vagisil ointment, Rendell's Cone and Ovule Spermicide, and the sexual lubricant called Elbow Grease.
- Diaphragm, IUD, spermicidal foam, gel, film, suppository, natural family planning (NFP), or any hormonal method may be used in combination with condoms.
- After intercourse, remove the condom immediately while the penis is still erect, holding on to the base of the condom to prevent spilling. Dispose of properly after use.
- Check the condom for tears, then throw it away. If tears are detected, immediately insert spermicidal gel or cream into the vagina.
- Use each condom only once.

THE FEMALE CONDOM

The first female condom was approved by the FDA in 1993 for over-the-counter sale in the United States. The female condom consists of a polyurethane sheath with an outer ring and inner ring. Each condom is prelubricated with silicone, and a container of water-based lubricant is supplied for those who prefer more lubrication. It is inserted vaginally, like a diaphragm, and held in place by the pubic bone. The closed upper tip is anchored near the cervix by a flexible inner ring that holds the device in place, preventing expulsion. The condom covers the surfaces of the vaginal wall, allowing the penis to move freely inside the condom. An external ring at the outer opening of the pouch remains outside the vagina and partially covers the labia. It is used for one act of intercourse only. If used correctly with every sex act, the female condom also helps to prevent the spread of STD. It is approved by the FDA for prevention of pregnancy and STDs.

Mechanism of Action

This device serves as a mechanical barrier to prevent sperm from entering the vagina or cervix. The polyurethane female condom also has the ability to prevent transmission of most STDs, including HIV.

Effectiveness

The typical failure rate in U.S. studies was similar to that for diaphragm, sponge, and cervical cap during typical use. The female condom is impermeable to various STD organisms and HIV (Speroff & Darney, 2011) (see Table 12–3).

Advantages

- Use controlled by the woman.
- Available without a prescription or examination.
- Easily reversible.
- Considered medically safe.
- Little danger of systemic effects.
- May provide protection against STIs.
- May be worn prior to intercourse.
- Not dependent on male arousal.
- May be used while pregnant or menstruating.
- May be used during lactation.
- May be removed immediately after intercourse.
- Provides improved sensation for man and woman and allows transfer of body heat.
- Eliminates postcoital drainage of semen.

Disadvantages

- Expensive for frequent use (about three times the price of the male condom).
- For single use only.
- Cumbersome; insertion can be difficult.
- Can slip or be pushed out of place.
- May make noise during use.
- Unsightly ring dangles outside the vagina.
- Breakage, tearing can occur (though rarely).

Contraindications

- Allergy of man or woman to polyurethane.
- Anatomic abnormalities that interfere with proper placement.
- Inability to master insertion technique.

Client Counseling

The following instructions will be helpful to the client:

- Practice wearing and inserting the female condom before depending on it for protection.
- Be careful not to tear the condom with sharp objects such as rings or long fingernails.
- Extra spermicidal lubricant may be used if desired.
- Refer to the package inserts for detailed use and insertion instructions.
- Insert inner ring high in the vagina, against the cervix.
- Place the outer ring properly outside the vagina.
- During intercourse, be sure the penis is placed inside the female condom.
- After intercourse, remove the female condom carefully to avoid spilling semen.
- Female and male condoms should not be used together.

SPERMICIDES

Spermicides are chemical substances that immobilize and kill sperm. The spermicidal agent available in the United States is nonoxynol-9. This is a surfactant that destroys the sperm cell membrane. Nonoxynol-9 formulations, available in creams, jellies, suppositories, and film, are inserted into the vagina prior to intercourse. When used alone, they are inserted vaginally near the cervix, forming a chemical barrier. Spermicides are also essential components of vaginal barrier methods of contraception (diaphragm, cervical cap, and sponge). Surfaces of male condoms may be coated with spermicide to enhance the effectiveness of this method as a contraceptive.

When used alone, all spermicidal products provide protection for up to 1 hour and for one episode of intercourse only. Additional acts of intercourse, or intercourse occurring more than 1 hour after insertion, require repeated application of the product. Spermicides are ineffective as microbicides, thus do not recommend the use of spermicide alone to prevent STIs. Furthermore, frequent use (more than twice daily) of spermicide causes more vulvovaginal epithelial disruption, which theoretically could increase susceptibility of HIV (see Chapter 15).

Foams, Jellies, Creams

These can be used alone or with a condom, diaphragm, or cervical cap. Foams are available in multidose aerosol containers or in small, single-use, prefilled cartridges. Creams and jellies come in multidose tubes with reusable applicators. Some jellies are sold in single-use packets.

Suppositories

Referred to as *spermicidal vaginal tablets*, the suppositories are of a small ovoid shape. They can be used alone or with a condom but must be inserted 10 to 15 minutes before intercourse in order to melt and disperse the spermicide.

Vaginal Contraceptive Film

Vaginal contraceptive film (VCF), which can be used alone or with a condom or diaphragm, is a paper-thin sheet of film containing nonoxynol-9, measuring 2 × 2 in. The sheet is inserted on or near the cervix (or inside a diaphragm) 15 minutes prior to intercourse in order to melt and disperse the spermicide.

Mechanism of Action

Spermicides contain a chemical surfactant that immobilizes and kills sperm (by destroying sperm cell membrane) and vehicle ingredients to keep the spermicide in place around the cervix. The active ingredient in spermicidal products sold in the United States is nonoxynol-9.

Effectiveness

Spermicides used alone are low to moderately effective at preventing accidental pregnancy (see Table 12–3). Spermicides are the least effective of modern contraceptives. Failures are most frequently attributed to inconsistent use. Proper use, including placement of the product deep inside the vagina against the cervix, is essential. Efficacy is much greater if used with a condom or diaphragm. Data is not available comparing the efficacies of the various spermicidal products (Best, 2000a; Hatcher et al., 2011).

Advantages

- Widely available without a prescription or examination.
- Relatively inexpensive.
- Medically safe.
- Readily available as a backup method in a variety of circumstances:
  - In the event of condom rupture.
  - To augment other methods during midcycle, when a woman is most fertile.
  - When a woman begins using oral or other hormonal contraceptives.
  - When a woman taking oral contraceptives misses one or more pills.
- Completely reversible.
- No effect on the return to fertility.
- Women can decide independently to use it.
- Can provide lubrication during intercourse.
- Can be used during lactation.
- Convenient, useful method of contraception after delivery and before the first postpartum visit, and when changing from one method to another.

Disadvantages

- May interfere with sexual spontaneity (requires forethought and preparedness).
- Must be on hand at or near the time of intercourse.
- Suppositories and film require time to disperse before intercourse can take place.
- Perceived as messy by some individuals (drainage of the substance from the vagina occurs after intercourse).
- Incomplete dissolution of suppositories can cause an uncomfortable, gritty sensation for either partner and may impair contraceptive effectiveness.
- Some users experience a warm sensation; some feel that the suppository burns.
- For couples engaging in oral-genital sex, the taste of spermicides is unpleasant. Spermicide may be inserted after this activity, but before penis-vagina contact takes place.

- Skin irritation of the vulva or penis can result from frequent use of spermicides or from allergy or sensitivity to the spermicide or base ingredients. Another product may be tried.
- Not protective against STIs.

Contraindications

- Allergy of either partner to spermicide or its other ingredients.
- Inability to learn the proper insertion technique.
- Anatomic abnormalities of the vagina that might interfere with the correct placement or retention of the spermicide.

Client Counseling

The following instructions will be helpful to couples using a spermicide:

- The spermicide must be used every time intercourse occurs; must be in place prior to penis-vagina contact.
- Store spermicides in a cool, clean, and dry place.
- Wait the specified time after insertion so that the spermicide is adequately dispersed (for film and suppositories).
- One application is good for 1 hour after insertion and for one act of intercourse only. Additional application is needed if 1 hour has passed since insertion or before each additional act of intercourse.
- All spermicides must be left in place for at least 6 hours after the last act of intercourse. Do not douche or rinse the product out for at least 6 hours.
- Instructions for specific products include the following:
  - *Foam:* Shake vigorously at least 20 times before dispensing. Insert the applicator as far into the vagina as it will go comfortably. Holding the applicator in place, push the plunger to release the product.
  - *Jelly or cream:* Fill applicator by squeezing the tube from the bottom. Insert as for foam (see earlier point).
  - *Suppository (vaginal tablet):* Remove the wrapper and insert as far as possible so that the tablet rests on or near the cervix. Wait the specified time before intercourse.
  - *Film:* Fingers must be completely dry. Place one sheet of film on a fingertip and slide it along the back wall of the vagina as far as possible, so that the film rests on or near the cervix. Wait 15 minutes before intercourse.
- If burning or irritation occurs, stop use of the product. Changing brands or the form of spermicide may diminish reactions. If a reaction persists, discontinue use.

VAGINAL BARRIER METHODS: DIAPHRAGMS, CERVICAL CAPS, SPONGE

Diaphragm

A *diaphragm* is a dome-shaped cup made of silicone with a flexible-spring metal rim. It is inserted vaginally prior to intercourse, so that the posterior rim rests in the posterior fornix and the anterior rim fits snugly behind the pubic bone. Spermicidal cream, jelly, or film is applied inside the dome of the diaphragm and around the rim before insertion. The most commonly used diaphragm in the United States is the Ortho All-Flex®, an arcing spring diaphragm made from silicone and available in four sizes (65, 70, 75, and 80 mm). The sturdy rim of this type of diaphragm imparts firm spring strength. Furthermore, the arcing rim facilitates insertion. Most women can use it comfortably, and it can be retained in the presence of cystocele and/or rectocele or relaxed vaginal muscle tone. Another option is the Milex Wide Seal® diaphragm. This type has a thin, flexible flange approximately 1.5 cm wide attached to the inner edge of the rim to keep spermicide in place inside the dome and to enhance the seal between the rim and the vaginal wall. It is made in two styles: arcing and coil spring. It is considered to provide a better seal for some women and is also made of silicone. It is available from the manufacturer only and has a range of eight sizes from 60 to 95 mm (sized in 5 mm increments). Two new one-size-fits-all diaphragms, SILCS® and BufferGel Duet®, are being evaluated for efficacy and may be available in the near future. Both these diaphragms have the advantage of not needing to be fit by a provider (Hatcher et al., 2011).

Fitting the Diaphragm

- Insert index and middle finger into the vagina until your middle finger reaches the posterior wall of the vagina.
- Use the tip of your thumb to mark the point at which your index finger touches the pubic bone.
- Extract your fingers.
- Place the rim on the tip of your middle finger. The opposite rim should lie just in front of your thumb.
- Insert a sample diaphragm of the size you have selected.

The diaphragm should fit snugly between the posterior fornix and the symphysis pubis, touching lateral vaginal walls and covering the cervix. There should be just enough space to insert one fingertip comfortably between the inside of the pubic arch and the anterior edge of the diaphragm rim. Check for displacement when the client bears down. Have her walk around the room, sit, and squat. Check again for displacement and client comfort. If the client feels the diaphragm while walking around, it may be too large. If it is easily displaced with a finger or with moving/walking, it can be displaced during intercourse. If in doubt about fit, try the next larger size. Two or three different sizes should be tried before a final decision is made. Instruct the client to practice removal and insertion three times, while you verify proper placement each time (Hatcher et al., 2011).

Vaginal Contraceptive Sponge

The Today vaginal contraceptive sponge was introduced in the United States in 1983. It is a small, soft, pillow-shaped disposable polyurethane sponge that is impregnated with nonoxynol-9. After it is moistened with water and inserted high into the vagina, the sponge is immediately effective for the next 24 hours, without need to add more spermicide, even for repeated acts of intercourse. The concave dimple on one side fits over the cervix. A woven polyester loop on the other side facilitates removal. The sponge must be left in place for 6 hours after the last act of intercourse. It may then be removed and discarded. Maximum recommended wear time is 30 hours (Mayer Laboratories, 2009).

Cervical Cap

The cervical cap is a soft, rubber, cup-shaped device, resembling a small diaphragm with a deep dome (much like a thimble). It fits over the cervix and is held in place by a seal that forms between its flexible rim and the outer surface of cervix. A small amount of spermicide is placed inside the cap, but not on the rim, which would interfere with forming the seal. The only cervical cap currently available in the United States is the FemCap.

The FemCap is made of durable silicone rubber, is flared to prevent dislodgement, and has a strap to aid in removal. The FemCap is held in place by the muscular walls of the vagina and does not have to be snug around the cervix or hinge behind the pubic bone. The FemCap has a brim that flares outward like an inverted funnel to direct sperm toward the groove that traps the sperm and exposes it to the stored spermicide; this is the major difference between the FemCap and the diaphragm.

The FemCap does not require precise measurements or custom fitting. It comes in three easy-to-fit sizes (the inner diameter of the rim determines its size):

- The smallest rim diameter (22 mm) cap is intended for women who have *never* been pregnant.
- The medium (26 mm) cap is intended for women who have been pregnant, but did not have a vaginal delivery (miscarriage, C-section, or abortion).
- The largest (30 mm) cap is intended for women who have had a vaginal delivery of a full-term baby (FemCap, 2011).

Fitting the FemCap

- Perform pelvic exam to exclude any contraindication, and determine the size of the cervix.
- Provide the woman with her FemCap size, according to her obstetrical history, and the pelvic exam.
- Allow her ample time to learn how to insert and remove the FemCap.
- She should feel her cervix, then practice insertion and removal of the FemCap *on her own*.
- Check the FemCap for correct placement by digital exam to ensure that the FemCap is covering her cervix completely (FemCap, 2011).

Mechanism of Action

- The contraceptive effect of the diaphragm is related to the barrier effect, which prevents sperm entry into the cervix, and to the sperm-killing action of spermicide used with all diaphragms.
- Similar in action to the diaphragm, the cervical cap serves as a barrier to the cervix and holds spermicide within its dome.
- The sponge has the barrier effect, the sperm-killing action of spermicide, and the additional action of trapping and absorbing semen before sperm can enter the cervix.

Effectiveness

Contraceptive efficacy among these methods is comparable (see Table 12–3). Some cervical cap failures are attributed to cap dislodgement during intercourse and to deterioration of rubber after prolonged use and/or storage.

Vaginal barrier methods depend largely on extremely conscientious use, although individual fertility characteristics are probably equally important. These methods must be used correctly and consistently. They are used with more success by women 30 years of age or older, who have intercourse fewer than four times weekly, and who may have slightly lower fertility than their younger counterparts. Many women who experience accidental pregnancy with these methods report misuse (including inconsistent use). Users must be highly motivated to prevent or delay pregnancy. The role of the clinician can be very significant in assisting women to use these products successfully (Best, 2000b; Hatcher et al., 2011).

Advantages

- Attractive method for women needing contraception on an irregular basis and whose sexual patterns are fairly predictable.
- Does not require partner involvement.
- Considered medically safe.
- Little danger of systemic effects.
- Easily reversible.
- Provides significant protection against STIs and PID.
- Can be used during lactation.
- Diaphragm may provide some protection against cervical neoplasia.
- Sponge available over the counter; one size fits all.

Disadvantages

- The diaphragm requires accurate fitting by a professional clinician.
- May interfere with sexual spontaneity if not readily available.
- Learning insertion and removal techniques may be difficult for some.
- Perceived as aesthetically objectionable or messy by some individuals.
- Silicone rubber, polyurethane, or spermicide could cause irritation or allergy in either partner.
- Foul odor or vaginal discharge may occur if the product is left in place more than a few days.
- Silicone lubrication can damage the silicone diaphragm or cervical cap.
- Potential for vaginal trauma associated with difficult insertion or removal of the device.
- Increased risk of UTI in diaphragm users.
- Potential for toxic shock syndrome (TSS).
- Sponge and the cervical cap are somewhat less effective in parous women.

Contraindications

- Allergy to silicone, rubber, polyurethane, or spermicide.
- Delivery in prior 6 weeks or abortion in prior 2 weeks (for cap or sponge).
- Anatomic abnormalities that interfere with proper fitting of the cap or diaphragm.
- Inability to master insertion or removal techniques.
- Recurrent UTIs with use of the diaphragm.
- History of cervical malignancy or abnormal Pap that has not been evaluated.
- History of TSS.

Client Counseling

A critical aspect of successful use of either the diaphragm or the cervical cap is that sufficient time be offered to the client for teaching and practice at the office visit. The following points should be part of client teaching:

- Devices may be inserted immediately prior to intercourse; however, some experts recommend waiting 30 minutes after cervical cap insertion to be sure that the seal has formed between the rim and the cervix.
- Devices must be left in place for a minimum of 6 hours after the last act of intercourse.
- Diaphragm may not be reliable if coitus is to take place in water because spermicide could wash away.
- The danger signs of TSS include sudden high fever, vomiting, diarrhea, dizziness, faintness, weakness, sore throat, aching muscles or joints, rash.
- The diaphragm or cap should be inspected prior to insertion for cracks, holes, tears, or drying of rubber or silicone.
- After using a cap or diaphragm, wash the device with soap and water, dry thoroughly, and store in its container.
- Follow up with a health care provider if experiencing recurrent UTIs or yeast infections.

Specific Instructions for Diaphragm Use

- Place approximately one tablespoon of spermicidal cream or jelly in the dome and around the rim of the diaphragm.
- Insert the diaphragm *up to* 6 hours prior to intercourse.
- The diaphragm must remain in place for 6 to 8 hours following each act of coitus. If coitus does not take place within 6 hours of insertion, remove the diaphragm and reapply spermicide. For subsequent acts of coitus, spermicide is added with an inserter, without removing diaphragm.

Specific Instructions for Sponge Use

- Wet the sponge thoroughly with water. Gently squeeze the sponge to produce suds. Fold the sponge with dimple side facing upward and insert deeply into the vagina, sliding it along the posterior wall of the vagina. The dimple should be up against the cervix.

- The sponge may be inserted up to 24 hours prior to intercourse.
- Six hours after the last act of intercourse, the sponge may be removed by inserting a finger into the vagina and reaching up to find the string loop. Hook the finger around the loop and gently pull the sponge from the vagina. Relaxing and bearing down can facilitate removal. Package instructions are well illustrated (Mayer Laboratories, 2009).

Specific Instructions for Cervical Cap Use

- To use a cervical cap, the woman should be at least 6 weeks postpartum or 2 weeks postabortion.
- Unlike the diaphragm, the bulk of the spermicide is stored in the groove between the dome and brim of the FemCap, facing the vaginal opening, to expose sperm to the spermicide upon deposition into the vagina.
- Cap may be left in place up to 48 hours without regard to frequency of intercourse during that period. It is not necessary to insert additional spermicide.

INTRAUTERINE DEVICES

IUDs are small objects, usually plastic, that are placed inside the uterus. They contain either copper or levonorgestrel. Two strings are attached that protrude into the vagina to enable the user to check placement and remove the device. IUDs are packaged in individual sterile units that include the device, insertion barrel, and manufacturer literature. Insertion may take place at any time during the menstrual cycle as long as it is certain that the client is not pregnant. The IUD may be inserted at 6 weeks postpartum.

Currently in the United States, two IUDs are available: the copper ParaGard-T-380A marketed by Teva Women's Health and the LNG-IUS (brand name: Mirena by Bayer Healthcare Pharmaceuticals), which releases levonorgestrel.

The Dalkon Shield, associated with a high rate of pelvic infections and septic abortions, was removed from the U.S. market in 1975. There is no doubt that the problems with the Dalkon Shield were due to defective construction. The multifilamented tail (porous material) of the Dalkon Shield provided a pathway for bacteria to ascend into the uterus (Speroff & Darney, 2011).

By 1986, most U.S. companies had voluntarily withdrawn IUDs from the U.S. market, not for medical or scientific reasons, but primarily because of decreased popularity, negative consumer perception, increasing litigation costs, and subsequent difficulty obtaining liability insurance. Fears of side effects or complications hampered widespread acceptance of IUDs among potential users, physicians, and other family planning providers.

The modern IUDs, however, are safe, highly effective, and convenient. A landmark case-control study from Mexico City showed that among nulligravid women, use of a copper IUD was not associated with tubal infertility; in contrast, prior exposure to *Chlamydia trachomatis* was associated with a significant increase in risk (Hubacher, Lara-Ricalde, Taylor, Guerra-Infante, & Guzman-Rodriguez, 2001). IUDs are an excellent alternative for women considering sterilization who might be at risk for later regret (see Voluntary Sterilization, later in this chapter). In many countries of the world, IUDs are the most popular reversible method of birth control.

ParaGard-T-380A

ParaGard was approved in the United States in 1984. It is a T-shaped polyurethane device with barium sulfate added (for x-ray visibility). A very fine copper wire is wound around a vertical stem and crossbar. A white polyethylene string attached through a hole in the "T" creates a double string effect that, after insertion, protrudes into the vagina. ParaGard-T-380A is approved for 10 years of use, and may be effective for 12 or more years (Duramed, 2006; Hatcher et al., 2011).

Levonorgestrel Intrauterine System (Mirena)

Approved by the FDA for use in the United States in December 2000, the levonorgestrel intrauterine system (LNG-IUS) consists of a T-shaped polyethylene frame with a steroid reservoir that contains LNG. The IUS releases a low dose of LNG, 20 mcg per day, into the uterine cavity for at least 5 years and may be effective up to 7 years. It has a double thread tail. It is distributed in the United States by Bayer Healthcare Pharmaceuticals. It has a success rate nearly equal to sterilization (ARHP, 2011; Hatcher et al., 2011).

In addition to its effective contraception, this system has several noncontraceptive benefits including prevention of anemia, therapy for menorrhagia, and dysmenorrhea. It protects against uterine fibroid development and growth. Ectopic pregnancy is rare. The antiproliferative effect of the LNG-IUS on the endometrium can also offer therapy against the proliferative action of estrogen during postmenopausal hormone replacement therapy. Occasionally, users experience facial, androgenic skin changes, breast tenderness, or benign follicular cysts.

Mirena will alter bleeding patterns. During the first 3 to 6 weeks of use, the number of bleeding and spotting days may be increased and bleeding patterns may be irregular. Thereafter, the number of bleeding and spotting days usually decreases, but bleeding patterns remain irregular. Within a year, many women experience little or no bleeding, and 20 percent will experience amenorrhea. Overall, there is a 90 percent decrease in menstrual blood loss (Hubacher & Grimes, 2002; Pakarinen, Toivonen, & Luukkainen, 2001).

Mechanism of Action

IUDs appear to work primarily by preventing sperm from fertilizing ova. There are effects on both fertilization and the endometrium. When a foreign body is in the uterus, the endometrium reacts by releasing white blood cells, enzymes, and prostaglandins. These endometrial reactions appear to prevent sperm from reaching the fallopian tubes.

Contrary to previous belief, IUDs are not abortifacients. Normally cleaving, fertilized ova cannot be obtained in tubal flushing in women with IUDs in contrast to noncontraceptors, indicating the failure of sperm to reach the ovum. Thus, fertilization does not occur. In women using copper IUDs sensitive assays for human chorionic gonadotropin do not find evidence of fertilization. This is consistent with the fact that IUDs protect against intrauterine and ectopic pregnancies (Segal et al., 1985; Speroff & Darney, 2011; Wilcox, Weinberg, Armstrong, & Canfield, 1987).

The local mechanism by which continuously released levonorgestrel enhances contraceptive effectiveness of Mirena has not been conclusively demonstrated. Levonorgestrel contributes to several mechanisms that prevent pregnancy: thickening of cervical mucus preventing passage of sperm into the uterus, inhibition of sperm capacitation or survival, and alteration of the endometrium.

Copper-bearing IUDs release copper ions into the fluids of the uterus and the fallopian tubes, enhancing debilitating effects on sperm. The copper releases free copper and copper salts that have a biochemical and morphologic impact on the endometrium and also produce alterations in cervical mucus and endometrial secretions. There is no measurable increase in serum copper levels. Copper has many specific actions, including the enhancement of prostaglandin production and the inhibition of various endometrial enzymes (Speroff & Darney, 2011).

Effectiveness

IUDs are highly effective in preventing pregnancy. Users exhibit high compliance and high continuation rates. Effectiveness is impacted by IUD characteristics, such as size, shape, expulsion rates, presence of copper, or progesterone; and by user characteristics, such as age and parity. Also influential are medical variables, such as experience of the clinician inserting the device, the ease of insertion, placement of the device at the top of the fundus of the uterus, and likelihood that expulsion will be detected (see Table 12–3) (Andersson et al., 1994; Hatcher et al., 2011; Sieven, Stern, Coutnho, Mattos, & Diaz, 1991).

Advantages

- Once inserted, an IUD requires no continuing action, equipment, or motivation on the part of the user. Is immediately effective.
- Highly effective.
- Continuously effective.
- Very safe for carefully selected users.
- Allows for sexual spontaneity.
- Cost-effective.
- Mirena (LNG-IUS) has several noncontraceptive benefits.
- Return to fertility immediate.
- Can be used during lactation.
- Protective against ectopic pregnancy.
- Long-term method.

Disadvantages

- Insertion requires a trained professional.
- Menstrual disturbances may occur.
- User may experience pain or nausea during insertion.
- Provides no protection against STIs.
- Device can be expelled without the user's being aware.
- String may be felt by the partner.
- Risks of insertion are perforation of the uterus and infection.

Contraindications

Carefully screen potential IUD users for contraindications. Include general, contraceptive, and menstrual histories, a physical examination, and chlamydia and gonorrhea testing. Use of this product before menarche is not indicated (Andersson et al., 1994; ARHP, 2001; Intrauterine Devices, 2000; Ronnerdag & Odlind, 1999).

Absolute Contraindications (IUD Not Recommended)

- Current PID or PID in past 3 months.
- Known or suspected pregnancy.
- Uterine anomaly.
- Allergy to copper (for ParaGard).
- Current purulent cervicitis, chlamydia, or gonorrhea.
- Cervical cancer (awaiting treatment).

Strong Relative Contraindications (Strongly Encourage Choice of Another Contraceptive Method)

- Undiagnosed, abnormal vaginal bleeding.
- High-risk sexual behavior.
- Past postpartum endometritis; infection following abortion in past 3 months.
- Unresolved, abnormal Pap smear.
- Known or suspected bleeding disorder.
- Anatomic variations that make insertion or retention difficult (e.g., diethylstilbestrol exposure, fibroids).

Client Counseling

- Advise the patient about what to expect during and after IUD insertion.
- Teach how and when to check for the IUD string.
- Discuss likely bleeding patterns.
- Warn of signs of infection.
- Encourage prophylactic administration of NSAIDS for the first few menstrual cycles post insertion (ARHP, 2011; Hatcher et al., 2011).
- Give each IUD user an identification card with the name and a picture of the IUD, the day of insertion, and the recommended removal date printed on it. Written informed consent is needed.

Managing Problems and Complications

- Spotting or bleeding may occur at the time of insertion or at anytime after, especially during the first 3 to 6 months following insertion.
- Cramping or pain also may occur at the time of insertion or at anytime after. If treatment with NSAIDS fails, evaluate for infection, pregnancy, and/or expulsion.
- The IUD may be expulsed or partially expulsed. Two to 10 percent of IUDs will spontaneously expel. Most often, expulsion occurs during the first few weeks to months after insertion. For partial expulsion, remove the IUD and check for pregnancy. If no further problems are identified, another IUD may be inserted if no contraindications exist.
- The IUD can become embedded. If it cannot be removed after reasonable attempts, refer the client to a gynecologist.
- The IUD string may become lost. Attempt to determine whether the device has been partially or completely expulsed. Insertion of a Pap smear cytobrush into the endocervical canal and rotating it while withdrawing the brush will often extract the strings. If unable to locate strings within the endocervical canal, order a pelvic ultrasound to verify placement.
- At the time of insertion, uterine perforation can occur. Perforation is rare and happens between 1 in 1,000 and 1 in 2,000.
- If the person becomes pregnant, confirm that the pregnancy is intrauterine and not ectopic, remove the IUD promptly, regardless of her plans for the pregnancy. Early removal reduces the risk of spontaneous miscarriage.
  - If the IUD is left in place, severe pelvic infection resulting in death could occur.
  - Five percent will have an ectopic pregnancy.
  - Inform the client of the above; assist her to determine whether to continue the pregnancy.
- Potential for increased risk of PID during the first 20 days. This is believed to be due to introduction of bacteria into the uterus during the insertion procedure. *Appropriate* IUD users are at no greater risk of developing PID than nonusers. The following are signs of PID (see also Chapter 16).
  - Fever of 101°F or higher.
  - Purulent discharge from the vagina/cervix.
  - Abdominal/pelvic pain.
  - Dyspareunia.
  - Cervicitis.
  - Suprapubic tenderness or guarding.
  - Cervical motion tenderness.
  - Tenderness on bimanual examination.
  - Adnexal tenderness or mass (ARHP, 2001; Hatcher et al., 2011; Intrauterine Devices, 2000).

VOLUNTARY STERILIZATION

Female Sterilization

Female sterilization is accomplished by bilateral occlusion of the fallopian tubes, commonly referred to as bilateral tubal ligation (BTL). The fallopian tubes are ligated and cut; occluded with clips, rings, or microinserts; electrocoagulated; or plugged to prevent the ovum from moving toward the uterus and joining with sperm. Sterilization is considered to be a safe operative procedure. A hysterectomy (removal of the uterus) accomplishes sterilization, but should *never* be performed solely for that purpose.

Nonincision Sterilization Procedures for Females

There are two nonincision female sterilization procedures commonly used in the United States: Essure and Adiana.

Essure is considered a permanent method of birth control that is 99.8 percent effective in preventing pregnancy after 2 years of study (Conceptus, 2010). Microinserts of polyester fibers and metals are placed in the fallopian tubes during hysteroscopy in a 35-minute outpatient procedure. Women generally are able to go home 45 minutes after the procedure is completed, and resume normal activities within 1 to 2 days. No general anesthesia is required. A backup contraceptive method is used for 3 months until the inserts are totally enmeshed with tissue and block the tubes. At that time, a hysterosalpingogram is done to be sure the inserts are properly placed and are totally blocking the tubes. Surgery would be required to remove the inserts but there is no guarantee of future fertility.

Adiana's mechanism of action is similar, but has an additional step. The first step is delivery of bipolar radiofrequency energy to create a superficial lesion within the fallopian tube. The creation of this lesion will initiate an acute wound healing response. The second step is the deployment of a matrix within the area of the superficial lesion. The tissue in-growth response will lead to occlusion of the fallopian tube along the length of the matrix. The patient must use a reliable form of contraception until bilateral tubal occlusion is confirmed by the hysterosalpingogram 3 months after placement. Bilateral tubal occlusion must be confirmed before the patient can be advised that she can rely on it for pregnancy prevention (Hologic Inc, 2009).

Sterilization Techniques for Females Requiring Incision

Sterilization techniques may be performed using general or local anesthesia with sedation. Local anesthesia with light sedation has definite safety advantages over general anesthesia.

Tubal sterilization can be performed postpartum, postabortion, or as an interval procedure (unrelated to pregnancy). Performing sterilization during the early follicular phase of the menstrual cycle is desirable to prevent risk for presence of luteal-phase pregnancy. Pregnancy testing should be performed and effective contraception used until after the sterilization procedure.

Tubal occlusion methods include unipolar or bipolar electrocoagulation with or without tubal excision, ligation, and excision by various surgical techniques (Pomeroy, Irving, Prichard/Parkland, fibriectomy, Uchida), or use of various rings, bands, or clips (Silastic bands or rings, Falope rings, Hulka or Filshie clips) (ACOG, 2003; Hatcher et al., 2011).

Suprapubic Minilaparotomy. Performed at 4 weeks or more postpartum or 4 weeks or more postabortion, that is, interval BTL (when the uterus is fully involuted). Usually it is performed in lithotomy position. The procedure involves a small (2–5 cm) abdominal incision just above the pubic hairline. The uterus is elevated so that the uterus and tubes are close to the incision. The tubes are lifted, identified, and ligated by any of several occlusion techniques; the incision is sutured.

Laparoscopy. Laparascopic BTL is generally used for an interval procedure. A laparoscope consists of a viewing instrument, light source, and operating channel. *Single puncture technique* involves a small subumbilical incision. The abdomen is insufflated with a gaseous combination of nitrous oxide, carbon dioxide, and room air; the laparoscope is inserted, and the tubes are grasped and occluded through the operating channel of the instrument. With *double puncture technique*, a second tiny incision is made in the suprapubic region through which the operating channel is inserted and the procedure performed. Following bilateral tubal occlusion, the organs are inspected, the scope removed, gas gently expelled, and the incisions closed.

Subumbilical Minilaparotomy. Most frequently used during the immediate postpartum/postabortion period, when the uterus and tubes remain high in the abdomen. A small (1.5–3.0 cm) incision is made just below the umbilicus. Oviducts are usually easily reached for the occlusion procedure. Lithotomy position is not needed, and organ manipulation and instrumentation are less extensive, facilitating a rapid recovery.

BTL by Laparotomy. BTL using an abdominal incision greater than 5 cm, or during cesarean section, is associated with slightly higher morbidity and complication rates. BTLs performed during cesarean section, however, are relatively common.

Vaginal Approach. For interval BTL, direct visualization of the pelvic organs can be accomplished through an incision high in the vagina, posterior to the cervix (called a colpotomy). The tubes can be reached and directly sutured or cut. This method is rarely used, being less safe and less effective than other methods described earlier. Infection is more common and the technique is difficult to learn and perform.

Male Sterilization

Vasectomy is an operative procedure that blocks the vas deferens to prevent the passage of sperm into ejaculated seminal fluid. Considered a simple procedure, it can be performed quickly, safely, and inexpensively in an office or clinic setting (Hatcher et al., 2011).

Each vas deferens is cut between two ligated sections, preventing sperm from mingling with ejaculate. Local anesthetic is injected into each side of the scrotum, where a small incision is made to isolate, occlude, and usually resect the vasa. Closure of the incision(s) requires one or two sutures. A no-scalpel technique for performing vasectomies is now widely used throughout the world and the United States. This requires an instrument that punctures the scrotal skin and vas sheath. Once this is accomplished, the procedures to isolate, occlude, and resect are the same as for the scalpel technique. Little bleeding occurs, and no sutures are required. About 20 ejaculations are required for existing sperm in the vasa deferentia to be cleared (Hatcher et al., 2011). Approximately 50 percent of men will reach azoospermia at 8 weeks. However, the time to achieve azoospermia is highly variable, reaching only about 60 to 80 percent after 12 weeks (Griffin, Tooher, Nowakowski, Lloyd, & Maddern, 2005).

Effectiveness

See Table 12–3.

Advantages

- One-time decision provides permanent sterility.
- Highly effective, convenient.
- Highly acceptable.
- Considered safe; low complication and morbidity rates.
- Following procedure and recovery, very few or no systemic side effects occur.
- BTL has some protective effect against ovarian cancer and PID.
- Partner cooperation not required.
- Short recovery time.
- Certain techniques can be performed immediately after childbirth or abortion.
- BTL immediately effective.
- Not coitus linked.
- Low long-term risks.
- Cost-effective.
- Can be performed while lactating.
- Vasectomy is equally effective, simpler, safer, much less expensive than BTL.

Disadvantages

- Carries risks inherent in any surgical procedure (infection, injury to other organs, hemorrhage, complications of anesthesia).
- Procedures are difficult to reverse.
- Initial cost may be high.
- Some pain/discomfort during and right after procedure.
- Vasectomy is not immediately effective.
- Some states and third-party payors require a waiting period between time of counseling/consent and actual procedure.
- Provides no protection against STIs.
- Chance of regret.
- Uterine perforation is possible.
- Some women report menstrual pattern changes, increased dysmenorrhea, PMS following BTL (Peterson et al., 2000).
- If BTL fails, there is high probability of ectopic pregnancy.

Contraindications

- Known or suspected pregnancy.
- Existing infection of the reproductive tract.
- Client ambivalence about future pregnancy or sterilization.

Client Counseling

For several reasons, client teaching and counseling are especially important when an individual is considering sterilization. Sterilization is a surgical procedure, thus involving some risk; there are legal implications, and it is meant to be permanent. Postoperative regret about the sterilization decision is a serious concern. Indicators for risk of future regret include young age (under age 34), poverty, having a BTL postpartum or at the time of a cesarean section, change in marital status, decision was made during a time of personal or family crisis, children very young at the time of procedure, or pressure from partner to have the procedure. Reversal procedures often fail and are very costly. In lieu of sterilization or to postpone the decision for women at risk for later regret, women should be informed about and offered long-term reversible contraceptive options such as IUDs, implants, or DMPA. Documentation of adequate teaching/counseling about sterilization is essential. In addition to the points in the counseling process that follow, also refer to Guidelines for Client Education and Informed Consent at the beginning of this chapter (Baill, Cullins, & Pati, 2003; Hatcher et al., 2011).

- Assess client's interest in and readiness for sterilization, especially risk factors for later regret.
- When federal funds, and in some cases, state funds are used to reimburse for sterilization, the client must have signed informed consent at least 30 days prior to the procedure or before delivery or abortion, if sterilization is planned to immediately follow one of these procedures. The client must also be 21 years of age or older and mentally competent.
- Emphasize permanence; discuss possibility of failure; provide alternative reversible method information.
- Explain procedure using visual aids; discuss risks/benefits.
- Women who undergo sterilization are much less likely to use condoms or other barriers for prevention of STIs than nonsterilized women. Should be counseled to protect themselves and their partners.
- Have client read and sign informed consent form.
- Schedule appointment; provide copy of necessary forms.
- Discuss cost and payment.
- Provide pre- and postoperative instructions.
- Schedule postoperative follow-up visit.
- The client should have someone accompany her or him home following the procedure.
- The client should rest for a few days following the procedure.
- Sexual activity may be resumed after about 1 week for women and after 2 to 3 days for men.
- Men must be reminded that they are not sterile initially. Another method of contraception must be used until microscopic examination of semen ascertains that sterility has been achieved.

FERTILITY AWARENESS METHODS

Fertility awareness methods (FAM)—also referred to as menstrual cycle charting, NFP, or periodic abstinence—involve making observations and charting of scientifically proven fertility signs that determine whether a woman is fertile on any given day. The three primary fertility signs are (1) waking temperature (basal body temperature), (2) cervical mucus/fluid, and (3) cervical position. These are normal physiological changes caused by hormonal fluctuations during the menstrual cycle that can be observed and charted so that fertile and infertile periods can be identified.

FAM are used in combination with coital abstinence or barrier methods during fertile days, when the desire is to prevent pregnancy. Fertility awareness also helps a couple understand how to achieve pregnancy, detect probable pregnancy, detect impaired fertility, or manage PMS. The term *natural family planning* implies exclusive use of these methods and that absolute abstinence is maintained during the fertile phase. The charting of observed changes is an important component for successful use of these methods. The techniques of FAM include basal body temperature (BBT) method, cervical mucus/fluid (Billings or ovulation) method, and symptothermal method. At least two of these techniques should be used simultaneously. Figure 12–1 is an example of an NFP chart for recording fertility signs. Clients may design their own charts or adapt the one shown for their own use. There are several software applications available to download to personal electronic devices that assist in charting of the menstrual cycle (see Web Resources at end of chapter).

The calendar (rhythm) method is the original method based on periodic abstinence and is still widely used around the world. It is much less reliable than the newer methods listed earlier, however, because it relies on a statistical prediction based on past cycles to predict fertility in future cycles. With newer, more effective, and well-researched methods available, the calendar (rhythm) method is no longer recommended.

Modern FAM are considered reliable and are acceptable to diverse population groups with varied religious and ethical beliefs and to couples who do not wish to use other methods for medical or personal reasons (Hatcher et al., 2011).

Mechanism of Action

Pregnancy is prevented by avoidance of unprotected intercourse during times that a woman is determined to be fertile.

BBT Method. BBT refers to the lowest temperature reached by the body of a healthy person, taken upon wakening. A digital thermometer should be used that records

Natural Family Planning Chart

Name

Age

Chart #

Month & Year

CYCLE LENGTH

of days in shortest of last six cycles

minus 19 =

Draw a vertical line before this day

Length of this cycle =

TEMPERATURE

Time of taking temperature:

Basal Body Temperature (Fahrenheit)

.1
99.0
.9
.8
.7
.6
.5
.4
.3
.2
.1
98.0
.9
.8
.7
.6
.5
.4
.3
.2
.1
97.0
.9

MENSTRUAL CYCLE DAY	Circle day of intercourse	1	2	3	4	5	6	7	8	9	10	11	12	13	14	15	16	17	18	19	20	21	22	23	24	25	26	27	28	29	30	31	32	33	34	35	36	37	38	39	40
	Date																																								
CERVICAL SECRETIONS (Feel, look & touch	Wet, slippery, transparent or sketchy																																								
	Thick, cloudy or sticky																																								
	Dry, no secretions seen or felt																																								
	Period																																								
CERVIX	High, soft, open																																								
	Low, firm, closed																																								
COMMENTS	Disturbances, schedule changes, etc.																																								

FIGURE 12–1. Natural Family Planning Chart. *Source: Used with permission of the Institute for Reproductive Health at Georgetown University.*

temperature to the 0.1 degree. The temperature is taken daily after a minimum of three consecutive hours of sleep, before rising, eating, or drinking and is recorded on the chart (see Figure 12–1). The preovulatory temperatures are suppressed by estrogen, whereas postovulatory temperatures are increased by 0.4° to 0.8°F under the influence of heat-inducing progesterone. Temperatures typically rise within a day or two *after* ovulation has occurred and remain elevated for 12 to 16 days, until menstruation begins. If the woman were to become pregnant, the temperatures would remain elevated throughout the pregnancy. Based on the patterns observed, one should be able to predict the end of the fertile phase and the beginning of the safe, luteal phase of the cycle. If using BBT method as only method of contraception, the client should avoid unprotected intercourse from the beginning of the menstrual cycle (or at least from day 4) until the BBT has been elevated for 3 days. Using other FAM along with BBT should allow for shortening of the abstinent period.

It is important to know that numerous factors can delay or even prevent ovulation, thus prolonging the follicular (estrogenic) phase. These may include stress, travel, illness, medication, strenuous exercise, and sudden weight changes. Once ovulation occurs and the temperature rises, however, it is usually a standard 12 to 16 days until menses (Hatcher et al., 2011).

Cervical Mucus (Billings or Ovulation) Method. This method assesses the character of cervical mucus. The mucus secreted by exocrine glands lining the cervical canal changes in character during the menstrual cycle in response to hormonal levels. The woman is taught to begin checking cervical mucus the first day the period is over and to check it prior to urinating about three times each day. She should first note whether there is a sensation of wetness or dryness in the vaginal area. Then the woman should obtain fluid from the vaginal opening and feel it with her fingers to note changes in the physical properties of the mucus.

During a normal menstrual cycle, a woman experiences menses, then a few days of a dry sensation, then early mucus (may be milky white, translucent, yellow or clear, sticky at first and then smooth). As ovulation approaches, the mucus becomes more abundant, clear, slippery, and smooth. The mucus can be stretched between two fingers without breaking. This is called *spinnbarkeit* and closely resembles egg whites. The vaginal sensation is one of lubrication, being wet and slippery. These characteristics correspond to the peak in estrogen occurring immediately prior to ovulation. This mucus is more permeable to sperm and can prolong the life of sperm.

It is now known that sperm can live up to 5 days in the environment of wet-quality cervical mucus. The *peak day* is the last day of egg white–quality cervical mucus, or the lubricative vaginal sensation, or any midcycle spotting. Before ovulation, the only days that are considered safe are those dry days in which there is no cervical fluid present. Postovulation, a woman is considered infertile the evening of the fourth consecutive day after the peak day. Charting must be done, noting observed cervical mucus characteristics.

In addition to visually monitoring cervical mucus, women can purchase low-cost microscopes to identify their most fertile days. A woman's saliva and cervical mucus begin to form a distinct fern-like pattern when viewed under a microscope. This ferning pattern begins to appear 3 days prior to ovulation, allowing the user to predict fertility (see Web Resources at end of chapter).

Cervical Position Assessment

Cervical position is an optional fertility sign that can be assessed to augment or confirm the changes in temperature and cervical mucus/fluid. The woman should insert one finger into her vagina and feel the conditions of the cervix, beginning when menses has ended. She palpates the cervix for height in the vagina (low, midway, high), softness (firm, medium, soft), openness (closed, partly open, open), and wetness (nothing, sticky, creamy, egg white). Near ovulation, the cervix feels high/deep in the vagina, soft, open, and wet. These observations should be noted on the chart as well (Boston Women's Health Book Collective, 2011; Hatcher et al., 2011).

Symptothermal Method. This method merely connotes that at least two indicators are being combined to identify the fertile period. The term *fertility awareness methods* also implies that more than one indicator is used. The symptothermal method usually combines the BBT and cervical mucus methods. It may also incorporate the changes in the cervix (position, texture, openness) described earlier, as well as secondary fertility signs that a woman might observe, such as breast tenderness, libido changes, midcycle pain, spotting, and fluid retention.

Standard Days Method. This method is only appropriate for women with menstrual cycles between 26 and 32 days long. For these women, days 8 through 19 of their cycles are the days when pregnancy is likely to occur, so unprotected intercourse is avoided. On all other days, the probability of becoming pregnant is very low. Most women using the Standard Days Method utilize CycleBeads®, a string of color-coded beads that help her keep track of the fertile and infertile days. No calculations or observation are involved, making it easy for providers to teach and for clients to understand (The Standard Days Method, 2003).

Calendar (Rhythm) Method. This involves calculation of a woman's fertile period based on three assumptions:

- Ovulation occurs on the 14th day, plus or minus 2 days, prior to next menses.
- Sperm are viable for 3 days.
- The ovum is viable for 24 hours.

The client must chart the length of her menstrual cycles for a minimum of 8 months. The earliest day in the cycle she is likely to be fertile is determined by subtracting 18 days from the length of the shortest cycle occurring during that 8-month period. The latest day of potential fertility is obtained by subtracting 11 days from the longest cycle. These two numbers represent the beginning and end of the fertile period. For example, if the client's shortest cycle was 27 days, subtract 18 from 27; on the 9th day (27 minus 18) the client must begin to abstain from sexual intercourse. If her longest cycle was 34 days, on the 23rd day (34 minus 11) abstinence may be ended. She must abstain from day 9 through day 23, a total of 14 days, during each cycle. This technique is most effective when menstrual cycles are regular. With less variable cycles, the period of required abstinence is shorter. The abstinent period cannot be less than 7 days.

As noted earlier, the calendar (rhythm) method is not based on tested scientific principles, relying on information from past cycles to predict fertile patterns in future cycles. Couples should instead be encouraged to utilize the more reliable methods discussed in the chapter (Hatcher et al., 2011).

Home Test Kits and Monitors. Home test kits and monitors that predict when ovulation occurs are available from most pharmacies. Most kits/devices measure LH, which can be detected the day before or the day of ovulation. Most were developed to help women achieve conception. For NFP, intercourse should be avoided until 4 days after ovulation has occurred. Kits and monitors are being developed to help couples who wish to avoid pregnancy by identifying the beginning and the end of the fertile time.

Effectiveness

FAM are considered moderately effective for preventing pregnancy (see Table 12–3). It is extremely unforgiving, however, of imperfect use. These techniques require high levels of commitment and participation by both partners. High motivation to prevent pregnancy and ability to learn the necessary concepts are needed. Failures are often related to poor understanding or improper teaching and poor use of methods. Some pregnancies result from couples having trouble coping with periods of abstinence. Pregnancy must be an acceptable possible outcome of use of these methods (Speroff & Darney, 2011).

Advantages

- No damaging side effects.
- No interruption of normal body functions.
- Immediate return to fertility.
- No external or internal devices or chemicals.
- Acceptable to most religious groups.
- Low cost.
- Increases awareness of normal female body processes and fertility.
- Encourages communication between partners.
- The concepts and charting skills learned can also be applied to planning conception, detecting pregnancy, diagnosis and treatment of fertility problems, and mapping symptoms of PMS.
- Use of Standard Days Method with CycleBeads® is easily understood by most clients.

Disadvantages

- High failure rate with incorrect use.
- Interferes with sexual spontaneity.
- Requires meticulous recordkeeping and intensive, ongoing teaching, and partner cooperation.
- Couples may have difficulty learning the techniques.
- Periodic abstinence is difficult for some couples.
- Is a less reliable method if infection is present.
- Is a less reliable method if menstrual periods are irregular.
- No identifiable BBT pattern is seen in some women's cycles, even when ovulating.
- Emotional and physiological stress, shift work, and travel can alter the timing of ovulation.
- No protection provided against STIs.
- Methods are unreliable during lactation and perimenopausal periods.
- Intermenstrual bleeding can impede accurate observation of cervical mucus.

Contraindications

There are no absolute contraindications to FAM; however, if unplanned pregnancy would be unacceptable or inadvisable for a client or her family, for any reason, a more reliable contraceptive method should be considered. Relative contraindications include the following:

- Irregular menses.
- History of anovulatory cycles.
- Inability to keep careful records.
- Lack of partner cooperation.
- Frequent or persistent vaginal infections.

Client Counseling

Clients must receive teaching by a trained fertility awareness counselor. They may need assistance with interpreting charts. It is recommended that health care professionals be familiar with the available community resources for teaching these techniques and with the philosophy and teaching/learning resources used by the counselor. Teaching and counseling involves several aspects:

- Explanation of the normal menstrual cycle.
- Explanation of how the methods work.
- Selection of the methods.
- Techniques involved in the methods selected (e.g., how and when to take BBT, how to evaluate cervical mucus).
- Procedures for charting.
- How to determine fertile periods.
- Alternative sexual activity for fertile periods.

LACTATIONAL AMENORRHEA METHOD

The lactational amenorrhea method (LAM) is a highly effective temporary family planning method for breastfeeding women. LAM is based on the utilization of lactational infertility for protection from pregnancy. LAM can provide women with natural protection against pregnancy for up to 6 months after a birth, and following the guidelines for this method encourages the timely introduction of complementary methods of birth control while breastfeeding continues beyond 6 months. In the first 6 months following birth, women who meet the criteria for the method have a less than 2 percent pregnancy rate (Hatcher et al., 2011).

If the woman answers "no" to all the following questions, the LAM is a good method for her. If she answers "yes" to even one question, it most likely is not the appropriate method for her. Some method of contraception should be incorporated with LAM for backup while she is breastfeeding, and a method should be provided for use when she starts to give the baby food, other milk supplement, when the baby is 6 months old, and/or when she has her period for the first time (Labbock, Cooney, & Coly, 1994) (see also Chapter 22).

- Have your menses returned?
- Are you supplementing regularly or allowing long periods without breastfeeding, either day or night?
- Is your baby more than 6 months old?

Mechanism of Action

The physiology of LAM is based on the hypothalamic-pituitary-ovarian feedback system. The hypothalamus reacts to the suckling at the breast by reducing the pulsatile release of GnRH. This, in turn, changes the pulsatile secretion of prolactin and the gonadotropin hormones, FSH, and LH. The return of menses is the most important indication of the return of fertility (Hatcher et al., 2011).

Effectiveness

Studies have demonstrated that women who met the LAM criteria had only a 1 to 2 percent chance of pregnancy during the first 6 months postpartum. The LAM should not extend beyond 6 months. Research has emphasized the importance of full or nearly full breastfeeding patterns. If the woman is concerned that she is at risk for pregnancy, EC may be used while breastfeeding (Hatcher et al., 2011). LAM is less effective for women who are separated from their infants by returning to work, even when they are expressing their milk and exclusively breastfeeding (Valdes, Labbock, Pugin, & Perez, 2000).

Advantages

- Highly effective (when used perfectly—see criteria).
- No supplies, low cost.
- Not coitus linked.
- Controlled by the woman.
- Gives women time to choose which complementary family planning method they will use.
- Acceptable to many religious groups.
- No chance of synthetic hormone excretion into breast milk.

Disadvantages

- Temporary method, only effective in the postpartum months.
- If mother and baby are separated for extended periods, efficacy as a family planning method decreases.

Contraindications

- Does not fit above listed criteria

Client Counseling

In addition to teaching women the criteria for successful use of the LAM, several points should be considered in client teaching and counseling.

- Emphasize that if there are disruptions in patterns of breastfeeding, resumption of ovulation and fertility cannot be accurately predicted. A woman can become pregnant while breastfeeding and before the first menstrual period occurs.
- Women who are uncertain about whether they can continue to meet the specified criteria for LAM, and wish to avoid the risk of pregnancy, should begin using a reliable method of birth control immediately. For some women, this may be at the time of the 6-week postpartum examination or even sooner.
- If the client wishes to rely on LAM for contraception, she must breast-feed her infant on demand over each 24-hour period, with no formula or food supplementation. When the infant reaches 6 months or menses return, she should begin another method of birth control.

WITHDRAWAL (COITUS INTERRUPTUS)

Coitus interruptus, withdrawal, or "pulling out" involves the man removing his penis from the vagina before ejaculation so that ejaculation occurs away from the vagina and external genitalia. The man must rely on his own sensations to determine when he is about to ejaculate. Though not popular in the United States, withdrawal is one of the most common methods of preventing pregnancy in many countries and cultures of the world. Adolescents frequently use this method. Withdrawal is often used in conjunction with FAM.

Mechanism of Action

Coitus interruptus prevents conception when sperm-containing ejaculate is deposited away from the woman's genitalia, preventing contact between sperm and ovum. The man must interrupt intercourse and withdraw his penis from his partner's vagina before ejaculation occurs.

Effectiveness

Among typical users, about 19 percent experience method failure in the first year of use (see Table 12–3). Low success rates with this method may be due to the following:

- Presence of sperm in the preejaculate fluid that is emitted without sensation to the man.
- It is difficult for the man to predict when he will ejaculate.
- The required self-control is difficult to achieve (Boston Women's Health Book Collective, 2011; Hatcher et al., 2011).

Advantages

- Coitus interruptus involves no artificial devices or chemicals.
- Costs nothing.
- Has no systemic side effects.
- Can be used during lactation.
- It is a backup method that is always available.

Disadvantages

- Has a high failure rate.
- Requires considerable self-control by the man.
- Can diminish enjoyment for the couple.
- Depends solely on the cooperation of the man.
- Puts the woman in a dependent role.
- Provides no protection against STIs.
- Diminished pleasure could develop, as couples must remain alert, concentrate on timing, and interrupt the excitement or plateau phase of sexual response.

Contraindications

There are no absolute contraindications; however, if unplanned pregnancy is unacceptable or inadvisable, a more reliable method should be used. Relative contraindications include (1) questionable commitment of either partner to the method and (2) lack of effective communication between partners.

Client Counseling

The method should be taught as part of contraceptive counseling, especially for those who tend to use this method. Counseling and instruction should include several topics.

- Before intercourse, the man should urinate and wipe off any fluid on the tip of the penis; it may contain sperm. This is especially important if the couple intends to have more than one act of intercourse, because semen may be present in clear fluid at the tip of an erect penis.
- When a man feels impending ejaculation, he must immediately remove his penis from the vagina so that

ejaculation occurs well away from the vagina and external genitalia.

- Condom use with this method would greatly increase its effectiveness and provide protection against STIs.
- A supply of spermicide may be kept on hand in case withdrawal is not accomplished in time. An application could be inserted immediately, although this measure probably would not prevent some sperm from entering the uterus.
- Always advise to have EC on hand.

ABSTINENCE

Abstinence refers to refraining from penis-vagina intercourse. It is the most effective form of birth control and may be chosen at any stage of life. Abstinence does not preclude sexual intimacy. Partner cooperation, however, is critical. Health care providers can assist couples in communicating about this choice and in achieving intimacy that is satisfactory to both of them. Be sure the woman is informed about EC.

POSTCOITAL EMERGENCY CONTRACEPTION

Postcoital contraception, also called EC, refers to intervention taken to prevent pregnancy after a single act of unprotected intercourse. Indications for use include sexual assault, condom breakage, dislodgement of a cervical cap, diaphragm or sponge, missed OC, incorrect method use, or any unprotected intercourse. The treatment can be used if the woman has had unprotected intercourse within the last 120 hours (5 days) and does not wish to become pregnant. If a woman is already pregnant, treatment is ineffective, but will not cause harm to a pregnancy. EC provides a last chance to prevent pregnancy. EC is an ideal backup method of birth control, especially for those using barrier methods. Ideally, EC should be available in advance of need, just in case. Emergency contraception has the potential to reduce the number of unintended pregnancies each year by half, as well as reduce the need for abortion by half. EC is highly cost-effective.

Historically, the combined estrogen/progestin (Yuzpe method) was used as EC; this was soon replaced with POPs because of increased effectiveness and less side effects. The Yuzpe method consists of the estradiol equivalent of 100 to 120 mcg dosage of a COC (e.g., two Ovral tablets) taken for two doses 12 hours apart (Fritz & Speroff, 2011). The estrogen from this dosage caused significant nausea. The Yuzpe method, while still effective, is not typically used as a first line of treatment. POPs have

TABLE 12–9. Emergency Postcoital Contraceptive Options

Product	Tablets Taken Within 72 Hours of Unprotected Intercourse	Repeat Dose Taken 12 Hours Later
Combined oral contraceptives		
Preven	1 tablet	1 tablet
Ovral	2 tablets	2 tablets
Lo-Ovral; Nordette; Levlen; Levlite; Alesse	4 tablets	4 tablets
Triphasil (yellow tablet only); Tri-Levlen (yellow tablet only); Trivora (pink tablet only)	4 tablets	4 tablets
Progestin-only pills		
Plan B	1 tablet	1 tablet
Ovrette	20 tablets	20 tablets
IUD (copper containing such as ParaGard-T-380A)	Insert up to 7 days after unprotected intercourse. May be left in place for long-term contraception	
For all methods, review contraindications. Evaluate for pregnancy if no menses by 3 weeks		

Sources: ACOG Practice Bulletin, 2010; Finger, 2001.

also been used as EC, but 20 pills in two separate doses are required, which may be cumbersome and costly. The dosage regime when using POPs called for 20 pills of Ovrette (0.075 mg of norgestrel each pill; equivalent to 0.0375 mg of levonorgestrel each pill) each dose. The first dose is to be taken within 72 hours of unprotected intercourse, the second dose 12 hours later (see Table 12–9).

Currently, EC methods available in the United States include levonorgestrel, ulipristal acetate, and the postcoital insertion of a copper-T IUD. In 2006, the FDA approved EC for over-the-counter sale for women age 17 and older, and by prescription for those under 17 (Dickey, 2010; Finger, 2001; Speroff & Darney, 2011).

Levonorgestrel

Levonorgestrel (Plan B™) does not interrupt an established pregnancy. Patients and providers must also be aware that a small risk of ectopic pregnancy exists if EC fails (Neilson & Miller, 2000). It may be taken as a single dose of two tablets (1.5 mg total dose) rather than two doses of one tablet (0.75 mg each dose) 12 hours apart. The one-dosage regime is being manufactured as a single pill called Plan B One-Step™.

Mechanism of Action

Levonorgestrel is believed to work by all or some of the following mechanisms:

- Inhibition or delay of ovulation.
- Luteal-phase dysfunction.

- Histologic or biochemical alterations in the endometrium, making the endometrium less receptive to implantation.
- Thickening of cervical mucus.
- Alterations in tubal transport of sperm, egg, or embryo.
- Direct inhibition of fertilization.

Effectiveness

The use of levonorgestrel reduces the risk of pregnancy between 59 and 94 percent, with efficacy improved when taken promptly after unprotected intercourse. Ideally, levonorgestrel should be discussed and/or dispensed at every contraceptive visit so that it can be used as soon as possible (Hatcher et al., 2011).

Contraindications

Contraindications to EC are few, but they should not be used with a known or suspected pregnancy, hypersensitivity to any component of the product, or undiagnosed abnormal genital bleeding.

Client Counseling

- Instruct the patient to take Plan B™ as soon as possible, within 120 hours of unprotected intercourse.
- If menses does not start within 3 weeks, the patient should take a pregnancy test.
- The next period may start a few days earlier or later than usual.
- Advise the patient not to have unprotected intercourse in the days or weeks following treatment.
- Patients need to continue or start another method of contraception immediately.
- Remind patients EC is not as effective as other methods, and are meant for one-time emergency protection.

ULIPRISTAL ACETATE

Mechanism of Action

Ulipristal acetate (Ella™) prevents progesterone from binding to the progesterone receptor. It postpones follicular rupture when administered prior to ovulation, thereby inhibiting or delaying ovulation. It may also alter the normal endometrium, impairing implantation.

Effectiveness

A large prospective clinical trial conducted in the United States showed that ulipristal acetate was effective and well tolerated as a single 30-mg dose for EC when used 48 to 120 hours following unprotected intercourse. Two prospective randomized EC trials compared the efficacy of ulipristal acetate to levonorgestrel. The first included women up to 72 hours following unprotected intercourse and the second up to 120 hours. When these two studies were combined in a meta-analysis, ulipristal acetate was found to have a pregnancy rate 65 percent lower than levonorgestrel when taken in the first 24 hours following unprotected intercourse and 42 percent when taken within 72 hours. In the second randomized study, ulipristal acetate prevented significantly more pregnancies than did levonorgestrel in the 72-to-120-hour subgroup, which is consistent with the increased effectiveness of ulipristal acetate in delaying ovulation during the preovulatory period as described previously (Fine, 2011).

Contraindications

- Known pregnancy.
- Breastfeeding.

Client Counseling

- Instruct the patient to take with or without food.
- Should be taken within 120 hours after unprotected intercourse.
- If vomiting occurs, within 3 hours of taking the drug, a repeat dose should be considered.
- If decreases the efficacy of CHCs, a backup method should be used for the remainder of the cycle.
- Irregular bleeding, spotting, early or late menses may occur.
- Pregnancy testing should be done if menses is greater than 7 days late.

POSTCOITAL IUD INSERTION

Mechanism of Action

The copper IUD insertion alters the endometrium, producing an inflammatory response that makes the endometrium unsuitable for implantation, and interferes with fertilization (Hatcher et al., 2011).

A recent meta-analysis concluded that the IUD is very effective for EC. The copper IUD is appropriate for EC in women who meet standard criteria for IUD insertion and is most effective if inserted within 5 days after unprotected intercourse. If immediate IUD placement is not available, the patient should be offered levonorgestrel or ulipristal. This method is particularly useful for women who desire long-term contraception and who are otherwise appropriate candidates for IUD use. The LNG-IUS is not effective as an emergency contraceptive (ACOG Practice Bulletin, 2010).

Effectiveness

This approach probably has a pregnancy rate of no higher than 0.2 percent (Hatcher et al., 2011).

Contraindications

- Known pregnancy.
- IUDs should be avoided by women at risk for STDs.
- The LNG-IUS has not been studied for EC insertion and is not recommended (Hatcher et al., 2011).

Client Counseling

- Side effects after postcoital IUD insertion are similar to those seen after routine insertion and include abdominal discomfort, vaginal bleeding, or spotting.

INDUCED ABORTION

Induced abortions are voluntary interruptions of pregnancy and may be performed as elective or medically therapeutic procedures. Induced abortions involve the expulsion or extraction of the products of conception from the uterus by medical or surgical intervention.

- *Elective reasons* do not relate to the health of the mother or fetus. They could be because the pregnancy was a result of rape or incest, but more commonly, because of unreadiness to start or expand one's family, lack of money to support a pregnancy and a child, lack of a supportive relationship, or other personal crisis.
- *Maternal indications* are reasons for which the mother's health would be jeopardized if the pregnancy were to continue, such as heart disease, severe depression, or cancer.
- *Fetal indications* most commonly are congenital defects, or exposure to a teratogenic agent.

The number of abortions in the United States has been declining since 1981, with the greatest decrease among teenagers. This is partly because the number of pregnancies has been decreasing and the proportion of reproductive-age women under 30 is also decreasing. However, better use of effective contraception has made a major contribution to the decline of the abortion rate (Centers for Disease Control and Prevention, 2002; Deardorff, Montgomery, & Hollmann, 1996; Henshaw & Van Vort, 1994; Jones, Darrock, & Hensaw, 2002).

The 1973 U.S. Supreme Court decision *Roe v. Wade* allows women to choose to terminate pregnancy in the first trimester; after that point, individual state laws become effective. Many states have placed restrictions on access to abortion services in certain circumstances (Boston Women's Health Book Collective, 2011; Hatcher et al., 2011).

For poor and minority women who wish to obtain abortion services, barriers to access to safe and affordable abortion often exist. The Hyde Amendment prohibits federal Medicaid funds to be used to pay for abortion except in rare circumstances. Difficulty in making financial arrangements is a commonly cited reason for delay in obtaining abortion that results in poor women having later, and therefore, less safe abortion procedures. Poor women are more likely to carry an unintended pregnancy to term (Dehlendorf, Rodriguez, Levy, Borrero, & Steinauer, 2010).

Death as a result of legal induced abortion is unusual; in fact, maternal mortality associated with carrying a pregnancy to term is 16 times higher than the risk of death due to abortion. Risk of complications and death from induced abortion vary according to weeks of gestation, method used, and type of anesthesia. Later abortions and general anesthesia are more hazardous. Many of the first trimester abortions in the United States are performed by vacuum aspiration and curettage (Fritz & Speroff, 2011). This is a very safe method of induced abortion. The number of U.S. women reported as dying from abortion declined from nearly 300 deaths in 1961 (mostly illegal abortions), to only 6 in 1987, or 0.4 deaths for every 100,000 legal abortions. Currently, mortality per 100,000 legal abortions is 0.6 deaths (Fritz & Speroff, 2011). Major and minor complications associated with the procedures do occur. Major complications include retained tissue, sepsis, uterine perforation, hemorrhage, incomplete abortion. Minor complications include mild infection, reaspiration (same day or later), cervical stenosis, cervical tear, underestimated gestation, convulsions/seizure. Major complications are 2.5 times higher for instillation methods than with instrument evacuation procedures in the second trimester. Use of general anesthesia during any abortion procedure carries a significantly higher risk of serious complications and death than use of local anesthesia (Hatcher et al., 2011).

Risk of long-term complications after having one or more legal abortions is low. Subsequent problems with fertility, spontaneous abortion, premature delivery, and low birth rate have not been found to be associated with first trimester abortions, or for later abortions when performed by skilled and well-trained abortion providers. Concurrent abortion and sterilization procedures are not recommended due to higher rates of morbidity and mortality.

CLIENT EVALUATION AND PREPARATION COUNSELING

Counseling can assist a woman in decision making and prepare her to give informed consent. When a woman finds out she is pregnant with an undesired conception, it is essential that she (and her partner or other supportive person, if appropriate) has the opportunity to discuss concerns and needs in a nonjudgmental atmosphere. Women seeking abortions may experience feelings of anxiety, conflict, isolation, or fear. Situations involving sexual abuse or rape will require referral for further counseling and support. Abortion counselors should convey the characteristics of empathy, warmth, and genuineness while helping women to work through confusion, ambivalence, or guilt before or after the procedure is performed. Sensitivity to cultural differences among clients is essential. In addition, clients must be made to feel safe, considering today's volatile environment related to abortion.

The client should be given the opportunity to discuss her current and future life situations, plans and expectations, and the possible impact of the pregnancy and/or abortion. The counselor must be able to provide other referrals that may be indicated such as social services and group or individual support.

It is the responsibility of the counselor to explain—in a kind, thorough, and objective manner—all aspects of the procedures, including options, risks, preparations for the procedures, techniques and their effects, pain management, and guidance in what to expect. Postabortion contraceptive options also need to be discussed.

Health History

The following historical data is needed.

- Menstrual history, especially last and previous menstrual periods.
- Contraceptive history and what methods the client wants to use in the future.
- Obstetric history.
- Reproductive system disease and/or prior surgery.
- Drug/anesthesia allergies.
- Other illnesses affecting health, past or present.
- Current medications.

Physical Examination

The *physical exam* may be brief (heart, lungs, abdomen, vital signs); however, the *reproductive exam* should be thorough to estimate the size and position of the uterus, to estimate the state of the conceptus, and to determine any abnormality, such as a mass or anatomical variation (Hatcher et al., 2011).

Diagnostic Tests

Several diagnostic tests may be done.

- *Pregnancy test:* A urine test for first screening; if test is negative but pregnancy suspected, a sensitive serum test is done.
- *Ultrasound evaluation*
- *Hemoglobin/hematocrit*
- *Blood type:* Necessary to determine if a woman is Rh negative. Rh negative women will need to receive Rh(D) immunoglobulin (RhoGAM) after the procedure.
- *Vaginitis/STD screening:* Chlamydia, gonorrhea, saline wet mount, and other if indicated.

METHODS OF INDUCED ABORTION

Early Medication Abortion Methods (First 9 Weeks of Pregnancy)

The following two methods of medical abortion are carried out only in early pregnancy. Women choose medical abortion in the first trimester for reasons of greater privacy and autonomy, less invasiveness, and a more natural process than surgery. The first to be discussed is the use of methotrexate (a folic acid analog that completely inhibits dihydrofolate reductase, an enzyme necessary for DNA synthesis) given intramuscularly followed by misoprostol in vaginal or oral form 3 to 7 days later. Methotrexate induces abortion because of its toxicity to trophoblastic tissue and is most successful as an abortifacient when used at 8 or fewer weeks' gestation. When used in abortion, misoprostol, a prostaglandin, works by causing contractions of the uterus, helping to expel the uterine contents. If abortion does not occur within 7 to 10 days, a second dose of misoprostol is given. Side effects of methotrexate used in this way are minimal. Misoprostol side effects include diarrhea, nausea, vomiting. This method is 90 to 98 percent successful in accomplishing completed abortion. Incomplete abortions may require a surgical procedure to complete. Follow-up evaluation to be certain abortion is complete is important because of the potential teratogenicity of the drug, should the pregnancy continue (Hatcher et al., 2011; *What Is Medical Abortion?* 2000).

A second method of induced first trimester abortion involves use of mifepristone (Mifeprex, also known as RU-486) followed by administration of the prostaglandin misoprostol. Mifepristone is a potent oral antiprogestogen. Mifepristone blocks the action of the natural hormone progesterone, which prepares the lining of the uterus for the fertilized egg and then maintains the pregnancy. Without progesterone, the lining of the uterus softens, breaks down, and bleeding begins. The pregnancy is thus interrupted in its early stages. The actions of misoprostol cause contractions of the uterus and expulsion of uterine contents.

This method of medical abortion is approved for the termination of intrauterine pregnancy with a duration of 49 or fewer days (counting from the last menstrual period). A follow-up visit 14 days later is required to determine if termination of pregnancy has occurred. If not complete, vacuum curettage is performed. This method is 95 percent effective. Five percent of women may require surgical completion of the abortion.

Clinicians prescribing mifepristone must have a referral plan in place for surgical intervention if necessary. Side effects of the mifepristone are minimal, though some nausea, headache, weakness, and fatigue may occur. The misoprostol has possible side effects of cramping, abdominal pain, nausea, vomiting, diarrhea, and uterine bleeding. Contraindications to mifepristone include confirmed or suspected ectopic pregnancy, adrenal failure, current corticosteroid therapy, allergy to prostaglandins, and bleeding disorders (Fielding, Lee, & Schaff, 2001).

Early Surgical Abortion Methods (Up to 14 Weeks of Pregnancy)

Vacuum aspiration or suction curettage is the most commonly used abortion procedure in the United States. It is an ambulatory care procedure and may be done through week 14 of gestation. The procedure is done under local anesthesia or a para-cervical block. Sometimes a mild sedative is also given. Prior to surgery, the cervix is dilated either by graduated instrumentation or by osmotic dilators. The products of conception are removed by suction evacuation. Completion may be confirmed by curettage. The procedure takes about 10 minutes.

Potential complications include incomplete abortion, cervical laceration, seizure, cardiac arrest, allergic reaction, uterine atony, uterine perforation, bleeding, and infection. Advantages of the procedure are that it costs less than procedures performed during later gestation and little time is lost from work. It also requires only one visit to the clinic (Hatcher et al., 2011).

Later Trimester Surgical Abortion (14–22 Weeks)

Other surgical methods include dilatation and curettage (D&C), though this is rarely used because of potential complications. Dilatation and evacuation (D&E), also known as dilatation and extraction, is a commonly used procedure for second trimester abortions, after about 14 weeks. (This is the procedure misleadingly referred to as "partial birth abortion" by those who oppose abortion.) This involves dilatation of the cervix (to about 1.5 to 2 cm) by various possible means and evacuation of the products of conception with specially designed forceps, followed by curettage, then suction. The D&E procedure is considered safer, faster, and less expensive for second trimester abortions than previously used instillation methods and can be carried out under local anesthesia (Hacker, Moore, & Gambone, 2004; Hatcher et al., 2011).

POSTABORTION COUNSELING

Clients who undergo vacuum aspiration or suction curettage need to expect menstrual cramping during and after the procedure and some vaginal bleeding that will taper over the next week. Analgesia may be needed after the abortion for cramping and/or breast engorgement.

Abortions later in pregnancy may require hospital stays of 1 to 3 days. The patient may experience severe cramping, necessitating analgesia. Instruct all clients not to put anything in the vagina for 7 days after their procedure. They should expect to feel fatigue and breast tenderness for a few days. A return visit should be scheduled for 2 to 4 weeks.

Advise clients that fertility can return as early as 10 days following an abortion procedure. Contraceptive options must be discussed and decided on. An IUD may be inserted at the same time as a surgical abortion or otherwise as soon as termination is confirmed (Fritz & Speroff, 2011).

POSTABORTION CLINIC VISIT

A postabortion clinic visit is not mandatory, but may serve many purposes: confirmation of pregnancy termination, assessment of physical and emotional well-being, identification of any complications, discussion of feelings about the abortion experience, education, provision of contraception, and reinforcement of the need for future preventative care.

Many women appreciate reassurance that pregnancy has been terminated; however, urine pregnancy tests may show positive up to 8 weeks post abortion. Pelvic exams at 2 to 3 weeks should be consistent with complete involution (Cappiello, Beal, & Simmonds, 2011).

WEB RESOURCES

FERTILITY AWARENESS

Fertile-Focus
www.fertile-focus.com

The Couple to Couple League
www.ccli.org/

The National Fertility Awareness and Natural Family Planning Service for the United Kingdom
www.fertilityuk.org

The Natural Family Planning Site, BYG publishing Inc.
www.bygpub.com/natural

The Fertility Awareness Center
www.fertaware.com

LAM

The Academy of Breastfeeding Medicine
www.bfmed.org

The Linkages Project
www.linkagesproject.org

WHO Medical Eligibility Criteria for Contraceptive Use
http://www.who.int/reproductivehealth/publications/family_planning/9789241563888/en/index.html

Medical Eligibility Criteria Wheel for Contraceptive Use
http://www.who.int/reproductivehealth/publications/family_planning/9789241547710/en/index.html

CONTRACEPTION (GENERAL)

Association of Reproductive Health Professionals
www.arhp.org/patienteducation

EngenderHealth
www.engenderhealth.org

Planned Parenthood Federation of America
www.ppfa.org

World Health Organization
www.who.int/health_topics/contraception

EMERGENCY CONTRACEPTION

Emergency Contraception Website & Hotline
1-888-NOT-2-LATE
http://not-2-late.com

ADOLESCENT SEXUAL HEALTH

Scarleteen
www.scarleteen.com

REFERENCES

ACOG Committee Opinion #450. (2009). Increasing use of contraceptive implants and intrauterine devices to reduce unintended pregnancy. Retrieved February 24, 2012, from http://www.acog.org/Resources_And_Publications/Committee_Opinions/Committee_on_Gynecologic_Practice/Increasing_Use_of_Contraceptive_Implants_and_Intrauterine_Devices_To_Reduce_Unintended_Pregnancy

ACOG Practice Bulletin No. 46. (2003). Clinical management guidelines for obstetrician-gynecologists. *Obstetrics and Gynecology, 102*(3), 647–658.

ACOG Practice Bulletin No. 112. (2010). Emergency contraception. *Obstetrics and Gynecology, 115*(5), 1100–1109.

Advisor Forum. (2002, May). Depo-Provera and topical estrogen: A risky combination. *Clinician Advisor*, 98.

Alan Guttmacher Institute. (2011). *National reproductive health profile*. Retrieved February 25, 2011, from http://www.guttmacher.org/datacenter/profiles/US.jsp

American College of Obstetricians and Gynecologists [ACOG]. (2009). *Adolescent facts: Pregnancy, births and STDs*. Retrieved February 24, 2012, from http://www.acog.org/~/media/Departments/Adolescent%20Health%20Care/AdolescentFactsPregnancyAndSTDs.pdf?dmc=1&ts=20120224T0317272704

Andersson, K., Odlind, V., & Rybo, G. (1994). Levonorgestrel-releasing and copper-releasing (Nova T) IUDs during five years of continuing use: A randomized comparative trial. *Contraception, 49,* 56–72.

Association of Reproductive Health Professionals [ARHP]. (2001, February). New developments in contraception featuring the levonorgestrel intrauterine system. *ARHP Clinical Proceedings,* 6–16.

Association of Reproductive Health Professionals [ARHP]. (2011). *Position statement on contraception*. Retrieved July 1, 2011, from http://www.arhp.org/about-us/position-statements#11

Baill, C., Cullins, V.E., & Pati, S. (2003). Counseling issues in tubal sterilization. *American Family Physician, 67*(6), 1287–1294.

Best, K. (2000a). How effective are spermicides? *Network: FHI, 20*(2), 11–15.

Best, K. (2000b). New barrier devices may be easier to use. *Network, FHI, 20*(2), 16–17.

Borgelt-Hansen, L. (2001). Oral contraceptives: An update on health benefits and risks. *Journal of the American Pharmaceutical Association, 41*(6), 875–886.

Boston Women's Health Book Collective. (2011). *Our bodies, ourselves*. New York: A Touchstone Book Simon & Schuster.

Cappiello, J.D., Beal, M.W., & Simmonds, K.E. (2011). Clinical issues in post abortion care. *Nurse Practitioner, 36*(5), 35–40.

Centers for Disease Control and Prevention (CDC). (2002). Abortion surveillance: United States, 1999. *Morbidity and Mortality Weekly Report, 52,* 1.

Centers for Disease Control and Prevention (CDC). (2011). Update to CDC's U. S. Medical eligibility criteria for contraceptive use, 2010, revised recommendations for the use of contraceptive methods during the postpartum period. *MMWR, 60*(26), 878–883.

Conceptus Inc. (2010). *Essure instructions for use*. Retrieved May 13, 2011, from http://www.essuremd.com/portals/essuremd/PDFs/TopDownloads/L3002%2009_09_09%20smaller.pdf

Deardorff, K.E., Montgomery, P., & Hollmann, F.W. (1996). *U.S. population estimates by age sex, race and Hispanic origin: 1990–1995*. Washington, DC: U.S. Department of Commerce, Economics and Statistics Administration, Bureau of the Census.

Dehlendorf, C., Rodriguez, M.I., Levy, K., Borrero, S., & Steinauer, J. (2010). Disparities in family planning. *American Journal of Obstetrics and Gynecology, 202,* 214–220.

Dickerson, V. (2001). Contraception in the perimenopause. *The Female Patient, 26*(3), 12–16.

Dickey, R. (2010). *Managing contraceptive pill patients* (14th ed.). Dallas, TX: EMIS, Inc.

Duramed. (2006). *ParaGard prescribing information*. Pomona, NY: Duramed Pharmaceuticals Inc.

Edelman, A., Gallo, M.F., Jensen, J.T., Nichols, M.D., & Grimes, D.A. (2010). *Continuous or extended cycle vs. cyclic use of combined hormonal contraceptives for contraception*. Retrieved February 24, 2012, from http://onlinelibrary.wiley.com/doi/10.1002/14651858.CD004695.pub2/full

Faculty of Family Planning and Reproductive Healthcare Clinical Effectiveness Unit. (2005). Faculty statement from the CEU on a new publication: WHO selected practice recommendations for contraceptive use update. Missed pills: New recommendations. *Journal of Family Planning Reproductive Health Care, 31*(2), 153–155.

FemCap, Inc. (2011). *FemCap product information*. Retrieved March 18, 2011, from http://www.femcap.com/clinician-information.html

Fielding, S., Lee, S., & Schaff, E. (2001). Professional considerations for providing mifepristone-induced abortion. *Nurse Practitioner, 26*(11), 44–54.

Fine, P. (2011). A new option in emergency contraception. *Female Patient, 36,* 41–44.

Finger, W. (2001). Contraception after intercourse. *Network: FHI, 21*(1), 185.

Fritz, M., & Speroff, L. (2011). *Clinical gynecologic endocrinology and infertility* (8th ed.). Philadelphia: Lippincott Williams & Wilkins.

Griffin, T., Tooher, R., Nowakowski, K., Lloyd, M., & Maddern, G. (2005). How little is enough? The evidence for post-vasectomy testing. *Journal of Urology, 174,* 29–36.

Grimes, D. (1999). DMPA good choice for women with sickle cell. *Network: FHI, 19*(2), 10–11.

Hacker, N.F., Moore, J.G., & Gambone, J. (2004). *Essentials of obstetrics and gynecology* (4th ed.). Philadelphia: Saunders.

Hatcher, R., Trussell, J., Nelson, A.L., Cates, W., Jr., Kowal, D., & Policar, M.S. (2011). *Contraceptive technology* (20th rev ed.). New York: Ardent Media.

Henshaw, S.K., & Van Vort, J. (1994). Abortion services in the United States, 1991–1992. *Family Planning Perspectives, 26,* 100.

Hologic Inc. (2009). *Adiana permanent contraception: Instructions for use and radiofrequency (RF) generator operator's manual*. Retrieved April 1, 2011, from http://www.adiana.com/pdf/hcp/adiana-instructions-for-use.pdf

Hubacher, D., & Grimes, D.A. (2002). Non-contraceptive health benefits of intrauterine devices: A systematic review. *Obstetric-Gynecologic Survey, 57*(2), 120–128.

Hubacher, D., Lara-Ricalde, R., Taylor, D.J., Guerra-Infante, F., & Guzman-Rodriguez, R. (2001). Use of copper intrauterine devices and the risk of tubal infertility among nulligravid women. *New England Journal of Medicine, 345,* 561–567.

Intrauterine devices. (2000). *Network: FHI, 20*(1), 1–19.

Jick, S., Kaye, J.A., Li, L., & Jick, H. (2007). Further results on the risk of nonfatal venous thromboembolism in users of the contraceptive transdermal patch compared to users of oral contraceptives containing norgestimate and 35 microg of ethinyl estradiol. *Contraception, 76,* 4–7.

Jick, S.S., & Jick, H. (2007). The contraceptive patch in relation to ischemic stroke and acute myocardial infarction. *Pharmacotherapy, 27,* 218.

Jick, S.S., Kaye, J.A., Russman, S., & Jick, H. (2006). Risk of nonfatal venous thromboembolism in women using a contraceptive transdermal patch and oral contraceptives containing norgestimate and 35 microg of ethinyl estradiol. *Contraception, 73,* 223–228.

Jones, R.K., Darrock, J.E., & Hensaw, S.K. (2002). Patterns in the socioeconomic characteristics of women obtaining abortions in 2000–2001. *Perspectives in Sexual Reproductive Health, 34,* 226.

Kupecz, D., & Berandinelli, C. (2002). Drugs and device approval highlights from 2001. *Nurse Practitioner, 26*(2), 16.

Labbock, M., Cooney, K., & Cole, S. (1994). *Guidelines: Breastfeeding, family planning and the lactational amenorrhea method*. Washington, DC: Institute for Reproductive Health, Georgetown University.

Lidegaard, O., & Kreiner, S. (2002). Contraceptives and cerebral thrombosis: A five year national case controlled study. *Contraception, 65*(3), 197–205.

Lynaugh, J. (1991). The death of Sadie Sachs . . . Margaret Sanger. *Nursing Research, 40*(2), 124–125.

Mantel-Teeuwisse, A., Kloosterman, J., & Maitland-Van der Zee, A. (2001). Drug induced lipid changes: A review of the unintended effects of some commonly used drugs on serum lipid levels. *Drug Safety, 24,* 443–456.

Marchbanks, P.A., McDonald, J.A., Wilson, H.G., Folger, S.G., Mandel, M.G., Daling, J.R., et al. (2002). Oral contraceptives and the risk of breast cancer. *New England Journal of Medicine, 346*, 2025–2032.

Mayer Laboratories Inc. (2009). *Today sponge consumer information leaflet*. Retrieved May 13, 2011, from http://www.TodaySponge.com

Milne, R.L., Knight, J.A., John, E.M., Dite, G.S., Balbuena, R., Ziogas, A., et al. (2005). Oral contraceptive use and risk of early-onset breast cancer in carriers and noncarriers of BRCA1 and BRCA2 mutations. *Cancer Epidemiology Biomarkers Preview, 14*(2), 350–356.

National vital statistics report. (2009). Retrieved February 25, 2011, from http://www.cdc.gov/nchs/about.htm

Neilson, C., & Miller, L. (2000). Ectopic gestation following emergency contraceptive pill administration. *Contraception, 62,* 275–276.

New approach to prescribing oral contraception. (2001). *Clinical Reviews* [Online]. Retrieved from http://www.Medscape.com/viewarticle/407324

Norplant effective for seven years. (2000). *Network: FHI, 20*(3), 2.

Pakarinen, P., Toivonen, J., & Luukkainen, T. (2001). Therapeutic use of the LNG-IUS and counseling. *Seminars in Reproductive Medicine, 19*(4), 365–372.

Peterson, H.B., Jeng, G., Folger, S.G., Hillis, S.A., Marchbanks, P.A., & Wilcox, L.S. (2000). The risk of menstrual abnormalities after tubal sterilization: U.S. collaborative review of sterilization working group. *New England Journal of Medicine, 343*(23), 1681–1687.

Pymar, H., & Creinin, M. (2001). The risks of oral contraceptive pills. *Seminars in Reproductive Medicine, 19*(4), 305–312.

Rawlins, S.I.C., & Smith, D.M. (2002). Innovative contraception: New options in hormonal contraception. *American Journal of Nurse Practitioners, 6*(1), 20–28.

Ronnerdag, M., & Odlind, V. (1999). Health effects of long-term use of the intrauterine levonorgestrel-releasing system: A follow-up study over 12 years of continuous use. *Acta Obstetricia et Gynecologica Scandinavica, 78*(8), 716–721.

Schering-Plough. (2009). *Implanon (etonogestrel implant): Prescribing information*. Retrieved February 24, 2012, from http://www.drugs.com/pro/implanon.html

Schwartz, S., Petitti, D., Siscovick, D., Longstreth, W.T., Sidney, S., Raghunathan, T.E., et al. (1998). Stroke and use of oral contraceptives in young women: A pooled analysis of two U.S. studies. *Stroke, 29*(11), 2274–2284.

Secura, G.M., Allsworth, J.E., Madden, T., Mullersman, J.L., & Peipert, J.F. (2010). The contraceptive CHOICE project: Reducing barriers to long-acting reversible contraception. *American Journal of Obstetrics and Gynecology, 203,* 115.e1–115.e7.

Segal, S.J., Alvarez-Sanchez, F., Adejuwon, C.A., Brache De Mejla, V., Leon, P., & Faundes, A. (1985). Absence of chorionic gonadotropin in sera women who use intrauterine devices. *Fertility and Sterility, 44,* 214.

Sieven, I., Stern, J., Coutnho, E., Mattos, C.E.R., & Diaz, S. (1991). Prolonged intrauterine contraception: A seven year randomized study of the levonorgestrel 20 mcg/day (LNG20) and the copper T 380A IUDs. *Contraception, 44*(5), 473–480.

Speroff, L., & Darney, P.D. (2011). *A clinical guide for contraception* (5th ed.). Philadelphia: Lippincott Williams & Wilkins.

Srikanthan, A., & Reid, R.L. (2008). Religious and cultural influences on contraception. *Journal of Obstetrics Gynaecology Canada, 30*(2), 129–137.

The Standard Days Method. (2003). *Institute for Reproductive Health, Georgetown University* [Online]. Retrieved January 14, 2003, from http://www.irh.org

Trussell, J. (2007). Contraceptive efficacy. In R.A. Hatcher, J. Trussell, A.L. Nelson, W. Cates, F.H. Stewart, & D. Kowal (Eds.), *Contraceptive technology* (19th revised ed.). New York: Ardent Media.

U.S. National Center for Health Statistics. (2009). *Vital statistics of the United States*. Retrieved April 1, 2011, from http://www.cdc.gov/nchs/

Valdes, V., Labbock, M., Pugin, E., & Perez, A. (2000). The efficacy of the lactational amenorrhea method (LAM) among working women. *Contraception, 62*(5), 217–219.

Vandenbroucke, J.P., Rosing, J., Bloemenkamp, K.W., Middeldorp, S., Helmorhorst, F.M., Bourma, B.N., et al. (2001). Oral contraceptives and the risk of venous thrombosis. *New England Journal of Medicine, 334*(20), 1527–1535.

What is medical abortion? (2000). Washington, DC: National Abortion Federation.

Wilcox, A.J., Weinberg, C.R., Armstrong, E.G., & Canfield, R.E. (1987). Urinary human chorionic gonadotropin among intrauterine device users: Detection with a highly specific and sensitive assay. *Fertility and Sterility, 47,* 265.

World Health Organization. (2009). *Medical eligibility criteria for contraceptive use* (4th ed.). Geneva, Switzerland: WHO Press.

Wright, J. (2010). A history of contraception. *British Journal of School Nursing, 5*(7), 356–357.

Zieman, M., Hatcher, R.A., Cwiak, C., Darney, P., Creinin, M., & Stosur, H. (2010). *A pocket guide to managing contraception*. Tiger, Georgia: Bridging the Gap Foundation.

CHAPTER ❖ 13

INFERTILITY

Michelle J. Valentine ◆ *Jennifer R. Gardella*

The etiology of infertility can be identified in 85 to 90 percent of couples: 30 percent have male factor infertility, 35 percent have female factor infertility, and 20 percent have a combination of male and female factor infertility.

Highlights

- Factors Affecting Fertility
- Diagnostic Infertility Evaluation
- Female Infertility: Causes, Diagnoses, and Interventions
- Recurrent Pregnancy Loss
- Male Infertility: Causes, Diagnoses, and Interventions
- Combined Factors of Male and Female Infertility
- Selected Infertility Treatments
- Alternative Family Building
- Future Trends and Controversies
- Resources

❖ INTRODUCTION

Infertility is generally defined as 1 year of unprotected, frequent intercourse without attaining conception. Infertility may also result from recurrent miscarriage. Primary infertility, meaning a couple has never conceived, is a potentially more ominous diagnosis than secondary infertility, or difficulty conceiving after any prior conception. Today, couples are more aware of specific causes of infertility and of the sophisticated treatments available. Also, the number of available infertility services is increasing. However, in many cases health insurance may not share the burden of treatment costs to diagnose or treat infertility.

Infertility is a widespread problem that often is initially identified in the obstetric/gynecologic, or less commonly, the urologic practice. It is imperative that the nurse practitioner recognize infertility and understand its causes and treatment options. Prevention of infertility, through patient education, can also be incorporated into the nurse practitioner's practice. Evaluation and treatment may be initiated in the general practice setting with referral to a reproductive endocrinologist when necessary.

With the advent of in vitro fertilization (IVF) and other assisted reproductive technologies (ART) in the late 1970s, an increase in media attention focused on infertility, increased public awareness of the availability of fertility services, and increased social acceptance of the use of ART. There has also been an increase in the proportion of women over 35 seeking medical attention for infertility. The rate of infertility in the United States, however, has not risen but has decreased slightly over time. The National Survey of Family Growth by the National Center for Health Statistics has been performed several times since 1960. In the most recent survey, it was reported that 7.4 percent of women in the reproductive-age group, 15 to 44 years, were infertile in the United States (U.S. Department of Health and Human Services, 2009). But, despite the availability of medical treatment, only 11.9 percent of childless couples ever seek infertility services. One out of five U.S. women has her first child after age 35. Yet about one fourth of women who defer pregnancy until the mid-to-late 30s will have an infertility problem.

The reproductive endocrinologist and nurse practitioner in an infertility practice collaborate closely as they would in any medical setting. Their roles are multifaceted: to diagnose and treat; to identify multiple impacts on an individual, couple, and significant others; to provide information, support, and counseling; and to refer to appropriate specialties. Roles also include research, community education, and advocacy.

FACTORS AFFECTING FERTILITY

There are multiple known and unknown factors that impact fertility. The most important factors that reflect current research and practice are discussed in this section.

MATERNAL AGE

Maternal age is one of the most important factors to influence a couple's fertility, although it is important to remember that biological age is more important than chronological age. Some women will be unable to conceive in their 20s while others become pregnant in their 40s. However, generally a woman's fertility begins to decline by the age of 34. Risk of spontaneous abortion increases from 10 percent under age 30, to 20 percent in the late 30s, to 55 percent at age 44 (Centers for Disease Control and Prevention [CDC], 2008). The frequency of both euploid (chromosomally normal) and aneuploid (chromosomally abnormal) spontaneous abortions increases with age (see Table 13–1). Studies performed on embryos resulting from IVF have confirmed an increased incidence of aneuploidy in embryos obtained from older women (Munne, Alikani, Tomkin, et al., 1995). The urgency of the fertility evaluation and treatment increases after age 35. Advanced maternal age also presents risks to both mother and fetus in pregnancy including gestational diabetes, pregnancy-induced hypertension, premature labor, stillbirth, and placental problems (March of Dimes, 2011). Every woman over the age of 42 should undergo a medical evaluation and counseling by an obstetrician prior to undergoing fertility therapies.

BODY WEIGHT

Extremes of body weight are associated with altered ovarian function. A threshold body weight and fat content are necessary to establish and maintain normal ovarian

TABLE 13–1. Chromosomal Abnormalities in Liveborn Infants and Maternal Age

Maternal Age	Risk for Down Syndrome	Total Risk for Chromosomal Anomalies[a]
20	1/1667	1/526
21	1/1667	1/526
22	1/1429	1/500
23	1/1429	1/500
24	1/1250	1/476
25	1/1250	1/476
26	1/1176	1/476
27	1/1111	1/455
28	1/1053	1/435
29	1/1000	1/417
30	1/952	1/385
31	1/909	1/385
32	1/769	1/322
33	1/602	1/286
34	1/485	1/238
35	1/378	1/192
36	1/289	1/156
37	1/224	1/127
38	1/173	1/102
39	1/136	1/83
40	1/106	1/66
41	1/82	1/53
42	1/63	1/42
43	1/49	1/33
44	1/38	1/26
45	1/30	1/21
46	1/23	1/16
47	1/18	1/13
48	1/14	1/10
49	1/11	1/8

[a]The other chromosomal anomalies that are increased with maternal age in addition to 47,+21 (Down syndrome) are 47,+18; and 47,+13; 47,XYY (Klinefelter's syndrome); 47,XYY and 47,XXX. The incidence of 47,XXX for women between the ages of 20 and 32 years is not available.

Source: Modified from Hook, 1981; Hook, Cross, & Schreinemachers, 1983.

function. If body weight is reduced below the 10th percentile for a particular height (body mass index [BMI] < 17) or the body fat content is reduced to less than 22 percent, altered menstrual function and ovulatory dysfunction can develop (Fritz & Speroff, 2011). An increased incidence of amenorrhea in some female athletes and in anorexic women has been well described. Increased body weight can also be associated with ovulatory dysfunction. Obesity also increases the risk of complications in pregnancy and delivery. The most important endocrine change in obesity is elevation of the basal body insulin level, leading to increased insulin resistance. Insulin resistance, hyperandrogenism, and anovulation are hallmarks of the polycystic ovary syndrome (PCOS). Obese women are also at increased risk for miscarriage and experience decreased success with fertility therapies (American Society for Reproductive Medicine [ASRM], 2008).

SMOKING

Smoking has been shown to be a reproductive toxin in both women and men. Cigarette smoking reduces fertility, increases the rate of spontaneous abortion, and increases the incidence of abruptio placentae, placenta previa, bleeding during pregnancy, and premature rupture of placental membranes (Fielding, 1987). Smoking has clearly been associated with decreased fertility in several large studies (Bolumar, Olsen, & Boldsen, 1996; De Mouzon, Spira, & Schwartz, 1988). Women who smoke generally go through an earlier menopause by 1 to 5 years, suggesting that the metabolic products of cigarette smoke may be directly toxic to the ovaries (American College of Obstetricians and Gynecologists, 1997). Tobacco use by men may also have a detrimental impact on their fertility (Bayer, Alper, & Penzias, 2012). Tobacco use decreases sperm motility and density (Aubuchon, Burney, Schust, & Yao, 2012).

ALCOHOL

Alcohol is a known human teratogen, and it is known to be embryotoxic. Any degree of alcohol intake in a woman can decrease her chance for conception. Alcohol consumption was shown to reduce the ability to conceive in a dose-dependent fashion in two large studies (Hakim, Gray, & Zacur, 1998;Jensen et al., 1998). Alcohol consumption of more than two drinks per day is associated with a risk of spontaneous abortion twice that in non-alcohol-consuming controls (Harlap & Shiono, 1980). Moderate drinking also may be associated with an increased risk for spontaneous abortion in the second and third trimesters (see Table 13–2). Alcohol should be eliminated from the diet in women attempting to achieve pregnancy. There are no published data, however, that suggest that low to moderate alcohol use affects male reproduction.

TABLE 13–2. Alcohol Effects on Fetal Development

Amount of Absolute Alcohol per Day	Fetal Effect
≥ 4 oz	FAS is induced
2–3 oz	Birth weight reduction
1.5 oz	IQ deficits (reduction of 5–7 points)
Five drinks/occasion, at least once per week	Memory and attention deficits
Amount necessary to induce spontaneous abortion	Unknown

Source: Gardella & Hill, 2000.

CAFFEINE

Several reports link a woman's caffeine intake to decreased fertility (Bolumar, Olsen, Rebagliato, & Bisanti, 1997; Hatch & Bracken, 1993). A dose-dependent relationship of more than one serving of caffeine has been confirmed to be detrimental to fertility. Caffeine in excess of 300 mg/day (three cups of coffee) is also associated with an increase in risk for spontaneous abortion (Gardella & Hill, 2000).

RECREATIONAL DRUG USE

Combined effects of substances of abuse may be additive with those related to alcohol consumption and cigarette smoking (Jacobson, Jacobson, & Sokol, 1994). Males who use marijuana on a regular basis have decreased sperm motility and, therefore, are also at risk for fertility problems (Aubuchon et al., 2012; Bayer et al., 2012).

ENVIRONMENTAL HAZARDS

Many toxins (including lead, mercury, and organic solvents) encountered by women in the environment and workplace may affect reproductive health by decreasing fertility or lead to spontaneous abortion, fetal malformation, or developmental abnormalities. Men are also susceptible to environmental toxins because spermatogenesis is an ongoing and dynamic process. DBCP (a pesticide), lead, ethylene glycol ethers, kepone (an insecticide), organic solvents, and other chemicals have been shown to impact male fertility (Gardella & Hill, 2000). Currently, the Longitudinal Investigation of Fertility and the Environment (LIFE) study is following 800 couples to help determine the contribution of environmental contaminants to human fertility and associated health conditions.

PSYCHOLOGICAL STRESS

Infertility is associated with an intense psychological component, which can produce feelings of anger, anxiety, guilt, inadequacy, and overt depression. In addition, the experience of infertility can lead to isolation from social support systems. There are no adequate studies indicating that psychological stress actually causes infertility. Nevertheless, the benefit of relaxation techniques in reducing stress has been reported to potentially improve fertility (Domar et al., 2000). Further research is needed to clarify the association of stress and fertility and the benefits of intervention.

Many couples take for granted that they are fertile and hence are not emotionally prepared for the psychological impact of a diagnosis of infertility. Emotional distress may be no less severe for couples who experience secondary infertility. A couple's ability to admit that they may have a fertility problem is an important first step, but they may also feel threatened as potential causes are identified and treatment recommended. The many complex feelings associated with loss and infertility involve self-image, self-esteem, and sexuality (see Table 13–3). Infertility is a couple's problem, not an individual's. Both partners need to be involved in diagnostic and treatment choices and to accompany each other to appointments when possible. The health care provider can assist the couple experiencing grief by giving accurate information; supporting or making referrals for individual, group, or sex therapy; and encouraging couples to use support services. Couples may also need to be given permission to stop treatment.

DIAGNOSTIC INFERTILITY EVALUATION

Expedite the evaluation and treatment of a couple in which (1) the female partner is over the age of 35, (2) she has a history of oligo/amenorrhea, (3) she has known or suspected uterine/tubal disease or endometriosis, or (4) the male partner is known to be subfertile (ASRM, 2011). The etiology of infertility is believed to be roughly equally divided between male and female causes, with approximately one third of affected couples experiencing a combined problem. Multiple factors of infertility are more difficult to overcome. Unfortunately, 15 to 30 percent of infertility remains unexplained, despite a thorough evaluation (Quaas & Dokras, 2008).

The infertility evaluation must be couple-oriented and evaluation of both partners should begin at the same time (ASRM, 2011) (see Figure 13–1). The evaluation can become an extremely stressful and dehumanizing experience if not performed by a caring and thoughtful clinician. Providing preconception care and counseling is an important part of the assessment and treatment of the infertile couple. The goal of fertility therapy is not only to establish a pregnancy, but to conceive a pregnancy that is uncomplicated and results in the delivery of a healthy baby (see Chapter 19).

After an initial consultation with a couple, which includes a complete history of the female and male partners (see Tables 13–4 and 13–5), physical examination of the female partner (see Table 13–6), preconception counseling, and instruction on how timing of intercourse might be optimized, the remainder of the infertility evaluation can usually be completed within two menstrual cycles (ASRM, 2011; Cowan, 2002). Physical examination of the male

TABLE 13–3 Common Emotional Responses to Infertility and Coping Mechanisms (the manifestation of these may differ significantly between men and women)

Emotional Response	Coping Mechanisms
Guilt	Avoidance Coping
One or both partners assume blame for the infertility. Self-reproach increases and self-esteem decreases. Problems with self-esteem and self-blame are more significant for women.	Impacts personal, marital, and social distress. Use of this is directly related to personal marital and social distress. Use of this mechanism by one partner increased personal and social distress for the other. Increased use of this mechanism by men increased marital distress for women.
Depression	Active-confronting coping
One or both partners develop a sense of hopelessness, loss and despair cry often, fatigue, anxiety, problem with sleep or eating disturbances, or an inability to concentrate. The onset of menses can often trigger a depression in many infertile couples. Women have significantly more anxiety. Men and women experience depression equally.	Women's increased use of this mechanism was related to marital distress for men over time
Anger	Passive-avoidance coping
The infertile couple often feels that life has not been fair for them. They may feel out-of-control, resentful, and angry with others, including family, friends, and medical personnel.	Impacts personal distress for men and women. Women using this over time had an increased partner effect. Also impacts marital distress. Men's use of this mechanism increases marital distress for women.
Isolation	Meaning-based coping
Sense of social aloneness and not belonging. Feeling "left out" of the mainstream of life. Social stigma of childlessness impact women more than men. Emotional and social isolation negatively impacts self-confidence and self-esteem.	Use of this mechanism decreased personal distress for women. Use of this did not impact personal distress for men. However, use of this mechanism by women decreased marital distress for both men and women. Increased use of this by men increased their social distress.

Adapted from: Anderson et al., (2003) Distress and concerns in couples referred to a specialist infertility clinic. *Journal of Psychosomatic Research, 54.* 353–355; *Applegarth, L.D. (1995). The psychological aspects of infertility. In W. R. Keye, Jr. R. J. Chang, R. W. Rebar, & M. R. Soules (Eds.),* Infertility: Evaluation and treatment. *Philadelphia: W. B. Saunders Company. Peterson et al. (2009)* The longitudinal impact of partner coping in couples following 5 years of unsuccessful fertility treatments. *Human Reproduction, 24*(7), 1656–1664.

partner and referral to a urologist is initiated with abnormal semen analyses (see Table 13–7). Depending on the setting and practice protocols, a nurse practitioner may initiate the infertility evaluation, educate and support the couple, prescribe initial interventions, and refer to a specialist.

Years ago, the standard infertility evaluation involved the performance of several tests, including endometrial biopsy (EMB), postcoital test, and a laparoscopy. Studies performed in the past decade confirmed that EMB and postcoital testing are not always reliable and do not always differentiate between fertile and infertile populations (Bayer et al., 2012). Moreover, often the findings at the time of a laparoscopy, if done as an initial part of the infertility workup, do not change the recommended course of treatment. Therefore, the infertility evaluation has become more practical, efficient, informative, and cost-effective (see Table 13–8).

SEMEN ANALYSIS

In 2001, the American Urological Association (AUA) and the ASRM recommended that the initial screening evaluation of the male partner include, at a minimum, a male reproductive history (see Table 13–5) and two semen analyses. Their recommendations have not changed. If possible, the two semen analyses should be separated by 1 month. In practice however, if the first semen analysis is normal, many clinicians do not require a second. A full evaluation by a urologist or other specialist in male reproduction should be done if the initial screening evaluation demonstrates an abnormal male reproductive history or an abnormal semen analysis.

Early in a woman's evaluation, her partner, after 2 to 3 days of abstinence, collects a semen specimen by means of masturbation or, less commonly, by use of a special condom. The semen is deposited directly into a sterile container and evaluated microscopically within an hour of collection. Semen analyses vary in different labs.

Normal semen analysis parameters per the World Health Organization (WHO) (AUA, 2010; Aubuchon et al., 2012) are the following:

- *Volume:* > 1.5 mL.
- *pH:* 7.2 to 7.8.
- *Count:* Equal to or greater than 15 million per mL.
- *Motility:* Equal to or greater than 32 percent.
- *Forward progression:* Greater than 2 (on a 0–4 scale with 0 = no movement, to 4 = excellent forward progression).
- *Morphology:* Greater than 30 percent normal oval heads, midpiece, and tail.

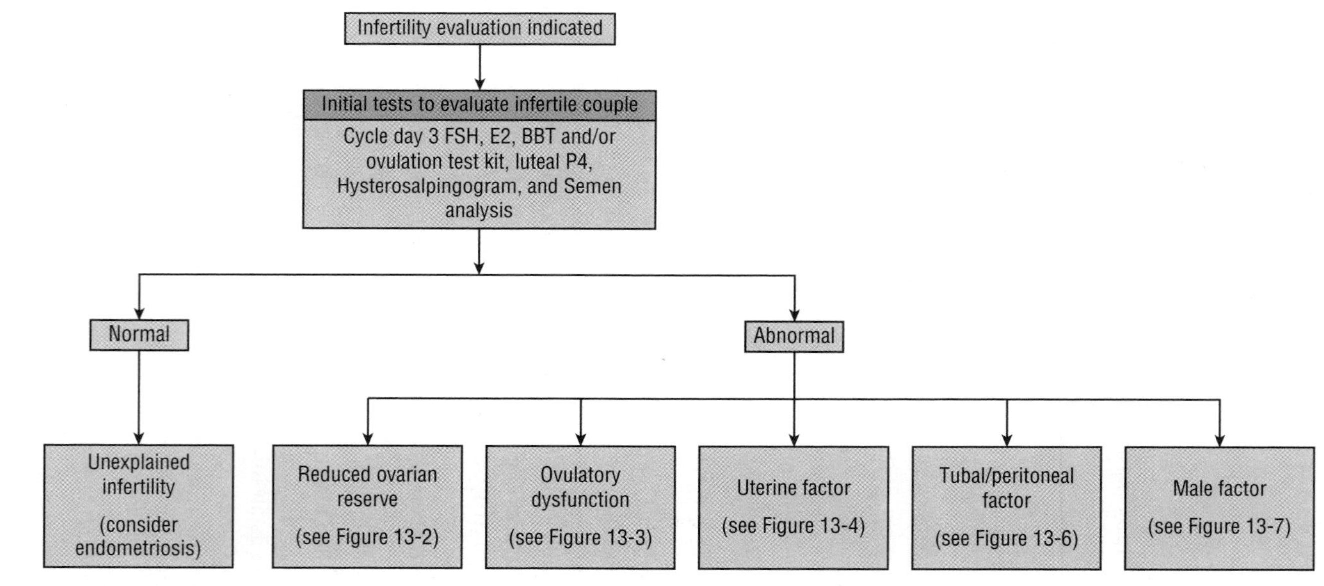

FIGURE 13–1. Infertility Evaluation. *Source:* Adapted from Aubuchon et al. in Berek, J.S., 2012, pp. 1136–1141; Bayer et al., 2012, p. 52; & Wright & Johnson, pp. 705–715 in Gibbs et al., 2008.

TABLE 13–4. Female History: Summary of Pertinent Data

Age of client
Menstrual history (age at menarche, cycle length, duration/amount of flow, onset/severity of dysmenorrhea, other moliminal symptoms. If amenorrhea present, duration.)
Obstetric history (gravidity, parity, pregnancy outcome, associated complications, time to conception)
Contraceptive history (current or past oral contraceptive use, IUD use, duration)
Sexual history (coital frequency, sexual dysfunction, number of partners, sexual orientation, history of sexually transmitted diseases and treatment)
Duration of infertility and results of any previous evaluation and treatment
Medical/surgical history (past surgeries, indications and outcomes, previous hospitalizations, serious illnesses or injuries, pelvic inflammatory disease, or exposure to sexually transmitted diseases)
Symptoms of thyroid disease, pelvic or abdominal pain, galactorrhea, hirsutism, and dyspareunia
Previous abnormal Pap smears and any subsequent treatment (LEEP, cryotherapy)
Current medications and allergies
Social and occupation history (use of tobacco, alcohol, recreational drug use, caffeine intake, workplace exposures)
Nutrition history (BMI, vitamin supplementation, herbal remedies)
Family history of birth defects, mental retardation, reproductive failure, and other inheritable disorders

Source: Adapted from ASRM, 2011.

TABLE 13–5. Male History: Summary of Pertinent Data

Duration of couple's infertility.
Previous paternities, including time to conceive.
General health, pubescence, disorders of the urogenital tract.
Frequency and timing of coitus, sexual practices.
Contraceptive methods (condoms, vasectomy).
Exposure to toxins, excessive warmth, or irradiation.
Drugs (chemotherapy, anabolic steroids, hypertensive medications, caffeine, nicotine, alcohol, recreational drugs).
Developmental characteristics, e.g., onset of secondary sex characteristics, descent of the testes, and abnormalities of general development. (This may indicate endocrinological causes of reproductive dysfunction.)
Histories of any sexually transmitted diseases, systemic febrile illnesses, or genital infections such as mumps, chickenpox, or other forms of orchitis.
Surgical history, e.g., inguinal herniorrhaphy, injuries to the vas or bladder neck, retroperitoneal node dissection, testicular cancer, or circumcision.
Testicular torsion or general trauma.
Gynecomastia or anosmia.

Source: Adapted from Edwards, R.G., & Brody, S.A. (1995). *Principles and practice of assisted human reproduction.* Philadelphia: W.B. Saunders Company.

TABLE 13–6. Female Physical Exam: Summary of Pertinent Data

Height, weight, body mass index (BMI)
Thyroid enlargement, nodule, or tenderness
Breast exam (note masses, Tanner stage, any secretions and their character)
Signs of androgen excess (such as hirsutism, cliteromegaly, acanthosis nigricans)
Pelvic exam (note abdominal tenderness, organ enlargement, masses)
Adnexal mass or tenderness
Cul-de-sac mass, tenderness, or nodularity
Uterine size, shape, position, and mobility
Vaginal or cervical lesions, stenosis, secretions, or discharge

Source: Adapted from ASRM, 2011.

TABLE 13–7. Male Physical Exam: Summary of Pertinent Data

State of virilization (hair pattern, body proportions, muscle development).
Neurological symptoms (libido, headache, visual symptoms, papilledema, olfactory dysfunction).
Thyroid size, consistency, presence of nodules.
Presence of gynecomastia and/or galactorrhea.
Penis, circumcised, Tanner staging.
Testicular location, size, volume, and consistency.
Presence of epididymis and vas deferens.
Varicocele.
Prostate size, consistency.

Sources: Adapted from Sherins, R.J. (1995). How is male infertility defined? How is it diagnosed? Epidemiology, causes, work-up (history, physical, lab tests). In The American Society of Andrology (Ed.), *Handbook of andrology.* Lawrence, KS: Allen Press, Inc.; Edwards, R.G., & Brody, S.A. (1995). *Principles and practice of assisted human reproduction.* Philadelphia: W.B. Saunders Company.

TABLE 13–8. Past and Present Tests Used for Evaluation of Infertility

Past	Present
Semen analysis	Semen analysis
Endometrial biopsy	Assessment of ovarian function (cycle day 3 FSH/estradiol or CCCT)
Hysterosalpingogram	Hysterosalpingogram
Postcoital test	Laparoscopy (optional)
Laparoscopy	

CCCT—clomiphene citrate challenge test
FSH—follicle-stimulating hormone
Source: Bayer et al., 2012.

- *Kruger's strict criteria:* Kruger developed strict criteria for morphology, which have proven to be more predictive of fertilization in IVF cycles. This system identifies greater than 15 percent normal forms as "normal or good prognosis," 5 to 14 percent as "fair to good prognosis," and less than 4 percent as "poor prognosis," and usually requires IVF with intracytoplasmic sperm injection (ICSI) (Kruger et al., 1988.). Greater than 4 percent normal forms are now considered a normal sperm morphology percentage when using *strict criteria* (Aubuchon et al., 2012).

- Abnormal semen analysis requires that the test be repeated in 4 to 6 weeks. If time is not critical, 3 months should be allowed to complete a sperm cycle if a viral illness, hot bath, or toxicants could have caused poor semen parameters (AUA, 2010). Normal semen parameters indicate no further male evaluation is necessary unless infertility persists (AUA, 2010; Bayer et al., 2012) (see Figure 13–7).

ASSESSMENT OF OVARIAN FUNCTION

Ovulatory dysfunction will be identified in approximately 15 percent of all infertile couples and accounts for up to 40 percent of infertility in women (ASRM, 2011). Ovulatory dysfunction can result in gross menstrual disturbances (oligo/amenorrhea, dysfunctional uterine bleeding), but it is also often more subtle (polymenorrhea, short luteal phase). It is important to discover the underlying cause (e.g., thyroid disease, hyperandrogenism, pituitary tumor, eating disorder, extremes of weight loss or exercise, hyperprolactinemia, obesity) because the correct diagnosis will lead to specific treatment and many conditions have long-term consequences on general health.

Menstrual History

If a woman is having regular menstrual cycles that are 25 to 35 days in length, then she is ovulating. Ovulation may further be supported by the presence of moliminal symptoms (fluid retention/bloating, breast tenderness, mood changes).

Basal Body Temperature

A daily record of the basal body temperature (BBT) may provide a simple and inexpensive method for confirming ovulation, with a biphasic pattern characteristic of ovulation. BBT charts, however, can sometimes be difficult to interpret, some ovulatory women exhibit monophasic BBT patterns, and the test cannot reliably define the time of ovulation (see Chapter 12).

Urinary Luteinizing Hormone

Urinary ovulation predictor kits can identify the midcycle luteinizing hormone (LH) surge. These kits can provide reliable, if still indirect, evidence of ovulatory function and can help define the interval in which conception is most likely (intercourse or insemination the day of and the day after the LH surge). Results correlate well with the peak in serum LH.

TABLE 13–9. Clomiphene Citrate Challenge Test

Step 1: Draw serum FSH and estradiol (E2) levels on menstrual cycle day 2, 3, or 4.
Step 2: Administer clomiphene citrate 100 mg (50 mg, 2 tabs po qd) on cycle days 5 through 9.
Step 3: Draw serum FSH level on cycle day 10.
Interpretation: If either of the FSH levels are > 10–12 mIU/mL or the day 3 E2 level is greater than 70–80 pg/mL, the test confirms reduced ovarian reserve. If either of the FSH levels are greater than 15, the test is considered abnormal. If either (day 3 or day 10) FSH level is ≥ 20, direct the patient toward alternatives such as egg donation or adoption. An FSH level > 40 is menopausal.

Assessment of Ovarian Reserve

The maximum number of oocytes a woman will have in her lifetime is present in utero at 20 weeks' gestation. There is a developmental and progressive decrease in the number of oocytes from this point forward. Evaluation of the ovarian reserve by measurement of cycle day 3 serum follicle-stimulating hormone (FSH) and estradiol levels is the gold standard for testing. Common criteria for normal ovarian reserve are an early follicular-phase FSH level of ≤ 10 mIU/mL and an estradiol level of ≥ 80 pg/mL (ASRM, 2005a).

Performing an *antral follicle count* early in the follicular phase is commonly used to predict the number of oocytes that may be recruited for ovulation induction. An antral follicle count consists of counting the number of follicles between the size of 2 mm and 10 mm. A low number of follicles have been directly correlated with poor ovarian response to stimulation medications.

Recently, the testing of AMH (anti-Müllerian hormone) levels has gained popularity due to the flexibility of the timing of the test. AMH is produced by the granulosa cells of follicles that are microscopic and peaking in follicles around 4 mm in size. There is essentially no AMH secreted in follicles 8 mm or larger. Because of this, AMH can be tested on any day in a woman's cycle. Currently, a value of 1.0 ng/mL or greater has been associated with normal ovarian reserve (LaMarca & Volpe, 2006).

The clomiphene citrate challenge test (CCCT) (see Table 13–9) is also an easy test that provides an assessment of the number and quality of the remaining oocytes (Bayer et al., 2012).

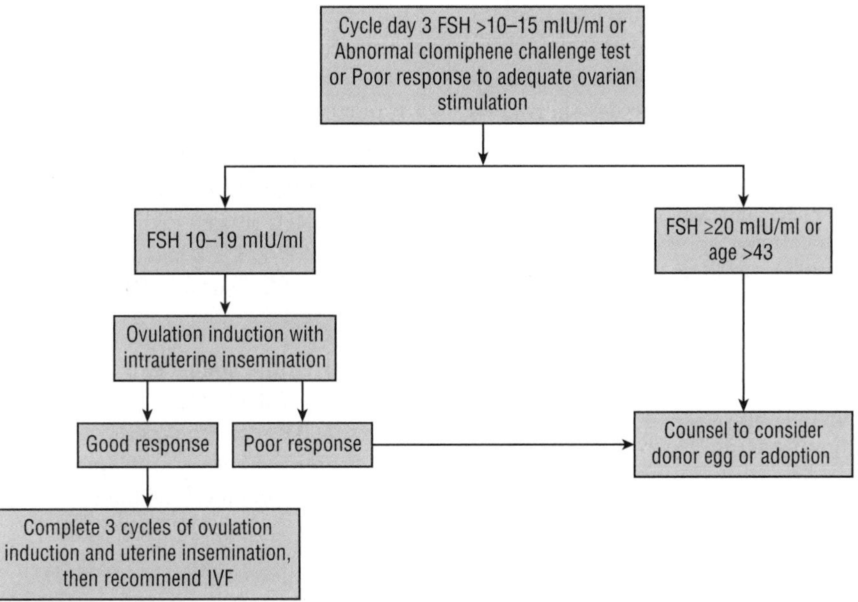

FIGURE 13–2. Reduced Ovarian Reserve. *Source:* Adapted from Aubuchon et al. in Berek, J.S., 2012, pp. 1136–1141; Bayer et al., 2012, p. 53; & Wright & Johnson, pp. 705–715 in Gibbs et al., 2008.

Reduced ovarian reserve is associated with reduced fertility and increased risk of miscarriage (ASRM, 2005a). The routine assessment of ovarian reserve reflects the current practice of most reproductive endocrinologists. Any woman who has evidence of reduced ovarian reserve should be referred for counseling and offered aggressive treatment (see Figure 13–2).

ASSESSMENT OF UTERINE CAVITY AND ENDOMETRIUM

Hysterosalpingogram

An x-ray test is performed after menses but before ovulation. Radioactive dye is placed in the uterus to outline the uterine cavity and determine the patency of the fallopian tubes. This process can push out mucus in the fallopian tubes, which may have been blocking them. Cramping may occur with this procedure and can be reduced by use of 600 to 800 mg of ibuprofen taken 1 hour prior to the test. The client may have a paracervical block and/or be given a sedative, such as midazolam HCl (Versed®), which will virtually eliminate discomfort. If a sedative is used, advise the client that someone must accompany her home. Recommend use of a sanitary pad after the procedure for fluid leakage and spotting. Prophylactic antibiotic therapy may be given prior to hysterosalpingogram (HSG) if the client has any prior history of sexually transmitted infections (STIs) or pelvic inflammatory disease (PID).

Endometrial Biopsy

Histologic documentation of secretory endometrial development implies that ovulation has taken place. Until recently, luteal-phase insufficiency was thought to cause infertility and recurrent miscarriages. Controversies, however, persist regarding the accuracy of the diagnostic criteria, the prevalence, and the clinical relevance of a "luteal-phase defect" (ASRM, 2011). Because the chances are small of discovering a significant abnormality, many specialists omit this step, except in patients at high risk of poor response, including women who have received chemotherapy or pelvic radiation or who have a history of severe intrauterine adhesive disease or significant prior uterine surgery (Sauer, 2002).

Pelvic Ultrasound/Sonohysterogram

A pelvic ultrasound, and if possible, a 3D ultrasound should be done with the initial infertility workup. This can identify fibroids, polyps, and some uterine congenital anomalies, such as a septated uterus. An ovarian evaluation and follicle count to help assess ovarian reserve is obtained at this time. Vaginal ultrasounds performed throughout a cycle, natural or stimulated, will help determine ovarian response and confirm endometrial changes. Ideally, the midcycle endometrial stripe should measure ≥ 7 mm.

A sonohysterogram is a simple in-office procedure in which sterile saline is injected into the uterine cavity to separate the uterine walls while a vaginal ultrasound is being performed. This process is better able to determine uterine abnormalities, which may inhibit a pregnancy such as submucosal fibroids, polyps, and Asherman's syndrome.

ASSESSMENT OF THE PELVIS

Laparoscopy—Diagnostic or Therapeutic

Laparoscopy is performed early in the cycle after menses as an outpatient surgery, usually under general anesthesia. It is recommended after other tests have been completed, unless a woman is experiencing severe pelvic pain, which would be an indication to perform laparoscopy earlier in the evaluation. The laparoscope is inserted through the navel to visualize the pelvis. Laser or cautery can be used to treat endometriosis, pelvic adhesions or scarring, and some tubal diseases at the time of the diagnostic laparoscopy, thereby avoiding the need for major abdominal inpatient surgery. Usually, the client can return home in several hours (see Chapter 16).

When uterine anomalies have been identified (abnormal HSG or sonohysterogram), laparoscopy is performed in conjunction with hysteroscopy. Hysteroscopy delineates the internal and external uterine contour, thus differentiating between a bicornuate and a septate uterus. Laser or cautery can be used at hysteroscopy to lyse adhesions, repair septa, and remove polyps or fibroids.

FEMALE INFERTILITY: CAUSES, DIAGNOSES, AND INTERVENTIONS

Female infertility may be caused by ovulatory dysfunction, uterine factors, and/or tubal or peritoneal factors.

OVULATORY DYSFUNCTION

Ovulatory dysfunction, in which ovulation occurs infrequently (oligoovulation) or not at all (anovulation), may be related to normal reproductive development (aging), a variety of endocrine disorders, premature ovarian failure (POF), or gonadal dysgenesis (see Figure 13–3).

HYPOTHALAMIC, PITUITARY, AND ADRENAL DISORDERS

Hyperprolactinemia is a common pituitary disorder; it requires extensive evaluation and referral. Hypogonadotropic hypogonadism and Sheehan's syndrome are rare causes of pituitary disorders (Fritz & Speroff, 2011).

Hyperprolactinemia

Serum prolactin (PRL) levels are greater than 20 ng/mL. Elevated PRL interferes with gonadotropin-releasing hormone (GnRH) release, which in turn results in lowered levels of FSH/LH. Elevated PRL may directly inhibit the gonads (Fritz & Speroff, 2011).

Subjective Data. Take a complete history: infertility; cyclic, irregular menses, or amenorrhea; spontaneous milky breast discharge; headache/visual field disturbances; and stress are commonly reported. Medications such as antipsychotics, antidepressants, clonidine, reserpine, metoclopramide, and cimetidine can cause an elevation in PRL (LaTorre & Falomi, 2007).

Objective Data

- *Physical examination:* This must include a thorough neurological exam. Note any milky breast discharge or abnormal neurological findings, especially visual field disturbances.
- *Diagnostic tests and methods:* The following are indicated:
  - Pregnancy test.
  - PRL level (must be elevated on more than one sample at least several days apart, before a breast exam, or any nipple stimulation, and prior to 11 A.M.).
  - SH and T_3, total T_4, free T_4 to rule out thyroid disease (see Appendix D for normal values).
  - Magnetic resonance imaging (MRI) of the sella turcica to rule out pituitary adenoma.

Differential Medical Diagnoses. Galactorrhea, oligo/amenorrhea, ovarian dysfunction, hypothalamic lesions, pituitary lesions (tumors, acromegaly, Cushing's disease, empty sella syndrome), hypothyroidism, physiological conditions (pregnancy, breast stimulation), pharmacological effects (reserpine, cimetidine, tricyclic antidepressants, estrogens), idiopathic conditions.

Plan

- Refer the client who desires fertility to a reproductive endocrinologist for continued evaluation and ovulation induction.
- Refer the client to a medical endocrinologist, neurologist, ophthalmologist, or surgeon as indicated.
- Provide the client with information, anticipatory guidance, stress management, and counseling for anxiety and body image disturbance.

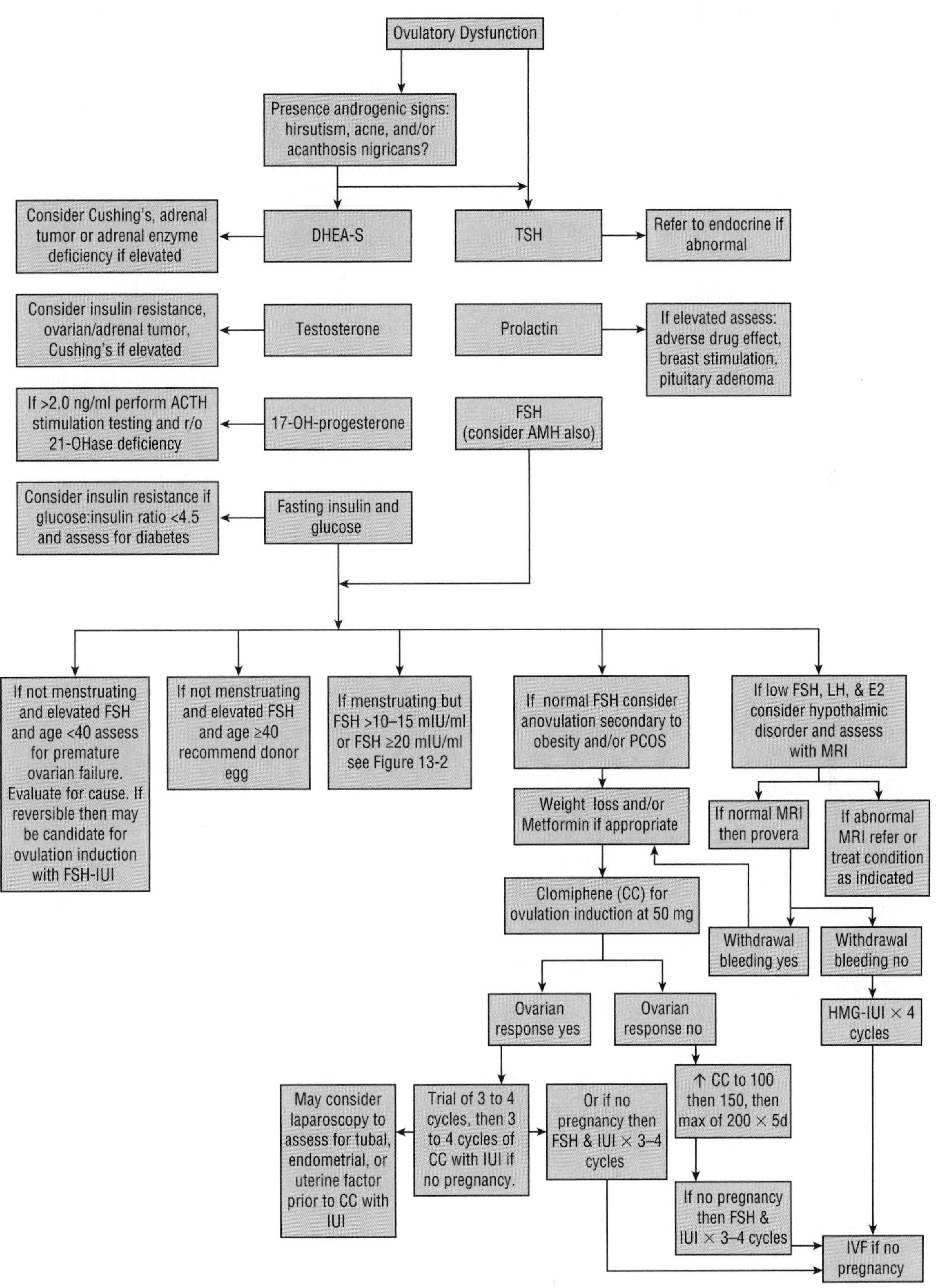

FIGURE 13–3. Ovulatory Dysfunction. *Source:* Adapted from Aubuchon et al. in Berek, J.S., 2012, pp. 1136–1141; Bayer et al., 2012, p. 54; & Wright & Johnson, pp. 705–715 in Gibbs et al., 2008.

Hypogonadotropic Hypogonadism

A hypoestrogenic woman has a negative progesterone withdrawal (i.e., no menstrual bleeding after the administration of progesterone), normal or slightly lower than normal FSH/LH levels, and normal PRL levels (Fritz & Speroff, 2011). Amenorrhea can be caused by GnRH pulse suppression, which in turn inhibits pituitary function.

Subjective Data. Obtain an accurate menstrual history and determination of pubertal milestones. Inquire specifically about Crohn's disease, connective tissue disorders, hepatitis, galactorrhea, stress, adequacy of nutrition (take a dietary history to assess for eating disorders), exercise, and medications. Clients commonly report absent menses, monophasic BBT, history of excessive dieting or exercise, altered eating habits, and/or a stressful lifestyle.

Objective Data

- *Physical examination:* Assess for low body weight, low fat, little breast tissue, normal secondary sex characteristics, and hair patterns. The vagina may be dry with decreased rugae, and the uterus may be small. If the client has primary amenorrhea, assess the patency of the cervix.
- *Diagnostic tests and methods:* The following are indicated:
  - Serum pregnancy test (quantitative): Negative.
  - Serum multiphasic analysis-12 (SMA-12): Results are evaluated for indications of systemic illnesses that could affect hypothalamic function; may be normal or abnormal.
  - E2 (estradiol): Low.
  - FSH/LH: Low to normal.
  - Thyroid studies (TSH, T_3, T_4, free T_4): May be abnormal.
  - PRL: If elevated, complete workup of pituitary is required.

Differential Medical Diagnoses. Primary or secondary amenorrhea, anovulation, hyperprolactinemia, psychiatric disorder.

Plan

- Refer the client with primary amenorrhea (see Chapter 11).
- Medical therapy as indicated.
- Refer the client to a reproductive endocrinologist for evaluation and ovulation induction as indicated.
- Ovulation induction in clients with hypothalamic disorders is best managed with the GnRH pump, although clomiphene, menotropin, or urofollitropin are often used. Bromocriptine is used to treat hyperprolactinemia. If no ovulation results, then clomiphene is used. If this does not result in ovulation, menotropin or urofollitropin is used (see Table 13–9).

Androgen Excess

Adrenal gland or ovarian dysfunction may result in androgen excess. Androgen excess is a common cause of ovulatory dysfunction and may also be an indicator of adrenal or ovarian tumor. Careful evaluation and referral are required. The three primary androgens in females are dehydroepiandrosterone sulfate (DHEA-S), androstenedione (A), and testosterone (T). Androgen excess interferes with feedback mechanisms and results in increased FSH/LH levels. Adrenal disorders result in the production of sex steroids that interact with GnRH, FSH/LH, and PRL.

Rapid progression of hirsutism, virilization, and changes in menstrual patterns are suggestive of a tumor. An adrenal tumor is suspected if serum DHEA-S levels are > 700 μg/dL. Ovarian tumors are suspected if total female serum testosterone is > 200 μg/dL (Levy, 1995).

Polycystic Ovary Syndrome

Women who experience PCOS frequently are oligomenorrheic, hirsute, obese, and infertile. The components of PCOS are hyperandrogenism and oligoovulation or anovulation in the absence of other hyperandrogenic disorders such as androgen-secreting tumors or nonclassical adrenal hyperplasia. Clinical evidence of hyperandrogenism includes hirsutism, acne, acanthosis nigricans, numerous acrochordons (skin tags), and polycystic-appearing ovaries on ultrasound. In a population of women of reproductive age, the prevalence of PCOS is approximately 4 to 10 percent, although this figure might not reflect the true prevalence as there has been no population-based studies and the criteria for diagnosis is varied (Cahill, 2009).

Current studies suggest that 50 to 70 percent of women with PCOS have some level of insulin resistance (Diamanti-Kandarakis, 2006). A compensatory increase in insulin production contributes to excess androgen production and chronic anovulation. In addition to reproductive problems, women with PCOS are at an increased risk for developing metabolic syndrome that includes abdominal obesity, hypercholesterolemia, hypertension, and insulin resistance

(ASRM, 2005b). If the patient is overweight, weight loss should be encouraged. Even a 5 percent weight loss can have positive effects on insulin resistance, impaired glucose tolerance, and the metabolic syndrome (American College of Obstetricians and Gynecologists, 2003). If weight loss does not help with ovulation, clomiphene, gonadotropins, and insulin-sensitizing drugs such as Glucophage (metformin), may be used to help induce ovulation.

Subjective Data. Note BMI, hirsutism, and menstrual history. Ask the client about any use of danazol (Danocrine), progestins, glucocorticoids, anabolic steroids, phenytoin, or minoxidil. The client may reveal concern about a history of excessive body hair, oily skin or acne, being overweight, and having irregular menses.

Objective Data

- *Physical examination:* A complete physical exam is indicated. Assess the client's face, chin, and abdomen for male hair patterns (fine to coarse); note frontal balding, increased muscle mass, clitoral enlargement, decreased breast size, and voice changes. Also note if obesity is present, and evaluate for ovarian mass.
- *Diagnostic tests and methods:* Several may be indicated (see Figure 13–3):
  - *FSH:* Low or normal.
  - *LH:* Elevated.
  - *LH–FSH ratio: Greater than 3.*
  - *Testosterone:* Free. Normal is 100–200 pg/dL.
  - *DHEA-S:* Normal is 80–350 mcg/mL; normal ranges may decrease with age (Fritz & Speroff, 2011).
  - *17-Hydroxyprogesterone (17-OHP):* Screens for androgen excess due to PCOS, enzyme deficiency, or congenital adrenal hyperplasia (normal in follicular phase is 15–70 ng/dL; normal in luteal phase is 35–290 ng/dL). Significant elevation suggests adrenal hyperplasia.
  - *Dexamethasone suppression:* Dexamethasone 1.0 mg is given orally at 11 P.M. Plasma cortisol is measured at 8 A.M.; if suppressed to less than 5 mcg/mL, Cushing's disease is ruled out (Fritz & Speroff, 2011).
  - *Corticotropin (ACTH) Stimulation Test:* At 8 A.M., an intravenous bolus of synthetic ACTH 0.25 mg is administered; blood samples for 17-OHP and cortisol are obtained prior to the bolus and at 60 minutes (normal random cortisol levels are 5–25 mcg/dL; normal morning levels are 5–25 mcg/dL; normal evening levels are 2–12 mcg/dL). Significant elevation suggests enzyme deficiency or adrenal hyperplasia.
  - *Glucose Tolerance Test:* (3° GTT)
  - *Fasting insulin*
  - *BUN/creatinine:* Normal renal function is critical to treatment with metformin. Decreased renal blood flow increases metformin toxicity.

Differential Medical Diagnoses. Ovarian disorders (PCOS, hyperthecosis, androgen-producing tumors, virilization of pregnancy). Adrenal disorders (congenital adrenal hyperplasia, androgen-producing tumors, Cushing's disease, drug related, obesity, post menopause, incomplete testicular feminization, idiopathic conditions).

Plan

- Weight loss, counseling about improved nutrition and an exercise routine that can be incorporated into a major change in lifestyle.
- Refer the client to an endocrinologist or to a reproductive endocrinologist for evaluation and treatment.
- Psychosocial interventions include anticipatory guidance regarding treatment and medication. Offer the client support and referral to a psychologist and referral to a respected weight loss program or nutritionist.
- Review risks of endometrial cancer secondary to endometrial hyperplasia resulting from persistent anovulation. Review risks related to overweight such as non-insulin-dependent diabetes mellitus, hypertension, and cardiovascular disease.

Metformin (Glucophage) is an antihyperglycemic drug that improves tissue sensitivity to insulin while decreasing insulin levels and inhibiting hepatic glucose production. When used in patients with PCOS, metformin reduces LH, sex hormone-binding globulin, and ovarian androgens and corrects hyperinsulinemia. In 2007, a consensus paper between ASRM and ESHRE (European Society of Human Reproduction and Embryology) offered a bleak view of the use of metformin in infertility, recommending that "Metformin use in PCOS should be restricted to women with glucose intolerance" (Nestler, 2008; Thessaloniki, ESHRE/ASRM, 2008).

Start metformin at 500 mg qhs for 1 week. Increase the dose to 500 mg bid for 1 week, and then increase the dose to 500 mg tid for 1 week. Once the client is on a tolerable regimen of metformin 500 mg tid, continue the full dose therapy for 5 weeks. During the last 21 days of therapy, obtain a progesterone level every 10 days. If the patient does not ovulate on metformin alone, add clomiphene in a regular regimen. Obtain progesterone levels or other testing to ensure that ovulation is occurring. Consider using metformin for up to 6 months in a solo therapy if it is producing ovulation or in combination with clomiphene. Metformin is a category B drug. The most common side effects are gastrointestinal disturbances, including diarrhea, nausea, vomiting, and abdominal bloating. A gradual increase in the dose over time will minimize gastrointestinal discomfort. Caution the client to discontinue metformin with severe dehydration of any cause; metformin's toxicity is increased with compromised renal blood flow.

In addition, start folic acid 1 to 4 mg daily. Risk of neural tube defects is increased with obesity.

Premature Ovarian Failure

In POF, failure of ovarian estrogen production results in elevated FSH levels (greater than 40 mIU/mL) on more than one serum sample (see Figure 13–2). The ovaries do not produce enough estrogen to inhibit hypothalamic release of GnRH. Continued release of GnRH results in elevated FSH/LH levels as ovulation ceases. Failure may occur at any age between menarche and 40 years and requires careful endocrine evaluation. POF can be caused by autoimmune disease (Fritz & Speroff, 2011).

Subjective Data. These include amenorrhea, hot flashes/night sweats, vaginal dryness.

Objective Data. A complete physical examination is indicated: assess for signs of hypoestrogenicity (refer to Table 13–2). Several diagnostic tests are indicated:

- Cycle day 3 *FSH/LH* or CCCT elevated (see Figure 13–2).
- *TSH,* T_3, T_4, *free* T_4: Rule out thyroid disease.
- *PRL:* Rule out hyperprolactinemia.

Additional tests to rule out autoimmune disorders include complete blood count with differential and sedimentation rate, total serum protein, albumin to globulin ratio, rheumatoid factor, antinuclear antibodies, antithyroid globulin, antimicrosomal antibodies, fasting blood sugar, A.M. cortisol, and serum calcium and phosphorus. If the woman is younger than 30 years, a karyotype is indicated (assessment of normal female versus presence of Y chromosome, which is associated with increased risk of malignant gonadal tumor) (Fritz & Speroff, 2011).

Differential Medical Diagnoses. Chromosome abnormality, autoimmune disease (polyendocrinopathy type I or II, myasthenia gravis, idiopathic thrombocytopenic purpura, hemolytic anemia), thyroid dysfunction (hypoparathyroidism, thyroiditis), adrenal insufficiency/failure, 17-hydroxylase deficiency, gonadal tumor.

Plan

- Medical therapy as indicated.
- Hormone replacement as necessary.
- Refer the client who desires fertility to a reproductive endocrinologist.
- Psychosocial interventions involve providing information and anticipatory guidance about the physical and emotional changes that accompany loss of ovarian function, including disturbances in body image, personal identity, self-esteem, grief process, and sexual dysfunction. The client may need to be referred for individual/marital counseling and possible sex therapy. Review nutrition, including calcium and red meat intake, need for weight-bearing exercise, as well as the risks of osteoporosis, cardiovascular disease, and endometrial cancer.
- Medication may include estrogen/progesterone replacement, lubricants, estradiol vaginal cream.
- IVF with donor oocytes.
- Adoption.
- Childfree living.

Gonadal Dysgenesis

Gonadal dysgenesis is a broad term for clients with female genitalia, normal Müllerian structures, and streak gonads (Fritz & Speroff, 2011).

Dysgenesis results from the gonads undergoing partial or complete regression, which leads to abnormal sexual development (Nestler & Jakubowicz, 1996). Fibrous gonads caused by complete regression do not produce hormones. This syndrome is associated with a broad range of genetic patterns. Surprisingly, some women with pure gonadal dysgenesis have a normal XX chromosome pattern. A majority of clients with dysgenesis have only one X chromosome; others have multiple cell lines of varying sex chromosome composition (mosaicism). Women with XY chromosome patterns (usually mosaic) are at risk for neoplastic changes in the gonads, thus requiring gonad removal (Fritz & Speroff, 2011).

Turner's syndrome is a gonadal dysgenesis condition in which a woman has only one X chromosome, a structural abnormality in one X chromosome, or mosaicism with an abnormal X. The fetus has a normal complement of ova at 20 weeks' gestation; however, they have totally or partially disappeared by birth. The ovaries appear as streak gonads. The incidence of Turner's syndrome is 1 in 2,500 to 5,000 liveborn girls (Fritz & Speroff, 2011).

Subjective Data. Scant or absent pubic or axillary hair; primary or secondary amenorrhea; absent or arrested secondary sex development.

Objective Data. A complete physical examination is necessary (see Table 13–2).

Gonadal Dysgenesis Clients May Have Any of the Following

- Normal height or short stature.
- Scant or absent pubic/axillary hair.
- Normal appearing female external genitalia.
- Normal or no breast development.
- Ambiguous genitalia (intra-abdominal testes often found in hernia), blind vaginal pouch, and absent or arrested secondary sex characteristics.
- May have no secondary sex characteristics but normal appearing external female genitalia *or* ambiguous external genitalia.

Turner's Syndrome Clients Classically Have the Following

- Short stature.
- Scant or absent pubic/axillary hair.
- Webbing of the neck.
- Broad shield-type chest with laterally placed nipples.
- Lack of breast development.
- Vagina and uterus present but infantile.
- Ovaries absent.
- Diagnostic tests:
  - Karyotype—Abnormal chromosome pattern.
  - FSH/LH—Elevated.
  - Testosterone—Normal or elevated.
  - Additional studies to detect cardiac malformations (coarctation of the aorta) and renal abnormalities may be indicated in clients with Turner's syndrome.

Differential Medical Diagnoses. Turner's syndrome, testicular feminization, Swyer-James syndrome, coarctation of the aorta, kidney dysfunction.

Plan

- Refer the client to a reproductive endocrinologist and for genetic counseling.
- Medical therapy as indicated.
- During psychosocial interventions, information and anticipatory guidance are provided regarding physical differences and the emotional impacts of body stature, impaired sexual development, and lack of reproductive capacity. Refer the client for individual/marital counseling and, possibly, sex therapy.
- Client teaching is related to estrogen deficiencies: review nutrition, exercise, hormone replacement and risks of osteoporosis, cardiovascular disease, glucose intolerance, and thyroid dysfunction.
- Medication in the management of Turner's syndrome includes oral cyclic administration of estrogen and progesterone. Oral contraceptives are not indicated for this client, as there are only streak gonads and the estrogen dose is not adequate to protect the bones and cardiovascular system.
- IVF with donor eggs is an option for the client with Turner's desiring fertility.

UTERINE DISORDERS

Uterine causes of infertility are due to anatomic abnormalities or infection (see Figure 13–4). Congenital anomalies result from arrested uterine development, abnormal formation of the uterus, or incomplete fusion of the Müllerian ducts, diethylstilbestrol (DES) exposure, pelvic irradiation, adhesions, infection, fibroids, and polyps can interfere with conception, sperm migration, and implantation.

Müllerian Anomalies

Such abnormalities may result from genetic patterns of inheritance or spontaneous mutations, such as trisomy 13 and 15, which would have been diagnosed as a neonate. Women who are presenting with a history of infertility or recurrent pregnancy loss (RPL) may be found to have a subtle Müllerian anomaly. Fortunately, uterine structural defects, except those caused by DES exposure, are often amenable to surgical correction (see Figure 13–5 and Table 13–10).

Subjective Data. May include a history of infertility and/or pregnancy loss, abnormal uterine bleeding, primary amenorrhea, dysmenorrhea, dyspareunia.

Objective Data

- A physical exam is indicated to assess for abnormal anatomic structures.
- Diagnostic tests and methods including ultrasound, HSG, laparoscopy/hysteroscopy, and/or pelvic MRI are used to detect structural abnormalities. Karyotype is performed to rule out chromosomal abnormalities.

Differential Medical Diagnoses. Congenital anomalies, endometriosis, urinary tract anomalies.

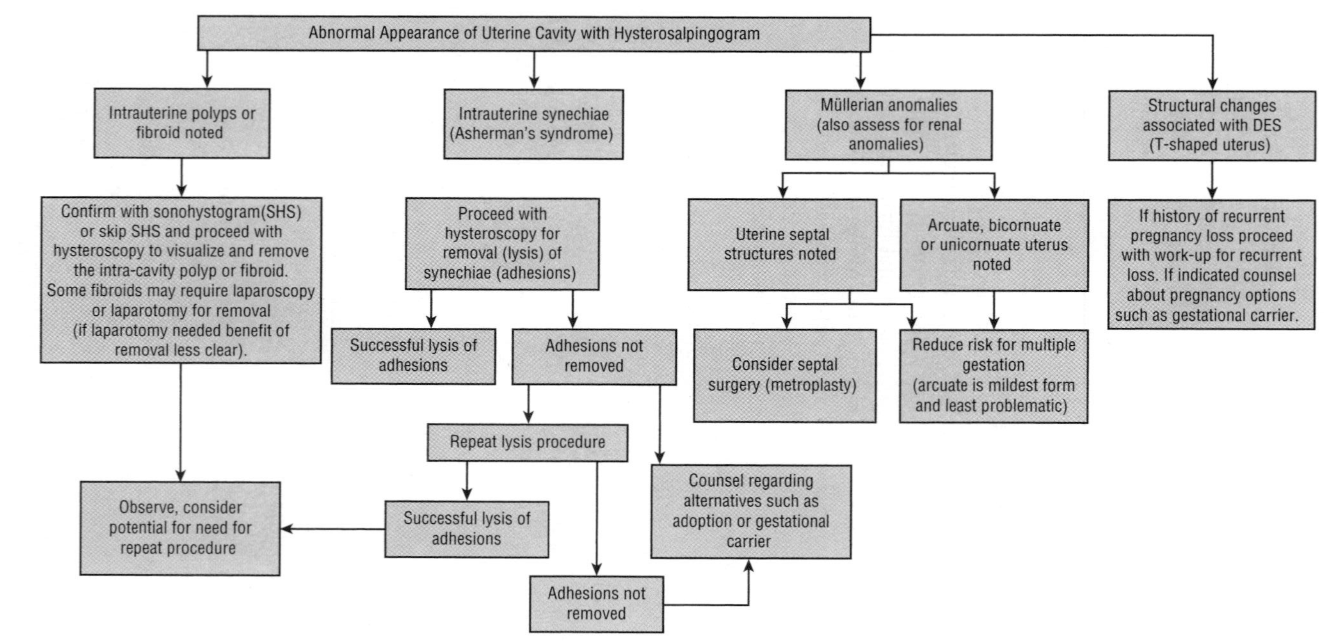

FIGURE 13–4. Uterine Disorders. *Source:* Adapted from Aubuchon et al. in Berek, J.S., 2012, pp. 1136–1141; Bayer et al., 2012, p. 55; & Wright & Johnson, pp. 705–715 in Gibbs et al., 2008.

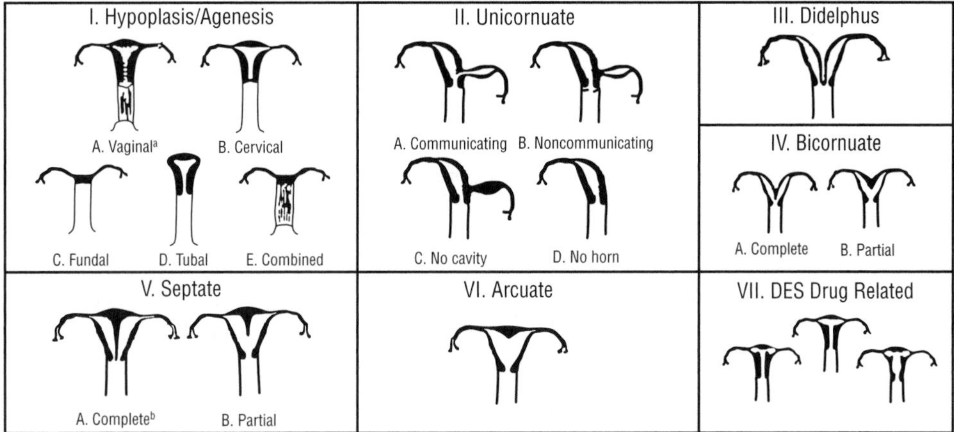

FIGURE 13–5. The American Society for Reproductive Medicine Classification of Müllerian Anomalies. [a]Uterus may be normal or take a variety of abnormal forms. [b]May have two distinct cervices. *Source:* Adapted from The American Society for Reproductive Medicine classifications of adnexal adhesion, distal tubal occlusion secondary to tubal ligation, tubal pregnancies, müllerian anomalies and intrauterine adhesions. (1988). *Fertil Steril, 49* (6), 944–955. Reproduced with permission of the American Society for Reproductive Medicine.

TABLE 13-10 Classification of Müllerian Anomalies

Hypoplasia or agenesis malformation: Abnormal development of the caudal portion of the uterovaginal primordium. Malformations range from a transverse membrane in the vagina, to vaginal atresia with normal or abnormal uterine shapes, to hypoplasia of the endometrium, to segmental agenesis of the fallopian tubes. Infertility may be the presenting symptom. Obstetrical (OB) complications depend on the anomaly.

Unicornais uterus: Unilateral abnormality caused by arrested development of one Müllerian duct. If implantation occurs in a rudimentary horn pregnancy wastage or tubal pregnancy can be the result. OB complications include malpresentations, intrauterine growth retardation, premature labor, and incompetent cervix.

Uterus didalphus: The Müllerian ducts never fused, so there are two uteri, two cervices, and possibly two vaginas. Outflow from one uterus may be obstructed and cause symptoms. OB complications include malpresentations and premature labor.

Bicornuate uterus: Partial lack of fusion of the two Müllerian ducts produces a single cervix with a varying degree of separation in the two horns. OB complications include early abortions, preterm labor, and breech presentations.

Septate uterus: Lack of resorption of the midline septum between the two Müllerian ducts resulting in defects varying from a slight midline septum to a septum dividing the uterus and vagina. OB complications depend on the severity of the defect, but can include recurrent pregnancy loss, preterm labor, and breech presentations.

Arcuate uterus: A mild form of septate uterus (heart-shaped cavity) not associated with pregnancy loss.

Diethylstilbestrol (DES)-related anomaly: Due to in utero DES exposure. T-shaped uterus, small cavity, constriction rings may present in any combination. Cervical defects include anterior cervical ridge, a cervical collar, a hypoplastic cervix, or a pseudopolyp. All may lead to an incompetent cervix.

Source: Sims & Gibbons, 1996; Speroff et al., 1999. *Clinical gynecology endocrinology and infertility* (6th ed.). Baltimore: Williams and Wilkins.

Plan

- Refer the client to a reproductive endocrinologist.
- Psychosocial interventions include providing information, anticipatory guidance, and support.
- If indicated, refer the client to a counselor for individual, group, or sex therapy.
- Laparoscopy/hysteroscopy (metroplasty) is done to correct vaginal and uterine abnormalities and to restore the uterine cavity or endometrium.

Follow-Up. Follow-up depends on the extent of the abnormalities and the procedures needed to correct them.

Diethylstilbestrol Exposure

Exposure of the female fetus to DES is associated with uterine cavity abnormalities, including T-shaped uteri, hypoplastic cavities, intrauterine adhesions, and cervical stenosis. In addition, DES exposure in utero is linked with ectopic pregnancy, pregnancy loss, and preterm birth (Fritz & Speroff, 2011). Later cellular abnormalities (adenosis) in vaginal or ectocervical epithelium are associated with DES exposure during fetal life, resulting in susceptibility to carcinogenic effects of endogenous estrogens (clear cell adenocarcinomas). (see Diethylstilbestrol Exposure Sequelae in Chapter 16.)

DES was synthesized in 1938 and used by several million women from 1945 through 1971 to prevent pregnancy loss, toxemia, stillbirth, and preterm labor (Sims & Gibbons, 1996). Research has documented an increased occurrence of clear cell adenocarcinoma in DES-exposed women between 14 and 22 years of age, with a peak incidence at age 19. Currently, studies are beginning on examining DES effects on the third generation; however, because those women are just entering the reproductive years, it may be many years before statistical data is available.

Subjective Data. Data reveals a history of maternal DES treatment and a client history of menstrual abnormalities, miscarriage, lower fertility rate, ectopic pregnancy, premature delivery, incompetent cervix, or abnormal Pap smears.

Objective Data. A complete physical examination is indicated to detect abnormalities of anatomic structure. DES-exposed women need to begin having pelvic examinations soon after the onset of menses and to have them at least annually. Common abnormalities include vaginal adenosis (ridge, septum, malformation), cervical adenosis (collar, hood, polyp, malformation, stenosis), and Müllerian anomalies.

Diagnostic tests and methods include a Pap smear of the cervix to screen for squamous cell carcinoma, and a colposcopy and biopsy of abnormal vaginal and cervical tissue. Other methods may be indicated to evaluate anatomic abnormalities (ultrasound, HSG, laparoscopy/hysteroscopy, pelvic MRI).

Differential Medical Diagnoses. Congenital anomalies, chromosomal abnormalities.

Plan. Psychosocial interventions include providing information, anticipatory guidance, and support. No medication is recommended. No treatment is indicated unless complications—such as abnormal Pap smears, pregnancy complications, or infertility arise.

Follow-Up. Referrals for individual, group, or sex therapy may be indicated; or an infertility specialist may be indicated if the client is unable to become pregnant or has a history of pregnancy loss. Careful follow-up for clear cell adenocarcinoma and squamous cell carcinoma is required; immediate referral is made if suspicious findings occur.

Intrauterine Adhesions (Asherman's Syndrome)

The syndrome results from damage to the endometrium after excessive curettage, cesarean birth, metroplasty, pelvic irradiation, myomectomy, as well as infections (Sims & Gibbons, 1996). It interferes with fertility by disrupting sperm migration, mechanically obstructing tubal ostia, and impeding blastocyst implantation. Pregnancy loss may result from decreased functional intrauterine volume and endometrial fibrosis and inflammation (Fritz & Speroff, 2011).

Subjective Data. The client may report a history of menstrual abnormalities (scant flow, secondary amenorrhea, dysmenorrhea), or normal menses, dyspareunia, uterine infection, pregnancy losses, surgical procedures, cancer therapies.

Objective Data

- A complete physical examination is indicated. Often, findings are normal. Assess for cervical stenosis; cervical discharge; signs of cervical, vaginal, or uterine infection; and abnormal uterine contour, firmness, immobility, tenderness.
- Diagnostic tests and methods include EMB to diagnose endometritis; HSG to determine abnormalities in uterine contour; laparoscopy and hysteroscopy (when indicated). Repeat HSG may be indicated after surgical correction if conception does not occur. (An EMB may diagnose fibrosis, but a normal result does not rule out fibrosis in another area of the uterus.)

Differential Medical Diagnoses. Amenorrhea, dysmenorrhea, cervical stenosis.

Plan

- Provide the client with information, anticipatory guidance, and support.
- Medication may include cyclic high-dose estrogen/progesterone replacement to help restore normal endometrium after surgical correction. Postoperative pain is usually managed with acetaminophen or nonsteroidal anti-inflammatory agents.
- Laparoscopy and hysteroscopy may be indicated for lysis of adhesions and cervical dilation.
- Following lysis of adhesions, high-dose estrogen therapy is sometimes used to build the endometrium in an attempt to keep the uterine walls from adhering to each other.

Follow-Up. Refer the client to a reproductive endocrinologist and for psychological counseling. Repeat procedures to lyse adhesions are indicated if normal menses is not established.

Endometritis

Endometritis is an endometrial inflammation due to infection caused by pathogens. It may result from ascending infection, use of an intrauterine device (IUD), endometrial trauma, or as a secondary infection associated with cancer. Common pathogens include aerobic/anaerobic bacteria, mycoplasma, chlamydia, gonorrhea, viruses, toxoplasmas, parasites, and rarely mycobacterium tuberculosis. Treatment is controversial when no pathogen is identified because resolution may occur spontaneously. Infertility may be associated with an unfavorable endometrial environment that results from a heightened immune response and interferes with blastocyst implantation (Winkel, 1995).

Tuberculosis endometritis is rare. Infertility occurs due to extensive tubal scarring and uterine adhesions. Diagnosis is made by curettage and culture of the premenstrual endometrium. Antituberculosis medications are used until repeat curettage is normal.

Subjective Data. The client may report uterine tenderness, dyspareunia, dysmenorrhea, foul odor, or an abnormal vaginal discharge. She may also report a history of dilation and curettage or trauma to the cervix decreasing secretion of cervical mucus (Winkel, 1995). Infertility may be the only sign of chronic endometritis.

Objective Data. Physical examination will reveal tenderness on bimanual examination, especially if it is acute endometritis.

Diagnosis of chronic endometritis is accomplished by follicular-phase EMB with culture, as well as histologic evaluation of the biopsy tissue (Winkel, 1995). (See Pelvic Inflammatory Disease in Chapter 16 for tests to diagnose acute infection.)

Differential Medical Diagnoses. Urinary tract infection, acute pyelonephritis, appendicitis, pelvic abscess, thromboembolism, gastrointestinal disease, endometriosis, uterine adhesions.

Plan

- Psychosocial interventions include teaching the client about the causes, treatment, prevention, and effects of infection. Provide support and counseling, and encourage support from significant others.
- Medication specific to the identified organism is prescribed for recurrent endometrial/pelvic infections because the inflammation, abnormal endometrium, and adhesion formation associated with infection decrease fertility (see Chapter 14).
- EMB (follicular phase) is indicated after antibiotic treatment to determine resolution of endometritis.
- Pain management is often indicated.

Follow-Up. Refer the client to a reproductive endocrinologist for continued evaluation and infertility treatment. Diagnostic evaluation and treatment will be affected by a history of recurrent infection and the degree of pelvic and tubal pathology.

- Once the infection is resolved, HSG, laparoscopy, laparoscopy/hysteroscopy, and laparotomy for lysis of adhesions and tubal repair may be indicated. After tubal repair, clients are at risk for ectopic pregnancy. IVF may be necessary if other corrective therapies cannot restore normal tubal function. If scarring or adhesions lead to an atrophic endometrium, treatment may involve the use of a gestational carrier.

Uterine Leiomyomas (Fibroids)

Leiomyomas are common tumors occurring in approximately 20 to 50 percent of reproductive-age women (ASRM, 2008). Fibroids are classified as subserosal, intramural, or submucosal, depending whether they are located just beneath the serosa, within the myometrium, or adjacent to the endometrium, respectively. Depending on the fibroid size, number, and location, if the uterine cavity is partially obliterated or the contour is significantly altered, the fibroid may result in poorly vascularized endometrium and interfere with implantation or otherwise compromise placental development. Some studies suggest that uterine myomas have no effect on IVF outcomes unless they distort or displace the uterine cavity, while other investigators suggest IVF rates are lower in women with intramural myomas, particularly when larger than 5 cm in diameter (Fritz & Speroff, 2011).

Hysteroscopic myomectomy has been shown to improve clinical pregnancy rates and decrease risk of spontaneous abortion. In a large review ($N = 1941$), Buttram and Reiter (1981) reported that in women who underwent an abdominal myomectomy, the subsequent spontaneous abortion rate dropped from 41 percent preoperatively to 19 percent postoperatively. In women with submucous fibroids and either infertility or RPL, hysteroscopic myomectomy is recommended because the abdominal approach has been associated with longer anesthesia time, higher blood loss, higher risk for postoperative adhesion formation and infection, and the need for elective cesarean delivery in subsequent pregnancies (Goldenberg et al., 1995).

Subjective Data. The client may report pain (dysmenorrhea or dyspareunia) increased, prolonged, or irregular menstrual flow. Small fibroids may be asymptomatic.

Objective Data. A complete physical exam may reveal an enlarged, irregularly shaped, firm uterus.

- Diagnostic tests and methods may include ultrasound, HSG, or hysteroscopy to access the uterine cavity.

Plan

- Refer the client to a gynecologist.
- *Preoperative medication:* Surgery may be necessary for a successful pregnancy. Use of Lupron Depot® (leuprolide acetate) or other GnRH analogue preoperatively may be indicated with large tumors to impose anovulation and thereby decrease tumor size, risk of hemorrhage, and trauma to the uterus. Medications such as leuprolide acetate suppress the growth of the fibroid tumor, but as it causes a medical menopause, the risk of osteoporosis increases, and consequently cannot be given on a long-term basis. When the drug is stopped, the tumor starts to grow again, so usually Lupron is used on a short-term (3- to 6-month) basis to shrink the tumor prior to surgery.
    - Common transient side effects include hot flashes, night sweats, breakthrough bleeding, vaginal dryness.
    - Protected intercourse is indicated during entire course of therapy.
- Laparotomy is required to remove large fibroids; small fibroids may be removed with laparoscopy/hysteroscopy.
- Pain (dysmenorrhea) management includes acetaminophen and nonsteroidal anti-inflammatory agents.

TUBAL AND PERITONEAL DISORDERS

Sequelae of PID, postoperative adhesions, and endometriosis are involved in the pathogenesis of impaired fertility (see Figure 13–6).

Pelvic Inflammatory Disease

Every year, more than 750,000 women in the United States are treated for PID (CDC, 2011). Westrom's (1980) classic study demonstrated that the incidence of tubal occlusion after one episode is 11.4 percent, after two episodes, 23.1 percent, and after three or more episodes, 54.3 percent. Early diagnosis of acute PID and aggressive antimicrobial treatment decreases the chances of resulting sequelae (Rogers, 1995).

Tubal pathology is one of the most common causes of infertility in women. Sexually transmitted diseases caused by *Neisseria gonorrhoeae* and *Chlamydia trachomatis* are the major source of tubal disease. Other infectious agents include aerobic/anaerobic bacteria, toxoplasmosis, and parasites. Tubal repair may be accomplished by laser or cutting laparoscopy or laparotomy (salpingostomy, fimbrioplasty, reanastomosis). The success of tubal repair depends on the extent of disease and, due to the delicate microsurgery involved, the skill of the surgeon. Further fertility treatment if repair is unsuccessful may include IVF. A repeat surgery usually does not result in functional tubes (see Figure 13–6 and Chapter 16).

Tubal Reversal

Success rates of tubal reversal are difficult to assess, as it can be measured threefold: operative success rates, pregnancy rates, and birth rates. Pregnancy rates are between 45 and 82 percent, with an increase of ectopic rates between 1 and 7 percent (Fritz & Speroff, 2011). Success rates depend on the type of sterilization procedure performed, the site of anastomosis, and postoperative tubal length. Because randomized studies have not been done on IVF compared to tubal reconstructive surgery, it is important to individualize patient options. A quick overview of female age, ovarian reserve, and semen analysis should also be reviewed with the patient prior to a final recommendation. Many insurance companies will not pay for the cost of tubal reversals, so this should also be considered when discussing this option.

Pelvic Adhesions

Pelvic adhesions that interfere with pickup/transport of the oocyte are a major cause of infertility in women. Meticulous surgical technique, minimal tissue handling, stringent hemostasis, constant irrigation, avoidance of abrasion between raw surfaces (adhesion barriers), and microsurgery using unipolar fine wire cautery or laser will reduce adhesion formation and preserve fertility (Strickler, 1995).

Subjective Data. The client may report a history of chronic pelvic pain, dyspareunia, menstrual disorders, or pelvic surgery. In half of all cases, a history of infertility with no history of antecedent disease is the presentation.

Objective Data. An examination is indicated. Tenderness and a fixed uterus on bimanual examination are common. Diagnostic methods are a HSG and a laparoscopy to diagnose and treat pelvic pathology.

Differential Medical Diagnoses. Chronic salpingitis, residual inflammatory disease, tubal blockage, PID.

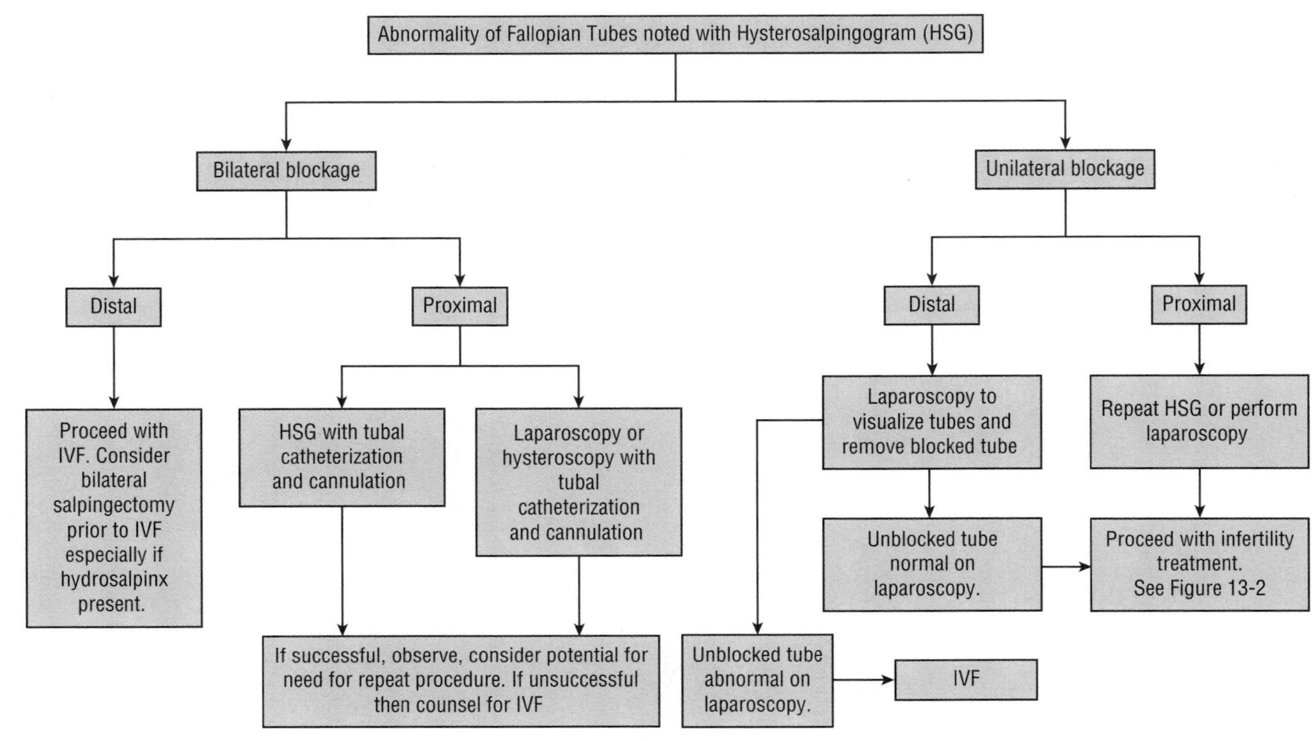

FIGURE 13–6. Tubal/Peritoneal Factor. *Source:* Adapted from Aubuchon et al. in Berek, J.S., 2012, pp. 1136–1141; Bayer et al., 2012, p. 55; & Wright & Johnson, pp. 705–715 in Gibbs et al., 2008.

Plan

- Psychosocial interventions include providing information and support. Relaxation techniques, biofeedback, and pain management may also be indicated.
- Antibiotic and pain therapy may be used prior to invasive procedures.
- Other possible interventions include laser or cautery laparoscopy for lysis of adhesions; tubal repair (salpingostomy, neosalpingostomy, fimbrioplasty) as indicated; laparotomy to treat severe pelvic disease (adhesion lysis; microscopic tubal or cornual reanastomosis); IVF if indicated.
- Refer the client to a reproductive endocrinologist.

Hydrosalpinges

The presence of large hydrosalpinges has been shown to be associated with decreased clinical pregnancy rates with IVF, decreased implantation rates, increased spontaneous abortions, and increased ectopic pregnancy rates (Cohen, Lindheim, & Sauer, 1999; Nackley & Muasher, 1998). In a large meta-analysis, the effect of salpingectomy was to increase implantation rates, clinical pregnancy rates, and live birth rates with IVF, while decreasing rates of spontaneous abortion and ectopic pregnancies (Johnson, Mak, & Sowter, 2002).

Endometriosis

Endometriosis, a major cause of infertility, is a condition in which endometrial tissue, glands, and stroma are located outside of the uterine cavity. The tissue responds to cyclic hormones like the endometrial lining (see Chapter 16). Fertility is impaired by mechanical factors interfering with ovum pickup and tubal transport; by ovulatory dysfunction; and by interference with sperm function, fertilization, and implantation. Endometriosis is a chronic disease and can be associated with chronic pelvic pain (see Resources, later in this chapter). Treatment depends on the severity of symptoms and the desire for fertility. Infertility management may include both laparoscopy and medical management with GnRH agonists. In mild cases, conservative management (doing nothing), or laser or cautery laparoscopy may be the only treatment needed. Moderate disease may be treated with medication such as Lupron Depot and nafarelin acetate or danazol for 6 months. These medications suppress estrogen and progesterone production so that atrophy of the endometrial implants occurs. Symptoms often return after the medications are stopped. Severe cases, however, may also require either preoperative or postoperative danazol, Lupron Depot, or nafarelin acetate (Synarel®) (Lewis & Bernstein, 1996). Further infertility treatment may include ovulation induction intrauterine insemination (IUI) or IVF.

RECURRENT PREGNANCY LOSS

The most common obstetrical complication is spontaneous abortion, which is seen in 15 to 20 percent of all clinically recognized pregnancies. *Recurrent abortion* is defined as three or more consecutive spontaneous pregnancy losses prior to 20 weeks' gestation. This is discouraging for both the couple and the provider. The good news is that almost 70 percent of women will eventually achieve a live birth in subsequent pregnancies without treatment. Treatment is designed to decrease the risk of subsequent pregnancy losses (Cramer & Wise, 2000). However, no explanation for RPL is found in 50 to 75 percent of couples.

Evaluation of a couple experiencing recurrent abortion should begin after three pregnancy losses or after two if the woman is over 35 years of age. Pregnancy loss may be caused by anatomic, endocrine, genetic, or immunologic variations; infection; chronic illness; or environmental toxins.

Hormonal, metabolic, and uterine abnormalities are some of the most common reasons of RPL. These three areas are also the most common to be reviewed in an initial infertility workup. Inherited genetic or chromosomal causes are found in less than 5 percent of couples. However, 60 percent of early miscarriages are caused by a random chromosomal abnormality. Anticardiolipin antibodies and lupus anticoagulant may be a cause for 3 to 15 percent of recurrent miscarriages (ASRM, 2008). Pregnancy outcomes in patients with this type of antiphospholipid syndrome may be improved with the use of aspirin and heparin. Studies are currently being performed on sperm DNA and miscarriage rates, but data is very preliminary at this time.

Subjective Data. The client may report a history of recurrent abortion. A detailed history of occupational exposures, cigarette smoking, alcohol consumption, and substances of abuse should be obtained.

Objective Data. A complete physical examination is indicated. Assess for anatomic uterine abnormalities during pelvic exam. Diagnostic tests include anticardiolipin antibodies, lupus anticoagulant, antiphospholipids, and possibly karotyping.

Differential Medical Diagnoses

- *Anatomic abnormalities (uterus):* Müllerian defects, fibroids, septum defects, Asherman's syndrome, incompetent cervix.
- *Endocrine abnormalities:* Thyroid (hypothyroid), hyperprolactinemia, ovulatory dysfunction/luteal-phase defect, ovarian reserve testing.
- *Infection:* Chlamydia, TORCH (T, toxoplasmosis; O, other infections [varicella, listeria, syphilis]; R, rubella; C, cytomegalovirus; H, herpes simplex virus), ureaplasma/mycoplasma.
- *Chronic illness:* Wilson's disease, heart/renal disease, blood dyscrasias.
- *Genetic abnormality:* Aneuploidy of products of conception; balanced translocation, sex chromosome mosaicism, chromosome inversions, and ring chromosomes of the couple (Adashi, 2000).
- *Thrombophilias*
- *Immunologic disorders:* Systemic lupus erythematosus, parental histocompatibilities.
- *Environmental toxins:* Radiation, chemotherapy, recreational drugs, smoking, ethyl alcohol abuse, caffeine.

Plan

- Provide the client with information and psychological support; be available for questions and listening. Evaluate the client's stage of crisis and grief, communication patterns, relationships, coping abilities, and use of support systems.
- Collaborate with medical (reproductive endocrinology) and mental health specialists.
- Medication or surgery is determined by the cause of the RPL.

Follow-Up. As appropriate, provide information about counseling, RESOLVE, or Compassionate Friends (see Resources).

MALE INFERTILITY: CAUSES, DIAGNOSES, AND INTERVENTIONS

Male factor infertility is found alone in approximately 30 percent of couples, and is involved in another 20 percent where there is also a female problem. Thus, male factor may be implicated in up to 50 percent of infertile cases. Male factor infertility may result from a variety of causes, such as endocrine disorders, varicocele, antisperm antibodies, occupational and environmental practices, and sexual dysfunction. Evaluation of male fertility should be coordinated with the evaluation of his female partner. Evaluation may be initiated in the general practice or gynecology office (see Figure 13–7). Referral is made to a urologist when abnormalities are identified. Frequently, medical therapies are unsuccessful, but surgery has often been successful in treating post-testicular and ductal disorders.

Subjective Data. A detailed history is essential to identify factors that may affect sperm production (see Table 13–5). For normal spermatogenesis, a delicate balance must exist between the neuroendocrine system and testes (Fritz & Speroff, 2011).

Objective Data

- A thorough physical examination (see Table 13–7) and Doppler evaluation are indicated when sperm parameters are abnormal.
- Diagnostic tests begin with a semen analysis (performed twice) (see Figure 13–7).

Semen culture is obtained if there are five or more white blood cells per high power field or if agglutination of sperm indicates a need for culture. Other tests may include TSH, T_3, T_4, free T_4; FSH (normal is 5–25 mIU/mL); LH (normal is 6–26 mIU/mL); testosterone (normal is 250–1,200 ng/dL); PRL; CT Scan/MRI of sella turcica; karyotyping. Tests may be used to identify a male factor contributing to unexplained infertility or for selecting therapy such as ART, sperm viability tests, and sperm penetration assays.

Endocrine Disorders

Such disorders constitute rare causes of male infertility, and therefore, endocrine evaluation is indicated when sperm concentration is very low or if there is a clinical suspicion (AUA, 2010). A basic endocrine evaluation measuring FSH and total testosterone will detect the vast majority of clinically significant endocrinopathies (Fritz & Speroff, 2011). Some specific endocrine problems with usual test results are the following:

- *Germ cell aplasia:* elevated FSH/LH.
- *Testicular failure:* elevated FSH/LH.
- *Pituitary adenoma/impotence:* elevated PRL.

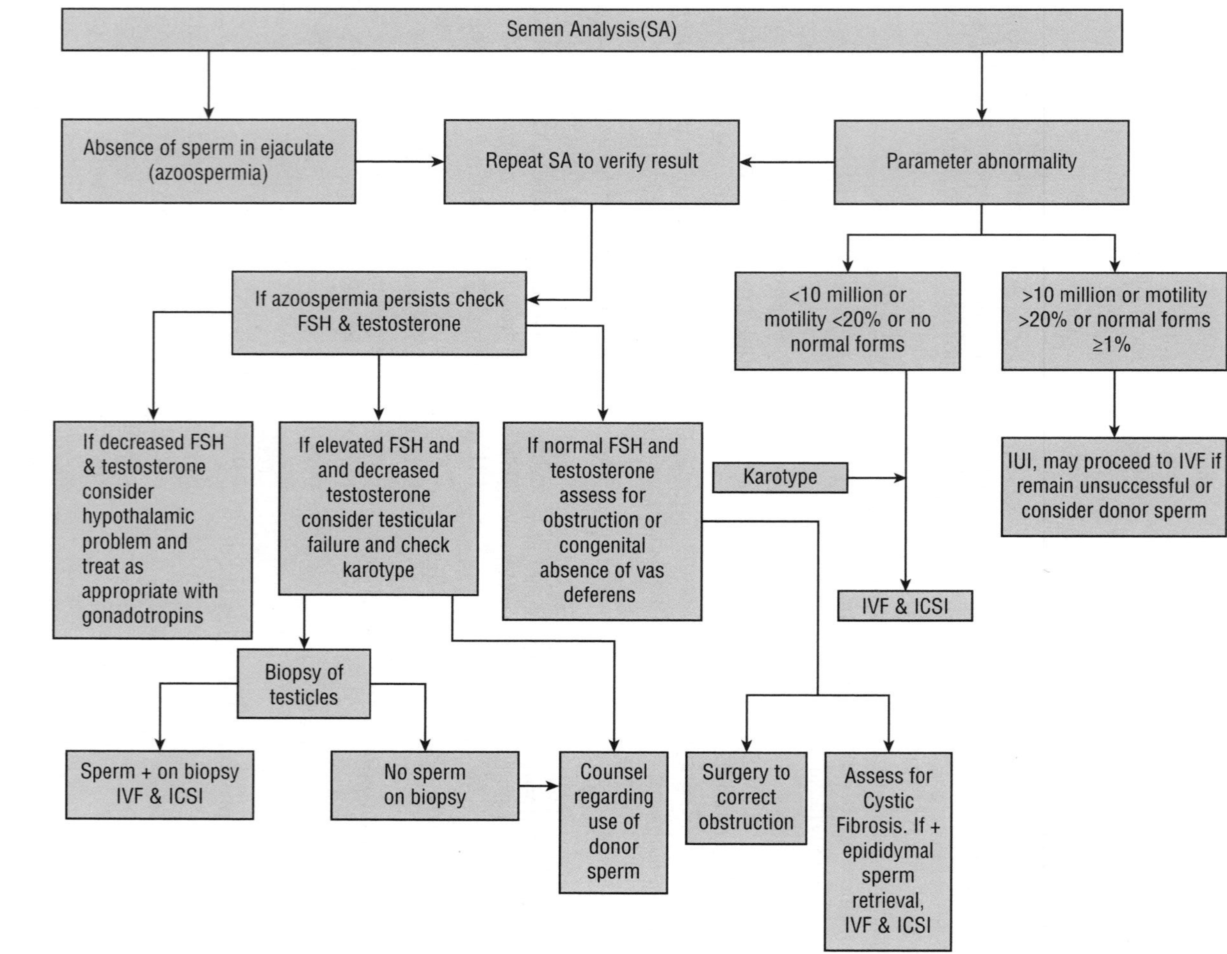

FIGURE 13–7. Male Factor. *Source:* Adapted from Aubuchon et al. in Berek, J.S., 2012, pp. 1136–1141; Bayer et al., 2012, p. 56; & Wright & Johnson, pp. 705–715 in Gibbs et al., 2008.

- *Thyroid dysfunction:* elevated or low TSH, T_3, T_4, free T_4.
- *Hypogonadotropic hypogonadism (Kallmann's syndrome):* low FSH/LH, testosterone (Matsumoto, 1995).

VARICOCELE

This varicosity of the internal spermatic vein is usually on the left side and found in both fertile and infertile men. It impairs infertility by raising testicular temperature, thus killing sperm. Surgical correction is beneficial in some cases (Fritz & Speroff, 2011).

DISORDERS OF SPERM TRANSPORT

Sperm transport can be caused by congenital disorders, such as absence of major portions of the epididymis, vas deferens, and seminal vesicles in males with cystic fibrosis, or acquired disorders due to infections, surgery, or trauma. Such conditions may be surgically corrected.

Functional obstruction occurs in clients with spinal cord injuries, in diabetic males with autonomic neuropathy, and with medications such as tranquilizers, antidepressants, and antihypertensives.

SPERM TRANSPORT DYSFUNCTION

Clients with hypospadias, retrograde ejaculation, or sexual dysfunction are unable to deliver sperm to cervical mucus. Sperm collection by means of masturbation for cervical insemination may be indicated. Sperm may also be retrieved from alkalinized urine and prepared for IUI in the client with retrograde ejaculation.

INTERVENTIONS

- *Medications:* Clomiphene citrate, human menopausal gonadotropins (hMG), human chorionic gonadotropin (hCG), and the GnRH pump have been used in men to increase sperm count and motility, and to provide normal gonadotropin pulsatility to increase spermatogenesis. Refer to a reproductive endocrinologist or urologist for these therapies.
- Surgery (varicocelectomy, removal of obstruction, vasectomy reversal).
- Artificial insemination.
- Donor insemination.
- Electroejaculation.
- IVF.
- ICSI where one sperm is injected directly into each oocyte with IVF.
- Psychosocial support must be assessed, as self-esteem issues are often dramatic when the diagnosis of male infertility is made. Referral may be indicated for counseling.

COMBINED FACTORS OF MALE AND FEMALE INFERTILITY

Combined factors of male and female infertility may be more difficult to overcome. It is critically important to assess each partner's fertility status before the other undergoes corrective surgery. For example, IVF may be indicated instead of surgical intervention for couples with tubal pathology and a severe male factor. Individual and couple factors determine the choice of therapy. To maximize chances of conception, evaluation and intervention are coordinated, for example, using varicocele repair and endometriosis surgery.

UNEXPLAINED INFERTILITY

For many infertile couples, no specific cause of infertility can be identified by any of the standard tests. Some couples with unexplained infertility will conceive at an unpredictable time, but many will not. They have multiple needs; although they have the biologic potential to conceive, efforts have been unsuccessful, resulting in frustration for the couple, and there is nothing identified to treat.

Subjective Data. The couple reports a history of infertility.

Objective Data. A complete infertility evaluation is performed resulting in normal findings.

Plan

- Refer the couple to a reproductive endocrinologist.
- Laparoscopy or hysteroscopy may be considered to rule out a tubal or peritoneal factor.
- Psychosocial interventions include providing information and, as treatment becomes more complex, using a variety of educational strategies, such as written information, videotape, demonstration, and individual and group sessions. It is important to be available to answer questions and provide psychosocial support for the individual and couple. Explore all

treatment options and allow the couple to regain control by decision making.

- *Medication:* If the female partner is under 35 years of age and the duration of infertility is less than 12 months, then consider observation alone, or ovulation induction with clomiphene citrate and intercourse for three cycles, or clomiphene citrate and IUI for three cycles. If the female partner is older than 35, consider three cycles of ovulation induction with recombinant FSH (rFSH) and IUI.
- IVF.
- Referral may be made for the individual or couple for counseling for psychological support.

SELECTED INFERTILITY TREATMENTS

OVULATION INDUCTION

This therapy may be used alone with timed intercourse or in combination with inseminations or ART. Ovarian response to hMG or rFSH determines dose and duration of therapy. The most common initial medication used is clomiphene citrate. This is a low-cost, relatively risk-free medication if monitored regularly. If pregnancy does not occur after six ovulatory cycles, medications should be changed. Injectable gonadotropins should be used in conjunction with ultrasound monitoring to assess ovarian response. It is recommended to refer the couple to a reproductive endocrinologist when beginning this treatment.

There is some controversy in the field regarding the taking of fertility drugs and the risk of ovarian cancer. A study released in 2009 followed 54,362 Danish women treated between 1963 and 1998. Four groups of fertility medications (gonadotropins, clomiphene citrate, hCG, and GnRH) were studied. Analyses with cohort showed no overall increased incidence of ovarian cancer using any of the four groups of fertility medications regardless of the number of cycles of use, length of follow-up, or parity (Jensen, Sharif, Frederiksen, & Kjaer, 2009).

In the first 5 years of data collection in the National Institutes of Health–supported "Health Surveillance of Women Treated for Infertility by In Vitro Fertilization," no cases of ovarian cancer were reported among approximately 3,100 women (Marrs & Hartz, 1993). This study has been stopped. In addition, there appears to be no increased risk of breast cancer associated with ovarian stimulation with exogenous gonadotropins for IVF (Venn et al., 1995). In 2002, the ASRM (Rebar, 2002) concluded that women taking ovulation-inducing drugs face no greater cancer risk than the general population. Clients should be made aware of the potential ramifications of ovulation induction. Because parity is a protective factor, conception and delivery at term may provide protection. Each client must balance the risks, benefits, and her own needs to make a decision.

ARTIFICIAL INSEMINATION

Husband or donor sperm may be used for artificial insemination. Insemination enables sperm to be deposited closer to the oocyte, which improves the chances of conception. Therapeutic insemination with donor sperm provides hope of parenthood for many single women, lesbian women, and infertile couples. Due to the large amount of variables, insemination success rates are difficult to determine (Fritz & Speroff, 2011) (Table 13–11).

TABLE 13–11. Indications for IUI

I. Normal Semen Analysis
- A. Anatomic male causes
  - 1. Retrograde ejaculation
    - a. Surgery
    - b. Trauma
    - c. Systemic disease
    - d. Medications
- B. Female causes
  - 1. Cervical stenosis (conization, cauterization, diethylstilbestrol exposure)
  - 2. Deficiencies in cervical mucus
  - 3. Defects in sperm transport or survival
- C. Coital dysfunction
  - 1. Impotence
  - 2. Premature ejaculation
  - 3. Vaginismus
- D. Unexplained infertility

II. Abnormal Semen Analysis
- A. Oligospermia
- B. Asthenospermia
- C. Volume disorders
- D. Immune mediated disorders
- E. Multiple male factor disorders

III. Frozen Sperm
- A. Husband (sperm stored prior to vasectomy, chemotherapy, or radiation)
- B. Donor (azoospermia, genetic disease, Rh incompatibility, single woman)

Source: Byrd, 1995. Used with permission and adapted from Garner, C. (1995). Infertility. In C.L. Fogel & N.F. Woods (Eds.), *Women's health care: A comprehensive handbook.* Thousand Oats, CA: Sage Publications, Inc.

Procedures

- *IUI:* Performed using washed partner's specimen or thawed, cryopreserved sperm. The sperm is separated from the seminal fluid to prevent the proteins, prostaglandins, and bacteria in semen from being deposited in the uterus (Fritz & Speroff, 2011).
- *Therapeutic donor insemination (TDI):* Must be performed according to the ASRM's *Guidelines for Gamete and Embryo Donation: 2000–2002*. Consent forms are signed and donors selected. Female evaluation includes current history and physical examination, including Pap smear, chlamydia and gonorrhea cultures, rubella titer, cytomegalovirus (CMV) titer, serologic test for syphilis, hepatitis profile, and human immunodeficiency virus (HIV) test. Both partners have blood type and Rh determinations in donor matching. Donors are extensively screened, with cryopreserved specimens quarantined for at least 6 months, and donors are rescreened for HIV prior to release for use. Laboratory tests include serologic tests for syphilis, hepatitis profile, CMV titer, HIV test, and chlamydia and gonorrhea cultures. Specimens are thawed prior to use.

Timing of insemination is determined by using urine LH ovulation predictor kits or ultrasounds for follicular growth and serum LH or estradiol monitoring. Unstimulated IUI is performed the day after the LH surge. Stimulated ovulation induction IUIs are performed approximately 18 and 40 hours after ovulation is induced by administration of hCG or once at 36 hours after administration of hCG.

If conception with unstimulated IUI/TDI does not occur within three cycles, then treatment should proceed to stimulated ovulation induction IUI/TDI for three to six cycles.

ASSISTED REPRODUCTIVE TECHNOLOGIES

When other treatment options have been exhausted or when other therapies have a poor prognosis, ART are used. Options include IVF, gamete intrafallopian transfer (GIFT), embryo cryopreservation, assisted hatching, and ICSI. IVF counts for 99 percent of ART procedures with 64 percent of patients also using ICSI. ART may include the use of donor gametes or donated embryos (see Table 13–12).

Success Rates

Success rates vary from practice to practice. An overall live birth rate of 47.5 percent (under age 35) to 17.0 percent (age 41–42) per IVF embryo transfer using fresh, nondonor eggs and embryos was reported in 2009 in the United States. A live birth rate of 55.1 percent per embryo transfer was obtained with fresh donor egg IVF cycles in the same report (Society for Assisted Reproductive Technology [SART], 2009).

PREIMPLANTATION GENETIC DIAGNOSIS/SCREENING

Preimplantation genetic diagnosis (PGD) is a technique used during IVF procedures to test embryos for specific genetic disorders and/or chromosomal abnormalities prior to their transfer into the uterus. PGD makes it possible for couples or individuals with serious inherited disorders to decrease the risk of having a child who is affected by the same problem (also see Chapter 21).

Preimplantation genetic screening (PGS) is recommended for patients with unexplained infertility, recurrent miscarriage, and unsuccessful IVF cycles to rule out chromosomal abnormalities from presumed chromosomally normal genetic parents.

There are over 200 disorders that can potentially be prevented by the gender selection of embryos. Currently, PGD can detect the following single-gene disorders and chromosomal abnormalities: alpha-1-antitrypsin deficiency, cystic fibrosis, fragile X syndrome, Lesch-Nyhan syndrome, Charcot-Marie-Tooth disease, Down syndrome, Tay-Sachs disease, Duchenne muscular dystrophy, hemophilia A, retinitis pigmentosa, and Turner's syndrome.

PGD/PGS is performed during IVF by isolating embryos at the 4- to 12-cell stage, usually on the third day of development, when all the cells of the embryo are omnipotent, removing a single blastomere (cell) under microscopic guidance and analyzing the chromosomal material. A diagnosis is obtained within a day of the biopsy, and only the unaffected embryos are transferred to the uterus.

High-Order Multiple Gestation

A high incidence of multiple births continues to be a major concern in relation to ovulation induction and IVF treatment. In the United States in 2008, of the 46,326 pregnancies conceived through ART, 68.4 percent were singletons, 29.8 percent twins, 1.8 percent triplets or greater. Thus, fully 32 percent of all IVF-conceived pregnancies were with a multiple gestation (CDC, 2008). Not all of these pregnancies resulted in live births. Many of these spontaneously reduced or the parents decided, with the advice of

TABLE 13–12. Summary of Procedure and Indications for Assisted Reproductive Technologies

Assisted Reproductive Technologies	Procedure	Indications
In vitro fertilization (IVF)	Oocytes are fertilized in the laboratory. Resulting embryos are transferred to the uterus.	Tubal factor. Male factor. Endometriosis. Unexplained infertility.
Gamete intrafallopian transfer (GIFT)[a]	Gametes (oocytes and sperm) are transferred to the fallopian tubes.	Religious proscription against IVF. Unexplained infertility.
Intracytoplasmic sperm injection (ICSI)	One sperm is injected directly into the cytoplasm of the oocyte.	Male factor infertility.
Assisted hatching	A hole is made in the zona pellucida with a microinjection needle, laser or acidic Tyrode's solution to enhance embryo hatching.	Failed IVF cycle. Woman 35 years or older. Frozen embryos.
Donor oocytes	Oocytes are retrieved from a donor, inseminated and resulting embryos are transferred to a recipient in an IVF cycle.	Premature ovarian failure. Loss of gonadal function due to surgery, radiation, or chemotherapy. Congenital absence of ovaries. Genetic disorder carrier (X-linked or autosomally dominant). Repeated, unexplained pregnancy loss. Poor response to gonadotropins.
Gestational carrier	Oocytes are fertilized in the laboratory. Resulting embryos are transferred to the uterus of another woman, who will carry the pregnancy.	Uterine absence or anomaly (surgical or congenital, distortion of cavity, trauma, cancer). Medical contraindication to pregnancy.
Embryo cryopreservation	Freeze extra embryos from an IVF, GIFT, or ZIFT cycle.	To allow for a subsequent attempt at pregnancy without ovarian stimulation or retrieval.
Embryo donation	Previously cryopreserved embryos are transferred to the uterus prepared with estrogen and progesterone.	Infertility (must have an intact uterus).

[a]Absolute contraindication for GIFT or ZIFT is not having an open fallopian tube.

Source: Adapted from Broer, K.H., & Turanli, I. (Eds.). (1996). *New trends in reproductive medicine.* Berlin, Germany: Springer.

their clinician, to opt for a multifetal pregnancy reduction. In a recent review, ovulation induction accounted for 10 to 69 percent of triplet gestations, compared to approximately 24 to 30 percent associated with ART and 7 to 18 percent arising spontaneously. Quadruplet and greater multiple gestations were associated with ovulation induction in 5 to 72 percent of cases (ASRM, 2006). The SART and the ASRM have jointly published guidelines recommending an optimal number of embryos to transfer based on patient characteristics and embryo quality (ASRM & SART, 2009). In addition, there has been a movement to consider transferring only one embryo to a select group of clients, in order to limit risks to mother and fetuses. Clients should be aware of the risks of high-order multiple gestation and encouraged to balance these health concerns with their desire for pregnancy.

Stress Management

The complex psychological stressors and emotional impacts of infertility therapies may heighten a couples' feeling of loss of control and intensify over time as the couple undergoes treatment. Stressors are physical, emotional, social, religious, ethical, legal, and financial. Both couples and individuals benefit from counseling, stress management, and assistance with grief resolution (Applegarth, 1995).

Treatment Selection

The risks and benefits of each treatment regimen as well as the couple's prognosis versus their desire of a biologic child need to be carefully weighed before treatment protocols are selected. Treatment choice is often dictated by finances and insurance coverage. Information about clinics in the United States may be obtained from the ASRM (Birmingham, Alabama) at www.asrm.org (see Resources).

ALTERNATIVE FAMILY BUILDING

NONTRADITIONAL FAMILY BUILDING

Lesbian and gay couples experience the same stressors and decision-making difficulties as their heterosexual counterparts, but they also experience additional social (coparenting), financial (insurance), and legal (adoption-by-partner) concerns (see Chapter 8). In addition, they are coping and must help their children cope with a variety of social stigma that face families with same-sex parents. Family building for lesbian women may require treatment as straightforward as artificial insemination with donor sperm, but becomes increasingly complex if either partner has an additional infertility diagnosis. Gay male couples are parenting through the use of donor eggs and a gestational carrier. Multiple social, financial, and legal obstacles face these couples. As single-parent families are increasingly socially accepted, single women are also increasingly turning to fertility therapies to become pregnant.

EGG DONATION

Oocyte (egg) donation is an increasingly common option offered to couples when the female partner has poor or absent ovarian function. Indications for egg donation are POF (cessation of ovarian function prior to age 40), congenitally or surgically absent ovaries, ovarian failure induced by chemo- or radiation therapy, developmental ovarian failure (menopause), or decreased ovarian function demonstrated by multiple failed IVF or ovulation induction cycles (ASRM, 2009). Many philosophical and legal issues related to egg donation are similar to those of sperm donation, yet there are obvious differences. The technical difficulties related to ovulation induction and egg retrieval in the donor and the difficulty in synchronizing the menstrual cycles of the donor and recipient make the process logistically more complicated. Egg donation in the human has been used quite successfully and has provided many couples with an opportunity to experience pregnancy, childbirth, and breastfeeding who would otherwise not have been able to.

Candidates for egg donation must be in good physical health and have a uterus with a normal endometrial cavity. A potential recipient of donated eggs requires medical clearance for estrogen and progesterone replacement and must be considered to be an acceptable risk for carrying a pregnancy. Egg donors should be healthy, ideally between the ages of 21 and 33, and free of infectious disease. Known egg donors include sisters, relatives, friends, or colleagues. Anonymous egg donors may be recruited by word of mouth, by advertising, through recruiting agencies, or over the Internet. Most women who become egg donors express an altruistic desire to help another woman, although financial compensation may be a motivating factor for anonymous egg donors. Payments for anonymous egg donors can range from \$2,500 to over \$10,000 per cycle. All egg donors, whether anonymous or known, must be screened to ensure that their motivation appears reasonable and voluntary. Egg donation presents a number of unique legal and emotional issues, which need to be carefully considered. Most egg donation programs require psychological counseling for both recipients and donors, and many programs also recommend legal counsel for both parties and a contract between recipient and donor.

GESTATIONAL CARRIER

Use of a gestational carrier is indicated when the uterus of the female partner is surgically or congenitally absent, when the uterine cavity is distorted by uterine anomalies or trauma, or when the endometrial lining is unreceptive to implantation such as after multiple surgical repairs, Asherman's syndrome, or after chemo- or radiation therapies. Use of a gestational carrier is also indicated if the female partner has a medical contraindication to pregnancy.

Traditional surrogacy implies that a woman is inseminated with the intended father's sperm and at the time of delivery relinquishes her rights to the child. This relationship raises many ethical and legal difficulties. These difficulties can be avoided through the use of a gestational carrier. Utilizing ART, embryos created from the gametes of the intended parents, or donor gametes, are transferred to the uterus of another woman, who will carry the pregnancy. Prior to the embryo transfer, extensive psychological counseling of the intended parents and the potential gestational carrier and her spouse is required. In addition, a legal contract between the intended parents and the gestational carrier is critical. A contract establishes intent, so that, at the time of delivery, it is clear who intends to parent the child. Laws regarding this relationship vary tremendously from state to state, and prior to treatment it is important for the couple to seek legal counsel from an expert in reproductive law.

ADOPTION

The decision to adopt may be difficult and is almost always come to gradually. Guide couples toward adoption resources during their infertility treatment if they are interested. Beginning the adoption process does not always resolve a couple's grief over the loss of their own fertility. This process occurs over time with the support of each other, significant others, and professionals (Johnston, 1992). Options for adoption are by means of a private arrangement (parental placement) or through an agency or international organization. Many adoption agencies insist that all infertility treatment be complete and neither partner over 40 years old. Waiting lists may be years long. Adoptive children may have special needs or be an older child. The process can be complicated, time consuming, and costly. Many couples, however, once their child has found their adoptive home, are able to find fulfillment, happiness, and resolution of their desire for biologic children. Adoptive parents often express wonder at how long it took them to take this step and wish that they had begun the process sooner.

CHILDFREE LIVING

Infertile couples are faced with many difficult decisions. They must take into consideration their motivation in pursuing fertility therapies, their energy and resources, and the value of continuing treatment. Choosing to remain without children may be painful, and many couples must come to terms with a tremendous sense of loss. In the end, however, there may be some relief in finding their family complete without children. A couple may no longer feel pressured to perform on demand, put their lives on hold, or conform to medical therapies. They are able to regain privacy, control their lives, and focus their energies on themselves, each other, their relationship, and future life goals (Carter & Carter, 1989; Robertson 1994).

FUTURE TRENDS AND CONTROVERSIES

OOCYTE CRYOPRESERVATION

To date, there are over 1,000 births worldwide as the result of egg freezing. Rapid advances in oocyte preservation are allowing some women, especially those who are facing chemotherapy or radiation, the opportunity to preserve their fertility. Fertile women may also take advantage of this advancement to delay childbearing. In the late 1990s to early 2000s, live birth rates were 2 to 10 percent. Currently, some IVF centers advertise pregnancy rates up to 50 percent. However, it is important to keep in mind that because this is a new program for many centers, most have done less than 50 cycles so success rates may be skewed. Currently, neither the CDC nor the SART collects data on the success rates for egg freezing.

HUMAN CLONING

In a position statement made April 5, 2002, the ASRM stated opposition to any attempt at reproductive cloning of a human being.The ASRM has maintained this position to this day. At present, despite claims to the contrary, there is no scientific evidence to justify an attempt to clone a human being. The ASRM urges the media, the public, and policy makers to meet such claims with skepticism rather than alarm, unless they are accompanied by peer-reviewed scientific evidence. In addition, the ASRM finds it unconscionable to recruit patients to participate in these efforts. Because infertility can be emotionally devastating, the ASRM states that any effort that offers false hope to couples with infertility is irresponsible and unethical.

RESOURCES

American Society for Reproductive Medicine
1209 Montgomery Highway
Birmingham, Alabama 35216-2809
Phone: 205-978-5000
Fax: 205-978-5005
www.asrm.org

Patient education booklets, fact sheets, guidelines are available. Nurses' Professional Group of ASRM has developed protocols and procedures to provide nursing care.

The Compassionate Friends
P.O. Box 3696
Oak Brook, IL 60522-3696
Phone: 877-969-0010
Fax: 630-990-0246
www.compassionatefriends.org

National self-help group is to provide support to families who have experienced the death of a child. National newsletter for parents and grandparents and a newsletter for siblings are available. National and regional conferences are held annually.

RESOLVE: The National Infertility Association
1760 Old Meadow Rd, Suite 500
McLean, VA 22102
Phone: 703-556-7172
Fax: 703-506-3266
www.resolve.org

National lay organization with local chapters dedicated to providing education, support, and advocacy for couples experiencing infertility. Newsletter and fact sheets are available.

American Infertility Association
666 Fifth Ave., Suite 278
New York, NY 10103
Phone: 203-740-7874
www.americaninfertility.org

Endometriosis Association International
8585 North 76th Place
Milwaukee, WI 53223
Phone: 414-355-2200
www.endometriosisassn.org

The endometriosis association is a nonprofit, self-help organization dedicated to providing information and support to women and girls with endometriosis.

REFERENCES

Adashi, E.Y. (2000). Recurrent pregnancy loss: State of the art. *Seminars in Reproductive Medicine, 18*, 327–443.

American College of Obstetricians and Gynecologists. (2003). ACOG practice bulletin: Polycystic ovary syndrome. *International Journal of Gynecology and Obstetrics, 80,* 335–348.

American Society for Reproductive Medicine (ASRM). (2005a). *Polycystic ovarian syndrome.* Retrieved June 30, 2011, from http://www.asrm.org

American Society for Reproductive Medicine (ASRM). (2005b). *Prediction of fertility potential (ovarian reserve) in women.* Retrieved July 1, 2011, from http://www.asrm.org

American Society for Reproductive Medicine (ASRM). (2006). *Multiple pregnancy associated with infertility therapy.* A Practice Committee Report: An Educational Bulletin. Retrieved June 9, 2011, from http://www.asrm.org

American Society for Reproductive Medicine (ASRM). (2008). *Obesity and reproduction.* A Practice Committee Report: An Educational Bulletin. Retrieved July 7, 2011, from http://www.asrm.org

American Society for Reproductive Medicine (ASRM). (2009). *Guidelines for gamete and embryo donation.* A Practice Committee Report: Guidelines and Minimum Standards. Retrieved June 9, 2011, from http://www.asrm.org

American Society for Reproductive Medicine (ASRM). (2011). *Optimal evaluation of the infertile female.* A Practice Committee Report: A Committee Opinion. Retrieved June 9, 2011, from http://www.asrm.org

American Society for Reproductive Medicine Statement on Attempts at Human Cloning. (2002, April 5). *Statement attributable to William Keye, M.D., President, American Society for Reproductive Medicine.* Retrieved January 7, 2002, from http://www.asrm.org

American Society for Reproductive Medicine (ASRM) & Society for Assisted Reproductive Technology (SART). (2009). Guidelines on number of embryos transferred. *Fertility and Sterility, 92*(5), 1518–1519.

American Urological Association (AUA). (2010). *Infertility: Report on optimal evaluation of the infertile male: An AUA best practice policy and ASRM practice committee report* (Vol. 1, ISBN 0-9649702-7-9). Retrieved February 28, 2012, from http://urology.ucsf.edu/patientGuides/pdf/maleInf/Optimal%20Evaluation%20of%20Infertile%20Male.pdf

Anderson, K.M., Sharpe, M. Rattray, A., & Irvine, D.S., (2003) Distress and concerns in couples referred to a specialist infertility clinic. *Journal of Psychosomatic Research, 54.* 353–355

Applegarth, L.D. (1995). The psychological aspects of infertility. In W.R. Keye, Jr., R.J. Chang, R.W. Rebar, & M.R. Soules (Eds.), *Infertility: Evaluation and treatment* (pp. 19–24). Philadelphia: W. B. Saunders Company.

Aubuchon, M, Burney, R.O., Schust, D.J., & Yao, M.W.M. (2012). Infertility and assisted reproductive technology. In J.S. Berek (Ed.), *Berek & Novak's gynecology* (15th ed., pp. 1133–1189). Philadelphia: Lippincott Williams & Wilkins.

Bayer, S.R., Alper, M.M., & Penzias, A.S. (2012). *The Boston IVF handbook of infertility* (3rd ed.). New York: Informa Healthcare.

Bolumar, F., Olsen, J., Boldsen, J., & European Study Group on Infertility Subfecundity. (1996). Smoking reduces fecundity: A European multicenter study on infertility and subfecundity. *American Journal of Epidemiology, 143,* 578–587.

Bolumar, F., Olsen, J., Rebagaliato, M., & Bisanti, L. (1997). Caffeine intake and delayed conception: A European multicenter study in infertility and subfecundity. *American Journal of Epidemiology, 145*(14), 324–334.

Buttram, V.C., & Reiter, R.C. (1981). Uterine leiomyomata: Etiology, symptomatoloty, and management. *Fertility & Sterility,* 36(4), 433–445.

Byrd, W. (1995). Sperm preparation and homologous insemination. In W.R. Keye, Jr., R.J. Chang, R.W. Rebar, & M.R. Soules (Eds.), *Infertility: Evaluation and treatment* (pp. 696–711). Philadelphia: W. B. Saunders Company.

Cahill, D. (2009). *PCOS.* Retrieved January 15, 2009, from BMJ Clinical Evidence: http://www.clinicalevidence.com

Carter, J., & Carter, M. (1989). *Sweet grapes: How to stop being infertile and start living again.* Indianapolis, IN: Perspective Press.

Centers for Disease Control and Prevention (CDC). (2008). *Assisted reproductive technologies success rates.* Retrieved from www.cdc.gov/ncadphp/drh/art.htm

Centers for Disease Control and Prevention (CDC). (2011). *Pelvic inflammatory disease.* Retrieved from http://www.cdc.gov/std/pid/stdfact-pid.htm

Cohen, M.A., Lindheim, S.R., & Sauer, M.V. (1999). Hydrosalpinges adversely affect implantation in donor oocyte cycles. *Human Reproduction, 14,* 1087–1089.

Cowan, B.D. (2002). Evaluation of the female for infertility. In D.B. Seifer & R.L. Collins (Eds.), *Office-based infertility practice* (pp. 1–9). New York: Springer-Verlag.

Cramer, D.W., & Wise L.A. (2000). The epidemiology of recurrent pregnancy loss. In E.Y. Adashi, R.M. Silver, & J.A. Hill (Eds.), *Seminars in Reproductive Medicine. Recurrent Pregnancy Loss: State of the Art, 18*(4), 331.

De Mouzon, J., Spira, A., & Schwartz, D. (1988). A prospective study of the relation between smoking and fertility. *International Journal of Epidemiology, 17,* 378–384.

Diamanti-Kandarakis, E. (2006). Insulin resistance in PCOS. *Endocrine, 301*(1), 13–17.

Domar, A.D., Clapp, D., Slawsby, E.A., Dusek, J., Kessel, B., & Freizinger, M. (2000). Impact of group psychological interventions on pregnancy rates in infertile women. *Fertility and Sterility, 73,* 805–811.

Fielding, J.E. (1987). Smoking and women: Tragedy of the majority. *New England Journal of Medicine, 317,* 1343–1345.

Fritz, M., & Speroff, L. (2011). *Clinical gynecologic endocrinology and infertility* (8th ed.). Philadelphia: Lippincott Williams & Wilkins.

Gardella, J.R., & Hill, J.A. (2000). Environmental toxins associated with recurrent pregnancy loss. In E.Y. Adashi, R.M. Silver, & J.A. Hill (Eds.), *Seminars in Reproductive Medicine. Recurrent Pregnancy Loss: State of the Art, 118*(4), 407–424.

Goldenberg, M., Sivan, E., Sharabi, Z., Bider, D., Rabinovici, J., & Seidman, D.S. (1995). Outcome of hysteroscopic resection of submucous myomas for infertility. *Fertility and Sterility, 64,* 714–716.

Hakim, R.B., Gray, R.H., & Zacur, H. (1998). Alcohol and caffeine consumption and decreased fertility. *Fertility and Sterility, 70,* 632–637.

Harlap, S., & Shiono, P.H. (1980). Alcohol, smoking, and incidence of spontaneous abortions in the first and second trimester. *Lancet, 2,* 173–178.

Hatch, E.E., & Bracken, M.B. (1993). Association of delayed conception with caffeine consumption. *American Journal of Epidemiology, 138*(12), 1082–1092.

Hook, D.B., Cross, P.K., & Schreinemachers, D.M. (1983). Chromosomal abnormality rates at amniocentesis and in live-born infants. *Journal of the American Medical Association, 249,* 2034–2038.

Hook, E.B. (1981). Rates of chromosome abnormalities at different maternal ages. *Obstetrics and Gynecology, 58,* 282–285.

Jacobson, J.L., Jacobson, S.W., & Sokol, R.J. (1994). Effects of alcohol use, smoking and illicit drug use on fetal growth in black infants. *Journal of Pediatrics, 124,* 757–764.

Jensen, A., Sharif, H., Frederiksen, K., & Kjaer, S.K. (2009, February). Use of fertility drugs and risk of ovarian cancer: Danish Population Based Cohort Study. *British Medical Journal, 338,* b249.

Jensen, T.K., Hjollund, N.H.I., Henriksen, T.B., Scheike, T., Kolstad, H., Giwercman, A., et al. (1998). Does moderate alcohol consumption affect fertility? Follow up study among couples planning first pregnancy. *British Medical Journal, 317,* 505–510.

Johnson, N.P., Mak, W., & Sowter, M.C. (2002). Laparoscopic salpingectomy for women with hydrosalpinges enhances the success of IVF: A Cochrane review. *Human Reproduction, 17*(3), 543–548.

Johnston, P. (1992). *Adopting after infertility.* Indianapolis, IN: Perspective Press.

Kruger, T.F., Acosta, A.A., Simmons, K.F., Swanson, R.J., Matta, J.F., & Oehninger, S. (1988). Predictive value of abnormal sperm morphology in in vitro fertilization. *Fertility and Sterility, 49,* 112–117.

LaMarca, A., & Volpe, A. (2006). AMH as a marker of ovarian reserve in patients undergoing assisted reproductive technology (ART). *Clinical Endocrinology, 64*(6), 603–610.

LaTorre, D., & Falomi, A. (2007). Pharmacological causes of hyperprolactinemia. *Therapeutics and Clinical Risk Management, 3*(5), 929–951.

Levy, M.J. (1995). Hirsutism. In W.R. Meyer (Ed.), *Infertility and Reproductive Medicine Clinics of North America, 6*(1), 215–227. Philadelphia: W. B. Saunders Company.

Lewis, J.A., & Bernstein, J. (1996). *Women's health: A relational perspective across the life cycle.* Boston: Jones and Bartlett Publishers.

Marrs, R.P., & Hartz, S.C. (1993, January). *Comments on the possible association between ovulation inducing agents and ovarian cancer (Statement from the American Fertility Society to its members).* Birmingham, AL: American Fertility Society.

Matsumoto, A.M. (1995). Pathophysiology of male infertility. In W.R. Keye, Jr., R.J. Chang, R.W. Rebar, & M.R. Soules (Eds.), *Infertility: Evaluation and treatment* (pp. 555–579). Philadelphia: W. B. Saunders Company.

Munne, S., Alikani, M., Tomkin, G., Grifo, J., & Cohen, J. (1995). Embryo morphology, developmental rates, and maternal age are correlated with chromosome abnormalities. *Fertility and Sterility, 64,* 382–391.

Nackley, A.C., & Muasher, S.J. (1998). The significance of hydrosalpinx in in vitro fertilization. *Fertility and Sterility, 69,* 373–384.

Nestler, J.E. (2008). Metformin for the treatment of the polycystic ovary syndrome. *New England Journal of Medicine, 358,* 47–54.

Nestler, J.E., & Jakubowicz, D.J. (1996). Decreases in ovarian cytochrome P450c17 activity and serum free testosterone after reduction of insulin secretion in polycystic ovary syndrome. *New England Journal of Medicine, 335,* 617–623.

Peterson, B.D., Pirritano, M. Christensen, U., Boivin, J., Block, J. & Schmidt. L. (2009) The longitudinal impact of partner coping in couples following 5 years of unsuccessful fertility treatments. *Human Reproduction, 24(7),* 1656–1664

Quaas, A., & Dokras, A. (2008, Spring). Diagnosis and treatment of unexplained infertility. *Review Obstetrics and Gynecology, 1*(2), 69–76.

Rebar, R. (2002). *ASRM statement on risk of cancer associated with fertility drugs.* Retrieved January 24, 2002, from http://www.asrm.org

Robertson, J.A. (1994). *Children of choice: Freedom and the new reproductive technologies.* Princeton, NJ: Princeton University Press.

Rogers, S.F. (1995). Pelvic inflammatory disease: Effects on future fertility. In W.R. Meyer (Ed.), *Infertility and Reproductive Medicine Clinics of North America, 6*(1), 95–101. Philadelphia: W. B. Saunders Company.

Sauer, M.V. (2002). *Milestones in oocyte donation: A 20-year review.* Fourth annual ART of Donor Oocytes and Third Party Reproduction conference, Charleston, SC.

Sims, J.A., & Gibbons, W.E. (1996). Treatment of human infertility: The cervical and uterine factors. In E.Y. Adashi, J.A. Rock, & Z. Rosenwaks (Eds.), *Reproductive endocrinology, surgery, and technology* (pp. 2141–2169). Philadelphia: Lippincott-Raven.

Society for Assisted Reproductive Technology (SART). (2009). *IVF success rates.* Retrieved from http://www.sart.org/frame/detail.aspx?id=3893

Strickler, R.C. (1995). Factors influencing fertility. In W.R. Keye, Jr., R.J. Chang, R.W. Rebar, & M.R. Soules (Eds.), *Infertility: Evaluation and treatment* (pp. 8–18). Philadelphia: W. B. Saunders Company.

Thessaloniki, ESHRE/ASRM-Sponsored PCOS Consensus Workshop Group. (2008). Consensus on infertility treatment related to polycystic ovary syndrome. *Fertility and Sterility, 89*(3), 505–522.

U.S. Department of Health and Human Services. (2009). *Fertility, family planning, and women's health.* (New data from the 1995 National Survey of Family Growth; Centers for Disease Control and Prevention/National Center for Health Statistics, Series 23, No. 19). Washington, DC: Author. Retrieved February 28, 2012, from http//www.cdc.gov/nchs/nsfg.htm

Venn, A., Watson, L., Lumley, J., Giles, G., King, C., & Healy, D. (1995). Breast and ovarian cancer incidence after infertility and in vitro fertilization. *Lancet, 346,* 995–1000.

Westrom, L. (1980). Incidence, prevalence, and trends of acute pelvic inflammatory disease and its consequences in industrialized countries. *American Journal of Obstetrics and Gynecology, 138*(7), 880–892.

Winkel, C. (1995). Lesions affecting the uterine cavity. In W.R. Keye, Jr., R.J. Chang, R.W. Rebar, & M.R. Soules (Eds.), *Infertility: Evaluation and treatment* (pp. 387–411). Philadelphia: W.B. Saunders Company.

World Health Organization (WHO). (1995). *Physical status: The use and interpretation of anthropometry* (Report of a WHO expert committee. WHO Tech. Rep. Ser. 854). Geneva: Author.

CHAPTER ❖ 14

VAGINITIS AND SEXUALLY TRANSMITTED DISEASES

Susan D. Schaffer ◆ *Jane F. Houston*

First-void urine tests and self-obtained vaginal swabs have the potential to simplify screening and diagnosis of many sexually transmitted infections. Outside of lifelong monogamy with an uninfected partner, consistent latex condom use provides the best risk reduction for STDs. However, appreciable risk remains.

Highlights

- Sexually Transmitted Diseases and the Centers for Disease Control and Prevention
- Vaginitis
- Cervicitis
- Ulcerative Genital Infections
- Epidermal Diseases
- Hepatitis B

❖ INTRODUCTION

Vaginitis and sexually transmitted diseases (STDs) are frequently occurring problems among women. These conditions occur most often during the reproductive years; in fact, many reach their peak incidence during adolescence and young adulthood.

Women bear the greatest burden of STDs, suffering more frequent and more serious complications than men. Gonorrhea and chlamydia can cause pelvic inflammatory disease (PID), with resultant infertility or ectopic pregnancy. Infection with some types of human papillomavirus (HPV) is associated with cervical cancer. Bacterial vaginosis (BV) and herpes virus infections are associated with adverse pregnancy outcomes, and most STDs have been shown to increase the risk of acquiring human immunodeficiency virus (HIV).

Early diagnosis and appropriate treatment can prevent many adverse STD outcomes. But diagnosis and treatment are not enough. Preventing the spread of STDs requires providers to determine the sexual history of all women in their care and to deliver prevention messages when risky behaviors are identified. Counseling skills such as respect, compassion, and a nonjudgmental attitude are essential to the effective delivery of prevention messages as well as STD care. Prevention messages should include a description of actions to avoid acquiring or transmitting STDs. Consistent condom use provides the best STD risk reduction for women outside of a lifelong monogamous relationship with an uninfected partner (see Table 14–1 for condom usage guidelines). Consistent and correct use of latex condoms reduces HIV risk by 85 percent in men and women; has been shown to reduce the risk of transmission of gonorrhea, chlamydia, and herpes simplex virus (HSV) in both men and women (Steiner & Cates, 2006); and also reduces HPV risk in women (Winer et al., 2006).

Table 14–2 provides an overview of general information that should be provided to women with vaginitis or an STD. For STD screening guidelines, see Table 14–3.

TABLE 14–1. How to Use a Condom Consistently and Correctly

- Use a new condom for every act of vaginal, anal, and oral sex throughout the *entire* sex act (from start to finish).
- Before any genital contact, put the condom on the tip of the erect penis with the rolled side out.
- If the condom does not have a reservoir tip, pinch the tip enough to leave a half-inch space for semen to collect. Holding the tip, unroll the condom all the way to the base of the erect penis.
- After ejaculation and before the penis gets soft, grip the rim of the condom and carefully withdraw. Then gently pull the condom off the penis, making sure that semen doesn't spill out.
- Wrap the condom in a tissue and throw it in the trash where others won't handle it.
- If you feel the condom break at any point during sexual activity, stop immediately, withdraw, remove the broken condom, and put on a new condom.
- Ensure that adequate lubrication is used during vaginal and anal sex, which might require water-based lubricants. Oil-based lubricants (e.g., petroleum jelly, shortening, mineral oil, massage oils, body lotions, and cooking oil) should not be used because they can weaken latex, causing breakage.

Source: Reproduced from CDC. (2011). *Condom fact sheet in brief.* Accessed from http://www.cdc.gov/condomeffectiveness/brief.html#Consistent

SEXUALLY TRANSMITTED DISEASES AND THE CENTERS FOR DISEASE CONTROL AND PREVENTION

Some STDs, but not all, are reportable by state agencies to the Centers for Disease Control and Prevention (CDC) in Atlanta, Georgia. The CDC is part of the U.S. Public Health Service and charged with, among other functions, assisting states to identify and control certain diseases. The actual mandate to report specific diseases comes from individual states through their legislative bodies. The CDC can recommend which diseases should be reported; however, the final decision rests with the states. The following STDs are reportable by all states to the CDC: HIV, gonorrhea, hepatitis A, hepatitis B, hepatitis C, *Chlamydia trachomatis*, chancroid, and syphilis (CDC, 2011). In addition, some states also require the reporting

TABLE 14–2. General Information Needed in the Care of Women With Vaginitis and Sexually Transmitted Diseases

Provide both written information and verbal explanations to the client.

Disease process	Etiology, incubation, risk factors, diagnosis, management, follow-up.
Treatments	Medications and their side effects; signs of allergic response; discomfort; time commitments; simultaneous partner treatment; the need to keep appointments for treatment and thereby control growth and spread of lesions and worsening of disease and symptoms; avoidance of douching and tampon use (unless medically directed) until healing is complete.
Transmission	A description of all possible modes; the need to suspend genital and oral sexual relations, foreign body insertion, and manual manipulation until healing is complete; use of lubricated latex condoms until partners are examined and determined disease-free; the dangers of multiple partners and the principles of "safer sex."
Comfort measures	Sitz baths and oral analgesics may help some conditions.
Hygiene	The importance of cleanliness and dryness to enhance healing. Use of a hair dryer on low setting to aid drying. Avoidance of powders, douches (especially perfumed or deodorized), perfumed sprays. Discussion of secondary infection and how it may occur. Wearing clean cotton underwear, loose clothing, and fabrics that "breathe"; washing hands thoroughly before and after touching genitalia; not wearing underwear more than 1 day; not wearing anyone else's underwear; not allowing anyone other than oneself to wear one's underwear or tight fitting trousers; changing out of moist clothing as soon as possible.
Other prevention	Decreasing smoking in infection with human papillomavirus (HPV); self-monitoring of the vulva (HPV); client examination of partner and asking about past exposure; empowerment of client (through role playing) to be motivated and skillful in talking about sensitive issues with her partner; caution in new sexual liaisons; avoidance of alcohol and drugs that limit inhibitions; an agreement ("contract") with her partner that they have a mutually monogamous relationship; for their mutual safety, an agreement between the two partners in the relationship to tell each other if either one has sexual relations with someone else.

TABLE 14–3. STD Screening Guidelines

Population	Test
Pregnant women	HIV, syphilis (serologic test), hepatitis B (surface antigen)
	If at risk, *Chlamydia trachomatis*, hepatitis C
Young women (≤ age 25)	*Chlamydia trachomatis* (annually), HIV
	If at risk, *Neisseria gonorrhoeae*, syphilis, hepatitis B & C
Women > 25 to 64	HIV (unless live in area of < 1 in 1,000 infected)
	If at risk, *Chlamydia trachomatis, Neisseria gonorrhoeae,* syphilis, hepatitis B & C
Women > 64	If at risk, HIV, *Chlamydia trachomatis, Neisseria gonorrhoeae,* syphilis, hepatitis B & C

Source: Adapted from CDC, 2010a.

of neonatal herpes simplex, granuloma inguinale, lymphogranuloma venereum (LGV), PID, and nonspecific urethritis (NC Communicable Disease Branch, 2008).

Three factors are considered in determining which diseases should be reported:

Ability to test: If no reasonable test for a condition is readily available (e.g., herpes), then that disease is unlikely to become reportable.

Ability to cure: Especially important to report are readily curable diseases (e.g., gonorrhea) in order to control epidemics.

Public awareness: Diseases that gain widespread public attention and represent a public health threat (e.g., HIV) are usually reportable.

In addition to compiling STD statistics, the CDC recommends treatment for individual diseases. Approximately every 4 to 5 years, it publishes STD treatment guidelines. The most recent of these guidelines, published in 2010, are used throughout this chapter when discussing medication, although some other evidence-based newer research-based recommendations are also included. These guidelines are freely available through the CDC website at www.cdc.gov/std/treatment/2010/default.htm.

The remainder of this chapter is organized according to clinical syndromes. This facilitates clinical decision making when the clinician is faced with vaginitis or a possible STD. First, the clinician must determine the type of clinical syndrome based on presenting symptoms. Then the possible causes of that syndrome can be considered. Although HIV infection is primarily sexually transmitted, it is discussed in Chapter 15 because of the complex psychosocial and medical management required by persons with this infection.

VAGINITIS

The vagina is a dynamic ecosystem. Vaginal discharge is usually without odor and white or clear. Lactobacilli proliferate, but many other organisms can be present including potential pathogens at lower levels. The presence of lactobacilli is an important factor in maintaining a normal acidic pH. Vaginitis occurs when the vaginal ecosystem has been disturbed, either by the introduction of an organism, or by a disturbance that allows the pathogens normally residing in this environment to proliferate. It is characterized by pruritus, irritation, and sometimes external dysuria. Vaginal odor may be present with excessive discharge. Factors that may alter the vaginal ecosystem include antibiotics, hormones, contraceptive preparations (oral and topical), douches, vaginal medication, sexual intercourse, STDs, stress, and changes in sexual partners. Diagnosis of vaginitis is made by close inspection of the external genitalia, determination of the pH of the vaginal discharge (normally 3.8–4.2), and microscopic examination of the discharge. Although BV, vulvovaginal candidiasis (VVC), and trichomoniasis are the most common causes of abnormal vaginal discharge, other etiologies such as gonorrhea, chlamydia, herpes virus infection, foreign body, allergies, and hormonal deficiency should also be considered. Quan (2010) notes that > 10 percent of office visits for women's health care are related to vaginitis, adding that making a definitive diagnosis requires skillful performance of laboratory procedures including the vaginal wet mount, vaginal pH determination, and the whiff test. Syed and Braverman (2004) indicate that vaginitis is also common among adolescent females and can cause extreme distress with recurrent symptoms.

Sometimes more than one disease may be present (CDC, 2010a). The CDC estimates that approximately 19 million new sexually transmitted infections occur annually. Women are hit hardest in relation to chlamydial infections. The sequelae for females are much more serious than for males. For African American women, the rate is eight times higher than among whites, nearly half of all new chlamydial infections are reported in this group. Gonorrhea, which historically had higher rates among males than females, has now become more common among the latter group in the past 6 years according to the CDC (2010a).

BACTERIAL VAGINOSIS

Bacterial vaginosis is a clinical syndrome characterized by alterations in vaginal flora. It is the most prevalent form of vaginitis among childbearing women. BV is a syndrome in which normal H_2O_2-producing lactobacilli in the vagina are replaced with high concentrations of anaerobic bacteria (e.g., *Gardnerella vaginalis*, *Mobiluncus* species, *Mycoplasma hominis*, *Ureaplasma urealyticum*, and *Prevotella* species [CDC, 2010a]). Current recommendations on the screening and risk of BV among pregnant women vary widely. The U.S. Preventive Services Task Force (USPSTF) reviewed published research to evaluate the benefits and harms of screening asymptomatic pregnant women. The authors discovered that no studies directly showed that screening for BV improves pregnancy outcomes for women at low or high risk for preterm delivery (USPSTF, 2008).

However, certain studies do suggest an association with preterm labor, chorioamnionitis, and PID (Yudin & Money, 2008). They indicate that in symptomatic pregnant women, testing for and treatment of BV is recommended for symptom resolution. Diagnostic criteria are the same for pregnant and nonpregnant women. The authors note that treatment with either oral or vaginal antibiotics is acceptable for achieving a cure in pregnant women with symptomatic BV who are at low risk of adverse obstetric outcomes. Asymptomatic women and women without identified risk factors for preterm birth should not undergo routine screening for or treatment of BV. Women at increased risk for preterm birth may benefit from routine screening for and treatment of BV. If treatment for the prevention of adverse pregnancy outcomes is undertaken, it should be with metronidazole 500 mg orally twice daily for 7 days or clindamycin 300 mg orally twice daily for 7 days. Topical (vaginal) therapy is not recommended for this indication. Testing should be repeated 1 month after treatment to ensure that cure was achieved.

Epidemiology

Etiology/Risk Factors. Longitudinal studies suggest that douching and multiple sexual partners are associated with acquisition of BV; however, women without these risk factors also acquire the infection. The presence of vaginal lactobacilli that produce H_2O_2 seems to confer protection (USPSTF, 2008).

Transmission. Research suggests a nonsexual mode of transmission, although BV occurs almost exclusively in sexually active women. The treatment of male partners does not reduce the risk of recurrence; however, consistent condom use does (Hutchinson, Kip, & Ness, 2007).

Incidence. BV prevalence ranges from 10 to 40 percent, depending on the population of women studied.

Subjective Data

Clients with BV may be asymptomatic or may have malodorous vaginal discharge. Often, clients report foul odor after intercourse. Symptoms such as pruritus, abdominal pain, dyspareunia, and dysuria do not reliably correlate with BV.

Objective Data

Physical Examination. Clinical diagnosis of BV requires that three of the following four criteria be met: thin, white homogeneous malodorous adherent vaginal discharge; pH level above 4.5; positive whiff test; and/or presence of clue cells on wet-mount microscopic examination. Cultures are not recommended (CDC, 2010a).

Diagnostic Tests and Methods

- *Saline wet mount:* Diagnostic evaluation for clue cells—characteristic epithelial cells with bacteria adherent to the cell wall, giving it a stippled, granular appearance. Cell margins become blurred, and few white blood cells are noted.
  The test procedure is to mix a sample of vaginal secretions (obtained from the vaginal pool or posterior blade of the speculum) with normal saline, place on a slide, and cover with a coverslip. Examine microscopically under low and high power. Explain the procedure to the client. Advise her that an immediate diagnosis is possible.
- *Whiff test:* Diagnostic evaluation for a fishy amine odor. The test procedure is to mix vaginal secretions with 10 percent potassium hydroxide (KOH); the characteristic odor is readily emitted. Advise the client of the test purpose.
- *Vaginal pH:* Diagnostic evaluation for acidity of vaginal secretions. In BV, pH is greater than or equal to 4.5, but this is not specific for BV alone. The test procedure is to dip appropriate pH paper (pH range 4.0 to 6.0) into vaginal secretions and observe the color change. The sample may be obtained by swabbing the lateral and posterior fornix and applying directly to pH paper, or by dipping pH paper into the posterior blade of the speculum after removal from the vagina. Advise the client of the purpose of the test.

Differential Medical Diagnoses

Trichomoniasis vaginitis, foreign body vaginitis, monilia.

Plan

Psychosocial Interventions. BV is considered to be a polymicrobial disease that is not sexually transmitted, and the etiology is uncertain (McPhee & Papdakis, 2011). For this reason, a client's confusion is understandable. Counsel clients about what is currently known and what is being suggested. Treatments for BV vary in efficacy and adverse effects (Oduyebo, Anorlu, & Ogunsola 2009). Clindamycin and oral metronidazole are effective treatments for BV. Oral metronidazole can cause nausea, vomiting, and a metallic taste in the mouth.

Medication

Metronidazole Oral Tablets/Metronidazole Vaginal Gel

- *Indications:* Oral metronidazole is recommended for BV (including during pregnancy) (CDC, 2010a). Vaginal gel and cream preparations may be used in the first half of pregnancy also.
- *Administration:* Oral tablets—500 mg bid for 7 days. The CDC (2010a) also recommends metronidazole 250 mg orally tid in pregnant women. Other options include metronidazole gel (0.75%), one full applicator (5 g) intravaginally, once a day for 5 days.
- *Side effects and adverse reactions:* All alcohol products must be avoided with any metronidazole regimen because profuse nausea and vomiting (disulfiram reaction) may occur. Therefore, patients should be advised to avoid consuming alcohol during treatment with metronidazole and for 24 hours thereafter. Transient nausea and a metallic taste have also been reported. Because metronidazole has a broad antimicrobial spectrum, normal vaginal flora may be suppressed with subsequent monilial infection. Vaginal gel is used for vaginal candidiasis, occasional genitourinary/perineal itching, irritation, swelling, and gastrointestinal (GI) complaints.
- *Contraindications:* Known allergy to metronidazole.
- *Anticipated outcomes on evaluation:* Symptoms clear rapidly after treatment. A test for cure is not routinely indicated. Some authors suggest retesting pregnant clients at 1 month post treatment (Nygren et al., 2008).
- *Client teaching and counseling:* Stress the need to avoid alcohol. If symptoms return, reexamination is indicated. Treatment of the sexual partner with recurrent infection is recommended. Sexual abstinence or use of condoms during treatment is recommended. Advise the client about side effects.

Clindamycin

- *Indications:* Alternative treatment of BV; may be useful in recurrent cases and orally during pregnancy.

- *Administration:* Clindamycin cream (2%), one full applicator (5 g) intravaginally, at bedtime for 7 days. Clindamycin may be used orally 300 mg bid for 7 days, but this is less effective and severe side effects are more common with this regimen (CDC, 2010a).
- *Side effects and adverse reactions:* Colitis may be severe (more common with oral form). Vaginitis from *Candida albicans* is more common with clindamycin use.
- *Contraindications:* Known sensitivity to clindamycin. Clindamycin cream is oil based and might weaken latex condoms and diaphragms for up to 5 days after use.
- *Anticipated outcomes on evaluation:* Symptoms resolve rapidly. Test for cure is not necessary.
- *Client teaching and counseling:* The regimen of medication must be completed.
- *Follow-up and referral:* No follow-up is necessary.

VULVOVAGINAL CANDIDIASIS

According to Chibana and Magee (2009), *C. albicans* is the most important human fungal pathogen. Candidal vulvovaginitis accounts for approximately one third of all vaginitis cases. About 30 percent of women with a healthy vaginal environment harbor *Candida*, usually *C. albicans.* An upset in the homeostatic balance in the vagina leads to an overgrowth of this organism and symptoms of infection. VVC is a common, irritating, and recurrent cause of vaginitis that is not generally sexually transmitted. Predisposing factors include antibiotic use, obesity, diabetes, HIV infection (or other immunosuppressive conditions), and pregnancy. Other names for the condition are monilia and yeast infection.

Epidemiology

C. albicans is a fungal species that is responsible for 75 to 85 percent of infections. *C. tropicalis* and *C. glabrata* are responsible for the remainder of infections. As many as 75 percent of women will experience at least one episode of VVC during their lifetime; 40 to 50 percent of women will experience two or more infections (CDC, 2010a). The organism gains access to the vaginal mucosa primarily from the perianal area.

C. albicans can be transmitted from infected mother to newborn at delivery. Neonates develop an oral infection known as thrush.

Subjective Data

VVC presents with vaginal itching, burning, and irritation. Dysuria (burning when urine hits the involved tissue) is common. Vaginal discharge, which may be scanty or profuse, is white and thick. Symptoms frequently worsen prior to menses. Most clients report an acute onset of symptoms that rapidly clear with treatment. A small subset of women experience persistent chronic infection that does not respond well to classic treatment. Around 3 to 6 percent of women will experience episodes of VVC occurring four or more times per year. This is termed recurrent VVC (RVVC) (CDC, 2010a) and current recommendations for care of these clients are noted at the end of this section.

Candida can be found in the vaginas of normal women, and differentiating between colonization and infection may be difficult (Rosenfeld, 2009).

Objective Data

Physical Examination. The vulva may be red and inflamed and edematous or appear normal. Excoriations may be present. Typically, a white discharge with the consistency of cottage cheese is adherent to the vaginal mucosa, which may also be inflamed and edematous. Odor is absent and the pH is normal.

Diagnostic Tests and Methods. Microscopic examination of vaginal solution diluted with saline (wet mount) or 10 percent KOH preparations will demonstrate hyphal forms or budding yeast cells in 50 to 70 percent of infected women. The test procedure involves mixing a sample of vaginal secretions with saline, covering with coverslip, and viewing under microscope. A wet mount prepared with 10 percent KOH will obliterate cellular material so that yeasts may be seen more easily.

Some cases of VVC are not detected in a wet mount because there are relatively few organisms or because of poor smear technique. Additionally, nonalbicans species tend not to form pseudohyphae.

Focus client teaching on explaining that immediate diagnosis is possible.

- *Vaginal culture:* Although routine culture is not cost-effective, cultures may be helpful in RVVC. Cultures are prepared by placing a sample of vaginal secretions on Nickerson's medium or Sabouraud's agar. Accurate culture is only possible using the appropriate medium. Advise the client that the yeast culture is the most sensitive test but results take up to 72 hours to obtain.

Differential Medical Diagnoses

Bacterial vaginosis, trichomonas, allergic contact dermatitis, pediculosis pubis.

Plan

Psychosocial Interventions. Advise the client that infection is not sexually transmitted and treatment of her partner is unnecessary unless pruritic balanitis is present in her partner. Rigorous, immediate treatment in pregnancy is recommended to avoid neonatal thrush. Women with chronic moniliasis need intensive counseling to cope with discomfort and long-term medication regimens. Often chronic infection leads to chronic dyspareunia, which can stress relationships. Advise clients to wear cotton underwear, avoid tight fitting nylons and slacks, wipe the perineum from front to back, and use mild soaps. Douching should be avoided. Clients should be advised that topical vaginal creams or ointments formulated with petrolatum will weaken latex; latex condoms and diaphragms may not be reliable if used within 72 hours of treatment.

Medication. Many effective topical azole drugs are available over the counter (OTC). Self-treatment with OTC medications should be reserved for women who have been previously diagnosed with VVC and experience the same symptoms. Uncomplicated VVC (mild, sporadic symptoms in a normal host) will respond to short-term treatments. Women with severe or recurrent symptoms, women with uncontrolled diabetes, or women who are immunosuppressed should be treated for 7 to 14 days (CDC, 2010a).

Miconazole (Monistat). 2 percent cream, 100 mg vaginal suppository, 200 mg vaginal suppository. Available OTC.

- *Indications:* Acute and chronic infections. Safe during pregnancy (category B).
- *Administration:* One applicator of 2 percent cream in vagina qhs for 7 nights, *or* one 100 mg vaginal suppository qhs for 7 nights, *or* one 200 mg suppository qhs for 3 nights (CDC, 2010a).
- *Side effects and adverse reactions:* Few reactions are reported. Occasional burning after application may occur.
- *Contraindications:* Known hypersensitivity to miconazole.
- *Anticipated outcomes on evaluation:* Symptoms will rapidly resolve. Routine test for cure (wet mount) is not recommended for acute infection but is advised with chronic recurrent vaginitis.
- *Client teaching and counseling:* Advise the client that medication is to be completed as prescribed. Symptoms often will abate before medication is finished, but it must be completed to avoid recurrence. Cream or suppositories should be inserted immediately before retiring or lying down. Some may leak out on arising. Panty liners are helpful during the daytime to prevent moist underwear. Avoid tampon use with cream or suppository because tampons absorb medication, interfering with delivery of the therapeutic dose.

Clotrimazole (Gyne-Lotrimin, Mycelex). 1 percent cream, 100 mg vaginal tablet (OTC), 500 mg vaginal tablet.

- *Indications:* Acute and chronic infections. Safe during pregnancy (category B).
- *Administration:* One applicator of 1 percent cream in vagina qhs for 7 to 14 nights, *or* one vaginal tablet qhs for 7 nights, *or* two vaginal tablets qhs for 3 nights, *or* one single 500 mg vaginal suppository once (CDC, 2010a).
- *Side effects and adverse reactions:* Same as miconazole.
- *Contraindications:* Known hypersensitivity to miconazole or clotrimazole.
- *Anticipated outcomes on evaluation:* Symptoms will rapidly resolve. Routine test for cure (wet mount) is not recommended for acute infection but is advised with chronic recurrent vaginitis.
- *Client teaching and counseling:* Same as miconazole.

Terconazole (Terazol). 0.4 or 0.8 percent vaginal cream; 80 mg vaginal suppository.

- *Indications:* Acute infection; suspected *C. tropicalis* and *C. glabrata* may respond better to terconazole than to miconazole or clotrimazole. Not recommended in pregnancy (category C).
- *Administration:* One applicator of 0.4 percent cream intravaginally qhs for 7 days, *or* one application of 0.8 percent cream intravaginally qhs for 3 days, *or* one vaginal suppository qhs for 3 days (CDC, 2010a).
- *Side effects and adverse reactions:* Same as miconazole.
- *Contraindications:* Same as miconazole.
- *Anticipated outcomes on evaluation:* Same as miconazole.
- *Client teaching and counseling:* Same as miconazole.

Fluconazole (Diflucan). 150 mg oral tablet.

- *Indications:* Acute infection with *Candida* (not recommended for noncandidal species) for clients who prefer not to use topical vaginal medications. Not recommended in pregnancy (pregnancy category C).

- *Administration:* One 150 mg oral tablet.
- *Side effects and adverse reactions:* Most common side effects include headache, nausea, and abdominal pain. Hepatic toxicity has been associated with azole antifungals (not dose related) (*Mosby's drug consult*, 2007).
- *Contraindications:* Hypersensitivity to fluconazole. There is no information related to cross hypersensitivity between fluconazole and other azoles. Avoid with other hepatoxic drugs.
- *Drug interactions:* Clinically significant hypoglycemia may be precipitated by the use of Diflucan with oral hypoglycemic agents. Prothrombin time may be increased in patients receiving fluconazole with coumarin-type anticoagulants. Diflucan increases the plasma levels of Dilantin, cyclosporin, and theophylline. Rifampin enhances the metabolism of fluconazole (may require increased dose of Diflucan when given with rifampin). Fluconazole may inhibit the metabolism of ethinyl estradiol and levonorgestrel. The clinical significance of these effects is unknown (*Mosby's drug consult*, 2007).
- *Anticipated outcomes on evaluation:* Symptoms will improve.
- *Client teaching and counseling:* Client should be advised of possible drug interactions.

Ketoconazole (Nizoral). 200 mg oral tablet.

- *Indications:* Should be reserved for long-term suppression of chronic infection with *C. albicans* (resistance, however, has been associated with chronic use).
- *Administration:* Suppressive therapy—one tablet po daily for 6 months (CDC, 2010a).
- *Side effects and adverse reactions:* Hepatotoxic—monitor hepatic function before and during treatment.
- *Contraindications:* Known sensitivity to ketoconazole. Hepatic dysfunction. Pregnancy category C.
- *Drug interactions:* Potentiates triazolam, midazolam, possibly oral anticoagulants, and oral hypoglycemics. Avoid antacids, anticholinergics, and H2 blockers within 2 hours of ketoconazole. Avoid rifampin, isoniazid. Monitor digoxin, phenytoin, cyclosporine, and tacrolimus. Caution with other hepatically metabolized drugs (Clinical Pharmacology Online, 2010).
- *Anticipated outcomes on evaluation:* Symptoms will improve.
- *Client teaching and counseling:* Once long-term therapy is completed, rebound infection may result. Oral absorption may be impaired by antacids, cimetidine, or rifampin.

Other Medications. Other intravaginal formulations that may be used include butoconazole 2 percent cream qd for 3 days or tioconazole 6.5 percent ointment once intravaginally in one single dose (now available OTC) (CDC, 2010). Both are pregnancy category C.

Nontraditional Interventions. Boric acid 600 mg in size 0 gelatin capsules inserted into the vagina nightly for 5 days has been reported to be effective, but should be avoided in pregnancy. Boric acid has not gained widespread acceptance, perhaps because so many other preparations are readily available and it usually has to be obtained from a compounding pharmacy (De Seta, Schmidt, Vu, Essman, & Larsen, 2008).

Follow-Up and Referral

Clients with simple, acute candidiasis do not require a follow-up visit.

Recurrent Vulvovaginal Candidiasis. RVVC is usually defined as four or more episodes of symptomatic VVC in 1 year and affects a small percentage of women (< 5), according to the CDC (2010a). The pathogenesis of RVVC is poorly understood, and the majority of women with RVVC have no apparent predisposing or underlying conditions. Vaginal cultures should be obtained from patients with RVVC to confirm the clinical diagnosis and to identify unusual species, including nonalbicans species, particularly *C. glabrata* (does not form pseudohyphae or hyphae and is not easily recognized on microscopy). *C. glabrata* and other nonalbicans *Candida* species are observed in 10 to 20 percent of patients with RVVC. Conventional antimycotic therapies are not as effective against these species as against *C. albicans*.

Medication. Each individual episode of RVVC caused by *C. albicans* responds well to short duration oral or topical azole therapy. However, to maintain clinical and mycologic control, some specialists recommend a longer duration of initial therapy (e.g., 7–14 days of topical therapy or a 100 mg, 150 mg, or 200 mg oral dose of fluconazole every third day for a total of three doses [day 1, 4, and 7] to attempt mycologic remission before initiating a maintenance antifungal regimen).

Oral fluconazole (i.e., 100 mg, 150 mg, or 200 mg dose) weekly for 6 months is the first line of treatment. If this regimen is not feasible, some specialists recommend topical clotrimazole 200 mg twice a week, clotrimazole (500 mg dose vaginal suppositories once weekly), or other topical treatments used intermittently.

In addition, long-term use of topical and oral antifungal drugs have significant adverse effects including local irritation and pain, hepatotoxicity, interactions with some contraceptives, and oral hypoglycemic agents (Mehta, Ozick, & Gbadehan, 2010).

Suppressive maintenance antifungal therapies are effective in reducing RVVC. However, 30 to 50 percent of women will have recurrent disease after maintenance therapy is discontinued. Routine treatment of sex partners is controversial. *C. albicans* azole resistance is rare in vaginal isolates, and susceptibility testing is usually not warranted for individual treatment guidance (CDC, 2010a).

A vaccine against RVVC caused by the pathogenic form of *C. albicans* indicated for women with a history of RVVC is now in phase I of clinical trials. Preliminary phase I data shows immunogenicity in humans even at low dose (Pevion, 2010).

TRICHOMONIASIS

In this common form of vaginitis, women may be markedly symptomatic or asymptomatic. Men are asymptomatic carriers. Although this infection is localized, there is increased incidence of premature delivery and postpartum endometritis in women infected with *Trichomonas vaginalis* (CDC, 2010a).

Epidemiology

T. vaginalis, a flagellated, anaerobic protozoan, is the causative organism. Sexual contact is the primary means of transmission. Although nonsexual transmission via fomites is theoretically possible, clinically it is rare. The organism lives in the vagina, urethra, Bartholin's, and Skene's glands in women and in the urethra and prostate gland of men. It is transmitted during vaginal-penile intercourse, and transmission rates are high. There is no finite incubation period. The prevalence of *T. vaginalis* infection in the United States is estimated to be 2.3 million (3.1%) among women ages 14 to 49. It is more common among African American women than white or Mexican American women (Sutton et al., 2007).

Prevalence is highest in STD clinics and lowest in the private sector.

Subjective Data

Foul-smelling, yellow-green, frothy vaginal discharge may be profuse or scanty. Vaginal odor is the primary presenting symptom. Infrequently, women report dyspareunia and dysuria. However, some women have minimal or no symptoms. Rarely, men have symptoms of urethritis or prostatitis.

Objective Data

Physical Examination. Infection is often detected on routine examination in the absence of subjective complaints. In addition to discharge as previously described, physical examination reveals vulvar erythema and edema and occasionally petechial lesions on the cervix (sometimes called "strawberry cervix"). The pH will be elevated. Signs and symptoms alone are insufficient to make the diagnosis.

Diagnostic Tests and Methods. A culture is the most sensitive and specific diagnostic method, but it is expensive and not widely available. Wet mount using saline is the most clinically useful test. Diagnosis is made when a motile flagellated trichomonad is visualized. In addition, an increased number of white blood cells may be evident in the wet mount. Pap smear results often include reporting of trichomonads, but the sensitivity of the method is low (65%).

Differential Medical Diagnoses

Bacterial vaginosis, candidiasis, foreign body vaginitis.

Plan

Psychosocial Interventions. The client may experience anxiety and fear with the knowledge that trichomoniasis is sexually transmitted. Reassure her that the infection is curable. Counseling should include the need to treat male partners.

Medication

Metronidazole

- *Indications:* Symptomatic and asymptomatic clients and partners; it is the drug of choice for *Trichomonas* infection.
- *Administration:* Metronidazole 2 g po, in a single dose for both partners. If treatment fails, nonpregnant clients should be retreated with metronidazole 500 mg bid for 7 days. Symptomatic pregnant women should be treated with 2 g orally in a single dose (CDC, 2010a). Data on the treatment of pregnant women with trichomoniasis who fail on the 2 g dose is not clearly stated by the CDC. Consultation is advised with a specialist.

- *Side effects and adverse reactions:* Avoid alcohol during and for 3 days after use. May potentiate oral anticoagulants, phenytoin, and lithium. Antagonized by phenytoin, phenobarbital, and other hepatic enzyme inducers. Potentiated by cimetidine. Use reduced dose in hepatic disease. Rare seizures, peripheral neuropathy, pancreatitis (Clinical Pharmacology Online, 2010). Transient nausea and a metallic taste have also been reported. Because metronidazole has a broad antimicrobial spectrum, normal vaginal flora may be suppressed with subsequent candidal infection.
- *Contraindications:* Known allergy to metronidazole.
- *Anticipated outcomes on evaluation:* Symptoms clear rapidly after treatment. A test for cure is not routinely indicated.
- *Client teaching and counseling:* Stress the need to avoid alcohol 24 hours before and 72 hours after treatment. If symptoms return, reexamination is indicated. Routine treatment of the sexual partner is recommended, and the client should be sexually abstinent or use condoms until her partner is treated.

CERVICITIS

Although many sexually transmitted pathogens may gain entry through the vagina, vulva, or cervix, infections characterized by cervicitis primarily use the cervix as a portal of entry. Thus, barrier methods such as condoms and diaphragms are particularly effective in the prevention of cervicitis. Clinical syndromes characterized by cervicitis are considered when mucoid or purulent discharge is observed in the cervical os or when cervical bleeding can be easily induced. Women with cervicitis may have vaginal discharge and dysuria, although many women with cervicitis (perhaps most) are asymptomatic.

CHLAMYDIA TRACHOMATIS INFECTIONS

C. trachomatis is the most common STD in the United States, with more than 1.2 million estimated new cases in 2009. Asymptomatic infection is common among both men and women. Men primarily develop urethritis. In women, chlamydia is associated with cervicitis, acute urethral syndrome, salpingitis, PID, infertility, and perihepatitis. Some women with apparently uncomplicated cervical infection have been shown to have subclinical upper reproductive tract infection. All women with chlamydia should be tested for gonorrhea before treatment is begun because both are reportable and a specific diagnosis may enhance partner notification and treatment (CDC, 2010a).

Newborns delivered to infected mothers may develop conjunctivitis or pneumonitis. In the adult population worldwide, chlamydia is the etiologic agent of trachoma, the leading cause of preventable blindness. Trachoma is not endemic to the United States, however.

Epidemiology

C. trachomatis is an obligate intracellular parasite that displays some bacterial properties and some viral properties. Unable to produce its own energy, it depends on the host for survival. Risk factors parallel those of gonorrhea. Transmission may be sexual, requiring direct contact with an infected individual, or it may be congenital, acquired at birth when delivery occurs through an infected birth canal. Transplacental transmission does not occur. The incubation period is 10 to 30 days.

The infection is particularly prevalent among adolescents and young adults, so testing sexually active adolescent women should be routine during gynecologic examination. If the availability of chlamydial testing is limited, priority should be given to screening adolescents, high-risk pregnant women, and those with multiple sexual partners. See Chapter 3 for the proper sequencing of the Pap smear and chlamydia/gonorrhea tests. Women using oral contraceptives have been found to be at increased risk for chlamydia, possibly because oral contraceptive–induced ectopy exposes more susceptible cells to infection (Neinstein, Gordon, Katzman, Rosen, & Woods 2007).

Incidence ranges from 3 to 5 percent among asymptomatic women and 20 percent among women attending STD clinics.

Subjective Data

Women may be asymptomatic. Subjective symptoms are similar to those seen with gonorrhea and relate to the site of infection. They include vaginal discharge, pelvic pain (dull or severe), fever, and dysuria (frequency and urgency). Men may report a penile discharge and burning with urination.

Objective Data

Physical Examination. The physical examination may reveal nothing abnormal, or the cervix may show mucopurulent discharge, hypertrophic ectopy, and friability.

There may be mild to severe adnexal tenderness and/or cervical motion tenderness.

Diagnostic Tests and Methods. A wet mount of the discharge may show numerous white blood cells but also may be negative in the presence of infection. Urine culture may be sterile in the presence of urinary symptoms.

Selection of a diagnostic test for chlamydia depends on availability, local expertise, and prevalence of chlamydia in the test population. Nucleic acid detection assays and ligase chain reaction assays are more sensitive than culture or antigen tests. Explain to the client that minor discomfort may occur with endocervical sampling. Testing first-void urine specimens has shown that amplification tests are as sensitive as test with endocervical swabs. Excess secretions should be removed prior to endocervical sampling to ensure that cellular material is obtained for testing (CDC, 2010a).

Differential Medical Diagnoses

Gonorrhea, mucopurulent cervicitis (MPC), salpingitis, PID.

Plan

Psychosocial Interventions. Encourage clients to have chlamydia screening if they are in a risk group. Those with multiple partners or a new sexual partner are especially at risk. Partners of individuals diagnosed with chlamydia should be tested and treated; if testing is unavailable, the partners should be treated presumptively. High-risk pregnant women need screening and treatment to prevent congenital transmission. Individuals with chlamydia should be tested for other STDs because of the high rate of concurrent disease. Instruct the client that all medication must be taken. Partners should be treated concurrently and should abstain from intercourse until the treatment is completed.

Medication

Azithromycin

- *Indications:* Treatment of uncomplicated urethral, endocervical, and rectal infections in women and men. Useful if compliance may be a problem. Expense must be considered.
- *Administration:* 1 g once po (CDC, 2010a).
- *Side effects and adverse reactions:* GI side effects, photosensitivity, and overgrowth of vaginal candida are common; hepatic changes (cholestatic jaundice), renal changes, headache, dizziness, rash, and angioedema are less common. Caution should be used in patients with impaired hepatic function. Although not reported with azithromycin, the following reactions/interactions have been observed with other macrolides: ventricular arrhythmias; increased serum levels of theophylline; increased anticoagulant effects with coumarins; elevated digoxin levels; elevated ergot levels; increased pharmacologic effect of triazolam; and elevated levels of Dilantin, carbamazepine, cyclosporine, and hexobarbital. Because of the long half-life of azithromycin, allergic reactions may be persistent and should be carefully monitored.
- *Contraindications:* Sensitivity to macrolides. Clinical experience and preliminary data suggests that azithromycin is safe and effective although efficacy and safety data in pregnancy and lactation is not fully established (CDC, 2010a).
- *Anticipated outcomes on evaluation:* Test of cure unnecessary.

Erythromycin

- *Indications:* Chlamydial infection during pregnancy.
- *Administration:* 500 mg po qid for 7 days (CDC, 2010a).
- *Side effects and adverse reactions:* GI distress.
- *Contraindications:* Sensitivity to erythromycin.
- *Anticipated outcomes on evaluation:* Because experience in treating with erythromycin is limited, a test for cure 3 weeks after completion of medication is recommended. Retesting should be done at 3 weeks to allow time for antigen to clear.
- *Follow-up and referral:* Necessary only if the client was nonresponsive to the medication.

Doxycycline

- *Indications:* Treatment of uncomplicated urethral, endocervical, and rectal infections in women and men.
- *Administration:* Doxycycline 100 mg po bid for 7 days (CDC, 2010a). Avoid antacids during treatment.
- *Side effects and adverse reactions:* GI upset, rash, photosensitivity. Overgrowth of vaginal candida.
- *Contraindications:* Known pregnancy, sensitivity to tetracyclines. Not for use in children.
- *Anticipated outcomes on evaluation:* Antimicrobial resistance to this treatment has not been observed. Provided that treatment is completed, test for cure is not recommended.

Other Medications. Ofloxacin 300 mg po bid for 7 days has been recommended by the CDC (2010a), but is expensive and cannot be used in pregnancy or with adolescents age 17 years and under.

GONORRHEA

Gonorrhea, the second most commonly reported notifiable disease, is a cause of cervicitis, urethritis, and PID in women. *Neisseria gonorrhoeae* is becoming more complicated to treat due to its ability to develop antimicrobial resistance. Rectal transmission is common with anal intercourse, and pharyngeal transmission with oral sex is possible but rare. Gonorrhea can be transmitted during birth and cause conjunctivitis and blindness in neonates. Other rare manifestations of gonorrhea include arthritis, meningitis, perihepatitis, and disseminated gonococcal infection. In pregnancy, gonorrhea has been associated with chorioamnionitis, premature labor, premature rupture of membranes, and postpartum endometritis.

Epidemiology

In 2009, a total of 301,174 cases of gonorrhea were reported (CDC, 2010a). The causative agent is *N. gonorrhoeae*, a gram-negative intracellular diplococcus. Risk factors include low socioeconomic status, urban residency, nonmarried status, and multiple sexual partners. Infection rates in African Americans are over 20 times higher than those in whites. More females are now diagnosed yearly than males, however the number of cases among both sexes have been decreasing since 2005. Often, gonorrhea and chlamydia coexist (CDC, 2010a). This finding has led to the recommendation that patients treated for gonococcal infection also be treated routinely with a regimen that is effective against uncomplicated genital *C. trachomatis* infection (Newman, Moran, & Workowski, 2007). Direct sexual contact with mucosal surfaces of an infected individual is required for the transmission of gonorrhea. Although the organism has been recovered from inanimate objects artificially inoculated with the bacteria, there is no evidence that natural transmission occurs this way. The incubation period is 3 to 7 days.

Subjective Data

Among women, asymptomatic infection can be present in the urethra, endocervix, rectum, or pharynx. Symptoms may include vaginal discharge, pelvic pain, fever, menstrual irregularities, and dysuria.

Objective Data

Physical Examination. The examination may be normal. Some women exhibit MPC, erythema, and friability of the endocervix. Bartholin's abscess is infrequent. Other infections, among them chlamydia, trichomonas, monilia, and herpes, are frequently seen with gonorrhea and may confound the clinical picture.

Diagnostic Tests and Methods. Although gram stains showing intracellular gram-negative diplococci are reliable in males with gonorrhea, gram stains are not reliable in females. Culture, nucleic acid hybridization tests, and nucleic acid amplification tests are available for the detection of genitourinary infection with *N. gonorrhoeae* (CDC, 2010a). Specimens may be obtained with endocervical swabs or with first-void urine samples.

Guidelines for the laboratory agnosis of gonorrhea, chlamydia, and syphilis are available at http://www.aphl.org/aphlprograms/infectious/std/Pages/stdtestingguidelines.aspx.

Differential Medical Diagnoses

C. trachomatis infection, MPC.

Plan

Psychosocial Interventions. Advise the client that persons with untreated gonorrhea risk the development of PID and subsequent infertility. Sexual partners must be treated concurrently and abstain from intercourse during their treatment. With appropriate treatment gonorrhea is curable. Clients must be checked for other STDs before treatment, especially chlamydia and syphilis, as multiple infections are common. Pregnant clients should be screened at the first prenatal visit, and those at high risk should be rescreened in the third trimester.

Medication. CDC (2010a) recommends that persons treated for gonorrhea also be treated routinely with a regimen effective against uncomplicated C. trachomatis infection if chlamydia has not been ruled out. Due to increasing antimicrobial resistance, only one class of antimicrobials, the cephalosporins, is recommended and available for the treatment of gonorrhea in the United States (Newman et al., 2007). Effective drugs for chlamydia include doxycycline 100 mg bid for 7 days or 1 g azithromycin orally. In pregnant women, doxycycline may not be used, but azithromycin 1 g orally may be given (see section on chlamydia).

Ceftriaxone

- *Indications:* This is the treatment of choice for uncomplicated urethral, endocervical, pharyngeal, and rectal infection.
- *Administration:* Ceftriaxone 250 mg IM once (CDC, 2010a). Ceftriaxone is the most effective drug for pharyngeal infection and anal infection in males.
- *Side effects and adverse reactions:* Although usually well tolerated, ceftriaxone has occasionally been associated with pain at injection site, diarrhea, rash, and headache. See discussions of chlamydia for more information about drugs for concurrent treatment of chlamydia.
- *Contraindications:* Known sensitivity to cephalosporins. Patients with a history of IgE-mediated allergic reactions to penicillin (e.g., anaphylaxis, angioneurotic edema, immediate urticaria) should not receive cephalosporin.
- *Anticipated outcomes on evaluation:* Treatment failure is rare. Test for cure with this regimen is not essential.
- *Client teaching and counseling:* Advise the client to complete all oral medication and report any drug intolerance. If symptoms recur, retesting is needed. Stress the need for the partner's treatment.

Other Medications. Other recommended regimens for uncomplicated urogenital or rectal gonococcal infections in adults include cefixime 400 mg po in a single dose. Azithromycin 2 g orally is effective against uncomplicated gonococcal infection but concerns over the ease with which *N. gonorrhoeae* can develop resistance to macrolides should restrict its use to limited circumstances (CDC, 2010a).

MUCOPURULENT CERVICITIS

In about half of women with mucopurulent discharge, the diagnosis cannot be established. MPC is a syndrome with symptoms including this discharge and other inflammatory signs such as a friable cervix. Although *Ureaplasma urealyticum* and *Mycoplasma hominis* testing is not done routinely, these organisms have been recovered in women with nongonococcal/nonchlamydial MPC and in women with chronic-voiding symptoms. A finding of leukorrhea (>10 WBC per high-power field on microscopic examination of vaginal fluid) has been associated with chlamydial and gonococcal infection of the cervix. In the absence of inflammatory vaginitis, leukorrhea might be a sensitive indicator of cervical inflammation with a high negative predictive value (Lusk & Konecny, 2008).

Epidemiology

Ureaplasma urealyticum and *Mycoplasma hominis* are bacterial organisms that are sexually transmitted in adults. Colonization in infants may occur through an infected birth canal, although disease rarely results and colonization does not persist. The incidence of genital mycoplasma infections is unknown, but it is believed to be common. Infection is more common among low socioeconomic groups and minorities.

Subjective Data

May be asymptomatic or may present with dysuria, vaginal discharge, abnormal vaginal bleeding, and/or abdominal pain. Mycoplasma/ureaplasma infection may also be suspected in women who present with infertility or recurrent miscarriages.

Objective Data

Physical Examination. MPC is characterized by a yellow endocervical exudate visible in the endocervical canal or in an endocervical swab specimen (the yellow color of the exudate is apparent when contrasted with the white swab).

Diagnostic Tests and Methods. Tests for chlamydia, gonorrhea will be negative. Wet prep will contain many white blood cells, but no candida or trichomonads.

Culture. MPC may be treated empirically by many clinicians; however, confirmation of the diagnosis may be made by vaginal culture. Culture is particularly important when the client has infertility or recurrent miscarriage. The test procedure is to do a vaginal culture, which is better than an endocervical culture. An adequate sample from the vagina is necessary to enhance the yield. Obtain the specimens, place them immediately in medium, and transport them to the lab as soon as possible. Keep specimens refrigerated. Explain the procedure to the client.

Differential Medical Diagnoses

C. trachomatis infection, gonorrhea.

Plan

Psychosocial Interventions. Explain to the client the widespread nonspecific nature of genital mycoplasmas and the difficulty in establishing a definitive diagnosis. Partners should be treated empirically.

Medication. Consider empiric treatment for gonorrhea *and* chlamydia. Medications effective for chlamydia are also effective for ureaplasma and mycoplasma. Doxycycline 100 mg bid for 7 days (see chlamydia treatment for prescribing details) (CDC, 2010a). Azithromycin 1 g orally as a single dose (some ureaplasma strains are resistant to tetracyclines) (Sendag, Terek, Tuncay, Ozkinay, & Guven, 2000). May be used in pregnancy (see chlamydia treatment for prescribing cautions). Ofloxacin 300 mg bid for 7 days (treatment is expensive, but also effective for resistant strains) (CDC, 2010a). Should not be used in pregnancy or with adolescents under age 18.

ULCERATIVE GENITAL INFECTIONS

In the United States, most young, sexually active persons with genital and/or perianal ulcers have either HSV or syphilis; however, genital herpes is more prevalent. Chancroid and donovanosis are less common causes of genital ulcers. These conditions can coexist with each other and may also be found in conjunction with yeast, trauma, carcinoma, fixed drug eruption, or psoriasis. Diagnosis based on history and physical alone is often inaccurate. All persons with suspected genital herpes infection should be tested for HIV and syphilis and, where prevalent, for *Haemophilus ducreyi* (CDC, 2010a). Specific tests for evaluation of genital or perianal ulcers include (1) syphilis serology and darkfield examination; (2) culture for HSV (polymerase chain reaction [PCR] testing for HSV is available from some laboratories, but is not FDA approved); and (3) serologic testing for type-specific HSV antibody. In addition, biopsy can help to identify the cause of ulcers that are unusual or that do not respond to initial treatment. Because syphilis management is very complex, clinicians unfamiliar with diagnostic and treatment protocols should seek consultation for questions related to diagnostic and treatment strategies. Consultation is also recommended if one of the rare bacterial ulcerative diseases is suspected.

HERPES SIMPLEX VIRUS

No cure is known for this recurring viral disease. HSV-1 commonly produces oral lesions, and HSV-2 commonly primarily produces genital lesions; however, HSV-1 is causing an increasing proportion of initial genital HSV episodes in young women and men who have sex with men (Ryder, Jin, McNulty, Grulich, & Donovan, 2009). Many persons infected with HSV have mild or unrecognized infections, but shed virus intermittently in the genital tract. Thus, the majority of genital herpes infections are transmitted by persons unaware that they have the infection or who are asymptomatic when transmission occurs. Recurrences and subclinical shedding are much less frequent for genital HSV-1 infection than for genital HSV-2 (Engelberg, Carrell, Krantz, et al., 2003). A patient's prognosis and the type of counseling needed depend on the type of genital herpes (HSV-1 or HSV-2) causing the infection; therefore, the clinical diagnosis of genital herpes should be confirmed by laboratory testing (Scoular, 2002).

Characteristic painful lesions can occur in the mouth and genitalia of men and women, although virtually any skin or mucous membrane is vulnerable. Neonates who contract the virus congenitally develop infection of the central nervous system (CNS) and eyes. Significant perinatal morbidity and mortality are associated with congenital herpes simplex. Persons who are immunosuppressed are at risk for disseminated HSV, which often presents as meningitis/encephalitis. Once it enters the body, the herpes virus never leaves, although clinical manifestations disappear as the virus becomes dormant in sensory ganglia. When recurrence is triggered, the virus travels from nerve roots to the skin surface, where lesions develop. Reactivation of the virus is triggered by local or systemic stimuli such as trauma, fever, menstruation, ultraviolet light, and emotional stress (McKenzie, 2001).

Epidemiology

Herpes simplex virus is transmitted primarily by direct contact with an infected individual who is shedding the virus. At least 50 million persons in the United States are infected with HSV-2 (Xu, Sternberg, Kottiri, et al., 2006). Kissing, sexual contact, and vaginal delivery are means of transmission. Primary herpes in pregnancy may be passed to the neonate transplacentally or at birth. Autoinoculation is possible.

Most mothers of infants who acquire neonatal herpes do not have clinically evident genital herpes. The risk of vertical transmission is high among women who acquire genital herpes near the time of delivery (30–50%) and low among women with histories of recurrent herpes at term or who acquire herpes during the first half of pregnancy (1%) (Brown, Wald, Morrow, et al., 2003). The incubation period of HSV is 2 to 7 days.

Subjective Data

Primary herpes causes a prolonged clinical illness characterized by multiple painful vesicular lesions, fever, chills, malaise, and severe dysuria if the lesions are genital. Symptoms peak 4 to 5 days after onset and may last 2 to 3 weeks. *Recurrent herpes*, on the other hand, is a localized disease characterized by typical HSV lesions at the site of initial viral entry. Recurrent herpes lesions usually are fewer, are less painful, and resolve more rapidly than primary herpes lesions. Recurrent HSV lasts an average of 5 to 7 days, preceded by a prodromal symptom—frequently a burning, itching, or swelling sensation. Lesions will appear within 24 hours of prodrome.

Objective Data

Physical Examination. Characteristic lesions are visible on the vulva and/or cervix. They are vesicular, usually multiple, and exquisitely painful to touch. The vesicles will open and weep and finally crust over, dry, and disappear without scar formation. Clients with primary HSV may have low-grade fever and tender lymphadenopathy.

Diagnostic Tests and Methods

Virologic Tests. Cell culture and PCR are the preferred HSV tests for persons who seek medical treatment for genital ulcers or other mucocutaneous lesions. The sensitivity of viral culture is low, especially for recurrent lesions, and declines rapidly as lesions begin to heal. Viral culture isolates should be typed to determine which type of HSV is causing the infection (CDC, 2010a). The culture yield is best if the specimen is taken during the vesicular stage of disease; viral isolation is markedly reduced as lesions resolve. In primary episodes, viral shedding is prolonged and HSV more easily isolated. Failure to detect HSV by culture or PCR does not indicate an absence of HSV infection, because viral shedding is intermittent.

Advise the client that obtaining the culture will be painful because vigorous sampling is essential to collect adequate cells.

Serologic Testing for HSV Antibodies. Serologic testing (including recently developed point-of-care testing such as BioKit HSV-2) is sensitive, but not helpful for diagnosis of primary infection because of the delay in antibody development. Type-specific serologic testing may be particularly useful in symptomatic persons with negative HSV cultures or in the evaluation of a person whose sexual partner has genital herpes. Both type-specific and nontype-specific antibodies to HSV develop during the first several weeks after infection and persist indefinitely. Type-specific glycoprotein G (gG)-based assays should be requested because older assays cannot reliably distinguish HSV-1 from HSV-2 antibodies. Because nearly all HSV-2 infections are sexually acquired, the presence of type-specific HSV-2 antibodies implies anogenital infection. The presence of HSV-1 antibody alone is more difficult to interpret (CDC, 2010a).

Differential Medical Diagnoses

Primary syphilis, mucocutaneous manifestations of Crohn's disease, Behçet's syndrome, chancroid, LGV.

Plan

Psychosocial Interventions. Clients diagnosed with herpes require extensive counseling to understand the complex nature of the disease and its ramifications. Support groups may be helpful. Advise clients to abstain from intercourse during the prodrome and when lesions are present in any stage. Consistent condom use may reduce transmission rates. In addition, clients must know to wash their hands after touching lesions to avoid autoinoculation. Risk of acquiring HIV is higher in HSV-2 seropositive persons (CDC, 2010a). Clients with a history of genital HSV should know to advise their care provider of this history if they become pregnant.

There is no evidence that HSV causes cervical cancer. Clients with genital HSV, both primary and recurrent, will benefit from comfort measures such as nonconstricting clothes, lukewarm sitz baths, and air drying of lesions with a handheld hair dryer on medium setting. Clients with severe dysuria may benefit by urinating in water. Extremes of temperature such as ice packs or heating pads should be avoided, as should steroid creams, anesthetic sprays, and any type of lotion or gel (e.g., petroleum jelly).

Management of HSV in Pregnancy. Pregnant women should be asked whether they or their partners have had genital herpes lesions. Suspicious or recurrent lesions should be cultured to document HSV or a type-specific serologic test should be used.

The risk of herpes is high in infants of women who acquire genital HSV in late pregnancy; such women should be managed in consultation with an infectious disease specialist. At onset of labor, women with a history of recurrent HSV should be questioned about symptoms of genital herpes, including prodrome, and all women should be examined carefully for herpetic lesions. Women without symptoms or signs of genital herpes or its prodrome can deliver vaginally (CDC, 2010a). Women with genital herpes lesions at the onset of labor should deliver by cesarean section, although this does not eliminate risk.

Although the safety of antivirals in pregnant women has not been definitively established, available data does not indicate an increased risk of major birth defects in women treated with acyclovir during the first trimester (Stone, Reiff-Eldridge, White, et al., 2004). However, data related to prenatal exposure to valacyclovir and famciclovir is too limited to provide useful information on pregnancy outcomes (CDC, 2010a). Acyclovir can be administered orally to pregnant women with initial or recurrent genital herpes, and given late in pregnancy, reduces the frequency of recurrences at term (Sheffield, Hollier, Hill, Stuart, & Wendel, 2003).

Antiviral Therapy. Antiviral therapy is beneficial for most symptomatic patients and is the mainstay of therapy. Randomized trials have demonstrated the efficacy of three systemic drugs for genital herpes: acyclovir, valacyclovir, and famciclovir. Valacyclovir and famciclovir have enhanced oral absorption. Topical therapy with antiviral drugs offers minimal benefit (CDC, 2010a). Systemic antiviral drugs can partially control the signs and symptoms of HSV for initial episodes, recurrent episodes, or when used as daily suppressive treatment for patients with frequent recurrences of HSV-2. Suppressive therapy reduces the frequency of recurrent HSV by 70 to 80 percent. Safety and efficacy have been documented among those receiving daily acyclovir for as long as 6 years, and with valacyclovir and famciclovir for 1 year (Fife, Crumpacker, Mertz, Hill, & Boone, 1994). However, these drugs neither eradicate a latent virus nor affect the risk, frequency, or severity of recurrences after the drug is discontinued. The dosage of all antiviral drugs should be adjusted in patients with reduced creatinine clearance. When using antivirals for recurrent symptoms, they should be instituted as soon as the patient notices prodromal symptoms. Doses for different indications follow the general description.

- *Indications:* Primary herpes infection and recurrent disease.
- *Administration:* See specific indications.
- *Side effects and adverse reactions:* These are minimal, even with long-term use. Nausea, vomiting, and headache have been reported, however. Clients on long-term suppression can expect a rebound recurrence when therapy is stopped.
- *Contraindications:* Known hypersensitivity.
- *Anticipated outcomes on evaluation:* Accelerated healing and shortened course of the disease.
- *Client teaching and counseling:* The goals of counseling are to help patients cope with the infection and prevention of sexual and perinatal transmission. Patients with a first episode of genital herpes should be advised that suppressive therapy is available and effective in suppressing recurrent episodes and episodic treatment will shorten their duration. All infected persons should know about the potential for recurrent episodes, asymptomatic viral shedding, and the risks this poses for sexual transmission. Patients should abstain from sexual activity with uninfected partners when lesions or prodromal symptoms are present. Consistent use of latex condoms may reduce the risk of HSV transmission (Martin, Krantz, Gottlieb et al., 2009). Advise the client that short courses of antivirals neither eradicate HSV nor have an impact on the subsequent risk and frequency of recurrences. Daily suppressive therapy reduces the frequency and severity of recurrences, but this effect does not persist after medication is discontinued.

Initial Episode

Note: Treatment can be extended if healing is incomplete after 10 days

Acyclovir 400 mg orally three times daily for 7 to 10 days

Or

Acyclovir 200 mg orally five times daily for 7 to 10 days

Or

Famciclovir 250 mg orally three times daily for 7 to 10 days

Or

Valacyclovir 1 g orally twice daily for 7 to 10 days

Episodic Therapy for Recurrent HSV

Acyclovir 400 mg orally three times daily for 5 days

Or

Acyclovir 800 mg orally twice daily for 5 days

Or

Acyclovir 800 mg three times daily for 5 days

Or

Famciclovir 125 mg orally twice daily for 5 days

Or

Famciclovir 1,000 mg twice daily for 1 day

Or

Famciclovir 500 mg once, followed by 250 mg twice daily for 2 days

Or

Valacyclovir 500 mg twice daily for 3 days

Or

Valacyclovir 1 g orally once daily for 5 days

Daily Suppressive Therapy

Acyclovir 400 mg orally twice daily

Or

Famciclovir 250 mg twice daily

Or

Valacyclovir 500 mg orally once daily (may be less effective in patients with very frequent episodes)

Or

Valacyclovir 1 g orally once daily

SYPHILIS

Syphilis is a systemic STD that can lead to serious illness and even death if untreated. Infection manifests in distinct stages with diverse clinical manifestations. The disease has been divided into three stages based on clinical findings that are used to guide treatment and follow-up. The presentation begins with *primary syphilis*, which is characterized by a chancre at the site of bacterial entry. *Secondary syphilis* is recognized by flulike symptoms and a maculopapular rash of the palms and soles. Following secondary syphilis, *latency* occurs. Ultimately *tertiary* (*late*) *syphilis* occurs, characterized by irreversible cardiovascular, neurologic, dermatologic, or bony disease.

Clients with any STD or genital ulcer should be evaluated for syphilis. All pregnant women should have a nontreponemal serologic test for syphilis at the first prenatal visit. Women suspected of being at risk for syphilis should have the test repeated during the third trimester and at delivery. Clients who have been exposed to syphilis within the preceding 3 months may be infected but seronegative and thus should be treated for early syphilis (CDC, 2010a). All clients who have syphilis should be tested for HIV.

Epidemiology

Treponema pallidum, a bacterium in the spirochete family, is the causative organism. Direct sexual contact (or, less frequently, blood contact) with an infected individual transmits the disease. The risk of developing syphilis after one unprotected contact is up to 50 percent (Jacobs, 2001). Because the initial anorectal or vaginal chancres are not likely to be noticed, syphilis is infrequently diagnosed in the primary stage among women or homosexuals. Transplacental transmission of an infected mother to her fetus is also possible. Untreated syphilis during pregnancy, especially early syphilis, can lead to stillbirth, neonatal death, bone deformities, or neurological impairment (CDC, 2010c). Long-standing untreated disease is less contagious than the primary or secondary stage; however, evaluation and treatment of sexual contacts is necessary. The incubation period is from 10 to 90 days (3 weeks average).

After persistent declines during 1992–2003, the rate among women increased from 0.8 cases in 2004 to 1.4 cases in 2009 (CDC, 2009a).

Subjective Data

- *Primary syphilis:* Client may be an asymptomatic contact or may report a lesion.
- *Secondary syphilis:* Low-grade fever, headache, sore throat, rash on the palms and soles.
- *Tertiary syphilis:* Cardiovascular symptoms (chest pain, cough), neurological symptoms (headache, irritability, impaired balance, memory loss, tremor), skeletal symptoms (arthritis, myalgia, myositis), or skin symptoms (multiple nodules or ulcers).
- *Congenital syphilis:* See Objective Data.

Objective Data

Physical Examination

- *Primary syphilis:* Classic chancre is a painless, rounded, indurated ulcer with serous exudate. It may be genital or extragenital. Usually a single chancre occurs, but multiple chancres may be present. An extragenital chancre is likely to be atypical in appearance. Lymphadenopathy, which may accompany the chancre, will resolve spontaneously in 3 to 6 weeks. Must be distinguished from genital herpes, chancroid, lymphogranuloma, or neoplasm.
- *Secondary syphilis:* Classic maculopapular rash that gradually covers the body, including the palms and soles. Less common signs include patchy alopecia, generalized nontender lymphadenopathy, mucosal ulcers, and condyloma lata (flat broad wartlike papules on warm, moist skin surfaces). Spontaneous healing of all secondary manifestations occurs. Must be distinguished from infectious exanthems, pityriasis rosea, and drug eruptions.
- *Tertiary syphilis:* Manifestations are dependent on whether the client has neurosyphilis, cardiovascular syphilis, or other expressions of the disease. Aortic

diastolic murmur, aneurysms, and congestive failure characterize cardiovascular syphilis; meningeal irritation, unequal reflexes, irregular pupils with poor light response, wide-based gait, and personality deterioration characterize neurosyphilis. Must be distinguished from neoplasms of the skin, liver, stomach, or brain; other forms of meningitis; and primary neurologic lesions.

- *Congenital syphilis:* Premature birth, intrauterine growth retardation, mucocutaneous lesions, snuffles (serous nasal discharge), hepatosplenomegaly, condyloma lata, skeletal lesions, CNS involvement, ocular lesions, and others.

Diagnostic Tests and Methods. Diagnosis is largely dependent on testing of primary and secondary lesion tissue and serology during latency and late infection. Direct tissue examination is definitive; diagnosis of syphilis using serologic testing is considered presumptive. The use of only one type of serologic test is insufficient for diagnosis because each type of test has limitations, including the possibility of false positive results (CDC, 2010a). Persons with a positive nontreponemal test should receive a treponemal test to confirm the diagnosis of syphilis.

Direct Tissue Examination. Diagnostic evaluation for definitive identification of *T. pallidum* is possible when lesions (e.g., chancre, rash) are present. If antibiotics have been taken, the tests are not useful. If darkfield microscopy is not available, an immunofluorescent staining technique is available for demonstrating *T. pallidum* in fluid taken from suspicious lesions, spread on slides, fixed appropriately, and mailed to a reference lab. Some laboratories offer locally developed PCR tests for the detection of *T. pallidum.*

The test procedure is first to cleanse the lesion with sterile saline. Then gently abrade to produce oozing of serous fluid. Avoid active bleeding. Collect serous fluid on a slide and fix as directed by the laboratory. Advise the client that the testing procedure is not uncomfortable, but results will have to be obtained from the laboratory.

Serological Tests (Nontreponemal). Diagnostic evaluation for antilipid antibodies produced by the host exposed to *T. pallidum*. Examples are Venereal Disease Research Laboratory (VDRL) and rapid plasma reagin (RPR). Both of these are valid tests, but quantitative results from the two tests cannot be compared directly. Used for syphilis screening and follow-up after treatment. Nontreponemal tests may be negative in latent syphilis; however, treponemal tests will still be positive (Ratnam, 2005). Nontreponemal tests usually decline after treatment (a fourfold decline in titer is considered significant) and are used to assess treatment response. However, these may remain positive for the person's lifetime. Most persons with positive treponemal tests will have reactive tests for their lifetimes, regardless of treatment of disease activity.

The test procedure is to collect a blood sample in a dry tube without anticoagulant. Advise the client that venipuncture is required. Results are reported as either reactive (positive) or nonreactive (negative). *Reactive results* are quantitated in the form of a titer. The false positive rate is 1 to 2 percent in the general population, higher in low-risk groups. False positive reactions are encountered in connective tissue diseases, mononucleosis, Lyme disease, and periodontal disease (APHL, 2009). False negative results may occur when high antibody levels are present. If syphilis is strongly suspected and the nontreponemal test is negative, the laboratory should be instructed to dilute the specimen to detect a positive reaction.

All reactive results require confirmation by the treponemal test (description follows). Tests become reactive 14 days after the chancre appears. If results are equivocal, repeat testing is indicated. A rising titer is evidence of primary syphilis. If syphilis is suspected and the initial nontreponemal test is nonreactive, repeat in 1 week, 1 month, and 3 months. *Nonreactive results* after 3 months exclude the diagnosis of syphilis.

Serological Tests (Treponemal). Diagnostic evaluation to detect *T. pallidum*–specific antibodies. These tests are designed to confirm the diagnosis of a reactive nontreponemal test. Fluorescent treponemal antibody-absorption (FTA-ABS) test, the *T. pallidum* passive particle agglutination (TP-PA) assay, various enzyme immunoassays (EIAs), and chemiluminescent immunoassays are all serological tests. The test procedure is to collect a blood sample in a dry tube without anticoagulant.

If treponemal tests are used for screening, a nontreponemal test should be performed reflexively by the laboratory to guide treatment decisions. If the nontreponemal test is negative, diagnosis should be confirmed with a different treponemal test. Treponemal tests are also used if symptoms of tertiary syphilis are present. The results are reported as reactive or nonreactive. Pregnant patients who are allergic to penicillin should be desensitized and treated with penicillin (CDC, 2010a). Final decisions about the significance of serologic test results must be based on a total clinical appraisal of risks.

Plan

Psychosocial Interventions. Extensive counseling and support are needed. Explain the complex nature of the disease and its ramifications. Case finding and treatment of sexual partners are essential to epidemic control but difficult when the relationship is associated with crack or cocaine use. Persons who were exposed within the 90 days preceding the diagnosis of primary, secondary, or early latent syphilis in a sex partner should be treated presumptively, even if seronegative (CDC, 2010a). The need must be stressed for follow-up testing to ensure adequate treatment. Explain the meaning of test results, especially rising or falling titers and persistent reactive results. Clients with serological evidence of syphilis in any stage are best treated by practitioners experienced in the management of this complex disease. Suggest HIV counseling and testing.

Medication. Parenteral penicillin G (Bicillin L-A) is the treatment of choice for all clients with syphilis and the only proven therapy for syphilis during pregnancy and for congenital syphilis. Penicillin prevents congenital syphilis in 90 percent of cases, even when given late in pregnancy (Jacobs, 2001). Pregnant women with syphilis of any stage who report penicillin allergy should be desensitized and treated with penicillin (CDC, 2010a).

Benzathine Penicillin G

- *Indications:* Primary and secondary syphilis and early latent syphilis of less than a year's duration.
- *Administration:* 2.4 million units IM in one dose. Clients with syphilis of greater than a year's duration (latent or tertiary stages) require weekly treatment with 2.4 million units of benzathine penicillin G for 3 weeks. Neurosyphilis (diagnosed by lumbar puncture) requires intravenous treatment (CDC, 2010a).
- *Side effects and adverse reactions:* Penicillin adverse effects include wheezing, weakness, abdominal pain, nausea or vomiting, diarrhea, rash, fever, increased thirst, and seizures. In addition, Jarisch-Herxheimer reaction, an acute febrile illness with headache and flulike symptoms, may occur a few hours after antibiotic administration. It is probably due to treponemal lysis and subsides within 24 hours. It may be severe. Antipyretics may be used to manage symptoms (CDC, 2010a).
- *Contraindications:* A known sensitivity to penicillin.
- *Anticipated outcomes on evaluation:* Clients treated for syphilis must be followed with a nontreponemal test at 3 and 6 months. Titers should fall fourfold by 6 months in those treated for primary and secondary syphilis (CDC, 2010a).
- *Client teaching and counseling:* Provide the client with information about the possibility of the Jarisch-Herxheimer reaction and its treatment—rest, fluids, and antipyretics. Stress the importance of follow-up testing. Clients allergic to penicillin may be treated with doxycycline, tetracycline, erythromycin, or ceftriaxone (not single dose). Specific protocols are recommended by the CDC (2010a).

CHANCROID

Chancroid is an STD characterized by painful genital ulceration. Lesions are usually confined to the genitals and accompanied by inguinal lymphadenopathy. Systemic illness does not occur. The prevalence of chancroid has declined in the United States and worldwide, although infection may still occur in parts of Africa and the Caribbean. Ten percent of patients with chancroid have coinfection with HSV and/or syphilis. An increased rate of HIV infection has also been associated with chancroid, so those with suspected chancroid should be tested for HIV (CDC, 2010a).

Epidemiology

H. ducreyi, a gram-negative bacillus, is the causative agent. The incubation period is 3 to 5 days. The condition occurs most commonly in uncircumcised males; incidence among women is low. Transmission is by direct contact with an infected individual. Fomite transmission does not occur.

Subjective Data

The initial lesion is a vesicopapule that breaks down to form a painful soft ulcer. Multiple lesions may develop, spread by autoinoculation. These may rupture spontaneously. Fever, malaise, and chills may also develop. Women may have nonspecific symptoms such as dysuria, vaginal discharge, and dyspareunia, or they may be asymptomatic.

Objective Data

Physical Examination. A characteristic ulcerative lesion is seen on the genitalia with a necrotic base and surrounding erythema. In over 50 percent of the cases, a bubo will be present (a greatly enlarged, inflamed lymph node). This unilateral inguinal adenitis is tender and the overlying skin is inflamed. Buboes may spontaneously rupture. One or two lesions are the norm, although more may occur.

Diagnostic Tests and Methods. A definitive diagnosis requires the identification of *H. ducreyi* on special media that is not widely available. However, presumptive diagnosis for clinical and surveillance purposes may be made in a patient who has a painful genital ulcer with a typical appearance for chancroid in combination with negative darkfield examination for syphilis, negative syphilis RPR, and negative HSV test (CDC, 2010a).

Differential Medical Diagnoses

Genital herpes, syphilis, granuloma inguinale.

Plan

Psychosocial Interventions. Advise the client that her sexual partners within the past 10 days need examination and treatment. Symptoms improve within 3 days; ulcers heal within 7 days. Buboes resolve more slowly and may require aspiration. Scarring can result in advanced cases.

Medication

Azithromycin

- *Indications:* Suspected or culture-proven chancroid. A presumptive diagnosis is made if the clinical picture is clear. Single dose facilitates compliance.
- *Administration:* One gram orally as a single dose (CDC, 2010a).
- *Side effects and adverse reactions:* GI distress, rare angioedema, and cholestatic jaundice. Caution should be used in patients with impaired hepatic function. See also side effects listed under chlamydia.
- *Contraindications:* Known hypersensitivity to any macrolide drug.
- *Anticipated outcomes on evaluation:* Ulcerative lesions resolve.

Ceftriaxone

- *Indications:* Suspected or culture-proven chancroid. A presumptive diagnosis is made if the clinical picture is clear. Single dose facilitates compliance.
- *Administration:* 250 mg IM (CDC, 2010a).
- *Side effects and adverse reactions:* Although usually well tolerated, ceftriaxone is occasionally associated with pain at the injection site, diarrhea, rash, and headache.
- *Contraindications:* Known sensitivity to cephalosporins. Use with caution for clients sensitive to penicillin.
- *Anticipated outcomes on evaluation:* Treatment failure is rare. Test for cure with this regimen is not essential.

Erythromycin Base

- *Indications:* Suspected or culture-proven chancroid. A presumptive diagnosis is made if the clinical picture is clear.
- *Administration:* 500 mg po tid for 7 days (CDC, 2010a).
- *Side effects and adverse reactions:* GI distress. (See Azithromycin under chlamydia treatment for drug reactions/interactions that have been reported with macrolides.)
- *Contraindications:* Known hypersensitivity to erythromycin. Concomitant use of ketoconazole (Nizoral).
- *Anticipated outcomes on evaluation:* Ulcerative lesions resolve.
- *Client teaching and counseling:* Azithromycin must be taken 1 hour before or 2 hours after a meal. It should not be taken with food. If no improvement occurs within 2 to 3 days, diagnosis must be reconsidered. Infection with other STDs, including HIV, may also exist. Partners should be treated.

Treatment

Azithromycin 1 g orally in a single dose

Or

Ceftriaxone 250 mg IM (single dose)

Or

Ciprofloxacin 500 mg orally twice daily for 3 days

Or

Erythromycin base 500 mg orally three times daily for 7 days

Other Medications. Ciprofloxacin 500 mg po bid for 3 days (CDC, 2010a). With the exception of ciprofloxacin, which is contraindicated for pregnant and lactating women and children under 17, all of the regimens listed may be used in pregnancy.

Follow-Up/Referral

Only if nonresponsive to drug treatment.

GRANULOMA INGUINALE

A chronic, progressive bacterial infection of the genitals, granuloma inguinale presents with large, unsightly ulcers of the genitalia, inguinal region, and anus. Other names for the condition are donovanosis and granuloma venereum. Because other STDs frequently coexist, cultures for these and serological tests for syphilis and HIV must be performed.

Epidemiology

Calymmatobacterium granulomatis, a gram-negative bacterium, is the causative agent. Anal intercourse, often associated with homosexuality, is a particular risk factor. Transmission is by sexual or nonsexual trauma to infected sites, primarily the anus and penis. The disease is mildly contagious; repeated exposures are needed in order for clinical manifestations to develop. The incubation period is 8 days to 12 weeks (Schwartz, 2011).

Rarely reported in the United States, granuloma inguinale is epidemic in parts of Australia and common in India and many tropical and subtropical environments. Donovan bodies (bacteria encapsulated in mononuclear leukocytes) are found in tissue scrapings that are stained with Wright's stain.

Subjective Data

The disorder often begins as a papule, which then ulcerates, leaving a beefy-red, relatively painless granular area with sharply defined rolled edges. The ulcer is persistent, and satellite ulcers may unite to form a large ulcer. Inguinal swelling is common, with late formation of painful abscesses (buboes). Superinfection of the ulcer with spirochete and fusiform organisms is common; the ulcer then becomes purulent, painful, and foul smelling. Rarely, granuloma inguinale presents with granulomatous cervical lesions that must be distinguished from carcinoma.

Objective Data

Physical Examination. An examination reveals the characteristic lesions, as noted previously.

Diagnostic Tests and Methods. Diagnostic evaluation for pathognomonic Donovan bodies (common name for causative organism). The test procedure is to crush/smear a clean piece of granulation tissue on a slide. Air dry, and then stain using appropriate Wright's or Giemsa staining technique. Explain to the client that the test procedure is simple and reliable. Must be done by a laboratory familiar with these techniques.

Differential Medical Diagnoses

Chancroid, carcinoma, syphilis, amebiasis.

Plan

Medication. A variety of antibiotics are useful. The first-line treatment is doxycycline.

Doxycycline

- *Indications:* Positive diagnosis of granuloma inguinale.
- *Administration:* Doxycycline 100 mg bid for at least 3 weeks until lesions have healed (CDC, 2010a).
- *Side effects and adverse reactions:* GI upset, rash, photosensitivity. Overgrowth of vaginal candida.
- *Contraindications:* Pregnancy; allergy to tetracyclines.
- *Anticipated outcomes on evaluation:* Lesions will heal and Donovan bodies will disappear from the smears.
- *Client teaching and counseling:* Advise the client that compliance with treatment is critical. Medication must be continued until all lesions are healed. This may take up to 4 weeks. Discontinuing therapy early results in high recurrence rates.

Other Medications. Trimethoprim 160 mg/sulfamethoxazole 800 mg (Bactrim DS) tablets bid for at least 3 weeks or until lesions have healed. Ciprofloxacin 750 mg po bid daily for at least 3 weeks (not in pregnancy). Erythromycin base 500 mg qid for at least 3 weeks may be used in pregnancy (CDC, 2010a).

Follow-Up and Referral

The client should be seen 1 to 2 months after the initial diagnosis to ensure resolution. Partners must be treated.

LYMPHOGRANULOMA VENEREUM

This chronic bacterial STD initially presents as a vesiculopustular eruption that may go unnoticed. After the genital lesion disappears, the infection spreads to lymph channels and lymph nodes of the genital and rectal areas (in women, the genital lymph drainage is to the perirectal glands). This secondary invasion is characterized by painful ulceration, lymphedema, and draining abscesses (buboes). Early anorectal manifestations are proctitis with tenesmus and bloody purulent discharge; late rectal manifestations include inflammation, scarring, and stricture of rectal and vaginal tissue. Systemic symptoms (fever, headache, abdominal pain, chills, and arthralgias) may develop.

Epidemiology

The causative organisms are *C. trachomatis serovars:* L1, L2, and L3. LGV is rare in the United States. LGV is endemic in some tropical and developing areas, such as

Southeast Asia, the Caribbean, Latin America, and parts of Africa (McLean, Stoner, & Workowski, 2007). Men with the disease outnumber women by 5 to 1. The incubation period is 3 to 12 days or longer.

Subjective Data

LGV contacts are initially asymptomatic, or may report genital ulcers and painful groin nodes or abscesses. A wide variety of nonspecific symptoms may be present.

Objective Data

Physical Examination. Tender inguinal lymphadenopathy is the most common sign. A spectrum of other clinical symptoms may occur, including papules, ulcers, cervicitis, proctitis, bubo formation (tender abscesses), and genital edema. A hard cutaneous induration may also be present.

Diagnostic Tests and Methods. Serological tests using fixation, neutralizing antibody, or immunofluorescents are available. Because LGV is so rare in the United States, specific information should be obtained from the local laboratory when testing is required.

Differential Medical Diagnoses

Chancroid, genital herpes, syphilis. Lymph node involvement must be distinguished from that due to tularemia, tuberculosis, or neoplasm. Rectal strictures must be distinguished from neoplasm and ulcerative colitis.

Plan

Psychosocial Interventions. Prevention is critical. When LGV is diagnosed, all sexual contacts must be identified and treated to eliminate a reservoir of continued transmission. Surgical excision of lesions may be necessary after infection has been halted.

Medication. Clients should be referred to an infectious disease specialist if LGV is suspected. Antibiotic therapy is indicated, and adequate treatment and follow-up are essential.

Doxycycline

- *Administration:* Doxycycline 100 mg po bid for 21 days (CDC, 2010a).
- *Side effects and contraindications:* The same as those discussed in the section on tetracycline therapy for granuloma inguinale.
- *Anticipated outcomes on evaluation:* Resolution of symptoms. Relapse is common.
- *Client teaching and counseling:* Assist the client to complete the medication regimen, which is difficult because it lasts for 21 days.

Other Medications. Alternative treatment regimens include erythromycin 500 mg po qid for 21 days (may be used in pregnancy) (CDC, 2010a).

EPIDERMAL DISEASES

Clinical syndromes with epidermal manifestations vary in seriousness, persistence, and treatment approaches. HPV infections are unique in that different viral types have different clinical manifestations.

HUMAN PAPILLOMAVIRUS INFECTION

Human papillomavirus infection is the most prevalent viral STD in the United States (Carey & Rayburn, 2002). It is estimated that 50 percent of sexually active persons become infected in their lifetimes (CDC, 2009b). High-risk types (e.g., HPV types 16 and 18) are the cause of cervical cancers. These HPV types are also associated with other anogenital cancers in men and women and some oropharyngeal cancers. Low-risk types (e.g., HPV types 6 and 11) are the cause of genital warts (Cogliano, Baan, Straif, et al., 2005). However, prospective studies in young women screened for HPV DNA suggest that HPV is frequently a transient infection, with most initially positive DNA tests becoming negative within 1 year (CDC, 2007). Clinically evident genital warts are only present in 1 percent of women and men (Juckett & Hartman-Adams, 2010). Infection with high-risk HPV types, older age, cigarette smoking, parity, and long-term use of oral contraceptives are risk factors for persistent HPV infection that may in turn increase the risk for cervical squamous intraepithelial lesions (Castellsague & Munoz, 2003).

Individuals with clinical evidence of HPV in one genital site have a significant risk of other HPV manifestations in another genital site (vulva, vagina, cervix, urethra, perianal skin, and rectum) (Carey & Rayburn, 2002). Unlike the treatment goal for bacterial sexually transmitted infections, the goal of HPV treatment is to remove obvious lesions and prevent the progression of neoplasias, not to eradicate HPV. Intra-anal warts should be managed in conjunction with a specialist. Because rectal warts often accompany anal warts, inspection using digital exam or an anoscope is advised.

Screening for HPV can be done using liquid-based molecular tests that detect HPV DNA; however, screening is recommended only for women ages ≥ 30 in conjunction with cervical cytology screening (CDC, 2007).

Epidemiology

Human papillomavirus is a slow-growing DNA virus of the papovavirus family; more than 100 strains are identified, 40 of which have been associated with genital tract infections. Condyloma acuminata and low-grade neoplasias are usually associated with HPV types 6 and 11. Other HPV types in the anogenital area (16, 18, 31, 45, and 56) are strongly associated with higher grades of genital dysplasia and carcinoma (CDC, 2010a). More than one type may be present at one time.

HPV is most commonly spread by means of sexual or other intimate contact. The organism may have limited survival on fomites, but nonsexual transmission is rare and difficult to document. Autoinoculation and mother–child transfer at birth can occur. The incubation period is 3 weeks to 8 months or longer.

Subjective Data

Clinical HPV lesions are papular lesions with a warty, granular surface. They are usually painless; however, malodorous vaginal discharge, pain and burning with urination, pruritus, and bleeding during and after coitus may occur. The lack of visible lesions or complaints is not uncommon, however. A woman may have a history of an infected partner but have no evidence of infection. Lesions may grow so large in pregnancy as to affect urination, defecation, mobility, and descent of the fetus, although rarely is cesarean delivery necessitated (CDC, 2010a).

Objective Data

Physical Examination. Genitalia/reproductive tract shows one or more soft, pale, pink or flesh-colored, dry, irregular lesions on the external genitalia, perineum, or anus. The lesions, 1 mm or larger, may be flat, papular, or pedunculated papules on the vulva, introitus, vagina, cervix, perineum, urethra, and/or anus. Small condylomata should not be confused with vulval vestibular papillae that are normally located on the epithelium of both labia minora. In true condyloma acuminata, multiple papillae converge toward a single base, whereas each papilla has its own base in normal vulvar tissue (Ferenczy, 1995). Large lesions may be cauliflower-like in appearance, exist in coalesced clusters, and be friable. Areas most often traumatized during coitus are common sites for HPV infection.

Diagnostic Tests and Methods

Pap Smear (Cytology). It is imperative that women with vulvar HPV or partners with HPV have a cervical examination with a Pap smear because more than one type of HPV may be present. This screening evaluation will identify squamous intraepithelial lesions on Bethesda System reports. A Pap smear is a screening test and not diagnostic because the sample can miss the lesion. The severity of any cervical lesion reported on a Pap smear can be determined best by HPV molecular testing or colposcopically directed cervical biopsy. (See Chapters 3 and 16 for Pap smear techniques and management of abnormal Pap smears.) It is important to note that any grossly visible suspicious cervical lesion requires biopsy, regardless of the Pap smear findings.

Colposcopy With Directed Biopsy (Histology). Diagnostic evaluation for subclinical lesions, dysplasia, and malignancy, performed by trained, experienced colposcopist using colposcope. The procedure provides a magnified view of direct biopsy sites. An abnormal Pap report, cervical lesions, or extensive external lesions warrant referral for colposcopy and biopsy. Endocervical curettage should not be performed if the client is pregnant.

The test procedure included the application of a 3 to 5 percent solution of acetic acid to the tissue of the vulva or cervix. After several seconds, abnormal areas turn white. The tissue is then examined under magnification with the colposcope. Directed biopsy is done on the most abnormal sites (e.g., acetowhite with punctuation and mosaic pattern).

Explain the procedure to the client: no anesthesia required; lithotomy position; instrument introduced through wide speculum opening; uncomfortable stinging from acetic acid; pinching, cramping sensation when tissue is removed. Tell the client that no excessive bleeding should occur, although a blood-tinged discharge may continue for 2 to 3 days; no coitus, douching, tampon use, or putting other objects in the vagina for 3 days.

DNA Typing (Nucleic Acid Hybridization Tests). Diagnostic evaluation to determine the specific HPV strain; may be useful to discriminate between low-risk and high-risk HPV types when Pap smear reveals atypical squamous cells of undetermined significance (ASCUS) or low-grade squamous intraepithelial lesions (LGSIL) in women over age 21. If test is positive for high-risk types, the client is referred for colposcopy. If low-risk HPV types are identified, the Pap should be repeated in 12 months (Wright et al. 2007).

A specimen for testing can be obtained with a fluid-phase collection system such as Thin Prep®. Explain to the client that HPV typing may identify particularly virulent strains of the virus. The use of HPV tests is not indicated for the routine diagnosis or management of visible genital warts.

Differential Medical Diagnoses

Condyloma lata; molluscum contagiosum; carcinoma; concomitant STDs.

Plan

If left untreated, genital warts may resolve on their own, remain unchanged, or increase in size or number. The effect of treatment on future transmission of HPV infection is unclear. The primary goal of treating visible genital warts is removal for cosmetic reasons; however, recurrences are frequent (CDC, 2007). The presence of genital warts is not associated with the development of cervical cancer in women. Therefore, the presence of genital warts is not an indication for colposcopy or a change in the frequency of Pap tests for women (CDC, 2007). Clients should be advised that persistent hypopigmentation or hyperpigmentation occurs commonly with ablative modalities and has also been described with immune-modulating therapies (imiquimod).

Psychosocial Interventions. Implications for counseling include relationship dissatisfaction, depression, and fear related to the seriousness of the diagnosis (dysplasia or cancer). Referral may be indicated. Discuss treatment options with the client (and partner, if appropriate); fully involve her in the therapy plans.

Anxiety associated with knowing one has a potentially malignant disease and lack of a definitive cure may necessitate referral for psychological counseling and support. Partners may also be involved in counseling. Through education about HPV, anxiety may be reduced. Involvement in controlling decisions empowers the client by decreasing her dependency.

Medication. There is no evidence that the use of more than one therapy at a time will improve efficacy. With any topical application, an alternative treatment should be tried if lesions have not resolved in four to five treatments. Clients should be referred for biopsy of any nonresponsive or atypical lesions.

Trichloracetic Acid. 80 to 90 percent.

- *Indications:* To reduce the size of external genital and vaginal lesions.
- *Administration:* Apply trichloracetic acid (TCA) solution sparingly to lesions, using a cotton swab and avoiding the surrounding tissue. Calcium alginate swabs may be preferred because they are smaller and decrease damage to surrounding tissue. Treated areas will turn white. A mixture of baking soda and water may be applied to neutralize the acid after application or to prevent damage from solution inadvertently applied to normal skin. A burning sensation occurs for several minutes following application but may be avoided by pretreatment spraying of topical anesthetic. Applications are repeated once weekly; may be repeated twice weekly if the client can tolerate it.
- *Side effects and adverse reactions:* Burning sensation on application should resolve quickly. There may be erythema, tenderness, swelling, and sloughing of tissue in the area for a few days after application. No systemic effects.
- *Contraindications:* TCA is contraindicated with severely irritated tissues. The medication has been used safely in pregnancy.
- *Anticipated outcomes on evaluation:* Lesions will become smaller and finally disappear after a few applications. If no visible improvement occurs after three treatments, use another method. If lesions persist or are multiple or internal, refer the client to a gynecologist.
- *Client teaching and counseling:* Tell the client that it is not necessary to wash off the acid. Persistent leukorrhea, increased pain, and redness may indicate infection. Spotting or bleeding may occur if the healing tissue is jarred. In addition, lidocaine (Xylocaine) ointment may be given, or warm sitz baths and a baking soda/water mixture may soothe.

Liquid Nitrogen Cryotherapy

- *Indications:* External warts. For internal lesions, the client is referred to a gynecologist.
- *Administration:* Application may be accomplished with a finely twisted cotton tip, or the wooden end of a cotton-tipped applicator, or a special applicator jet. The lesion will turn white.
- *Side effects and adverse reactions:* The same as for TCA and podophyllin.
- *Contraindications:* None.
- *Anticipated outcomes on evaluation:* The lesions will disappear after one to four weekly treatments.
- *Client teaching and counseling:* Inform the client that the application of the drug may burn. For the discomfort, the same teaching and counseling as used for application of TCA or podophyllin are appropriate.

Imiquimod 5 Percent Cream (Aldara)

- *Indications:* Imiquimod is an immune response modifier indicated for external genitalia and perianal warts. Pregnancy category C.
- *Administration:* Clients apply a thin layer to warts and rub in three times weekly at bedtime. May be used for a total of 16 weeks.
- *Side effects and adverse reactions:* Causes mild to moderate skin erythema and erosion.
- *Contraindications:* Not for urethral, intravaginal, or intra-anal warts.
- *Anticipated outcomes on evaluation:* Gradual clearing of warts over the treatment period.
- *Client teaching and counseling:* Cream must be washed off with soap and water 6 to 10 hours after application. Cream is petrolatum based and will cause condoms and diaphragms to deteriorate. Sexual contact should be avoided while cream is on the skin. Avoid eyes.

Podofilox 0.5 Percent. Podofilox 0.5 percent gel or solution, a self-treatment, may be prescribed. Unlike podophyllin, this is a stable, purified product that does not need to be washed off. Advise the client to apply it twice a day (only to the warts) for 3 days with a cotton swab or fingertip (for the gel) followed by 4 days of no therapy. The treatment may be repeated for a total of four cycles. The health care provider must teach wart identification, proper medicine application, and avoidance of getting any solution on other areas. The total treatment area should be 10 cm^2 or less. No more than 0.5 mL of solution should be used daily. Pregnancy category C.

Podophyllin. 10 to 25 percent in tincture of benzoin compound.

- *Indications:* For external lesions only. Because of potential toxicity and variations in potency of this natural plant extract, podophyllin is not recommended as a first-line treatment.
- *Administration:* Compound is applied to the lesion using a cotton swab and avoiding normal tissue. Unaffected areas may be protected by applying petroleum or lubricant jelly to them. Podophyllin must be washed off 4 hours after application. Applications are repeated weekly; more frequent use may result in burning.
- *Side effects and adverse reactions:* Erythema, burning, swelling, tissue damage. Lesions may become tender several days after treatment.
- *Contraindications:* Pregnancy or presence of large warts. Absorption may cause toxicity.
- *Anticipated outcomes on evaluation:* The same as for TCA. Do not exceed four applications if no significant improvement results.
- *Client teaching and counseling:* Provide the client with information about the signs of toxicity: nausea, vomiting, lethargy, coma, paralysis. Repeated use may be carcinogenic. Instruct the client to wash off podophyllin 4 hours after application with mild soap and water, sooner if irritation causes discomfort.

Sinecatechin 15 Percent Ointment. A green-tea extract with an active product (catechins).

- *Indications:* For external lesions only.
- *Administration:* Patient-applied three times daily (0.5 cm strand of ointment to each wart) using a finger to ensure coverage with a thin layer of ointment until complete clearance of warts. This product should not be continued for longer than 16 weeks.
- *Side effects and adverse reactions:* Erythema, pruritis/burning, pain, ulceration, edema, induration, and vesicular rash. No clinical data is available regarding the efficacy or safety of sinecatechins compared with other available anogenital wart treatment modalities. The medication is not recommended for HIV-infected persons, immunocompromised persons, or persons with clinical genital herpes because the safety and efficacy of therapy in these settings has not been established. The safety of sinecatechins during pregnancy also is unknown.
- *Anticipated outcomes on evaluation:* Gradual clearing of warts over the treatment period.
- *Client teaching and counseling:* This medication may weaken condoms and diaphragms. The medication should not be washed off after use. Sexual (i.e., genital, anal, or oral) contact should be avoided while the ointment is on the skin.

Surgery and Other Interventions. Indications are internal lesions, large lesions, or external lesions unresponsive to prior therapy. The client is referred to a trained, experienced specialist.

HPV Prevention. Appropriate administration of HPV vaccines prevents up to 70 percent of cervical cancer cases. The quadrivalent vaccine (Gardasil®) protects against four HPV types (6, 11, 16, 18), which are responsible for 70 percent of cervical cancers and 90 percent of genital warts. The vaccine is administered through a series of three intramuscular injections over a 6-month period (at 0, 2, and 6 months) and is recommended for use in females, ages 9 to 26 (Markowitz et al., 2007). Gardasil® can be administered to males aged 9 to 26 years to prevent genital warts, but is not Advisory Committee on Immunization Practices (ACIP) recommended for routine use (CDC, 2010b). In 2009, a second HPV vaccine (Cervarix®) was approved for use in females aged 10 through 25 years. This vaccine provides protection only against HPV types 16 and 18. Dosing and administration schedules are the same as for Gardasil®. Regular cervical cancer screening is still necessary for vaccinated women because: (1) the vaccine will *not* provide protection against all types of HPV that cause cervical cancer; (2) women may not receive the full benefits of the vaccine if they do not complete the vaccine series; and (3) women may not receive the full benefits of the vaccine if they receive the vaccine after they have already acquired a HPV type included in the vaccine (CDC, 2007).

Given the efficacy of the vaccine in the prevention of cervical cancer, it is important for providers to be proactive in recommending this vaccine. A recent survey of 2,295 Los Angeles women revealed that only 5 percent of vaccine-eligible women had received the vaccine, and that Latina, black, and Asian/Pacific Islander women were only half as likely to have heard of the vaccine as white women (Cui, Baldwin, Wiley, & Fielding, 2010). Given that minority women have a higher risk of cervical cancer than white women (Ries et al., 2005), culturally appropriate educational campaigns about HPV immunization are needed, and should target high-risk populations. Appropriate strategies may include explicit provider endorsement, assurance of vaccine safety, and making vaccines affordable and available (Hopfer & Clippard, 2011).

MOLLUSCUM CONTAGIOSUM

This benign, viral, papular infection occurs on the abdomen, thighs, and genitals of adults and on the face, trunk, and extremities of children. Mollusca are common in persons infected with HIV and are difficult to eradicate in these persons. The infection is generally minor and self-limited. Another name for the condition is seed wart.

Epidemiology

Molluscum contagiosum virus (MCV), a member of the pox virus family, is the causative organism. In adults, transmission is primarily sexual; in children, it is nonsexual and via fomites. Autoinoculation may also occur. The incubation period ranges from 1 week to 6 months (2- to 3-month average).

Subjective Data

The client is generally asymptomatic, and diagnosis is often made when treatment is sought for some other reason.

Objective Data

Physical Examination. A firm, smooth, waxy, nontender, dome-shaped papule with a central umbilication is seen (may be single or multiple). Lesions contain a caseous material. Principal sites of involvement include face, upper thighs, lower abdomen, and genitals. In HIV-infected patients, the infection is often generalized.

Diagnostic Tests and Methods. Diagnosis is made upon sight of a characteristic lesion. Biopsy reveals molluscum bodies.

Differential Medical Diagnoses

Genital warts, genital herpes, dermatologic folliculitis, lichen planus, basal cell epithelioma.

Plan

Psychosocial Interventions. Reassure the client that MCV is benign, is self-limiting, and grows slowly. Clients with multiple or persistent lesions, however, should be questioned about risk factors for HIV. Many cases spontaneously resolve over a few months. Bacterial superinfection may require a systemic antibiotic, but such a condition is rare. Clients should avoid sharing razors. Advocate good handwashing.

Surgical Interventions. Unroofing the lesion with a fine gauge needle to remove the central core is effective and practical if there are only a few lesions. Multiple lesions have been successfully treated using cryotherapy with liquid nitrogen; direct destruction is achieved. Electrosurgery with a fine needle may be used.

PEDICULOSIS PUBIS

A species of human lice causes this common STD. Another name for this condition is pubic lice or crabs. Body and head lice also occur in humans but do not infect the pubic area. Pubic lice, however, have been found in axillae, beards, eyebrows, and eyelashes.

Epidemiology

Phthirus pubis is the crab louse. It requires human blood to survive. Off the host, pubic lice will die within

24 hours. Transmission is through infected humans, clothing, or bedding. The examination table and toilet used by the client will need to be washed with an appropriate disinfectant, or the rooms may be closed for the life span of the lice (24 hours) if this is feasible. Young adults (15 to 25 years old) have the highest incidence of pubic lice; prevalence declines after age 35.

Subjective Data

Itching is the primary symptom. It leads to scratching, erythema, and skin irritation. The client may be asymptomatic. The underwear of the client with pubic lice may be speckled with blood.

Objective Data

Physical Examination. Adult lice may be viewed moving along pubic hairs. Eggs (nits) appear as minute white dots adherent to pubic hair.

Diagnostic Tests and Methods. Characteristic lice and nits may be observed; microscopic examination confirms. Clients who report pubic lice do not need an office visit to confirm.

Differential Medical Diagnoses

If small white flakes are noted in the pubic hair, seborrheic dermatitis must be considered.

Plan

Psychosocial Interventions. Assist the client to deal with the anxiety and embarrassment that diagnosis causes. Tell her that pubic lice are usually curable and have no long-term consequences. In addition, advise her that contacts need to be checked and treated if they are infected. Clothing and household items require disinfection. Washable items may be laundered in hot water or dry cleaned. Nonwashable items can be treated with products that contain pyrethrin (Black Flag or Raid). These products should be used only on inanimate objects.

Medication. A variety of prescription and OTC medications are available. Ideally, medication should be lethal to both adult lice and eggs; however, there is some indication that head lice are developing resistance to usual treatments and this may be seen in the future with pubic lice.

Permethrin. 1 percent liquid (Nix).

- *Indications:* For treatment of pubic lice and eggs. This is an OTC preparation.
- *Administration:* Application is as a shampoo or liquid. Manufacturer's directions for application must be followed exactly. Repeat application is usually unnecessary but may be done 7 to 10 days after initial treatment if living lice are seen. Pregnancy category B.
- *Side effects and adverse reactions:* Minimal but minor skin irritation may occur. Avoid contact with mucous membranes.
- *Contraindications:* Sensitivity to pyrethrin or chrysanthemum—for these individuals, the solutions should be used with caution.
- *Anticipated outcomes on evaluation:* Destruction of pubic lice and eggs. Reexamination is needed 1 week after initial treatment to confirm positive outcome.
- *Client teaching and counseling:* Encourage the client to follow the directions exactly. Instruct her in the use of the fine-tooth comb usually provided with the medication; dead nits are combed out of the pubic hair.

Lindane. 1 percent (Kwell).

- *Indications:* This prescription solution is used in the treatment of pubic lice. It kills both adult lice and eggs. Should be reserved for second-line treatment due to potential neurotoxicity.
- *Administration:* Application is as a shampoo. Apply exactly according to the manufacturer's directions. One application is usually adequate, but the treatment may be repeated in 7 days.
- *Side effects and adverse reactions:* May include skin irritation, but it is usually minor. Lindane permeates human skin and has potential CNS toxicity. Care must be taken to avoid contact with the eyes.
- *Contraindications:* Known seizure disorders and known sensitivity to lindane. Do not use during pregnancy and lactation or on infants/children.
- *Anticipated outcomes on evaluation:* The same as that achieved with the use of permethrins.

HEPATITIS B

Hepatitis B, or serum hepatitis, is a viral inflammation of the liver that results in a broad spectrum of disease from mild illness to chronic carrier state with possible cirrhosis, liver cancer, and death secondary to liver failure. Most infected persons never become jaundiced; their illness is mistaken for a nonspecific viral syndrome unless liver biochemical tests are ordered. The primary risk factors associated with infection among adolescents and adults are unprotected sex with an infected partner, unprotected sex with more than one partner, men who have sex with men, history of other STDs, and illegal injection-drug use. Hepatitis B vaccination is recommended for all unvaccinated, uninfected persons being evaluated for an STD (CDC, 2006).

Women infected with hepatitis B may transmit the virus to their neonates at the time of delivery; the risk of chronic infection in the infant is as high as 90 percent (CDC, 2010a). Testing for hepatitis B is indicated for persons who are jaundiced, who have elevated liver transaminases (alanine aminotransferase [ALT] and aspartate aminotransferase [AST]), or who are sexual partners of a person diagnosed with hepatitis B. Persons with presumptive hepatitis B should also be tested for hepatitis A, hepatitis C, and hepatitis D. Hepatitis D is caused by a defective RNA virus that requires coinfection with hepatitis B. Further information about hepatitis A and C is beyond the scope of this chapter because their transmission is not primarily sexual.

Epidemiology

Hepatitis B virus (HBV) is the causative organism. Those at special risk include intravenous drug users, heterosexuals and homosexuals with multiple partners, sexual partners of HBV carriers, infants of HBV-infected mothers, health workers who have contact with blood, and people born in areas where HBV is endemic. Hepatitis B may occasionally be transmitted to household contacts. Hepatitis B may be transmitted parenterally, sexually, or perinatally. The incubation period ranges from 4 weeks to 6 months (average is 10 weeks). One to 2 percent of persons with hepatitis B become chronic carriers, remain capable of transmitting the virus, and may progress to cirrhosis or liver failure.

Universal vaccination against HBV for children in the United States was started in 1991. A NHANES analysis, done between 1999 and 2006, showed a 68 percent reduction in the incidence of HBV among children and a 79 percent decrease of chronic infection for this age group. This analysis also showed a smaller percentage decrease for those ages 20 to 49 and fewer females than males with chronic infection. The majority of current cases in the United States, estimated at 730,000, are in adults over age 50 (Wasley et al., 2010). Since 2008, the WHO reports that 177 countries have introduced vaccination against HBV for infants and adolescents (Romano, Paladina, Van Damme, & Zanetti, 2011).

Subjective Data

Many persons have asymptomatic infection and develop lifelong immunity. The symptoms, which may be mild or severe, include fatigue, loss of appetite, dark urine, light-colored bowel movements, nausea/vomiting, diarrhea, malaise, and myalgias. The onset of symptoms is usually gradual, and resolution is slow.

Objective Data

Physical Examination. Examination may reveal jaundice, low-grade fever, or the only sign may be mild right-upper quadrant pain.

Diagnostic Tests and Methods. Initial diagnostic workup for acute hepatitis should include a urinalysis (for bilirubin), a check of serum transaminases (ALT and AST), hepatitis B surface antigen (HBsAg), antibody to hepatitis B core antibody (anti-HBc IgM), antibody to hepatitis A (anti-HAV IgM), and antibody to hepatitis C (anti-HCV). Antibody to hepatitis D (anti-HDV) should be measured in all persons diagnosed with acute hepatitis B. If hepatitis B is diagnosed, prothrombin time and serum albumin should be measured. The test procedure is to obtain a blood sample. Advise the client that blood testing is highly accurate and can determine active infection.

Differential Medical Diagnoses

Hepatitis A, C, and D.

Plan

Medical Management. Treatment is symptomatic and avoidance of strenuous physical exertion and hepatotoxic agents (such as alcohol) is recommended. Pronounced nausea and vomiting may be treated with intravenous 10 percent glucose (Dienstag, 2006). Clients should be followed weekly in the acute phase to monitor symptom management.

Prothrombin time, serum bilirubin, albumin, and aminotransferases should be rechecked weekly if there is suspicion of worsening. At 3 months, transaminases should be repeated along with serum bilirubin, albumin, and prothrombin time. HBsAg should be rechecked to determine antigen status. If symptoms and laboratory evidence of activity persist after 3 months, evaluations should be repeated monthly. If antigen persists 6 months after acute infection, referral for liver biopsy should be considered (Dienstag, 2006).

Psychosocial Interventions. Advise the client that there is no specific treatment for hepatitis B. Rest and nutritious diet are important. Alcohol should be restricted, but oral contraceptives need not be stopped (Dienstag, 2006). Activity restrictions are based on how the individual feels. Household contacts should be vaccinated. Sexual partners should receive hepatitis B immune globulin (HBIG) as well as vaccination if susceptible. In addition to vaccination, general counseling to prevent transmission of HBV includes information about using latex condoms, and not sharing needles, razors, or toothbrushes.

Medication

Hepatitis B Immune Globulin

- *Indications:* Sexual contacts of clients with acute HBV, those who have sexual contact with HBV carriers, nonimmunized health care workers with needlesticks from patients with hepatitis B, and newborns of mothers with HBV. HBIG should be followed by HBV immunization.
- *Administration:* Intramuscular injection, 0.06 mL/kg. In neonates, 0.5 cc IM at birth.
- *Side effects and adverse reactions:* Minimal, local irritation at the injection site.
- *Contraindications:* None known.
- *Anticipated outcomes on evaluation:* Highly effective, immediate immunity, although temporary.
- *Client teaching and counseling:* HBIG should be given within 14 days of HBV exposure. Three-dose immunization with hepatitis B vaccine should follow.

Hepatitis B Vaccination

- *Indications:* Persons with multiple sexual partners, homosexual/bisexual men, illicit intravenous drug users, prison inmates and other institutionalized individuals, prostitutes, health care workers with exposure to blood products, infants of HBV-infected mothers, clients attending STD clinics, and household or sexual contacts of HBV carriers. Universal vaccination of newborns and previously unvaccinated children through age 18 is now recommended (CDC, 2010a).
- *Administration:* Requires three intramuscular injections—an initial injection, another 1 month later, and the third at 6 months. The deltoid muscle should be used. May give first dose concurrently with HBIG.
- *Side effects and adverse reactions:* Minimal, local soreness at injection site.
- *Contraindications:* None.
- *Anticipated outcomes on evaluation:* Active immunity to HBV, lasting 5 years or longer. Postvaccination testing to confirm immunity is not routinely recommended.
- *Client teaching and counseling:* Educate the client that prevaccination HBV testing is recommended only for very high-risk groups where the presence of HBV antibodies would negate the necessity of vaccination. The cost-effectiveness of such testing in moderate risk groups must be considered. HBsAg positive individuals who receive the vaccine are unharmed.

REFERENCES

Association of Public Health Laboratories (APHL). (2009). *Laboratory diagnostic testing for Treponema pallidum expert consultation meeting summary report, Atlanta, Georgia.* Retrieved May 8, 2011, from http://www.aphl.org/aphlprograms/infectious/std/Documents/LaboratoryGuidelines-TreponemapallidumMeetingReport.pdf

Brown, Z.A., Wald, A., Morrow, R.A., Selke, S., Zeh, J., & Corey, L. (2003). Effect of serologic status and cesarean delivery on transmission rates of herpes simplex virus from mother to infant. *Journal of the American Medical Association, 289,* 203–209.

Carey, J.C., & Rayburn, W.F. (2002). *Obstetrics and gynecology* (4th ed., p. 127). Philadelphia: Lippincott Williams & Wilkins.

Castellsague, X., & Munoz, N. (2003). Cofactors in human papillomavirus carcinogenesis—Role of parity, oral contraceptives, and tobacco smoking. *Journal of the National Cancer Institute Monographs, 31,* 20–28.

Centers for Disease Control and Prevention (CDC). (2006). A comprehensive immunization strategy to eliminate transmission of hepatitis B virus infection in the United States: Recommendations of the Advisory Committee on Immunization Practices (ACIP) Part II: Immunization of adults. *Morbidity and Mortality Weekly Report, 55*(RR-16). Retrieved from http://www.cdc.gov/mmwr/pdf/rr/rr5516.pdf

Centers for Disease Control and Prevention (CDC). (2007). *Human papillomavirus: HPV information for clinicians.* Retrieved from http://www.cdc.gov/std/hpv/common-clinicians/ClinicianBro.txt

Centers for Disease Control and Prevention (CDC). (2009a). *Genital HPV infection–Fact sheet.* Atlanta, GA: U.S. Department of Health and Human Services, Centers for Disease Control and Prevention. Retrieved November 24, 2009, from http://www.cdc.gov/STD/HPV/STDFact-HPV.htm

Centers for Disease Control and Prevention (CDC). (2009b). *Sexually transmitted disease surveillance, 2009.* Atlanta, GA: U.S. Department of Health and Human Services, Centers for Disease Control and Prevention.

Centers for Disease Control and Prevention (CDC). (2010a). Congenital syphilis-United States, 2003–2008. *Morbidity and Mortality Weekly Report, 59*(14), 413.

Centers for Disease Control and Prevention (CDC). (2010b). FDA licensure of quadrivalent human papillomavirus vaccine (HPV4, Gardasil) for use in males and guidance from the Advisory Committee on Immunization Practices (ACIP). *Morbidity and Mortality Weekly Report, 59,* 630–632.

Centers for Disease Control and Prevention (CDC). (2010c). Sexually transmitted diseases treatment guidelines, 2010. *Morbidity and Mortality Weekly Report, 59*(RR-12), 1–110.

Centers for Disease Control and Prevention (CDC). (2011). *Nationally notifiable infectious conditions: United States 2011.* Retrieved January 26, 2011, from http://www.cdc.gov/ncphi/diss/nndss/PHS/infdis2011.htm

Chibana, H., & Magee, P. (2009). The enigma of the major repeat sequence of Candida albicans. *Future Epidemiology, 4*(2), 171–179.

Clinical Pharmacology Online. (2010). *Advancing healthcare through medication management solutions.* Retrieved April 25, 2011, from http://www.clinicalpharmacology.com/?epm=2_1

Cogliano, V., Baan, R., Straif, K., Grosse, Y., Secretan, B., & El Ghissassi, F. (2005). Carcinogenicity of human papillomaviruses. *Lancet Oncology, 5*(6), 204.

Cui, Y., Baldwin, S.B., Wiley, D.J., & Fielding, J.E. (2010). Human papillomavirus vaccine among adult women: Disparities in awareness and acceptance. *American Journal of Preventive Medicine, 39*(6), 559–563.

De Seta, F., Schmidt, M., Vu, B., Essman, M., & Larsen, B. (2008). Antifungal mechanisms supporting boric acid therapy of Candida vaginitis. *Journal of Antimicrobial Chemotherapy, 16*(2), 325–336.

Dienstag, J.L. (2006). Management of hepatitis. In A.H. Gorroll & A.G. Mulley (Eds.), *Primary care medicine: Office evaluation and management of the adult patient* (5th ed.). Philadelphia: Lippincott Williams & Wilkins.

Engelberg, R., Carrell, D., Krantz, E., Corey, L., & Wald, A. (2003). Natural history of genital herpes simplex virus type 1 infection. *Sexually Transmitted Diseases, 30,* 174–177.

Ferenczy, A. (1995). Epidemiology and clinical pathophysiology of condyloma acuminata. *American Journal of Obstetrics and Gynecology, 172*(4), 1331–1339.

Fife, K.H., Crumpacker, C.S., Mertz, G.J., Hill, E.L., & Boone, G.S. (1994). Acyclovir study group. Recurrence and resistance patterns of herpes simplex virus following cessation of ≥6 years of chronic suppression with acyclovir. *Journal of Infectious Disease, 169*(6), 1338–1341.

Hopfer, S., & Clippard, J.R. (2011). College women's HPV vaccine decision narratives. *Qualitative Health Research, 21*(2), 262–277.

Hutchinson, K.B., Kip, K.E., & Ness, R.B. (2007). Condom use and its association with bacterial vaginosis and bacterial vaginosis-associated vaginal microflora. *Epidemiology, 18*(6), 702–708.

Jacobs, R.A. (2001). Infectious diseases: Spirochetal. In L.M. Tierney, S.J. McPhee, & M.A. Papadakis (Eds.), *Current medical diagnosis and treatment 2001.* New York: Lange Medical Books/McGraw Hill.

Juckett, G., & Hartman-Adams, H. (2010). Human papillomavirus: Clinical manifestations and prevention. *American Family Physician, 82*(10), 1209–1214.

Lusk, M.J., & Konecny, P. (2008). Cervicitis: A review. *Current Opinions in Infectious Diseases, 21,* 49–55.

Markowitz, L.E., Dunne, E.F., Saraiya, M., Lawson, H.W., Chesson, H., & Unger, E.R. (2007). Quadrivalent Human Papillomavirus Vaccine: Recommendations of the Advisory Committee on Immunization Practices (ACIP). *Morbidity and Mortality Weekly Report, 56*(RR-02), 1–24.

Martin, E.T., Krantz, E., Gottlieb, S.L., Magaret, A.S., Langenberg, A., Stanberry, L., et al. (2009). A pooled analysis of the effect of condoms in preventing HSV-2 acquisition. *Archives of Internal Medicine, 169,* 1233–1240.

McKenzie, J. (2001). Sexually transmitted diseases. *Emergency Medicine Clinics of North America, 19*(3), 723–743.

McLean, C.A., Stoner, B.P., & Workowski, K.A. (2007). Treatment of lymphogranuloma venereum. *Clinical Infectious Diseases, 44,* S147–S152.

McPhee, S., & Papadakis, M. (Eds.). (2011). *Current medical diagnosis and treatment.* New York: McGraw-Hill.

Mehta, N., Ozick, L., & Gbadehan, E. (2010). *Drug-induced hepatotoxicity.* Retrieved March 10, 2011, from http://emedicine.medscape.com/article/169814-overview

Mosby's drug consult (pp. II-539–II-540). (2007). St. Louis, MO: Mosby.

NC Communicable Disease Branch. (2008). *Sexually transmitted disease protocols/reporting/reporting and partner notification.* Retrieved from http://www.epi.state.nc.uf/epi/hiv/stdmanual/Management%20Protocols/Reporting%20and%20Partner%20

Neinstein, L., Gordon, C., Katzman, D., Rosen, D., & Woods, E. (2007). *Adolescent health care* (5th ed.). Hagerstown, MD: Lippincott Williams & Wilkins.

Newman, L.M., Moran, J.S., & Workowski, K.A. (2007). Update on the management of gonorrhea in adults in the United States. *Clinical Infectious Diseases, 44*(Suppl.), 84–101.

Nygren, P., Fu, P., Freeman, M., Bougatsos, C., Klebanoff, M., & Guise, J.M. (2008). Evidence on the benefits and harms of screening and treating pregnant women who are asymptomatic for bacterial vaginosis: An update review for the U.S. Preventive Services Task Force. *Annals of Internal Medicine, 148*(3), 130.

Oduyebo, O., Anorlu, R., & Ogunsola, F. (2009). The effects of antimicrobial treatment on bacterial vaginosis in non-pregnant women. *Cochrane Database of Systematic Reviews, 3,* CD006055. doi:10.1002/14651858.CD006055.pub2

Pevion. (2010). *PEV 7. Subunit vaccine against RVVC.* Retrieved March 10, 2011, from http://pevion.com/images/content/Pevion%20PEV7%20candida%20vaccine.pdf

Quan, M. (2010). Vaginitis: Diagnosis and management. *Journal of Postgraduate Medicine, 122*(6), 117–127.

Ratnam, S. (2005). The laboratory diagnosis of syphilis. *Canadian Journal of Infectious Diseases and Medical Microbiology, 16*(1), 45–51.

Ries, L., Harkins, D., Krapcho, M., Mariotto, A., Miller, B.A., Feuer, E.J., et al. (Eds.). (2005). *SEER Cancer Statistics Review, 1975–2004.* Bethesda, MD: National Cancer Institute. Retrieved November 2005, from http://seer.cancer.gov/csr/1975_2004/

Romano, I., Paladina, S., Van Damme, P., & Zanetti, A.R. (2011). The worldwide impact of vaccination on the control and protection of viral hepatitis B. *Digestive and Liver Disease, 43,* S2–S7.

Rosenfeld, J., (Ed.). (2009). *Handbook of women's health.* Retrieved from http://lib.myilibrary.com/Open.aspx?id=238643&loc=&srch=undefined&src=0

Ryder, N., Jin, F., McNulty, A.M., Grulich, A.E., & Donovan, B. (2009). Increasing role of herpes simplex virus type 1 in first-episode anogenital herpes in heterosexual women and younger men who have sex with men, 1992–2006. *Sexually Transmitted Infections, 85,* 416–419.

Schwartz, B.S. (2011). Bacterial & chlamydial infections. In S.J. McPhee, M.A. Papadakis, & M.W. Rabow (Eds.), *2011 Current medical diagnosis and treatment.* New York: McGraw-Hill Lange.

Scoular, A. (2002). Using the evidence base on genital herpes: Optimising the use of diagnostic tests and information provision. *Sexually Transmitted Infections, 78,* 160–165.

Sendag, F., Terek, C., Tuncay, G., Ozkinay, E., & Guven, M. (2000). Single dose oral azithromycin versus seven day doxycycline in the treatment of non-gonococcal mucopurulent endocervicitis. *Australian and New Zealand Journal of Obstetrics and Gynecology, 40,* 44–47.

Sheffield, J.S., Hollier, L.M., Hill, J.B., Stuart, G.S., & Wendel, G.D. (2003). Acyclovir prophylaxis to prevent herpes simplex virus recurrence at delivery: A systematic review. *Obstetrics and Gynecology, 102,* 1396–1403.

Steiner, M.J., & Cates, W. (2006). Condoms and sexually-transmitted infections. *New England Journal of Medicine, 354,* 2642–2643.

Stone, K.M., Reiff-Eldridge, R., White, A.D., Cordero, J.F., Brown, Z., Alexander, E.R., et al. (2004). Pregnancy outcomes following systemic prenatal acyclovir exposure: Conclusions from the international acyclovir pregnancy registry, 1984–1999. *Birth Defects Research. Part A, Clinical and Molecular Teratology, 70,* 201–207.

Sutton, M., Sternberg, M., Koumans, E.H., McQuillan, G., Berman, S., & Markowitz, L. (2007). The prevalence of Trichomonas vaginalis infection among reproductive-age women in the United States, 2001-2004. *Clinical Infectious Diseases, 45*(10), 1319–1326.

Syed, T.S., & Braverman, P.K. (2004). Vaginitis in adolescents. *Adolescent Medical Clinics, 15*(2), 235–251.

U.S. Preventive Services Task Force. (2008). Screening for bacterial vaginosis in pregnancy to prevent preterm delivery: U.S. Preventive Services Task Force recommendations. *Annals of Internal Medicine, 148,* 214–219.

Wasley, A., Kruszon-Moran, D., Kuhnert, W., Simard, E., Finelli, L., McQuillan, G., et al. (2010). The prevalence of hepatitis B virus infection in the United States in the Era of Vaccination. *Journal of Infectious Diseases, 202,* 192–201.

Winer, R.L., Hugnes, J.P., Feng, Q., O'Reilly, S., Kiviat, N.B., Holmes, K.K., et al. (2006). Condom use and the risk of genital human papillomavirus infection in young women. *New England Journal of Medicine, 354,* 2645–2654.

Wright, T.C., Massad, S.J., Dunton, C.J., Spitzer, M., Wilkinson, E.J., & Solomon, D. (2007). 2006 consensus guidelines for the management of women with abnormal cervical screening tests. *Journal of Lower Genital Tract Disease, 11*(4), 201–222.

Xu, F., Sternberg, M.R., Kottiri, B.J., McQuillan, G.M., Lee, F.K., Nahmias, A.J., et al. (2006). Trends in herpes simplex virus type 1 and type 2 seroprevalence in the United States. *Journal of the American Medical Association, 296,* 964–973.

Yudin, M., & Money, D.M. (2008). Infectious diseases committee. Screening and management of bacterial vaginosis in pregnancy. *Journal of Obstetrics and Gynaecology Canada, 30*(8), 702–708.

CHAPTER ❖ 15

WOMEN AND HIV

Susan D. Schaffer ◆ Donna Treloar

The advent of highly active antiretroviral therapy has transformed HIV infection from an inevitably fatal illness to a controllable chronic disease; however, gender-based differences that include female-specific complications, psychosocial impact of the disease, and access to quality care require careful attention by health care providers.

Highlights

- Epidemiology of HIV
- Diagnostic Testing
- Pre- and Posttest Counseling
- Initial Evaluation of a Woman With HIV
- Management of Early HIV Infection
- Management of Late HIV Infection

❖ INTRODUCTION

Acquired immunodeficiency syndrome (AIDS), first identified in 1981, is a viral infection caused by the human immunodeficiency virus (HIV). Although once inevitably fatal, HIV infection is now a highly treatable chronic infection with the advent of highly active antiretroviral therapy (HAART). The spectrum of HIV disease ranges from asymptomatic to full-blown infection (AIDS). Through a loss of cell-mediated immune function and the depletion of T4 lymphocytes, individuals who do not receive antiviral treatment progress from HIV infection to death in about 11 years (Bartlett & Gallant, 2002). The deterioration of the immune system confers susceptibility to rare opportunistic infections (OIs) and malignant tumors. These phenomena, along with dementia and a wasting syndrome, signal the end stage of HIV infection (AIDS). HIV infection has a profound effect on women both as an illness and as a social and economic challenge. HIV affects women's caregiving role in the family; women must deal with their own life-threatening illness while they also deal with the impact of disease on their families. Women who become pregnant while HIV infected or who contemplate pregnancy while infected need information on risks to the fetus as well as information on caring for themselves. The stigma attached to HIV/AIDS can subject women to discrimination, job loss, social rejection, and other violations of their rights. Although primarily sexually transmitted, AIDS is covered in a separate chapter from other sexually transmitted infections because of the devastating effect HIV/AIDS has on infected women and their families and because of the complex psychosocial and medical management that is required to delay the effects and to promote a high quality of life in infected women.

Because there is no cure for HIV infection, primary prevention remains the most important strategy for primary care providers. Well-known measures that women can take to prevent acquisition of HIV include abstaining from intercourse, selecting low-risk partners, negotiating partner monogamy, and male/female condom use. However, the rising HIV incidence of women in the United States speaks to the prevention barriers women face in heterosexual relationships (NIAID, 2008). Advances in the use of antiviral agents to prevent debilitating OI highlight the importance of early diagnosis and treatment. Women with HIV require diagnostic evaluation, periodic physical examinations, monitoring of prognostic markers (CD4 counts and viral load tests), antiviral and prophylactic therapy, therapy for HIV-related complications and supportive counseling. As the disease progresses, women require assistance with pain control and durable power of attorney. Because of the complexity of initiating, maintaining, and adjusting HAART, only a practitioner with a specialty in HIV/AIDS should provide this type of service. Specialty care providers are physicians, nurse practitioners, and physician assistants who have been trained in initiating and monitoring antiretroviral therapy. Strategies to combat HIV infection depend on understanding the epidemiology of the virus.

EPIDEMIOLOGY OF HIV

VIRAL LIFE CYCLE

HIV, a retrovirus, is an intracellular parasite that interacts with the host cell's CD4 T lymphocyte cells. T lymphocytes play a central part in the immune system by destroying infected cells and helping B cells make antibodies. T4 helper cells (CD4+ cells) are specialized T lymphocytes that do little to repel intruding substances themselves but instead become activated to alert B cells, killer cells, and phagocytes to the presence of a bacterial, fungal, or viral antigen. When HIV is introduced into the bloodstream, the virus joins the host T4 cell's DNA and awaits activation of the cell. Only after the HIV-infected T4 cells are activated by some non-HIV antigen do the T4 cells manufacture HIV viral RNA strands, replicating the virus and destroying themselves in the process. Over 1 billion virions are produced daily. With ongoing destruction and replacement of the T4 cells, the body gradually loses its ability to mount an immune response and ward off pathogens. When the CD4 lymphocyte populations decline to less than 500 cells/mm^3, minor infections, such as vaginal candidiasis, occur. When the CD4 lymphocyte count declines to less than 200 cells/mm^3, increasingly serious infections, such as *Pneumocystis carinii* pneumonia (PCP), are seen. It is difficult to eradicate the virus entirely because HIV hides out in places such as the lymphoid tissue and the central nervous system (Fauci & Lane, 2008).

Thus, management of HIV requires a lifetime of controlling the virus through adherence to medications.

INCIDENCE AND ACCESS

As of December 2009, 33.3 million people are estimated to be living with HIV/AIDS worldwide (UNAIDS, 2010). In the United States, over 1,100,000 people are currently estimated to be living with HIV, including nearly 280,000 women (Centers for Disease Control and Prevention [CDC], 2009a). One in five (21%) of those people living with HIV is unaware of their infection (CDC, 2010a). The rate of diagnosis in black/African American women is 47.8/100,000 compared with 11.9/100,000 in Latino women and 2.4/100,000 in white women (CDC, 2011a). Race and ethnicity are not risk factors, but serve as markers of socioeconomic status and access to medical care. Access to health care is a problem for many Americans especially those who are impoverished or disenfranchised. Financial barriers are certainly significant, but there are also a number of other factors that prevent lower socioeconomically situated individuals from seeking care including preventive screening. The stigma of HIV precludes conversation about its prevalence in many communities, including those of people of color. Other issues include difficulties with transportation, lack of childcare, employment obstacles, denial, depression, and fear of the unknown.

Primary care practitioners often interact with women during annual examinations and can use this encounter as an opportunity for counseling about the prevalence of HIV, methods to prevent transmission, and reasons for HIV testing in themselves and their partners. Most women are receptive to screening during annual examinations and especially during prenatal visits. Some states have "opt-out" regulations in place for pregnant women in order to increase detection early in the pregnancy when therapy to prevent vertical transmission will be most effective.

The benefits of early intervention in preventing vertical transmission of HIV with antiretroviral medications were evident in 1994 in Pediatric AIDS Clinical Trials Group Protocol 076 (Connor et al., 1994). This landmark study has been supported with additional research-supporting combination therapy during pregnancy. With the implementation of recommendations for universal prenatal HIV counseling and testing, combination antiretroviral prophylaxis, scheduled cesarean delivery, and avoidance of breastfeeding, the rate of perinatal HIV transmission has dramatically diminished to less than 2 percent in the United States and Europe (National Institutes of Health [NIH], 2010). The primary care provider facilitates compliance and, therefore, successful pregnancy outcomes by supporting prescribed therapies and maintaining contact with the woman during the pregnancy. Encouragement and coaching from a trusted medical contact may provide the support that is needed for a young female to accept the challenges of the diagnosis in an unfamiliar setting.

TRANSMISSION

Three main routes of HIV transmission have been documented: (1) sexual contact with infected body fluids; (2) contact with infected blood or blood products via transfusion, organ transplants, shared needles, or accidental needlestick injury (health care workers); and (3) transmission from an infected woman to her infant prenatally, at birth, or during breastfeeding. With current use of antibody screening for donated blood, only 0.02 percent of HIV diagnoses in the United States through 2009 were related to hemophilia, blood transfusions, and perinatal transmission combined (National Center for HIV/AIDS, 2009). Transmission via casual contacts, fomites, and insect bites does not occur. Transmission via artificial insemination is possible; however, current safeguards make this unlikely. Oral-genital contact is less risky than vaginal or anal sex, but there have been reports of documented HIV transmission resulting solely from receptive fellatio and insertive cunnilingus (Fauci & Lane, 2008). Gum infection and bleeding increases the risk of acquiring HIV through this route (CDC, 2009b). Receptive anal intercourse is especially risky because traumatic lacerations of the delicate rectal mucosa provide direct bloodstream access for HIV. The presence of concomitant sexually transmitted infections in the source partner, particularly ulcerative diseases, increases the risk of transmission due to the presence of inflammatory cells (CDC, 2010b).

Women are at far greater risk of contracting HIV during heterosexual intercourse than are men. Semen has greater quantities of lymphocytes that may be infected than does vaginal fluid. Women have a larger mucosal surface area available for HIV penetration (vagina and cervix) while the only exposed mucosal surface in men is the urethra. Vaginal mucosa can suffer microscopic abrasions during intercourse, increasing susceptibility to HIV penetration. It has been hypothesized that women have increased risk for acquisition of HIV during the 7 to 10 days each month when humoral and cell-mediated immunity are suppressed by estradiol and/or progesterone

(Wira & Fahey, 2008). Women are often devastated at the news that they have been infected by someone whom they trusted. Depression and denial are common reactions after diagnosis.

TESTING FOR HIV

HIV-infected individuals may be relatively asymptomatic or asymptomatic for 10 years or longer (Fauci & Lane, 2008). Diagnosis while asymptomatic provides optimal opportunities to slow disease progression. Testing for antibodies to HIV is an important first step in establishing a diagnosis. The CDC (2010b) recommends routine counseling and voluntary testing for all pregnant women in the United States. Recommendations for testing of nonpregnant women are based on the guidelines from CDC urging universal testing as a part of routine clinical care and including an opt-out provision (CDC, 2006). High-risk individuals, such as intravenous drug users, persons who exchange sex for money or drugs, and those with multiple partners, warrant frequent repeat testing. Partners of HIV-infected individuals and men who have sex with men also require repeat testing. Such testing can occur after the patient is notified and the encounter is documented in the medical record. Women have the right to refuse testing but the practitioner is in a pivotal position to educate, persuade, and convince. General medical consent is adequate under most of these circumstances. However, clinicians should always defer to state policies that may differ in certain circumstances. Providers should make sure women who refuse testing at the time of care are aware of local testing centers.

DIAGNOSTIC TESTING

HIV antibody becomes detectable in the blood between 2 and 12 weeks after exposure. However, incubation periods may vary. The enzyme-linked immunosorbent assay (ELISA) is the initial screening test and may be repeated by the reference lab before results are reported. The positive ELISA is then confirmed with the Western blot test prior to reporting. There may rarely be false positives for the ELISA if there is underlying liver disease, autoantibodies, recent influenza vaccine, or acute viral infection (Fauci & Lane, 2008). The Western blot is usually negative in these cases. When ELISA and Western blot tests are combined, they have greater than a 99 percent accuracy rate (Bartlett, Gallant, & Pham, 2009). Women may deny the accuracy of the testing procedure and reinforcement and repeat testing may be necessary for confirmation. The diagnosis is obviously difficult to accept and there is a period of grieving that may occur before there is acceptance. Primary care nurse practitioners can reinforce the need for valid, scientific confirmation in an accepting environment.

Certain women may refuse blood testing but agree to salivary testing. OraSure® is an example of a collection kit that uses saliva and is sent to a lab for testing. OraQuick® is a Clinical Laboratory Improvement Amendments (CLIA)-waived in-office testing kit that uses saliva and can provide results during a visit (20 minutes). Positive results must be confirmed by Western blot testing. In addition to available HIV antibody tests, direct quantification of viral load can be performed. This testing occurs by polymerase chain reaction, nucleic acid sequence-based amplification, or branched chain DNA signal amplification. Nucleic acid testing is used to diagnose acute retroviral syndrome (ARS), which may occur in the first few weeks after HIV transmission. ARS may be characterized by fever, pharyngitis, malaise, lymphadenopathy, and headache. The symptoms are similar to influenza. This is called the "window" period as antibody testing will be negative, but transmission risk is increased due to high viral loads. Positive nucleic acid tests require referral to an infectious disease specialist.

PRE- AND POSTTEST COUNSELING

It is recommended that all women being tested for HIV receive extensive pretest counseling about viral transmission, implications for pregnancy, modes and prevention of transmission, personal risk, possibility of positive test results, and available support mechanisms. Again, the clinician should be aware that some states have specific policies and guidelines regarding pre- and posttest counseling. It is generally preferable for all HIV test results to be presented in person.

Persons testing negative for HIV can probably be reassured that they are virus free if it has been 6 months since their last possible exposure to HIV. They should be counseled about primary prevention strategies, however, and should be encouraged to have the test repeated if they have had more recent possible exposure.

Women testing positive for HIV require extensive counseling. Disclosure should consider social, cultural, and psychological characteristics of the person tested. Immediate interventions should include assessing the woman for the potential for violence to herself or others, ensuring access to a comprehensive medical evaluation, scheduling the next appointment, prevention of further HIV transmission, assessing the availability of key support persons, and providing information on local and national sources of support. Referral should be made for any services not available on site.

Later counseling should also include the natural history of HIV infection and available treatments. Disclosure of HIV status to sexual and needle-sharing partners by the woman should be encouraged so they can be tested. At the same time providers must be aware of the potential for domestic violence that may be triggered by this disclosure. Women should be advised that discrimination based on HIV status or AIDS regarding matters of employment, housing, state programs, or public accommodations is illegal. It should also be recommended that children born after acquisition of maternal infection be tested.

HIV-infected pregnant women should additionally be advised of the risk for perinatal HIV transmission (15–25%), ways to reduce this risk (including not breastfeeding), and the prognosis for infants who become infected. They should be given information concerning combination antiretroviral therapy to reduce the risk for perinatal transmission. Information about treatment should include addressing the potential benefit and short-term safety of and the uncertainties regarding risks of therapy and effectiveness. A woman's decision not to accept treatment should not result in punitive action or denial of care. The following guidelines for testing are from CDC (2010b, pp. 14–15). Practitioners may find these guidelines useful in clinical practice.

- HIV testing must be voluntary and free from coercion. Patients must not be tested without their knowledge.
- HIV screening after notifying the patient that an HIV test will be performed (unless the patient declines) is recommended in all health care settings.
- Specific signed consent for HIV testing should not be required (be aware of specific state policy in regard to need for signed consent). In most settings, general informed consent for medical care is considered sufficient to encompass informed consent for HIV testing.
- Use of rapid HIV tests should be considered, especially in clinics where a high proportion of patients do not return for HIV test results.
- Positive screening tests for HIV antibody must be confirmed by a supplemental test before the diagnosis of HIV infection can be established.

INITIAL EVALUATION OF A WOMAN WITH HIV

SUBJECTIVE DATA

The comprehensive surgical and medical history for all HIV-infected women should include the following: sexual, smoking, and drug use history and history of exposure to bacterial, viral, parasitic, and fungal infections such as tuberculosis, syphilis, herpes simplex and other sexually transmitted diseases (STDs), or *Giardia lamblia*. Immunization history as well as the presence of household pets (cat litter boxes transmit toxoplasmosis and reptiles transmit salmonella) should be determined. A social history should include family system history, occupational history, socioeconomic needs (insurance, disability benefits, etc.), and psychiatric history (medications and potential for suicide). Travel history includes time spent in geographic locations that may predispose to certain fungal infections, such as histoplasmosis in the Ohio River valley region or coccidiomycosis in the southwest.

Review of Systems

A careful review of all symptoms should precede the physical examination. Clues to conditions may be revealed by this review, such as shortness of breath, dysphagia, visual disturbances, and skin lesions.

Symptoms

Most symptoms reported by women with HIV or AIDS are caused by decline of the immune system and related to established disease. Early in the disease process, when the CD4 count is greater than 200 but less than 500 cells/mm^3, the symptoms will be vague and may be attributable to normal maladies such as a vaginal itching from a yeast infection. Any women with repeated vaginal or oral candidiasis should be tested for HIV. Complaints of shortness of breath, fevers, exercise intolerance, skin lesions, weight loss, headaches, visual disturbances, gait abnormalities, or night sweats are harbingers of more serious disease and immunocompromise and demand a thorough evaluation.

Flu-like symptoms within weeks to 1 month after exposure, unexplained fever or weight loss, severe fatigue, pharyngitis, shingles, swollen glands, diarrhea, and other nonspecific symptoms may indicate ARS. If the patient has had a new sexual partner or been engaging in risky activities, such as IV drug use or trading sex for money or drugs, the practitioner should look for an early HIV infection with the use of nucleic acid testing.

Signs

Signs that should alert practitioners to possible HIV infection include persistent or recurrent vaginal candidiasis, weight loss, lymphadenopathy, oral candidiasis or oral hairy leukoplakia of the tongue, and skin lesions such as varicella zoster, psoriasis, seborrheic dermatitis, or folliculitis. Persistent or recurrent genital herpes simplex infection, recurrent cervical neoplasia (despite treatment), and nonspecific genital ulcers may suggest HIV infection. Recurrent (nonpneumocystis) pneumonias, recurrent or particularly severe pelvic inflammatory disease (PID), and persistent urinary tract infections unresponsive to standard treatments may also be markers for early HIV infection. Hepatosplenomegaly and/or mental status changes may also be suspicious.

OBJECTIVE DATA

A complete physical examination should be done, including weight, height, body mass index, and nutritional status; blood pressure and temperature; oral cavity and tongue; skin and nails (lesions and clubbing); funduscopic exam (for exudates associated with cytomegalovirus [CMV] retinitis); ears, nose, and sinuses; neurological status (including mental status, cranial nerves, reflexes, gait, and fine motor skills); lymph nodes; heart and lungs; extremities (muscle mass, myositis); and abdominal exam (hepatomegaly, splenomegaly, or tenderness). A breast exam and complete vaginal and perirectal exam should also be done.

Recommended baseline labs for newly diagnosed persons with HIV include a CD4 lymphocyte count and percentage panel, baseline HIV genotype, viral load assay, complete blood count with differential and platelets, *Toxoplasma gondii* IgG, CMV serology, chemistry panel including liver function, lipid profile, serology for syphilis, hepatitis screen (for A, B, and C), and tuberculosis skin testing (purified protein derivative [PPD]) (Bartlett, 2010). The PPD should be repeated in 6 months if CD4 count was < 200 cells/μL initially, but increases to > 200 cells/μL (AIDS Education and Training Centers [AETC], 2006). A Pap smear, specimens for gonorrhea and chlamydia, and wet mounts for bacterial vaginosis, trichomonas, white blood cells, and *Candida* should be obtained at baseline. Cervical cytology should be repeated 6 months after diagnosis, then annually provided initial testing is normal (American College of Obstetricians and Gynecologists [ACOG], 2010). Robinson (2011) recommends that ACOG guidelines for annual cervical cytology be followed only if the two negative Pap smears were accompanied by a negative human papillomavirus (HPV) test; women with HIV and high-risk HPV DNA should have repeat cervical cytology every 6 months.

Recommended health maintenance, including appropriate testing for any comorbid conditions, such as hypertension, chronic obstructive pulmonary disease, and diabetes, should also be done. Routine screening mammography should be scheduled in age-appropriate women.

MANAGEMENT OF EARLY HIV INFECTION

It has been demonstrated that HIV-infected persons who are followed in a comprehensive program of care survive longer than those who present for care only according to their symptoms. The establishment of trust in a nonjudgmental care provider and sufficient time to express concerns are crucial. Specialty care providers for HIV-infected women should refer them for comprehensive case management services if they are unable to provide such services.

The CD4 cell count is a standard test to stage HIV, determine immune reconstitution, and make decisions regarding antiviral treatment and prophylaxis for OIs. Viral load is a better predictor of the progression of the disease and the therapeutic effectiveness of antiviral therapy. However, when to start treatment may not be related to CD4 count in the future. A large international study, HPTN 052, provided evidence that beginning antiretroviral treatment immediately upon diagnosis, even when CD4 counts are less than 250 cells/mm^3, significantly prevented transmission of the virus and introduced the concept of *treatment as prevention* (Alcorn, 2011).

Women with asymptomatic HIV infection should be followed by a specialty care provider every 3 to 6 months as long as their CD4+ counts remain normal. In addition to measuring CD4 counts and viral load, each visit should include monitoring for mental disorders, alcohol and drug abuse, measurement of weight and temperature, neurological status (including mental status and mood), abdominal examination, assessment of lymph nodes, and assessment of skin, oral cavity, and retina for characteristic lesions. Rescreening for sexually transmitted infection should be based on individual risk assessments. Additional strategies for ongoing care of HIV-infected women follow.

SELF-CARE STRATEGIES

Management of early HIV infection requires extensive teaching in health maintenance and in the avoidance of infectious disease risks. Latex condoms (or latex dental dams) should be encouraged for all vaginal, oral, and anal intercourse for the protection of HIV-infected persons and their partners (Hirschhorn, 2010). Smoking cessation decreases the risk of oral candidiasis, hairy leukoplakia, and bacteria pneumonia. Women who are abusing drugs or alcohol should be referred to treatment programs. HIV-infected persons experience several unique oral conditions, including frequent oral lesions and rapidly progressive periodontal disease, and should receive twice yearly dental prophylaxis.

HIV-infected persons should avoid pet reptiles that may carry salmonella; they should avoid young animals with diarrhea that may carry enteric pathogens; and they should avoid contact with cat feces that may be infected with *T. gondii.* Because *Toxoplasma* may be present in soil, hands should be washed after gardening, and raw fruits and vegetables should be washed before eating. Poultry and meats should be well cooked (>165°), and uncooked meats should not come into contact with foods that will be eaten raw. Patients should not drink unpasteurized dairy products. Gloves should be worn while cleaning aquariums to avoid the risk of *Mycobacterium marinum* infection (Pollack & Libman, 2011).

HIV-infected persons should be counseled about avoidance of *Cryptosporidium* transmitted through contact with stools of infected adults and diaper-age children, infected animals, contaminated drinking water, contaminated lake and river water, and uncooked or unwashed foods. Using drinking water purified through reverse osmosis or through distillation may be considered by HIV-infected persons whose municipal water supply is known to be contaminated by *Cryptosporidium.*

IMMUNIZATIONS

The Advisory Committee on Immunization Practices recommends that no live vaccines be given, with the exception of MMR. However, persons who are severely immunosuppressed should not receive MMR. Inactivated polio, pneumococcal, and influenza vaccines should be administered. Clinicians should also make sure that tetanus immunization is up-to-date and that immunization for hepatitis A and B is given as appropriate. Pneumococcal vaccine should be readministered every 5 years and influenza vaccine yearly (AETC, 2006). Vaccination with Gardasil® may also be considered.

GYNECOLOGIC CARE

Cervical dysplasia, vaginal candidiasis, and PID are more common in HIV-infected women and tend to follow more aggressive courses. The incidence of cervical intraepithelial abnormalities is four to five times higher in HIV-positive women, with risk increasing with degree of immunosuppression (Ellerbrock et al., 2000). Referral for colposcopy and biopsy is recommended for HIV-infected women with atypia or any grade of cervical intraepithelial neoplasia. Colposcopic evaluation should include the anal canal. Standard excisional or ablative treatment is recommended, although HIV-infected women have a high rate of recurrence (50%). Conization may be associated with less treatment failure than loop electrical excision procedure (Reimers et al., 2010).

Vaginal candidiasis, although not life-threatening, is not a trivial condition in HIV-infected women. Severe pruritus and excoriation can be disabling. Extension of candida to vulvae and thighs is common. Symptoms can often be controlled with topical antifungals, which may be more effective if used for 7 days. Single-dose fluconazole 150 mg may be used. Recurrent candidiasis may require maintenance therapy: fluconazole 150 mg for two or three sequential doses 72 hours apart (i.e., one dose would be taken every 3 days) has been shown to be effective (Pappas et al., 2009). Although the bacteriology remains the same, PID is more common in HIV-infected women and is often more severe. Accordingly, inpatient management should be considered (Hirschhorn, 2010). Genital herpes simplex infections occur more frequently, tend to be more severe, and are more likely to disseminate in immunocompromised hosts. Because of the risk of progressive disease, all herpes simplex should be treated with acyclovir 400 mg three times a day for 5 to 10 days, or famciclovir 500 mg twice daily for 5 to 10 days, or valacyclovir 1 g bid for 5 to 10 days (all orally). Daily suppressive therapy reduces clinical manifestations of HSV in persons with frequent recurrence. Recommended regimens include acyclovir 400 to 800 mg two to three times daily, famciclovir 500 mg twice daily, or valacyclovir 500 mg orally twice daily (CDC, 2010b). There have been reports of thrombotic thrombocytopenic purpura/hemolytic uremic syndrome with valacyclovir in persons with advanced AIDS, suggesting that alternative regimens may be considered in this setting (Hirschhorn, 2010). If lesions persist, HSV resistance should be suspected and a viral isolate should be obtained for sensitivity testing. Such persons should be managed in conjunction with an HIV specialist. Foscarnet, 40 mg/kg IV every 8 hours until clinical resolution is attained, is frequently effective for treatment of acyclovir-resistant genital herpes (CDC, 2010b).

CONTRACEPTION

For HIV-positive women, serostatus is one of many factors that influence reproductive decision making. Providers should advise about relative risks and therapeutic options and dangers and refrain from directive counseling where moral judgment is involved. The decision to initiate a pregnancy or to continue a pregnancy must remain a choice of the woman and her partner. The message conveyed to women must be that contraception and protection against STDs are separate issues. Properly and consistently used male condoms are the only means shown to prevent STDs, including HIV. Female condoms have less evidence of STD prevention efficacy. Condoms are helpful in protecting uninfected partners and also protect HIV-infected women from increased HIV viral load and new viral strains from HIV-positive partners. Polyurethane male condoms or polyurethane or nitrile female condoms may be recommended for persons who are allergic to latex as laboratory evidence has documented their impermeability to HIV (CDC, 2010b).

Vaginal spermicides (nonoxynol-9) used with latex condoms enhance prevention of pregnancy; however, they are ineffective for the prevention of HIV and other STDs. Also nonoxynol-9 has been shown to increase the transmission of HIV, possibly due to local irritative effects and ulceration of vaginal mucosa (CDC, 2010b). The use of spermicides alone should be discouraged in women with HIV, and risks of spermicide use with condoms should be discussed.

Hormonal contraceptives are highly effective and should not be denied to women who wish to use them. Although conflicting results have been published on the effects of hormonal contraception on disease progression and on susceptibility to HIV, the balance of the evidence suggests no increased risk. Efficacy of oral contraceptives may be compromised by interactions between estrogen and antiretroviral medications, including efavirenz and nevirapine, protease inhibitors, and other medications (rifampin) commonly used for HIV-infected patients (CDC, 2010c).

Previously, intrauterine devices (IUD) were not recommended for use in HIV-positive women; however, they appear to be safe and effective (CDC, 2010c). One large randomized controlled trial in Zambia reported only one woman with PID during 2-year follow-up (Stringer et al., 2007). Although they can be used in women with HIV and in women with disease well controlled on HAART, they should not be initiated in women whose disease has progressed to AIDS (Castano, 2007; CDC, 2010c). There are no medication interactions and they are easily reversible. Of course, barrier protection is still required when using an IUD for contraception.

Diaphragms and cervical caps have been associated with microabrasions, and they leave most of the woman's vaginal vault unprotected. Use of spermicides and/or diaphragms (with spermicide) can disrupt the cervical mucosa, which may increase viral shedding and HIV transmission to uninfected sex partners. These problems make these methods less desirable for HIV-infected women; they should be used only when no other contraceptive option is available (CDC, 2010c).

Certain antiretroviral medications, such as efavirenz, carry a pregnancy risk for teratogenic effects and should not be used in women who are capable of childbearing. If efavirenz is used for women of childbearing age, a specific consent for its use should be obtained. Pregnancy with HIV is a sensitive subject and requires additional counseling with a trusted practitioner. Although the chance of a successful pregnancy outcome has increased with adherence to perinatal antiretroviral drug guidelines, childbearing with HIV requires knowledge and commitment (NIH, 2010).

MYCOBACTERIUM TUBERCULOSIS PREVENTION

Because immunosuppression caused by HIV can cause rapid progression of *M. tuberculosis* infection to an active state, PPD-positive persons with negative x-rays should receive isoniazid (INH) therapy, usually 300 mg po daily for 9 months (CDC, 2009a). See www.hivatis.org for alternative medications. The addition of 50 mg of pyridoxine (vitamin B_6) po daily will prevent peripheral neuritis. Because INH is hepatotoxic, persons taking it should be monitored monthly for the development of adverse effects such as nausea, anorexia, fever, rash, visual problems, or jaundice. Monthly hepatic enzymes should be monitored in those over age 35. INH should be avoided in pregnant women (preventive therapy should be deferred until after delivery). A PPD reaction of 5 mm or greater is considered positive in a person with HIV infection. Women should be assessed for health and social conditions (alcoholism, mental illness, or failure to keep appointments) that may affect their ability to complete a course of INH treatment. Case management and directly observed therapy should be used when needed to ensure successful completion of INH treatment (CDC, 2009a).

Women presenting with weight loss, hemoptysis, night sweats, or fever should receive an immediate chest x-ray and a sputum smear should be examined. Those who are coughing with symptoms of tuberculosis should be placed on respiratory isolation until active tuberculosis has been ruled out. Active tuberculosis or infection with possibly drug-resistant organisms should be managed by an infectious disease specialist.

MONITORING IMMUNE STATUS

The assessment of immune status is a key element in the ongoing management of early HIV infection. Measurement of plasma viral load should be used with physical findings and CD4+ cell counts to stage patients and to determine appropriate time for initiating antiretroviral therapy and prophylaxis for PCP and other OIs. CD4+ cells and viral load should be measured every 3 to 6 months upon entry to care and before HAART is initiated. CD4+, viral load, and viral resistance testing should be done upon initiation of HAART and viral load should be rechecked 2 to 8 weeks post HAART initiation or modification. In clinically stable patients with suppressed viral load, viral load can continue to be measured every 3 to 6 months, but CD4+ count can be monitored every 6 to 12 months (U.S. Department of Health and Human Services [USDHHS], 2011).

MANAGEMENT OF LATE HIV INFECTION

HIV infection is termed AIDS with a CD4+ count of less than 200 cells/mm^3 (14% lymphocytes) or one or more of the conditions in the 1993 expanded surveillance case definition for AIDS (see Table 15–1).

Although recurrent vaginal candidiasis, pulmonary tuberculosis, bacterial pneumonia, and persistent generalized lymphadenopathy may occur during early HIV infection, most of the conditions associated with AIDS occur when the CD4+ count falls below 500 cells/μL according to the CDC (USDHHS, 2011). All states except Hawaii and Vermont require reporting of HIV diagnosis by name and all states require reporting of AIDS cases by name (CDC, 2011b). Persons with AIDS should be managed in conjunction with an infectious disease specialist and may also require referral to oncology or other subspecialty care.

TABLE 15–1. 1993 Expanded Surveillance Case Definition for AIDS

HIV Seropositivity *and* CD4+ Count < 200 Cells/mm^3 *or* One or More of the Following Conditions:
Candidiasis of bronchi, trachea, esophagus, or lungs; invasive cervical cancer; coccidioidomycosis (disseminated or extrapulmonary), cryptococcosis (extrapulmonary), cryptosporidiosis, cytomegalovirus (CMV) disease (other than spleen, liver, and nodes), or CMV retinitis; encephalopathy; herpes simplex virus (chronic ulcers, esophagitis, or bronchitis); histoplasmosis; isosporiasis; Kaposi's sarcoma; lymphoma (Burkitt's, immunoblastic, or primary); mycobacterium tuberculosis (any site); *Mycobacterium avium* complex, *Mycoplasma kansasii*, or other species (disseminated or extrapulmonary); *Pneumocystis carinii* pneumonia, any recurrent pneumonia, progressive multifocal leukoencephalopathy, *Salmonella septicemia* (recurrent), toxoplasmosis of brain, or wasting syndrome due to HIV.

Source: Centers for Disease Control and Prevention. (1992). 1993 revised classification system for HIV infection and expanded surveillance case definition for AIDS among adolescents and adults. *Morbidity and Mortality Weekly Report, 41*, 1–19.

HIGHLY ACTIVE ANTIRETROVIRAL THERAPY

The goal of antiretroviral therapy is to maximize suppression of viral load, restore and preserve the immune system (CD4 count), improve the quality of life, and reduce HIV-related morbidity and mortality. Antiretroviral drugs do not cure HIV or prevent transmission of HIV. The time for initiating HAART is controversial, and depends on symptoms, cell counts, and patient readiness to adopt a lifelong drug regimen (USDHHS, 2011). The most recent guidelines recommend starting HAART in all patients with a CD4 count of 350 or less cells/mm^3. Persons with renal disease, hepatitis B, who require treatment and all pregnant women should also be started on HAART. Persons with CD4 counts between 350 and 500 cells/mm^3 should be considered for HAART, although the evidence is less clear. Developments supporting earlier initiation of HAART include (1) recognition that HIV disease may be associated with non-HIV-associated diseases such as heart disease and malignancies, (2) availability of treatment regimens that are more effective, more convenient, and better tolerated than older regimens, and (3) recognition that effective antiviral treatment decreases HIV transmission. However, drug-related complications affecting quality of life, nonadherence to treatment in asymptomatic patients, and the potential for drug resistance may offset benefits of earlier treatment. Delaying treatment may preserve treatment options and delay drug resistance. However, treatment delay risks the possibility that damage to the immune system will be irreversible and suppression of viral replication may be more difficult at a later stage of disease (USDHHS, 2011).

A high level of adherence is necessary for optimal success of HAART, requiring client understanding and commitment to the treatment plan. Clinicians should inform clients in advance about potential side effects, provide them with treatment for expected side effects, and inform them when to contact the clinician. Daily or weekly pillboxes, timers, pagers, and other devices may be useful along with discussion of compliance at each client encounter. Results of HAART are evaluated primarily with plasma HIV RNA levels and secondarily with CD4 cell count (USDHHS, 2011).

There are currently five classifications of antiviral therapy drugs for oral use and one category for parenteral use. The oral categories include the nucleoside reverse transcriptase inhibitors (NRTIs), protease inhibitors (PIs), non-nucleoside reverse transcriptase inhibitors (NNRTIs), integrase strand transfer inhibitors (INSTI), and CCR5 antagonists (entry inhibitors [EIs]). In general, the various classes attack the virus from different directions and in different ways. There is one drug that is subcutaneously administered, enfuvirtide (Fuzeon) (Table 15–2). Current HAART recommendations for initial therapy are for three different drugs to be initiated simultaneously from different classes. Monotherapy should not be used because it rapidly leads to drug resistance. Drug resistance occurs when viral mutations occur during viral replication rendering the drug ineffective. Multiple mutations severely limit options for pharmacologic success. Updated HIV drug management strategies are provided on the website maintained by the panel on clinical practices for treatment of HIV infection convened by the DHHS and the Henry J. Kaiser Family Foundation (http://www.hivatis.org). Because developing drug regimens should be left to HIV specialists, drug choices are not discussed further. Major side effects, adverse reactions, and drug interactions are common and clinicians who provide primary care for women with HIV should be familiar with these aspects of using HAART.

The primary care clinician should review all medications with patients at every visit. Encourage women to maintain and carry a list of all prescribed and over-the-counter medications. Discourage use of herbal products unless interaction safety has been documented. Clinicians should use electronic medication regimen monitors to check for interactions before prescribing new medications. The Health Resources and Services Administration has a *warmline* that clinicians can call. It is listed on its AETC page at http://hab.hrsa.gov/abouthab/partfeducation.html. A full listing of medication

TABLE 15–2. Medications for HIV (generic name first) and Combination Products

Nucleoside/Nucleotide Reverse Transcriptase Inhibitors	Non-nucleoside Reverse Transcriptase Inhibitors	Protease Inhibitors	Entry Inhibitors	Integrase Inhibitor	Combination Products
Abacavir (ABC)	Delavirdine (DLV)	Atazanavir (ATV)	Enfuvirtide (ENF,T-20)	Raltegravir (RAL)	Efavirenz, emtricitabine, tenofovir
Ziagen	Rescriptor	Reyataz	Fuzeon (fusion inhibitor)	Isentress	Atripla
Didanosine (DDI)	Efavirenz (EFV)	Darunavir (DRV)	Maraviroc (MVC)		Zidovudine, lamivudine
Videx EC	Sustiva	Prezista	Selzentry (CCR5 inhibitor)		Combivir
Emtricitavine (FTC)	Etravirine (ETR)	Fosamprenavir (FPC)			Abacavir, lamivudine
Emtriva	Intelence	Lexiva			Epzicom
Lamivudine (3TC)	Nevirapine (NVP)	Indinavir (IDV)			Zidovudine, lamivudine, abacavir
Epivir	Viramune	Crixivan			Trizivir
Stavudine (D4T)		Lopinavir/Ritonavir (KAL, LPV/r)			Tenofovir, emtricitabine
Zerit		Kaletra			Truvada
Tenofovir (TDF)		Nelfinavir (NFV)			
Viread		Viracept			
Zidovudine (AZT)		Ritonavir (RTV)			
Retrovir		Norvir			
		Saquinavir (SQV)			
		Invriase			
		Tipranavir (TPV)			
		Aptivus			

interactions, contraindications, and adverse reactions are available at http://www.aidsinfo.nih.gov/ContentFiles/AdultandAdolescentGL.pdf.

Long-Term HAART-Associated Complications

Although HAART improves immune functioning and prolongs life, it can have consequences. Women, in particular, can experience changes that cause concern. Changes in body fat distribution (central obesity, peripheral fat wasting, breast enlargement, facial thinning, and dorsocervical fat accumulation) occur in 60 to 80 percent of persons receiving HAART, particularly with PIs and NRTIs. Hyperlipidemia and insulin resistance occur in up to 17 percent and are frequently associated with this lipodystrophy. The effects of lifestyle in reversing these changes are not clear, but exercise and weight maintenance should be encouraged. Concurrent use of statin drugs with PIs must be undertaken with caution, due to the potential for enhanced statin toxicity that may cause muscle pain and rhabdomyolysis (see Table 15–3).

Potentially severe adverse drug reactions include the abacavir hypersensitivity reaction; however, this has been decreased due to preliminary screening for the HLA-B 5701 antigen. Other reactions include severe skin reactions (nevirapine), peripheral neuropathy (zalcitabine), bone marrow suppression, anemia, and neutropenia (zidovudine). Hepatotoxicity (a three- to fivefold elevation in serum transaminases) has been associated with all of the NNRTIs and with PIs. Coinfection with hepatitis C, hepatitis B, alcohol abuse, and other use of other hepatotoxic drugs increases this risk. Close monitoring of clinical symptoms and liver enzymes is required. Although rare, lactic acidosis/hepatic steatosis has been demonstrated with NRTIs and is related to the effect of these drugs on mitochondrial DNA. Risk factors for this adverse effect include female gender, obesity, and prolonged use of NRTIs. Clinical presentation is diarrhea, abdominal pain, vomiting weight loss, dyspnea, respiratory failure, tachypnea, and elevated liver enzymes. Other manifestations of drug-related mitochondrial dysfunction may include pancreatitis, peripheral neuropathy, myopathy, and cardiomyopathy. Raltegravir can cause myopathy and any complaint of muscle pain or weakness should be investigated.

Decreased bone density has been demonstrated with more potent antiretroviral therapy. Skin rash is common with NNRTIs and is seven times more frequent in women (USDHHS, 2011).

PREVENTING OPPORTUNISTIC INFECTIONS

Life-threatening infection with pathogens that pose little threat to persons with normal immune systems is characteristic of full-blown AIDS. These infections become more evident when the CD4 count drops below 200 cells/mm^3. Although HAART is effective in preserving and even restoring CD4 cells, some persons are unable or unready to take HAART, some initiate HAART with CD4 counts below 200 cells/mm^3, and others have failed antiretroviral treatment. For these persons, medication to prevent OIs remains appropriate. Preventing OIs with antibiotics is called primary prophylaxis. Preventing a recurrence of an OI after treatment is called secondary prophylaxis. In persons who demonstrate CD4 cell rebound after starting HAART, it may be appropriate to discontinue OI prophylaxis (CDC, 2009a).

P. Carinii Pneumonia Prophylaxis

P. carinii pneumonia is the most common OI in persons with AIDS. Prophylaxis with the preferred agent trimethoprim/sulfamethoxazole (TMP/SMX), one double strength tablet daily or three times a week, not only prevents this common infection but also prolongs life (CDC, 2009a). PCP prophylaxis is recommended for adults and adolescents with a CD4+ count below 200 cells/mm^3, a prior episode of PCP, oral candidiasis, or unexplained fever lasting 2 weeks or more.

For those unable to tolerate TMP/SMX, dapsone 50 mg po bid or 100 mg qd, or dapsone 50 mg qd plus pyrimethamine 50 mg po weekly, plus leucovorin 25 mg po weekly may be used (CDC, 2009a).

Another alternative is atovaquone (Mepron) dosed at 1,500 mg daily. Atovaquone will also prophylax against toxoplasmosis if the woman is toxoplasmosis IgG positive. This means she has antibodies (IgG) against toxoplasmosis indicating a prior infection that is dormant but could become reactivated when the CD4 count declines to 100 or less cells/mm^3. TMP/SMX and pyrimethamine are also used for treatment and prophylaxis of toxoplasmosis. Prior to initiation of dapsone, it is necessary to document a normal G6PD level in the blood with testing. When TMP/SMX is used, it is necessary to monitor for anemia, neutropenia, and agranulocytosis. Severe dermatologic reactions such as Stevens-Johnson syndrome, erythema nodosum, erythema multiforme, or epidermal necrolysis are possible with TMP/SMX and dapsone (CDC, 2009a).

When the CD4+ T cell count rises above 200 cells/mm^3 and has remained stable for 3 months, prophylaxis maybe

TABLE 15–3. Drugs That Should Not Be Used With PI, NNRTI, or CCR5 Antagonist

	Drug Categories									
Antiretroviral Agents[a,b]	Cardiac Agents	Lipid-lowering Agents	Antimycobacterials	Gastro-intestinal Drugs	Neuroleptics	Psychotropics	Ergot Derivatives (vasoconstrictors)	Herbs	Antiretroviral Agents	Others
ATV +/– RTV	None	Lovastatin Pitavastatin Simvastatin	Rifampin Rifapentine[c]	Cisapride[d]	Pimozide	Midazolam[e] Triazolam	Dihydroergotamine Ergonovine Ergotamine Methylergonovine	St. John's wort	ETR NVP	Alfuzosin Irinotecan Salmeterol Sildenafil for PAH
DRV/r	None	Lovastatin Pitavastatin Simvastatin	Rifampin Rifapentine[c]	Cisapride[d]	Pimozide	Midazolam[e] Triazolam	Dihydroergotamine Ergonovine Ergotamine Methylergonovine	St. John's wort	None	Alfuzosin Salmeterol Sildenafil for PAH
FPV +/– RTV	Flecainide Propafenone	Lovastatin Pitavastatin Simvastatin	Rifampin Rifapentine[c]	Cisapride[d]	Pimozide	Midazolam[e] Triazolam	Dihydroergotamine Ergonovine Ergotamine Methylergonovine	St. John's wort	ETR	Alfuzosin Salmeterol Sildenafil for PAH
LPV/r	None	Lovastatin Pitavastatin Simvastatin	Rifampin[f] Rifapentine[c]	Cisapride[d]	Pimozide	Midazolam[e] Triazolam	Dihydroergotamine Ergonovine Ergotamine Methylergonovine	St. John's wort	None	Alfuzosin Salmeterol Sildenafil for PAH
RTV	Amiodarone Flecainide Propafenone Quinidine	Lovastatin Pitavastatin Simvastatin	Rifapentine[c]	Cisapride[d]	Pimozide	Midazolam[e] Triazolam	Dihydroergotamine Ergonovine Ergotamine Methylergonovine	St. John's wort	None	Alfuzosin Sildenafil for PAH
SQV/r	Amiodarone Dofetilide Flecainide Lidocaine Propafenone Quinidine	Lovastatin Pitavastatin Simvastatin	Rifampin[f] Rifapentine	Cisapride[d]	Pimozide	Midazolam[e] Triazolam Trazodone	Dihydroergotamine Ergonovine Ergotamine Methylergonovine	St. John's wort Garlic supplements	None	Alfuzosin Salmeterol Sildenafil for PAH
TPV/r	Amiodarone Flecainide Propafenone Quinidine	Lovastatin Pitavastatin Simvastatin	Rifampin Rifapentine[c]	Cisapride[d]	Pimozide	Midazolam[e] Triazolam	Dihydroergotamine Ergonovine Ergotamine Methylergonovine	St. John's wort	ETR	Alfuzosin Salmeterol Sildenafil for PAH

	Drug Categories									
Antiretroviral Agents[a,b]	Cardiac Agents	Lipid-lowering Agents	Antimycobacterials	Gastro-intestinal Drugs	Neuroleptics	Psychotropics	Ergot Derivatives (vasoconstrictors)	Herbs	Antiretroviral Agents	Others
EFV	None	None	Rifapentine[c]	Cisapride[d]	Pimozide	Midazolam[e] Triazolam	Dihydroergotamine Ergonovine Ergotamine Methylergonovine	St. John's wort	Other NNRTIs	None
ETR	None	None	Rifampin Rifapentine[c]	None	None	None	None	St. John's wort	Unboosted PIs ATV/r, FPV/r, or TPV/r Other NNRTIs	Carbamazepine. Phenobarbital Phenytoin Clopidogrel
NVP	None	None	Rifapentine[c]	None	None	None	None	St. John's wort	ATV +/– RTV Other NNRTIs	Ketoconazole
MVC	None	None	Rifapentine[c]	None	None	None	None	St. John's wort	None	None

ATV +/– RTV—atazanavir +/– ritonavir
DLV—delavirdine
DRV/r—darunavir/ritonavir
EFV—efavirenz
ETR—etravirine
FDA—Food and Drug Administration
FPV +/– RTV—fosamprenavir +/– ritonavir
HIV—human immunodeficiency virus
IDV—indinavir
LPV/r—lopinavir/ritonavir
MVC—maraviroc
NFV—nelfinavir
NNRTI—non-nucleoside reverse transcriptase inhibitor
NVP—nevirapine
PAH—pulmonary arterial hypertension
PI—protease inhibitor
RPV—rilpivirine
RTV—ritonavir
SQV/r—saquinavir/ritonavir
TB—tuberculosis
TPV/r—tipranavir/ritonavir

[a]DLV, IDV, and NFV are not included in this table. Refer to the FDA package insert for information regarding DLV-, IDV-, and NFV-related drug interactions.

[b]Certain listed drugs are contraindicated based on theoretical considerations. Thus, drugs with narrow therapeutic indices and suspected metabolic involvement with CYP450 3A, 2D6, or unknown pathways are included in this table. Actual interactions may or may not occur in patients.

[c]HIV-infected patients treated with rifapentine have a higher rate of TB relapse than those treated with other rifamycin-based regimens; an alternative agent is recommended.

[d]The manufacturer of cisapride has a limited-access protocol for patients who meet specific clinical eligibility criteria.

[e]Use of oral midazolam is contraindicated. Parenteral midazolam can be used with caution as a single dose and can be given in a monitored situation for procedural sedation.

[f]A high rate of Grade 4 serum transaminase elevation was seen when a higher dose of RTV was added to LPV/r or SQV or when double-dose LPV/r was used with rifampin to compensate for rifampin's induction effect, so these dosing strategies should not be used.
This table lists only drugs that should not be coadministered at any dose and regardless of RTV boosting.

Source: http://www.aidsinfo.nih.gov/ContentFiles/AdultandAdolescentGL.pdf, Table 14, p. 134.

discontinued. If prior pneumonia, history of thrush, or wasting syndrome is present, prophylaxis should be continued (CDC, 2009a).

Mycobacterium Avium Complex

Mycobacterium avium complex (MAC) typically occurs at CD4+ counts below 50 cells/mm^3. Drugs for disseminated MAC prophylaxis are generally started at CD4+ counts of 75 cells/mm^3 for those with previous infections and at CD4+ counts of less than 50 to 100 cells/mm^3 for those without previous infections. Prophylaxis for MAC includes clarithromycin or azithromycin. Azithromycin is usually better tolerated. Prophylaxis therapy can be discontinued if the CD4+ T cell count remains elevated above 100 cells/mm^3 for 3 months. However, persons with a prior episode of disseminated MAC should receive prophylaxis indefinitely (CDC, 2009a).

Cytomegalovirus Infection

Cytomegalovirus retinitis is a common OI associated with visual loss in HIV-infected persons. Although oral valganciclovir may be used to prevent the occurrence of CMV disease in those with CD4+ counts less than 50 cells/mm^3, prophylactic use is not recommended as prophylaxis may invoke resistance. Those with visual symptoms suggestive of CMV retinitis should be immediately referred to an ophthalmologist for confirmation of possible diagnosis (CDC, 2009a).

Immune Reconstitution Syndrome

When HAART is initiated, the immune system usually rebounds and if an OI is present or incubating, the immune response may exacerbate symptoms and cause a clinical deterioration. This syndrome is particularly likely to occur with mycobacterial infections, but it can occur with other OIs. There may be worsening of symptoms accompanied by fever, and this syndrome is usually seen in the first 4 to 8 weeks after starting HAART. Practitioners should be aware of this event and refer the woman back to the infectious disease specialist for consultation. Sometimes it may be difficult to differentiate between immune reconstitution syndrome and adverse reactions to HAART. In general, although HAART indicated as the definitive treatment for complications of HIV/AIDS, in the face of a fulminant OI, it is prudent to wait for at least 2 weeks to start therapy (USDHHS, 2011).

CONCLUSION

Managing a female patient with HIV is challenging for primary care practitioners, especially those in remote areas. The female patient may see an infectious disease provider only once or twice a year and she relies on her nurse practitioner for closer management of this complex condition. The practitioner can provide local support, assisting the woman with adherence to complex regimens and serve as a liaison with specialists. The practitioner should also establish a close working relationship with the infectious disease specialists in the region and call frequently with questions or problems. Attention to housing, mental health status, birth control, substance abuse, and childcare may alleviate obstacles to adherence. The local practitioner is usually familiar with the community and has access to resources in the area.

Additional resources for practitioners include all the guidelines available through the DHHS. Guidelines are available in hard copy or online. A relationship with an infectious disease pharmacist may also be helpful. Electronic drug management programs can provide immediate information about drug doses, interactions, precautions, monitoring, and adverse reactions. These would be available even at the most remote locations.

In general, the role of the nurse practitioner in managing the needs of a female patient with HIV focuses on drug management and adherence, laboratory monitoring, health maintenance, symptom control, identifying potential infections, and referral for care. The female patient is often constrained by family pressures and would have difficulties visiting a specialist on a regular basis. By offering local care, the practitioner establishes a bond that facilitates confidence in her care and offers compassion with cultural sensitivity. Although difficult, the role is extremely rewarding.

REFERENCES

ACOG Committee on Practice Bulletins—Gynecology. (2010). ACOG practice bulletin no. 117: Gynecologic care for women with human immunodeficiency virus. *Obstetrics and Gynecology, 116,* 1492–1509.

AIDS Education and Training Centers (AETC). (2006). *Clinical manual for management of the HIV infected adult.* Retrieved May 15, 2011, from http://www.aidsetc.org/pdf/AETC-CM_071007.pdf

Alcorn, K. (2011). Treatment as prevention works! *HAITiP, 177,* 2.

Bartlett, J.G. (2010). *Screening laboratory tests in HIV-infected individuals.* Retrieved May 21, 2011, from UpToDate Database: http://www.uptodate.com

Bartlett, J.G., & Gallant, J.E. (2002). *The 2002 abbreviated guide to medical management of HIV infection* [Electronic version]. Baltimore: Johns Hopkins University School of Medicine. Retrieved December 12, 2002, from http://hopkins-aids.edu/publications/abbrevad.html

Bartlett, J.G., Gallant, J.E., & Pham, P. (2009). *Medical management of HIV infection* (15th ed.). Durham, NC: Knowledge Source Solutions.

Castano, P. (2007). Use of intrauterine devices and systems by HIV-infected women. *Contraception, 75,* S51–S54.

Centers for Disease Control and Prevention (CDC). (2006). Revised recommendations for HIV testing of adults, adolescents, and pregnant women in health-care settings. *Morbidity and Mortality Weekly Report: Recommendations and Reports, 55*(RR-14), 1–17.

Centers for Disease Control and Prevention (CDC). (2009a). Guidelines for prevention and treatment of opportunistic infections in HIV-Infected adults and adolescents. *Morbidity and Mortality Weekly Report, 58*(RR-4), 1–206.

Centers for Disease Control and Prevention (CDC). (2009b). *Oral sex and HIV risk.* Retrieved May 15, 2011, from http://www.cdc.gov/hiv/resources/factsheets/oralsex.htm

Centers for Disease Control and Prevention (CDC). (2010a). *HIV in the United States.* Retrieved May 15, 2011, from http://www.cdc.gov/hiv/resources/factsheets/us.htm

Centers for Disease Control and Prevention (CDC). (2010b). Sexually transmitted disease guidelines 2010. *Morbidity and Mortality Weekly Report, 59*(RR-12), 2–61.

Centers for Disease Control and Prevention (CDC). (2010c). U.S. Medical eligibility criteria for contraceptive use, 2010. *Morbidity and Mortality Weekly Report, 59,* 1–88.

Centers for Disease Control and Prevention (CDC). (2011a). *HIV prevalence by race/ethnicity through 2009.* Retrieved May 15, 2011, from http://www.cdc.gov/hiv/topics/surveillance/index.htm

Centers for Disease Control and Prevention (CDC). (2011b). *Nationally notifiable infectious conditions: United States 2011.* Retrieved May 23, 2011, from http://www.cdc.gov/ncphi/diss/nndss/PHS/infdis2011.htm

Connor, E.M., Sperling, R.S., Gelber, R., Kiselev, P., Scott, G., O'Sullivan, M.J., et al. (1994). Reduction of maternal-infant transmission of human immunodeficiency virus type 1 with ziduvidine treatment. *New England Journal of Medicine, 331,* 1173–1180.

Ellerbrock, T.V., Chaisson, M.A., Bush, T. J., Sun, X.W., Sawo, D., Brudney, K., et al. (2000). Incidence of cervical squamous intraepithelial lesions in HIV-infected women. *Journal of the American Medical Association, 283,* 1031–1037.

Fauci, A.S., & Lane, H.C. (2008). Human immunodeficiency virus disease: AIDS and related disorders. In A.S. Fauci, E. Braunwald, D.L. Kasper, S.L. Hauser, D.L. Longo, J. Jameson, & J. Loscalzo (Eds.), *Harrison's principles of internal medicine-online* (Chapter 182, 17th ed.). New York: McGraw-Hill. Retrieved May 15, 2011, from http://accessmedicine.com/resourceTOC.aspx?resourceID=4

Hirschhorn, L. (2010). *HIV and women.* Retrieved May, 21, 2011, from UpToDate Database: http://www.uptodate.com

National Center for HIV/AIDS, Viral Hepatitis, STDs and TB Prevention. (2009). *Epidemiology of HIV infection through 2009.* Retrieved May 15, 2011, from http://www.cdc.gov/HIV/topics/surveillance/resources/slides/general/slides/general.pdf

National Institute of Allergy and Infectious Disease (NIAID). (2008). *HIV infection in women overview.* Retrieved May 15, 2011, from http://www.niaid.nih.gov/topics/HIVAIDS/Understanding/Population%20Specific%20Information/Pages/womenHiv.aspx

National Institutes of Health (NIH). (2010). *Recommendations for use of antiretroviral drugs in pregnant HIV-1-infected women for maternal health and interventions to reduce perinatal HIV transmission in the United States* (pp. 1–117). Retrieved May 15, 2010, from http://aidsinfo.nih.gov/ContentFiles/PerinatalGL.pdf

Pappas, P.G., Kauffman, C.A., Andes, D., Benjamin, D.K., Jr., Calandra, T.F., Edwards, J.E., Jr., et al. (2009). Clinical practice guidelines for the management of candidiasis: 2009 update by the Infectious Diseases Society of America. *Clinical Infectious Diseases, 48,* 503–535.

Pollack, T.M., & Libman, H. (2011). *Primary care of HIV-infected adults.* Retrieved May 21, 2011, form UpToDate Database: http://www.uptodate.com

Reimers, L.L., Sotardi, S., Daniel, D., Chiu, L.G., Van Arsdale, A., Wieland, D.L., et al. (2010). Outcomes after an excisional procedure for cervical intraepithelial neoplasia in HIV-infected women. *Gynecologic Oncology, 119,* 92–97.

Robinson, W.R. (2011). *Screening for cervical cancer in HIV infected women.* Retrieved May 21, 2011, from UpToDate Database: http://www.uptodate.com

Stringer, E.M., Kaseba, C., Levy, J., Sinkala, M., Goldenberg, R.L., Chi, B.H., et al. (2007). A randomized trial of the intrauterine contraceptive device vs hormonal contraception in women who are infected with the human immunodeficiency virus. *American Journal of Obstetrics and Gynecology, 197,* 144.e1–144.e8.

UNAIDS. (2010). *UNAIDS report on the global AIDS epidemic, 2010.* Retrieved May 15, 2011, from http://www.unaids.org/globalreport/

U.S. Department of Health and Human Services (USDHHS). (2011). Panel on Antiretroviral Guidelines for Adults and Adolescents: Guidelines for the use of antiretroviral agents in HIV-1 infected adults and adolescents. Retrieved from http://www.aidsinfo.nih.giv/ContentFiles/AdultandAdolescentGL.pdf

Wira, C.R., & Fahey, J.V. (2008). A new strategy to understand how HIV infects women: Identification of a window of vulnerability during the menstrual cycle. *AIDS, 22,* 1909–1917.

CHAPTER ❖ 16

COMMON GYNECOLOGIC PELVIC DISORDERS

Jennifer M. Laubach ◆ *Reena P. Lorntson*

Frustrating for all health care providers is the client who presents with chronic pelvic pain, because in most cases a specific etiology cannot be determined and care is very difficult.

Highlights

- Endometriosis
- Pelvic Inflammatory Disease
- Adnexal Masses (Ovarian Tumors)
- Dyspareunia
- Nonmalignant Disorders of the Vulva
- Leiomyomas
- Adenomyosis
- Pelvic Organ Prolapse
- Chronic Pelvic Pain
- Chronic Cervicitis
- Bartholin's Gland Duct Cysts and Bartholinitis
- Cervical Polyps
- Gynecologic Cancers
- Diethylstilbestrol Exposure

❖ INTRODUCTION

A health care provider needs to be familiar with the diagnosis, management, and follow-up of common gynecologic pelvic disorders encountered in practice and must recognize when a client should be referred for further evaluation and management. With the changing health care climate where accountable care organizations, evidence-based practice, and cost-effectiveness are major influences, the practitioner must use sound clinical judgment in gathering pertinent history and physical examination data, selecting cost-efficient diagnostic tests, and implementing medical, nursing, and adjunct therapies. The population of older women is growing rapidly in the United States; quality-of-life issues are most important and should always be in the forefront of a clinician's mind. The clinician should be knowledgeable about those disorders more common in older women, such as pelvic organ prolapse, and the importance of screening for gynecologic cancers.

The evaluation of any complaint of pelvic symptoms begins with a thorough client history that includes the following:

- The onset and description of the pelvic symptoms and any associated abdominal symptoms.
- A description of the character, nature, location, and timing of any pain.
- A detailed menstrual and sexual history.
- A history of previous related surgeries or hospitalizations.
- An obstetric history.
- A thorough psychosocial history.

For clients with chronic pelvic pain, a thorough history, physical examination, and diagnostic evaluation are critical because the etiology is often elusive. Consultation with a gynecologist may be necessary.

Although a goal is to prevent unnecessary medical and surgical intervention, the fact remains that surgical intervention often is necessary to evaluate and manage pelvic disorders. The clinician has a responsibility to the client to review alternative therapies, to evaluate the severity of her symptoms and their impact on her lifestyle, to discuss the potential benefits of proposed surgery, and to assist her in seeking consultation with a qualified, reputable surgeon.

In many clinical situations, the clinician will find himself or herself in a unique position to thoroughly evaluate a chronic or ongoing problem. In the evaluation, management, and follow-up of nonmalignant vulvar disorders, especially vulvodynia, the clinician's most important role is to obtain a complete history, to offer emotional support, and to evaluate therapy.

This section cannot completely address all gynecologic disorders. It is intended to be a clinical guideline for current evaluation and management of common, more frequently seen problems.

ENDOMETRIOSIS

Endometriosis is a common benign gynecologic disorder characterized by endometrial glands and stroma outside the endometrial cavity (Hsu, Khachikyan, & Stratton, 2010). Endometriosis is associated with chronic pain and infertility. It is the third leading cause of gynecologic hospitalization in the United States (American College of Obstetricians and Gynecologists [ACOG], 2010; Missmer et al., 2010). Endometrial tissue responds cyclically to estrogen by swelling and producing local inflammation (Fritz & Speroff, 2011). Symptom severity varies widely; the stage of endometriosis correlates poorly with the extent and severity of the pain (Hsu et al., 2010). Some women with minimal disease have debilitating pain and other women with severe disease are asymptomatic. It is generally thought that the extent of the pain is influenced primarily by the location and depth of the endometriotic implant, with deep implants in highly innervated areas most consistently associated with pain. Endometriosis occurs mainly on the pelvic peritoneum, ovaries, and rectovaginal septum, and rarely on the diaphragm, pleura, and pericardium (Giudice, 2010).

EPIDEMIOLOGY

Several theories for the pathogenesis of endometriosis have been proposed. One theory is that the primary mechanism is associated with attachment and implantation of the endometrial glands and stroma on the peritoneum from retrograde menstruation. This theory was proposed by John Sampson in 1927. Sampson identified and named this condition, endometriosis, in 1921 (Fritz & Speroff, 2011). Other theories consider that disease could be caused by lymphatic transport or metaplastic transformation of endometrial cells (ACOG, 2010; Fritz & Speroff, 2011; Giudice, 2010).

There is an interaction between the expression of endometrial genes and an altered hormonal response, predisposing women to the formation of endometrial lesions. Key components of the development of endometriotic lesions include overproduction of prostaglandins and local estrogen. Progesterone resistance lessens the antiestrogenic effect of progesterone and increases the local estrogenic effect. Endometrial lesions can lead to a chronic inflammatory disorder due to increased numbers of macrophages and proinflammatory cytokines in the peritoneum that may cause pain and infertility. Nerve growth factor is also expressed in endometriotic lesions, leading to an increased density of nerve fibers. The mechanism by which endometriosis causes infertility at an early stage is not entirely understood, although there may be damage done to both sperm and oocyte function by the abnormal peritoneal environment of increased inflammatory cytokines and oxidative stress (ACOG, 2010).

Endometriosis is more likely to occur in women with menarche before age 11, cycle length less than 27 days, and heavy, prolonged cycles. Higher parity and increased length of lactation are related to a decreased risk of endometriosis. Women who exercise more than 4 hours per week regularly are also less likely to develop endometriosis. Additionally, consumption of animal fat and transfat is associated with an increased risk of laparoscopically confirmed endometriosis, whereas greater long-term intake of long-chain omega-3 fatty acid is associated with a decreased risk of laparoscopically diagnosed endometriosis (Giudice, 2010).

Endometriosis occurs in 6 to 10 percent of women of reproductive age. There is a 7- to 10-fold increased risk of developing endometriosis in those with an affected first-degree relative. Among women with infertility, 38 percent are affected and 71 to 87 percent of women with chronic pelvic pain are affected. The incidence of endometriosis does not appear to be on the rise, although there may be an increased rate of detection due to improved recognition of endometriotic lesions (ACOG, 2010). The actual prevalence is difficult to determine because of the difficulty of diagnosis (Fritz & Speroff, 2011). Endometriosis should be considered as a potential cause of chronic pain when an adolescent woman presents with this complaint. Early recognition is essential to preserve fertility.

SUBJECTIVE DATA

A complete medical, surgical, social, and family history should be collected from the patient (Giudice, 2010). Commonly reported symptoms include dysmenorrhea, chronic pelvic pain, and dyspareunia (ACOG, 2010). However, many women with endometriosis are asymptomatic. Women who exhibit typical symptoms of abdominal or pelvic pain, dysmenorrhea, menorrhagia, and dyspareunia are more likely to be diagnosed. The client may complain of dysmenorrhea (often beginning before the onset of menses), deep dyspareunia (more pronounced during menses), or sacral backache during menses. Commonly reported bowel and bladder symptoms include perimenstrual tenesmus, diarrhea or constipation, dyschezia, dysuria, hematuria, nausea, distention, and early satiety (Giudice, 2010). Endometriosis found in specific organs may result in pain or dysfunction of the affected organs; however, there may be symptoms without lesions affecting the specific organ. The most predictable symptoms of deeply infiltrating endometriosis are painful defecation during menses and severe dyspareunia (ACOG, 2010).

OBJECTIVE DATA

Physical Examination

The client should undergo a physical exam including a pelvic examination (Giudice, 2010). When focal pain or tenderness is detected on pelvic examination, it is associated with pelvic disease in 97 percent of patients and with endometriosis in 66 percent of patients. Pelvic mass, immobile pelvic organ, rectovaginal nodules, uterosacral ligament nodularity, and adnexal mass are well-recognized findings; however, they are not diagnostic because of their poor sensitivity and specificity (ACOG, 2010). In cases with associated infertility, both the female patient and her male partner should be evaluated (Giudice, 2010).

Diagnostic Tests and Methods

To date, the definitive, gold standard test to diagnose endometriosis is by direct visualization of classical or subtle lesions at time of laparoscopy or laparotomy and the histology of lesions removed during surgery (ACOG, 2010). Neither serum testing nor imaging studies have been able to replace diagnostic laparoscopy in diagnosis of endometriosis (ACOG, 2010).

Imaging. Ultrasonography, magnetic resonance imaging (MRI), and computed tomography appear useful only in the presence of pelvic or adnexal mass. Ultrasonography is the preferred choice in imaging when assessing for the presence of endometrial masses. Imaging studies do have high predictive accuracy in differentiating an ovarian endometrioma from other adnexal mass (ACOG, 2010). Doppler ultrasonography may be of value in establishing the diagnosis; characteristically there is little blood flow to the endometrioma, normal flow to normal ovarian tissue, and increased flow to an ovarian tumor (Giudice, 2010). Transvaginal ultrasound is preferred over MRI due to cost. MRI should be reserved for equivocal ultrasound results or in cases of suspected rectovaginal or bladder endometriosis (ACOG, 2010; Giudice, 2010).

CA-125 Assay. The clinical value of obtaining a CA-125 as a diagnostic marker for endometriosis is limited (ACOG, 2010). There may be elevated levels of CA-125 in patients with endometriosis; however, the test is not recommended for diagnostic purposes because of the poor sensitivity and specificity (Giudice, 2010).

Endometrial Biopsy. There is emerging data suggesting the role of endometrial biopsy as a diagnostic tool in endometriosis. Advantages for use of endometrial biopsy include being less invasive than laparoscopy and reducing lengthy delay in diagnosis of the condition. A study by Al-Jefout et al. (2009) found endometrial biopsy, with detection of nerve fibers, provided a reliability of diagnosis of endometriosis close to the accuracy of laparoscopic assessment. Endometrial biopsy is not a diagnostic tool in practice at this time and more research is necessary prior to its utilization for diagnosis.

Diagnostic Laparoscopy. The definitive method to diagnose and stage endometriosis is visualization at surgery (Giudice, 2010). The histological appearance of endometriotic lesions consists of endometrial glands and stroma and differing amounts of inflammation and fibrosis. Many surgeons rely on their visualization of typical lesions to make the diagnosis of endometriosis; however, recent studies have documented the presence of endometriosis in nontypical lesions. Classic endometriotic lesions are the powder-burn lesion or the endometrioma (chocolate cyst), whereas nonclassic endometriotic lesions are clear vesicles, red vesicles, and even microscopic lesions (Hansen, Chalpe, & Eyster, 2010).

Stage of endometriosis is determined based on a scoring system created by the American Society for Reproductive Medicine, ranging from I, indicating minimal disease, to IV, indicating severe disease. Staging from I to IV is determined by the type, location, appearance and depth of invasion of lesions, extent of disease, and adhesions. If there is suspicion of bladder endometriosis, cystoscopy with biopsy is recommended (ACOG, 2010).

Diagnostic laparoscopy requires the client be referred to a gynecologic surgeon with special training and experience using the laparoscope. Laparoscopy is usually performed as an outpatient procedure, with the client under general anesthesia. The laparoscope is inserted through a small incision just above the umbilicus after the abdomen has been inflated with carbon dioxide gas. The surgeon is able to visualize the pelvic organs directly.

Explain the procedure to the client in detail. In addition, discuss the risks. Complications, which are rare, may include bleeding or injuries to nearby organs. Anesthesia complications are rare. Discuss the recovery process. Usually, the client may return home the same day. Common discomforts are neck and shoulder pain from the carbon dioxide gas used to inflate the abdomen, mild nausea, pelvic discomfort at the incision site, mild cramps, and mild vaginal discharge. Instruct the client that she may usually shower or bathe in 24 hours and return to normal activities as soon as she feels able. Review the signs and symptoms of infection and explain how to keep the incision site clean and dry. To reinforce this discussion, provide the client with written information about the procedure and recovery.

DIFFERENTIAL MEDICAL DIAGNOSES

Diagnosis is challenging due to overlapping symptoms with many gynecologic and nongynecologic conditions, including pelvic inflammatory disease (PID), pelvic adhesions, ovarian cysts or masses, leiomyomas, adenomyosis, irritable bowel syndrome, inflammatory bowel disease, interstitial cystitis, myofascial pain, depression, and a history of sexual abuse (Giudice, 2010).

PLAN

Management of the client with endometriosis should be determined by one or more of the following factors:

- Severity of symptoms.
- Desire for fertility.
- Degree of disease.
- Client's therapeutic goals.

Medical management should be considered initially in clients with mild to moderate symptoms who wish to maintain their fertility potential. Conservative surgery is indicated when medical therapy fails, but fertility is still desired. Medical therapy and conservative surgery can be combined. Those clients who have severe endometriosis with debilitating pain should be counseled to complete their childbearing. Total abdominal hysterectomy and bilateral salpingo-oophorectomy represent definitive treatment of endometriosis.

There are a variety of therapeutic options. Assist the client in determining her desired therapeutic outcome. Monitor side effects of medications and response to therapy. Also, provide education and emotional support.

Psychosocial Interventions

Encourage active participation by the client and her significant other in treatment decisions. Assess the client's lifestyle and future plans, such as childbearing, marriage, education, and career. Discuss the impact of the disease on her life and which treatment option will best suit her lifestyle. Assess the client for depression, which can be initiated or worsened by chronic pain. Many of the hormonal therapies have side effects such as depression, loss of libido, and/or mood swings. Inform the client of these potential side effects. Sexual therapy should be offered if the disease has significantly impacted sexual relations (Jones, Kennedy, Barnard, Wong, & Jenkinson, 2001; Waller & Shaw, 1995).

There is some data that suggests diet, a potentially modifiable risk factor, may be important in the pathogenesis of endometriosis. Lower rates of laparoscopically confirmed endometriosis are found in women with higher long-chain omega-3 fatty acid (e.g., salad dressing, tuna, and dark fish) consumption, whereas trans-unsaturated fat (e.g., commercially produced foods, fried foods, margarine, and crackers) consumption and possibly a diet with greater animal fat consumption is associated with an increased risk of laparoscopically confirmed endometriosis. Interestingly, total fat intake was not associated with endometriosis. Particularly, red meat, containing the saturated fat palmitic acid, has been linked to greater likelihood of endometriosis (Missmer et al., 2010).

Medication

Medical therapy is commonly initiated empirically for pain control without surgical confirmation of endometriosis. The goal of medical therapy is intended to reduce pain through a variety of mechanisms, including reducing inflammation, suppressing ovarian hormone production, blocking the action and production of estradiol, and decreasing or completely suppressing menstrual bleeding (Giudice, 2010). Available medications include progestins, danazol, combined oral contraceptives, nonsteroidal anti-inflammatory drugs (NSAIDs), and gonadotropin-releasing hormone (GnRH) agonists (ACOG, 2010). A recent Cochrane review demonstrated that danocrine, medroxyprogesterone acetate, gestrinone, oral contraceptive pills, and GnRH analogs were equally effective in suppressing endometriosis-associated pain (Hansen et al., 2010). First-line therapies include oral contraceptives and NSAIDs; if these treatment modalities fail, then a 3-month course of GnRH agonist is appropriate. Progestins and androgens could also be considered after failure of oral contraceptives (ACOG, 2010).

NSAIDs. NSAIDs are the most commonly used first-line treatment for endometriosis because they have few side effects and are available over the counter. NSAIDs work to reduce pain in women experiencing endometriosis by acting on local cytokines within the ectopic endometrial lesions, as well as acting as analgesics. NSAIDs work to inhibit prostaglandin production, and prostaglandin-related, locally produced chemicals thought to cause the pain of endometriosis (Allen, Hopewell, Prentice, & Gregory, 2009).

There is a paucity of information in the literature of research comparing NSAIDs with placebo in the treatment of women with endometriosis. This is surprising given that NSAIDs are commonly prescribed and readily available over the counter. However, there is a great deal of literature suggesting efficacy for the use of NSAIDs in treatment of primary dysmenorrhea. It has been surmised that prostaglandins are involved in the physiologic mechanism of pain in both groups. However, it is worth noting the available information surrounding use of NSAIDs in treatment of primary dysmenorrhea is insufficient to suggest which individual NSAID is the most safe and effective treatment. It is also important that women know, although readily available, NSAIDs are not without side effects. Finally, NSAIDs may be taken in doses not high enough to be therapeutic and higher doses can cause side effects of nausea, diarrhea, headache, drowsiness, dizziness, and dry mouth (Allen et al., 2009).

Combined Oral Contraceptives. Dysmenorrhea-associated withdrawal bleeding can be eliminated with use of extended-cycle pills. When endometriosis-associated dysmenorrhea is not responsive to cyclic oral contraceptives, continuous combined oral contraceptives have been found to give significant decrease in pain from baseline. If empiric treatment with medication fails, it would be reasonable to trial an alternate medication or offer referral for diagnostic laparoscopy to confirm an endometriosis diagnosis (ACOG, 2010).

Progestogens. Oral norethindrone acetate and subcutaneous depot-medroxyprogesterone acetate (DMPA) have been approved by the U.S. Food and Drug Administration (FDA) for the treatment of endometriosis-associated pain. Subcutaneous DMPA has been shown to be equally effective in reducing endometriosis-associated pain in comparison to GnRH agonists and women incur substantially less decrease in bone mass. The disadvantage in using depot formulations is delay in return of ovulatory cycles; therefore, this may not be a viable option for women who desire pregnancy in the near future (ACOG, 2010).

The levonorgestrel intrauterine system has also been shown to be as effective in reducing endometriosis-associated pain as a GnRH agonist; however, it has not been approved by the FDA for treatment of endometriosis-associated pain. After 3 years of use, the levonorgestrel intrauterine system showed continued benefit; however, 40 percent of patients discontinued use due to irregular bleeding, persistent pain, or weight gain. In comparing the levonorgestrel intrauterine system with a GnRH agonist, there was no significant difference in control of pain (ACOG, 2010).

Danazol. Danazol is an androgenic drug that has been shown to be highly effective in treating endometriosis-associated pain (ACOG, 2010). However, the side effect profile includes acne, hirsutism, and myalgia, and therefore, is more undesirable than other available medication options (ACOG, 2010).

GnRH Agonists. Use of GnRH agonists is not recommended as a primary treatment approach because review of studies comparing GnRH agonists to other treatments has shown little or no difference in pain relief between GnRH agonists and other medical treatments, such as first-line therapy with combined hormonal contraceptives. However, GnRH agonists are highly effective in treating endometriosis-associated pain when first-line therapy has failed. Side effects with GnRH agonist use are significant and include hot flushes, vaginal dryness, and osteopenia. Short-term use of a GnRH agonist has shown osteopenia to be reversible. However, it may not be reversible with long-term use or with multiple cycles. The FDA has approved use of a 12-month course of GnRH agonist therapy. In patients who have responded well to previous GnRH agonist therapy, long-term therapy with add-back (see next) has been reported. Patients using long-term therapy should be monitored for physical findings, bone density, and serum lipids (ACOG, 2010).

Add-Back Therapy. For women achieving relief of pain with a GnRH agonist, the use of add-back therapy is indicated to mitigate bone loss and provide symptomatic relief (ACOG, 2010). The efficacy of GnRH agonist therapy for pain control has not been shown to be diminished by add-back therapy for 3 to 6 months; therefore, add-back therapy is recommended with multiple cycle use of a GnRH agonist. Add-back regimens have included progestins alone, progestins and bisphosphonates, low-dose progestins, and estrogens. Norethindrone 5 mg daily as add-back with a GnRH agonist has been approved by the FDA. GnRH and norethindrone with or without a low-dose estrogen (conjugated estrogen 0.625 mg daily) were found to decrease the side effect profile and maintain efficacy in treating pain. It is recommended all women using a GnRH agonist add 1,000 mg of calcium daily. There appears to be no disadvantage to use of an add-back regimen in combination with a GnRH agonist other than added cost.

Alternatively, in women unable to tolerate high-dose norethindrone, transdermal estradiol, 25 μg daily, plus medroxyprogesterone acetate, 2.5 mg orally daily, may be used. However, this add-back treatment has not been approved by the FDA and may not prevent bone loss.

Surgical Interventions

Conservative Surgery. Conservative surgery by removal of visible deposits of endometriosis is indicated for adnexal masses, symptoms unresponsive to medical therapy, severe endometriosis in a client who desires future fertility, and concomitant conditions such as leiomyomas or adhesions. Endometriosis is removed with surgical excision or ablation. A Cochrane review found that laparoscopic surgery in the treatment of subfertility related to minimal and mild endometriosis may improve future fertility. Additionally, laparoscopic surgery compared to diagnostic laparoscopy alone has also been found to improve pain outcomes in women with endometriosis. Surgery can be done at the time of diagnostic laparoscopy if this has been previously discussed and consent for possible ablation is obtained preoperatively. Alternately, a second laparoscopy for ablation of minimal to moderate endometriosis may be carried out after the initial diagnostic laparoscopy, although this is a more invasive approach (Jacobson, Duffy, Barlow, Koninckx, & Garry, 2010).

Uterosacral nerve ablation as an adjunct to surgical management has been found to be ineffective in treating pain associated with endometriosis. The exception is presacral neurectomy, which has been found to be beneficial for midline pain only. Constipation and urinary dysfunction are possible postoperative complications (ACOG, 2010).

Endometriomas are thought to be the progression of endometriotic lesions and form cystic structures. Removal of endometriomas involves risk that normal tissue will be removed. These cysts may cause pain and infertility and they are associated with risk of torsion, rupture, and rarely malignancy. Excision is recommended to confirm the cyst is benign. Recurrence is common (ACOG, 2010).

When explaining the procedure to the client, point out that conservative surgery is not curative. Review the postoperative instructions, addressing the client's return to activity, resumption of sexual relations, and signs and symptoms of infection. The possible adverse effects in conservative laparoscopic surgery include a reaction to anesthesia, incisional infection, bleeding, and injury to nearby organs. The anticipated outcomes on evaluation are the relief of pain and return to fertility.

Definitive Surgery. For women who do not desire future fertility and in whom conservative medical therapy and surgical management have failed, definitive surgery is indicated. Radical (and definitive) surgery for endometriosis includes hysterectomy, bilateral oophorectomy, and removal of all endometriotic implants. For women with endometriosis who have intractable pain and have completed childbearing, radical therapy is a reasonable treatment. For women with normal ovaries, a hysterectomy with preservation of the ovaries could be considered. If oophorectomy is not completed at the time of hysterectomy for endometriosis-related pain, women are more likely to have pain recurrence and may require additional surgery. In young women who are menopausal after surgical removal of their ovaries, consideration should be given to the addition of hormone therapy. Use of a progestin is not necessary; however, it needs to be considered and use is recommended by some experts in order to prevent unopposed estrogenic stimulation of residual endometriotic tissue (Hansen et al., 2010).

There are possible adverse effects, namely, bleeding, infection, wound infection, or damage to nearby organs. The anticipated outcome on evaluation is complete resolution of the disease, including relief of dysmenorrhea, dyspareunia, dyschezia, and/or dysuria.

Prepare the client by giving her a thorough explanation of the anatomy and physiology, surgical procedure, and risks and benefits. Reassure her that femininity remains unchanged by the surgery. Hormonal replacement therapy may be needed. Full recovery usually takes about 6 weeks. Review the postoperative instructions, including topics such as the return to activity, the expectation that vaginal bleeding will change to clear discharge, signs of infection, return to sexual activity, and dietary needs.

FOLLOW-UP AND REFERRAL

Follow-up of women with pelvic pain and laparoscopically identified endometriosis has shown that 17 to 19 percent of lesions resolve spontaneously, 24 to 64 percent progress, and 9 to 59 percent are stable over a 12-month period (Giudice, 2010). Appropriate follow-up intervals depend on the choice of therapy and the client's needs. An initial evaluation made at 3 months of therapy should report the incidence, severity, and cyclicity of pain, dysmenorrhea, and dyspareunia.

Review the side effects of any medications and their impact on the client. Inquire about the issue of pregnancy and provide emotional support and encouragement. Assess and treat or refer for reactive depression. Encourage the client to adopt healthy lifestyle habits with respect to diet, exercise, sleep, and stress management. Referral sources include the Endometriosis Association, RESOLVE, and the American Society for Reproductive Medicine. Personal or group counseling may also be helpful.

PELVIC INFLAMMATORY DISEASE

PID comprises a spectrum of inflammatory disorders of the upper female genital tract, including any combination of endometritis, salpingitis, tubo-ovarian abscess, and pelvic peritonitis (Soper, 2010). Sexually transmitted organisms, especially *Neisseria gonorrhoeae* and *Chlamydia trachomatis*, are implicated in many cases; however, microorganisms that comprise the vaginal flora (e.g., anaerobes, *Gardnerella vaginalis*, *Haemophilus influenzae*, enteric gram-negative rods, and *Streptococcus agalactiae*) also have been associated with PID. In addition, cytomegalovirus, *Mycoplasma hominis*, *Ureaplasma urealyticum*, and *Mycoplasma genitalium* might be associated with some cases of PID. All women who have acute PID should be tested for *N. gonorrhoeae* and *C. trachomatis* and should be screened for HIV infection (CDC, 2010).

EPIDEMIOLOGY

PID is thought to have a polymicrobial etiology including aerobic and anaerobic organisms. The two major organisms thought to cause PID include *C. trachomatis* and *N. gonorrhoeae*. The presence of organisms associated with bacterial vaginosis has been seen in many cases of proven PID. Recently, some studies have shown

M. genitalium to play a role in the development of PID as well (Ross, Brown, Saunders, & Alexander, 2009; Short et al., 2010; Soper, 2010). PID can affect upwards of 1 million women annually. Sexually transmitted infections (STIs) are the cause of nearly 85 percent of PID. Due to these staggering numbers, the U.S. Preventive Services Task Force recommends screening women under the age of 25 for chlamydia annually (Abatangelo et al., 2010). Women under the age of 25 are at the highest risk of development of PID, with a higher incidence in African American women. Other risk factors for the development of PID include multiple sex partners, sexual activity at a young age, vaginal douching, inconsistent condom use, smoking, alcohol use, prior history of PID infection, and exchange of sex for money or drugs (Abatangelo et al., 2010; Balamuth, Zhao, & Mollen, 2010). Other risk factors include insertion of an intrauterine device (IUD) within the past 3 to 4 weeks and breaking the barrier of the cervical mucosa during other medical procedures.

SUBJECTIVE DATA

PID can be difficult to diagnose due to a broad array of presenting symptoms. The diagnosis is usually based on clinical findings. A patient may present with complaints of one or more of the following symptoms: abdominal pain, lower abnormal vaginal discharge, postcoital bleeding, intermenstrual bleeding, fever, nausea, vomiting, symptoms of a urinary tract infection (UTI), or low back pain. The symptoms of PID can range from subtle to severe (Soper, 2010).

Clinicians should begin empiric treatment in women at risk for development of PID if there is pelvic or lower abdominal pain with no other identifiable cause for the symptoms and if one or more of the following minimum criteria is present on physical exam (Judlin, 2010):

- Cervical motion tenderness (CMT)
- Uterine tenderness
- Adnexal tenderness

OBJECTIVE DATA

- *Vital signs:* May reveal an elevated temperature >101° F
- *Abdominal exam:* May reveal guarding, rebound tenderness, pain with palpation over the lower quadrants
- *Speculum exam:* Purulent cervical or vaginal discharge
- *Bimanual exam:* CMT, uterine tenderness, adnexal tenderness or fullness

Diagnostic Tests and Methods

Pregnancy Test. Evaluation for pregnancy needs to be done to rule out unsuspected pregnancy or ectopic pregnancy. It is important to establish the patient's last menstrual period. If a pregnancy test is positive, an ultrasound should be considered to evaluate for ectopic pregnancy (Mol et al., 2010).

Vaginal Smears and Cervical Cultures. Evaluation to determine the causative agent of infection needs to be performed. A pH of vaginal secretions and whiff test along with saline wet mount need to be done to evaluate for trichomoniasis and bacterial vaginosis. Cervical testing for infection due to *C. trachomatis* and *N. gonorrhoeae* should also be performed (Soper, 2010).

Complete Blood Count, Erythrocyte Sedimentation Rate, and C-Reactive Protein. Serum screening should be obtained as part of a comprehensive workup. Many women will have a normal peripheral white blood cell (WBC) count. C-reactive protein, which can help detect inflammation, and erythrocyte sedimentation rate (ESR) are typically elevated, but are not always performed as part of a routine workup (Soper, 2010).

Urinalysis. The patient's urine should be evaluated to rule out UTI and pyelonephritis as the cause of abdominal pain.

Pelvic Ultrasound. Although pelvic ultrasound may have limited sensitivity for detection of PID, it may be considered useful in diagnosing upper genital infection, such as tubo-ovarian abscess in patients with pelvic mass on bimanual exam.

Laparoscopy. Laparoscopy is not routinely ordered for diagnosis of PID; however, it may be indicated if the patient has failed to respond to first-line therapy. It would assess for tubo-ovarian abscess, access for tubal factor infertility, or provide further evaluation of any pelvic mass.

DIFFERENTIAL MEDICAL DIAGNOSES

There are many other illnesses that have symptoms that may resemble PID and must be considered and effectively ruled out. These include acute appendicitis, ectopic pregnancy, ovarian torsion, UTI/pyelonephritis, vaginal infection, salpingitis, endometritis, ovarian cyst or mass, and degeneration of a leiomyoma (Abatangelo et al., 2010).

PLAN

Medications (Outpatient)

Most patients can be managed on an outpatient basis. See later for red flags that indicate need for hospitalization. The following treatment regimens are based on CDC revisions done in 2010.

Regimen A:

- Ceftriaxone 250 mg IM in a single dose
- Doxycycline 100 mg orally twice daily for 14 days
- Consider adding metronidazole 500 mg orally twice daily for 14 days (this will give treatment for bacterial vaginosis and trichomoniasis as well as anaerobic organism coverage, which is often the suspected etiology of PID)

Regimen B:

- Cefoxitin 2 g IM in a single dose and probenecid 1 g orally in a single dose administered together
- Doxycycline 100 mg orally twice daily for 14 days
- Consider adding metronidazole 500 mg orally twice daily for 14 days

Regimen C:

- Cefoxitin 2 g IM in a single dose and probenecid 1 g orally in a single dose administered together
- Doxycycline 100 mg orally twice daily for 14 days or azithromycin 500 mg orally followed by 250 mg orally daily for a total of 7 days
- Consider adding metronidazole 500 mg orally twice daily for 14 days

Regimen D:

- Ceftizoxime 2 g every 8 hours IV or cefotaxime 1 g every 12 hours IM or IV
- Doxycycline 100 mg orally twice daily for 14 days
- Consider adding metronidazole 500 mg orally twice daily for 14 days

Due to growing resistance to fluoroquinolones, this class of antibiotics is no longer routinely recommended for treatment of gonorrhea and, therefore, cannot be a primary option for treatment of PID. Further studies suggest that azithromycin may be superior to doxycycline in treatment of PID (Soper, 2010).

Patient Education

It is important to have an in-depth discussion regarding PID including importance of adhering to the medication regimen, side effects of medications, avoidance of intercourse until all antibiotics are finished, evaluation and treatment of partners, and risk for long-term health risks. Patient should be instructed on the importance of following up in clinic in 48 to 72 hours and then again in 10 to 14 days to monitor resolution of symptoms. The patient needs to be instructed on warning signs to monitor for and report immediately. It is routinely recommended for patients who were positive for gonorrhea and chlamydia to have repeat cultures for infection 3 to 6 months after completion of medication regimen (CDC, 2010). It is recommended that the patient be counseled on safe sexual habits and steps to prevent reinfection, especially consistent use of condoms (Chacko et al., 2010).

Red flags that may signal need for hospitalization:

- Any type of surgical emergency has not been ruled out
- Pregnancy
- No improvement after 14-day oral therapy
- The patient cannot or will not follow the oral antibiotic therapy
- The patient is severely ill, possibly presenting with high fever, nausea, vomiting
- Presence of tubo-ovarian abscess
- HIV positive or other immunodeficiency

Medications (Inpatient)

Inpatient IV treatments for PID include antibiotics such as cefotetan, cefoxitin, doxycycline, clindamycin, and gentamicin (CDC, 2010).

Surgical Interventions

If a patient does not respond to parental antibiotic therapy within 72 hours or a tubo-ovarian abscess ruptures, conservative therapy may be considered to remove abnormal tissue (Soper, 2010). Colpotomy or unilateral or bilateral salpingo-oophorectomy may be indicated in patients with tubo-ovarian abscesses if there is significant involvement of the tubes or ovaries.

FOLLOW-UP AND REFERRAL

Patients treated in an ambulatory setting need to be reevaluated 48 to 72 hours after initiation of antibiotic therapy. If there is not a significant improvement at that time, the patient needs to be considered for hospitalization. If there has been appropriate improvement in symptoms, the patient needs to be evaluated again in 1 to 2 weeks.

The risk of PID associated with IUD use is primarily confined to the first 3 weeks after insertion and is uncommon thereafter (CDC, 2010). No evidence suggests that IUDs should be removed in women diagnosed with acute PID. However, caution should be exercised if the IUD remains in place, and close clinical follow-up is mandatory. The rate of treatment failure and recurrent PID in women continuing to use an IUD is unknown. No data exists on antibiotic selection and treatment outcomes according to type of IUD (e.g., copper or levonorgestrel).

The current guideline does not recommend removal of IUD, but does recommend close follow-up of those with an IUD in place (CDC, 2010).

ADNEXAL MASSES (OVARIAN TUMORS)

An adnexal mass is an enlarged structure located within the uterine adnexa that is discovered on a pelvic exam or on radiologic imaging. It can be found on a patient that presents with symptoms or can be an incidental finding in a patient with no symptoms (Griffin, Grant, & Sala, 2010).

CATEGORIES OF OVARIAN TUMORS

Benign adnexal masses: functional cysts (follicular or corpus luteum), endometriomas, tubo-ovarian abscess, hydrosalpinx

Benign cystic ovarian tumors: dermoid cysts, serous and mucinous cyst adenomas

Benign solid ovarian tumors: fibrothecomas, adenofibromas, and Brenner tumors

Malignant ovarian tumors: serous and mucinous tumors, endometrioid carcinoma, clear cell carcinoma, granulosa cell tumors, Sertoli-Leydig cell tumors, germ cell tumors

EPIDEMIOLOGY

Adnexal masses can be present in women of any age. The majority of masses presenting during reproductive years are functional and will resolve spontaneously. The risk of malignancy rises with age, with nearly half of all adnexal masses in postmenopausal women being malignant (Bottomley & Bourne, 2009).

SUBJECTIVE DATA

Patients presenting with any of the following symptoms should be evaluated for an adnexal occurrence such as functional, inflammatory, metaplastic, or neoplastic ovarian tumors; menstrual irregularities; pelvic pain described as a dull ache that can be constant or intermittent and can radiate to the thighs or lower back; dyspareunia; pain with defecation; nausea; vomiting; fever; full or heavy feeling in the abdomen; pressure on the bladder; or loss of appetite.

OBJECTIVE DATA

A careful evaluation needs to be done including assessment of vital signs, abdominal exam, and pelvic exam. Vital signs may show an elevated temperature, tachycardia, and/or elevated blood pressure. Abdominal exam is performed to evaluate for guarding or rebound tenderness and localized or generalized tenderness with palpation. Bimanual pelvic exam should assess for CMT, adnexal tenderness, or a palpable adnexal or ovarian mass.

Diagnostic Tests and Methods

Urine Pregnancy Test. Any woman of childbearing age presenting with abdominal pain should receive a pregnancy test.

Complete Blood Count. Blood work should be done for evaluation of an elevated white count. This can indicate infection such as appendicitis or abscess.

Urinalysis. A urine test may be helpful in ruling out pathology due to a UTI or calculus. The absence of blood leucocytes and nitrites can essentially rule these out.

Cervical and Vaginal Cultures. Testing for gonorrhea and chlamydia should be considered in sexually active patients. A wet mount to assess for vaginal infection from candidiasis, gardnerella, or trichomoniasis should also be considered.

Transvaginal Pelvic Ultrasound. Imaging is still the gold standard for evaluation of a suspected adnexal mass. Imaging can differentiate between a solid and cystic adnexal mass and can also help characterize thickness, internal septations, or nodules. Ultrasound findings that are concerning for a malignancy include a mass with a total volume of greater than 50 mL, presence of a solid component, a wall or septal thickness that is greater than 3 mm, and tendency to have low-resistance Doppler waveform (Griffin, Grant, et al., 2010).

Pelvic MRI. Typically done as second-line imaging, an MRI can help characterize complex adnexal masses and can differentiate between benign and malignant better than pelvic ultrasound.

Laparoscopy. Patients with an adnexal mass larger than 7 cm, mass that is concerning for malignancy, or mass occurring in a postmenopausal patient should be referred to gynecologist for surgical management with laparoscopy and possible cystectomy or oophorectomy.

DIFFERENTIAL MEDICAL DIAGNOSIS

Gynecologic and nongynecologic causes need to be considered in a patient presenting with the symptoms discussed earlier. These include ectopic pregnancy, PID, tubo-ovarian abscess, uterine leiomyoma, appendicitis, diverticulitis, intestinal obstruction, UTI, and renal calculi (Bottomley & Bourne, 2009).

PLAN

Psychosocial Interventions

Patient education is vital in helping patients understand their diagnosis. Many will fear malignancy and reassurance and support is key in helping patients understand the differences between various adnexal masses and to reaffirm that not all masses are malignant. Make sure they understand the plan and the need for follow-up and continued monitoring.

Expectant Management/Referral Indications

Expectant management is preferable for masses that appear to be benign functional ovarian cysts—those that are smaller than 7 cm, mobile, and unilateral. These types of cysts should resolve spontaneously in one to two menstrual cycles and should be reevaluated with a repeat pelvic ultrasound. If the mass has not become smaller on follow-up, referral to a gynecologist should be considered (Levine et al., 2010). Patients being followed with expectant management, especially those with larger cyst size, should be educated on symptoms that may indicate torsion of the ovary. These symptoms include an increase in level of pain that is severe (doubling over) and persistent with or without nausea or vomiting. If these symptoms occur, the patient should be advised to seek evaluation in an emergency room setting. Torsion of the ovary, while rare, is a medical emergency. Patients should also be advised that sudden severe pain that resolves quickly may indicate rupture of the cyst. In this case, the patient does not need to be seen emergently. Finally, referral to a gynecologist is indicated for postmenopausal patients with any palpable adnexal mass or any adnexal mass that is seen on imaging.

Medication

Analgesics such as NSAIDs may be helpful for temporary management of pain associated with adnexal masses. The appropriateness of narcotic use can be determined by the individual practitioner.

Hormone management with a combination of estrogen and progesterone such as oral contraceptives, transdermal patches, or vaginal rings can help suppress ovarian function and help to resolve functional cysts. They can also help lower risks for development of ovarian cysts. Educate the patient on appropriate use of the medication and potential side effects, and ensure that she is an appropriate candidate without contraindications to hormonal use. Also, assess that the patient is not hoping for pregnancy in the near future. Educate the patient it may take a few cycles to suppress ovarian function completely (Bottomley & Bourne, 2009).

Surgery

Referral to a gynecologist is indicated for treatment of adnexal masses that are persisting beyond a few months, increasing in size, larger than 7 cm, or if any of these treatment regimens fails to control symptoms. The type of surgery performed may depend on factors such as patient's age, size of mass, or desire for future childbearing. Different types of surgery including ovarian cystectomy, unilateral or bilateral salpingo-oophorectomy, and hysterectomy may be considered in women over age 40 who are done with childbearing. Surgery can be done via laparoscopy, laparotomy, abdominally, or vaginally (usually only performed if hysterectomy is also being performed).

FOLLOW-UP AND REFERRAL

Expectant management for a functional ovarian cyst should be followed up in 6 weeks in clinic. Any suspicion of malignancy needs referral to gynecologist or gynecologic oncologist for intervention.

DYSPAREUNIA

Dyspareunia or painful coitus occurs either on intromission (entry) or on deep penetration of the penis. Painful coitus may result from any number of factors, such as infection, inflammation, anatomic abnormalities, pelvic pathology, atrophy or failure of lubrication, or psychological conflicts (Binik, 2010; van Lankveld et al., 2010). See Chapter 7 for more information.

EPIDEMIOLOGY

Intromission, introital, or superficial pain may be caused by vulvovaginitis (recurrent and chronic), provoked vestibulodynia (formerly vulvar vestibulitis) (see section Nonmalignant Disorders of the Vulva), urethritis/urethral syndrome, interstitial cystitis, cervicitis, lack of lubrication, levator spasm, or female circumcision.

Pain on deep penetration may be caused by uterine retroversion, pelvic relaxation, endometriosis, adhesions, adenomyosis, pelvic congestion syndrome, or lack of vaginal expansion due to insufficient arousal (Binik, 2010; Hyde, 2007; van Lankveld et al., 2010).

Physiological and psychological risk factors for dyspareunia include estrogen depletion–associated menopause, psychological factors (including restrictive sexual attitudes), relationship difficulties and history of sexual trauma, history of sexually transmitted disease (STD), recurrent infection (candidiasis), and poor hygiene (Binik, 2010; van Lankveld et al., 2010).

The incidence is unclear because clients tend not to report dyspareunia to health professionals. Of the reported cases, the most common cause is vulvo/vaginitis infection. Studies vary in reported incidence of dyspareunia ranging from 6.5 to 45 percent in older women, to 14 to 34 percent in younger women (ter Kuile, Both, & van Lankveld, 2010).

SUBJECTIVE DATA

A client's history is crucial to determining if the client has pain and, if so, the etiology of dyspareunia. One problem, such as vaginitis, may cause another problem, such as anxiety or fear about pain with intercourse, thus altering sexual response, decreasing lubrication, and increasing pain. Pain may occur on intromission or on deep penetration; it may occur after long pain-free intervals or with first intercourse. Vaginal discharge or irritation may be present. There may be a history of chronic pelvic pain. Relationship difficulties may be reported. The client may have been unable to use tampons previously or may have had difficult pelvic exams. Menopausal symptoms may be beginning (ACOG, 2011; Binik, 2010; Hyde, 2007; van Lankveld et al., 2010).

OBJECTIVE DATA

Physical Examination

Examination includes the genitalia and reproductive tract. The vulvar/vaginal mucosa may reveal irritation, inflammation, lesions, discharge, atrophy, hymenal remnants, Bartholin's cyst/abscess, or vestibulitis (focal irritation/inflammation of the vestibular glands; see section Nonmalignant Disorders of the Vulva). A decision may be made by the clinician and the patient to defer use of a speculum for the initial exam. When decision to use a speculum is made, use the smallest size possible. Involuntary contractions of the perineal muscles (vaginismus) may occur during a speculum or digital exam, prohibiting examination. Proceed carefully and allow the client control during pelvic exam. Bimanual exam may reveal uterine prolapse, pelvic mass, nodularity of endometriosis, CMT of PID, or loss of pelvic support (cystocele, rectocele) (van Lankveld et al., 2010).

Diagnostic Tests and Methods

Select tests discriminately as indicated by the findings of the history and physical examination. Review previous test results in order to avoid unnecessary and repetitive diagnostic testing.

Complete Blood Count and ESR. Diagnostic evaluation to detect any inflammatory process (see Pelvic Inflammatory Disease for test procedure). The WBC count and ESR are elevated in PID.

Urinalysis. Diagnostic evaluation to identify any urinary tract conditions that might be a source of pain. WBCs, bacteria, or red blood cells in the urine may indicate chronic or recurrent UTI.

Pregnancy Test (Urine or Blood Level of β-hCG). Diagnostic evaluation to detect unsuspected intrauterine pregnancy or suspected ectopic pregnancy (see Pelvic Inflammatory Disease for test procedure).

Vaginal Smears/Cervical Cultures. Diagnostic evaluation to determine whether infection is present. Wet mount with normal saline is used to detect bacterial vaginosis or trichomoniasis; potassium hydroxide preparation is used to detect candidiasis; and cervical tests can detect *N. gonorrhoeae* and *C. trachomatis* (see Chapter 3 or 14 for test procedures).

Ultrasound. Diagnostic evaluation using ultrasound may be useful if a bimanual exam is difficult, as with clients who are obese or unable to tolerate the exam. The procedure is most useful in diagnosing acute pelvic pain conditions, such as ruptured ovarian cyst, adnexal masses, or ectopic pregnancy; it should not be performed in clients with a clearly negative pelvic.

Diagnostic Laparoscopy. Diagnostic evaluation is accomplished by directly visualizing the pelvic pathology that may be causing dyspareunia (see Endometriosis for test procedure).

DIFFERENTIAL MEDICAL DIAGNOSES

Vulvovaginitis, atrophic vulvovaginitis, vulvar vestibulitis, urethritis, urethral syndrome, cystitis, cervicitis, muscle spasm, hymenal strands, scar tissue, episiotomy, vaginismus, pelvic relaxation, uterine prolapse, PID, endometriosis, adenomyosis, adhesions, pelvic masses, Bartholin's cyst. Consider possible contributing psychological factors, such as previous sexual trauma, conflictual relationships, stress, or restrictive sexual attitudes. Also consider inappropriate sexual technique, including lack of foreplay, or low estrogen in the oral contraceptive (ACOG, 2011; Binik, 2010; van Lankveld et al., 2010).

PLAN

The management of dyspareunia depends on the symptoms and etiology.

Psychosocial Interventions

Refer the client for psychotherapy or cognitive-behavioral therapy (CBT) if her history reveals the possibility of a psychological component to the dyspareunia or if significant discord is present in the couple's relationship. Select a therapist with special training in sexual problems. Discuss fully with the client the findings of the physical examination and diagnostic testing, and include her partner whenever possible. Address and discuss all client fears, concerns, and anxieties. Sexual attitudes may need to be addressed (ACOG, 2011; ter Kuile et al., 2010; van Lankveld et al., 2010).

Medication

The etiology of the dyspareunia determines whether medication is prescribed.

- *Vaginitis/STD:* See Chapter 14.
- *Atrophic vaginitis*
  - Hormonal therapy may be the treatment of choice for perimenopausal or menopausal women with atrophic vaginitis (see Chapter 18). Estrogen revitalizes atrophic tissues.
  - A water-based lubricant (e.g., K-Y Jelly or Replens) available over the counter is indicated for poor vaginal lubrication. The lubricant may be administered prior to or during intercourse to improve vaginal lubrication and enhance foreplay. Latex condoms should not be used with vegetable-based lubricants. Vaginal suppositories may be inserted three times weekly, without regard to intercourse. Instructing the client in the use of a lubricant is important.
  - Anticipated outcomes on evaluation are improved vaginal lubrication and relief of dyspareunia secondary to vaginal dryness. Local allergic irritation is a potential adverse reaction, however, that would contraindicate lubricant use.
- *Vulvodynia:* See Nonmalignant Disorders of the Vulva.
- *PID, endometriosis, adnexal mass, and leiomyoma:* Medications for these causes of dyspareunia are described in other sections of this chapter.

Surgical Intervention

The cause of dyspareunia determines whether surgery is necessary. In cases where surgical evaluation is needed, referral should be made to a gynecologist. For descriptions of specific surgical interventions, see the appropriate section in this chapter: Endometriosis, Pelvic Inflammatory Disease, Adnexal Masses, Leiomyomas, or pelvic relaxation syndrome. Other surgical interventions would depend on the specific cause, such as marsupialization of a Bartholin's cyst.

Progressive Dilation and Muscle Awareness Exercise for Vaginismus

This procedure, with appropriate counseling, is indicated for clients with vaginismus, an anatomically narrow introitus, hymenal remnants or scar tissue, or psychogenic factors.

Begin by reviewing the anatomy and physiology of the sexual organs and sexual response, stressing the normalcy of vulvar tissue. Using a mirror, have the client become familiar with her genitalia. Instruct the client on how to perform Kegel exercises to increase her awareness of the muscles involved. Involve the client's partner whenever possible.

Progressive digital dilation may be practiced by the client at home in order to familiarize her with her tissue, sensitization, and muscular control. Measured vaginal dilators are also available. These dilators may be used in the clinic setting by the clinician or at home by the client. Allow the client to stop at any point that pain occurs. Have her bear down on insertion and use water-soluble lubricant to alleviate discomfort.

CBT may also be used in combination with vaginal dilators. A CBT program for vaginismus may include relaxation techniques, sensate focus, and sexual fantasy (ACOG, 2011; Mandal et al., 2010; ter Kuile et al., 2010).

FOLLOW-UP AND REFERRAL

As with the entire evaluation and plan of care for clients with dyspareunia, follow-up will depend on the cause and the therapy selected. Follow-up evaluation is important, especially when dyspareunia is multifactorial. Stress to the client the importance of keeping follow-up appointments. Reassess the client frequently to determine whether psychological intervention is needed.

NONMALIGNANT DISORDERS OF THE VULVA

The client who presents with vulvar symptoms requires conscientious evaluation by the primary care provider. Knowledge of common nonmalignant disorders of the vulva is important in deciding whether to initiate careful medical therapy or to refer for further evaluation and management, including biopsy and/or surgical therapy. In this section, common vulvar conditions are presented. Pruritus and pain are two of the most common presenting symptoms of vulvar disorders in women. The client may complain of pruritus and vulvar pain when there is obvious dermatologic disease or in conditions with few visible skin changes (ACOG, 2008a). In evaluating women with vulvar pruritus, it is often helpful to group conditions into acute and chronic symptoms. It is helpful for the clinician to have available for reference a comprehensive textbook of genital dermatology and/or vulvar disorders.

Most clients who present with recurrent pain, itching, burning, or irritation are frustrated, are desperate for relief, and have previously used a variety of antifungal and/or steroid creams. Many will have already seen a variety of health care providers without resolution of symptoms. Psychological distress, depression, and anxiety may be present either as a risk factor for the current problem or as a result of the chronic discomfort.

The clinician is in a unique position to obtain a comprehensive, detailed history related to the problem, to identify possible causative factors, to initiate and evaluate therapy, and to provide emotional support. The more experience the clinician gains, the better she or he is able to evaluate and manage vulvar problems. It is most critical to recognize the need for referral to a knowledgeable specialist when necessary. Common conditions associated with vulvar pain and/or pruritus include vulvodynia, lichen sclerosis, chronic/cyclic fungal infections.

VULVODYNIA

Vulvodynia is defined as burning, stinging, rawness, or soreness, with or without pruritus, and can be further characterized by the site of the pain, either general or localized, and whether it is provoked, spontaneous, or both (ACOG, 2009b).

EPIDEMIOLOGY

In evaluating women with vulvar disorders, the most common etiologies are dermatologic and vulvodynia (ACOG, 2008a, 2009b).

The International Society for the Study of Vulvovaginal Disease defines vulvodynia as vulvar discomfort, usually described as burning pain, occurring in the absence of relevant visible findings or a specific, clinically identifiable, neurological disorder. Patients can be further stratified by the location of the pain (e.g., generalized vulvodynia, hemivulvodynia, clitorodynia) and additionally by whether the pain is provoked or unprovoked (Mandal et al., 2010).

A conservative estimate is that 16 percent of women will have chronic vulvar pain for 3 to 6 months at one point in their lifetime. This estimate is probably low because 40 percent of women who suffer from vulvar pain fail to seek treatment. Sixty percent of women who do seek treatment for vulvar pain see on average three care providers before an accurate diagnosis is established. Vulvar pain is most common in women of reproductive age, with onset typically between women 18 and 25 years of age. Vulvar pain tends to be intermittent (Danby & Margesson, 2010).

Diagnosis and treatment of vulvar pain requires a multidisciplinary approach. Vulvar pain can be a presenting complaint for many vulvar skin disorders. Given the complexity of vulvar pain, involving gynecology, urology, dermatology, psychology, physical therapy, and pain management in the evaluation of the client is often beneficial. A lead clinician may be prudent to triage patients and consider referral to other health professionals who have a role in vulvodynia management (Danby & Margesson, 2010).

SUBJECTIVE DATA

Pain is often acute in onset and is described as "burning, stinging, irritation, or rawness." Onset may be associated with recent episodes of vaginitis. Dyspareunia interferes with sexual function. Pain can be mild to severe, interfering with normal activities, and may be continuous or episodic.

Previous treatments have provided either partial or no relief. Clients will report having seen many different clinicians and will generally express frustration and anxiety.

A thorough history including a review of systems is essential and considered the cornerstone of workup for vulvar pain (Danby & Margesson, 2010). Invite the client to tell her story.

Gather the history of the vulvar pain:

- Social history (occupation and activity at work, marital status, sexual preference, and leisure activities)
- Duration
- Timeline (start, factors at onset, what happened then and now and course of pain)
- Site (localized area of vulva or entire vulva)
- Description (spontaneous or provoked, intermittent or constant; burning, rawness, stabbing, shooting, crawling, tearing, itching, irritation)
- Severity
- Aggravating and alleviating factors
- Treatments, both over-the-counter and prescription
- Other vulvovaginal diagnoses (yeast, bacterial vaginosis, STI, cystitis)
- Sexual history (age at first sexual activity, lifetime partners, sexual preferences, current sexual activity, frequency, lubricants, devices, contraception)
- Dyspareunia (pain on arousal, foreplay, touch, penetration, thrusting, post coital, last time pain-free intercourse)
- Obstetric history (pregnancies, mode of delivery, complications, lacerations)
- Menstrual history
- Trauma history (vulvar, obstetric, pelvic, back, sexual or physical abuse, motor vehicle, bicycle, equestrian)
- Family history (vulvovaginal, dermatologic, allergy, gastrointestinal disease)
- Past medical history (with specific attention to migraine headaches, irritable bowel syndrome, interstitial cystitis, temporomandibular joint disease, fibromyalgia, low back pain, depression, anxiety)
- Review of systems (atopy, hygiene practices, skin, gastrointestinal, gynecologic, genitourinary, musculoskeletal, and psychiatric) (Danby & Margesson, 2010).

OBJECTIVE DATA

Physical Examination

Begin the physical exam with a mucocutaneous inspection of the oral cavity, perineum, perianal area, and vagina. Having a detailed diagram of the normal vulva on hand may be helpful in documentation. Upon completion of the vulvar inspection, a sensory Q-tip examination should be done. Use a cotton swab to gently indent the vulva at locations either based on anatomy or by positions identifiable by the face of a clock, proceed in clockwise fashion noting pain. Have the patient rate the pain on a 0 to 10 scale, 0 being no pain and 10 being the most severe pain. A positive Q-tip test can signify underlying pathology, for example, vestibular epithelium (vulvitis, dermatoses), pathology of the vulva affected the vestibule (interstitial cystitis, bladder, bowel, sacroiliac), or pain from the C fibers (nociceptors) in localized vulvodynia (Danby & Margesson, 2010).

Following the Q-tip test, a speculum exam should be performed, using a pediatric speculum if necessary to evaluate the vaginal mucosa and to rule out erythema, erosions, or ulcerations. A wet prep should be performed, noting presence of WBCs, lactobacilli, visible yeast buds or hyphae, clue cells, or trichomonads. Following the speculum exam, perform a bimanual exam, noting any abnormalities and if pain is reproducible. Evaluation of pelvic floor muscles, hips, and back is included as these areas may be primarily or secondarily involved and, therefore, should be assessed. In some cases, x-ray, cystoscopy, colonoscopy, ultrasound, and MRI may be warranted (Danby & Margesson, 2010).

The diagnosis of vulvodynia is clinical and biopsies of symptomatic areas are not necessary to make a diagnosis. However, other problems may develop during treatment of vulvodynia requiring biopsy. Patch testing is also not indicated to exclude contact allergy (Mandal et al., 2010).

Differential Diagnoses of Vulvar Pain

Infectious causes with abnormal exam findings include candidiasis, herpes simplex virus, herpes zoster virus, streptococcus, and staphylococcus. Hormonal causes with abnormal exam findings include labial adhesions and atrophic vulvovaginitis. Inflammatory causes with abnormal exam findings include contact dermatitis (irritant, allergic), lichen sclerosis, lichen simplex chronicus, lichen planus, fissures, drug eruption, and desquamative inflammatory vaginitis. Neoplasms causing vulvar pain and abnormal appearance of the vulva include squamous cell carcinoma, vulvar intraepithelial neoplasia (VIN), and Paget's disease. Neurologic and neuropathic etiologies of vulvar pain also will present with abnormal exam findings and include postherpetic neuralgia, multiple sclerosis, pudendal neuralgia, or entrapment. Pain localized to the vulvar vestibule with a normal exam finding could include localized vestibulodynia, usually provoked, unprovoked, or mixed, primary or secondary. Pain generalized to the vulva: generalized vulvodynia, usually unprovoked, can be unprovoked or mixed (Danby & Margesson, 2010).

PLAN

Psychosocial Interventions

It is important to identify psychosexual morbidity as referral to psychosexual counseling may be appropriate to compliment medical treatments being offered. The presence of vaginismus, adequate lubrication during intercourse, anorgasmia, and partner problems should be inquired about if there are sexual problems. In women with vulvodynia compared with asymptomatic women, psychological morbidity is significantly higher. Research has shown high degrees of anxiety, depressive symptoms, somatization disorders, and hypochondriacal symptoms; however, there is no evidence for a primarily psychological cause for pain (Mandal et al., 2010).

Treatment of Labial Adhesions

- Common in prepubertal girls and typically spontaneously resolve by menarche.
- Observe unless symptomatic (i.e., urinary obstruction).
- First-line treatment: topical estrogen cream. To reduce risk of reagglutination of raw opposing surfaces, apply emollient nightly for 1 month. Under adequate anesthesia in the office setting, manual separation can be performed and surgical excision reserved for acute urinary obstruction.
- Side effects: Monitor girls for breast budding and vaginal bleeding (ACOG, 2008a).

Treatment of Vaginal Atrophy

- A variety of therapies including hormone applications are available to treat symptoms of vulvovaginal dryness, burning, pruritus, and dyspareunia.
- Management options include lifestyle modification, use of vaginal moisturizers, and low-dose topical estradiol preparations.
- Maintenance of regular vaginal sexual intercourse increases blood flow to the pelvic organs, thereby providing protection from atrophy.
- Local or systemic estrogen use may improve sexual function in women with vulvar atrophy, although this remains controversial. Some studies have shown improved circulation and sexual function.
- Side effects: All forms of topical estrogen therapy increase the risk of endometrial hyperplasia and overstimulation. It is currently unknown whether the use of long-term therapy with a topical estrogen requires prophylactic therapy with progesterone. Systemic treatment with estradiol may not be sufficient to treat the symptoms of urogenital atrophy and raises concern of additional health risk for many women (ACOG, 2008a).

Treatment of Lichen Sclerosus

- Recommended treatment: high-potency topical steroid; clobetasol propionate is the most studied.
- Women can anticipate complete or partial resolution of symptoms; skin color and texture will return to normal in some women; partial resolution of hyperkeratosis, purpura, fissuring, and erosions associated with the disorder.
- Recommended dosing is once daily application of ultrapotent topical steroid for 4 weeks, then alternate days for 4 weeks, and finally twice weekly for 4 weeks. Controversy remains whether ongoing maintenance therapy is necessary.
- Side effects include contact sensitization, skin changes, and secondary infection.

- Monitor at 3 and 6 months to evaluate initial response to therapy. For patients who are well controlled, annual examinations are suggested.
- Biopsy may be necessary of persistent lesions, erosions, hyperkeratotic or hyperpigmented areas to rule out intraepithelial neoplasia or invasive squamous cell cancer (ACOG, 2008a).
- Prognosis for spontaneous resolution of vulvovaginal lichen planus is poor. Lichen planus is a frustrating, chronic disease requiring long-term maintenance.
- Treatment options are numerous and include topical and systemic corticosteroids, topical and oral cyclosporine, topical tacrolimus, hydroxychloroquine, oral retinoids, methotrexate, azathioprine, and cyclophosphamide (ACOG, 2008a).

Antifungals

See Chapter 14.

Topical Agents

- A trial of local anesthetic agent may be considered in all subsets of vulvodynia. In general, topical agents should be prescribed with caution due to potential for irritancy. Topical lidocaine gels or ointments can be used in women with provoked vestibulodynia making penetrable intercourse possible. It is recommended the anesthetic be applied 15 to 20 minutes prior to sex and patients should be cautioned about irritancy. Oral contact should be avoided and male partners may want to wear condoms as penile numbness could occur (Mandal et al., 2010).
- Many other topical agents have been suggested such as capsaicin cream, ketoconazole cream, estrogen creams, steroid creams, interferon, and nifedipine, all with mixed results (Mandal et al., 2010).

Tricyclic Antidepressants

- Amitriptyline or nortriptyline is a reasonable initial treatment for unprovoked vulvodynia. Amitriptyline is the best studied tricyclic antidepressant (TCA) and should be increased according to the pain level of the patient. A starting dose of 10 mg per day has been suggested, increasing every week until the pain is controlled, with an average dose being 60 mg per day, although up to 100 mg per day can be used. Side effects should be reviewed with patients and may affect compliance. Gabapentin and pregabalin can be considered in addition to a TCA.

Surgical Intervention

After other measures have been tried, surgical excision of the vestibule may be considered in patients with local provoked vulvodynia. Only a minority of patients may be eligible candidates for surgery. If surgery is offered, adequate counseling and support should be offered both pre- and postoperatively (Mandal et al., 2010).

Physical Therapy

Patients with vulvodynia who have sex-related pain often have pelvic floor muscle dysfunction. Techniques to desensitize the pelvic floor muscles are likely to be beneficial. Physical therapy may help to address the vaginismus "response." Patients can be taught pelvic floor exercises, external and internal soft tissue self-massage, trigger point pressure, biofeedback, and use of vaginal trainers (Mandal et al., 2010) (see section Dyspareunia).

Acupuncture

Acupuncture may be considered in the treatment of unprovoked vulvodynia.

Intralesional Injections

Various injection drugs have been suggested in treatment of vulvodynia. Subcutaneous injections of 40 mg methylprednisolone acetate and lidocaine in 10 mL of normal saline into the vestibule have been shown to be beneficial in some women with provoked vulvodynia. Betamethasone and lidocaine infiltration as well as Botox injections have also been found beneficial (Mandal et al., 2010).

FOLLOW-UP AND REFERRAL

Continuing, consistent follow-up is extremely important in managing vulvar pain syndromes. Careful observation for visible improvement or worsening of vulvar tissue is crucial. Offer continued emotional support. Clients may need to be seen biweekly when initiating therapy, monthly during active medical therapy, and perhaps every 1 to 2 months as improvement occurs.

If improvement does not occur or if the clinician is unsure of the diagnosis, referral to a specialist with knowledge of vulvar disorders is mandatory.

LEIOMYOMAS

Leiomyomas or myomas (uterine fibroids) are the most common gynecological neoplasm and the most common cause of uterine enlargement in nonpregnant women. Fibroids are benign tumors of smooth muscle origin separated by fibrous connective tissue. They derive from a single progenitor myometrial cell. Forty percent of these cells have a chromosomal mutation that is thought to enhance the cellular response to steroid and growth factors. Myomatous tissue has a higher concentration of estrogen and progesterone receptors than normal myometrial tissue. This gives an explanation for growth of fibroids during pregnancy and in response to hormonal contraception (Griffin, Sudigali, & Jacques, 2010).

Most uterine fibroids originate from the uterine corpus. Occasionally, they are discovered in the fallopian tube, round ligament, or cervix. They can be single but are usually multiple (Griffin, Sudigali, et al., 2010).

Fibroids are classified by their location:

- Intramural, within the myometrial wall, and the most common uterine fibroid.
- Submucosal, located just below the endometrium, in 5 to 10 percent of cases. Submucosal fibroids can cause infertility by interfering with embryo transfer and implantation.
- Subserous, occur just below the serosa.
- Pedunculated, classified by further growth of subserousal myoma into the peritoneal cavity.
- Broad ligament myoma, lateral growth of myoma, can be difficult to differentiate from an adnexal mass on clinical exam (Griffin, Sudigali, et al., 2010).

Leiomyomas grow in response to sex steroid hormones. Some women with uterine leiomyomas are asymptomatic while others are symptomatic and require treatment. Hysterectomy is the most common surgical treatment because it is definitive and the possibility of recurrence is eliminated. However, for women who desire future childbearing or to maintain their uteri, alternatives are available. The most common symptoms women present with are abnormal uterine bleeding and pelvic pressure. The most common kind of irregular bleeding is heavy and prolonged, often leading to iron deficiency anemia and significant interruption to a woman's daily activities. Often the pelvic or abdominal discomfort caused by leiomyomas is described as pressure and can lead to dyspareunia and difficulties with urination and defecation (ACOG, 2008b).

ETIOLOGY/EPIDEMIOLOGY

Although leiomyomas are benign tumors, they share many characteristics with malignant neoplasms. As previously mentioned, leiomyomas arise from a single smooth muscle cell. It has been hypothesized that, similar to malignant tumors, leiomyomas result from genetic mutations that lead to the dysregulation of the cell cycle and unchecked growth. Leiomyomas are sensitive to hormonal influence and exhibit an exaggerated response to estrogen and progesterone (Tarnawa, Sullivan, Underwood, Richardson, & Spruill, 2011).

Leiomyomas are two to three times more common in African American women (Tarnawa et al., 2011). Uterine leiomyomas are very common with some studies suggesting that by age 50, 70 percent of Caucasian women and 80 percent of African women are affected (ACOG, 2008b). They are typically discovered in the late reproductive period (Gupta, Sinha, Lumsden, & Hickey, 2009). The prevalence of clinically significant leiomyomas is estimated to be 50 percent in African women and 35 percent among Caucasian women (Van Voorhis, 2009).

SUBJECTIVE DATA

Symptoms of leiomyomas include menorrhagia, dyspareunia, bloating, pelvic pressure, urinary urgency, and frequency (Spies et al., 2010). Symptoms are affected by the size, number, and location of the leiomyomas (ACOG, 2008b).

OBJECTIVE DATA

Physical Examination

An abdominal exam may reveal a large mass if the leiomyoma has grown larger than a 12- to 14-week pregnant uterus. The absence of ascites and presence of rebound tenderness and normal bowel sounds should be noted.

The genitalia and reproductive tract are also examined. Examine the cervix for any extraneous tissue or distortion and note any bleeding or discharge. Prior to the pelvic exam, ask the client to empty her bladder to decrease risk of confusing the tumor with the bladder. The pelvic exam may reveal an enlarged uterus that is firm and irregular but not tender. Usually palpated at midline, a leiomyoma may feel very firm or soft and cystic. If it is situated laterally, it may be mistaken for an adnexal mass. If the mass moves with the cervix, then it is likely to be a leiomyoma. Size of the uterus should be described in terms of gestational size (Griffin, Sudigali, et al., 2010).

Diagnostic Tests and Methods

Hemoglobin. Evaluate to determine whether the client is experiencing clinically significant anemia.

Urinalysis. To identify urinary tract conditions that might account for any urinary tract symptoms. WBCs, bacteria, or red blood cells in the urine may indicate chronic or recurrent UTI. Hematuria may indicate the presence of renal stone or a tumor of the urinary tract. Further diagnostic testing may be indicated, specifically cystoscopy or intravenous pyelogram.

Pregnancy Test (Urine or Serum β-hCG). Evaluation for unsuspected intrauterine pregnancy.

Stool Guaiac (Colocare or Hemoccult). To detect gastrointestinal pathology that may be the source of a palpable abdominal mass, for example, an inflammatory diverticulum or an intestinal mass. A stool found to be positive for occult blood suggests gastrointestinal polyps or malignancy. Refer to a specialist for follow-up.

Ultrasound. The initial imaging of choice is ultrasound due to availability and cost. Transvaginal ultrasound allows better visualization of the endometrium and submucosal fibroids than transabdominal ultrasound, especially in obese patients or when overlying bowel gas is present. Ultrasound reveals uterine enlargement, contour abnormality, and focal masses with an echogenicity different from that of the myometrium. Shadowing from calcification may be present. Sensitivity with ultrasound diagnosis is operator dependent and varies from 63 to 99 percent. Limitations in transvaginal sonography include failure to identify small myomas and subserosal myomas. Also, with increasing size of the uterus and multiple fibroids, it becomes more difficult to map myomas (Griffin, Sudigali, et al., 2010).

Hysterosalpingogram. Myomas can be diagnosed with hysterosalpingogram; however, there is limited sensitivity for subserosal or small intramural fibroids and hysterosalpingogram also does not allow the ability to locate where the fibroids are within the uterus (Griffin, Sudigali, et al., 2010).

MRI. MRI allows for excellent soft tissue contrast resolution; therefore, pelvic MRI is superior to transvaginal ultrasound in the evaluation of location, number, and size of myomas. MRI is the preferred imaging modality for presurgical planning. In comparison to ultrasonography, MRI has a greater sensitivity for pedunculated submucosal fibroids, pedunculated subserosal fibroids, and large fibroids. Before uterine artery embolization, pelvic MRI is increasingly being performed (Griffin, Sudigali, et al., 2010).

Computerized Tomography. Computerized tomography (CT) is not helpful for diagnosis unless fibroids are calcified, because CT has limited tissue contrast for pelvic organ resolution (Griffin, Sudigali, et al., 2010).

Diagnostic Hysteroscopy. Hysteroscopy can aid in the diagnosis of submucosal fibroids (Griffin, Sudigali, et al., 2010). Hysteroscopy employs the use of endoscopic equipment to view the uterine cavity. It enables direct examination of the endocervical canal and lower uterine segment. Also, some fibroids may be amenable to resection during the hysteroscopy (Luciano, 2009).

The most common indications for hysteroscopy are evaluation of abnormal uterine bleeding and direct observation of intrauterine fibroids, polyps, adhesions, and location of IUDs. It enables the clinician to identify the exact presence, location, size, and number of fibroids and is helpful in treatment planning. Contraindications to the procedure include a recent or present episode of salpingitis or diagnosed cervical or uterine malignancy. The procedure should be performed with careful consideration in women who are bleeding heavily, are pregnant, or have cardiovascular or systemic disease.

Risks are infrequent and include possible cervical trauma, uterine perforation, and infection. See Chapter 3 for description of this procedure.

DIFFERENTIAL MEDICAL DIAGNOSES

Ovarian neoplasm, tubo-ovarian inflammatory mass, diverticular inflammatory mass, pregnancy, ectopic pregnancy, adenomyosis, pelvic kidney, malignancy, interstitial cystitis, irritable bowel syndrome, obstipation.

PLAN

Psychosocial Interventions

Provide the client with explanations and printed information about leiomyomas (fibroids). Reassure her that leiomyomas occur commonly, that they are rarely malignant, and that if she is asymptomatic or if symptoms are mild, treatment will be unnecessary. Assess her future reproductive plans and the extent of her symptoms. Stress the importance of regular monitoring and follow-up examinations.

If the client is or becomes pregnant, provide reassurance and support. Reassure her that in most pregnancies, fibroids do not grow enough to cause complication. Advise the client of the signs and symptoms of preterm labor later in the pregnancy.

Medical Management

Expectant Management. In asymptomatic women, expectant management is the norm. Previous thought was that increased uterine size alone could be indication for hysterectomy. Reasoning behind hysterectomy for large leiomyomas was that a large uterus made assessment of the ovaries and early surveillance of ovarian or uterine cancer impossible. Recently, the National Institutes of Health and National Cancer Institute Consensus Conference recognized the ineffectiveness of the routine pelvic exam in identification of early ovarian cancer. Historically, a second argument was made that because of increased rate of morbidity during surgery for a large uterus, that surgery is a safer option when the uterus is smaller. There is not a clear consensus about increased morbidity with increased uterine size; therefore, this currently is not indication for intervention. In rare cases, increased uterine size can cause compression of the ureters and affect renal function; this appears to be more of a concern if the uterus is greater than 12-week size. If there is concern that the mass is not a leiomyoma but instead a sarcoma, the major clinical sign to monitor for would be rapid growth in uterine size. However, sarcomas are rare. Endometrial biopsy and MRI are useful diagnostic tools in differentiating leiomyomas from sarcomas (ACOG, 2008b).

Medication

The goal of medical therapy is to reduce the symptoms and myoma size.

NSAIDs. NSAIDs are effective in decreasing dysmenorrhea. However, to date, no studies have shown improvement with use of NSAIDs in women with dysmenorrhea caused by leiomyomas (ACOG, 2008b).

Contraceptive Steroids. Combined hormonal contraceptives and progestin-only contraceptives are widely used to control abnormal menstrual bleeding and dysmenorrhea in women with and without leiomyomas. The literature suggests that medical therapies give short-term relief and many women ultimately seek surgical treatment. There is limited data on the effect of estrogen and progestin in treatment of leiomyomas. Treatment with estrogen and progestin, usually with oral contraceptive pills, may control bleeding symptoms without stimulating growth of leiomyomas. However, progestin-only methods have shown mixed results. Due to conflicting evidence of estrogen and progestin effect on leiomyoma growth, close monitoring of fibroid and uterine size is recommended when initiating contraceptives. The levonorgestrel intrauterine device has little systemic hormone effect and is beneficial for treatment of menorrhagia. Smaller studies suggest the levonorgestrel intrauterine device may be effective for treatment of menorrhagia in women with leiomyomas. However, these women may experience higher rates of expulsion and vaginal spotting (ACOG, 2008b).

GnRH Agonist. GnRH analogues bind to GnRH receptors resulting in a decrease in luteinizing hormone and follicle-stimulating hormone, which produces a hypoestrogenic effect.

Within 3 months of treatment, GnRH agonists lead to amenorrhea in most women and a 35 to 65 percent reduction in leiomyoma size (ACOG, 2009a).

The FDA has approved use of the GnRH agonist, leuprolide acetate, for preoperative therapy in women with leiomyoma who are anemic. Iron supplementation should also be used preoperatively. Leuprolide acetate has been found to be most useful in women with large leiomyomas. GnRH agonists provide temporary treatment, within several months of cessation the leiomyomas grow back to previous size. Due to the adverse effect of pseudomenopause associated with leuprolide acetate, it is recommended treatment be no longer than 6 months without addition of add-back hormonal therapy. Hypoestrogenism induces bone loss and vasomotor symptoms. The use of steroid hormone add-back in treatment of leiomyomas has been limited to low doses equivalent to menopausal hormone therapy, not higher doses associated with combined hormonal contraceptive pills used to treat other gynecologic disease states. This is in part due to studies showing the effect of progestin on leiomyomas, with add-back therapy. There is an increase in mean uterine volume to 95 percent of pretreatment size within 24 months of initiating the progestin. Best results may be achieved when add-back therapy is added after 1 to 3 months of treatment with the GnRH agonist (ACOG, 2008b).

Add-Back Therapy. See section Endometriosis.

Aromatase Inhibitors. These medications have not been approved by the FDA for use in treatment of leiomyomas; however, this is an intriguing area of future research and a potential treatment option. Aromatase inhibitors work by blocking ovarian and peripheral estrogen production with lower estradiol levels after 1 day of treatment. Due to their mechanism of action and rapid effect, these medications have fewer adverse effects compared to GnRH agonists. Small studies suggest aromatase inhibitors decrease leiomyoma size and symptoms (ACOG, 2008b).

Progesterone Modulators. Mifepristone is the most extensively studied progesterone-modulating compound with results indicating reduction of leiomyoma size. However, further study is needed before implementing into practice. High concentrations of progesterone receptors are found in the uteri of women with leiomyomas and antiprogesterone agents, such as mifepristone, bind to these receptors and thereby reduce the size of leiomyomas. The reduction in leiomyoma size is found to be similar to those with GnRH analogues. After cessation of mifepristone, the recurrent growth is slower. Unlike GnRH analogues, mifepristone does not decrease bone mass density. Additional side effects include amenorrhea, endometrial hyperplasia without atypia, and transient elevations in transaminase levels, requiring monitoring of liver function. The drug has limited availability as a compounding pharmacy is required to produce. If approved for clinical use, there may be a role for short-term use of mifepristone prior to surgical treatment (ACOG, 2008b).

Surgical Intervention

Abdominal Myomectomy. Myomectomy may be an option for women who wish to retain their uteri. The goal of surgery is to remove all leiomyomas, relieve symptoms, and increase fertility. Research has found risk of abdominal myomectomy and hysterectomy to be about the same. Abdominal myomectomy has been found to improve menorrhagia symptoms with an overall resolution rate of 81 percent and similar results for cessation of pelvic pressure symptoms. Abdominal myomectomy does carry the risk of recurrence; however, that risk is lessened with women who have subsequent childbirth. There is a greater risk of leiomyoma recurrence with women who have a greater number of leiomyomas present. Risks of myomectomy include risk of undergoing an unanticipated hysterectomy due to intraoperative complications. Other risks include blood loss and risk of need for blood transfusion (ACOG, 2008b).

Discuss the difficult surgery and its potential complications with the client. Inform her about the high rate of myoma recurrence and the possible later need for a hysterectomy. Warn her not to attempt pregnancy until 4 to 6 months after the procedure. Review the postoperative/discharge instruction.

Laparoscopic Myomectomy. Traditionally, myomectomy was performed via laparotomy; however, increasing endoscopic options are available. Benefits of laparoscopic myomectomy include less scarring and quicker recovery. Previously, it has been suggested to avoid laparoscopic myomectomy for leiomyomas larger than 5 to 8 cm, multiple leiomyomas, or the presence of deep intramural leiomyomas. Successful outcomes for laparoscopic myomectomy depend on the skill level and expertise of the surgeon. A large retrospective study reported recurrence rate of leiomyomas after laparoscopic resection being 11.7 percent after 1 year and 84.4 percent after 8 years and rate of reoperation being 6.7 percent at 5 years and 16 percent at 8 years. Fertility being an important outcome to measure, subsequent pregnancy rates have been found to be between 57 and 69 percent after laparoscopic myomectomy (ACOG, 2008b).

Hysteroscopic Myomectomy. Hysteroscopic myomectomy is an option for treatment of abnormal uterine bleeding caused by leiomyomas classified as submucosal. Submucosal leiomyomas are estimated to be the cause of 5 to 10 percent of cases of abnormal uterine bleeding, pain, subfertility, and infertility. Ability to surgically remove the entire leiomyoma is indicative of surgical success. Studies have demonstrated successful resection of the leiomyoma usually at a rate of 85 to 95 percent. As with abdominal leiomyomectomy, the effectiveness of the procedure decreases over time, with 5 to 15 percent of women requiring a second hysteroscopic procedure (ACOG, 2008b).

Potential complications associated with hysteroscopic myomectomy are between 1 and 12 percent, including fluid overload, pulmonary edema, cerebral edema, bleeding, uterine perforation, gas embolism, and infection (ACOG, 2008b).

Uterine Artery Embolization. Uterine artery embolization performed by an interventional radiologist is a procedure in which the uterine arteries are embolized through a transcutaneous femoral artery approach. Subsequently, the uterine leiomyoma devascularizes and involutes. Uterine artery embolization results in decreased menstrual duration, dysmenorrhea, urinary frequency, and urinary urgency. Short- and long-term outcomes have found uterine artery embolization to be safe and effective for appropriately selected women who wish to retain their uteri. Referral to an obstetrician-gynecologist is necessary to determine appropriateness of therapy and ensure optimal collaboration with the interventional radiologist. The effect of uterine artery embolization on pregnancy remains understudied and should be used with caution for women who desire future pregnancy (ACOG, 2008b). Current contraindications include pregnancy, infertility, future desire for pregnancy, and uterus greater than 20-to 24-week size.

MRI-Guided Focused Ultrasound Surgery. MRI was approved by the FDA in 2004 for the treatment of leiomyomas with focused ultrasound therapy. Benefits include noninvasive approach. The technique uses high-intensity ultrasound waves directed into a focal volume of soft tissue of a leiomyoma-causing protein denaturation, irreversible cell damage, and coagulative necrosis. This technique has shown short-term safety and efficacy; however, it is still being studied to determine long-term efficacy (ACOG, 2008b).

Hysterectomy. Hysterectomy is the definitive treatment of leiomyomas. Hysterectomy is indicated in women who have completed childbearing, or if menorrhagia worsens, leading to anemia. In addition, hysterectomy may be done to resolve any of the following: pelvic pain and secondary dysmenorrhea, urinary symptoms, or uterine growth after menopause. In comparing women treated for leiomyomas with hysterectomy, myomectomy, and uterine fibroid embolization, at 12 months posttreatment, women with hysterectomy reported significantly lower symptoms and better health-related quality-of-life outcomes compared to women receiving the other two therapies (Spies et al., 2010).

Hysterectomies can be performed vaginally, abdominally, or with laparoscopic or robotic assistance. When deciding on the route and method of hysterectomy, the surgeon should consider how the procedure will be performed most safely and cost-effectively to fulfill the medical needs of the patient. Research shows that generally, vaginal hysterectomy is associated with better outcomes and fewer complications than laparoscopic or abdominal hysterectomy. Salpingo-oophorectomy can be performed by any route. Data shows that 66 percent of hysterectomies are performed abdominally, 22 percent vaginally, and 12 percent with laparoscopic hysterectomy (ACOG, 2008b, 2009a).

FOLLOW-UP AND REFERRAL

For the client who is asymptomatic or has mild symptoms, the treatment of choice is expectant management (ACOG, 2008b). During pregnancy, rest and analgesics are appropriate if pain is present. Stress the importance of keeping appointments for close follow-up. If expectant management, medical therapy, or myomectomy is chosen as a treatment option, the client should be reexamined at 3- to 6-month intervals. It is generally accepted that cancer does not develop from leiomyomas. The client may be monitored without risk of the development of cancer. Rapid increase in uterine size raises the question of malignancy (ACOG, 2008b). Uterine size and the leiomyoma should be evaluated carefully by pelvic exam and, if necessary, ultrasound should be used. Discuss with the client any new or worsening symptomology. Alter the plan of care as necessary. Monitor hemoglobin and hematocrit frequently if menorrhagia or metrorrhagia is present. Refer for physician consultation if there is rapid increase in size, increase in menorrhagia or development, or increase in pain/pressure.

ADENOMYOSIS

Adenomyosis is a uterine disease where the endometrial glands and stroma penetrate into the myometrium. Women suffering from adenomyosis experience symptoms of dysmenorrhea and menorrhagia. The reason for growth of the glandular and stromal cells into the myometrium is not completely known. However, it is hypothesized that trauma during delivery or uterine abrasion causes a breakdown of the myometrial-endometrial border, and a reactive hyperplasia follows that penetrates the myometrium (But, Pakiz, & Rakic, 2011). Other hypotheses include a link with estrogen secretion; hypervascularity and the presence of ectopic endometrial lesions occurring within vascular channels; and inflammatory factors have all been implicated in the pathophysiologic pain response (Dietrich, 2010).

Adenomyosis is typically diagnosed in the fourth or fifth decade of life, among women who are perimenopausal and multiparous (Dietrich, 2010; Ozdegirmenci et al., 2010). Definitive treatment is through hysterectomy; therefore, the prevalence of disease can be estimated through hysterectomy specimens, which may vary between 15 and 25 percent. There may be a genetic link as well, with a 6.9 percent relative risk of adenomyosis if a first-degree relative has endometriosis (Dietrich, 2010). Adenomyosis is also frequently observed in women wishing future childbearing, therefore, requiring a more conservative approach to management (Kim, Yoon, et al., 2011).

One study compared women undergoing hysterectomy for the diagnosis of adenomyosis with the diagnosis of uterine leiomyoma, and found that adenomyosis was associated with younger age, history of depression, dysmenorrhea, and pelvic pain (Taran, Weaver, Coddington, & Stewart, 2010).

SUBJECTIVE DATA

Symptoms of adenomyosis are typically menorrhagia, chronic pelvic pain, dysmenorrhea, and infertility (Osada et al., 2011; Taran et al., 2010). Other symptoms are related to uterine enlargement, causing urinary frequency and pelvic heaviness (Kim, Yoon, et al., 2011).

OBJECTIVE DATA

Physical Examination

Bimanual examination may reveal an enlarged, symmetrical uterus (Taran et al., 2010).

Diagnostic Tests and Methods

Traditionally, diagnosis of adenomyosis is made histopathologically after routine hysterectomy. Recent improvements in imaging technology, MRI and ultrasound, have been helpful for earlier diagnosis. Earlier diagnosis results in opportunities for earlier treatment and prevention of endometriosis-related infertility as well as improvement in quality of life due to prevention of adenomyosis progression or regression (Dietrich, 2010).

Ultrasound. Three-dimensional transvaginal ultrasound has been found to be a good tool in diagnosis of adenomyosis as it allows accurate evaluation and measurement of the junctional zone. Overall accuracy of adenomyosis with three-dimensional ultrasound has been found to be 89 percent (Exacoustos et al., 2011).

MRI. Adenomyosis can be diagnosed using MRI with a diagnostic accuracy of 85 percent (Novellas et al., 2011). In making a diagnosis of adenomyosis, the most important finding on MRI is thickness of the junctional zone exceeding 12 mm. Limitations of MRI are mainly difficulty in defining the junctional zone on imaging that can occur in up to 20 percent of premenopausal women (Novellas et al., 2011). MRI has shown better sensitivity and specificity in diagnosis of adenomyosis abnormalities in comparison to ultrasound (Dietrich, 2010).

DIFFERENTIAL MEDICAL DIAGNOSES

Leiomyomas, endometriosis.

PLAN

Psychosocial Interventions

Women with adenomyosis may have an increased risk of depression and antidepressant use (Taran et al., 2010). Discuss the condition with the client and determine the impact of her symptoms. The severity of symptoms will determine therapy, which should be described to the client. Reassure her if necessary.

Medication

Medical management studies are limited for treatment of adenomyosis; currently reported cases have derived treatment for adenomyosis to be modeled after traditional endometriosis treatments. This rationale is based on similarity in the mechanism of disease in adenomyosis and endometriosis (Dietrich, 2010).

Combination Oral Contraceptive Pills. Hormonal suppression with combination oral contraceptive pills is considered initial first-line therapy for treatment of adenomyosis and is of particular importance for females desiring to preserve fertility (Dietrich, 2010).

NSAIDs, Medroxyprogesterone Acetate, Danazol, GnRH Agonists. See section Endometriosis.

Levonorgestrel Intrauterine System. One study found the levonorgestrel intrauterine system has shown comparable improvements in hemoglobin to hysterectomy in treating adenomyosis-associated menorrhagia. The levonorgestrel intrauterine system also showed greater improvements in quality of life in comparison to patients undergoing hysterectomy for treatment of adenomyosis (Ozdegirmenci et al., 2010).

Surgical Interventions

Adenomyosis presents a surgical challenge to women who wish to maintain their uterus, but require surgical intervention. The nature of adenomyosis is that there is no discrete border between the normal uterine tissue and the lesion, making it difficult to establish a clear plane (Osada et al., 2011).

Hysterectomy. In women who are post-childbearing, whose symptoms have been refractory to medical management, definitive surgical intervention with hysterectomy may be indicated (Dietrich, 2010).

Surgical Adenomyomectomy. In women who wish to retain their uterus or desire future childbearing, adenomyomectomy has been shown to result in a dramatic reduction in symptoms and allows over half of the women to conceive and go to term without uterine rupture. The procedure involves radical excision of adenomyotic tissue. The uterine wall is reconstructed by a triple-flap method, without overlapping suture lines, thus preventing uterine rupture in subsequent pregnancies. Prior conservative surgeries have been associated with frequent recurrence of adenomyosis and spontaneous uterine rupture in pregnancy (Osada et al., 2011).

Hysteroscopic Endometrial Ablation. Hysteroscopic rollerball endometrial ablation as a surgical management option for adenomyosis in women with menorrhagia and dysmenorrhea has been found to be effective and safe, thus reducing the need for the more radical surgery of hysterectomy (Preutthipan & Herabutya, 2010).

In terms of recurrence of chronic pain due to adenomyosis, no difference has been found between those undergoing ablation of lesions and excision (Dietrich, 2010).

Uterine Artery Embolization. Uterine artery embolization has been found to be safe and very effective in achieving complete necrosis of adenomyosis. Of patients who have achieved complete necrosis at 18-month follow-up, none experienced recurrent menorrhagia. Although hysterectomy is considered the only definitive treatment for adenomyosis, uterine artery embolization is an alternative that can yield a positive short-term outcome (Kim, Kim, et al., 2011).

FOLLOW-UP AND REFERRAL

Recurrence of adenomyosis is possible because it is a progressive disorder (Osada et al., 2011). If medical therapy is the initial treatment of choice, then the client needs to be evaluated in 3 to 6 months. Increasing pain or bleeding may necessitate referral to a gynecologic surgeon for possible hysterectomy. Sarcoma can be a complication.

PELVIC ORGAN PROLAPSE

Pelvic organ prolapse, also called genital prolapse, occurs when there is descent of one or more of the pelvic organs from its normal location toward the vaginal opening. Pelvic organ prolapse can involve a herniation of any combination of the pelvic organs (bladder, cervix, bowel, and rectum) (Kuncharapu, Majeroni, & Johnson, 2010).

There are six types of prolapse:

- *Uterine prolapse:* Occurs when the uterus and cervix descend down the vaginal canal as a result of weak or damaged pelvic support structures.
- *Vaginal vault prolapse:* Occurs when the top of the vagina descends further forward in the vaginal vault. This happens more commonly in women with a history of a hysterectomy.
- *Cystocele:* Occurs when the tissue that supports the wall between the vagina and posterior bladder weakens and allows a part of the bladder to descend into the vaginal wall.
- *Urethrocele:* Occurs when the urethra descends and presses into the vaginal wall. It is rare for this to occur by itself, but usually occurs with a cystocele. A cystourethrocele occurs when there is prolapse of both the bladder and the urethra.
- *Enterocele:* Occurs when the pouch of Douglas (the area located between the rectum and uterus) descends and presses into the vaginal wall.
- *Rectocele:* Occurs when the tissue that supports the wall between the rectum and vagina weakens, which allows the rectum to descend and press into the wall of the vagina.

EPIDEMIOLOGY

Prolapse of the pelvic organs is the leading cause of hysterectomy in postmenopausal women and accounts for up to 18 percent of hysterectomies in women of other age groups (Smith, Holman, Moorin, & Tsokos, 2010; Tinelli et al., 2010). Nearly 45 to 76 percent of patients seen for routine gynecological care complain loss of vaginal or uterine support (Jelovsek, Maher, & Barber, 2007). Pelvic organ prolapse has been shown to be due to multiple risk factors, which include vaginal birth including forceps delivery, macrosomic infant, and prolonged second stage of labor; increasing age; obesity; prior anal sphincter laceration; increased intra-abdominal pressure, which can be due to chronic coughing (related to factors such as smoking or chronic respiratory conditions); straining due to constipation; heavy lifting; race or ethnicity (Caucasian women are shown to be at greater risk for pelvic relaxation); and previous hysterectomy (Jelovsek et al., 2007; Kuncharapu et al., 2010; Salvatore, Siesto, & Serati, 2010).

SUBJECTIVE DATA

Common complaints from patients can include pelvic or vaginal pressure or heaviness; a feeling of something bulging from the vaginal area; seeing something bulging from the vaginal area; dyspareunia; urinary incontinence; urinary frequency, hesitancy, or urgency; a prolonged or weak urine stream; incomplete feeling of emptying; need to change positions to start or finish voiding; need to manually reduce a prolapse in order to begin or finish voiding; incontinence of stool or flatus; straining with defecation; urgent need to defecate; feeling of incomplete emptying during defecation; feeling of a blockage or obstruction during defecation; need to digitally evacuate bowels; and pushing the area around the vagina to begin or finish defecation (Eva, Gun, & Preben, 2005; Jelovsek et al., 2007).

OBJECTIVE DATA

A thorough pelvic and rectal exam is crucial in examining the patient with complaints of pelvic organ prolapse. Exam should be done in a supine and dorsal lithotomy position with the patient at rest and straining. First, it is important to assess the external genital area for signs of vulvar atrophy and obvious organ protrusion. To assess for anterior vaginal wall defect, the practitioner should insert the posterior blade of a speculum into the vagina, retract the posterior wall, and have the patient strain. Next, flip the blade to retract the anterior vaginal wall and have the patient bear down and assess posterior wall for defect. Observe for any leaking of urine. Bimanual exam is done to assess for degree of uterine prolapse. A rectovaginal exam should be performed to assess for a rectocele. If the patient has urinary symptoms, she should undergo a postvoid residual testing and possible bladder ultrasound. Careful note should be made of the degree of prolapse of each of the organs.

A staging system has been developed to document the degree of prolapse.

Stage 0: No prolapse is demonstrated.

Stage 1: The distal portion of the prolapse is >1 cm above the level of the hymen.

Stage 2: The distal portion of the prolapse is ≤1 cm proximal or distal to the level of the hymen.

Stage 3: The distal portion of the prolapse is >1 cm below the level of the hymen but protrudes not more than 2 cm less than the total length of the vagina, measured in centimeters.

Stage 4: Complete eversion of the total length of the lower genital tract.

DIFFERENTIAL MEDICAL DIAGNOSES

Missed or threatened abortion, ovarian cysts, ectopic pregnancy, UTI, vaginitis, tumors of the abdomen or pelvis.

PLAN

Psychosocial Interventions

It is important the patient has a thorough understanding of pelvic organ prolapse; illustrations or patient education models may be beneficial to show the different types of prolapse. It is also important to determine the degree that the prolapse is affecting quality of life for the patient—this may help determine the best type of management options for the patient. Lastly, it is important to reassure the patient that these interventions are very successful in restoring normal functioning.

Medication

Hormone estrogen therapy can provide some relief in symptoms by increasing the tone of the genital tissue. However, the benefits versus risks of estrogen use must be considered. The patient must be counseled on the potential health risks associated with use of hormone therapy. Vaginal estrogen therapy such as creams, suppositories, and rings can provide local estrogen treatment without systemic effects. There is no need for progesterone use with a local estrogen regimen.

Diet

For patients with constipation, pelvic organ prolapse can be a result of straining on a regular basis. Education and counseling relating to dietary changes such as increasing fiber and fluids, weight loss recommendations, and healthy diet choices may be beneficial.

Kegel Exercises

This exercise can be done as a way to strengthen pelvic floor muscles. For these pelvic floor muscle exercises to be effective in management of pelvic floor dysfunction, a patient will need to be able to isolate and contract the proper muscles with force and duration. Assessment can be done during a bimanual exam in which palpation of the pelvic floor muscles confirms that the patient can maintain proper contraction of the pelvic muscles for at least 3 seconds. Patients should be instructed on how to contract the proper muscles. A common way of doing this is to instruct the patient to use the same muscles she would to stop and start a flow of urine while voiding. Then, discuss a regimen of 10 to 20 muscle contractions each lasting 3 to 5 seconds. This should be done at least three times daily (Moen et al., 2007) (see also Chapter 22).

Pessaries

Vaginal pessaries are synthetic devices that can be inserted into the vagina and help to provide support to the pelvic organs as a management option for urinary incontinence and pelvic organ prolapse (Storey, Aston, Price, Irving, & Hemmens, 2009). Vaginal pessaries can be a useful alternative to surgery. There are nearly 20 different types of pessaries used today. Most are plastic or silicone and they come in different sizes and shapes including ring, ring with support, Gellhorn, donut, inflatable, Smith-Hodge, and cube. When choosing a proper pessary for a patient, factors to be considered include the type and extent of the prolapse, manual dexterity, cognitive functioning, and amount of sexual activity. Estimate the size of the vagina and the largest pessary that comfortably fits should be used to reduce the prolapse. Before the patient leaves the clinic, have her walk, stand, perform Valsalva maneuver, and bend to ensure that she can perform these activities without discomfort from the pessary. She should also be able to void without difficulty (Jelovsek et al., 2007). Pessaries require routine maintenance and the patient should be given the option to return to the clinic every 3 months for a pessary cleaning or shown how to do this herself if she is comfortable with care of the pessary.

Treatment of Chronic Cough

Treating conditions causing chronic cough, leading to increased intra-abdominal pressure, will help relieve symptoms of pelvic organ prolapse. Smoking cessation can be achieved using a number of different treatment modalities such as patches, lozenges, inhalers, gum, cognitive and behavioral therapies, and prescription smoking cessation medication. Referral to a primary care provider or specialist can be made for treatment of chronic respiratory conditions.

Physical Therapy

Referral can be made to a physical therapist who has special training in pelvic floor disorders. Patients can work with the therapist to strengthen the muscles of the pelvic floor. Biofeedback therapy is also used by physical therapists in conjunction with pelvic strengthening exercises.

Surgery

Women who either fail the above management options or decline pessary or physical therapy can be given surgery as a management option. Surgery can help to restore function and help the patient return to normal anatomy. Patients need to be finished with childbearing before undergoing surgery. The three major types of surgery can be done by an abdominal, vaginal, or laparoscopic approach. The type of surgery done depends on the cause of the prolapse (Jelovsek et al., 2007; McIntyre, Goudelocke, & Rovner, 2010).

Anterior colporrhaphy: Done for management of anterior prolapse—cystocele/urethrocele.

Posterior colporrhaphy: Done for management of posterior prolapse—rectocele/enterocele.

Vaginal hysterectomy: Done for management of any type of uterine prolapse.

Refer patient to a gynecologic surgeon. Potential adverse effects need to be explained to the patient prior to the procedure and can include abnormal bleeding, dyspareunia, UTI, incontinence, or a recurrence of the prolapse.

FOLLOW-UP AND REFERRAL

Follow-up needs to be based on the type of treatment the patient pursues. Patients who choose observation or Kegel exercises should be seen as needed with worsening symptoms or with a reduction of quality of life. Patients with pessaries need to be counseled on insertion and removal of pessary for cleaning. Patients who are not comfortable removing and inserting the pessary independently should be seen every few months in the clinic for cleaning. Surgical patients need annual monitoring to evaluate for recurrence of the prolapse.

CHRONIC PELVIC PAIN

Chronic pelvic pain is defined as cyclic or noncyclic pain in the lower abdomen or pelvis, lasting at least 6 months, arising continuously or intermittently, and impacting activities of daily living (Daniels & Khan, 2010). Etiology is usually multifactorial, requiring that etiologies of organic pathology, personal beliefs, coping skills, and social interactions are considered (Daniels & Khan, 2010). Chronic pelvic pain is a symptom rather than a disease and often has more than one underlying pathologic causes (Vercellini, Somigliana, et al., 2009). The condition may encompass dyspareunia, dyschezia, or worsening dysmenorrhea. In many women, an underlying cause cannot be determined. Gaining a woman's trust and establishing a strong patient–provider relationship is essential to long-term outcome and quality care.

EPIDEMIOLOGY

Following endometriosis, the most common causes of chronic pelvic pain are postoperative adhesions, pelvic varices, interstitial cystitis, and irritable bowel syndrome (Vercellini, Somigliana, et al., 2009). Other causes of chronic pelvic pain include chronic pelvic inflammatory infection and pelvic congestion syndrome. Musculoskeletal etiologies for pain include pelvic organ prolapse or adaptive posture as a result of lower back pain. One study showed no obvious pathological cause for chronic pelvic pain at time of diagnostic laparoscopy in 55 percent of women (Daniels & Khan, 2010).

In a U.S. population–based study, 61 percent of women with pelvic pain symptoms did not have a clear diagnosis. Even investigation of pain via laparoscopy often reveals no obvious etiology. When abnormality is discovered, it may be coincidental rather than causal and often the site of the lesion (e.g., adhesion) does not correlate with the site of the pain (Stones, Cheong, Howard, & Singh, 2010).

Known etiologies of pelvic pain include endometriosis (chronic in nature), primary dysmenorrhea (a recurrent acutely painful condition exclusively related to menstruation), pain due to active chronic PID (chronic low-grade sepsis in devitalized tubal tissue with acute exacerbations incompletely treated by antibiotics), and irritable bowel syndrome (Stones et al., 2010).

Another hypothesis is the vascular hypothesis in which pain is thought to originate from dilated pelvic veins that cause blood flow to be reduced. Others have speculated there is an alteration in processing of stimuli by the spinal cord and brain in women with chronic pelvic pain. Another neuropathic theory is one in which normal stimuli is perceived as painful (Stones et al., 2010).

Risk factors for chronic pelvic pain include the following:

- Drug or alcohol misuse
- Miscarriage
- Menorrhagia
- Previous cesarean surgery
- Pelvic pathology
- Experience of sexual abuse at any age
- Psychological comorbidities (Daniels & Kahn, 2010)

In the United States, the estimated direct medical cost of outpatient visits for chronic pelvic pain in women age 18 to 50 is $881.5 million annually (Dalpiaz et al., 2008). The incidence of chronic pelvic pain in women is about 8.5 to 15 percent (Neis & Neis, 2009). Women with chronic pelvic pain report lower general physical health compared to women without pain. Women also describe negative effects on relationships, loss, and social isolation. They also have a higher incidence of sleep disturbance and fatigue (Daniels & Khan, 2010).

SUBJECTIVE DATA

The patient's history is essential and generally considered central to correct diagnosis and may be more valuable than several diagnostic investigations. Specifically, women should be asked about the location and character of pain, exacerbating and relieving factors, the temporal course, and relationship with the menstrual cycle. Pain described as both ventral and dorsal often suggests an intrapelvic pathology, whereas pain located specifically in the dorsal low back suggests a musculoskeletal etiology. Women should be questioned where the pain occurs; women who identify a specific location of pain typically have an organic cause, whereas women with psychogenic chronic pelvic pain typically move their hand around all the lower abdominal quadrants versus locating precisely where the pain is (Vercellini, Somigliana, et al., 2009).

Ask about medical and surgical therapies and their effect on pain as well as side effects (Vercellini, Somigliana, et al., 2009). Reproductive history is important in that pregnancy and childbirth can be traumatic events to the musculoskeletal system and can cause chronic pelvic pain.

Cyclicity of the pain should raise suspicion of a gynecologic origin, although nongynecologic conditions such as interstitial cystitis and irritable bowel syndrome may worsen premensturally. Dyspareunia may be due to endometriosis, pelvic floor dysfunction, interstitial cystitis, and vulvodynia. In women with dyspareunia and infertility, a history of STI and low-grade fever could be due to chronic pelvic infection (Vercellini, Somigliana, et al., 2009).

Symptoms associated with pelvic congestion syndrome include changing location of pain, dysmenorrheal, deep dyspareunia, pain after intercourse, and dull pain worsened by standing for long periods; this pain is improved by lying down (Vercellini, Somigliana, et al., 2009).

Subjective symptoms suggestive of interstitial cystitis are dysuria, urgency, frequency, and laboratory confirmation with many negative urine cultures.

Irritable bowel syndrome is frequent in women with chronic pelvic pain with an incidence of 65 to 79 percent. Symptoms indicative of irritable bowel syndrome are alternating constipation and diarrhea, abdominal bloating, mucus per rectum, relief of pain after a bowel movement, and sensation of incomplete evacuation after a bowel movement (Vercellini, Somigliana, et al., 2009). However, these symptoms can also be associated with endometriosis.

A thorough social history is important. Investigate for abuse and domestic violence. Approach should be gentle and sympathetic. Referral to a mental health care provider for women identified with considerable psychosocial issues may be beneficial (Vercellini, Vigano, et al., 2009).

OBJECTIVE DATA

Physical Examination

The physical examination is frequently painful and emotionally stressful; therefore, it should be performed gently so as to establish trust and confidence (Vercellini, Somigliana, et al., 2009).

The clinician should begin with the abdominal exam inspecting for scars and palpating for masses. Determine the exact location of pain to verify correspondence with the distribution of the ilioinguinal and genitofemoral nerves. In patients with functional pain, the abdominal exam usually reveals mild to moderate tenderness that is diffuse or periumbilical. In contrast, pain suggestive of an organic pathology will reveal a more severe localized tenderness with guarding. Assess for possible hernia. The clinician should note distinct hyperirritable pain, elicited by pain with pressure (tender points), and localized areas of deep muscle tenderness in a tight band of a muscle (trigger points). Tender and trigger points often cause referred pain that is visceral. Abdominal wall trigger points may be localized using a single-digit palpation and mapped with a pen. When an area of abdominal tenderness is palpated, the patient should be instructed to tense the muscles by raising her head or legs. While maintaining palpation, an increase in pain suggests a myofascial origin, in contrast a decrease in pain suggests a visceral cause. Poor posture or body mechanics may cause repetitive stress and strain on these structures, leading to chronic pelvic pain. Leg-length discrepancy and lumbar vertebral or disc disease are causes of low back pain, and can cause referred pelvic pain (Vercellini, Somigliana, et al., 2009).

Inspection of the external genitalia should be performed noting any lesions and vulvar, vestibular, and urethral point tenderness. The vaginal exam should begin with insertion of the index finger only. Pelvic floor muscles should be inspected for painful spasm and trigger points. Pelvic floor pain may be a primary problem or the result of other pathologies such as interstitial cystitis or endometriosis. Interstitial cystitis or urethral syndrome may be suggested if an excruciating pain is provoked with palpation of the anterior vaginal wall. Pain elicited by deeper palpation of the cervix and vaginal fornices are suggestive of endometriosis or chronic pelvic infection. Uterine tenderness may be suggestive of adenomyosis, pelvic congestion syndrome, or chronic pelvic infection. A fixed retroverted uterus points to endometriosis or adhesions. Next, the traditional bimanual exam may be performed. Then a rectal or rectovaginal exam should be performed. Evaluate the perineum for areas of hypoesthesia or paresthesia and the anal sphincter tone. While performing the speculum exam, bacteriological specimens can be collected. Also assess the cervical and paracervical tissues (assess the vaginal cuff in case of hysterectomy) for tenderness with a cotton-tipped swab (Vercellini, Somigliana, et al., 2009).

Diagnostic Tests and Methods

Diagnostic tests should be selected discriminately as indicated by the findings of the history and physical examination (Vercellini, Somigliana, et al., 2009).

Lab Tests. In most women presenting with chronic pelvic pain, the following basic lab tests are considered prudent: CBC, serum chemistry, sedimentation rate, urine microscopy and culture, vaginal and endocervical swabs for microscopy, culture and chlamydia detection. A test to assess for occult blood in the stool is reasonable to screen for inflammatory bowel disease. If diarrhea is a significant symptom, a stool culture to evaluate for ova and parasites is indicated (Vercellini, Somigliana, et al., 2009).

Abdominopelvic Ultrasound. Abdominopelvic ultrasound may reveal ovarian masses, ovarian remnants, tubal dilatation, adenomyosis, or endometriosis. Ultrasound is also an aid to counseling and reassurance for women (Vercellini, Somigliana, et al., 2009).

Additional Imaging. In certain instances, sigmoidoscopy and/or colonoscopy, abdominal CT, small bowel radiographic series, MRI, or cystoscopy may be indicated (Vercellini, Somigliana, et al., 2009).

Laparoscopy. Laparoscopy has been identified as the gold standard in the diagnosis of chronic pelvic pain. Laparoscopy is the only diagnostic tool available to diagnosis peritoneal endometriosis and adhesions

(Ojha & Matah, 2008). It allows for direct visualization and is performed when pelvic pathology is not detectable by pelvic exam or other diagnostic methods. The goal of laparoscopy is to simultaneously treat a disorder causing the symptoms and improve health-related quality of life. Laparoscopy is useful in the diagnosis of acute or chronic salpingitis, ectopic pregnancy, hydrosalpinx, endometriosis, ovarian tumors and cysts, ovarian torsion, appendicitis, and adhesions. Notably 40 percent of diagnostic laparoscopies are performed with chronic pelvic pain being the indication and 40 percent show a normal pelvis. Clients may experience less anxiety about their symptoms when no serious pathology is found. When pathology is identified, 85 percent of the time endometriosis or adhesions are found. However, a negative laparoscopy does not mean there is no organic cause for the pain (Vercellini, Somigliana, et al., 2009).

Risks associated with laparoscopy include risk of death of approximately 1 out of 10,000 and risk of injury to bowel, bladder, or blood vessel of approximately 2.4 out of 1,000; two thirds of these cases necessitate laparotomy. Limitations include disease states such as irritable bowel syndrome and adenomyosis are not identifiable via laparoscopy and some forms of endometriosis are also not identified (Ojha & Matah, 2008).

DIFFERENTIAL MEDICAL DIAGNOSES

The evaluation of pelvic pain must differentiate between acute and chronic and gynecologic and nongynecologic etiologies. Table 16–1 summarizes common causes of pelvic pain.

Gynecologic causes of chronic pelvic pain include endometriosis, chronic pelvic infection, pelvic varicosities, ovarian remnant/retention. Urologic conditions include interstitial cystitis, detrusor dyssynergia and urethral syndrome. Gastrointestinal conditions include irritable bowel syndrome, inflammatory bowel diseases, diverticular disease, celiac disease, postsurgical dense adhesions. Musculoskeletal conditions include abdominal wall myofascial pain; fibromyalgia; pelvic floor myalgia; neuralgia of iliohypogastric, ilioinguinal, or genitofemoral nerve; coccygeal or lumbosacral back pain; and peripartum pelvic pain syndrome. Additional conditions include depression, visceral hyperalgesia, somatization disorders, psychosexual dysfunction, and porphyria (Vercellini, Somigliana, et al., 2009).

PLAN

Currently, the main approaches to treatment of chronic pelvic pain include counseling or psychotherapy, use of laparoscopy to exclude serious pathology, progestogen therapy such as with medroxyprogesterone acetate, and surgery to interrupt nerve pathways such as laparoscopic uterine nerve ablation and presacral neurectomy, or hysterectomy with or without removal of the ovaries. The risks and benefits must be considered; a psychological approach is less invasive, but is time consuming and may not be desired by all women. Hormonal therapy is associated with side effects and impairs fertility during use, and surgery, although it may definitively treat symptoms, may be associated with loss of reproductive capacity and is invasive (Stones et al., 2010).

TABLE 16–1. Common Causes of Acute and Chronic Pelvic Pain

Common GYN Causes of Acute Pelvic Pain	Common GYN Causes of Chronic Pelvic Pain
Ectopic pregnancy Salpingitis Abortion Ruptured ovarian cyst Adnexal torsion Endometriosis Menstruation Ovulation pain	Endometriosis Adenomyosis Uterine fibroids Chronic salpingitis Adhesions Dysmenorrhea Dyspareunia Pelvic relaxation Psychopathology/enigmatic (30–50%)
Common NonGYN Causes of Acute Pelvic Pain	**Common NonGYN Causes of Chronic Pelvic Pain**
Appendicitis Cystitis Diverticulitis Ureteral calculus Gastroenteritis/Spastic colon Trauma	Chronic appendicitis Irritable bowel syndrome Ulcerative colitis Diverticulosis Urinary tract disease Neuromuscular disorders

Source: ACOG, 2004, PB 51; Carter & Soper, 2001.

Psychosocial Interventions

When chronic pelvic pain symptoms are moderate to severe, it can negatively affect capacity to function in family, sexual, social, and occupational roles. Research demonstrates that when there is no obvious etiology for chronic pelvic pain, treatment outcomes are superior with a multidisciplinary team versus traditional treatment from gynecology alone (Vercellini, Vigano, et al., 2009). Writing therapy has shown some short-term benefit in treatment of chronic pelvic pain (Stones et al., 2010).

Medication

NSAIDs. Analgesics are often the first line of management, and women often try to manage their pain with over-the-counter pain medications prior to consulting with their primary care provider (Daniels & Khan, 2010). NSAIDs, with or without acetaminophen, may be useful in the context of chronic pelvic pain (Ojha & Matah, 2008).

Antidepressants. TCAs and venlafaxine provide pain relief for chronic pelvic pain with a neuropathic etiology (Daniels & Khan, 2010). The use of sertraline has been studied in treatment of chronic pelvic pain and has not been shown to be effective (Stones et al., 2010). See Table 25–5 for a comprehensive list of dosages and side effects.

Oral Contraceptives. Combined oral contraceptive pills are often used in the traditional manor with monthly cycles or continuously to suppress monthly periods and avoid associated pain. Oral contraceptive pills are commonly used in treatment of chronic pelvic pain despite no direct evidence for efficacy in chronic pelvic pain and limited evidence in dysmenorrhea (Daniels & Khan, 2010).

Oral contraceptives may be initiated after a successful 3-month trial with a GnRH agonist. Continuous oral contraceptives have been shown to be effective long-term therapy with a low-dose monophasic oral contraceptive. Alternatively, continuous use of a progestogen (e.g., oral norethisterone acetate, 2.5 mg/day) may be considered for long-term therapy (Vercellini, Vigano, et al., 2009).

Medroxyprogesterone Acetate. Medroxyprogesterone acetate has been shown to improve pain in women with pelvic congestion syndrome; however, pain relief has not been shown to be long term. Additionally, progestogens have side effects of weight gain and acne that may lead to discontinuation (Daniels & Khan, 2010).

GnRH Agonist. In women who have not undergone laparoscopy for investigation of endometriosis, the use of a GnRH agonist is based on the presupposition that the induced hypoestrogenic state will result in significant relief of symptoms in nearly all women with endometriosis. Therefore, a trial of 2 to 3 months of a GnRH agonist in women suspected to have endometriosis is reasonable. Use of a GnRH agonist may also be effective in the case of adenomyosis, pelvic varicosities, irritable bowel syndrome, and interstitial cystitis, because these conditions all typically have exacerbations associated with the menstrual cycle. Empiric treatment with a GnRH agonist for all women with cyclic components to their pain is reasonable prior to laparoscopy (Vercellini, Vigano, et al., 2009).

Progestogen. Medroxyprogesterone acetate has been shown to be beneficial in reduction of pain during treatment, although use of a GnRH agonist has been found to be more beneficial long term (Stones et al., 2010).

Surgical Interventions

Surgical management of chronic pelvic pain can be conservative or radical; laparoscopy allows for the most conservative approach (Ojha & Matah, 2008).

Laparoscopy. Indications are for therapeutic as well as diagnostic purposes. The goal of treatment is to restore normal anatomy and prevent or delay recurrence of disease. Due to advances in equipment, laparoscopy is the preferred surgical method and allows for less tissue trauma, improved visualization, less adhesion formation, and early recovery. Therapeutically, laparoscopy may be used for lysis of pelvic adhesions and ablation of endometrial implants. When investigating women with chronic pelvic pain, typically laparoscopy reveals adhesions 24 percent of the time, endometriosis 33 percent, and no clear pathology 35 percent (Ojha & Matah, 2008).

Endometriotic lesions can be removed during laparoscopy by surgical excision with scissors, bipolar coagulation, or laser methods (e.g., carbon dioxide laser, argon laser) (Ojha & Matah, 2008).

In the case of ovarian endometriosis, the size of the lesion determines how it is treated. Ovarian endometriomas can be vaporized, aspirated and irrigated, or stripped away (cystectomy) from the ovary.

Postoperative treatment with danazol or a GnRH agonist for 6 months after surgery decreases endometriosis-associated pain and delays recurrence at 12 and 24 months in comparison with placebo and expectant management (Ojha & Matah, 2008).

Laparotomy. Laparotomy is reserved for patients with advanced disease in whom laparoscopic procedure is not feasible and for those in whom it is not necessary to preserve fertility. Laparotomy may be indicated for the removal of a large endometrioma, extensive adhesiolysis, or bowel resection. If disease is severe, a multidisciplinary approach with a gynecologist, a colorectal surgeon, and a urologist may be necessary (Ojha & Matah, 2008).

Hysterectomy. Hysterectomy with bilateral salpingo-oophorectomy is generally indicated for women who are finished with childbearing, have debilitating symptoms, and have failed other therapies. If endometriosis is the cause of chronic pelvic pain, endometriotic lesions should be removed at the time of surgery. Performing salpingo-oophorectomy at the time of surgery results in better pain relief and decreased risk of future surgery. Hysterectomy is typically performed by laparotomy and sometimes laparoscopically. Hysterectomy is indicated for women with chronic pelvic pain related to endometriosis, adenomyosis, or pelvic congestion (Ojha & Matah, 2008).

Generally, hormone replacement therapy is indicated in young women following bilateral oophorectomy. There is small risk of recurrent disease while taking hormone replacement therapy. In this case, adding a progestogen is unnecessary. However, the argument has been made that for those with endometriosis the addition of a progestogen may protect against the effect of unopposed estrogen on any remaining disease. However, this may increase a woman's risk of breast cancer, as reported to be associated with combined estrogen and progestogen therapy. Therefore, hormone replacement therapy should be tailored on an individual basis (Ojha & Matah, 2008).

Alternative Interventions

Nonpharmacologic modalities such as transcutaneous nerve stimulation, acupuncture, and other complementary therapies may be beneficial in some women (Ojha & Matah, 2008). Two thirds of women who underwent physical therapy with internal manual therapy for myofascial trigger points in the pelvic floor have shown improvement in symptoms (Vercellini, Vigano, et al., 2009).

Dietary Interventions

Modifications in diet may be indicated when the client is experiencing constipation, bloating, edema, excessive fatigue, irritability, or lethargy, or is overweight. Dietary habits may contribute to the pain pattern, although not directly cause it.

Anticipated outcomes on evaluation are regular bowel movements without discomfort; decreased gas, bloating, and edema; improved energy level and stability of mood; and attainment and maintenance of ideal body weight.

Provide the client with information about the need for a high fiber diet and increased fluids to prevent constipation; explain how constipation can contribute to the pain pattern. In addition, less sodium, caffeine, and carbonated beverages reduce edema and abdominal bloating. Discuss with the client alternative cooking and seasoning methods, explain pertinent information on food labels, and suggest alternatives to soft drinks, coffee, and tea in order to limit intake of caffeine and carbonated beverages. Instruction may also include information about achieving stable blood sugar levels and weight loss by reducing refined carbohydrates and sugar in the diet and by eating low-fat foods with fewer calories. Reinforce the information with printed materials.

FOLLOW-UP AND REFERRAL

Referral to a gynecological pain specialist or gynecologist with access to a multidisciplinary pain team is recommended. Establishing trust and consistent communication with the patient is essential; women with chronic pelvic pain want to be taken seriously and attach a high value to identifying a cause for their pain (Daniels & Khan, 2010).

CHRONIC CERVICITIS

Chronic cervicitis is a chronic inflammation of the cervix. There is an inflammatory process in the mucosa and submucosa. An epithelial necrosis can exist (Eckert & Lentz, 2007). The presence of yellow exudate on the cervix, mucopurulent vaginal discharge, and cervical friability are common signs of cervicitis.

Cervical ectropion is considered to be a false cervicitis in the United States, but is treated as a true cervicitis in China with some manner of topical treatment to destroy the cells being utilized, including microwave tissue coagulation (Liu et al., 2007). Women with cervical ectropion may experience bleeding with intercourse and increased vaginal discharge because the mucus-secreting cells of the endocervix are everted onto the ectocervix. Some providers in the United States will also treat this condition with cryocautery or loop electrosurgical excision procedure (LEEP) if the increased vaginal discharge and postcoital bleeding caused by the condition is very bothersome to the woman and all evidence of infection has been eliminated (Northrup, 2010). Most cases of cervicitis are acute, asymptomatic, noninfectious and carry little clinical significance.

EPIDEMIOLOGY

Chronic cervicitis needs to be differentiated from acute cervicitis. Acute cervicitis is most commonly caused by one of two organisms: *C. trachomatis* and *N. gonorrhoeae*. Other organisms such as *M. genitalium*, *Trichomonas vaginalis*, and herpes simplex virus types 1 and 2 have been associated with nonchlamydial, nongonorrheal infectious cervicitis (Gaydos, Maldeis, Hardick, Hardick, & Quinn, 2009). Interestingly, *M. genitalium* was found to account for nearly 20 percent of the cases of cervicitis in the study by Gaydos and colleagues. Also, about 47 percent of the women who met the criteria for the diagnosis of cervicitis defined by the study criteria (cervical discharge or cervical friability) were culture negative for *C. trachomatis*, *N. gonorrhoeae*, *Trichomonas vaginalis*, and *M. genitalium* (Gaydos et al., 2009). Perhaps these women had what in the United States has been defined as false cervicitis.

Acute cervicitis can become chronic if left untreated or if the organism is resistant to antibiotic treatment. Human papillomavirus (HPV), associated with cervical cancer, can also play a role in development of chronic cervicitis. Risk factors for development of chronic cervicitis include sexual activity at an early age, exposure to STDs or previous STD, new or multiple sex partners, high-risk behaviors such as sale of sex for money or drugs, and use of oral contraceptive pills (Gaydos et al., 2009; Laine, Williams, & Wilson, 2009).

SUBJECTIVE DATA

The client will often present complaining of mucopurulent vaginal discharge, postcoital spotting, and/or dyspareunia.

OBJECTIVE DATA

Speculum exam reveals a cervix that can appear inflamed, swollen, and red. There may be yellowish discharge seen coming from the cervical os. The cervix can be easily friable (bleeds easily).

Diagnostic Tests and Methods

Wet Mount. A vaginal sample should be obtained to rule out acute cervicitis. This can assess for candida, trichomoniasis, bacterial vaginosis, and leukocytes.

Cultures. Specimens should be obtained for assessment of *N. gonorrhoeae* and *C. trachomatis*. Sampling should also be obtained for herpes simplex if lesions are visible. Cultures for *M. genitalium* and *U. urealyticum* may also be appropriate (Ross et al., 2009).

Papanicolaou Smear. Consider screening Papanicolaou (Pap) smear to assess for early cervical neoplasia. Colposcopy will need to be performed in follow-up to any abnormal Pap result or for persistent cervicitis that does not respond to medical therapy.

DIFFERENTIAL MEDICAL DIAGNOSIS

Consideration needs to be given to alternate medical conditions including benign cervical lesions (such as cervical polyps or nabothian cysts), candidiasis, cervical cancer, chancroid, chlamydia infection, gonococcal infection, herpes simplex virus, HPV, salpingitis, trichomoniasis, cervical tuberculosis, bacterial vaginosis, or retained foreign body.

PLAN

Psychosocial

Patient education is important in women with chronic cervicitis. It may be helpful to review the anatomy of the vagina, cervix, and uterus with the patient to make sure she truly understands her disease process. Education on the role of Pap smear screening and implications is important. Discuss common etiologies of development of cervicitis and include a discussion on safe sexual habits to help reduce chances that cervicitis can reoccur. Condom use should be encouraged.

Medication

Antibiotics for infection should be prescribed based on abnormal laboratory results. Client education regarding length of therapy, possible side effects, and importance of finishing the entire prescribed course of medication is important.

Surgery

Surgical intervention should be reserved for women in whom antibiotic therapy is unsuccessful. Cryocautery or LEEP should be done as needed to destroy abnormal tissue.

FOLLOW-UP AND REFERRAL

The client needs to be counseled on importance of routine follow-up to ensure adequate resolution. Complications of untreated chronic cervicitis include leukorrhea, cervical stenosis, and salpingitis. See Chapter 14 for further discussion of mucopurulent acute cervicitis and see section on cervical cancer, later in this chapter, for further discussion of treatment of HPV-related cervical abnormalities.

BARTHOLIN'S GLAND DUCT CYSTS AND BARTHOLINITIS

The Bartholin's glands are located on each side of the vaginal opening. The glands, which are approximately the size of a pea, provide moisture to the vulvar area. A Bartholin's gland cyst is a fluid-filled mass that can develop from a blockage of one or both of the glands. This may be from the duct that drains the gland, or the gland itself. These can be commonly seen in approximately 2 percent of reproductive-age women (Pancini et al., 2007). Bartholinitis occurs when the glands become inflamed and infected.

EPIDEMIOLOGY

- *Bartholin's gland cyst:* obstruction of the duct (infection, trauma, mucous)
- *Bartholinitis:* secondary infection from STI, *Streptococcus*, *Staphylococcus*, *Escherichia coli* (Hoosen, Nteta, Moodley, & Sturm, 2005).

SUBJECTIVE DATA

- Symptoms of an uninfected Bartholin's gland cyst can include a lump on one side of the vulvar area that is painless. Erythema or inflammation of the vulvar area may also be present.
- Symptoms of Bartholin's gland abscess can include increased inflammation in the vulvar area over a few days, purulent drainage from a cyst that can occur 4 to 5 days after inflammation begins, pain that can occur with sexual intercourse, physical activity, walking, sitting, fever, chills. Patient may complain of vaginal discharge, especially if the infection is related to an STD (Shlamovitz, 2010).

OBJECTIVE DATA

Pelvic examination of the patient may reveal a fluctuant mass located unilaterally, adjacent to the vestibule. There may also be tenderness, erythema, edema, purulent drainage, surrounding lymphadenopathy.

DIFFERENTIAL MEDICAL DIAGNOSIS

Mucous cyst of the vestibule, vulvar hematoma, vulvar fibroma, vulvar lipoma, epidermal inclusion or sebaceous cyst, or malignancy of the Bartholin's gland should be considered in the differential diagnosis.

PLAN

Psychosocial

Review with the patient the infectious process and have a thorough discussion of the management and treatment options.

Nonsurgical Treatment Options

Cyst. If there is a noninfected cyst present, treatment options include monitoring of the cyst, sitz baths or warm compresses, and over-the-counter pain medication to relieve discomfort.

Abscess. If an infection is present, treatment options include sitz baths, use of broad-spectrum antibiotics, over-the-counter or prescription-strength pain medication, incision and drainage of the abscess, placement of a Word catheter into the abscess to allow continued draining of infectious fluid, marsupialization, carbon dioxide laser to open the cyst and heat to its wall to prevent it from developing a sac and reoccurring, and removal of the Bartholin's gland cyst if it continues to reoccur (Shlamovitz, 2010).

Minor Surgical Procedure Treatment Options

Incision and Drainage. This procedure can be done by the clinician or the client can be referred to a gynecologist. Obtain client consent after explaining risks, benefits, complications, alternative management options, after care (Lorswell, 2008). Assist the client into the lithotomy position and retract the labia to allow visualization of the infected cyst. Clean the area with Betadine. Inject 2 to 3 mL of the 1 percent lidocaine under the mucosa of the area of the abscess. Once the area has been anesthetized, make an incision with the scalpel within the area of the hymenal ring. Gently express the contents of the abscess. A hemostat may be used to break up any adhesions that may have formed. If a Word catheter is going to be used, insert the catheter into the abscess and fill the balloon with 2 to 5 mL of normal saline. The catheter will ideally stay inserted for 2 to 4 weeks, but oftentimes will fall out on its own sooner. Leaving the catheter in place allows for epithelization of the tract of the abscess. If the catheter stays in place, deflate the balloon to remove it once healing has occurred (Shlamovitz, 2010).

The client should be placed on broad-spectrum antibiotics for at least 10 days and pain medication should be offered.

Marsupialization. Marsupialization of the Bartholin's gland is usually indicated only in clients with recurrent abscesses or the presence of a large abscess that may not be easily drained in clinic. Referral should be made to a gynecologic surgeon for this procedure in which the wall of the abscess is opened widely to allow the infectious material to fully drain. The membrane of the abscess is sutured to the mucosa of the vagina and to the surrounding skin to help with epithelization of the wound. The purpose of the surgery is to allow the abscess to become epithelized at the base (Speights, Harris, & Cowan, 2002).

FOLLOW-UP AND REFERRAL

Follow-up in clinic for nonsurgical intervention should be within 7 days. At this time, any pain, tenderness, swelling, and erythema should be resolved. If there was placement of a Word catheter and it is still in place, it may be removed at this time (Lorswell, 2008).

CERVICAL POLYPS

Cervical polyps are the most common cervical lesions and occur in up to 10 percent of women, recurring 6.2 percent of the time (Younis, Iram, Anwar, & Ewies, 2010).

EPIDEMIOLOGY

The etiology of cervical polyps is surmised to be the result of chronic inflammation causing focal hyperplasia, reaction to foreign bodies, a localized congestion of cervical vasculature, and/or an abnormal local response to estrogen stimulation. More than 60 percent of women presenting with cervical polyps are between the ages of 40 and 65, and 45 percent of them are postmenopausal (Younis et al., 2010).

SUBJECTIVE DATA

Women may present with complaint of intermenstrual bleeding, postcoital bleeding, postmenopausal bleeding, bleeding after trauma (e.g., gynecological examination or coitus), or vaginal discharge. In premenopausal women cervical polyps are more often symptomatic, whereas in postmenopausal women cervical polyps tend to be asymptomatic (Younis et al., 2010).

OBJECTIVE DATA

Physical Examination

Cervical polyps vary in size from 5 mm to 50 mm and arise from the endocervical canal or, less frequently, from the ectocervix. Cervical polyps are typically cherry red to purplish red in color, soft, pliable, fleshy, pedunculated, friable and bleed easily when touched (Younis et al., 2010).

Diagnostic Tests and Methods

Controversy exists around the management of cervical polyps. Recent studies suggest the removal of only symptomatic polyps, whereas asymptomatic cervical polyps do not require removal or referral to a gynecologist. Furthermore, a policy of removing polyps in symptomatic women or those with abnormal cervical cytology and limiting histological examination to these polyps would result in significant cost savings (Younis et al., 2010). A large retrospective study found the prevalence of malignancy and dysplasia in cervical polyps removed over a 7-year span was 0.1 and 0.5 percent, respectively. Cervical polyps can harbor disease from sources beyond the cervix. Based on these results, it appears unlikely cervical polyps progress to malignancy. Clinicians should reassure their patients of the benign nature of cervical polyps (Berzolla et al., 2007).

Pap Smear. See Chapter 3.

DIFFERENTIAL MEDICAL DIAGNOSES

Endometrial polyps, small prolapsed myomas, cervical malignancy.

PLAN

Psychosocial Interventions

Explain to the client what polyps are and that they are usually benign.

Surgical Interventions

Cervical polyps may be removed and sent to a pathology laboratory. The procedure can be performed in an office without anesthesia by any appropriately trained clinician as long as the stalk of the polyp is narrow. Refer the client whose polyp has a broad base to a gynecologist. Paint the cervix with povidone-iodine (Betadine); using ring forceps, grasp and twist the polyp at the base. Silver nitrate or Monsel's solution may be applied as needed to the site of removal to control bleeding. Excessive bleeding is a potential adverse effect.

Client teaching includes the need for pelvic rest for 24 hours to ensure that bleeding does not occur at the removal site. If excessive bleeding or excessive vaginal discharge does occur, the client must return for evaluation and possible endometrial sampling.

Treatment of Vaginal Infections

Accompanying vaginal infections must be treated appropriately (see Chapter 14).

FOLLOW-UP AND REFERRAL

Regular Pap smears and gynecologic exams are important, and this needs to be stressed to the client.

GYNECOLOGIC CANCERS

OVARIAN CANCER

Epidemiology

Ovarian cancer is commonly referred to as the silent killer because it is the most fatal gynecologic cancer. In 2010, it was estimated that nearly 21,900 women were diagnosed with ovarian cancer in the United States and nearly 13,900 die annually from this deadly disease. Unfortunately, at the time of diagnosis, nearly two thirds of the patients present with late-stage disease and metastasis due to a lack of good screening tools for ovarian cancer. Due to this, only 20 percent of ovarian cancers are caught in an early stage (Blewitt, 2010).

Risk Factors. According to the National Cancer Institute (2009), a woman without a family history of ovarian cancer has a 1 in 55 lifetime chance of developing ovarian cancer. This risk increases 10-fold when familial/hereditary conditions exist. The inherited gene mutations, BRCA1 and BRCA2, are responsible for a significant number of familial ovarian and breast cancers. Other risk factors include increased age (postmenopause), early menarche, late menopause, nulliparity, no time spent breastfeeding, obesity, high-fat diet, Caucasian race, past medical history of breast cancer, and prolonged estrogen use. Lowering the total number of ovulatory menstrual cycles in a women's life can help decrease her risk of ovarian cancer. Multiple pregnancies, breastfeeding, use of combined contraceptives such as oral contraceptive pills, transdermal patches, vaginal rings, maintaining a healthy weight, and obtaining regular physical activity can all help lower risk.

Subjective Data

Early warning signs often go undetected as they are vague and nonspecific. These include menstrual changes, constipation, dyspareunia, back pain, indigestion, fatigue, frequency of urination, early satiety, abdominal or pelvic pain, and abdominal pain. With these vague symptoms, it is important for the provider to consider the possibility of ovarian cancer in a differential diagnosis.

Objective Data

A bimanual exam may help detect any abnormalities or masses and should be done annually.

Screening. To date, there is no effective screening method for ovarian cancer. Patients may inquire about a CA-125 blood test for screening. They need to be counseled that this test has poor reliability and sensitivity. Pelvic ultrasound is not routinely recommended as a screening tool due to its high cost. These tests may be considered in women with a history of a first-degree relative with ovarian cancer or in those with other risk factors.

For those with a family history of ovarian and/or breast cancer, it may be helpful to be screened for genetic mutations such as the BRCA1 and BRCA2 genes. Meeting with a genetic counselor to discuss personal and family risks of genetic mutations as well as benefits and risks of testing is helpful in determining who should be screened. A woman with the BRCA gene mutation has a 16 to 60 percent increased chance of developing ovarian cancer. Usually, it is recommended that the family member with the history of cancer be screened first, and if positive, other family members should be screened (National Cancer Institute, 2009).

Follow-Up and Referral

Any patient with pelvic pain or ovarian mass needs pelvic imaging for evaluation. Postmenopausal women with palpable ovaries or ovarian mass on bimanual exam need referral to a gynecologist for surgical evaluation. Surgical exploration is commonly a first-line treatment for a patient with a suspected ovarian cancer (Blewitt, 2010).

VULVAR CANCER

Epidemiology

Vulvar cancer is responsible for 3 to 5 percent of gynecological cancers. In 2007, the American Cancer Society estimated that nearly 3,500 women were diagnosed with vulvar cancer and close to 900 women died from the disease. Vulvar cancer has been named 1 of 12 cancers increasing in incidence (Lanneau et al., 2009). There are two types of vulvar carcinoma that have emerged in recent years. The first, a keratinizing vulvar squamous carcinoma, is primarily seen in older women. The second is an HPV-related warty carcinoma, primarily seen in younger women. VIN often precedes the development of vulvar cancer. The old staging system for severity, VIN I-III, has been replaced with a more current staging system. The new system classifies VIN into a usual (VIN warty type, VIN basaloid type, and VIN mixed type), a differentiated, and an unclassified type (ASCCP, 2011).

Risk Factors. Over 50 percent of newly diagnosed vulvar cancers occur in women over 70 years of age, while there has been an increase in VIN developing in younger women (Lanneau et al., 2009). Other risk factors include infection with HPV, cigarette smoking, history of lichen sclerosis, history of other gynecological cancers, vulvar melanoma, or atypical moles on the vulva.

Subjective Data

Similar to other gynecological cancers, there are no specific symptoms of vulvar cancer. Some symptoms include vulvar itching that does not resolve, changes in skin color around the vulva, changes in the texture of the skin around the vulva, sores, ulcers, wart-like bumps, pain with urination, enlarged lymph noted or glands in the groin, or discharge or bleeding not related to menstrual cycle.

Objective Data

The two biggest tools for screening for vulvar cancer include visual inspection and biopsy. Women with risks for development of vulvar cancer should be thoroughly inspected for abnormalities and biopsy should be done on any suspicious areas.

Paget's disease of the vulva is a rare disorder but should be considered in women presenting with symptoms of long-standing pruritus and tenderness, red or scaly plaques often with a raised border. Biopsy is needed for accurate diagnosis.

Squamous cell hyperplasia is a growth of the skin around the vulva and can appear as a pink or red area of the vulva that is elevated and has white patches. Biopsy would provide accurate diagnosis. Verrucous carcinoma is a slow-growing, well-differentiated type of squamous cell carcinoma.

Vulvar melanoma is the second most commonly seen vulvar cancer. Suspicious lesions appear black or blue in color; have an irregular and fuzzy border; and are raised, ulcerated, and larger than 1 cm in diameter. Most are on the labia minora or clitoris. Biopsy is needed to confirm diagnosis.

Plan, Follow-Up, and Referral

Clients presenting with symptoms or that have exam findings suspicious for malignancy or precancerous changes need a vulvar biopsy for diagnosis and this can be done by any clinician that is comfortable with obtaining vulvar biopsy or the client should be given a referral to a gynecologist (Cormio et al., 2009).

Clients need to be advised on doing self-exam on a regular basis to detect lesions early. They need to be counseled regarding timely evaluation of long-standing pruritus, skin changes, or development of lesions. Educate patient on importance of condom use to decrease transmission of STDs.

VAGINAL CANCER

Epidemiology

Vaginal cancer is extremely rare, accounting for 3 percent of cancers of the reproductive tract in women. There are four main types of vaginal cancer. Squamous cell carcinoma accounts for about 90 percent of vaginal cancers and begin in the epithelial lining of the vagina. These tend to occur in the upper part of the vagina and can develop from vaginal intraepithelial neoplasia. It is usually found in women between 60 and 80 years old. Adenocarcinomas are common in women over age 50, but clear cell adenocarcinomas can be seen in younger women. Malignant melanoma typically develops from melanocytes and make up about 2 to 3 percent of vaginal cancers. This type is usually seen in the outer or lower portion of the vagina. Lastly, sarcomas make up the last 2 to 3 percent of vaginal cancers. They form deeper in the wall of the vagina (ASCCP, 2011).

Risk Factors. The main risk factors for development of vaginal cancer include age (this usually develops in women over 60), exposure to diethylstilbestrol (DES) in utero, a medication given to women in the mid 1940s through 1971 to prevent miscarriage. Women who were exposed to this drug in utero are more likely to develop adenocarcinoma. Other risk factors include exposure to HPV and a history of cervical cancer.

Subjective Data

Symptoms of vaginal cancer include abnormal vaginal bleeding or discharge—neither of which is related to menstrual cycles, painful urination, dyspareunia, pelvic pain, or a vaginal lump (ASCCP, 2011).

Objective Data

There are four main ways a provider may diagnose vaginal cancer. The first is a pelvic exam. A full pelvic exam assesses all of the reproductive structures for abnormalities. The other three methods are described next.

Diagnostic Testing. A Pap smear allows cells from the vagina and cervix to be collected and analyzed under a microscope for abnormalities. Colposcopy is an exam in which an instrument magnifies the vagina and cervix, allowing visualization of potentially abnormal cells (see Chapter 3). Lastly, a biopsy allows for a piece of tissue to be removed and evaluated under a microscope by a pathologist to identify any potentially cancerous cells.

Plan, Follow-Up, and Referral

Patients presenting with symptoms or that have exam findings suspicious for malignancy or precancerous changes need referral to gynecologist for biopsy and treatment. Patients with diagnosed vaginal cancer will then be referred to a gynecologic oncologist for surgery and treatment.

UTERINE CANCER

Epidemiology

Uterine, or endometrial, cancer is the most common gynecologic cancer in the United States. The American Cancer Society estimated in 2010 that there were nearly 43,500 new cases of endometrial cancer and nearly 8,000 deaths from this cancer. Cancer of the uterus is uncommon in women under 40 years old. Most women are over the age of 50 at the time of diagnosis. Endometrial cancer is more commonly diagnosed in white women; however, black women succumb to the disease more often. The 5-year survival rate for endometrial cancer is nearly 83 percent as most cancers are diagnosed at an early stage (American Cancer Society, 2009).

Risk Factors. Endometrial cancer is often thought to be linked to an overexposure of estrogen. Conditions that cause increased amounts of estrogen are common risk factors. These include estrogen replacement therapy (without concurrent progesterone use), the total number of menstrual cycles a woman has in her life, early age at menarche, late age at time of menopause, low number of pregnancies, no history of breastfeeding, obesity, use of tamoxifen, history of polycystic ovary syndrome, increasing age, poor diet, history of diabetes mellitus, family history of gynecological cancers, history of breast or ovarian cancers, and endometrial hyperplasia (Ewies & Musonda, 2010).

Subjective Data

Symptoms of endometrial cancer include abnormal vaginal bleeding—this may be a heavier flow, prolonged flow, bleeding between menstrual cycles, or postmenopausal bleeding; vaginal spotting or discharge; pain with urination; dyspareunia; and pelvic pain (Neves-Castro, 2008).

Objective Data

Women with symptoms and risk factors concerning for endometrial cancer need evaluation. A pelvic exam should be performed to assess for abnormalities of the reproductive structures, including an enlarged uterus, masses, or a change in shape.

Diagnostic Testing. The next step is a pelvic ultrasound to evaluate the uterus, ovaries, bladder, and cervix. Postmenopausal women with bleeding should undergo pelvic ultrasound to assess the thickness of her endometrial stripe. An endometrial thickness less than 5 mm is considered normal and an endometrial biopsy is not indicated to assess for cancer. Postmenopausal women with an endometrial thickness of 5 mm or greater need endometrial sampling performed (Ewies & Musonda, 2010; Jacons et al., 2011). An endometrial biopsy may be performed by any clinician trained in the procedure. See Chapter 3 for description of the procedure. The tissue is sent to pathology for review to determine if there are precancerous or cancerous cells present. The procedure may cause cramping, but typically is not otherwise painful. Occasionally, a dilation and curettage, with or without a hysteroscopy, is necessary to evaluate the endometrial tissue. This would require referral to a gynecologist.

Plan, Follow-Up, and Referral

Patients with a diagnosis of endometrial hyperplasia or endometrial cancer need referral to either a gynecologist or a gynecologic oncologist for further management. Patients with risk factors for development of endometrial cancers need intervention to lower their risk; this includes avoiding use of unopposed estrogen in postmenopausal patients, use of hormonal medications such as contraceptives in women with anovulation, irregular menstrual cycles, weight reduction, and close monitoring of abnormal bleeding.

CERVICAL CANCER

Epidemiology

Cervical cancer is the third most common type of cancer in women across the world; however, in the United States it has become less common due to routine screening with Pap smears. Cervical cancer starts out very slow and initially begins as a precancer, known as dysplasia. Women who have not had routine Pap screening or have not followed up on an abnormal Pap smear are more likely to develop cervical cancer. The majority of cervical cancers are caused by HPV. Some strains of HPV can cause cervical cancer and are usually spread through sexual intercourse. Other strains of the virus can lead to the development of genital warts. In 2010, it was estimated that upwards of 12,000 women were diagnosed with cervical cancer and just over 4,000 women died from the disease (American Cancer Society, 2009).

Prevention. Gardasil is a quadrivalent vaccine that is indicated for use in young women ages 9 to 26 and has been recently been approved for use in young men as well. The vaccine is a three-dose series and was first released in June 2006. Gardasil helps protect women against two types of HPV (type 16 and 18) that have been shown to cause about 75 percent of cervical cancers and two types of HPV (type 6 and 11) that have been shown to cause 90 percent of genital warts diagnosed in women (Gardasil Vaccine Information, 2011). Another vaccine on the market, Cervarix, is bivalent and protects against HPV types 16 and 18 only.

Risk Factors. Risks for HPV infection and development of cervical cancer include sexual activity at an early age, multiple sex partners, partners who partake in high-risk sexual activities, weak immune system, smoking, exposure to DES, oral contraceptive use for more than 5 years, age 35 to 54, family history of cervical cancer, lower socioeconomic status, and more than three pregnancies.

Subjective Data

Symptoms may be absent in the early stages of cervical cancer, but they can include a persistent vaginal discharge; abnormal bleeding between menstrual periods, after menopause, or after sexual activities; or longer or heavier menstrual periods. Some symptoms of advancing cancer can include a loss of appetite, weight loss, pelvic or back pain, swelling in one leg, fatigue, heavy vaginal bleeding, fractures, and urinary incontinence (ASCCP, 2011).

Objective Data

Pap smears are used as a screening tool to help detect abnormal cells of the cervix. Although they can help detect abnormal cervical cells, they do not diagnose cervical dysplasia or cancer. ThinPrep and SurePath Pap smear are most commonly used today and use a liquid-based cytology to help suspend cells in a fixative until they can be analyzed. Specimens are collected by using a cytobrush and spatula. HPV DNA typing can be done to assess for the presence of high-risk strains that are likely to cause precancerous or cancerous changes. This can be done in conjunction with a screening Pap smear or as further assessment of an abnormal test. HPV DNA testing is not recommended for women under the age of 30.

ACOG (2009c) released updated practice guidelines with the new changes related to cervical cancer screening with Pap smear.

- It is now recommended that initial screening be delayed until age 21, regardless of sexual activity history.
- Once screening begins, a Pap smear should be done every other year from age 21 to 29 as long as a woman has negative findings.
- Beginning at 30, women may increase interval between Pap smears to every 3 years as long as the prior three screenings have been negative. Or, women can be screened with a Pap smear and HPV test looking for high-risk types, and if both are negative, screening can be every 3 years.
- Women with a history of moderate or severe dysplasia (CIN II or III) need annual screening for 20 years from the time of the initial abnormal Pap test.
- Women with a history of DES exposure or who are immunocompromised need annual screening.
- Screening with Pap smear can stop at the age of 65 as long as there have been three consecutive negative Pap smears in the last 10 years.
- After hysterectomy, Pap testing can stop as long as there was no history of moderate or severe dysplasia or cancer at the time of the surgery (ACOG, 2009c, pp. 4–6).

Bethesda System for Reporting Abnormal Results. The Bethesda system was last revised in 2001 and is used to classify Pap smear results. Squamous intraepithelial lesion (SIL) is the term used to describe precancerous cervical cell changes. The test results include the following:

- Negative for intraepithelial lesion—this is a normal result.
- Atypical squamous cells of undetermined significance (ASC-US)—this result shows the presence of changes to the cervical cells and may indicate infection with HPV. HPV testing should be performed on this result to determine presence or absence of high-risk types of HPV.
- SIL—this term means there are abnormal cervical cell changes that may be precancerous. It can be low grade (LSIL) or high grade (HSIL). LSIL typically means a presence of HPV, causing mild precancerous changes to the cervix. This will often resolve spontaneously. HSIL can be a sign of a more severe abnormality of the cervical cells. One type of HSIL is carcinoma in situ (CIS) and this can potentially lead to cervical cancer.
- Atypical squamous cells, cannot exclude HSIL (ASC-H)—this result is less clear and means there may be doubt regarding the presence of HSIL.
- Atypical glandular cells (AGC)—this result is concerning for precancerous changes. These results can be further classified by type of cells: endocervical, endometrial, or glandular cells not otherwise specified.
- Squamous cell carcinoma—usually, a rare finding on Pap smear as this is not a diagnostic test. This usually indicates abnormal cervical cells may have developed in surrounding tissue (ACOG, 2009c, pp.7–8).

Plan

Management of Abnormal Results. A Pap smear result that is ASC-US should also have HPV DNA typing performed to determine if there is low- or high-risk HPV present. An ASC-US Pap smear that is negative for low- or high-risk HPV or that is positive for low-risk HPV only should be repeated in 12 months. The first step in follow-up on a Pap smear that is ASC-US and high-risk HPV positive, LSIL, HSIL, ASC-H, AGC is to perform a colposcopy. A colposcopy is a procedure done by someone with special training to perform colposcopy. See Chapter 3 for description of the procedure. If any abnormal tissue is seen, a biopsy of the abnormal tissue is obtained and sent to pathology to determine if any precancerous or cancerous cells are present. That is, dysplasia or CIS. An endocervical curettage may also be done with a special instrument to sample cells from the cervical canal (ACOG, 2009d). If no biopsies are indicated or if the biopsy reveals mild dysplasia, typical recommendation is for a repeat Pap smear in 6 months.

Treatment of Cervical Dysplasia. For patients with moderate or severe dysplasia, treatment is needed to prevent development into cervical cancer.

- *LEEP.* LEEP uses a thin wire loop that can work like a surgical knife. An electric current passes through the loop and can cut away a layer of the cervix that has the dysplastic cells. The layer of the cervix that is removed is sent to pathology to confirm all of the abnormal cells have adequately been removed. Patients may expect some vaginal bleeding, discharge, cramping after the procedure.
- *Cryocautery.* This is an ablative therapy. Nitrous oxide is used to freeze the abnormal areas identified on colposcopy. One limitation of this procedure is that it does not work well for treatment of large areas or if there is advanced disease present. It is used mostly for milder dysplasia. Patients may experience a watery vaginal discharge after the procedure.
- *Cold Knife Conization.* In the past, this was the main procedure used to treat cervical dysplasia, but in recent years, the LEEP has become more first-line treatment. The advantage of this procedure is the size and shape of the area to be sampled can be tailored as needed and a cone-shaped wedge containing the abnormal cells is removed and sent for pathology.
- *Hysterectomy.* Hysterectomy is usually the recommended treatment for invasive cervical cancer. It can be done for treatment of severe dysplasia or recurrence of dysplasia as well (ASCCP, 2011).

Clients with an abnormal Pap smear will need referral to a clinician skilled to performed colposcopy. If colposcopy reveals moderate or severe dysplasia or CIS, the client needs referral to gynecologist to perform one of these treatment modalities. Clients will need counseling about follow-up for repeat Pap smear. They will also need education regarding how to lower their risks for cervical cancer, such as limiting risks that can expose them to STDs, implementing use of barrier methods, smoking cessation, and routine Pap smear screening.

DIETHYLSTILBESTROL EXPOSURE

DES was used extensively in the United States during the 1940s and early 1950s to treat pregnancy complications, including bleeding, premature labor, diabetes, and preeclampsia. Although studies during the late 1950s proved its ineffectiveness, DES use continued through 1971. An estimated 5 to 10 million women were prescribed DES during pregnancy or were exposed to the drug in utero (Palmer, Anderson, Helmrich, & Herbst, 2000). These women exposed to DES are now on average 55 years old (Kaufman et al., 2000). However, many of the offspring of those exposed to DES in utero are just now entering emerging or young adulthood. This cohort of individuals is being followed to assess for any risks as discussed next.

DES EXPOSURE SEQUELAE

Women exposed to DES in utero may exhibit one or more of the following sequelae:

- Structural changes including transverse vaginal and cervical ridges (cocks, combs, collars, and pseudopolyps), abnormally shaped uterine cavity, uterine hypoplasia.
- Vaginal adenosis with columnar epithelium on or beneath the vaginal muscosa; it is self-limiting and gradually disappears.
- Clear-cell adenocarcinoma of the cervix or vagina (incidence rose at age 15 and median age at diagnosis was 19 years).
- Increased incidences of spontaneous abortion, ectopic pregnancy, premature cervical dilation, and premature rupture of membranes.
- Increased incidence of breast cancer.

Risk

Women who were born in the United States between 1945 and 1971 to mothers who had complicated pregnancies and received DES and possibly their offspring (Titus-Ernstoff et al., 2010).

Screening

All women born between 1940 and 1971 should be questioned about possible exposure to DES.

For those exposed in utero, the following screening techniques are employed:

- An initial examination was recommended following menarche or at age 14 if no menarche; routine examination to continue every 6 to 12 months thereafter and includes inspection, palpation, and cytology.
- Cytology requires vaginal scrapings taken from all four quadrants of the fornix and fixed on slides for cytological review.
- Careful inspection of the cervix and vagina using one-half strength of Lugol's solution and palpation of the entire vaginal wall.
- Colposcopy performed by an experienced colposcopist if the Pap smear is abnormal. Appropriate biopsies to be done for evaluation.
- DES daughters should be followed as high-risk obstetric patients because of the increased risk of spontaneous abortion, ectopic pregnancy, early cervical effacement, and premature labor (Kaufman et al., 2000).

Recent studies seem to demonstrate an absence of abnormalities in the lower genital tract in third generation offspring of DES daughters, but a possible increase in incidence of heart defects was noted in one study (Titus-Ernstoff et al., 2010). Also, the study by Kaufman and Adam in 2002, which found absence of abnormalities, included only 23 subjects. Research involving third-generation offspring of DES daughters continues. It has been hypothesized that reproductive tract changes may not become apparent in offspring until more of the third generation reach childbearing age. Mouse models have indicated that DES exposure in utero may cause epigenetic changes that are transmitted to offspring (Titus-Ernstoff et al., 2010). Therefore, it is currently unknown if the impact of exposure to DES in utero years ago may indeed continue on.

FOLLOW-UP AND REFERRAL

Any abnormal cytology or undiagnosed lesion requires referral to a gynecologist. Provide the client with information about DES and its possible effects. Stress the importance of having a regular examination and cytology. Allow time for the client to express her concerns.

REFERENCES

Abatangelo, L., Okereke, L., Parham-Foster, C., Parrish, C., Scaglione, L., Zotte, D., et al. (2010). If pelvic inflammatory disease is suspected empiric treatment should be initiated. *Journal of the American Academy of Nurse Practitioners, 22*, 117–122.

Al-Jefout, M., Dezarnaulds, G., Cooper, M., Tokushige, N., Luscombe, G.M., Markham, R., et al. (2009). Diagnosis of endometriosis by detection of nerve fibres in an endometrial biopsy: A double blind study. *Human Reproduction, 24*(12), 3019–3024.

Allen, C., Hopewell, S., Prentice, A., & Gregory, D. (2009). Nonsteroidal and anti-inflammatory drugs for pain in women with endometriosis. *The Cochrane Database of Systematic Reviews* (Issue 11). John Wiley & Sons, Ltd.

American Cancer Society. (2009). *Cancer facts and figures 2009.* Atlanta, GA: Author. Retrieved March 8, 2011, from http://www.cancer.org/acs/groups/content/@nho/documents/document/cffaa20092010pdf.pdf

American College of Obstetricians and Gynecologists (ACOG). (2004). Chronic pelvic pain. In *Compendium of selected publications* (Practice Bulletin 51). Washington, DC: Author.

American College of Obstetricians and Gynecologists (ACOG). (2008a). Diagnosis and management of vulvar skin disorders. In *Compendium of selected publications* (Practice Bulletin 93, pp. 1243–1253). Washington, DC: Author.

American College of Obstetricians and Gynecologists (ACOG). (2008b). Alternatives to hysterectomy in the management of leiomyomas. In *Compendium of selected publications* (Practice Bulletin 96, pp. 387–400). Washington, DC: Author.

American College of Obstetricians and Gynecologists (ACOG). (2009a). Choosing the route of hysterectomy for benign disease, CO 444. *Obstetrics and Gynecology, 114*(5), 1156–1158.

American College of Obstetricians and Gynecologists (ACOG). (2009b). Clinical updates in women's health care. *Vulvar Disorders, 8*(2), 67–73.

American College of Obstetricians and Gynecologists (ACOG). (2009c). Cervical cytology screening. In *Compendium of selected publications* (Practice Bulletin 109, pp. 1–8). Washington, DC: Author.

American College of Obstetricians and Gynecologists (ACOG). (2009d). *Colposcopy: Patient education pamphlet.* Washington, DC: Author.

American College of Obstetricians and Gynecologists (ACOG). (2010). Management of endometriosis: PB 114. *Obstetrics and Gynecology, 116,* 223–236. *Compendium of selected publications.* Washington, DC: Author.

American College of Obstetricians and Gynecologists (ACOG). (2011). Female sexual dysfunction: PB 119. *Obstetrics and Gynecology, 117,* 996–1007. *Compendium of selected publications.* Washington, DC: Author.

American Society for Colposcopy and Cervical Pathology (ASCCP). (2011). Compendium of Selected Publications: Practice Management: Invasive Cancer of the Cervix (2010). Diagnosis of HPV-Induced Diseases (2010). Vulva: HPV Infections & Vulvar Intraepithelial Neoplasia (2009). Vaginal Neoplasia (2009).

Balamuth, F., Zhao, H., & Mollen, C. (2010). Toward improving the diagnosis and the treatment of adolescent pelvic inflammatory disease in emergency departments. *Pediatric Emergency Care, 26*(2), 85–92.

Berzolla, C., Schnatz, P., O'Sullivan, D., Bansal, R., Mandavilli, S., & Sorosky, J. (2007). Dysplasia and malignancy in endocervical polyps. *Journal of Women's Health, 16*(9), 1317–1321.

Binik, Y.B. (2010). The DSM diagnostic criteria for dyspareunia. *Archives of Sexual Behavior, 39,* 292–303.

Blewitt, K. (2010). Ovarian cancer: Listen for the disease that whispers. *Nursing, 40*(11), 24–31.

Bottomley, C., & Bourne, T. (2009). Diagnosis and management of ovarian cyst accidents. *Best Practice and Research Clinical Obstetrics and Gynecology, 23,* 711–724.

But, I., Pakiz, M., & Rakic, S. (2011). Overactive bladder symptoms and uterine adenomysosis—Is there any connection? *European Journal of Obstetrics and Gynecology and Reproductive Biology, 156*(1), 109–112.

Carter, J.F., & Soper, D.E. (2001). Diagnosing and treating nongynecologic chronic pelvic pain; musculoskeletal causes, surgery, and "psychology." *Women's Health, Gynecology Edition, 1,* 166–174.

Centers for Disease Control and Prevention (CDC). (2010). *Sexually transmitted disease: Treatment guidelines 2010.* Retrieved from http://www.cdc.gov/std/treatment/2010/

Chacko, M., Wiemann, C., Kozinetz, C., von Sternberg, K., Velasquez, M., Smith, P., et al. (2010). Efficacy of a motivational behavioral intervention to promote chlamydia and gonorrhea screening in young women: A randomized controlled trial. *Journal of Adolescent Health, 46,* 152–161.

Cormio, G., Loizzi, V., Carriero, C., Cazzolla, A., Putignano, G., & Selvaggi, L. (2009). Groin recurrence in carcinoma of the vulva: Management and outcome. *European Journal of Cancer, 19,* 302–307.

Dalpiaz, O., Kerschbaumer, A., Mitterberger, M., Pinggera, G., Bartsch, G., & Strasser, H. (2008). Chronic pelvic pain in women: Still a challenge. *BJU International, 102,* 1061–1065.

Danby, C.S., & Margesson, L.J. (2010). Approach to the diagnosis and treatment of vulvar pain. *Dermatologic Therapy, 23,* 485–504.

Daniels, J.P., & Khan, K.S. (2010). Chronic pelvic pain in women. *British Medical Journal, 341,* 772–775.

Dietrich, J. (2010). An update on adenomyosis in the adolescent. *Current Opinion in Obstetrics and Gynecology, 22,* 388–392.

Eckert, L.O., & Lentz, G.M. (2007). Infections of the lower genital tract: Vulva, vagina, cervix, toxic shock syndrome, HIV infections. In V.L. Katz, G.M. Lentz, R.A. Lobo, & D.M. Gershenson (Eds.), *Comprehensive gynecology* (5th ed.). Philadelphia, PA: Mosby Elsevier.

Eva, U., Gun, W., & Preben, K. (2005). Prevalence of urinary and fecal incontinence and symptoms of genital prolapse in women. *Acta Obstetricia et Gynecologica Scandinavica, 82,* 280–286.

Ewies, A., & Musonda, P. (2010). Managing postmenopausal bleeding revisited: What is the best first line investigation and who should be seen within 2 weeks? A cross-sectional study of 326 women. *European Journal of Obstetrics and Gynecology and Reproductive Biology, 153,* 67–71.

Exacoustos, B., Brienza, L., Di Giovanni, A., Szabolcs, B., Romanini, M.E., Zupi, E., et al. (2011). Adenomyosis: Three-dimensional sonographic findings of the junctional zone and correlation with histology. *Ultrasound in Obstetrics and Gynecology, 37*(4), 471–479.

Fritz, M.A., & Speroff, L. (2011). *Clinical gynecologic endocrinology and infertility* (8th ed.). Philadelphia: Wolters Kluwer/Lippincott Williams & Wilkins.

Gardasil Vaccine Information. (2011). Retrieved September 3, 2011, from http://www.gardasil.com

Gaydos, C., Maldeis, N., Hardick, A., Hardick, J., & Quinn, T. (2009). Mycoplasma genitalium as a contributor to the multiple etiologies of cervicitis in women attending sexually transmitted disease clinics. *Sexually Transmitted Diseases, 36*(10), 598–606.

Giudice, L.C. (2010). Endometriosis. *New England Journal of Medicine, 362,* 2389–2398.

Griffin, N., Grant, L.A., & Sala, E. (2010). Adnexal masses: Characterization and imaging strategies. *Seminars in Ultrasound, CT, and MRI, 31,* 330–346.

Griffin, Y., Sudigali, V., & Jacques, A. (2010). Radiology of benign disorders of menstruation. *Gynecologic Imaging, 31*(5), 414–432.

Gupta, J.K., Sinha, A., Lumsden, M.A., & Hickey, M. (2009). Uterine artery embolization for symptomatic uterine fibroids. *The Cochrane Library,* John Wiley & Sons, Ltd. doi: 10.1002/14651858.CD005073.pub2.

Hansen, K.A., Chalpe, A., & Eyster, K.M. (2010). Management of endometriosis-associated pain. *Clinical Obstetrics and Gynecology, 53*(2), 439–448.

Hoosen, A., Nteta, C., Moodley, N., & Sturm, A. (2005). Sexually transmitted diseases including HIV infection in women with Bartholin's gland abscesses. *Genitourinary Medicine, 71,* 155–157.

Hsu, A., Khachikyan, I., & Stratton, P. (2010). Invasive and noninvasive methods for the diagnosis of endometriosis. *Clinical Obstetrics and Gynecology, 53*(2), 413–419.

Hyde, J.S. (2007). *Half the human experience: The psychology of women* (7th ed.). Belmont, CA: Wadsworth Cengage Learning.

Jacobson, T.Z., Duffy, J.M.N., Barlow, D., Koninckx, P.R., & Garry, R. (2010). Laparoscopic surgery for pelvic pain associated with endometriosis (Review). *The Cochrane Library* (Issue 1). John Wiley & Sons, Ltd.

Jacons, I., Gentry-Maharaj, A., Burnell, M., Manchanda, R., Singh, N., Sharma, A., et al. (2011). Sensitivity of transvaginal ultrasound screening for endometrial cancer in postmenopausal women: A case-control study within the UKCTOCS cohort. *Lancet Oncology, 12,* 38–48.

Jelovsek, J., Maher, C., & Barber, M. (2007). Pelvic organ prolapse. *Lancet, 369,* 1027–1038.

Jones, G., Kennedy, S., Barnard, A., Wong, J., & Jenkinson, C. (2001). Development of an endometriosis quality-of-life instrument: The endometriosis health profile-30. *Obstetrics and Gynecology, 98,* 258–264.

Judlin, P. (2010). Current concepts in managing pelvic inflammatory disease. *Current Opinion in Infectious Disease, 23,* 83–87.

Kaufman, R.H., & Adam, E. (2002). Findings in female offspring of women exposed in utero to diethylstilbestrol. *Obstetrics and Gynecology, 99,* 197–200.

Kaufman, R.H., Adam, E., Hatch, E.E., Noller, K., Herbst, A.L., & Palmer, J.R. (2000). Continued follow-up of pregnancy outcomes in diethylstilbestrol-exposed offspring. *Obstetrics and Gynecology, 96,* 483–489.

Kim, K.A., Yoon, S., Lee, C., Seong, S.J., Yoon, B.S., & Park, H. (2011). Short-term results of magnetic resonance imaging-guided focused ultrasound surgery for patients with adenomyosis: Symptomatic relief and pain reduction. *Fertility and Sterility, 95*(3), 1152–1155.

Kim, M.D., Kim, Y.M., Kim, H.C., Cho, J.H., Kang, H.G., Lee, C., et al. (2011). Uterine artery embolization for symptomatic adenomyosis: A new technical development of the 1-2-3 protocol and predictive factors of MR imaging affecting outcomes. *Journal of Vascular and Interventional Radiology, 22*(4), 497–502.

Kuncharapu, I., Majeroni, B., & Johnson, D. (2010). Pelvic organ prolapse. *American Family Physician, 81*(9), 1111–1117.

Laine, C., Williams, S., & Wilson, J. (2009). Vaginitis and cervicitis. *Annals of Internal Medicine*, ITC3, 2–16.

Lanneau, G., Argenta, P., Lanneau, M., Riffenburgh, R., Gold, M., McMeekin, S., et al. (2009). Vulvar cancer in young women: Demographic features and outcome evaluation. *American Journal of Obstetrics and Gynecology, 200,* 645.e1–645.e5.

Levine, D., Brown, D., Andreotti, R., Benacerraf, B., Benson, C., Brewster, W., et al. (2010). Management of asymptomatic ovarian and other adnexal cysts imaged at US. *Ultrasound Quarterly, 26*(3), 121–131.

Liu, Y., Yang, K., Wu, T., Roberts, H., Li, J., Tlan, J., et al. (2007, October). Microwave therapy for cervical ectropion. *Cochrane Database of Systematic Reviews*, (4), CD006227.

Lorswell, N. (2008). Management of Bartholin's gland abscesses. *Journal of Advanced Nursing, 61*(9), 2111–2113.

Luciano, A. (2009). Myomectomy. *Clinical Obstetrics and Gynecology, 52*(3), 362–371.

Mandal, D., Nunns, D., Byrne, M., McLelland, J., Rani, R., Cullimore, J., et al. (2010). Guidelines for the management of vulvodynia. *British Journal of Dermatology, 162,* 1180–1185.

McIntyre, M., Goudelocke, C., & Rovner, E. (2010). An update on surgery for pelvic organ prolapse. *Current Opinion in Urology, 20,* 490–494.

Missmer, S.A., Chavarro, J.E., Malspeis, S., Bertone-Johnson, E.R., Hornstein, M.D., Spiegelman, D., et al. (2010). A prospective study of dietary fat consumption and endometriosis risk. *Human Reproduction, 25*(6), 1528–1535.

Moen, M., Noone, M., Vassallo, B., Lopata, R., Nash, M., Sum, B., et al. (2007). Knowledge and performance of pelvic muscle exercises in women. *Journal of Pelvic Medicine and Surgery, 13*(3), 113–117.

Mol, F., Van Mello, N., Mol, B., van der Veen, F., Ankum, W., & Hajenius, P. (2010). Ectopic pregnancy and pelvic inflammatory disease: A renewed epidemic? *European Journal of Obstetrics and Gynecology and Reproductive Biology, 151,* 163–167.

National Cancer Institute. (2009). *BRCA1 and BRCA2: Cancer risk and genetic testing.* Retrieved August 22, 2011, from http://www.cancer.gov/cancertopics/factsheet/Risk/BRCA

Neis, K.J., & Neis, F. (2009). Chronic pelvic pain: Cause, diagnosis and therapy from a gynaecologist's and an endoscopist's point of view. *Gynecological Endocrinology, 25*(11), 757–761.

Neves-Castro, M. (2008). Association of ovarian and uterine cancers with postmenopausal hormonal treatments. *Clinical Obstetrics and Gynecology, 51*(3), 607–617.

Northrup, C. (2010). *Women's bodies, women's wisdom: Creating physical and emotional health and healing: Revised and updated.* New York: Bantam Books.

Novellas, S., Chassang, M., Delotte, J., Toullalan, O., Chevallier, A., Bouaziz, J., et al. (2011). MRI characteristics of the uterine junctional zone: From normal to the diagnosis of adenomyosis. *American Journal of Roentgenology, 196*(5), 1206–1213.

Ojha, K., & Matah, A. (2008). Surgical management of chronic pelvic pain. *Obstetrics, Gynaecology and Reproductive Medicine, 18*(9), 236–240.

Osada, H., Silber, S., Kakinuma, T., Nagaishi, M., Kato, K., & Kato, O. (2011). Surgical procedure to conserve the uterus for future pregnancy in patients suffering from massive adenomysosis. *Reproductive Biomedicine Online, 22,* 94–99.

Ozdegirmenci, O., Kayikcioglu, F., Akgul, M.A., Kaplan, M., Karcaaltincaba, M., Haeral, A., et al. (2010). Comparison of levonorgestrel intrauterine system versus hysterectomy on efficacy and quality of life in patients with adenomyosis. *Fertility and Sterility, 95*(2), 497–502.

Palmer, J.R., Anderson, D., Helmrich, S.P., & Herbst, A.L. (2000). Risk factors for diethylstilbestrol-associated clear cell adenocarcinoma. *Obstetrics and Gynecology, 95,* 814–820.

Pancini, P., Manci, N., Bellati, F., Di Donato, V., Marchetti, C., Calcago, M., et al. (2007). CO2 later therapy of the Bartholin's gland cyst: Surgical data and functional short- and long-term results. *Journal of Minimally Invasive Gynecology, 14,* 348–351.

Preutthipan, S., & Herabutya, Y. (2010). Hysteroscopic rollerball endometrial ablation as an alternative treatment for adenomyosis with menorrhagia and/or dysmenorrhea. *Journal of Obstetrics and Gynaecology Research, 36*(5), 1031–1036.

Ross, J., Brown, L., Saunders, P., & Alexander, S. (2009). Mycoplasma genitalium in asymptomatic patients: Implications for screening. *Sexually Transmitted Infection, 85,* 436–437.

Salvatore, S., Siesto, G., & Serati, M. (2010). Risk factors of recurrence of genital prolapse. *Current Opinion in Obstetrics and Gynecology, 22,* 420–424.

Shlamovitz, G. (2010). Drainage and treatment of Bartholin's gland abscess. *Gynecological Medicine, 12,* 128–132.

Short, V., Totten, P., Ness, R., Astete, S., Kelsey, S., Murray, P., et al. (2010). The demographic, sexual health, and behavioral correlates of Mycoplasma genitalium infection among women with clinically suspected pelvic inflammatory disease. *Sexually Transmitted Infection, 86,* 29–31.

Smith, F., Holman, C., Moorin, R., & Tsokos, N. (2010). Lifetime risk of undergoing surgery for pelvic organ prolapse. *Obstetrics and Gynecology, 116*(5), 1096–1100.

Soper, D. (2010). Pelvic inflammatory disease. *Obstetrics and Gynecology, 116*(2), 419–428.

Speights, S., Harris, R., & Cowan, B. (2002). Effectiveness of operative marsupialization for acute Bartholin's gland abscess. *Journal of Pelvic Surgery, 4*(5), 214–217.

Spies, J.B., Bradley, L.D., Guido, R., Maxwell, G.L., Levine, B.A., & Coyne, K. (2010). Outcomes from leiomyoma therapies: Comparison with normal controls. *Obstetrics and Gynecology, 116*(3), 641–652.

Stones, W., Cheong, Y.C., Howard, F.M., & Singh, S. (2010). Limited symptom relief is available for women with chronic pelvic pain. *Cochrane Summaries,* CD0003387.

Storey, S., Aston, M., Price, S., Irving, L., & Hemmens, E. (2009). Women's experiences with vaginal pessary use. *Journal of Advanced Nursing, 65*(11), 2350–2357.

Taran, F.A., Weaver, A.L., Coddington, C.C., & Stewart, E.A. (2010). Understanding adenomyosis: A case control study. *Fertility and Sterility, 94*(4), 1223–1228.

Tarnawa, E., Sullivan, S., Underwood, P., Richardson, M., & Spruill, L. (2011). Severe hypercalcemia associated with uterine leiomyoma in pregnancy. *Obstetrics & Gynecology, 117*(2), 473–476.

ter Kuile, M.M., Both, S., & van Lankveld, J.J.D.M. (2010). Cognitive behavioral therapy for sexual dysfunction in women. *Psychiatric Clinics of North America, 33,* 595–610.

Tinelli, A., Malvasi, A., Rahimi, S., Negro, R., Vergara, D., Martignago, R., et al. (2010). Age-related pelvic floor modifications and prolapse risk factors in postmenopausal women. *Journal of the North American Menopause Society, 17*(1), 204–212.

Titus-Ernstoff, L., Troisi, R., Hatch, E.E., Palmer, J.R., Hyer, M., Kaufman, R., et al. (2010). Birth defects in the sons and daughters of women who were exposed in utero to diethylstilbestrol (DES). *International Journal of Andrology, 33,* 377–384.

van Lankveld, J.J.D.M., Granot, M., Willibrord, C.M., Schultz, W., Binik, Y., Wesselmann, U., et al. (2010) Women's sexual pain disorders. *Journal of Sexual Medicine, 7,* 615–631.

Van Voorhis, B. (2009). A 41-year-old woman with menorrhagia, anemia, and fibroids: Review of treatment of uterine fibroids. *Journal of the American Medical Association, 301*(1), 82–93.

Vercellini, P., Somigliana, E., Vigano, P., Abbiati, A., Barbara, G., & Fedele, L. (2009). Chronic pelvic pain in women: Etiology, pathogenesis and diagnostic approach. *Gynecological Endocrinology, 25*(3), 149–158.

Vercellini, P., Vigano, P., Somigliana, E., Abbiati, A., Barbara, G., & Fedele, L. (2009). Medical, surgical and alternative treatment for chronic pelvic pain in women: A descriptive view. *Gynecological Endocrinology, 25*(4), 208–221.

Waller, J.G., & Shaw, R.W. (1995). Endometriosis, pelvic pain, and psychological functioning. *Fertility and Sterility, 63*, 796–800.

Younis, M.T.S., Iram, S., Anwar, B., & Ewies, A.A.A. (2010). Women with asymptomatic cervical polyps may not need to see a gynaecologist or have them removed: An observational retrospective study of 1126 cases. *European Journal of Obstetrics and Gynecology and Reproductive Biology, 150*(2), 190–194.

CHAPTER ❖ **17**

BREAST HEALTH

Linda Christinsen-Rengel

An understanding of both benign and malignant breast conditions is important for health care providers because both conditions are common and symptoms overlap.

Highlights

- Breast Examination and Assessment
- Benign Breast Disorders
- Malignant Breast Neoplasm (Breast Cancer)

❖ INTRODUCTION

The female breast has cultural and psychological significance to both men and women in American society. The lactation function plays a significant role in nurturing and motherhood. Psychologically, the breast is a source of sexual attraction and sensual pleasure for both men and women. Threats of injury or loss of the breast potentially influence a woman's perception of her body and her family/social relationships and role in society. The diagnosis of breast cancer with the threat of loss of a breast or loss of life is a fear for many women. Excluding nonmelanoma skin cancer, breast cancer is the most common cancer in women, with an average 12.5 percent (one in eight) lifetime risk of developing breast cancer (Siegel, Ward, Brawley, & Jemal, 2011). Early detection with breast cancer screening along with advances in treatment significantly reduced breast cancer mortality (U.S. Preventative Services Task Force [USPSTF], 2009). Benign breast conditions are also common, with signs and symptoms that overlap with malignant processes. Health care providers need an understanding of both benign and malignant conditions to diagnose and treat appropriately.

BREAST EXAMINATION AND ASSESSMENT

Breast examination is conducted both as a screening assessment for breast cancer and as a diagnostic tool in the assessment of breast symptoms. In the past 25 years, breast cancer screening programs have contributed to a nearly one-third reduction in mortality rates for breast cancer (Howlader et al., 2011). Screening programs have historically included clinical breast examination (CBE), patient breast self-examination (BSE), and mammography. In 2009, the USPSTF conducted a meta-analysis of research studies to determine risk/benefit by age group to establish screening recommendations. It found a 15 percent reduction in breast cancer–related mortality for women aged 39 to 69 who underwent screening mammography and insufficient evidence to demonstrate benefit for women aged 70 and older (Nelson et al., 2009). False-positive results were common in all age groups and led to additional imaging and biopsies, with women aged 40 to 49 experiencing the highest rate of additional imaging, but a lower rate of biopsy than older women. False-negative results were lower, especially among women aged 40 to 49 (Nelson et al., 2009). Balancing the risks/benefits, the USPSTF recommended biennial screening mammograms for women ages 50 to 74 and for women under the age of 50; biennial screening mammography should be individually determined taking into account the patient's values regarding specific benefits and harms. Annual or biannual mammographic screening in women over the age of 74 can be continued as long as there is reasonable life expectancy of at least 5 to 7 years because the mortality benefit begins to be seen 5 to 7 years after the onset of screening (Berg, 2009).

The USPSTF (2009) found that current evidence was insufficient to assess the additional benefits and harms of CBE in women 40 years or older and made no recommendation for or against CBE. It recommended against BSE, finding instruction in BSE resulted in additional imaging and biopsies with no significant decrease in breast cancer mortality. These recommendations have not been universally endorsed by other consensus groups with an interest in reducing breast cancer mortality such as the American Cancer Society (ACS), National Comprehensive Cancer Network (NCCN), and American College of Obstetricians and Gynecologists (ACOG) (see Table 17–1).

TABLE 17–1. Comparison of Breast Cancer Screening Recommendations for Normal Risk Women

Organization	Breast Self-Examination	Clinical Breast Examination	Mammogram
U.S. Preventative Services Task Force	Recommend against teaching BSE	Insufficient evidence to recommend for or against	Biennial ages 50–74 Biennial age <50 individual choice
American Cancer Society	BSE optional Breast awareness	Every 3 years in ages 20s and 30s. Annual age ≥40	Annual age ≥40 and continue as long as in good health
American College of Obstetricians and Gynecologists	Breast awareness Consider BSE for high-risk patients	Every 1–3 years in ages 20–39 Annual age ≥40	Annual age ≥40
National Comprehensive Cancer Network	Breast awareness	Every 1–3 years in ages 20–40 Annual age ≥40	Annual age ≥40

Source: ACOG, 2011; ACS, 2011; NCCN, 2010; USPSTF, 2009.

Health care providers can help their patients make decisions on appropriate screening based on identification and discussion of individual risk factors for breast cancer along with the potential risks and benefits of BSE and mammography. There are several risk assessment tools that can be used to identify women at high risk for breast cancer who may benefit from earlier or additional screening. The Gail model is weighted to hormonal risk: first-degree female relatives with breast cancer and breast biopsy. It is useful in white and African American women and can be accessed at http://www.cancer.gov/bcrisktool/ (National Cancer Institute [NCI], 2008). For women with a strong family history of breast cancer, the BRCAPRO model considers first- and second-degree relatives and their age at diagnosis (Berry et al., 2002). It was developed for use with women of Northern European and Ashkenazi Jewish culture, but has been shown to be of value in minority women, especially Hispanics (Huo et al., 2009). A free computer program is available at http://www4.utsouthwestern.edu/breasthealth/cagene/ (U.T. Southwestern Medical Center, 2004).

CLINICAL BREAST EXAMINATION

CBE is used as both a screening and diagnostic tool. The use of visual inspection and palpation of the breast and surrounding tissue can detect breast abnormalities that warrant further evaluation. Evidence suggests that CBE can detect a substantial proportion of cancers in areas where mammography is not available (USPSTF, 2009). The sensitivity and specificity of CBE varies substantially with age, breast density, experience of the provider, and time spent completing the examination. It has been suggested that a good CBE should take about 2 minutes to complete (Goodson, Hunt, Plotnik, & Moore, 2008). Recommendations for CBE vary depending on the organization. The sensitivity for CBE ranges from 40 to 70 percent, and specificity ranges from 86 to 99 percent (Nelson et al., 2009).

False-negative results may lead to a missed diagnosis and false-positive results may lead to unnecessary diagnostic workup with possible psychological consequences of anxiety, worry, and depression (Nelson et al., 2009). CBE is the only recommended screening modality in women with normal risk ages 20 to 39 and is generally recommended as an adjunct to mammographic screening in women aged 40 and older (Griffin & Pearlman, 2010).

Breast examination includes visual inspection and palpation. Healthy breast tissue demonstrates varying degrees of tenderness, nodularity, and density on examination. Breasts in premenopausal women are nodular with irregular texture, with most nodularity where breast tissue is more concentrated, such as the upper outer quadrants, inframammary ridge area, and subareolar region. Although clinicians have used the term *fibrocystic change* or *disease* to describe this normal breast finding, this is a pathology term and should not be used to describe clinical findings (Miltenburg &Speights, 2008). It is inaccurate to use the term *fibrocystic disease* to describe a normal condition (Marchant, 2002).Using descriptive terms such as *nodular, tender breast* describes the breast examination accurately and avoids identifying normal physiologic changes as disease.

A standardized approach and comparison can be helpful in detecting abnormalities. A dominant breast mass is three dimensional, the density differs from surrounding tissue, and a similar mass is not found in either breast. If a similar mass is found in the contralateral breast, no further evaluation is warranted. Documentation of physical and visual findings include dimpling of the skin; changes of the skin, areola, or nipple; nipple inversion or retraction; nipple discharge; associated tenderness; and the presence or absence of adenopathy. For any breast mass, note

- position in the breast (quadrant, distance from nipple)
- shape
- size
- smooth or irregular borders
- consistency
- discrete or indistinct thickening
- mobility, attachment to skin, or deep structures

For position documentation, the clock method uses tangents emanating from the nipple as numbers on the clock while facing the patient to more accurately indicate position and distance from the nipple. Use of a diagram along with a written description of the mass is recommended (Figure 17–1).

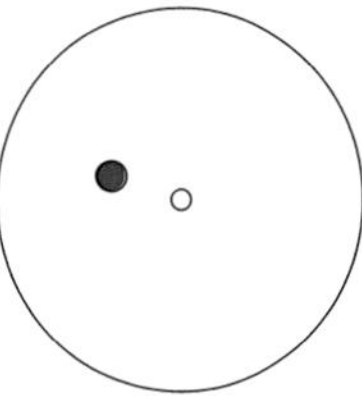

FIGURE 17–1. Graphic Method to Document Location of Breast Mass. For example, 10 o'clock, 2 cm from the nipple.

The optimal time for CBE for premenopausal women is within the first 5 to 10 days after the onset of menses. Breast examination should be included in the care of women during pregnancy and lactation (best performed 10 to 15 minutes after emptying the breast).

Method

A thorough breast examination begins with a comprehensive personal and family history, which include the elements in Table 17–2. An assessment of a patient presenting with a breast symptom should also include onset, associated breast symptoms, timing in relation to menstrual cycle, and aggravation and alleviation of symptoms. A suspicious mass found on clinical examination must be evaluated and explained even if mammography does not show an abnormality (Saslow et al., 2004).

Visual Inspection. Inform the patient in advance that the breast examination will include visual inspection and palpation of the breasts. Visual inspection technique includes the following:

- Inspection of the breasts while the patient is seated with her arms relaxed, comparing breast size and shape. If size discrepancy is noted, ask about chronicity. Recent changes require further evaluation. Alterations in breast shape such as bulges, dimpling, or retraction of the skin are suggestive of underlying tissue changes. Observe the skin of the breast and nipples. Edema of the breast has the appearance of orange peel skin (*peau d'orange*) and is usually caused by obstruction of the dermal lymphatics by tumor cells or obstruction of the lymph nodes by tumor cells, radiation, or surgical dissection (Robertson et al., 2010). Erythema may be caused by cellulitis, abscess, or inflammatory cancer. Observe the nipples for symmetry, retraction, or skin changes. Ask about onset of nipple retraction.
- Having the patient raise her arms over her head to observe the lower half of the breasts for dimpling or retraction of the skin.
- Having the patient sit with her hands pressed tightly against her hips, causing contraction of the pectoralis major muscles to highlight areas of dimpling or skin retraction.

TABLE 17–2. Breast History

Breast cancer risk
- Age at menarche
- Number of term pregnancies and age at first birth
- Lactation history
- Family history of breast and ovarian cancer, including affected relative, age of onset, and presence of bilateral disease (both maternal and paternal)
- Cultural ancestry, especially Ashkenazi Jews
- History of breast biopsy (histologic diagnosis)
- History of breast surgery
- Environmental factors—smoking, obesity, alcohol use
- Exposure to chest irradiation

Premenopausal
- Date of last menstrual period
- Use of oral or hormonal contraceptives

Postmenopausal
- Date of menopause
- Use of hormone therapy

Screening practices
- Breast self-examination
- Prior mammogram or other breast imaging

Breast changes
- Lumps
- Pain (focal, general, cyclic, or constant)
- Nipple discharge (spontaneous or expressed)
- Changes in appearance of skin or nipples (dimpling, rash, etc.)

Palpation. Appropriate palpation includes five key characteristics (Saslow et al., 2004).

- *Position:* The patient should be seated with the arm relaxed at the side for palpation of the axillary, supraclavicular, and infraclavicular lymph nodes. She should be lying down for breast palpation with the ipsilateral hand overhead to flatten the breast tissue against the chest wall. For larger breasts, place a small pillow under the shoulder of the breast to be examined to move the breast tissue over the chest wall.
- *Perimeter:* The area of breast to be examined is contained within the following landmarks—down the midaxillary line, across the inframammary ridge at the fifth/sixth rib, up the lateral edges of the sternum, across the clavicle, and back to the midaxillary line.
- *Pattern of search:* Use the vertical strip pattern starting at the axilla, including the chest wall, skin, and incision if a mastectomy was performed (see Figure 17–2).
- *Palpation:* Use the pads of the fingertips of the middle three fingers to palpate, using overlapping dime-sized circular motions. Palpate the entire perimeter of the breast including the upper outer

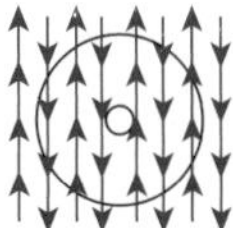

FIGURE 17–2. Vertical Strip Pattern. *Source:* Barton, Harris, and Fletcher, 1999, p. 1276.

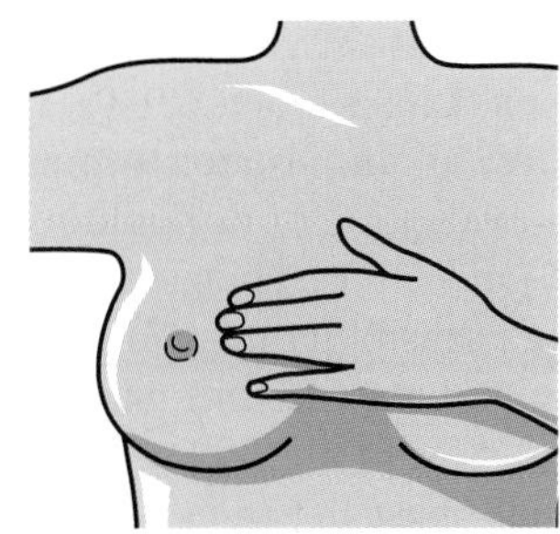

At each spot, make three small circles about the size of a dime.

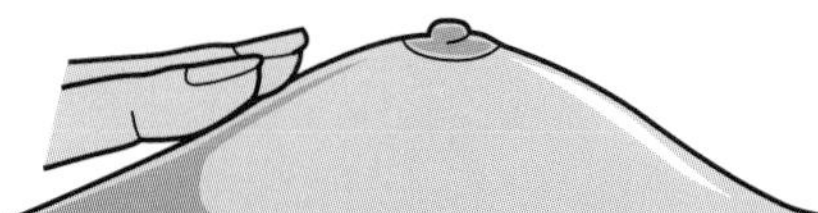

Use light pressure for the first circle.

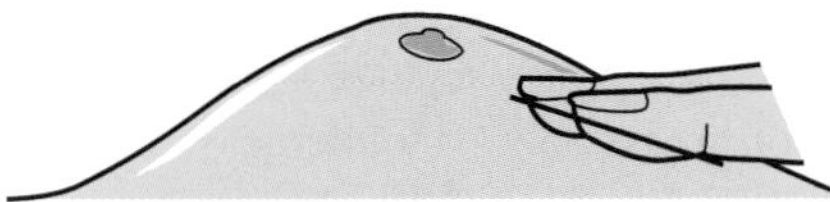

Use medium pressure for the second circle.

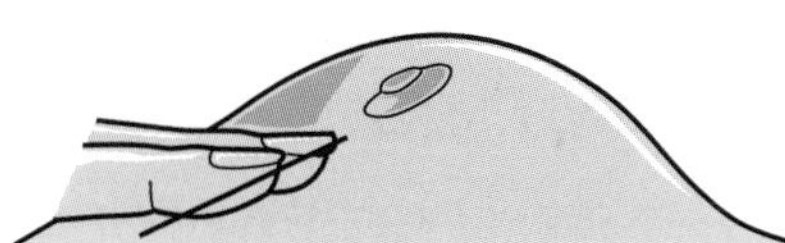

Use deep pressure for the third circle.

FIGURE 17–3. Levels of Pressure. *Source:* Barton, Harris, and Fletcher, 1999, p. 1277.

quadrant and under the areola and nipple, common sites for breast cancer to arise.

- *Pressure:* Three levels of pressure should be applied in sequence as each area of tissue is examined—light, medium, and deep. These levels correspond to subcutaneous, midlevel, and chest wall layers (see Figure 17–3).

BREAST SELF-AWARENESS

The 2009 USPSTF guidelines recommend against BSE based on lack of evidence of reduction in mortality and harms similar to CBE (Nelson et al., 2009). The ACS (2011) recommends women aged 20 and older be instructed on the benefits (increased awareness of breast changes leading to rapid evaluation and response) and limitations (false-positive results) of BSE and offered the option of scheduled step-by-step BSE or self-awareness. Patient instructions for step-by-step BSE are available on its website at http://www.cancer.org/Cancer/Breast-Cancer/MoreInformation/BreastCancerEarlyDetection/index. BSE is endorsed by NCCN and ACOG. NCCN (2010) describes BSE as women becoming familiar with the normal appearance and feel of their breasts and reporting changes promptly to their health care provider.

The CBE provides an opportunity to teach the patient breast awareness and the following signs that should be reported, regardless of whether the patient has had a recent negative CBE or mammographic screening (ACS, 2011).

- New lump or mass in breast or axilla
- Swelling of all or part of a breast (even if no distinct lump is felt)
- Skin irritation or dimpling
- Breast or nipple pain
- Nipple retraction (turning inward) or changes
- Redness, scaliness, or thickening of the skin of the nipple or breast
- A nipple discharge other than breast milk

BREAST IMAGING

Breast imaging can be used as a screening or as a diagnostic tool. Mammography is the primary breast cancer screening tool in low-risk women. Breast magnetic resonance imaging (MRI) is only used for screening in special cases, such as women at high risk for breast cancer. Women with breast symptoms or imaging abnormalities can be referred for diagnostic evaluation with mammography or ultrasound and, in special cases, with breast MRI or breast-specific gamma imaging (BSGI).

Mammography

There are two types of mammograms: screening and diagnostic. The purpose of a screening mammogram is detection of breast cancer at a preclinical or early stage to allow for greater treatment options and reduction in mortality by finding a higher percentage of localized disease and a lower incidence of positive regional nodes. Based on data from the NCI's Breast Cancer Surveillance Consortium (2009), mammography screening has an average overall sensitivity of 84.1 percent and specificity of 90.4 percent. Sensitivity of mammography is decreased in women with dense breast tissue or women of younger age. Mammography is not generally recommended for women under the age of 30. Hormonal status has no significant effect on the effectiveness of screening independent of breast density (Dongola et al., 2011).

Screening mammography consists of images taken in four views using compression plastic plates, which may produce temporary discomfort that can be relieved by oral analgesics. Scheduling the procedure at the end of the menstrual cycle may also decrease discomfort. Deodorant, body lotions, and powders containing aluminum, calcium, or zinc products should be avoided on the day of the examination or removed with soap and water before the mammogram.

Women who have undergone breast augmentation (mammoplasty) should still be referred for screening mammography to evaluate the native breast tissue. Although sensitivity is decreased, it does not affect breast cancer prognosis (Goodemote, Mitchell, & Nichols, 2008).

Diagnostic mammography is used to evaluate abnormal clinical findings, such as breast mass, thickening, or nipple discharge, and to obtain additional images of possible abnormalities identified on screening mammograms. In addition to the standard views taken with the screening mammogram, additional views at different angles with magnification of areas of concern are included (NCI, 2010). Radiologists use the American College of Radiology Breast Imaging Reporting and Data System to classify their mammography findings into assessment categories ranging from negative to highly suspicious of malignancy (D'Orsi et al., 2003).

Ultrasound

Ultrasound is best used to examine a targeted area of the breast and to differentiate a cystic from a solid mass. Sonography is the primary diagnostic tool in women with breast symptoms under the age of 30 and is used as an adjunct to mammography in women aged 30 and older with breast symptoms. An ultrasound also provides guidance for interventional breast procedures such as core needle biopsy and cyst aspiration.

Magnetic Resonance Imaging

Breast MRI is used as an adjunct to mammography for breast cancer screening in women identified at increased risk due to family history or genetic risk factors including a BRCA mutation or first-degree relative of an untested BRCA carrier (Saslow et al., 2007). Breast MRI is useful in defining the precise size of the tumor and detecting multifocal disease when assessing suitability for breast-conservation surgery (Lehman et al., 2007), in assessment of response to neoadjuvant chemotherapy for breast cancer (Yuan, Chen, Liu, & Shen, 2010), in evaluation of implant rupture, as an adjunct to mammography and ultrasound in evaluation of difficult lesions, and as guidance for MRI-guided breast biopsy.

MRI has a high sensitivity rate (71–100%), but low specificity, as benign breast lesions may produce false-positive results (Saslow et al., 2007). Timing the MRI during the follicular phase of the menstrual cycle minimizes false-positive results due to hormonal influences (Delille, Slanetz, Yeh, Kopans, & Garrido, 2005).

BSGI is a molecular breast imaging procedure that is as accurate as an MRI and may be more comfortable (Brem et al., 2010).

BENIGN BREAST DISORDERS

Benign breast disorders include all nonmalignant conditions of the breast, including benign tumors and infection. Clinical presentation may include a palpable mass, nipple discharge, or breast pain or tenderness. The same clinical presentation may occur with a breast malignancy. The role of the provider is to identify breast abnormalities and refer for appropriate diagnostic workup.

PALPABLE BREAST MASS

The breast mass is one of the most common breast symptoms. Although the majority of masses are benign, they cause anxiety for the patient with concern about breast cancer. Only 10 percent of women who present with a new breast lump have breast cancer. The younger the age of the woman with a new lump, the less likely a cancer diagnosis (only 1% in women age 40 or younger) (Heisey & McCready, 2010). The two most common benign breast masses are fibroadenoma and breast cysts. The "triple test" of palpation, imaging, and percutaneous biopsy is considered the gold standard in diagnosis of a breast mass (Rodden, 2009; Santen & Mansel, 2005).

Fibroadenoma

Epidemiology. Fibroadenomas are thought to be hyperplastic lesions that form during menarche and tend to grow slowly to 1 to 2 cm in size (Jayasinghe & Simmons, 2009). Fibroadenomas are most commonly found in women under the age of 30, although they may be discovered in women aged 30 to 50 due to changes in the surrounding breast tissue with involution or weight loss (Santen & Mansel, 2005). They change very little during the menstrual cycle, although they may grow rapidly in adolescence, pregnancy, and lactation and regress in size during perimenopause (Marchant, 2002). A fibroadenoma over 5 to 10 cm in size is called a giant or juvenile fibroadenoma and accounts for 10 percent of all fibroadenomas in adolescence (Jayasinghe & Simmons, 2009). Because 10 percent of malignant lesions in young women have features consistent with a fibroadenoma, a new palpable breast lump should be thoroughly evaluated (Foxcroft, Evans, & Porter, 2004). Simple fibroadenoma and complex fibroadenoma without atypia are associated with a nonsignificant increased risk for breast cancer (Kabat et al., 2010).

Subjective Data. The patient reports a small pea or marble-like, painless lump in one breast, which may have been present for months or years. It usually is found in the upper outer quadrant of the breast, but may occur anywhere in the breast (Jayasinghe & Simmons, 2009). No associated breast symptoms, such as nipple discharge or retraction, dimpling, or other skin changes are reported.

Objective Data

Physical Examination. Physical examination of the breast reveals a discrete, solitary, firm, mobile, well-circumscribed, nontender mass without supraclavicular or axillary lymphadenopathy. It is usually rubbery, but may feel firmer in the older patient (Miltenburg & Speights, 2008). In 20 percent of cases, multiple lesions occur, either in the same breast or bilaterally (Guray & Sahin, 2006).

Diagnostic Tests and Methods

MAMMOGRAPHY. See Breast Imaging.

ULTRASOUND. (See Breast Imaging.) Ultrasound along with clinical examination may be diagnostic of fibroadenoma in a woman under 30 years of age (Jayasinghe & Simmons, 2009).

CORE NEEDLE BIOPSY. In the triple-test evaluation for solid lesions, percutaneous biopsy is recommended if a mass is found as solid on imaging. Core needle biopsy is a minimally invasive procedure that is performed by a specialist under ultrasound or mammographic (stereotactic) guidance using a large-bore needle to provide a tissue sample for histologic evaluation (Pearlman & Griffin, 2010).

Differential Medical Diagnosis. Breast macrocyst, phyllodes tumor, adenoma, mammary hamartoma, breast carcinoma.

Plan

Psychological Interventions. Providing information about the usual benign status of solitary lumps found in women under the age of 50, along with a plan for diagnosis will help allay anxiety. Reassurance that fibroadenomas are not precancerous and will not impair ability to breast-feed may also be helpful.

Surgical Intervention/Excisional (Open) Biopsy. This procedure is done to remove or diagnose a breast lesion. It is indicated for initial diagnosis of a breast mass only if needle biopsy is not feasible for technical reasons such as location and implants. Surgical excision of a fibroadenoma is recommended with rapid growth in size or if the mass is greater than 5 cm in diameter (Jayasinghe & Simmons, 2009). Some women choose to have the fibroadenoma excised to decrease anxiety.

Conservative Treatment. In women with a benign diagnosis of fibroadenoma by triple test, serial examinations and imaging at 6-month intervals for 1 to 2 years is recommended to ensure stability and growth of the lesion (Miltenburg & Speights, 2008). The patient should be encouraged to return if she experiences anxiety or concern regarding the lesion. Small fibroadenomas in adolescence should be observed for signs of rapid growth or regression (Jayasinghe & Simmons, 2009).

Breast Cysts (Macrocyst/Gross Cyst)

Epidemiology. Breast cysts are commonly encountered fluid-filled lesions found in the terminal duct or lobule of the breast that form because of obstruction, involution, or aging of ducts within the breasts (Guray & Sahin, 2006). They may be palpable or nonpalpable, simple or complex. Cysts often fluctuate with the menstrual cycle and are more common during the luteal phase of the cycle. They often disappear with menopause but may persist with use of hormonal therapy (Heisey & McCready, 2010). Cysts that have filled rapidly with fluid may be tender. They are found in as many as one third of women between the ages of 35 and 50 (Guray & Sahin, 2006) and are uncommon in postmenopausal women unless they have received hormone therapy (Heisey & McCready, 2010). They do not undergo malignant change and are not associated with an increased risk for cancer (Morrow, 2000). However, complex cysts, even those that are not palpable, require aspiration or core biopsy to rule out malignancy (Miltenburg & Speights, 2008).

Subjective Data. The patient reports a single or multiple breast lumps in one or both breasts with or without associated tenderness. The patient may alternatively report a sudden onset of pain with point tenderness and a palpable mass.

Objective Data

Physical Examination. Physical examination of the breasts reveals a discrete, soft to firm, mobile, well-circumscribed mass that is most often tender to palpation and without supraclavicular or axillary lymphadenopathy or overlying skin changes (Heisey & McCready, 2010). It may be unilateral or bilateral, or there may be multiple masses. It is often difficult to distinguish a cyst from a solid mass, such as a fibroadenoma.

Diagnostic Tests and Methods

ULTRASOUND-GUIDED ASPIRATION/FINE NEEDLE ASPIRATION. Ultrasound-guided cyst aspiration by a trained provider is the preferred technique to diagnose and treat a presumed breast cyst. Fine needle aspiration (FNA) in the primary provider office may be an efficient, cost-effective diagnostic method to differentiate cystic or solid lesions. FNA may be attempted on lesions not clinically suspicious for malignancy (e.g., hard irregular mass, fixed to skin or chest, palpable ipsilateral nodes, or peau d'orange) (Heisey & McCready, 2010). Immediate pain relief may be obtained with aspiration of the fluid. Cystic fluid is typically white, yellow-green, or brown. If the aspirate is nonbloody or contains no debris, and the mass completely disappears with aspiration, the patient can be reassured of the low likelihood of cancer. If the fluid is bloody or cloudy, the mass is solid, or does not disappear with aspiration; a needle core biopsy is indicated for pathologic diagnosis. Routine aspiration of cysts in the absence of symptoms is not recommended (Miltenburg & Speights, 2008).

MAMMOGRAPHY. See Breast Imaging.

ULTRASOUND. See Breast Imaging.

Differential Medical Diagnosis. Fibroadenoma, phyllodes tumor, adenoma, mammary hamartoma, breast carcinoma.

Plan

Psychological Interventions. Reassurance that breast cysts are not precancerous and will not impair ability to breastfeed may allay anxiety.

Surgical Intervention/Excisional (Open) Biopsy. (See Fibroadenoma.) Surgical excision and biopsy of the breast cyst is recommended if there is refilling of the cyst or a residual mass is identified by clinical examination or ultrasound (Miltenburg & Speights, 2008).

Follow-Up. If ultrasound or aspiration demonstrates a simple cyst, which is asymptomatic, no intervention or follow-up is required (Miltenburg & Speights, 2008). Patients who have had aspiration of breast cysts should be instructed to return to clinic for follow-up with recurrence of symptoms.

Galactocele

Epidemiology. The galactocele is a discrete, milk-filled, cystic mass in the breast of a lactating or recently lactating woman that is thought to arise from dilation and obstruction of the lactiferous duct with retained milk and desquamated epithelial cells. It is most often found in the upper quadrants beyond the areolar border and there may be singular or multiple masses (Marchant, 2002).

Subjective Data. The client may report a lump or knot in her breast that may or may not be painful.

Objective Data

Physical Examination. Physical examination usually reveals a palpable, firm, round mass in one or both breasts (Marchant, 2002). Milk may be manually expressed from the nipple and pain may be elicited upon palpation.

Diagnostic Tests and Methods

ULTRASOUND-GUIDED ASPIRATION. (See Breast Cysts.) An ultrasound-guided aspiration or FNA can be performed to alleviate the symptoms and diagnose the galactocele. If the fluid is other than milky or if the galactocele does not disappear with aspiration, a needle core biopsy is indicated. Most often, no further treatment is needed if the mass disappears with aspiration, as aspiration is often curative.

MAMMOGRAPHY. See Breast Imaging.

ULTRASOUND. See Breast Imaging.

Differential Medical Diagnosis. Microcyst, fibroadenoma, malignant neoplasm.

Plan

Psychosocial Interventions. Once a definitive diagnosis is made, reassure the client that galactocele is a benign condition that usually will disappear within a few weeks. It rarely interferes with current or future lactation. If the patient is still breastfeeding, a referral to a breastfeeding support group, or breastfeeding consultant, may be beneficial.

Follow-Up. If the patient is breastfeeding, massage, warm moist packs, and a change in position or technique may be helpful. A galactocele that is aspirated while the patient is breastfeeding may refill. Schedule a follow-up visit in 1 to 2 months to assure the galactocele has resolved.

BREAST PAIN (MASTALGIA OR MASTODYNIA)

Mastalgia is one of the most common problems for which women consult health care providers with a concern that it is a sign of early breast cancer. In reality, the risk of breast cancer is very low when mastalgia is the only symptom. Breast pain may range from mild to severe, with significant interference with daily activities. Mastalgia can be divided into three categories: cyclic breast pain, noncyclic breast pain, and extramammary (nonbreast) pain (Smith, Pruthi, & Fitzpatrick, 2004). It may be related to infection, malignancy, or extramammary conditions. When these conditions are ruled out, mastalgia is considered a benign condition (Miltenburg & Speights, 2008).

Epidemiology

Both cyclical and noncyclical mastalgia are thought to be related to hormonal fluctuations, although direct relationships between serum progesterone, estradiol, and prolactin have not been identified (Miltenburg & Speights, 2008). Cyclical mastalgia typically occurs in premenopausal women 5 to 10 days before menstruation and is relieved with the onset of menses. This cyclic pain is more severe and prolonged than common minor premenstrual breast discomfort (Smith et al., 2004).

Noncyclical mastalgia is less common than cyclical mastalgia, is not associated with the menstrual cycle, and is constant or intermittent with irregular exacerbations. It generally affects women in their 30s, 40s, and 50s. Noncyclic pain may be caused by a variety of breast lesions, hormone therapy, pregnancy, Mondor's disease, or cancer but most often arises from unknown reasons (Smith et al., 2004). Extramammary pain is usually unilateral. It may be caused by musculoskeletal problems, cardiac disease, or a pulmonary etiology.

Subjective Data

The first step is careful history taking to rule out an infectious process or possible signs of malignancy (skin or nipple changes). The patient with cyclic pain reports bilateral dull, heavy, or aching breasts with pain that may radiate to the axilla or arm. It has a variable duration, but is usually resolved with menses. The patient with noncyclic pain typically reports a unilateral, sharp, burning pain that may be constant or intermittent with no relation to the menstrual cycle (Smith et al., 2004). With extramammary pain, she may report a new exercise regimen or new or past injury to the chest or breast.

Objective Data

Physical Examination. Evaluation of the breasts may reveal generalized thickening or lumpiness and tenderness (usually bilateral) without lymphadenopathy or a discrete mass or thickening at the site of pain. Breast pain associated with breast cancer is intense, unilateral, constant pain (Smith et al., 2004). However, most breast cancer is painless. Palpation of the chest wall may reveal pain and tenderness with extramammary pain. Move the breast away from the chest wall and palpate the breast separately to identify the source of the pain. Position patient on her side to facilitate differentiation of breast tissue from underlying chest wall muscles (Miltenburg & Speights, 2008).

Diagnostic Tests and Methods

Mammography. It is indicated in women presenting with a new symptom who are over the age of 30, and have not had mammography within the past 12 months to rule out any abnormalities (NCCN, 2010). Any breast lump requires triple-test evaluation.

Ultrasound. See Breast Imaging.

Lab. Pregnancy test, if appropriate for cyclical pain.

Differential Medical Diagnosis

Pregnancy, Tietze's syndrome or costochondritis, herpes zoster, Mondor's disease, cardiac disease, breast cyst, malignant breast mass, cervical (neck) radiculopathy, respiratory infection, rib fracture, peptic ulcer disease, or hiatal hernia.

Plan

Psychological Interventions. Perform a detailed history and thorough breast examination, explaining negative or positive findings, possible cause of the symptoms, natural history of the pain, and absence of increased risk for breast cancer with pain as the only symptom. In most women, mastalgia is a self-limiting condition that will resolve spontaneously over time (Miltenburg & Speights, 2008). Once any underlying pathology is ruled out, reassurance alone will resolve the problem in 86 percent of women with mild pain and 52 percent of women with severe breast pain (Barros, Mottola, Ruiz, Borges, & Pinotti, 1999).

Medication. Danazol, tamoxifen, and bromocriptine should be reserved for women with severe, persistent mastalgia, refractory to other measures. A daily diary should be maintained throughout the use of the medications. After assuring that the client is not pregnant, advise her to avoid pregnancy by consistent use of a barrier method of contraception.

Danazol reduces pain and tenderness by suppressing ovarian function, thereby reducing estrogen production and concentration in breast tissue and resulting in decreased pain, nodularity, and tenderness (Miltenburg & Speights, 2008; Smith et al., 2004). Recurring symptoms after discontinuation of danazol is common (Miltenburg & Speights, 2008).

Tamoxifen is not approved by the Food and Drug Administration (FDA) for treating mastalgia but may be effective in pain reduction in 57 to 96 percent of patients (Smith et al., 2004). Tamoxifen should be discontinued after 3 months if symptoms do not improve (Miltenburg & Speights, 2008).

Bromocriptine may be prescribed for breast pain associated with nodularity. However, this drug is primarily used for treatment of galactorrhea associated with elevated prolactin levels and is not a first-line therapy for breast pain (Smith et al., 2004).

Dietary Intervention

Caffeine. Although many women report that caffeine reduction or elimination alleviates their breast pain, clinical studies have shown a response no better than placebo (Smith et al., 2004).

Vitamin E and Evening Primrose Oil. Study findings are mixed on the effectiveness of vitamin E or evening primrose oil in reducing breast pain. A recent randomized study of vitamin E found a reduction in pain in 70 percent of women following a 4-month course of therapy (Parsay, Olfati, & Nahidi, 2009). Its method of action is unknown, although it is thought to have an antioxidant effect. Another small randomized pilot study showed a trend toward cyclical mastalgia improvement when vitamin E (1,200 IU) and evening primrose oil (3 g) were used in combination or separately for 6 months (Bayles & Usatine, 2009). Until larger randomized studies are completed, it is generally agreed that a short-term trial of either or both vitamin E and evening primrose oil using the recommended dosages may be suggested (Pruthi et al., 2010).

Practical Intervention. Good external support with a properly fit sports bra is recommended as a first-line intervention for breast pain. Application of heat or cold or gentle massage may be used for temporary pain relief. Nonsteroidal anti-inflammatory drugs (NSAIDs), acetaminophen, and topical NSAIDs are effective for the treatment of mastalgia and may be a choice for first-line treatment. Women with severe pain who are considering medication use can keep a daily breast pain diary for 6 weeks to document the occurrence and severity of pain, aggravating and alleviating factors, use of medications, and interference with lifestyle (Smith et al., 2004).

NIPPLE DISCHARGE

Nipple discharge is caused by factors outside the breasts.

Galactorrhea

Galactorrhea is a spontaneous milky nipple discharge unrelated to pregnancy or nursing, or occurring more than 1 year after weaning (Hussain, Policarpio, & Vincent, 2006). It is usually bilateral, comes from multiple ducts, and is most often found in women of childbearing age.

Epidemiology. Galactorrhea is usually caused by hyperprolactinemia that may be caused by medications, hypothalamic or pituitary disorder, hypothyroidism, renal disease, or breast or nipple stimulation (Colao, 2009). Medications that may cause hyperprolactinemia by dopamine antagonism or stimulation of prolactin-producing cells in the pituitary include tricyclic antidepressants, methyldopa, metoclopramide, phenothiazines, cimetidine, calcium channel blockers, prochlorperazine, butyrophenones, opiates, oral contraceptives, and amphetamines (Molitch, 2008). Prolactinomas, tumors of the pituitary gland, cause excessive endogenous production of prolactin resulting in galactorrhea (Colao, 2009). Hypothyroidism, with increased levels of thyrotropin-releasing hormone (TRH), results in stimulation of prolactin-producing cells in the pituitary. Hyperprolactinemia is often associated with menstrual abnormalities. Details about the incidence of galactorrhea are unknown.

Subjective Data. The client reports spontaneous milky white discharge from both nipples and says that she is not pregnant or lactating. She reports no nipple changes, breast lumps, or changes to her nipples. Amenorrhea is frequently the primary presenting symptom. Visual disturbances, headaches, temperature intolerance, seizures, polyuria, or polydipsia indicate pituitary or hypothalamic disease or tumor (Leung & Pacaud, 2004). Tiredness, cold intolerance, and constipation may indicate hypothyroidism (Reid, Middleton, Cossich, & Crowther, 2010). Additionally, patients with hyperprolactinemia have an altered body composition with increased fat mass and reduced lean mass. Increased prevalence of osteoporosis and osteopenia is also associated with prolactinomas due to decreased gonadal function. The result of this combination of symptoms is often a reduced quality of life (Colao, 2009).

Objective Data

Physical Examination. Physical examination of the breasts reveals a bilateral milky nipple discharge that is not expressed from any particular areolar quadrant or duct. No redness is visible. No tenderness, mass, or lymphadenopathy is palpated. Funduscopic examination of the eyes may be normal. Signs of hypothyroidism may be present. Hirsutism and acne may be observed with chronic hyperandrogenism.

Diagnostic Tests and Methods

PREGNANCY TEST. This diagnostic evaluation need to be performed to identify if an undiagnosed pregnancy is the etiology of the galactorrhea. See Chapter 3 for information about pregnancy testing.

SERUM PROLACTIN TEST. This diagnostic evaluation is performed to identify elevated prolactin, which may be indicative of a pituitary tumor. Values greater than 20 to 25 ng/mL are considered abnormal. A level of 20 to 100 ng/mL may represent a tumor or functional hyperprolactinemia and levels above 100 ng/mL are very suggestive of a tumor. The test is best done in the morning, and manual stimulation of the breast, including breast examination, should be avoided prior to performing the test to avoid misleading elevated results. Patients with levels suggestive of a tumor should be referred for further evaluation and management.

THYROID FUNCTION TEST. Because hypothyroidism is a relatively common problem, thyroid-stimulating hormone (TSH) should be drawn with the prolactin level (Colao, 2009).

MAMMOGRAPHY. See Breast Imaging.

Differential Medical Diagnoses. Drug-induced galactorrhea, pituitary tumor, prolactinoma, hypothyroidism, chest lesion, renal disease, nonpituitary prolactin-producing tumor.

Plan

Psychosocial Interventions. Help to allay the client's anxiety through teaching and providing literature about galactorrhea. Assure the client that galactorrhea is rarely associated with breast cancer.

Medication. Close consultation with the physician is essential while managing a client with galactorrhea.

BROMOCRIPTINE. Oral or vaginal bromocriptine is primary therapy to lower prolactin levels, cause tumor shrinkage of adenoma, end galactorrhea, and restore the menses to normal if they have been irregular.

CABERGOLINE. An alternative drug is cabergoline, a long-acting dopamine agonist, which may be better tolerated with fewer side effects than bromocriptine. Consistent use of a barrier method of birth control is important.

Follow-Up. If the TSH and serum prolactin are normal, no further testing is indicated and no treatment is required if the patient does not wish to conceive, shows no evidence of hypogonadism or reduced bone density, and is not bothered by the galactorrhea. In the patient with an elevated prolactin level who is on a medication that has been associated with hyperprolactinemia, a trial off the medication should be a first step, followed by a repeat prolactin level. If the prolactin is normal, the medication should be discontinued or an alternative medication trialed. If hypothyroidism is the cause of galactorrhea, then the disorder may be managed with thyroid hormone. Consultation with a physician is strongly recommended for medical management of galactorrhea.

NIPPLE DISCHARGE CAUSED BY DUCTAL SYSTEM DISORDERS

It is normal for many women to express with external pressure a few drops of sticky, gray, green, or black viscous fluid from the nipples. This fluid is physiologic secretion. It usually emanates from multiple ducts and discharge from each duct can vary in color. It is not spontaneous or bloodstained. Women may notice it after a warm shower or nipple manipulation. If no other condition is diagnosed, patients should be advised to avoid checking for discharge and offered reassurance. Physiologic discharge often resolves when the nipple is left alone (Hussain et al., 2006).

Pathologic nipple discharge tends to be spontaneous, unilateral, and from a single duct and is serous, serosanguineous, watery, or bloody. Malignancy is found in 7 to 15 percent of cases of nipple discharge (Louie et al., 2006). All pathologic nipple discharge requires further evaluation.

Intraductal Papilloma

Epidemiology. Intraductal papilloma accounts for more than 50 percent of all causes of nipple discharge. It is thought to be caused by proliferation and overgrowth of ductal epithelial tissue. It occurs most frequently in women 45 to 50 years of age and is the most common cause of bloody nipple discharge in the absence of a mass (Hussain et al., 2006).

Subjective Data. The client reports clear or bloody discharge on her clothing. The discharge may occur spontaneously or with nipple stimulation. If the papilloma is large, the client may report a nonpainful, mobile mass usually in the areola. She may complain of an associated feeling of fullness or pain beneath the areola. On rare occasions, the client may be able to palpate only the mass.

Objective Data

Physical Examination. Physical examination of the breasts reveals bloody, serous, serosanguineous, or watery discharge, which is expressed manually from the affected duct when the nipple is systematically massaged in quadrants. A soft, poorly delineated mass may be palpable near the nipple or a small, wart-like growth may be seen at the duct orifice on the nipple (Hussain et al., 2006).

Diagnostic Tests and Methods. Test for occult blood in breast fluids. The absence of bloody nipple discharge cannot reliably exclude an underlying carcinoma. Placing a sample of the nipple discharge on a small white gauze pad in order to see the true color of the discharge will frequently reveal the presence of blood in the nipple discharge.

MAMMOGRAPHY. See Breast Imaging.

ULTRASOUND. (See Breast Imaging.) Sonogram may reveal dilated ducts, but rarely identifies a lesion.

NEEDLE CORE BIOPSY. A needle core biopsy should be performed if a mass is seen. In some cases, the biopsy can completely remove the lesion and control the symptoms.

OTHER DIAGNOSTIC IMAGING TECHNIQUES. Ductography or galactography, ductoscopy, and ductal lavage are specialized imaging techniques that may be used to identify intraductal lesions and/or obtain cell samples for diagnostic purposes (Zervoudis, Iatrakis, Economides, Polyzos, & Navrozoglou, 2010).

Differential Medical Diagnoses. Intraductal papilloma, multiple papillomatosis, duct ectasia, breast abscesses, breast cancer, and Paget's disease of the nipple (Zervoudis et al., 2010).

Plan

Psychosocial Interventions. Counsel the client regarding the benign etiology of this diagnosis.

Surgical Intervention. Surgery is indicated for cases of spontaneous single-duct discharge that is confirmed on clinical examination and has one of the following characteristics: bloody fluid, persistent (over at least two occasions per week for 4–6 weeks), associated with a mass, or is a new development in a woman over 50 years of age. Papillomas diagnosed clinically or on biopsy should be completely excised and sent for pathologic diagnosis. Refer to a surgeon who specializes in breast surgery.

MICRODOCHECTOMY. Microdochectomy is removal of a single breast duct through an areolar incision centered over the discharging duct. It is the diagnostic and therapeutic treatment of choice for spontaneous, persistent single-duct discharge (Lantis et al., 2008). The patient will still be able to breast-feed.

TOTAL DUCT EXCISION OR DIVISION. Total duct excision is a surgical procedure in which the entire ductal system of the nipple is excised through a circumareolar incision and sent for pathologic diagnosis (Nelson & Hoehn, 2006). It is indicated for nipple eversion or multiple-duct pathologic nipple discharge. Inform the patient that she will no longer be able to breast-feed and she may experience significantly reduced nipple sensitivity.

Duct Ectasia

Epidemiology. Duct ectasia is a benign inflammatory condition of increased glandular secretion and dilation of the lactiferous ducts. It usually accompanies benign breast conditions (e.g., epithelial hyperplasia and papillomatosis), but may also be associated with breast cancer (Zervoudis et al., 2010).

It is typically seen in perimenopausal or postmenopausal women (Hari, Kumar, Kumar, & Chumber, 2007).

Subjective Data. The client reports a unilateral or occasionally bilateral, cheesy, viscous nipple discharge. She may also report a nipple retraction or a lump behind her nipple (Zervoudis et al., 2010).

Objective Data

Physical Examination. Physical examination of the breasts reveals unilateral or bilateral slit-like nipple retraction at the site of the shortened duct or ducts with nipple crusting and a firm stable mass behind the nipple (Zervoudis et al., 2010). Viscous discharge can be manually expressed from the one or several ducts when the nipple is systematically massaged in quadrants.

Diagnostic Tests and Methods

MAMMOGRAPHY. See Breast Imaging.

ULTRASOUND. See Breast Imaging.

Differential Medical Diagnoses. Intraductal carcinoma, periductal mastitis, Paget's disease.

Plan

Psychosocial Interventions. Provide information on the benign status of the disease to help alleviate the client's anxiety.

Medication. In women with a secondary infection, antibiotics may be prescribed (Zervoudis et al., 2010).

Surgical Intervention. Refer to a surgeon who specializes in breast surgery for microdochectomy or total duct excision as appropriate.

Follow-Up. In women with multiple-duct discharge with normal imaging and clinical examination and no distressing symptoms reassurance is the only indicated treatment.

Periductal Mastitis

Epidemiology. Periductal mastitis is a nonpuerperal mastitis characterized clinically by periareolar in inflammation with a mass or abscess or a mammary duct fistula. It predominately affects young women of reproductive age, of which 90 percent are smokers (Dixon & Khan, 2011).

Subjective Data. The patient reports a reddened, painful nipple or breast with or without a mass. Nipple retraction or a spontaneous creamy nipple discharge may also be reported (Dixon & Khan, 2011).

Objective Data

Physical Examination. Physical examination of the breasts may reveal subareolar warmth, tenderness on palpation, erythema, nipple retraction, dimpling, induration, or a fluctuant mass (Dixon & Khan, 2011). Purulent, uniductal nipple discharge may be observed or manually expressed, and/or a mammary duct fistula, an external opening at the areolar margin, may be present (Dixon & Khan, 2011).

Diagnostic Tests and Methods

CULTURE AND SENSITIVITY. Purulent nipple discharge or aspirate of abscess may be cultured to ensure appropriate antibiotic therapy.

MAMMOGRAPHY. (See Breast Imaging.) If mammography is not tolerated because compression of the inflamed breast is painful, ultrasound is an alternative imaging choice.

ULTRASOUND. See Breast Imaging.

Differential Medical Diagnoses. Inflammatory carcinoma, Paget's disease.

Plan

Psychosocial Interventions. Provide information on the benign status of the disease to help alleviate the client's anxiety. Discuss the association between smoking and periductal mastitis, assess patient's readiness to quit, and provide appropriate counseling.

Medication. Prescribe oral antibiotic therapy for 10 days with amoxicillin clavulanate or erythromycin with metronidazole for patients with a penicillin allergy.

Surgical Intervention. Aspiration or incision and drainage. If infection does not resolve after one course of antibiotics, ultrasound should be performed to determine if an abscess has formed. An abscess should be treated with aspiration or referral to a surgeon for incision and drainage under local anesthetic and a second course of antibiotics (Dixon & Khan, 2011). Recurrent episodes may be treated with total duct excision.

Practical Intervention. Warm packs to the breast may provide pain relief and will promote drainage of the abscess. NSAIDs may be used for pain relief.

Follow-Up. After resolution of the infection, women over 35 years of age should have mammography.

MALIGNANT BREAST NEOPLASM (BREAST CANCER)

Breast cancer, an overgrowth of neoplastic cells of the breast, is a life-threatening, and when diagnosed, a life-altering, disease. With improvements in early detection and treatment, death rates from breast cancer have been decreasing since 1990 (Siegel et al., 2011).

EPIDEMIOLOGY

Breast cancer has an enormous impact on women's health, accounting for 30 percent of all new cases of cancer in the United States. In 2011, an estimated 230,480 new cases of invasive breast cancer and an estimated 57,650 cases of in situ breast cancer were diagnosed. Breast cancer is the second only to lung cancer as the leading cause of cancer-related deaths in women, with an estimated 39,520 deaths in 2011 (Siegel et al., 2011).

The precise etiology of breast cancer is unknown; however, breast cancer risk can be attributed to three broad categories of risk factors: increasing age, lifetime exposure to estrogen, and genetic susceptibility. Increasing age is an uncontrollable risk fact for breast cancer. The median age at diagnosis is 61 years with 87.8 percent of breast cancers diagnosed in women aged 45 or greater (Howlader et al., 2011).

Estrogen exposure, both endogenous and exogenous, affects risk for breast cancer with 97 percent of breast cancer diagnosed in women. Prolonged exposure to endogenous estrogen with early menarche (at or before age 12) and late menopause (at or after age 55) increased the risk of breast cancer. Nulliparous women had a 38 percent increased risk of breast cancer compared to parous women who first gave birth before age 25 and an 11 percent increased risk compared to women who gave birth after age 25 (Schonfeld et al., 2011). There appears to be a transient increase in breast cancer risk immediately following a full-term pregnancy, especially for a first birth over the age of 35. Breastfeeding also reduces the risk of breast cancer, with greater benefit seen with longer duration (Stuckey, 2011).

Exogenous estrogen exposure also increases the risk of breast cancer. The results of the Women's Health Initiative, a randomized, controlled trial of estrogen plus progestin use in postmenopausal women, showed a statistically significant increased risk for invasive breast cancer. The risk was greatest in those with recent use (within the past 5 years) and long-term use (5 or more years) (Rossouw et al., 2002). The cancers are more commonly node positive with increased mortality (Chlebowski et al., 2010). Following the release of the study, postmenopausal estrogen and progestin use dropped, with a parallel decrease in breast cancer incidence from 1999 to 2003 (Howlader et al., 2011). The results of the California Teachers Study found an increase in breast cancer risk with both estrogen therapy (23–44% for ≤ 5 to 15+ years, respectively) and estrogen–progestin therapy (60–78% for ≤ 5 to 15+ years, respectively). Risk was increased with recent compared to prior use, and with increasing duration of use (Saxena et al., 2010). A review by Cibula et al. (2010) of all published cohort and case-control studies prior to 2009 indicated a slightly increased risk of breast cancer among current users of oral contraceptives, an effect that disappeared 5 to 10 years after stopping. The use of injectable or implantable progestin-only contraceptives in women age 35 to 64 is not associated with an increased risk of breast cancer (Strom et al., 2004).

Maternal or paternal family history is a risk factor for breast cancer. A meta-analysis reported risk ratios increased with increasing numbers of affected first-degree relatives. There were increased risk ratios of 1.8 (1.69–1.91), 2.93 (2.36–3.64), and 3.90 (2.03–7.49) for one, two, and three or more affected first-degree relatives, respectively. Risk was higher in younger women and in women with younger affected relatives (Collaborative Group on Hormonal Factors in Breast Cancer, 2001).

Only 5 to 10 percent of breast cancers are due to true hereditary risk. Most of these arise from mutations in the genes BRCA1 or BRCA2, which are inherited in an autosomal dominant pattern and are thought to act as tumor suppressor genes that function in the DNA repair process (Shulman, 2010). Women who are BRCA1 mutation carriers have a cumulative breast cancer risk at age 70, with 57 percent for breast cancer and 40 percent for ovarian cancer. For women with BRCA2 mutations, the risk is 49 percent for breast cancer and 18 percent for ovarian cancer (Chen & Parmigiani, 2007). Women with BRCA1 and BRCA2 mutations tend to be diagnosed with breast cancer at a younger age (premenopausal) and have a higher prevalence of bilateral breast cancer (Shulman, 2010). BRCA1 mutation–associated breast cancers are more frequently estrogen receptor (ER), progesterone receptor (PR), and HER2 negative (triple negative) and BRCA2 mutation–associated breast cancers are more likely to be high grade, ER positive, and HER2 negative (Honrado, Benitez, & Palacios, 2006).

Genetic counseling and evaluation for testing should be offered for individuals who are at high risk for BRCA1/BRCA2-associated hereditary breast cancer (USPSTF, 2005). The NCCN (2011b) guidelines criteria for referral include an individual with a personal history of breast cancer and one or more of the following: diagnosis ≤ 45 years; diagnosis ≤ 50 years with more than one close relative with breast cancer ≤ 50 years and/or with epithelial ovarian cancer; two primary breast cancer with first diagnosed at ≤ 50 years; more than two close relatives with breast and/or epithelial ovarian cancer; close male relative with breast cancer; personal history of epithelial ovarian cancer; Ashkenazi Jews. Individuals from a family with known BRCA1/BRCA2 mutation, who have a personal history of epithelial ovarian cancer, or who have a family history of male breast cancer or a first- or second-degree relative with any of these criteria should also be referred for genetic counseling and possible testing.

Genetic testing requires counseling on the risks and benefits of testing, cancer risk if tested negative, implications for family, and cancer risk if tested positive. If a family member tests negative for a known family mutation, the risk of cancer is the same as the general population. However, an individual with a strong family history with no known mutation and a negative BRCA test will still be at increased risk. A positive test result provides data for risk, but cannot predict if the individual will actually develop breast cancer.

Women treated with chest irradiation as a child or young woman have a significantly increased risk of a diagnosis of breast cancer at a young age, similar to women with a BRCA mutation (Henderson et al., 2010). Women with a pathologic diagnosis of atypical lobular hyperplasia (ALH) and atypical ductal hyperplasia (ADH) found on core breast biopsy have at least a fourfold increased risk for breast cancer (Degnim et al., 2007). Excisional biopsy should be performed because in up to 10 to 20 percent of ductal carcinoma in situ (DCIS) cases, an invasive cancer may be found (Margenthaler et al., 2006).

Modifiable factors that contribute to breast cancer risk include alcohol use and obesity. A meta-analysis of 98 studies comparing drinkers and nondrinkers found excess risk associated with alcohol drinking was 22 percent (95% CI: 9–37%); each additional 10 g of ethanol/day was associated with an additional 10% (95% confidence interval [CI]: 5–15%) risk (Key et al., 2006). Weight gain of 25 kg or more after age 18 or weight gain of 10 kg or more after menopause is associated with an increased risk of breast cancer, whereas weight loss of 10 kg after menopause is associated with a decreased risk of breast cancer (Eliassen, Colditz, Rosner, Willett, & Hankinson, 2006).

Incidence rates for breast cancer are highest in white women and lowest in Asian/Pacific Islanders. Although black women have a lower probability of developing breast cancer, the risk of dying from breast cancer is higher than white women with the mortality rate for black women at 32.4 versus 23.4 per 100,000 for white women. Black women have a lower 5-year survival rate than white women, which may be attributed to later stage at diagnosis (Siegel et al., 2011), as well as a higher prevalence of subtypes of breast cancer with a poor prognosis (Carey et al., 2006). Incidence rates and mortality rates for breast cancer are considerably lower for Hispanic, Asian/Pacific Islanders, and American Indian/Alaska Native women (Siegel et al., 2011).

BREAST CARCINOMAS

In Situ Cancers

In situ breast cancers may arise from ductal or lobular tissue. A proliferation of malignant epithelial cells confined within the terminal ductal lobular units with no lymphatic or vascular invasions.

Ductal Carcinoma In Situ. DCIS may present clinically as a palpable mass and/or as pathologic nipple discharge but is most commonly identified on screening mammogram. It is a direct precursor to invasive cancer, but it is uncertain what percentage of women will develop invasive cancer (Virnig, Tuttle, Shamliyan, & Kane, 2010). DCIS accounted for an estimated 20 percent of new cancers diagnosed in 2010 (Siegel et al., 2011).

Lobular Carcinoma In Situ. Lobular carcinoma in situ (LCIS) is usually an incidental finding on core biopsy and has no commonly associated clinical or mammographic abnormalities. It is characteristically multifocal and bilateral (Anderson, Calhoun, & Rosen, 2006). It was thought to be a risk factor for invasive cancer, but data suggests it may be a precursor lesion to contralateral or ipsilateral, multifocal invasive lobular or ductal carcinoma (Li, Malone, & Saltzman, Daling, 2006).

Invasive Carcinoma

Tumor cells usually arise from the terminal ductal lobular unit and extend into the breast parenchyma. There may be associated lymphatic or vascular invasion.

Invasive (Infiltrating) Ductal Carcinoma. The most common invasive breast cancer, accounting for an estimated 76 percent of cases (Li, Uribe, & Daling, 2005), may present as a palpable mass and/or mammographic abnormality. Average age at diagnosis is 62 years (Siegel et al., 2011).

Invasive (Infiltrating) Lobular Carcinoma. The second most common type of invasive breast cancer, accounting for an estimated 8 percent of cases (Li et al., 2005), often presents as a larger, less-distinct mass or mammographic abnormality in older women. There is an increased risk of multifocal and contralateral cancer, and metastases tend to be later than invasive (infiltrating) ductal carcinoma (IDC) and are more likely to the peritoneum, gastrointestinal tract, and ovaries (Arpino, Bardou, Clark, & Elledge, 2004).

Tubular Carcinoma. Presenting most often as a mammographic abnormality, it accounts for less than 2 percent of invasive breast cancers and is associated with limited metastasis and excellent prognosis (Li et al., 2005).

Mucinous (Colloid) Carcinoma. It usually presents as a palpable mass or mammographic abnormality in older women aged 70 to 80 with rare metastases and a highly favorable prognosis (Di Saverio, Gutierrez, & Avisar, 2008). It accounts for an estimated 2 percent of invasive breast cancers (Li et al., 2005).

Medullary Carcinoma. This relatively uncommon cancer, accounting for less than 2 percent of invasive cancers (Li et al., 2005), occurs more frequently in relatively young women, aged 40 to 50, and has been associated with BRCA1 mutations (Iau et al., 2004). It usually presents as a palpable mass in the upper outer quadrant of the breast and has a prognosis similar to IDC (Vo et al., 2007).

Other Invasive Carcinoma. These occur infrequently and include papillary carcinoma, invasive cribriform carcinoma, invasive carcinoma with ductal and lobular features, metaplastic carcinoma, adenoid cystic carcinoma, and apocrine carcinomas.

Paget's Disease

This uncommon presentation of cancer of the nipple is associated with underlying invasive or DCIS in more than 95 percent of cases (Seetharam & Fentiman, 2009). The main presenting symptom is eczema or ulceration of the nipple.

Inflammatory Breast Cancer

This is not a distinct cancer, but a rare and aggressive variant of locally advanced breast cancer with dermal lymphatic invasion with a 50 percent 5-year survival. There is a higher incidence in African American ethnicity, high body mass index (BMI), and younger age at disease. Nearly all women have nodal involvement (Robertson et al., 2010).

SUBJECTIVE DATA

Any of the following symptoms may be reported by the patient.

- A unilateral, fixed, poorly defined lump or mass that is often located in the upper outer quadrant of the breast. It is rarely painful.
- Spontaneous, unilateral, clear, bloody discharge.
- Persistent nipple irritation with erythema, itching, scaling, crusting, or ulceration of the nipple (associated with Paget's disease).
- Dimpling of the skin, nipple retraction, change in breast contour or size.
- Rapid onset (within 6 months) of inflammation of the breast with diffuse swelling and erythema, peau d'orange, warmth, and generalized pain. It is generally not associated with a discrete mass or fever (Robertson et al., 2010). (Signs and symptoms associated with inflammatory breast cancer.)
- Axillary adenopathy or supraclavicular/infraclavicular adenopathy (advanced metastatic disease).

OBJECTIVE DATA

Physical Examination

(See Clinical Breast Examination.) Observe and palpate for all subjective symptoms, starting with the nonaffected side. The classic sign of breast cancer is a solid, solitary, three-dimensional, dominant breast mass with indistinct borders. Sometimes, ill-defined unilateral thickening may be the only sign. The lesion may be fixed to the chest wall or skin and axillary or supraclavicular/infraclavicular adenopathy may be present.

Diagnostic Tests and Methods

Mammography. See Breast Imaging.

Ultrasound. See Breast Imaging.

MRI. See Breast Imaging.

Needle Core Biopsy. See Fibroadenoma.

Excisional Biopsy. See Fibroadenoma.

Hormone Receptor Assay. Assessment of ER and PR status of malignant breast tissue is done to determine dependency on estrogen or progesterone for tumor cell growth, to predict the likelihood of response to endocrine therapy, and to prognosticate survival and recurrence. Receptor-positive tumors usually exhibit less aggressive clinical behavior, including better disease-free and overall survival and longer survival after recurrence (Bartlett et al., 2011). Bone is the most common site for metastasis (Kennecke et al., 2010).

Human Epidermal Growth Factor (ERBB2/HER2/NEU). HER2 oncogene is a growth factor receptor that controls cell growth and repair. Overexpression of HER2 by tumor cells is a prognostic indicator of poor outcome with increased rate of metastasis, decreased time to recurrence, and decreased overall survival (Callahan & Hurvitz, 2011; Slamon et al., 1987). HER2-positive tumors have a relatively high rate of metastasis to the brain, liver, lung, and bone (Kennecke et al., 2010). It is an important predictive marker of responsiveness to chemotherapy. Tumors with HER2 overexpression are responsive to anti-HER2-targeted therapies such as trastuzumab, resulting in decreased disease recurrence and increase in survival. Trastuzumab (Herceptin) is a monoclonal antibody that binds to extracellular HER2 protein and inhibits cellular growth. Herceptin is used initially in combination with chemotherapy, followed by monotherapy for a total of 52 weeks. The major risk of cardiotoxicity with Herceptin is increased with concurrent treatment with doxorubicin (Viani, Afonso, Stefano, De Fendi, & Soares, 2007).

Staging of Breast Cancer

Staging refers to grouping of patients according to extent of their disease for the purposes of determining treatment and estimating prognosis. It can be based on clinical or pathological findings. The American Joint Committee on Cancer determines cancer staging based on tumor size and extension, node number and extent, and distant metastasis. Staging is grouped as 0 through IV, with DCIS as stage 0 and any tumor with distant metastasis as stage IV. Stage I cancers are smaller or less deeply invasive with negative nodes. Stage II and III cancers have increasing tumor or nodal extent (Edge et al., 2010).

DIFFERENTIAL MEDICAL DIAGNOSES

Fibroadenomas, intraductal papilloma, eczema, mastitis.

PLAN

Women awaiting results of a breast biopsy are understandably anxious. Provide the patient with clear expectations of when and how results will be reported. It is not helpful to discuss treatment options concurrently with giving news about diagnosis because most women will hear very little after the word *cancer*. Provide an appointment with a breast surgeon, oncologist, or breast cancer team to discuss treatment options. Recommend bringing a supportive significant other to the appointment to provide support and to hear the information. Assess coping, psychological response, and social support of the patient as well as of her identified family system and recommend support groups and/or counseling as appropriate. Anxiety and/or depressive symptoms may surface or become more acute requiring medication management. A collaborative approach to caring for this patient and her family is vital.

Local and Regional Control

Surgical Treatment

Breast-Conservation Surgery (Lumpectomy, Quadrantectomy). Breast-conservation surgery followed by whole breast irradiation is an appropriate option for locoregional treatment of early stage (stages I and II) breast cancer; achieving equivalent long-term survival to mastectomy (Fisher et al., 2002). Breast-conservation surgery requires a tumor small enough to be resected with a tumor-free surrounding margin of tissue and acceptable cosmesis. There is risk of recurrence with a resultant need for completion mastectomy, although radiation therapy reduces the risk by about 70 percent (Clarke et al., 2005). Absolute contraindications to breast-conservation therapy include previous radiation therapy to the chest or breast, radiation therapy required during pregnancy, and inability to achieve a negative margin on resection. It is generally contraindicated with multicentric cancer or active connective tissue disease (NCCN, 2011a). Potential complications include wound infection, poor cosmesis due to position or size of tumor, and need for re-excision or completion mastectomy with close margins.

Mastectomy. Mastectomy may be indicated in situations where there are absolute or relative contraindications to breast-conservation surgery or it may be a woman's choice for treatment following discussion of risks and benefits of treatment options. Total or simple mastectomy is removal of the entire mammary gland and generally the nipple areolar complex. If no reconstruction is to be performed, enough skin is removed to leave the chest wall flat. A skin-sparing incision preserves the breast skin envelope and inframammary fold for breast reconstruction. In a select group of patients with low risk for nipple areolar recurrence, nipple-sparing mastectomy may be an option (Reefy et al., 2010). Modified radical mastectomy includes the removal of axillary nodes when there is positive nodal involvement. Radical mastectomy includes resection of muscle as well and is reserved for gross tumor invasion only. All women should be offered the opportunity to meet with a reconstruction surgeon to discuss options for breast reconstruction. Because reconstruction can limit the ability to deliver optimal radiation therapy in some patients, those with known or at high risk for postmastectomy radiation therapy should discuss options prior to making surgical decisions (Reefy et al., 2010). Postsurgical complications include wound infection, seroma, and lymphedema. Locoregional recurrence after mastectomy for early stage breast cancer is approximately 5 percent (Vaughan et al., 2007).

Axillary Lymph Node Dissection/ Sentinel Lymph Node Biopsy. Axillary lymph node status is the single most important prognostic factor in women with early stage breast cancer. Histologic examination of axillary lymph nodes assesses spread of disease to the lymph nodes for staging and to guide systemic treatment. Current standard of care is sentinel lymph node (SLN) biopsy in women with clinically negative axillary lymph nodes with invasive or microinvasive breast cancer. Axillary lymph node dissection (ALND) is the removal of level I and/or II axillary lymph nodes and is indicated in women with preoperative diagnosis of axillary metastasis by FNA or core biopsy, neoadjuvant chemotherapy, or positive SLN biopsy (Lyman et al., 2005).

SLN biopsy is based on the idea that malignant cells metastasize in an orderly way from the primary tumor to the SLNs, then to other nearby lymph nodes. If the SLN is negative, ALND is not indicated because a negative SLN accurately stages the axilla and is associated with isolated recurrence in the axilla in less than 1 percent of cases (Naik et al., 2004). Current research is examining recurrence and survival outcomes in ALND versus radiation therapy and systemic therapy in women with positive lymph nodes (Guiliano et al., 2011). The rate of adverse events, such as lymphedema, is considerably less in women undergoing SLN biopsy versus ALND (Guiliano et al., 2011).

Breast Reconstruction. All women undergoing surgical treatment for breast cancer should be offered the opportunity to discuss breast reconstruction with a reconstructive surgeon at the time of initial surgical decision making. In the United States, the Women's Health and Cancer Rights Act of 1998 mandates insurance coverage of reconstruction if the insurance plan provides mastectomy coverage. The law also mandates coverage of breast symmetry procedures (such as augmentation, reduction, and mastopexy), prostheses, and physical complications of mastectomy (U.S. Department of Labor, 2009). Although the primary goal of breast reconstruction is to correct the anatomic defect created by mastectomy, it can also improve the psychosocial well-being and quality of life of patients who have breast cancer. Reconstruction options involve the use of implants or the patient's own tissue (autologous tissue reconstruction) and can be done at the time of mastectomy (immediate) or any time thereafter (delayed) (Hu & Alderman, 2007).

Immediate reconstruction is a good option for women with early stage breast cancer who do not anticipate radiation therapy or adjuvant chemotherapy (Hu & Alderman, 2007). It is associated with low morbidity and high levels of patient satisfaction (Reefy et al., 2010). Delayed reconstruction usually starts after wound healing and/or healing following radiation therapy or adjuvant chemotherapy (Hu & Alderman, 2007). There continues to be controversy about timing of reconstruction and radiation therapy. In patients with a high likelihood of requiring radiation therapy, delayed autologous reconstruction may be a better option. The reconstructive surgeon evaluates patient preference, cancer treatment, body habitus, and comorbidities in determining the best surgical option and timing for breast reconstruction.

Implant-based reconstruction using a tissue expander followed by permanent placement of saline or silicone implant is the most common form of breast reconstruction. In 2006, following a 14-year moratorium for safety concerns, the FDA (2006) approved the use of silicone implants for breast reconstruction in women of all ages. This two-stage process starts with placement of an expander in a submuscular pocket following a skin-sparing mastectomy. Saline is added weekly to overexpand the pocket and then the implant is placed in a second operation. Although the initial operation and recovery period is shorter, the expansion and final placement of the implants may take 6 to 9 months or longer (Hu & Alderman, 2007).

Autologous tissue reconstruction provides the most natural texture and appearance. The procedures include transverse rectus abdominis myocutaneous (TRAM) flap, deep inferior epigastric perforator, and superficial inferior epigastric artery flaps. Women need adequate extra soft tissue in the donor site, usually the abdominal wall. Tissue is transferred from the abdominal wall through a tunnel under the skin and extended through an excision in the breast area to create the new breast. The blood supply remains attached in a pedicled flap or is separated and reattached in a free flap. Latissimus dorsi myocutaneous flap procedure is used primarily in candidates who cannot undergo TRAM procedures and uses skin, fat, and muscle from the back. These procedures involve a second surgical site, longer operation, and 2- to 4-month recovery period, with the potential for abdominal wall laxity or hernia (Hu & Alderman, 2007).

The final stage of total breast reconstruction is nipple areolar reconstruction. This is a separate procedure done at least 6 to 8 weeks after reconstruction. Areolar reconstruction is done using skin grafting or tattooing.

Nipple reconstruction can be accomplished with a free nipple graft from the contralateral nipple or with a local flap. The patient should understand that although it will look like a nipple, sensation and function will not be restored.

In women undergoing unilateral mastectomy and reconstruction, modifications to the shape or size of the contralateral breast may be required to maintain symmetry. The most common procedures necessary are reduction mammoplasty, mastopexy, or augmentation mammoplasty.

Mastopexy. Mastopexy (breast lift) is performed to improve the appearance of ptotic (sagging) breasts. The breast, nipple, and areola are lifted to match the reconstructed breast. Adverse outcomes may be loss of sensation in the nipple and areolar, scar formation or fat necrosis, and the inability to breast-feed (De Benito & Sanchez, 2010).

Reduction Mammoplasty. Breast-reduction surgery is performed to reduce breast size and relieve back and shoulder pain caused by heavy pendulous breasts. Women may complain of neck strain, low back pain, occipital headache, shoulder pain, self-consciousness, and difficulty participating in exercise or sports activities. Reduction is also preformed for women undergoing a unilateral mastectomy with reconstruction or lumpectomy to provide symmetry to the contralateral breast. Adverse outcomes are dependent on type of surgery and may include loss of sensation in the nipple and areola, scar formation or fat necrosis, and loss of the ability to breast-feed (Noone, 2010).

Augmentation Mammoplasty. Breast-augmentation surgery is performed to improve the cosmetic appearance of the breast by increasing its size. Augmentation of the contralateral breast may be necessary for women with very small breasts undergoing mastectomy and reconstruction to maintain symmetry between the two breasts. A submuscular implant is used and can also give lift to the breast (Thorne, 2010). Women with implants may have a higher incidence of lactation insufficiency (Michalopoulos, 2007).

Radiation Therapy. Whole breast irradiation is used in conjunction with breast-conservation therapy to eradicate residual, subclinical disease, thereby decreasing recurrence and improving survival (Hulvat, Hansen, & Jeruss, 2009). Usual therapy is 5 to 6 weeks. Radiation therapy is also indicated for treatment of microscopic disease in regional lymph nodes and postmastectomy with four or more positive nodes (Lee & Jagsi, 2007). Accelerated partial breast irradiation is currently being investigated as an option to shorten radiation therapy (Beitsch, Shaitelman, & Vicini, 2011). Refer to a radiation oncologist for management. Side effects include fatigue, skin changes, lymphedema, and atrophy of breast tissue. Cardiac complications and development of a secondary cancer are rare events (Meric et al., 2002). Fatigue varies among individuals and returns to normal within a month after treatment. Posttreatment skin changes may persist for months and protection from sun exposure is recommended.

Systemic Control

The cause of death in breast cancer is organ dysfunction causes by distant metastases. Adjuvant systemic therapy is the administration of chemotherapy, endocrine therapy, or other targeted therapies following primary surgery for early stage invasive breast cancer to eliminate or inhibit the growth of micrometastases, thereby preventing recurrence and improving survival. Neoadjuvant therapy uses the same therapies except it is given before surgery to shrink the primary tumor as well as eliminate micrometastases. Refer to an oncologist for management. Some women may desire a second opinion before starting treatment.

Endocrine Therapy. Endocrine therapy is the most effective systemic treatment for hormone receptor–positive breast cancer. It prevents cancer cells from receiving stimulation from endogenous estrogen by lowering the level of estrogen with ovarian ablation (chemical and surgical) and aromatase inhibitors (AIs) or blocking the ER pathway with selective estrogen receptor modulators (SERMs) (Burstein et al., 2010). Treatment is usually begun after completion of chemotherapy and radiation therapy.

SERM. Tamoxifen, the most commonly prescribed SERM for breast cancer treatment, has estrogen antagonist effect in the breast and favorable estrogen agonist effect on bone mineral density and blood lipid profiles (Burstein et al., 2010). Tamoxifen taken for 5 years prolongs disease-free and overall survival in premenopausal and postmenopausal women (Early Breast Cancer Trialists' Collaborative Group, 2005). Raloxifene is approved for the prevention of breast cancer in high-risk women (Vogel et al., 2010). In postmenopausal women, optional treatment is with 2 years of tamoxifen, followed by 3 years of an AI (Burstein et al., 2010). Discuss menopausal side effects and management as well as risk of endometrial hyperplasia or cancer. Encourage yearly gynecologic examination and endometrial biopsy of any reported vaginal discharge or bleeding.

Aromatase Inhibitors (Anastrozole, Letrozole, or Exemestane). AIs block the synthesis of estrogen in tissues containing the enzyme and lower serum and tumor estrogen. They are indicated only for postmenopausal women and may be used alone or sequentially with tamoxifen, especially in women whose menopausal status is in question (Rugo, 2008). They are usually prescribed for 5 years or for 3 to 5 years following tamoxifen therapy (Burstein et al., 2010). Common adverse effects include joint pain and stiffness, hot flashes, lipid disorders, bone loss, ischemic cardiovascular disease, venous thromboembolism. Patients who are unable to tolerate the adverse effects of one medication may trial another AI.

Chemotherapy. The cytotoxic chemotherapeutic agents used most commonly in breast cancer include antimitotic agents, anthracyclines, alkylating agents, and antimicrotubules. Drugs are usually used as combination therapy for invasive breast cancer. The preferred regimens are docetaxel/doxorubicin/cyclophosphamide, doxorubicin/cyclophosphamide (AC), followed by pacltaxel, docetaxel/cyclophosphamide, and AC (NCCN, 2011a). Cytotoxic agents may also be used in combination with endocrine therapy or trastuzumab. The oncologist considers biologic features of the tumor, stage, comorbid conditions, and patient preferences in making the decision to start treatment and selecting the appropriate treatment regimen. Molecular genomic testing, such as Oncotype DX™, is useful in determining the benefit of chemotherapy in node negative ER positive patients. Side effects vary with the chemotherapeutic agent and tend to be moderate in severity. They may include alopecia, nausea, fatigue, myelosuppression, anemia, neuropathy, and myalgias. Cardiotoxicity has been associated with anthracyclines (NCCN, 2011a).

Targeted Therapies. Targeted cancer therapies block the growth and spread of cancer by interfering with specific molecules involved in tumor growth and progression. Bevacizumab, an angiogenesis inhibitor, and lapatinib, which targets a cell growth factor, are examples of agents already being used in the treatment of breast cancer. Agents such as PARP inhibitors and insulin-like growth factor in research development and clinical trials hold promise for breast cancers unresponsive to standard treatment (NCCN, 2011a).

Survivorship Care

It is estimated there are over 2.5 million breast cancers survivors in the United States (Howlader et al., 2011). Follow-up care for these women requires coordinated care between specialists and primary care providers to monitor for the development of recurrent disease. The optimal surveillance for breast cancer recurrence is routine history and physical examination observing for signs and symptoms of a new mass or skin change in the breast, chest, or axilla; axillary discomfort; nipple discharge; bone, chest, or abdominal pain; shortness of breath; or persistent headache (Khatcheressian et al., 2006). Breast cancer recurrences are most common in bone, soft tissue, lung, liver, and brain. Because the highest risk of recurrence is in the first 5 years, exams should be every 3 to 6 months for 3 years, then every 6 to 12 months for 2 years, then annually thereafter (Hayes, 2007). Annual mammography and self-breast exams of the contralateral and ipsilateral breast if conserved are recommended by the American Society of Clinical Oncology guidelines (Khatcheressian et al., 2006). Annual screening mammograms should be continued in elderly breast cancer survivors as long as there is reasonable functional status and life expectancy (Schootman, Jeffe, Lian, Aft, & Gillanders, 2008). Mammogram is not indicated following breast reconstruction.

Complementary and Alternative Medicine

Breast cancer survivors endure a multitude of symptoms and late effects during and following treatment for breast cancer. The Women's Healthy Eating and Living Study surveyed breast cancer survivors about the use of complementary and alternative medicines (CAM) to improve symptoms and quality of life. Of the 2,527 women who completed the survey, 80 percent reported CAM use, including naturopathy (85%), homeopathy (74%), acupuncture (71%), and chiropractic medicine (47%) (Saxe et al., 2008). CAM may have adverse or positive effects. Some herbal preparations react adversely with chemotherapeutic agents and should be avoided. Other complementary therapies may provide a beneficial effect. Blaes, Kreitzer, Torkelson, and Haddad (2011) reviewed evidence in support of CAM for symptom management in breast cancer survivors. They found evidence demonstrating physical exercise was effective in relief of fatigue; cognitive-behavioral therapy was beneficial in relief of insomnia; mindfulness-based stress reduction and yoga were effective in quality-of-life changes; and acupuncture was effective in relief of hot flashes, fatigue, and arthralgias. Complementary and integrative therapies should be offered to patients as options for managing symptoms and stress of cancer treatment.

REFERENCES

American Cancer Society. (2011). *Breast cancer: Early detection.* Retrieved from http://www.cancer.org/Cancer/BreastCancer/MoreInformation/BreastCancerEarlyDetection/

American College of Obstetricians and Gynecologists. (2011, August). *Practice bulletin, number 122: Breast cancer screening.* Retrieved from http://www.acog.org/publications/educational_bulletins/pb122.cfm

Anderson, B.O., Calhoun, K.E., & Rosen, E.L. (2006). Evolving concepts in the management of lobular neoplasia. *Journal of the National Comprehensive Cancer Network, 4*(5), 511–522.

Arpino, G., Bardou, V.J., Clark, G.M., & Elledge, R.M. (2004). Infiltrating lobular carcinoma of the breast: Tumor characteristics and clinical outcome. *Breast Cancer Research, 6*(3), R149–R156. doi:10.1186/bcr767

Barros, A.C., Mottola, J., Ruiz, C.A., Borges, M.N., & Pinotti, J.A. (1999). Reassurance in the treatment of mastalgia. *Breast Journal, 5*(3), 162–165.

Bartlett, J.M., Brookes, C.L., Robson, T., van de Velde, C.J., Billingham, L.J., Campbell, F.M., et al. (2011). Estrogen receptor and progesterone receptor as predictive biomarkers of response to endocrine therapy: A prospectively powered pathology study in the tamoxifen and exemestane adjuvant multinational trial. *Journal of Clinical Oncology: Official Journal of the American Society of Clinical Oncology, 29*(12), 1531–1538. doi:10.1200/JCO.2010.30.3677

Barton, M.B., Harris, R., & Fletcher, S.W. (1999). The rational clinical examination. Does this patient have breast cancer? The screening clinical breast examination: Should it be done? How? *Journal of the American Medical Association, 282*(13), 1270–1280.

Bayles, B., & Usatine, R. (2009). Evening primrose oil. *American Family Physician, 80*(12), 1405–1408.

Beitsch, P.D., Shaitelman, S.F., & Vicini, F.A. (2011). Accelerated partial breast irradiation. *Journal of Surgical Oncology, 103*(4), 362–368. doi:10.1002/jso.21785;10.1002/jso.21785

Berg, W. (2009). Tailored supplemental screening for breast cancer: What now and what next? *American Journal of Roentgenology, 192*(2), 390–399. doi:10.2214/AJR.08.1706

Berry, D.A., Iversen, E.S., Gudbjartsson, D.F., Hiller, E.H., Garber, J.E., Peshkin, B.N., et al. (2002). BRCAPRO validation, sensitivity of genetic testing of BRCA1/BRCA2, and prevalence of other breast cancer susceptibility genes. *Journal of Clinical Oncology, 20,* 2701–2712.

Blaes, A.H., Kreitzer, M.J., Torkelson, C., & Haddad, T. (2011). Nonpharmacologic complementary therapies in symptom management for breast cancer survivors. *Seminars in Oncology, 38*(3), 394–402. doi:10.1053/j.seminoncol.2011.03.009

Brem, R.F., Shahan, C., Rapleyea, J.A., Donnelly, C.A., Rechtman, L.R., Kidwell, A.B., et al. (2010). Detection of occult foci of breast cancer using breast-specific gamma imaging in women with one mammographic or clinically suspicious breast lesion. *Academic Radiology, 17*(6), 735–743. doi:10.1016/j.acra.2010.01.017

Burstein, H.J., Prestrud, A.A., Seidenfeld, J., Anderson, H., Buchholz, T.A., Davidson, N.E., et al. (2010). American Society of Clinical Oncology clinical practice guideline: Update on adjuvant endocrine therapy for women with hormone receptor-positive breast cancer. *Journal of Clinical Oncology: Official Journal of the American Society of Clinical Oncology, 28*(23), 3784–3796. doi:10.1200/JCO.2009.26.3756

Callahan, R., & Hurvitz, S. (2011). Human epidermal growth factor receptor-2-positive breast cancer: Current management of early, advanced, and recurrent disease. *Current Opinions in Obstetrics and Gynecology, 23*(1), 37–43.

Carey, L.A., Perou, C.M., Livasy, C.A., Dressler, L.G., Cowan, D., Conway, K., et al. (2006). Race, breast cancer subtypes, and survival in the Carolina Breast Cancer Study. *Journal of the American Medical Association, 295*(21), 2492–2502. doi:10.1001/jama.295.21.2492

Chen, S., & Parmigiani, G. (2007). Meta-analysis of BRCA1 and BRCA2 penetrance. *Journal of Clinical Oncology: Official Journal of the American Society of Clinical Oncology, 25*(11), 1329–1333. doi:10.1200/JCO.2006.09.1066

Chlebowski, R.T., Anderson, G.L., Gass, M., Lane, D.S., Aragaki, A.K., Kuller, L.H., et al. (2010). Estrogen plus progestin and breast cancer incidence and mortality in postmenopausal women. *Journal of the American Medical Association, 304*(15), 1684–1692. doi:10.1001/jama.2010.1500

Cibula, D., Gompel, A., Mueck, A.O., La Vecchia, C., Hannaford, P.C., Skouby, S.O., et al. (2010). Hormonal contraception and risk of cancer. *Human Reproduction Update, 16*(6), 631–650. doI:10.1093/humupd/dmq022

Clarke, M., Collins, R., Darby, S., Davies, C., Elphinstone, P., Evans, et al. (2005). Effects of radiotherapy and of differences in the extent of surgery for early breast cancer on local recurrence and 15-year survival: An overview of the randomized trials. *Lancet, 366*(9291), 2087–2106. doi:10.1016/S0140-6736(05)67887-7

Colao, A. (2009). Pituitary tumours: The prolactinoma. *Best Practice and Research. Clinical Endocrinology and Metabolism, 23*(5), 575–596. doi:10.1016/j.beem.2009.05.003

Collaborative Group on Hormonal Factors in Breast Cancer. (2001). Familial breast cancer: Collaborative reanalysis of individual data from 52 epidemiological studies including 58,209 women with breast cancer and 101,986 women without the disease. *Lancet, 358*(9291), 1389–1399. doi:10.1016/S0140-6736(01)06524-2

De Benito, J., & Sanchez, K. (2010). Key points in mastopexy. *Aesthetic Plastic Surgery, 34*(6), 711–715. doi:10.1007/s00266-010-9527-5

Degnim, A.C., Visscher, D.W., Berman, H.K., Frost, M.H., Sellers, T.A., Vierkant, R.A., et al. (2007). Stratification of breast cancer risk in women with atypia: A Mayo cohort study. *Journal of Clinical Oncology: Official Journal of the American Society of Clinical Oncology, 25*(19), 2671–2677. doi:10.1200/JCO.2006.09.0217

Delille, J.P., Slanetz, P.J., Yeh, E.D., Kopans, D.B., & Garrido, L. (2005). Physiologic changes in breast magnetic resonance imaging during the menstrual cycle: Perfusion imaging, signal enhancement, and influence of the T1 relaxation time of breast tissue. *Breast Journal, 11*(4), 236–241. doi:10.1111/j.1075-122X.2005.21499.x

Di Saverio, S., Gutierrez, J., & Avisar, E. (2008). A retrospective review with long term follow up of 11,400 cases of pure mucinous breast carcinoma. *Breast Cancer Research and Treatment, 111*(3), 541–547. doi:10.1007/s10549-007-9809-z

Dixon, J.M., & Khan, L.R. (2011). Treatment of breast infection. *British Medical Journal, 342,* d396. doi:10.1136/bmj.d396

Dongola, N., Lewin, J.M., Coombs, B.D., Azavedo, E., Krasny, R.M., & Davis, L.M. (2011). Mammography in breast cancer. *Medscape Reference*. Retrieved from http://emedicine.medscape.com/article/346529-overview?src=emailthis

D'Orsi, C.J., Bassett, L.W., Berg, W.A., et al. (2003). BI-RADS: Mammography. In C.J. D'Orsi, E.B. Mendelson, D.M. Ikeda, et al. (Eds.), *Breast imaging reporting and data system: ACR BI-RADS—Breast imaging atlas* (4th ed.). Reston, VA: American College of Radiology.

Early Breast Cancer Trialists' Collaborative Group (EBCTCG). (2005). Effects of chemotherapy and hormonal therapy for early breast cancer on recurrence and 15-year survival: An overview of the randomized trials. *Lancet, 365*(9472), 1687–1717. doi:10.1200/JCO.2009.23.1274

Edge, S.B., Byrd, D.R., Compton, C.C., Fritz, A.G., Greene, F.L., & Trotti, A. (Eds.). (2010). *AJCC cancer staging manual* (7th ed.). New York: Springer.

Eliassen, A.H., Colditz, G.A., Rosner, B., Willett, W.C., & Hankinson, S.E. (2006). Adult weight change and risk of postmenopausal breast cancer. *Journal of the American Medical Association, 296*(2), 193–201. doi:10.1001/jama.296.2.193

Fisher, B., Anderson, S., Bryant, J., Margolese, R.G., Deutsch, M., Fisher, E.R., et al. (2002). Twenty-year follow-up of a randomized trial comparing total mastectomy, lumpectomy, and lumpectomy plus irradiation for the treatment of invasive breast cancer. *New England Journal of Medicine, 347*(16), 1233–1241. doi:10.1056/NEJMoa022152

Food and Drug Administration. (2006). *FDA approves silicone gel-filled implants after in-depth evaluation*. Retrieved from http://www.fda.gov/NewsEvents/Newsroom/PressAnnouncements/2006/ucm108790.htm

Foxcroft, L.M., Evans, E.B., & Porter, A.J. (2004). The diagnosis of breast cancer in women younger than 40. *Breast, 13,* 297–306.

Goodemote, P., Mitchell, D., & Nichols, W. (2008). What is the best way to screen for breast cancer in women with implants? *Journal of Family Practice, 57*(7), 482–483.

Goodson, W.H., Hunt, T.K., Plotnik, J., & Moore, D.H. (2008). *A prospective evaluation of the utility of clinical breast examination*. Poster Session V presented at the 31st Annual San Antonio Breast Cancer Symposium, San Antonio, TX.

Griffin, J., & Pearlman, M.D. (2010). Breast cancer screening in women at average risk and high risk. *Obstetrics and Gynecology, 116*(6), 410–1421.

Guiliano, A.E., Hunt, K.K., Ballman, K.V., Beitsch, P.D., Whitworth, P.W., Blumencranz, P.W., et al. (2011). Axillary dissection vs no axillary dissection in women with invasive breast cancer and sentinel node metastasis: A randomized clinical trial. *Journal of American Medical Association, 305*(6), 569–575.

Guray, M., & Sahin, A.A. (2006). Benign breast diseases: Classification, diagnosis, and management. *Oncologist, 11*(5), 435–449. doi:10.1634/theoncologist.11-5-435

Hari, S., Kumar, J., Kumar, A., & Chumber, S. (2007). Bilateral severe mammary duct ectasia. *Acta Radiologica, 48*(4), 398–400. doi:10.1080/02841850701230226

Hayes, D.F. (2007). Clinical practice: Follow-up of patients with early breast cancer. *New England Journal of Medicine, 356*(24), 2505–2513. doi:10.1056/NEJMcp067260

Heisey, R.E., & McCready, D.R. (2010). Office management of a palpable breast lump with aspiration. *Canadian Medical Association Journal = Journal De l'Association Medicale Canadienne, 182*(7), 693–696. doi:10.1503/cmaj.090416

Henderson, T.O., Amsterdam, A., Bhatia, S., Hudson, M.M., Meadows, A.T., Neglia, J.P., et al. (2010). Systematic review: Surveillance for breast cancer in women treated with chest radiation for childhood, adolescent, or young adult cancer. *Annals of Internal Medicine, 152*(7), 444–455, W144–W154. doi:10.1059/0003-4819-152-7-201004060-00009

Honrado, E., Benitez, J., & Palacios, J. (2006). Histopathology of BRCA1- and BRCA2-associated breast cancer. *Critical Reviews in Oncology/Hematology, 59*(1), 27–39. doi:10.1016/j.critrevonc.2006.01.006

Howlader, N., Noone, A.M., Krapcho, M., Neyman, N., Aminou, R., Waldron, W., et al. (2011). *SEER cancer statistics review, 1975-2008*. Bethesda, MD: National Cancer Institute. Retrieved from http://seer.cancer.gov/csr/1975_2008/

Hu, E., & Alderman, A.K. (2007). Breast reconstruction. *Surgical Clinics of North America, 87*(2), 453–467. doi:10.1016/j.suc.2007.01.004

Hulvat, M.C., Hansen, N.M., & Jeruss, J.S. (2009). Multidisciplinary care for patients with breast cancer. *Surgical Clinics of North America, 89*(1), 133–176. doi:10.1016/j.suc.2008.10.002

Huo, D., Senie, R.T., Daly, M., Buys, S.S., Cummings, S., Ogutha, J., et al. (2009). Prediction of BRCA mutations using the BRCAPRO model in clinic-based African American, Hispanic, and other minority families in the United States. *Journal of Clinical Oncology: Official Journal of the American Society of Clinical Oncology, 27*(8), 1184–1190. doi:10.1200/JCO.2008.17.5869

Hussain, A.N., Policarpio, C., & Vincent, M.T. (2006). Evaluating nipple discharge. *Obstetrical and Gynecological Survey, 61*(4), 278–283. doi:10.1097/01.ogx.0000210242.44171.f6

Iau, P.T., Marafie, M., Ali, A., Sng, J.H., Macmillan, R.D., Pinder, S., et al. (2004). Are medullary breast cancers an indication for BRCA1 mutation screening? A mutation analysis of 42 cases of medullary breast cancer. *Breast Cancer Research and Treatment, 85*(1), 81–88. doi:10.1023/B:BREA.0000021049.61839.e5

Jayasinghe, Y., & Simmons, P. (2009). Fibroadenomas in adolescence. *Current Opinions in Obstetrics and Gynecology, 21*(5), 402–406.

Kabat, G.C., Jones, J.G., Olson, N., Negassa, A., Duggan, C., Ginsberg, M., et al. (2010). A multi-center prospective cohort study of benign breast disease and risk of subsequent breast cancer. *Cancer Causes and Control, 21*(6), 821–828. doi:10.1007/s10552-010-9508-7

Kennecke, H., Yerushalmi, R., Woods, R., Cheang, M.C., Voduc, D., Speers, C.H., et al. (2010). Metastatic behavior of breast cancer subtypes. *Journal of Clinical Oncology: Official Journal of the American Society of Clinical Oncology, 28*(20), 3271–3277. doi:10.1200/JCO.2009.25.9820

Key, J., Hodgson, S., Omar, R.Z., Jensen, T.K., Thompson, S.G., Boobis, A.R., et al. (2006). Meta-analysis of studies of alcohol and breast cancer with consideration of the methodological issues. *Cancer Causes and Control, 17*(6), 759–770. doi:10.1007/s10552-006-0011-0

Khatcheressian, J.L., Wolff, A.C., Smith, T.J., Grunfeld, E., Muss, H.B., Vogel, V.G., et al. (2006). American society of clinical oncology 2006 update of the breast cancer follow-up and management guidelines in the adjuvant setting. *Journal of Clinical Oncology: Official Journal of the American Society of Clinical Oncology, 24*(31), 5091–5097. doi:10.1200/JCO.2006.08.8575

Lantis, S., Filippakis, G., Thomas, J., Christofides, T., Al Mufti, R., & Hadjiminas, D.J. (2008). Microdochectomy for single-duct pathologic nipple discharge and normal or benign imaging and cytology. *Breast, 17*(3), 309–313.

Lee, M.C., & Jagsi, R. (2007). Postmastectomy radiation therapy: Indications and controversies. *Surgical Clinics of North America, 87*(2), 511–526.

Lehman, C.D., Gatsonis, C., Kuhl, C.K., Hendrick, R.E., Pisano, E.D., Hanna, L., et al. (2007). MRI evaluation of the contralateral breast in women with recently diagnosed breast cancer. *New England Journal of Medicine, 356*(13), 1295–1303. doi:10.1056/NEJMoa065447

Leung, A.K., & Pacaud, D. (2004). Diagnosis and management of galactorrhea. *American Family Physician, 70*(3), 543–550.

Li, C.I., Malone, K.E., Saltzman, B.S., & Daling, J.R. (2006). Risk of invasive breast carcinoma among women diagnosed with ductal carcinoma in situ and lobular carcinoma in situ, 1988-2001. *Cancer, 106*(10), 2104–2112. doi:10.1002/cncr.21864

Li, C.I., Uribe, D.J., & Daling, J.R. (2005). Clinical characteristics of different histologic types of breast cancer. *British Journal of Cancer, 93*(9), 1046–1052. doi:10.1038/sj.bjc.6602787

Louie, L.D., Crowe, J.P., Dawson, A.E., Lee, K.B., Baynes, D.L., Dowdy, T., et al. (2006). Identification of breast cancer in patients with pathologic nipple discharge: Does ductoscopy predict malignancy? *American Journal of Surgery, 192*(4), 530–533. doi:10.1016/j.amjsurg.2006.06.004

Lyman, G.H., Giuliano, A.E., Somerfield, M.R., Benson, A.B., Bodurka, D.C., Burstein, H.J., et al. (2005). American Society of Clinical Oncology guideline recommendations for sentinel lymph node biopsy in early-stage breast cancer. *Journal of Clinical Oncology, 23*(30), 7703–7720.

Marchant, D.J. (2002). Benign diseases of the breast. *Obstetrics and Gynecology Clinics of North America, 29*(1), 1–20.

Margenthaler, J.A., Duke, D., Monsees, B.S., Barton, P.T., Clark, C., & Dietz, J.R. (2006). Correlation between core biopsy and excisional biopsy in breast high-risk lesions. *American Journal of Surgery, 192*(4), 534–537. doi:10.1016/j.amjsurg.2006.06.003

Meric, F., Buchholz, T.A., Mirza, N.Q., Vlastos, G., Ames, F.C., Ross, M.I., et al. (2002). Long-term complications associated with breast-conservation surgery and radiotherapy. *Annals of Surgical Oncology, 9*(6), 543–549.

Michalopoulos, K. (2007). The effects of breast augmentation surgery on future ability to lactate. *Breast Journal, 13*(1), 62–67.

Miltenburg, D., & Speights, V.O. (2008). Benign breast disease. *Obstetrics and Gynecology Clinics of North America, 35*(2), 285–300.

Molitch, M.E. (2008). Drugs and prolactin. *Pituitary, 11*(2), 209–218. doi:10.1007/s11102-008-0106-6

Morrow, M. (2000). The evaluation of common breast problems. *American Family Physician, 61*(8), 2371–2378, 2385.

Naik, A.M., Fey, J., Gemignani, M., Heerdt, A., Montgomery, L., Petrek, J., et al. (2004). The risk of axillary relapse after sentinel lymph node biopsy for breast cancer is comparable with that of axillary lymph node dissection: A follow-up study of 4008 procedures. *Annals of Surgery, 240*(3), 462–468.

National Cancer Institute. (2008). *Breast cancer risk assessment tool*. Retrieved from http://www.cancer.gov/bcrisktool/

National Cancer Institute. (2010). *Fact sheet: Mammograms*. Retrieved from http://www.cancer.gov/cancertopics/factsheet/detection/mammograms

National Cancer Institute's Breast Cancer Surveillance Consortium. (2009). *Performance benchmarks for screening mammography*. Retrieved from http://breastscreening.cancer.gov/data/benchmarks/screening

National Comprehensive Cancer Network. (2010). *Clinical practice guidelines in oncology: Breast cancer screening and diagnosis* (Version 1.2011). Retrieved from http://www.nccn.org/professionals/physician_gls/pdf/breast-screening.pdf

National Comprehensive Cancer Network. (2011a). *Clinical practice guidelines in oncology: Breast cancer* (Version 2.2011). Retrieved from http://www.nccn.org/professionals/physician_gls/pdf/breast.pdf

National Comprehensive Cancer Network. (2011b). *Clinical practice guidelines in oncology: Breast cancer risk reduction* (Version 3.2011). Retrieved from http://www.nccn.org/professionals/physician_gls/pdf/breast_risk.pdf

Nelson, H.D., Tyne, K., Naik, A., Bougatsos, C., Chan, B., Nygren, P., et al. (2009). *Screening for breast cancer: Systematic evidence review update for the US Preventative Services Task Force* (Evidence syntheses, No. 74). Rockville, MD: Agency for Healthcare Research and Quality (US). Retrieved from http://www.ncbi.nlm.nih.gov/books/NBK36392

Nelson, R.S., & Hoehn, J.L. (2006). Twenty-year outcome following central duct resection for bloody nipple discharge. *Annals of Surgery, 243*(4), 522–524. doi:10.1097/01.sla.0000205828.61184.31

Noone, R.B. (2010). An evidence-based approach to reduction mammaplasty. *Plastic and Reconstructive Surgery, 126*(6), 2171–2176. doi:10.1097/PRS.0b013e3181f830d7

Parsay, S., Olfati, F., & Nahidi, S. (2009). Therapeutic effects of vitamin E on cyclic mastalgia. *Breast Journal, 15*(5), 510–514.

Pearlman, M.D., & Griffin, J.L. (2010). Benign breast disease. *Obstetrics and Gynecology, 116*(3), 747–758.

Pruthi, S., Wahner-Roedler, D.L., Torkelson, C.J., Cha, S.S., Thicke, L.S., Hazelton, J.H., et al. (2010). Vitamin E and evening primrose oil for management of cyclical mastalgia: A randomized pilot study. *Alternative Medicine Review, 15*(1), 59–67.

Reefy, S., Patani, N., Anderson, A., Burgoyne, G., Osman, H., & Mokbel, K. (2010). Oncological outcome and patient satisfaction with skin-sparing mastectomy and immediate breast reconstruction: A prospective observational study. *BMC Cancer, 10,*171–182. doi:10.1186/1471-2407-171

Reid, S.M., Middleton, P., Cossich, M.C., & Crowther, C.A. (2010). Interventions for clinical and subclinical hypothyroidism in pregnancy. *Cochrane Database of Systematic Reviews,* (7), CD007752. doi:10.1002/14651858.CD007752.pub2

Robertson, F.M., Bondy, M., Yang, W., Yamauchi, H., Wiggins, S., Kamrudin, S., et al. (2010). Inflammatory breast cancer: The disease, the biology, the treatment. *CA: A Cancer Journal for Clinicians, 60,* 351–375. doi: 10.3322/caac.20082

Rodden, A. (2009). Common breast concerns. *Primary Care: Clinics in Office Practice, 36,* 103–113.

Rossouw, J.E., Anderson, G.L., Prentice, R.L., LaCroix, A.Z., Kooperberg, C., Stefankick, M.L., et al. (2002). Risks and benefits of estrogen plus progestin in healthy postmenopausal women: Principal results from the women's health initiative randomized controlled trial. *Journal of the American Medical Association, 288*(3), 321–333.

Rugo, H.S. (2008). The breast cancer continuum in hormone-receptor-positive breast cancer in postmenopausal women: Evolving management options focusing on aromatase inhibitors. *Annals of Oncology: Official Journal of the European Society for Medical Oncology, 19*(1), 16–27. doi:10.1093/annonc/mdm282

Santen, R.J., & Mansel, R. (2005). Benign breast disorders. *New England Journal of Medicine, 353*(3), 275–285. doi:10.1056/NEJMra035692

Saslow, D., Boetes, C., Burke, W., Harms, S., Leach, M.O., Lehman, C.D., et al. (2007). American Cancer Society guidelines for breast screening with MRI as an adjunct to mammography. *CA: A Cancer Journal for Clinicians, 57*(2), 75–89.

Saslow, D., Hannan, J., Osuch, J., Alciati, M.H., Baines, C., Barton, M., et al. (2004). Clinical breast examination: Practical recommendations for optimizing performance and reporting. *CA: A Cancer Journal for Clinicians, 54*(6), 327–344.

Saxe, G.A., Madlensky, L., Kealey, S., Wu, D.P., Freeman, K.L., & Pierce, J.P. (2008). Disclosure to physicians of CAM use by breast cancer patients: Findings from the women's healthy eating and living study. *Integrative Cancer Therapies, 7*(3), 122–129.

Saxena, T., Lee, E., Henderson, K.D., Clarke, C.A., West, D., Marshall, S.F., et al. (2010). Menopausal hormone therapy and subsequent risk of specific invasive breast cancer subtypes in the California Teachers Study. *Cancer Epidemiology, Biomarkers and Prevention: A Publication of the American Association for Cancer Research, Cosponsored by the American Society of Preventive Oncology, 19*(9), 2366–2378. doi:10.1158/1055-9965.EPI-10-0162

Schonfeld, S.J., Pfeiffer, R.M., Lacey, J.V., Jr., Berrington de Gonzalez, A., Doody, M.M., Greenlee, R.T., et al. (2011). Hormone-related risk factors and postmenopausal breast cancer among nulliparous versus parous women: An aggregated study. *American Journal of Epidemiology, 173*(5), 509–517. doi:10.1093/aje/kwq404

Schootman, M., Jeffe, D.B., Lian, M., Aft, R., & Gillanders, W.E. (2008). Surveillance mammography and the risk of death among elderly breast cancer patients. *Breast Cancer Research and Treatment, 111*(3), 489–496.

Seetharam, S., & Fentiman, I.S. (2009). Paget's disease of the nipple. *Women's Health, 5*(4), 397–402. doi:10.2217/whe.09.23

Shulman, L.P. (2010). Hereditary breast and ovarian cancer (HBOC): Clinical features and counseling for BRCA1 and BRCA2, Lynch syndrome, Cowden syndrome, and Li-Fraumeni syndrome. *Obstetric and Gynecology Clinics of North America, 37*(1), 109–133.

Siegel, R., Ward, E., Brawley, O., & Jemal, A. (2011). Cancer statistics, 2011: The impact of eliminating socioeconomic and racial disparities on premature cancer deaths. *CA: A Cancer Journal for Clinicians, 61*(4), 212–236. doi:10.3322/caac.20121

Slamon, D.J., Clark, G.M., Wong, S.G., Levin, W.J., Ullrich, A., & McGuire, W.L. (1987). Human breast cancer: Correlation of relapse and survival with amplification of the HER-2/neu oncogene. *Science, 235*(4785), 177–182.

Smith, R.L., Pruthi, S., & Fitzpatrick, L.A. (2004). Evaluation and management of breast pain. *Mayo Clinic Proceedings, 79*(3), 353–372.

Strom, B.L., Berlin, J.A., Weber, A.L., Norman, S.A., Bernstein, L., Burkman, R.T., et al. (2004). Absence of an effect of injectable and implantable progestin-only contraceptives on subsequent risk of breast cancer. *Contraception, 69*(5), 353–360. doi:10.1016/j.contraception.2003.12.015

Stuckey, A. (2011). Breast cancer: Epidemiology and risk factors. *Clinical Obstetrics and Gynecology, 54*(1), 96–102. doi:10.1097/GRF.0b013e3182080056

Thorne, C.H. (2010). An evidence-based approach to augmentation mammaplasty. *Plastic and Reconstructive Surgery, 126*(6), 2184–2188. doi:10.1097/PRS.0b013e3181f83102

U.S. Department of Labor. (2009). *Your rights after a mastectomy… Women's Health & Cancer Rights Act of 1998*. Retrieved from http://www.dol.gov/ebsa/publications/whcra.html

U.S. Preventive Services Task Force. (2005). Genetic risk assessment and BRCA mutation testing for breast and ovarian cancer susceptibility: Recommendation statement. *Annals of Internal Medicine, 143*(5), 355–361.

U.S. Preventive Services Task Force. (2009). Screening for breast cancer: U.S. Preventive Services Task Force recommendation statement. *Annals of Internal Medicine, 151*(10), 716–726, W-236. doi:10.1059/0003-4819-151-10-200911170-00008

U.T. Southwestern Medical Center. (2004). *CancerGene*. Retrieved from http://www4.utsouthwestern.edu/breasthealth/cagene/

Vaughan, A., Dietz, J.R., Aft, R., Gillanders, W.E., Eberlein, T.J., Freer, P., et al. (2007). Scientific Presentation Award. Patterns of local breast cancer recurrence after skin-sparing mastectomy and immediate breast reconstruction. *American Journal of Surgery, 194*(4), 438–443. doi:10.1016/j.amjsurg.2007.06.011

Viani, G.A., Afonso, S.L., Stefano, E.J., De Fendi, L.I., & Soares, F.V. (2007). Adjuvant trastuzumab in the treatment of her-2-positive early breast cancer: A meta-analysis of published randomized trials. *BMC Cancer, 7,* 153. doi:10.1186/1471-2407-7-153

Virnig, B.A., Tuttle, T.M., Shamliyan, T., & Kane, R.L. (2010). Ductal carcinoma in situ of the breast: A systematic review of incidence, treatment, and outcomes. *Journal of the National Cancer Institute, 102*(3), 170–178. doi:10.1093/jnci/djp482

Vo, T., Xing, Y., Meric-Bernstam, F., Mirza, N., Vlastos, G., Symmans, W.F., et al. (2007). Long-term outcomes in patients with mucinous, medullary, tubular, and invasive ductal carcinomas after lumpectomy. *American Journal of Surgery, 194*(4), 527–531. doi:10.1016/j.amjsurg.2007.06.012

Vogel, V.G., Costantino, J.P., Wickerham, D.L., Cronin, W.M., Cecchini, R.S., Atkins, J.N., et al. (2010). Update of the National Surgical Adjuvant Breast and Bowel Project Study of Tamoxifen and Raloxifene (STAR) P-2 Trial: Preventing breast cancer. *Cancer Prevention Research, 3*(6), 696–706. doi:10.1158/1940-6207.CAPR-10-0076

Yuan, Y., Chen, X.S., Liu, S.Y., & Shen, K.W. (2010). Accuracy of MRI in prediction of pathologic complete remission in breast cancer after preoperative therapy: A meta-analysis. *American Journal of Roentgenology, 195*(1), 260–268.

Zervoudis, S., Iatrakis, G., Economides, P., Polyzos, D., & Navrozoglou, I. (2010). Nipple discharge screening. *Women's Health, 6*(1), 135–151. doi:10.2217/whe.09.81

CHAPTER ❖ 18

THE MENOPAUSAL TRANSITION

Catherine Juve

Women today can expect to live one third of their lives after their reproductive years.

Highlights

- Attitudes and Beliefs About the Menopausal Transition
- Physiology of Menopause
- Hypoestrogenic Changes
- Sexuality and the Menopause Transition
- Alterations in Mood
- Cognitive Function/Memory Loss/Alzheimer's Disease
- Sleep Disorders
- Overview of Current Hormone Replacement Therapy Research and Implications for Practice

❖ INTRODUCTION

Menopause, defined as the final menstrual period (FMP) and the end of reproductive life for women, is a universal event that is experienced by all women who live to be middle aged and older. As our population ages and life expectancy lengthens, we can expect an unprecedented increase in the number of peri- and postmenopausal women. The average age at menopause in the United States is 51 years with a normal range from 40 to 58 years of age. Despite a decline in the average age at puberty, the average age for menopause has remained consistent. Age at menopause is influenced by multiple factors that contribute to individual differences across and within cultures and environments. Actual age at menopause is influenced by genetics, health, environmental exposures, and behaviors such as smoking and diet. Although norms are helpful in guiding clinicians, understanding the unique feature of the menopausal transition experienced by individual women is critical to providing comprehensive, holistic, and individualized care that addresses health promotion, prevention, and optimal treatment for symptoms that are likely to accompany the menopausal transition (North American Menopause Society [NAMS], 2010).

In order to provide holistic care, a comprehensive understanding of the physical changes and the emotional and sociocultural dynamics that accompany the menopausal transition is essential for clinicians. Understanding the sociocultural and psychological meaning of menopause for individual women and their attitudes and beliefs about menopause provides an important context for offering optimal and holistic care.

ATTITUDES AND BELIEFS ABOUT THE MENOPAUSAL TRANSITION

Although the menopause transition is primarily thought of as a normal physiological transition, it also has psychosociocultural meaning in women's lives. A substantial body of research provides evidence that the meaning of menopause is socially and culturally contextual with symbolic meanings. The meaning attributed to menopause is significantly related to the experience of menopause, including any related distress and symptoms. Although cultural beliefs and attitudes are related to symptoms and beliefs about symptom management, there are vast individual menopausal experiential differences within every culture. Avoiding stereotyping based on cultural background is critical for health care providers (Hall, Callister, Berry, & Matsumura, 2007). However, a basic understanding of how cultural beliefs, perceptions, and attitudes about menopause and its meaning in the context of life experiences is important for clinicians to understand in order to effectively work with menopausal women from various cultural backgrounds with differing belief systems.

In societies where menopause is associated with increased privileges for women, perceptions about menopause are typically more positive and symptoms are fewer. Privileges may encompass greater participation in cultural ceremonies, increased status, and a "wise woman" position. In contrast, in societies where fertility defines femininity and is associated with the value of women, attitudes about menopause may be more negative. Traditionally, patriarchal societies are unlikely to confer status on women as they move through the menopausal transition. When menopause has negative connotations for women, it is not surprising that both emotional and physical symptoms are more pronounced. Women immigrating to a culture in which menopause has a negative connotation may feel the compounded effects of loss of status through menopause at the same time they are struggling with other major life transitions.

In modern western cultures, the menopausal transition is often marked by ambivalence. In cultures that value youth and beauty, menopause is a reminder to women that they are aging. The medicalization of menopause also delivers a message to women that something is wrong with them as they experience the menopause transition. The title of the book published in the 1960s that launched the surge of interest in hormone replacement therapy (HRT) for women was *Feminine Forever* (Wilson, 1966). This book equated femininity with premenopausal hormonal status.

Modern women in cultures that value youth and beauty may grieve for the loss of youth as they contend with bothersome symptoms that interfere with their quality of life and are reminders that they are aging.

Loss of control may also contribute to negative feelings about menopause. Disruption in life attributed to menopausal symptoms is portrayed in the media via pharmaceutical ads as an unwelcome annoyance that can be controlled with medications or supplements. Rather than messages about tolerating symptoms and reframing menopause as an important and positive life transition, the media tends to emphasize interventions to maintain youth and eliminate any reminders that a woman is in the midst of the menopausal transition (Avis et al., 2003; Ayers, Forshaw, & Hunter, 2010; Melby & Lampl, 2011).

DEFINITIONS

Having a standardized vocabulary for terminology associated with the menopausal transition is important to promote effective communication among clinicians and female patients.

The *menopausal transition* encompasses the period of time when women are experiencing changes in their menstrual cycle that are reflective of endocrine changes. In 2001, representatives from key American governmental and professional organizations gathered in Park City, Utah, at a workshop titled the Stages of Reproductive Aging Workshop (STRAW). The purpose of this workshop was to develop a staging model for the last 10 to 15 years of reproductive aging along with a standardized approach to menopause terminology (Soules et al., 2001). In 2011, the STRAW model was revised based on research findings published after 2001. According to the 2011 STRAW+10 model, the stages of the menopausal transition range from [–2 or *early menopausal transition* to –1 or *late menopausal transition*. The term *perimenopause* is similar and often used interchangeably with *menopause transition*. However, *perimenopause* generally encompasses at least 1 year *postmenopause* as well as the time leading to the FMP. *Postmenopause* includes the time span after the FMP and divided that period into *early postmenopause* (within 1 year of the FMP) and *late postmenopause* as any time after the first year postmenopause. The STRAW+10 model affirms that objective menstrual data reported by women is the most important criterion for determining menopausal status. Biomarker assays are not internationally standardized, as well as being costly and invasive. Biomarker data may provide supportive evidence, but is not required for menopausal transition diagnosis (Harlow et al., 2012).

STRAW+10 definitions include:

- *Early menopausal transition (stage –2):* This stage is marked by increased variability in the menstrual cycle, defined in a persistent difference of 7 days or more in the length of consecutive cycles. Persistent is defined as recurring variability within 10 cycles of the initial variable cycle. This stage is also marked by elevated, but variable, increases in the follicle-stimulating hormone (FSH) level during the follicular phase of the menstrual cycle.
- *Late menopausal transition (stage –1):* Specific indicators of this stage include amenorrhea for 60 days or longer, increased variability in cycle length, increased frequency of anovulatory cycles, and extreme fluctuations in hormonal levels.
- *Early postmenopause (stages +1a, +1b, +1c):* FSH levels continue to increase and estradiol levels continue to decrease for approximately 2 years after the FMP. After 2 years, the levels stabilize. Stage +1a lasts for 1 year after the FMP and marks the end of perimenopause and meets the official criteria for the definition of menopause. During stage +1b, hormonal levels continue to fluctuate. During stages +1a and +1b, lasting approximately 2 years after the FMP, vasomotor symptoms are most likely to occur.
- *Late postmenopause (stage +2):* Hormonal levels stabilize during this stage. Urogenital and vaginal symptoms typically become more prominent.

Evidence indicates that STRAW+10 criteria apply to most women. Although smoking and body mass index (BMI) may influence menopausal age, the trajectory of bleeding patterns and hormonal changes remains consistent (Harlow et al., 2012) (see Figure 18–1).

Other important terminology includes:

- *Induced menopause:* Cessation of menstruation that follows surgical removal of the ovaries (bilateral oophorectomy) with or without hysterectomy or ablation of ovarian function by radiation or chemotherapy. Nonsurgical-induced menopause may be temporary and may occur over a period of several months. The term *surgical menopause* refers to bilateral oophorectomy (NAMS, 2010).
- *Premature menopause:* Naturally occurring menopause at or below the age of 40 years. This age criterion is frequently used as an arbitrary cutoff date

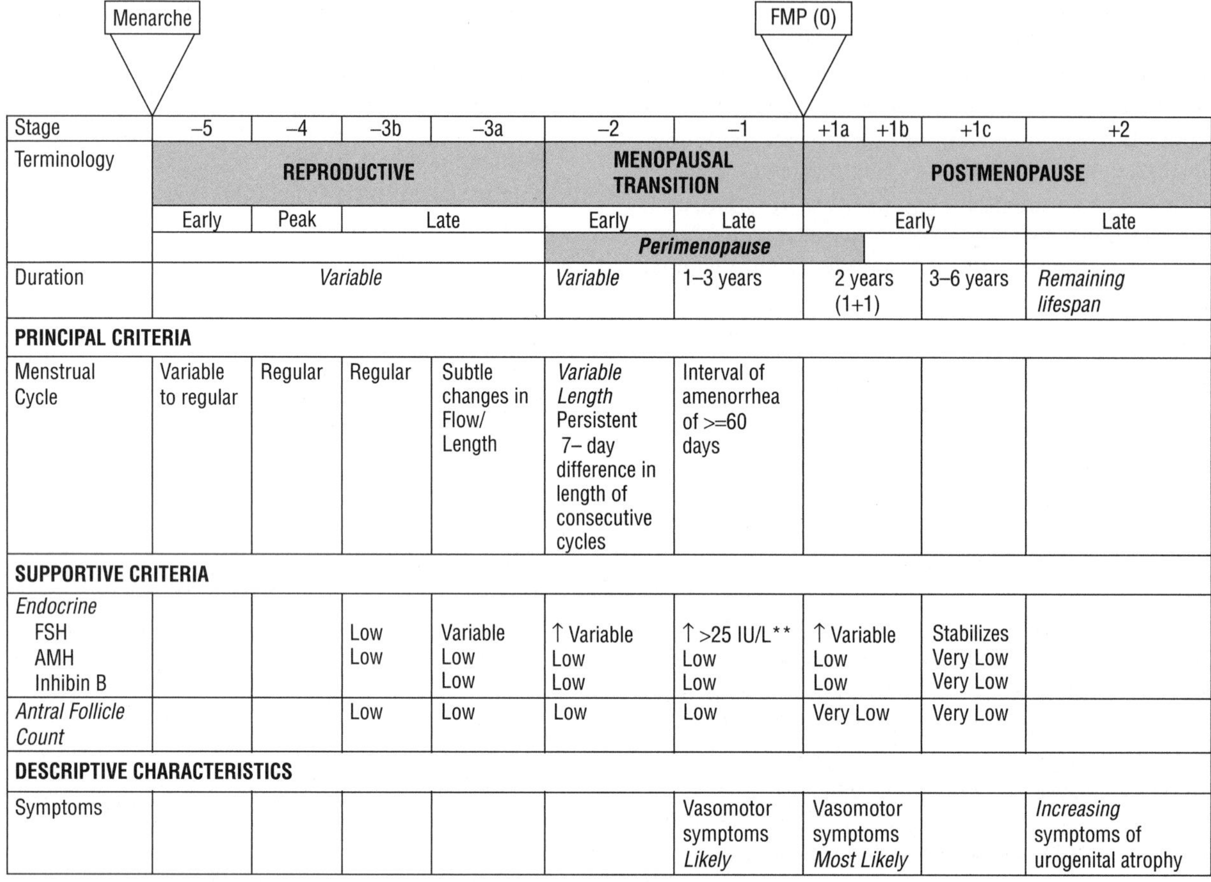

	Menarche					FMP (0)				
Stage	−5	−4	−3b	−3a	−2	−1	+1a	+1b	+1c	+2
Terminology	**REPRODUCTIVE**				**MENOPAUSAL TRANSITION**		**POSTMENOPAUSE**			
	Early	Peak	Late		Early	Late	Early			Late
					Perimenopause					
Duration	*Variable*				*Variable*	1–3 years	2 years (1+1)		3–6 years	*Remaining lifespan*
PRINCIPAL CRITERIA										
Menstrual Cycle	Variable to regular	Regular	Regular	Subtle changes in Flow/ Length	*Variable Length* Persistent 7– day difference in length of consecutive cycles	Interval of amenorrhea of >=60 days				
SUPPORTIVE CRITERIA										
Endocrine FSH AMH Inhibin B			Low Low	Variable Low Low	↑ Variable Low Low	↑ >25 IU/L** Low Low	↑ Variable Low Low		Stabilizes Very Low Very Low	
Antral Follicle Count			Low	Low	Low	Low	Very Low		Very Low	
DESCRIPTIVE CHARACTERISTICS										
Symptoms						Vasomotor symptoms *Likely*	Vasomotor symptoms *Most Likely*			*Increasing* symptoms of urogenital atrophy

* Blood draw on cycle days 2–5 ↑ = elevated

**Approximate expected level based on assays using current international pituitary standard[67–69]

FIGURE 18–1. Stages of Reproductive Aging. *Sources:* NAMS, 2010a; Soules et al., 2001.

for premature menopause. This term may also refer to induced menopause that occurs at or below the age of 40 years (NAMS, 2010).

- *Early menopause:* Natural or induced menopause that occurs before the average age of menopause, age 51. The term encompasses premature menopause (NAMS, 2010). Menopause between ages 31 and 40 is considered early and, because of the increased incidence of autoimmune disorders in those with early menopause, requires referral for medical endocrine evaluation. Smoking, earlier menarche, lower parity, and lower BMI are also each associated with earlier menopause.
- *Premature ovarian failure (POF):* Premature ovarian insufficiency leading to amenorrhea among women younger than age 40. POF may be transient but usually leads to permanent loss of ovarian function with permanent elevations of luteinizing hormone (LH) and FSH. This may be due to iatrogenic interventions (radiation, chemotherapy), genetics, autoimmune disorders, or other health conditions. POF should not be confused with hypothalamic amenorrhea (HA), which can be caused by eating disorders or intense exercising. HA results in lowered levels of LH and FSH that return to normal levels with the resumption of a healthier lifestyle (NAMS, 2010).

PHYSIOLOGY OF MENOPAUSE

Menopause results from a series of changes initiated in the ovary. General atresia of ovarian follicles begins with the onset of puberty and becomes more significant after age 35 when the ovary contains fewer follicles that are responsive to FSH. Eventually, the atresia leads to a decline in ovarian production of estrogen and progesterone and changes in the hypothalamic-pituitary-ovarian axis that leads to the FMP.

CHANGES IN THE HYPOTHALAMIC-PITUITARY-OVARIAN AXIS

In the normal premenopausal menstrual cycle, rising levels of FSH stimulate the developing dominant follicle to secrete increasing amounts of estradiol. The increasing level of pituitary FSH as well as declining ovarian inhibin production exerts a negative feedback on the hypothalamus and results in decreasing pituitary FSH. After menopause, there is an increase in FSH because of the reduction in pituitary gonadotropin inhibition of estrogen and progesterone. This change in ovarian steroid production is often gradual and variable, resulting in anovulatory bleeding patterns. FSH levels continue to rise and then plateau within 1 year of the FMP. Eventually, the ovaries are completely unable to respond to FSH and LH, and the level of gonadotropin hyperactivity stabilizes. FSH levels decrease somewhat after several years, but never return to premenopausal levels. During the menopause transition, LH levels remain stable and within normal premenopausal range or slightly elevated. After menopause, LH levels rise and then plateau after about 1 year. The subsequent postmenopausal decline in FSH and LH suggests that additional hypothalamic-pituitary changes occur with aging that are independent of the loss of ovarian feedback (NAMS, 2010).

DIAGNOSIS OF MENOPAUSE

Menopause is diagnosed retrospectively after 12 months of amenorrhea than cannot be attributed to another cause. Measuring ovarian hormonal levels to diagnose menopause is not a reliable diagnostic tool because of the variability in FSH levels during the menopause transition. A single measurement of FSH > 30 IU/mL cannot confirm menopause. Multiple measurements over several months may be necessary. All endogenous hormone use, including estrogen-containing contraception, must be discontinued for a minimum of 6 weeks to obtain accurate FSH measurements (Parker, 2004). For sexually active women, use of reliable contraception is essential to avoid unwanted pregnancy. Progestogen-only or nonhormonal contraception will not interfere with FSH measurement accuracy. It is important not to assume that amenorrhea for less than 1 year is an indication that menopause has occurred (NAMS, 2010).

FACTORS RELATED TO AGE AT MENOPAUSE

There is conflicting evidence regarding ethnic/racial variation in age of menopause. Educational level and socioeconomic status have also been inconsistently associated with age at menopause, suggesting the probable involvement of a complex interplay of genetic and environmental factors in determining age at menopause (Henderson, Bernstein, Henderson, Kolonel, & Pike, 2008). A model to predict age of menopause has been proposed that incorporates number of full-term pregnancies, BMI, history of breast surgery, and presence of two specific single nucleopeptide polymorphisms or estrogen metabolizing genes (CYP17 or CYP1B1-4). In various studies, late menopause has been associated with oral contraceptive (OC) use, Japanese ethnicity, increased BMI, and the experience of sexual or physical violence or assault (NAMS, 2010). Cultural background and practices have been studied in relationship to timing of menopause and frequency and severity of menopausal symptoms (Melby & Lampl, 2011). Although cultural differences may, in large part, be attributable to attitudes and perceptions about the meaning and acceptability of menopause, there are also significant differences in objective measures of hormonal levels and body temperature that are not data artifacts (Avis et al., 2003). Anti-Müllerian hormone levels measured 6 years prior to actual natural menopause have also been shown to successfully predict age of menopause for individual women (Tehrani, Shakeri, Solaymani-Dodaran, & Azizi, 2011).

POSTMENOPAUSAL ESTROGEN SOURCES

There are three types of estrogen: estradiol, estrone, and estriol. The major source of estrogen prior to menopause is from the ovarian follicle in the form of estradiol. Estradiol is produced cyclically, and the ovary accounts for over 90 percent of total body production. Relatively constant production of estrone by adrenal glandular secretion and peripheral conversion of androstenedione, the major circulating androgen in women, also occurs. Postmenopausally, little estradiol is produced in the ovarian follicles. Ovarian stroma, under stimulation by LH, continues to produce androstenedione and testosterone, which, along with androstenedione produced by adrenal glands, are converted to estrone in peripheral adipose tissue. Thus, the body weight of the woman contributes to her overall postmenopausal level of circulating estrogen. Initially, both the ovary and the adrenal glands are major sources of androstenedione. With advanced age, however, the ovarian stroma ceases production of androstenedione and is unable to maintain sufficient estrone production. Estriol is produced in significant amounts during pregnancy by the placenta. Levels of estriol in nonpregnant women remain stable throughout the menopause transition. Estriol has not been documented as having an important role in menopausal symptomatology (NAMS, 2010).

HYPOESTROGENIC CHANGES

Changes in the urogenital system that occur with declining estrogen levels may be benign or may cause severe discomfort and interference with daily activities.

- *Vulva:* With the loss of estrogen, the vulva undergoes atrophy, and subcutaneous tissues diminish. The labia majora become small and the labia minora almost nonexistent. The skin becomes thinner, and pubic hair loss is progressive. Dystrophies and pruritus are more frequent (Farague & Maibach, 2006).
- *Vagina:* Epithelial maturation decreases. The failure to produce glycogen-containing superficial cells causes an increase in the vaginal pH, which may predispose the woman to infection. The vagina becomes shortened, thinned, and narrowed, with obliteration of the vaginal fornices and eventual loss of vaginal rugae. Sebaceous gland secretions decrease and the vagina loses most of its lubricating ability, especially in response to sexual stimulation. Changes may be prevented or slowed by the continuation of regular intercourse (Farague & Maibach, 2006).
  Over time, the uterus decreases in size and the endometrium atrophies. The cervix pales and shrinks with loss of the fornices so that the external os is nearly flush with the vaginal wall. The endocervix becomes atrophic and the cervical canal stenotic. The ovaries and fallopian tubes atrophy and are usually not palpable on examination; in fact, any adnexal mass in a woman over age 50 is considered malignant until proven otherwise.
- *Pelvic floor:* The muscular tissue loses tone after menopause, causing increases in uterine prolapse, cystocele, and rectocele. This loss of tone may be heightened by past pregnancy and vaginal delivery. This heightened problem of loss of tone affects up to 50 percent of parous women (Tinelli et al., 2010).
- *Breast:* With aging, a woman's breasts lose tissue and subcutaneous fat, reducing breast size and fullness. There is also a decrease in the number of mammary glands, which the body replaces with fat tissue. These changes make the breast less firm. The breasts lose support. Aging breasts commonly flatten and sag. The nipple may turn in slightly. The areola also becomes smaller and may nearly disappear (National Cancer Institute, 2011).

The loss of estradiol with decreasing ovarian function results in a host of changes among postmenopausal women. The incidence and severity of complaints vary greatly, but most frequently include menstrual irregularity, vasomotor instability, and vaginal dryness/discomfort. Other associated concerns include sexual issues, cognitive decline, mood, sleep disturbances, weight gain, and changes in skin and hair. Research suggests that menstrual cycle changes, vasomotor instability, and genitourinary changes are clearly related to the physiologic changes of menopause. However, the impact of psychological, social, and cultural factors on other associated symptoms is less clear.

MENSTRUAL CYCLE CHANGES

As the number of ovarian follicles capable of producing estrogen decreases, a woman experiences irregularities of the menstrual cycle. During the menopause transition, hormonal levels have increasing variability with resulting inconsistent ovulation. Follicular atresia increases rapidly with age resulting in decreased fertility. Changes in the menstrual flow and frequency of menses are primary characteristics of the menopause transition and are considered normal. Ideally, her periods are shorter and less frequent, but often they are a mix of heavy, longer bleeding episodes that are closer together due to anovulation. With anovulation, the epithelium builds from unopposed estrogen stimulation with no progesterone to transpose it to a secretory state. Although irregular bleeding is common, it cannot be ignored and endometrial cancer must be ruled out (NAMS, 2010) (see Chapter 11).

Subjective Data

The client's history indicates a change in the regularity of cycles and characteristics of menses or the absence of menses, and, often, other symptoms of hypoestrogenism. Frequently reported changes in menstrual flow and cycle frequency include the following:

- oligomenorrhea and/or hypomenorrhea
- menorrhagia and metrorrhagia or hypermenorrhea
- sudden amenorrhea

Women may report fatigue, headaches, and pica (unusual cravings) when heavy and frequent bleeding results in anemia. Embarrassment, restriction of social activity, a decline in libido, and overall quality of life may also be reported as being related to menstrual irregularity. A woman may also report concerns about pregnancy with extended spacing of menses.

Objective Data

Physical Examination. The physical and pelvic exam should be normal, and may or may not reveal changes suggestive of approaching menopause (see section on vulvar and vaginal changes associated with menopause).

Diagnostic Tests and Methods. A pregnancy test must be used to rule out pregnancy as a cause of the bleeding or missed periods. Endometrial abnormalities (hyperplasia and carcinoma) may be ruled out with an endometrial biopsy or ultrasound. If anemia is suspected, a hemoglobin and hematocrit may be done. Because of the variability and inconsistency in ovarian hormone levels during the menopause transition, serum estradiol and FSH levels are not recommended as diagnostic tests.

Differential Medical Diagnoses

Pregnancy, spontaneous abortion, anovulation, hyperplasia, endometrial carcinoma, infection, abnormalities of the uterus such as fibroids or polyps, endometriosis, adenomyosis, injury, ovarian abnormalities such as tumors or cysts, abnormal (dysfunctional) uterine bleeding. (See Chapter 11 for comprehensive discussion of dysfunctional uterine bleeding and other conditions that contribute to abnormal bleeding patterns.)

Abnormal uterine bleeding patterns in a perimenopausal woman include the following:

- Menorrhagia, especially with clots, and average blood loss > 80 mL per cycle
- Menses lasting longer than 7 days or 2 days greater than usual
- Less than 21 days between onset of menses
- Intermenstrual bleeding (spotting or bleeding)
- Bleeding after sexual intercourse (NAMS, 2010)

Plan

Psychosocial Interventions. Reassure the client that bodily changes are normal, explain the physiology of menopause, and educate regarding methods of treatment, if indicated.

Medication

Hormonal Therapy. Treatment selection will depend on need for contraception and concerns about preserving fertility. For the perimenopausal woman who is ovulating, recommended treatment for establishing predictable cycling or cessation of menses is combined low-dose oral, vaginal, implantable, or transdermal contraceptives. Combined OCs and the contraceptive ring may be used continuously if amenorrhea is desired. Continuous progestins in the form of progestin-only contraceptive pills, injectable Depo-Provera, or the progestin intrauterine system (IUS) are also recommended to regulate menstrual cycles. Progestin-only contraception may be supplemented with a postmenopausal dosage of estrogen if vasomotor or vaginal symptoms are not well controlled. (See Chapter 12 for a discussion of contraindications to hormonal contraceptives and management of side effects.)

For women who do not need contraception, a cyclic progestogen may be used for 12 to 14 days each month to regulate the menstrual cycle. If other perimenopausal symptoms occur, a postmenopausal dosage of estrogen may be added for those with no contraindications to estrogen use. For a comprehensive review of other hormonal, nonhormonal, and surgical management options for dysfunctional uterine bleeding, see Chapter 11.

Endometrial Biopsy/Transvaginal Ultrasound. Office-based endometrial biopsy or transvaginal ultrasound (TVU) is important to rule out pathology versus normal menopause transition bleeding pattern.

Follow-Up

Any bleeding that does not respond to usual therapy or any abnormal findings from the endometrial biopsy or TVU requires that the client be referred. Postmenopausal uterine bleeding always requires further evaluation unless the bleeding is consistent with expected bleeding patterns related to use of hormonal therapy. Medication therapy requires follow-up to assure that the treatment is effective in regulating bleeding.

VASOMOTOR SYMPTOMS

Vasomotor instability, better known as hot flashes, hot flushes, or night sweats, coincides with a surge of LH and decrease in estrogen level and is followed by a measurable increase in body surface heat and a fall in core temperature. The hot flash is a transient and recurrent episode characterized by an intense feeling of heat that begins in the upper chest or neck and proceeds up the face and head. Hot flashes typically last from 1 to 5 minutes. Skin temperature rises as a result of peripheral vasodilation. The sensation is a sudden wave of heat, especially over the upper body that corresponds to the rising skin temperature. Heart rate may rise along with an increased metabolic rate that occurs simultaneously with sweating and peripheral vasodilation. Core body temperature decreases after the hot flash subsides, probably due to sweating and vasodilation, which may result in chills. Hot flashes can occur at any time of day and may be infrequent or daily occurrences. An individual's circadian rhythm may predict the timing of hot flashes, with a tendency for more hot flashes to occur in the early evening (Avis et al., 2003; NAMS, 2010). Vasomotor instability can have a profound effect on quality of life (Avis et al., 2009; Burleson, Todd, & Trevathan, 2010; Williams, Levine, Kalilani, Lewis, & Clark, 2009). See Table 18–1 for treatment options.

TABLE 18–1. Options for Treatment of Vasomotor Symptoms

Life style changes and complementary therapies
- Reducing body temperature
- Maintaining a healthy weight
- Smoking cessation
- Relaxation response techniques
- Acupuncture
- Yoga

Botanical therapies[a]
- Phytoestrogens
  - Soy/Soy isoflavones
  - Red clover
- Black cohosh
- Vitamin E
- Herbal therapies (dong quai, ginseng, chasteberry, and others)

Nonhormonal prescription medications[b]

SSRIs/SNRIs
- Paroxetine (10–20 mg/d, controlled release 12.5–25 mg/d)
- Venlafaxine (extended release 37.5–75 mg/d)
- Fluoxetine (20 mg/d)

Other
- Gabapentin (300 mg three times daily)
- Clonidine (0.1 mg weekly transdermal patch)

Hormone therapy
- Estrogen therapy
- Progestogenn alone[b]
- Combination estrogen-progestogen therapy

[a]Efficacy greater than placebo unproven.

[b]Not approved by U.S. Food and Drug Administration for treatment of vasomotor symptoms.

Source: Adapted from Schifren and Schiff, 2010, and NAMS, 2010a.

Epidemiology

After irregular menses, hot flashes are the most consistently reported symptom of menopause; for example, as many as 75 percent of women in the United States report having experienced hot flashes. Hot flashes typically increase during perimenopause and peak during the first 2 years postmenopause, then decline over time. Most women experience hot flashes from 6 months to 2 years, although some women continue to have hot flashes for 10 or more years postmenopause (Col, Guthrie, Politi, & Dennerstein, 2009).

Prevalence

Reported prevalence rates of vasomotor symptoms vary widely based on international studies. Variation may be related to different definitions of the menopause transition and to factors such as climate, diet, lifestyle, attitudes about menopause, and aging. In the United States, among women between the ages of 41 and 55 who participated in the Study of Women's Health Across the Nation, almost 46 percent of African American women have reported experiencing hot flashes in comparison to Hispanic women (35%), Caucasian women (31%), Chinese women (20.5%), and Japanese women (17.6%). BMI may be important confounding factor. Prevalence of severe and frequent flashes is higher among women who have had a bilateral oophorectomy (up to 90%) and those who have had chemotherapy (46%) (Fan et al., 2010; Jin et al., 2008; NAMS, 2010).

Subjective Data

Evaluate the client's menstrual history for changes suggestive of perimenopause, such as decreasing or increasing intervals between menses and dysfunctional/anovulatory bleeding patterns. The client will report episodes of feeling extreme warmth rising from the chest up to the face and head, followed by perspiration and sometimes chills. If these vasomotor symptoms occur at night, they disrupt sleep—causing insomnia, exhaustion, and irritability. Hot flashes can occur frequently during a 24-hour period; hence, the client may report the need to change clothing and bed linens often.

Objective Data

Physical Examination. Findings are frequently absent, but may include vasodilation of peripheral blood vessels in the skin coupled with mild increase in pulse, but without alteration in blood pressure, increased digital temperature, and decreased intracore temperature with chills.

Diagnostic Tests and Methods

- *Serum hormonal testing* is not recommended for diagnosing menopause as the cause of vasomotor symptoms. FSH levels are highly variable during the perimenopause and are not a reliable indicator of menopause (NAMS, 2010).
- *Thyroid-stimulating hormones* should be measured to document thyroid function as possible cause of vasomotor symptoms along with fatigue, sleep disorders, and weight changes.
- *Client diary of vasomotor symptoms* confirms oral history.

Differential Medical Diagnoses

Hypothalamic/pituitary tumor, infection (viral illness, tuberculosis, systemic infection with fever, human immunodeficiency virus [HIV]), alcoholism, thyroid disease.

Plan

Psychosocial Interventions/Lifestyle Changes. Reassure the client that vasomotor symptoms are normal during the menopause transition. Explain the physiology of menopause. Offer adaptive measures as follows:

- Adjust the room temperature; leave a window open; use a portable fan to accommodate an office environment.
- Wear clothing in layers for ease of removal; wear more cotton.
- Try stress management techniques such as relaxation exercises, meditation, and yoga.
- Refrain from smoking.
- Maintain healthy body weight.
- Exercise regularly.
- Avoid personal triggers such as spicy foods, caffeine, and alcohol; avoid hot drinks and foods.

Prescription Therapies: Hormonal. HT, including estrogen-progestin therapy (EPT) and estrogen therapy (ET) for women who have had a hysterectomy, is the most effective intervention for controlling vasomotor symptoms and improving quality of life in menopausal women (NAMS, 2012). Controversy about the Women's Health Initiative (WHI) study (Roussouw et al., 2002) results has raised concerns among clients and clinicians about the safety of HT. Clinicians need to be familiar with current evidence regarding the risks and benefits of HT and current practice guidelines related to HT use. Current guidance from national organizations (ACOG, NAMS) is consistent; use the lowest effective dose for the shortest period of time to manage symptoms (ACOG, 2002; NAMS, 2012). HT is appropriate for managing vasomotor symptoms, but should not be used for chronic disease prevention or management. There are numerous types of HT pharmaceutical formulations on the market that are either synthetically produced or natural such as plant (soy, Mexican yams) or animal (pregnant mare's urine) derived. A further distinction is that some preparations are bioidentical or nonbioidentical. Bioidentical refers to the structure of the hormones; bioidentical hormones and endogenous hormones have exactly the same chemical and molecular structure. The term *natural* is often used to describe bioidentical hormones. However, this term is misleading because all hormonal preparations require processing to convert them to a form that can be effectively utilized by humans. Bioidentical hormones may be produced by pharmaceutical companies or compounding pharmacies. A confusing issue is that plant- or animal-based hormones are not necessarily bioidentical and vice versa. Compounding pharmacies prepare bioidentical hormonal preparations to prescriber specifications using U.S. Pharmacopeia (USP)-grade hormone ingredients. However, compounded formulations are not FDA approved. It would not be feasible for every possible compounded formulation to be FDA approved. The USP standards ensure quality, purity, strength, and consistency of compounded hormones, but individual error and lack of consistency in preparation between batches of compounded hormones may occur. Labeling hormones as *bioidentical* or *natural* does not mean that they are safer than standardized dosage hormonal therapies produced by pharmaceutical companies (ACOG, 2005). Noncompounded bioidentical hormones of USP grade are routed to pharmaceutical companies where they are packaged into standard dose preparations as oral or vaginal tablets, transdermal patches, creams, spays, or sprays. This array of somewhat confusing terminology and the accompanying information and misinformation make for an environment where both clinicians and women feel less than confident about HT options (Hill & Hill, 2010; Sood, Shuster, Smith, Vincent, & Jatoi, 2011).

Hormone Therapy Regimens

A variety of regimens for taking EPT are marketed by pharmaceutical companies. The decision about which regimen to be used should be individualized to address symptoms and eliminate side effects. Continuous regimens have gained popularity because they eliminate regular uterine withdrawal bleeding. Continuous cycles also eliminate problems associated with fluctuating hormone levels. However, cyclic regimens may be preferred by women in early postmenopause who wish to avoid unpredictable breakthrough bleeding that may be associated with continuous regimens. Cyclic regimens may also be helpful to women who experience persistent progestogen side effects by limiting the number of days of progestogen exposure (Mitchell, Walsh, Wang-Cheng, & Hardman, 2003; NAMS, 2010).

Cyclic Estrogen/Progestin Therapy. Start with a low-dose estrogen (see examples in Table 18–2). If hypoestrogenic symptoms persist after 30 days, increase the daily dosage incrementally. If the client has an intact uterus, add a progestogen on days 1 to 12 or days 13 to 25 of the month. A dosage equivalent to 5 to 10 mg of medroxyprogesterone acetate (MPA) is advised. A progestin or progesterone may also be given at 2-, 3-, or 6-month intervals to aid in preventing endometrial hyperplasia. Prolonged withdrawal bleeding more than 10 days may indicate the need for endometrial biopsy or ultrasound. If bleeding begins before day 10 of the progestin administration and is cyclic, increase dosage or duration of progestin to see if this regulates the bleeding pattern.

Advantages. Cyclic therapy is effective for relief of hypoestrogenic symptoms and prevention of osteoporosis in recently menopausal women, especially those who experience unwanted breakthrough bleeding.

TABLE 18–2. Hormone Therapy Options Available in the United States

	Composition	Type of Preparation and Route of Administration
Estrogen products[a]	Conjugated estrogens (formerly conjugated equine estrogens)	Oral Vaginal cream and ring IM (for excessive bleeding)
	Synthetic conjugated estrogen	Oral
	Esterified estrogens	Oral Vaginal cream
	17 βestradiol[b]	Oral Transdermal reservoir and matrix patch Transdermal topical gel, emulsion, and spray Vaginal cream
	Estradiol acetate	Oral Vaginal ring
	Estropipate	Oral
	Estradiol hemihydrate	Vaginal tablet
	Estradiol valerate	IM
	Estradiol cypionate	IM
Progestogen products[a]	Medroxyprogesterone acetate (progestin)	Oral
	Norethindrone (progestin)	Oral
	Norethindrone acetate	Oral
	Norgestrel	Oral
	Norgestrel acetate	Oral
	Micronized progesterone[b]	Oral (peanut oil suspension)
	Levonorgestrel	Intrauterine system
	Progesterone	Vaginal gel
Combined estrogen-progestin therapy products[a]	Conjugated estrogens + medroxyprogesterone acetate	Oral—continuous cyclic[c] Oral—continuous combined[d]
	Ethinyl estradiol + norethindrone acetate	Oral and transdermal—continuous combined[c] Transdermal—continuous sequential[e]
	17β estradiol + norethindrone acetate	Oral—continuous combined[d]
	17β estradiol + drospirenone	Oral—continuous combined[d]
	17β estradiol + norgestimate	Oral—intermittent[f]

[a]Consult North American Menopause Society website for current listings of products and dosing recommendations; generic formulations are available for many products.
[b]May be prepared by compounding pharmacies.
[c]Cyclic—estrogen days 1 to 25; progestogen last 10 to 14 days of estrogen cycle.
[d]Continuous combined—estrogen and progestogen daily.
[e]Continuous sequential—daily estrogen; progestogen 10 to 14 days every month.
[f]Intermittent—daily estrogen; repeated cycles of 3 days on and 3 days off of progestogen.

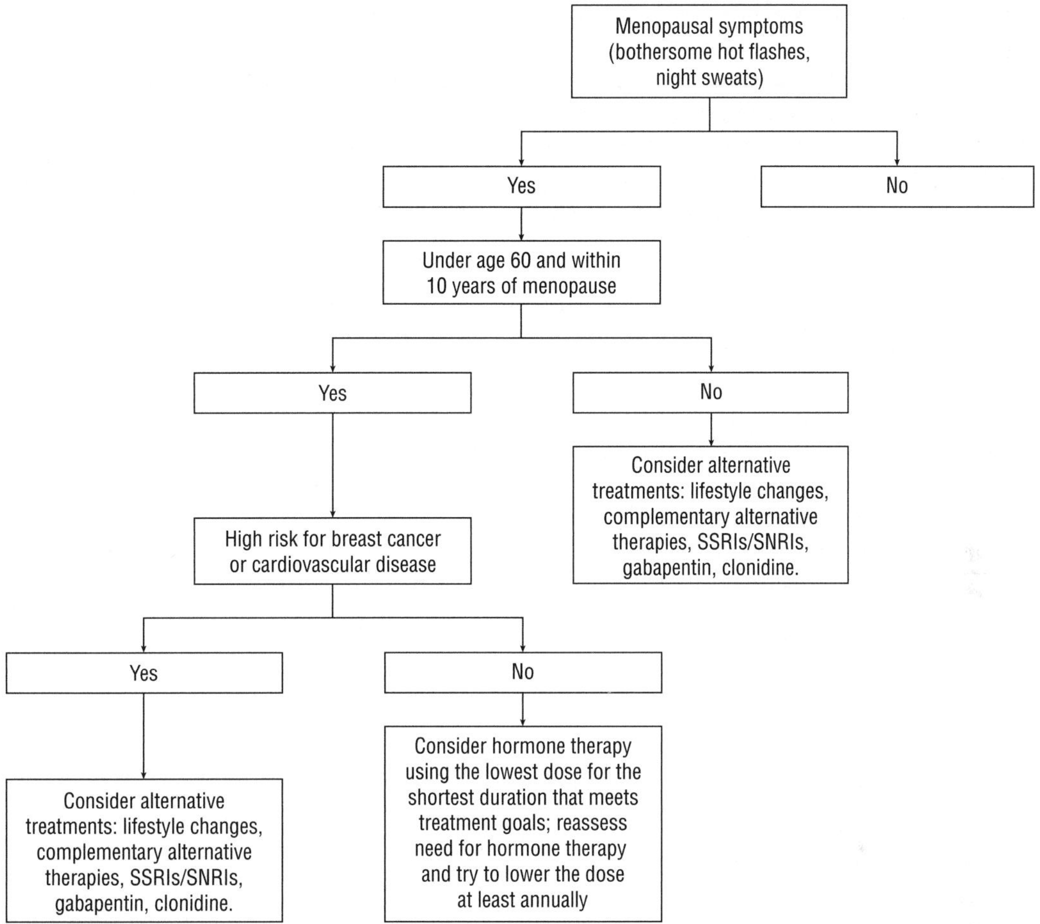

FIGURE 18–2. Systemic Hormone Therapy Decision Tree. *Source:* Shifren & Schiff, 2010.

Disadvantages. Withdrawal bleeding after the progestin is stopped may lead to decreased client compliance; however, dosing with a progestogen every 3 months may be less problematic (10 mg per day for 12–14 days) (Mitchell et al., 2003; NAMS, 2010).

Continuous Daily Estrogen/Progestin Therapy. Start with a low-dose estrogen once daily. If the uterus is intact, a continuous progestin should be added. If hypoestrogenic symptoms persist after 30 days, increase the estrogen incrementally. If the estrogen is increased, the progestin may need to be increased.

Advantages. Cyclic bleeding ends with continuous therapy, and therapy is effective in preventing osteoporosis.

Disadvantages. The client may have irregular bleeding during the first few months; this usually resolves by 6 months. This unpredictable bleeding pattern unacceptable may be unacceptable; if so, switch to cyclic HT, and try to convert to the continuous after several months. Endometrial evaluation by biopsy or ultrasound is required for prolonged and persistent bleeding, or if bleeding occurs once, amenorrhea is established. Even slight staining calls for evaluation (Mitchell et al., 2003; NAMS, 2010).

Types of Menopausal Estrogen Products

Conjugated Estrogen. Most clinical studies, including the WHI, used conjugated estrogens (CE), formerly called conjugated equine estrogen (CEE). The WHI study (2002) included CE 0.625 mg and MPA 2.5 mg and CE 0.625 mg alone for participants without a uterus. As a result, more is known about the safety and efficacy of CEE than any other estrogen product. The standard dosage of CE has been 0.625 mg daily. However, it has been established than many women require a lower dosage (0.45 mg or 0.3 mg daily) for relief of menopausal symptoms and bone protection (Mitchell et al., 2003; NAMS, 2010; Shifren & Schiff, 2010).

Estradiol. 17β estradiol requires processing (micronization) in order to be absorbed from the gastrointestinal (GI) tract. A variety of FDA-approved oral and transdermal products are available including patches, gels, a spray, and a topical emulsion. Vaginal preparations are also available as a cream and a ring. Evidence suggests that very low dosages of 17β estradiol are effective in treating vasomotor symptoms and preventing and treating osteoporosis in many women. 17β estradiol is the only commercially available FDA-approved estrogen product that is bioidentical (Mitchell et al., 2003; NAMS, 2010).

Synthetic and Other Estrogens. A variety of synthetic and other estrogen formulations are FDA approved for treating menopausal symptoms and, in some cases, prevention of osteoporosis. Synthetic hormones include synthetic CEs, esterified estrogens, and ethinyl estradiol. Estropipate is an oral form of estrone sulfate (NAMS, 2010).

Dosage equivalencies between different types of estrogen products are not standardized. For example, 0.625 mg of CE is approximately equivalent to 1.0 mg of micronized 17β estradiol. Providers must be aware of the lack of equivalency and consult trusted references for current information about standard dosages for different types of estrogens (Nelson, 2004).

Routes of Administration

Women have a variety of options to select from for the optimal route of administration to meet individual needs and lifestyle.

Oral

Advantages. Oral estrogen preparations are the most widely studied and used in North America. They are readily available in a wide variety of dosages and formulations, with several options that include both estrogen and progestogen in one tablet. Due to first-pass hepatic metabolism, high-density lipoprotein cholesterol (HDL-C) levels are raised with oral estrogen. Since the release of the WHI findings, research has verified that low-dose (0.45 mg or 0.3 mg) oral estrogen products are as effective as standard dose (0.625 mg) oral estrogen in managing menopausal symptoms (NAMS, 2010, 2011).

Disadvantages. Due to first-pass liver metabolism, oral estrogen has a greater stimulating effect than transdermal estrogen products on hepatic globulins, coagulation factors, and some inflammatory markers, including C-reactive protein, with implications for cardiac health. Oral preparations are also associated with a 25 percent increase in triglycerides. Recent data suggests that oral ET, but not transdermal ET, increases the risk of venous thromboembolism (VTE) and stroke. Further research comparing the risks and benefits of oral versus transdermal administration is needed before definitive conclusions can be drawn (NAMS, 2010).

Transdermal Estrogen

Advantages. Transdermal estradiol delivers 17β estradiol directly to the bloodstream, without first-pass liver metabolism or GI absorption. Bypassing the liver is an advantage because of the avoidance of a negative impact on coagulation factors and inflammatory markers, resulting in a decreased risk of VTE (Canonico et al., 2010; Shifren et al., 2008). Lower dosages are required for transdermal administration because of elimination of GI absorption. In addition, triglyceride levels are not increased by transdermal administration. Serum levels of estrogen remain more stable with transdermal products than with oral products, resulting in decreased incidence of some estrogenic side effects such as migraine headaches. Transdermal products provide protection from osteoporosis that is equal to that of oral estrogen products (NAMS, 2010, 2011; Shifren & Schiff, 2010).

Disadvantages. Possible side effects that are associated specifically with transdermal products include skin irritation from the patch adhesive component and the possibility of transfer of a small amount of a gel or emulsion product through skin-to-skin contact within 2 hours of application of the topical estrogen.

To avoid skin irritation:

- Make sure that the application area is clean, dry, and free of oil, powder, perfume, and soap.
- Leave the system open to the air (with protective covering off) for 10 to 15 minutes prior to application to allow some of the alcohol to evaporate.
- Rotate the patch with each change. Apply to upper outer quadrants of buttocks (less sensitive). Do not use on breasts (NAMS, 2010).

Transvaginal Estrogen. Vaginal estrogen preparations, in the form of creams, have been able for decades. Estrogen-containing rings and tablets are newer.

Advantages. The effect is primarily localized with minimal systemic estrogen effects. However, depending on dosage and type of product, there may be some systemic absorption with mild estrogenic side effects such as breast tenderness. However, side effects are typically much less pronounced than those associated with oral or transdermal preparations. Side effects can be addressed by lowering the dosage and/or changing the type of vaginal estrogen product prescribed. Low dosages are effective in treating vaginal atrophy and are ideal for women with primarily vaginal symptoms. Vaginal estrogen exerts a potent local effect by enhancing revascularization of the vaginal epithelium. One applicator of estrogen cream inserted twice weekly usually is adequate to relieve symptoms. The estradiol acetate ring is the only vaginal estrogen product that is used to treat systemic menopausal symptoms. The addition of a progestogen to low-dose vaginal ET is typically not recommended. However, a progestogen should be added with the use of the estradiol acetate vaginal ring or if higher than standard dosages of vaginal estrogen are prescribed (NAMS, 2007, 2010).

Disadvantages. Women with systemic vasomotor symptoms will usually not experience relief with vaginal ET. Some women find the cream to be messy and inconvenient to use. The ring may be inserted by the client, but may be difficult for some women to comfortably insert and remove. Health conditions that limit physical movement and agility may interfere with ability to use vaginal estrogen products (NAMS, 2007, 2010).

The selection of route of administration should be based on a woman's needs and preferences. Medical factors may dictate the optimal route of administration. For example, a woman with hypertriglyceridemia should avoid oral estrogen products and a woman with only vaginal symptoms should select a vaginal estrogen product. Cost and insurance coverage are other factors to consider in prescribing menopausal ET.

Types of Menopausal Progestogen Products. Progestogen therapy is an option for treating menopausal symptoms, but its primary use in menopausal women is to prevent endometrial cancer associated with unopposed systemic ET. As with menopausal estrogen products, there is a wide variety of progestogen formulations and options for routes of administration.

Terminology. Progestogen includes micronized progesterone and progestins.

- *Progesterone* is the steroid hormone produced by the ovaries. Exogenous progesterone is identical to endogenous progesterone. *Micronized progesterone* is the only FDA-approved bioidentical exogenous progesterone product.
- *Progestins* are synthetic products that act like progesterone, but are not identical to the progesterone produced by the human body. Progestins may more closely resemble progesterone or testosterone.

Progestins that are produced from the plant precursor, diosgenin, are not technically "natural" products because they undergo multiple chemical processes during synthesis in laboratories. Wild yam added to a cream has no progesterone activity (NAMS, 2010). Progestogen products may be provided in combination estrogen-progestin formulations or in progestogen-only formulations. Progestogen-only products allow for more dosing flexibility than the combined products. A summary of the most commonly prescribed and frequently studied progestogen products is provided here.

- *MPA* is the most widely used and most studied type of progestogen formulation that is used to protect the endometrium. There are metabolic advantages of using a low-dose transdermal progestogen formulation rather than a higher dosage of an oral progestogen (NAMS, 2010).
- The PEPI study (Writing Group for the PEPI Study, 1995) established that oral *micronized progesterone* is less likely to raise low-density lipoprotein (LDL) lipid levels than MPA. Micronized progesterone is the preferred progestogen, especially for women with elevated LDL lipid levels. Because micronized progesterone is provided in a peanut oil suspension in an oral preparation, a peanut allergy is a contraindication to micronized progesterone use. Custom compounded progesterone can be prepared without peanut oil in oral, transdermal, and other forms. However, compounded formulations are not FDA approved and the exact dosage of MP for endometrial protection has not been established. Over-the-counter progesterone creams should not be used for endometrial protection. Several FDA-approved vaginal micronized progesterone products are available and preliminary evidence shows adequate protection of the endometrium with these products. However, FDA approval is pending for vaginal micronized progesterone products to be used for endometrial protection. Progestogen side effects tend to be less with micronized progesterone, especially vaginal micronized progesterone, in comparison to MPA (NAMS, 2010).
- The *levonorgestrel progestin-releasing IUS* effectively delivers adequate endometrial protection directly to the lining of the uterus. At this time, the IUS is not approved for endometrial protection. However, ongoing studies provide support for the effectiveness of the IUS in providing adequate endometrial protection. Minimal amounts of levonorgestrel are absorbed systemically, thus decreasing the risk of progestin related side effects.
- The vaginal route of administration is appealing because of the avoidance of systemic effects.

Micronized progesterone is delivered through a sustained and controlled dose and is absorbed through the vaginal tissue to provide endometrial protection. Cyclic use of *vaginal progesterone* to protect the endometrium is currently being studied and preliminary results are promising. Compounded formulations of vaginal progesterone are available to meet individual dosage needs when standard formulations do not provide the desired results.

Androgens. Although androgens are typically associated with male sexual development and maintenance of secondary male characteristics and sexuality, they are important for women as well. In women, androgens affect sexual desire, muscle mass, strength, bone mineral density (BMD), and distribution of adipose tissue. Female androgens are synthesized primarily in the ovaries and the adrenal glands with significant peripheral conversion. On average, the level of free, circulating, bioactive testosterone in women is about 10 percent of that in men. Levels of androgen production decline with age, but there is not an abrupt decline at menopause as there is with ovarian estrogen production. An exception is with surgical menopause. There is an approximately 50 percent decline in androgen levels after a bilateral oophorectomy (NAMS, 2010). Other conditions and drugs may also decrease the level of bioavailable androgens. Corticosteroid use, adrenal insufficiency, and any drug that decreases sex hormone binding globulin levels (such as oral ET) can lead to a decline in circulating androgen levels. The primary androgens in women are testosterone, androstenedione, and dehydroepiandrosterone (DHEA) (Wierman et al., 2006).

Advantages. The potential benefits of androgen therapy include increased sexual desire and satisfaction as well as maintenance of BMD and body composition. Studies of a combination of estrogen and testosterone compared to estrogen alone found that the addition of testosterone yielded significantly greater BMD increases and increases in fat-free body mass (Davis, Davison, & Donath, 2005).

Disadvantages. Androgenic side effects are acne, hirsutism, alopecia, and clitoromegaly. Androgens may lower HDL levels. Side effects are infrequent and dose related and usually resolve after discontinuation of therapy or a decrease in dosage (Shufelt & Braunstein, 2009).

Androgen Products. There are no U.S. FDA-approved androgen-containing products for treating sexual dysfunction in women. Testosterone and DHEA are the most frequently used androgen products for menopausal symptoms and sexual concerns. Applications for FDA approval have been submitted, but have not been approved. Compounded creams and ointments are available that may be applied directly to the vaginal, clitoral, or other skin area. Skin absorption of testosterone cream is good and anecdotal evidence supports the effectiveness of these products in improving libido, arousal, and orgasmic function. Controlled studies are lacking (Somboonparn, Davis, Seif, & Bell, 2005). Oral DHEA is available over the counter as a nutritional supplement. Intravaginal DHEA shows promise in improving sexual desire and function.

Assessment Before Prescribing HT

Take a complete client history. Special emphasis is placed upon a personal history of heart disease, stroke, hypertension, diabetes, breast or reproductive system cancer, biliary disease, liver disease, tendency to have blood clots, other significant conditions, and symptoms of vasomotor dysfunction as well as any family history of osteoporosis, heart disease, hypertension, stroke, diabetes, clotting disorders, colon cancer, breast cancer, or other major disease. Personal characteristics that put the woman at risk for a condition that could be impacted by EPT or ET would be important, such as a history of smoking or drinking alcohol. However, smoking and alcohol use are not contraindications to menopausal hormone therapy. A complete physical examination is indicated. Note signs of hypoestrogenism in the presence or absence of menses. Note any abnormalities that would contraindicate hormone replacement use.

Diagnostic Tests and Methods

Complete evaluation per midlife and late-life protocol as recommended by the American College of Obstetricians and Gynecologists (ACOG) is indicated (ACOG Committee on Gynecologic Practice, 2011).

- Bone density evaluation (DEXA scan) is advised for all women with risk factors for osteoporosis. All women over 65 years of age, regardless of risk factors, should have a baseline DEXA. See Chapter 4 for further information. May be indicated if the reason for initiating therapy is to prevent osteoporosis.
- Endometrial biopsy or pelvic ultrasonography is indicated if dysfunctional bleeding is present.
- A menstrual diary and an accurate record of other bleeding episodes over several months may provide insights for diagnosis and treatment. The diary may also be helpful after HT is begun.

Ovarian/pelvic ultrasound is indicated if there is a suspected enlarged ovary or pelvic mass, or if there is a family history of ovarian cancer.

Warnings and Contraindications to Hormone Therapy Use

Providers should be familiar with the product information before prescribing any EPT/ET regimen. Product warnings about HT use included on the product insert are extensive and should be discussed with women to assure that any concerns are addressed prior to prescribing HT. All HT products include the same warnings whether the product is systemic or local, regardless of current evidence about differences in systemic absorption levels. A black-box warning on all HT products is that a progestogen should be included in therapy to protect the endometrial lining for women with an intact uterus. Other black-box warnings on all EPT and ET products include findings from the WHI study including an increased risk of stroke and deep vein thrombosis (DVT) for HT users between 50 and 79 years of age compared to placebo. Providers are also cautioned that EPT/ET should not be used for the prevention of cardiovascular disease (CVD) or dementia. There is an additional warning, based on the WHI Memory Study (WHIMS), that the risk for developing dementia may be increased among HT users aged 65 and older (Shumaker et al., 2003). Other information included in labeling are statements about the type and dosage of EPT/ET used in the WHI and recommend that providers assume that other HT preparations have similar risks. Prescribing the lowest possible effective dosage for the shortest duration is also recommended along with close clinical surveillance and follow-up of any undiagnosed vaginal bleeding. It should be assumed that compounded HT preparations carry similar risks as those that are FDA approved (NAMS, 2010). Contraindications to EPT/ET use that are listed in the package insert are provided in Table 18–3.

Management of Common Hormone Therapy Side Effects

Side effects associated with EPT or ET use will vary depending on dosage, regimen and route of administration, and type of estrogen or progestogen. Discontinuation of HT is frequently associated with side effects.

TABLE 18–3. Contraindications for Estrogen Therapy/Estrogen-Progestin Therapy (listed in product literature)

- Abnormal genital bleeding (undiagnosed)
- Breast cancer (history, current, suspected except in appropriately selected patients)
- Estrogen dependent neoplasia (known, suspected)
- Deep vein thrombosis or pulmonary embolism (history or current)
- Stroke, myocardial infarction (within past year, current)
- Liver dysfunction or disease
- Hypersensitivity to estrogen therapy/estrogen-progestin therapy

TABLE 18–4. Common Side Effects of Hormone Therapy

Possible Side Effects	Interventions
Uterine bleeding	Manipulate dosage; rule out other gynecologic disorders
Breast tenderness	Lower estrogen dose; change estrogen and/or progestogen[a]; limit salt, chocolate, caffeine
Nausea	Take dosage with meals or at bedtime; change or lower dose of estrogen and/or progestogen[a]
Fluid retention (primarily extremities)	Limit salt; change or lower dose of estrogen and/or progestogen[a]
Bloating (abdominal gaseous)	Switch or lower estrogen or progestogen level[a]; change to micronized progesterone
Changes in shape of cornea	May require change or discontinuation of contact lens use
Headaches (may be migraine)	Change route of administration to patch for lower and steadier dose of estrogen
Dizziness	Take dosage at bedtime; change or lower dose of estrogen/progestogen[a]
Mood changes (progestogen related)	Asses for other causes of depression; change or lower dose of estrogen and/or progestogen[a]

[a]Assure that progestogen dosage is adequate to protect endometrial lining of uterus.

Uterine Bleeding. Cyclic regimens are associated with regular withdrawal bleeding in women with a normal secretory endometrium. Breakthrough, or unpredictable bleeding, is common during the first 3 to 6 months of continuous-combined therapy, especially among women who have been amenorrheic for 12 or fewer months. Breakthrough bleeding may be diminished by switching from a continuous-combined to a cyclic-combined regimen for the first year after menopause. Other approaches are to switch the type of progestogen used or to lower the dosage of estrogen. Typically, 19-nortestosterone derivative progestogens, micronized progesterone, and intrauterine progestogen therapy (IUS) are associated with less bleeding that MPA (Ettinger, 2005; NAMS, 2010). Having unpredictable bleeding is one of the most common reasons for discontinuing HT. The provider must always rule out alternative causes of irregular uterine bleeding such as endometrial cancer, and not assume that postmenopausal breakthrough bleeding is a HT side effect.

Breast Tenderness. Breast tenderness symptoms may respond to a change in the type of estrogen or progestogen used. Other lifestyle approaches include limiting salt, caffeine, and chocolate intake. Regular yearly clinical breast exams and mammograms should be encouraged. More frequent exams are warranted in women with persistent breast symptoms.

Nausea. Changing from an oral to a nonoral route of delivery may eliminate nausea. Other approaches are to change the type and/or dosage of estrogen and taking oral estrogen with meals. A change in the dosage and type of progestogen may also be needed.

Fluid Retention/Bloating. Nonoral preparations are less likely to cause fluid retention and bloating than oral preparations. Decreasing the dosage and changing the type of progestogen may eliminate or substantially decrease abdominal bloating and fluid retention in the extremities. Oral micronized progesterone is associated with fewer bloating problems than other oral progestogens. However, the dosage of progestogen must remain at a level that will effectively protect the uterus (NAMS, 2010).

Headaches. Changing from a cyclic to a continuous regimen may eliminate headaches associated with changes in circulating hormone levels. Switching types of estrogens and progestogens may also be helpful. Micronized progesterone and 19-nortestosterone derivatives are associates with fewer headaches than MPA. Ensure adequate fluid intake and decrease salt and alcohol intake (NAMS, 2010).

Mood Changes. Changing the type, dosage, and route of delivery of the progestin component of EPT is advised. Micronized progesterone (oral) and IUS may be helpful in addressing EPT-associated mood changes. Evaluation for underlying depressive disorders is always warranted (NAMS, 2010).

Initiating HT and Follow-Up

Provide the client with written and oral information about HT. Explain the risks and benefits as they apply to the client's own situation. Request that the client keep a menstrual calendar; educate her concerning what constitutes abnormal bleeding. Advise the client to telephone the health care provider immediately if she experiences any of the following:

- Unexpected bleeding.
- Abdominal pains, bloating.
- An increase in headaches.
- Symptoms not relieved or that increase.
- Visual disturbances.
- Shortness of breath or chest pain.
- Calf pain.

Adequate follow-up is critical in maximizing compliance and to evaluate the response to medications and side effects. A reasonable approach is to call the client in a month, and schedule a 2- to 3-month visit after therapy is initiated. Inform clients that it may take 2 to 3 months for desired vasomotor symptoms control. Clients should be encouraged to call with questions or concerns at any time. Stress to the client that even if she experiences no problems, annual exams, routine tests, and communication are important. Follow-up assessment on an annual basis for all clients on HT should include the following: interim history; complete medical examination, including breast and pelvic examinations; mammography; and Papanicolaou smear, if indicated. Endometrial evaluation is indicated for clients on ET without progestin, and those with prolonged bleeding (>10 days) or persistent, irregular bleeding. Office-based endometrial biopsy and pelvic ultrasound are the standard methods of evaluation.

PERIMENOPAUSAL HORMONE THERAPY

Clients who are still ovulating may need contraception as they approach menopause, yet have indications for supplemental ET as their estrogen level declines. Therapy options to regulate anovulatory cycles for perimenopausal women include oral contraceptives containing less than 35 mcg of estrogen or low-dose progestational treatment. These may be used if no contraindications exist. Low-dose oral CE and an estradiol patch are options if contraception is not an issue. Progestin is added when the uterus is intact. Management includes screening as recommended based on national guidelines and individual risk factors. Exams allay the fears of older clients about the increased risks of heart disease and stroke (NAMS, 2010). Communicate to the client the contraindications to OC use: smoking, hypertension, diabetes, thromboembolic disorders, impaired liver function, and known or suspected estrogen dependent neoplasm (refer to Chapter 12).

OPTIONS AFTER HYSTERECTOMY/ OOPHORECTOMY

Posthysterectomy (Without Oophorectomy)

Hysterectomy promotes earlier ovarian failure; the surgery itself may compromise blood supply to the ovaries or the underlying condition that led to surgical intervention may be associated with the timing of menopause. Measure the FSH level every 1 to 2 years. Ten-year follow-up of women in the ET-only arm of the WHI showed no increased risk of stroke, coronary heart disease (CHD), DVT, colon cancer, or all cause mortality (LaCroix et al., 2011).

Postoophorectomy

An abrupt, drastic fall in estradiol occurs following oophorectomy (no gradual adaptation is possible, as with natural menopause). The symptoms are often severe, particularly hot flashes and intestinal symptoms. Surgical menopause is a predisposing factor to osteoporosis, and it is known that bone is maintained by ET. ET is generally begun immediately postoperatively; higher than usual dosages of estrogen may be needed for up to a year postoperatively (LaCroix, Chlebowski, & Manson, 2011).

CHANGING DOSAGE OR DISCONTINUATION OF THERAPY

Adjustment of HT dosage may be needed to provide symptom relief. The dosage is increased gradually to find the minimum level needed for symptom relief. There are no guidelines about the optimal approach to discontinuing HT. Tapering use over a period of several weeks to several months is frequently recommended. However, when outcomes such as resuming HT use and recurrence of vasomotor symptoms are evaluated, there is no indication that slow tapering is more effective than abrupt cessation of HT (Suffoletto & Hess, 2009).

Prescription Therapies: Nonhormonal.

If HT is contraindicated or a woman prefers nonhormonal treatment, the following drugs may be offered.

- *Clonidine:* Oral and transdermal clonidine have been shown to be effective in treating daily hot flashes, especially in women with breast cancer. Side effects include dry mouth, drowsiness, and dizziness. The transdermal route is preferable to avoid side effects (Ghufran, 2011).
- *Selective Serotonin Reuptake Inhibitors (SSRIs) and Serotonin and Norepinephrine Reuptake Inhibitors (SNRIs):* Several studies of low-dose SSRIs and SNRIs have demonstrated significant efficacy in managing hot flashes compared to placebo. Fluoxetine, citalopram, venlafaxine, and paroxetine reduce hot flashes by as much as 50 to 60 percent at a range of therapeutic dosages (Albertazzi, 2007). Venlafaxine, an SNRI, has been shown to be especially effective (Evans et al., 2005). Hot flash resolution is usually rapid (within 2–4 weeks), whereas the antidepressant effect of these drugs may take up to 6 to 8 weeks. SSRIs and SNRIs are also effective in reducing hot flashes among breast cancer survivors. Lower dosages are preferred to minimize side effects including nausea, dry mouth, drowsiness, dizziness, and decreased libido (Loibl, Lintermans, Dieudonne, & Neven, 2011). Caution is warranted in prescribing SSRIs or SNRIs for women taking tamoxifen due to recent concerns regarding the possibility of decreased effectiveness of tamoxifen with concomitant treatment with SSRIs or SNRIs (NAMS, 2010).
- *Gabapentin (Neurontin):* Gabapentin is an antiseizure drug. A meta-analysis found that gabapentin reduced hot flash frequency and severity by 20 to 30 percent in four randomized controlled trials (RCTs) with heterogeneity of findings between studies. Side effects including dizziness, unsteadiness, fatigue, and somnolence often resolve by the fourth week of treatment (Toulis, Tzellos, Kouvelas, & Goulis, 2009).

Follow-Up

- Evaluate the effectiveness of therapy in relieving symptoms and monitor dosages based on efficacy, safety, and side effects.
- At least yearly visits, as indicated by current screening guidelines. Assess need for continuation of therapy.

COMPLEMENTARY AND ALTERNATIVE THERAPIES

Perimenopausal and postmenopausal women are among the highest users of botanical and nutritional supplement products for symptoms management. However, 70 percent of women do not tell their health care providers about their use of these products and providers are unlikely to ask about use of complementary alternative therapies, largely because they have not been exposed to alternative medical practices in their training and are unfamiliar with these products (Geller & Studee, 2005). Unfortunately, there is limited information about the effectiveness of complementary therapies in the treatment of vasomotor symptoms. The existing studies have small sample sizes and inconsistent findings (Newton et al., 2006; Smith & Carmady, 2010). Women should be consistently asked about their use of both prescription and complementary alternative therapies to manage menopausal symptoms. Some of the most popular complementary alternative therapies are described.

- Soy foods, isoflavone supplements, black cohosh, omega-3 fatty acids, and vitamin E are commonly used and recommended alternatives used for managing hot flashes. Black cohosh is the most studied nonprescription remedy for hot flashes. Evidence for effectiveness is contradictory and especially limited regarding longer safety and efficacy.
  - Isoflavones are found in soy products and red clover preparations. Scientific studies show mixed results regarding the efficacy of soy-based food and supplements in treating hot flashes. Based on reviews of many studies, soy-based isoflavones have been shown to be modestly effective in relieving menopausal symptoms; supplements providing higher proportions of genistein or increased S(Y)-equol may provide more benefits (Coon, Pittler, & Ernst, 2007; D'Anna et al., 2009; NAMS, 2011; Tice et al., 2003; Vitolins et al., 2010). Neither isoflavones derived from soy products nor red clover has been consistently found to significantly reduce the number of hot flashes (Lethaby et al., 2007; Nelson, Vesco, & Haney, 2006).
  - Black cohosh is the most studied nonprescription remedy for hot flashes. Evidence for effectiveness is contradictory. However, a meta-analysis demonstrated a significant improvement in vasomotor symptoms (overall reduction of 26%) despite heterogeneity of the black cohosh products (Shams et al., 2010). In contrast, a randomized controlled study comparing the effectiveness of black cohosh, red clover, and HT (CEE/MPA) preparations found that neither black cohosh nor red clover preparations reduced the frequency of hot flashes in comparison to HT (Geller et al., 2009; NIH Office of Dietary Supplements, 2008a).
  - Omega-3 fatty acids in the form of fish oil capsule supplements have increased in popularity over recent years due to publicity about the potentially positive effects on heart health and depressive disorders (Wu et al., 2007). Studies that address the efficacy of omega-3 fatty acids in treating vasomotor symptoms are scarce, but have yielded promising findings that need to be confirmed by clinical trial data (Campagnoli et al., 2005; Lucas, Asselin, Mérette, Poulin, & Dodin, 2009).
  - Overall, clinical data does not support the efficacy of vitamin E in treating hot flashes. However, vitamin E 400 IU daily is frequently recommended as a safe alternative that may be marginally helpful in providing relief from hot flashes, especially for breast cancer survivors. Although some observational study data is promising (Ziaei, Kazemnejad, & Zareai, 2009), reviews of published studies have concluded that the benefits of vitamin E in controlling hot flashes are minimal, at best (Dennehy & Tsourounis, 2010).
- *Chinese medicine and acupuncture:*
  - Acupuncture is a form of traditional Chinese medicine has increased in popularity among all age groups but especially among women during perimenopause and early postmenopausal years (Smith & Carnady, 2010). A small number of well-designed RCTs have been conducted to study the effectiveness of acupuncture in treating vasomotor symptoms. A review of six RCTs found that only one RCT found a significant difference in treatment efficacy between the acupuncture and control groups (Lee, Shin, & Ernst, 2009). Further research is ongoing, indicating promising results related to hormonal shifts following 3 months of weekly traditional acupuncture treatments (Painovich et al., 2012). A small study of acupuncture treatment among women who were taking tamoxifen for breast cancer showed promising results in diminishing the intensity of hot flashes as well as supporting improvement in mood and decreasing anxiety (deValois, Young, Robinson, McCourt, & Maher, 2009).
  - Chinese herbal preparations have also been used for centuries to treat vasomotor symptoms. Examples of Chinese herbal preparations that are frequently recommended and used for hot flashes include dong quai, ginseng, vitex (chasteberry), and tea tree oil. Effectiveness has been primarily anecdotally reported with an absence of RCT data. Further research is needed.
- *Mind/body therapies:* High-quality studies are lacking. However, a systematic review of relaxation and slow-paced breathing suggested overall improvement in vasomotor symptoms. Two small studies have

also found that hypnosis may improve vasomotor symptoms. An advantage of mind/body therapies is the lack of side effects and risks (Warnecke, 2011). There is evidence to suggest that yoga degrees stress and has psychological benefits for perimenopausal and postmenopausal women. A recent systematic review of three RCTs and five uncontrolled studies found symptom improvement with yoga and other meditation-based programs (Innes, Selle, & Vishnu, 2010).

In a climate where women and their providers are searching for effective and safe alternatives to HT for management of vasomotor symptoms, it is critical that well-designed studies are conducted. The National Institutes of Health, National Center for Complementary and Alternative Medicine (NIH, NCCAM, 2011) is an excellent resource for current evidence about a wide variety of complementary and alternative therapy options to HT.

Follow-Up

- Monitor for effectiveness and side effects.
- Ask about complementary and alternative therapy use at all follow-up visits.
- At least yearly visits, as indicated by current screening guidelines. Assess need for continuation of therapy.

VULVOVAGINAL SYMPTOMS

In premenopausal women, the vagina, introitus, and vestibule are lined with glycogen-rich squamous epithelium during the reproductive years. Normal vaginal fluid is clear to white in appearance and usually homogenous and odorless. Normal fluid does not cause irritation or pruritus.

Epidemiology

Decreased estrogen levels during the menopause transition lead to thinning and vaginal and vulvar tissues that are more fragile and more prone to infection, trauma, and discomfort. The vaginal pH is altered from acidic to alkaline. Lactobacilli levels decrease and are replaced with more diverse flora, some of which are pathogenic and may cause vaginal and urinary tract infections. *Vaginal atrophy* describes the process that results in pale, thinning, fragile tissue and often inflamed walls of the vagina that are characteristic of *atrophic vaginitis*. This environment makes the tissue more vulnerable to trauma during speculum exams and sexual intercourse. Dyspareunia during vaginal penetration may be a woman's presenting symptom during the menopause transition. However, vaginal dryness and irritation may be present regardless of sexual activity, leading to a decreased quality of life (NAMS, 2010). Vulvar tissues are also affected by decreased estrogen levels, leading to a variety of uncomfortable benign or invasive conditions.

Subjective Data

A menstrual history will reveal symptoms of vulvovaginal change, possibly including vaginal dryness, loss of lubrication with intercourse, pain or soreness during intercourse, unusual vaginal discharge, infection, and postcoital bleeding. Other associated symptoms may include dysuria, urethral discomfort, and stress incontinence (Tan, Bradshaw, & Carr, 2012).

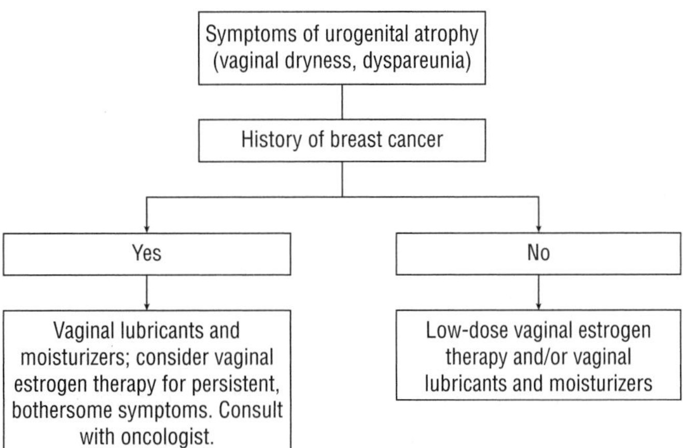

FIGURE 18–3. Hormonal Treatment of Vulvovaginal Symptoms Decision Tree. *Source:* Shifren & Schiff, 2010.

Objective Data

Note: Postmenopausal bleeding is not normal and should always be evaluated.

Physical Examination. Findings include thinning and paleness of vaginal epithelia, bloody vaginal discharge, brittle and thinning pubic hair, disappearance of rugae, and infection. Vaginal tissue may be friable and bleed easily with the speculum exam and vaginal/cervical specimen collection. The prepuce and clitoris may also show signs of atrophy. Examine vulvar tissue for atrophy and/or lesions. The vaginal tissue may appear to be smooth and shiny with patchy erythema. The vaginal epithelia become thin and pale with increased friability. Vaginal rugae disappear and the vaginal mucosa becomes less elastic. The volume of vaginal secretions decreases leading to increased time for lubrication during sexual intercourse with the potential for greater discomfort. The loss of estrogen that leads to urogenital atrophy also causes weakness of the vaginal walls and associated organ prolapse. Tissue may bleed easily with the speculum exam and vaginal/cervical specimen collection. A vaginal scraping may be done. Expected findings in menopausal woman would be a predominance of parabasal cells rather than superficial squamous cells due to estrogen depletion. Vaginal pH may also be measured and would be expected to be elevated in the absence of estrogen stimulation of the vaginal tissues (Tan, Bradshaw, & Carr, 2012).

Differential Medical Diagnoses

Vaginitis and sexually transmitted diseases (bacterial, viral, fungal infection), leukoplakia, lichen sclerosis, malignancy, postmenopausal uterine bleeding, diabetes mellitus, Sjögren's syndrome, side effect of antihistamines or antiestrogenic medications, side effect of radiation or chemotherapy.

Plan

Psychosocial Interventions. Teach the client about the normal physiological changes of menopause, aging, and sexuality that may occur.

Vaginal Hormonal Medication

Given the direct relationship between estrogen levels and vulvovaginal atrophy, ET, systemic or locally administered, unless contraindicated, is the standard of care for treatment. If hot flashes are also a concern, systemic ET, oral or transdermal, is the treatment of choice. If the primary concern is vaginal dryness, dyspareunia, or incontinence, local ET is indicated (NAMS, 2012).

Vaginal Hormonal Medication

Vaginal topical estrogens are indicated to reverse vaginal atrophic changes and reduce the discomfort associated with atrophic vaginal dryness. Topical vaginal estrogen restores tissue integrity and pH balance in the vagina, thus aiding in the prevention of vaginal infections, urinary incontinence, and urinary tract infections.

- *Vaginal CE cream* may be used continuously (0.5 g twice weekly) or cyclically (0.5–2 g daily for 21 days).
- *Estradiol cream 0.01%:* 2 to 4 g daily for 1 to 2 weeks, then 1 g thereafter.
- *Estradiol vaginal tablets:* 10 or 25 μg doses can be used once daily for 2 weeks and then one tablet twice weekly.
- *Estradiol vaginal rings* can be inserted by the client (one ring vaginally for 3 months).

Ongoing therapy for chronic vulvovaginal atrophy should be provided in the lowest possible effective dosage. Once vulvovaginal atrophy symptoms have improved, the dosage may be tapered for long-term therapy. Current data indicates that treatment may be continued indefinitely, although more long-term studies are needed that investigate safety beyond 1 year of continuous use. ET is the most effective treatment for relieving moderate to severe vaginal atrophy that may lead to dyspareunia and avoidance of sexual intercourse (NAMS, 2007, 2012). In addition, local ET may increase sexual satisfaction by increasing lubrication and blood flow to the area (Tan, Bradshaw, & Carr, 2012).

Local vaginal estrogen treatment is contraindicated for the same reasons as oral estrogen. Thus, a comprehensive history and individualized evaluation is very important. Adding a progestogen to low-dose vaginal ET is not typically recommended. Systemic absorption of estrogen is limited and endometrial hyperplasia is typically not a concern. However, if higher than usual dosages are used to treat systemic symptoms, either cyclic or continuous progestogen therapy is recommended to protect the endometrium (NAMS, 2010). However, some systemic absorption does occur in a dose-response manner and any unexpected postmenopausal bleeding should be investigated.

Other Interventions

Selective estrogen receptor modulators (SERMs), including raloxifene and tamoxifen, have not been shown to be effective in relieving vulvovaginal atrophy symptoms. However, investigational SERM preparations and tissue-selective estrogen complexes that are not yet FDA approved show some promise (Tan, Bradshaw, & Carr, 2012).

Intravaginal DHEA therapy is being tested with promising results. DHEA is a hormone precursor to testosterone. Recent studies show that intravaginal DHEA increases vaginal pH and may decrease pain with intercourse (Labrie et al., 2010; Tan, Bradshaw, & Carr, 2012).

Treat any vaginal infection as indicated, and educate the client about safer sex (see Chapters 11 and 12). Teach her Kegel exercises, as these may help with arousal. Offer the client suggestions or readings on sexual pleasuring to increase arousal (see Chapter 7). Advise her to use a water-soluble vaginal lubricant with intercourse to prevent trauma from penile thrusting and alleviate the discomfort of friction (lubricants will not reverse epithelial changes). Lubricant jellies, creams, and suppositories are available over the counter (without prescription). Nonprescription bioadhesive vaginal moisturizers help to maintain vaginal moisture and lower pH.

Women With History of Breast or Reproductive Organ Cancer

Oophorectomy and chemotherapy are associated with severe vulvovaginal symptoms and associated sexual dysfunction due to the induction of premature menopause. Vaginal testosterone cream use has been investigated and shown to be a promising treatment. However, further safety data is needed before FDA approval is given. Ongoing research is underway. Vaginal estrogens are commonly used to treat vaginal atrophy among breast cancer survivors. More long-term safety and efficacy data is needed, but current data suggests that vaginal estrogens do not adversely affect outcomes (Tan, Bradshaw, & Carr, 2012; Trinkhaus, Chin, Wolfman, Simmons, & Clemons, 2008).

Complementary and Alternative Therapies for Vulvovaginal Atrophy and Associated Sexual Dysfunction

Acupuncture, herbal supplements, and plant estrogens are frequently used among peri- and postmenopausal women to treat vulvovaginal atrophy. Soy, chasteberry, and ginseng are popular products. Studies of efficacy and safety are limited. A small study indicated that vitamin D supplementation may be more effective than placebo in treating vulvovaginal symptoms. In contrast, a study of supplementation with a soy-based phytoestrogen product did not show improvement in vulvovaginal symptoms when compared to placebo treatment (Tan, Bradshaw, & Carr, 2012).

Follow-Up

Advise the client to return to the health care provider if no relief occurs. Referral for sexual therapy may be indicated if the problem seems unrelated to physical changes in the vagina. Ongoing anticipatory guidance and education regarding normal physiological changes associated with menopause and aging are indicated.

SEXUALITY AND THE MENOPAUSE TRANSITION

Sexuality continues as an important component of a woman's life until her death. It represents a need to be accepted, a need for intimacy and companionship. During the menopause transition, ovarian secretion of androgens decreases markedly; androgens, especially testosterone, are thought to play a role in the maintenance of sexual desire, and therefore, this decrease may have an adverse impact on desire (NAMS, 2010). Another factor impacting desire is vulvovaginal changes. Vulvovaginal changes that occur as a result of hypoestrogenism during the menopause transition include, but are not limited to, the following:

- Thinning of vaginal walls
- Vaginal lubrication volume smaller
- Decreased labial sensation
- Dyspareunia from vaginal irritation, tissue friability, and anxiety
- Loss of elasticity, length, and width of vagina

Changes caused by hypoestrogenism may be lessened with estrogen or testosterone therapy. The use of testosterone to treat decreased sexual desire in women has also been considered and is frequently prescribed to treat sexual dysfunction in postmenopausal woman. However, testosterone is not FDA approved for this purpose and recommendations regarding its use vary. Custom-compounded testosterone creams are available from compounding pharmacies. Sexuality is often neglected in the counseling of midlife and aging women, yet women in this age group have a variety of concerns and information needs (see Chapter 7). Although indirect effects of hormonal therapy may improve female sexual function by increasing lubrication, blood flow, and sensation in vaginal tissues, there is no evidence that HT should be prescribed for other sexual problems including a diminished libido (NAMS, 2012).

ALTERATIONS IN MOOD

A significant number of women report that changes in mood and concentration, irritability, nervousness, and depression occur during midlife. A number of psychosocial changes occur at this time of life, including relationship changes, loss of partner, bodily changes of aging, parents and/or children needing care, and role changes that may also impact mood. The relationships between hormonal changes and anxiety and depression in the perimenopausal woman remain to be clarified, however. Both the central and peripheral nervous systems contain 17β estradiol sensitive cells, and the brain responds to withdrawal or absence of ovarian steroids. Estrogen influences the concentrations and availability of neurotransmitters, including serotonin, in the brain.

EPIDEMIOLOGY

No single cause for mood alterations has been identified. Hormonal deficiency may play a role, but consideration must be given to other factors in the client's life, such as aging and how she feels about it. U.S. society reveres youth, and the reality of lost youth and changes in body image may upset some women. Other major life changes that are common for a woman of perimenopausal and menopausal age include one's children leaving home, death or disability of a spouse or partner, helping aging parents, realization that one may not have achieved all of one's life goals, loss of childbearing capacity, and concerns about retirement and finances. Psychological symptoms, including decreased concentration and memory, mood changes, mild and transient depression, and decreased sexual desire not related to vaginal changes, have been attributed to menopause. Many of these symptoms may be interrelated to the physical symptoms of menopause, such as hot flashes causing insomnia, leading to loss of concentration from loss of sleep. The interrelationships among hormone levels, affective symptoms, and lifestyle factors need further examination.

SUBJECTIVE DATA

The client's history may reveal periods of crying, anger, sadness, irritability, depression, anxiety attacks, family members' reports of mood swings, and expressions of suicide. If a psychological disorder is suspected, a referral to a mental health professional is indicated.

OBJECTIVE DATA

Physical Examination

Findings on physical examination may include decreased affect, lethargy, inappropriate responses, and crying. A complete examination is indicated to rule out systemic diseases, drug use, or other conditions that could affect physiological function and cause symptoms.

Diagnostic Tests and Methods

General diagnostic tests, such as complete blood count (CBC), thyroid studies, FSH/LH, urinalysis, and blood chemistry analysis, are indicated to determine normal baselines and deviations. Drug testing may also be indicated. Routine screening for depression is indicated in all women during the menopause transition to aid in differentiating menopausal symptoms from major depressive disorders (Clayton & Ninan, 2010).

DIFFERENTIAL MEDICAL DIAGNOSES

Depression, anxiety disorders, neurological impairment, sexual dysfunction, psychiatric disorder.

PLAN

Psychosocial Interventions

Refer the client for psychological evaluation as appropriate; protect if the client is suicidal.

Life transitions, grief work, and affective and physical changes associated with perimenopausal transitions may require individual or group therapy and support. Educational programs focused on midlife and menopause that emphasize accurate information, positive attitudes, and connection with other women may reassure the client.

Medication

Although women seek HT to help with their mood, concentration, or depressive symptoms, no hormone is FDA approved for these symptoms without other indications for use. Evidence is insufficient to support the use of HT as an anti-depressant. The progestogen component of HT may worsen depressive symptoms (NAMS, 2012).

Exercise

Advise the client to engage in regular aerobic exercise and resistance training to improve muscle strength, unless contraindicated. Exercise may improve the client's psychological outlook and reduce mood swings.

Balanced Diet

Advise the client to maintain a nutritionally balanced diet and to avoid simple carbohydrates, which can induce hypoglycemic reactions.

Stress Reduction Techniques

Relaxation exercises, yoga, meditation, and regular physical exercise may reduce stress.

FOLLOW-UP

If the client does not respond to lifestyle changes and/or medication therapy, she should be referred to an appropriate mental health professional for additional treatment.

COGNITIVE FUNCTION/ MEMORY LOSS/ALZHEIMER'S DISEASE

Cognition encompasses the entire range of human intellectual functions, including learning and memory. Estrogen may enhance or preserve cognitive function by improving cholinergic function, neuronal survival, and cerebral blood flow. Some studies suggested that estrogen may be associated with a decreased risk or delayed age of onset of Alzheimer's disease, but several others found that it has no protective effects and is ineffective in delaying the progression of Alzheimer's disease. More recently, ET or EPT use by postmenopausal women was found to not result in a reduced risk of declined cognitive function or risk of developing Alzheimer's disease (Resnick et al., 2006). Thus, HT as a treatment to prevent or slow the progression of dementia or Alzheimer's disease is not recommended (NAMS, 2012). There are a variety of reasons why women may experience episodic difficulty with cognitive tasks during the perimenopausal years. Normal cognitive aging, stress, fatigue, vasomotor symptoms, sleep disorders, depression, medication side effects, and concurrent medical conditions such as thyroid dysfunction may all contribute to cognitive concerns in midlife.

SUBJECTIVE DATA

The client, or significant other, may report signs and symptoms of declining mental functioning, for example, forgetfulness, decreased concentration and attention, getting lost in familiar environments, and expressive or receptive language impairment.

OBJECTIVE DATA

A comprehensive history, physical examination, and review of prescribed and over-the-counter medications are done to rule out reversible and potentially treatable causes of cognitive impairment.

DIFFERENTIAL MEDICAL DIAGNOSES

Mild cognitive impairment, vascular dementia, Alzheimer's disease, alcohol dementia, depression, delirium, toxic effects of medications, malignancy, infection, thyroid disorders.

PLAN

Psychosocial Interventions

Depending upon the duration and severity of cognitive impairment, refer the client for consultation with a medical specialist for further evaluation. If symptoms are mild and screening, is normal, reevaluate in 6 to 12 months, and reassure the client about benign senescent forgetfulness. Individual and group therapy may be considered. Women can be reassured that cognitive concerns during the perimenopause may be time limited and related to life stress and menopausal symptoms (NAMS, 2012).

SLEEP DISORDERS

With aging, sleep stages 3 (early phase of deep sleep) and 4 (deep sleep and relaxation) decrease and brief arousals become more frequent (Espiritu, 2008). Alterations in sleep patterns may be the result of hot flushes and night sweats. The need for overall sleep diminishes slightly with age; the average adult needs 5 to 7 hours of sleep each day.

EPIDEMIOLOGY

Any number of factors may contribute to sleep disturbances in addition to estrogen decline: lack of exercise, excessive napping during the day, stress, depression, anxiety, illness, restless sleep partner, uncomfortable sleeping accommodations, excessive activity prior to bedtime, and stimulant drugs. Sleep disorders are common among the general population and increase in the perimenopausal and postmenopausal years. The exact incidence is unknown.

SUBJECTIVE DATA

The client reports signs and symptoms of menopause, as well as irritability, interrupted sleep, and feelings of tiredness.

OBJECTIVE DATA

Findings on physical examination include lethargy, dark circles under the eyes, and possible altered response time. Diagnostic tests are used to rule out other diseases that cause lethargy, fatigue, and insomnia, such as anemia, sleep apnea, or hypothyroidism.

DIFFERENTIAL MEDICAL DIAGNOSES

Neurological disorders, psychological disturbances. Obstructive sleep apnea is associated with significant daytime sleepiness and increased motor vehicle accidents.

PLAN

Reassure and educate the client about causes and remedies of sleep disorders. Referral to a sleep therapy specialist may be indicated. Consult current pharmacological therapy references for information on sedatives and sleeping medications, but only after giving nonpharmacological interventions a fair trial of several months.

Nonpharmacological Interventions

- *Evaluate naps:* Encourage 10- to 30-minute naps during the daytime if the client is severely sleep deprived. If napping is interfering with night sleep, however, urge decreasing naps if possible.
- *Avoid caffeine:* Foods and beverages containing caffeine should be decreased or eliminated, especially after 5 p.m. Evaluate prescription and over-the-counter medications that might contain caffeine, for example, some cold remedies.
- *Limit alcohol intake:* Alcohol consumption should be less than 4 oz per day or, preferably, eliminated altogether.
- *Avoid smoking:* Encourage the client to stop smoking. Offer literature and referral to a group for support.
- *Exercise before or in the early evening:* Exercising should occur no later than 7 p.m. (Aerobic exercise in late evening increases wakefulness.)
- *Arrange for a comfortable sleep environment:* Make suggestions concerning mattress comfort, soundproofing or earplugs, room darkening, sleeping clothes, room temperature, elimination of distractions.
- *Arrange quiet activity prior to bedtime:* Reading or listening to soothing music or environmental sounds may encourage sleep.
- *Avoid sleeping medications:* If the client is unable to sleep, advise her to get up and read or watch television, then try again in 30 to 60 minutes. Learning relaxation techniques, such as slow breathing from the diaphragm or playing mental games, and using them at bedtime may be beneficial. By setting aside a time to review concerns and activities of the day and coming up with solutions to problems before going to bed, the client may succeed in separating worries from the act of going to bed. (The bed should not be used as an office.) Taking warm baths, drinking milk (but not too much), and eating light (nonsugar) snacks before bedtime may also be helpful.
- *Limit food intake:* Heavy meals interfere with sleep; light snacks closer to bedtime are better.
- *Herbal remedies:* Valerian root has sedative-hypnotic qualities shown to improve sleep quality and the time it takes to fall asleep (NIH, Office of Dietary Supplements, 2008b). Short-term use is recommended. Effects may take several days to weeks before relief. Ingestion as a tea, tablet, or capsule about 60 minutes before bedtime is suggested.

FOLLOW-UP

The client may require referral to a sleep disorder program.

OVERVIEW OF CURRENT HORMONE REPLACEMENT THERAPY RESEARCH AND IMPLICATIONS FOR PRACTICE

The use of hormone therapy for the treatment of menopausal symptoms and chronic health conditions has been the topic of ongoing controversy for several decades.

In order to better understand the issues involved in this controversy, a more detailed discussion of HT use and research is included. Because the WHI research has been a critical turning point in provider and client attitudes and beliefs about hormone therapy, this section is divided into three time periods: (1) pre-WHI, (2) WHI, and (3) post-WHI (Roussouw et al., 2002).

PRE-WHI

Treatment of vasomotor symptoms with estrogen and progesterone is not a recent phenomenon. Since the 1930s, estrogen has been recognized as an effective treatment for hot flashes and other menopausal symptoms. However, in the 1960s, with the publication of the book, *Feminine Forever*, by Robert Wilson, ET became known as the miracle cure for menopausal symptoms and aging, in general. Wilson went so far as to claim that women who were not treated with hormones postmenopausally were no longer feminine. As a popular speaker, Wilson claimed that, "Every woman alive today has the option to remain feminine forever." Estrogen was promoted as the fountain of youth for all women.

In the decades that followed the publication of Wilson's book, hormone therapy was promoted and prescribed for a growing number of women until it became the most frequently prescribed drug in the United States. Hormone replacement therapy was prescribed for a broad range of conditions associated with aging ranging from wrinkles and general aches and pains to Alzheimer's disease, depression, and heart attack (Boston Women's Health Book Collective, 2011). The FDA initially approved estrogen treatment for hot flashes and other problems associated with menopause, not for disease prevention. However, by the late 1980s and the 1990s, observational studies suggested that hormone treatment may protect women against heart disease. In 1986, the FDA reviewed the evidence and found that hormone treatment was effective for treatment of osteoporosis. In 1990, the FDA found that the research done to date was not adequate to support adding heart disease prevention to the list of approved uses. But doctors are allowed to prescribe drugs for uses that are not approved by the FDA. Encouraged by the research suggesting that hormone treatment might be helpful for new uses, as well as by extensive drug company marketing efforts, many health care providers did just that. Such off-label prescribing is common practice in medicine when research to support new claims has not been completed, though in many cases it means that people are taking drugs that haven't been adequately proven to be safe or effective for the purposes for which they are being used (Boston Women's Health Book Collective, 2011).

In the mid-1970s, research findings about the link between estrogen and endometrial cancer were published. It was determined that adding a progestogen to estrogen ("combined treatment") would reduce the risk of endometrial cancer. After the publication of these findings, it became routine practice to prescribe combined therapy for women who still had a uterus and estrogen only for women who had a hysterectomy.

In the 1990s, two important studies were published that, once again, changed hormone therapy prescribing practices. The PEPI trial findings, published in 1995, showed that estrogen alone provided greater cardiac protection (measured as improved HDL-C lipid levels) than estrogen plus progestin. In addition, women who took oral micronized progesterone rather than oral MPA had lower HDL-C levels (Writing Group for the PEPI Trial, 1995). Prescriptions for oral micronized progesterone for women with a uterus rose substantially after the PEPI trial findings were released. The Heart and Estrogen/Progestin Replacement Study (HERS) findings, published in 1998, found that women with existing cardiac disease who used hormone estrogen/progestin therapy had worse outcomes than those who didn't take hormones. However, the results of the HERS were questioned regarding their applicability to healthy women. A warning that resulted from the HERS findings was that women with an existing cardiac condition should not be prescribed postmenopausal hormone therapy (Hulley et al., 1998).

WHI

The widespread use of hormone treatment did not change significantly until 2002, when the large-scale WHI findings revealed evidence that taking hormones did not protect healthy women against heart disease and stroke (Anderson et al., 2004).

The WHI trial had two arms: one in which the health benefits of combined hormone replacement therapy with 0.625 mg CEE and 2.5 mg MPA were being studied, and the other in which the benefits of ET alone (0.625 mg CEE) was studied among women without a uterus. The primary outcomes of interest of both arms of the WHI were cardioprotective benefits and breast cancer.

The *EPT arm* of the study was ended in 2002, 3 years before the planned 2005 completion. Writing about the EPT arm, the investigators concluded that the "overall health risks exceeded benefits . . . for an average 5.2 year follow-up," according to Rossouw et al. (2002, p. 321). Approximately half of the over 16,000 healthy postmenopausal women in the EPT arm, aged 50 to 79, were randomly assigned to oral EPT and the rest to oral placebo. Increased relative risks of 29 percent for CHD, 26 percent for breast cancer, 113 percent for pulmonary embolism (PE), and 41 percent for stroke were identified in the women using combined therapy compared to placebo. These findings equated to "absolute excess risks per 10,000 person-years attributable to estrogen plus progestin" of "7 more CHD events, 8 more strokes, 8 more PEs, and 8 more invasive breast cancers" (p. 321).

The *ET arm* of the WHI was stopped in 2004, 1 year prematurely, after 7 years. The reason for discontinuing the ET arm was failure to find cardioprotective benefit and an increased risk of stroke. The risk of stroke was found to be similar to that found in the EPT arm results (eight additional occurrences of stroke per 10,000 woman years). No increased risk of breast cancer was found during the 7-year study including 11,000 women who had a hysterectomy (Rossouw et al., 2002).

Publication of the WHI data leads to a rapid decline in hormone therapy use. Many women stopped using their hormone prescriptions immediately and many providers discontinued prescribing menopausal hormone therapy (Tsai, Stefanick, & Stafford, 2011).

POST-WHI

The early ending of the WHI EPT and ET studies was a turning point for both women and providers in their decision making about using HT during the menopause transition to treat symptoms and prevent other health problems. Staying current with evidence regarding the safety and efficacy of HT for symptom relief and disease prevention is a challenge for health care providers with the ongoing publications of findings based on the reanalysis of WHI data and new research. The following section summarizes evidence about the probable benefits and risks of HT (EPT and ET) related to specific diseases, health conditions, and symptoms, based on the WHI findings, the post-WHI reanalysis of the WHI data, and other research evidence published since the WHI study. NAMS (http://www.menopause.org/) and the Endocrine Society (http://www.endo-society.org/) are excellent resources for health care providers who wish to remain current about changes in guidelines and expert analysis of study findings.

Urinary Tract Health

An additional benefit of localized vaginal ET is urinary tract health. The estradiol ring has been found to effectively treat overactive bladder symptoms. Systemic estrogen may worsen these symptoms and transdermal estrogen has been shown to have a neutral effect on overactive bladder symptoms. A large study showed a decreased incidence of urinary tract infections among women who used intravaginal estrogen compared to placebo (NAMS, 2012).

Osteoporosis

Bone loss begins in the third or fourth decade of a woman's life, and accelerates rapidly with estrogen loss in the first postmenopausal decade. Standard-dose HT reduces postmenopausal osteoporotic hip, spinal, and nonspinal fractures, regardless of preexisting osteoporosis. The WHI trials confirmed a 33 percent reduction in hip fractures in healthy postmenopausal women receiving HT after an average follow-up of 5.6 years. Studies have confirmed that even very low-dose ET is effective in increasing BMD. Unfortunately, the BMD increase and fracture reduction seen with HT does not persist after discontinuation of HT. Five years after stopping HT, users have BMDs similar to those of never users (Ettinger et al., 2004; Greendale, Espeland, Slone, Marcus, & Barrett-O'Connor, 2002; International Menopause Society, 2007; NAMS, 2012; Shifren & Schiff, 2010; Yates et al., 2004). HT has been approved by the FDA for prevention of postmenopausal osteoporosis, but not for treatment of osteoporosis. Women who experience early menopause and require bone loss prevention are excellent candidates for HT or oral contraceptive until they reach the usual age of menopause. However, the data supports the effectiveness of HT in preserving bone mass and preventing osteoporotic fractures among women with early menopause, including those who had a hysterectomy with or without an oophorectomy (NAMS, 2012).

Cardiovascular Health

CHD. Most CHD data from observational studies supports the potential benefits of HT. In contrast, randomized clinical trial data, including data from the WHI, does not provide similar support. These differing results are probably related to characteristics of women participating in these studies with women in observational studies being younger and closer to the age of natural menopause than participants in RCTs. In the WHI, those in EPT group experienced a small increased risk of CHD events compared to women receiving a placebo and those receiving ET alone (Manson et al., 2003). Data from the PEPI study and HERS in the 1990s plus a meta-analysis of 22 trials led the American Heart Association to recommend that ET and EPT not be prescribed for secondary prevention of CVD or for primary prevention (Mosca et al., 2011).

Overall, WHI data indicated an increase of eight additional cases per 10,000 women per year in the EPT arm and a decrease of three cases per 10,000 women per year in the ET arm. Further analysis of the WHI data that included the subgroup of women between the ages of 50 and 59 showed a CHD risk that was substantially less than those who started HT several years postmenopause. These analyses have resulted in a "timing hypothesis," which predicts that the CVD benefit of HT is only evident if HT is initiated near the time of menopause and prior to the development of atherosclerotic plaques (Taylor & Manson, 2011). The timing hypothesis has been supported by several subsequent studies and there is ongoing research that will investigate this hypothesis further in order to clarify and guide treatment decisions (Bray et al., 2009; Harman et al., 2005; NAMS, 2012; Rossouw et al., 2007; Salpeter, Cheng, Thabane, Buckley, & Salpeter, 2009).

Stroke. The WHI study found that taking EPT and ET significantly increased the risk of ischemic stroke, with no effect on the risk of hemorrhagic stroke (Goldstein et al., 2011). Subsequent subanalysis of the WHI data for the EPT arm of the study showed that the increased risk of ischemic stroke disappeared when only the participants between the ages of 50 to 59 years were included in the analysis. However, a significant increased risk remained for women in the same age group in the ET arm. This result is not consistent with other data and may be an artifact of characteristics of women in the WHI ET arm. Evidence from the Nurses' Health Study suggests that women within 4 years of menopause and taking a lower than traditional dose of HT did not have a similar elevated risk of stroke (Grodstein, Manson, Stampfer, & Rexrode, 2008). However, other observational studies have yielded contradictory findings.

VTE. The risk for DVT and PE is increased significantly in postmenopausal women taking EPT or ET without other risk factors for VTE being present (Grady et al., 2001; Hulley et al., 1998). Numerous studies have suggested that venous thromboembolic risk is lowered with the use of transdermal hormone preparations compared to oral therapy (Heiss et al., 2008). However, further evidence is required. Clotting factors and triglycerides are raised to a greater degree with oral compared to transdermal therapy. In contrast, oral therapy provides more long-term benefits in reducing atherosclerotic risk by lowering overall and LDL cholesterol and increasing HDL (Taylor & Manson, 2011). The increased risk of VTE with HT use appears within the first 1 to 2 years after HT initiation and the magnitude of the risk declines over time. HT users with an increased baseline risk for VTE, including those who are obese (BMI > 30 kg/mg^2), have factor V Leiden mutation, or a history of VTE has an even greater risk than others for VTE while using HT. HT doubles the risk of VTE for women at any BMI. However, the risk level returns to baseline soon after HT discontinuation (Canonico, Plu-Bureau, & Lowe, 2008; NAMS, 2012).

Glucose Tolerance and Type 2 Diabetes Multiple studies have found that one type of ET (CEE) with or without a progestogen is associated with improved glucose tolerance and decreased risk of type 2 diabetes independent of any effects of HT on BMI (Kalish, Barrett-Connor, Laughlin, & Gulanski, 2003; Pentti et al., 2009; Santen et al., 2010).

Reproductive Tract and Breast Cancer

Endometrial Cancer. Unopposed systemic ET in postmenopausal women with an intact uterus causes an increased risk of endometrial cancer. The risk is directly related to the dosage and duration of ET use. The risk persists for several years after ET discontinuation. Concomitant use of a progestogen is recommended for women with an intact uterus using systemic HT. Estrogen use is contraindicated for women with a history of endometrial cancer. A progestogen alone may be helpful for long-term therapy of vasomotor symptoms. However, long-term data is not available (NAMS, 2012).

Ovarian Cancer. Published studies related to HT use and ovarian cancer risk have yielded conflicting findings (NAMS, 2012). Several studies have demonstrated a small but significant increased risk of epithelial ovarian cancer in current and recent users of ET (Rossing, Cushing-Haugen, Wicklund, Doherty, & Weiss, 2007). A consistent finding is that longer use (greater than 5 years) is associated with an increased risk of ovarian cancer. The increased risk did not persist 2 years after discontinuation. The increased risk found in the WHI was not statistically significant. Further study is needed because ovarian cancer is not typically an estrogen responsive tumor (Taylor & Manson, 2011). Based on these findings, women with an increased baseline risk for ovarian cancer (e.g., BRCA positive) should be counseled about the current study findings.

Breast Cancer. Fear about breast cancer is the most common reason for avoiding or discontinuing HT. The WHI confirmed that EPT increases breast cancer risk but, surprisingly, ET alone was not significantly associated with an increased risk (Prentice et al., 2008). Overall, the WHI results resulted in an absolute increased incidence of eight additional breast cancers per 10,000 women after 5 or more years of EPT use. Women diagnosed with breast cancer while taking EPT have a better prognosis than those who are not on EPT (Taylor & Manson, 2011). Both the timing of the initiation and the length of use of EPT are related to breast cancer risk. The risk for developing breast cancer increases with EPT use greater than 3 to 5 years (Chlebowski, Hendrix, & Langer, 2003; Stefanick et al., 2006). A marked decrease in the rate of breast cancer diagnosis was seen within the first 2 years after discontinuation of EPT in the WHI. After that time period, breast cancer rates are similar between users and nonusers (Calle et al., 2009; Chlebowski et al., 2009; Christiante et al., 2008; Ravdin et al., 2007). Multiple observational studies and clinical trials have consistently found that breast cancer risk is increased when EPT is initiated at the time of or within 3 years of menopause (Anderson, Chlebowski, & Rossouw, 2006; Fournier, Mesrine, Boutron-Ruault, & Clavel-Chapelon, 2009; Beral, Reeves, Bull, & Green, 2011). Later (more than 3 years postmenopause) initiation of EPT does not confer a similar increased risk. It has been suggested that the increased risk associated with early initiation of EPT may be the result of hormonal stimulation of preexisting tumors that were too small to be diagnosed by imaging studies or clinical exams prior to participation in the WHI. It is possible that some of these tumors may not have progressed without hormonal stimulation. This increased risk disappeared within 3 years of cessation of EPT. However, WHI follow-up data analysis of EPT users 11 years after the study began demonstrated a slight increase in breast cancer mortality among EPT users. Two additional breast cancer deaths per 10,000 women years were documented (Cheblowski, Anderson, & Gass, 2010). Findings that early initiation of EPT carries an increased risk of a breast cancer diagnosis are in direct contrast to the findings related to CVD including stroke and VTE. Based on observational study results, it has been suggested that cyclic or sequential use of EPT rather than continuous use may attenuate the breast cancer risk (Lyytinen, Pukkala, & Ylikorkala, 2009). It is unclear whether the type of progestogen used in EPT therapy has an impact on risk of a breast cancer diagnosis. Results of a large observational study suggest that short-term use of micronized progesterone carries a low risk of breast cancer. However, long-term (greater than 5 years) use of any progestogen formulation is associated with an increased risk of breast cancer (Fournier, Berrino, & Clavel-Chapelon, 2008; Fournier, Mesrine, Boutron-Ruault, & Clavel-Chapelon, 2009).

Women in the ET arm of the WHI did not have a similar pattern of risk for breast cancer as those in the EPT arm of the study. A small decrease in risk of both invasive and ductal breast carcinoma was demonstrated. However, the Million Woman Study found an increased risk of breast cancer among women who initiated ET use within 5 years after menopause. The older age and greater length of time since menopause of the women in the WHI study compared to those in the Million Woman Study may account for difference in findings. Differences in mammographic surveillance, study population characteristics, and types of ET used may also contribute to conflicting results regarding ET use and breast cancer risk (Beral, Reeves, Bull, & Green, 2011; Chen et al., 2006; Jordan & Ford, 2011).

Studies regarding the safety of use of HT following breast cancer treatment have yielded similarly conflicting results with observational studies suggesting that HT does not promote reoccurrence. However, clinical trials have had less promising results and indicate that HT is associated with an increased risk of reoccurrence (Col, Kim, & Chlebowski, 2005; Holmberg et al., 2008; NAMS, 2012).

Other Cancers

Colon Cancer. Observational studies and the EPT arms of the WHI have found a reduction in the risk of colon cancer among women who used EPT. In the post-WHI phase, the rate of detection of colon cancer was no longer decreased. Thus, the decrease appears to be associated with current use of EPT only (Taylor & Manson, 2011).

Lung Cancer. Subgroup analyses from the WHI indicate an increase in the diagnosis of small cell lung cancer among women over age 60 who were previous or current smokers. Because the WHI was not designed to include lung cancer as a study outcome, important baseline data related to lung health is not available. Other studies have had mixed results. However, the WHI findings underscore the importance of smoking cessation counseling and caution in prescribing HT to women over the age of 60, especially those with a history of or current tobacco use (Chlebowski et al., 2009, 2012; Greiser, Greiser, & Dören, 2010; NAMS, 2012; Oh, Myung, Park, Lym, & Ju, 2010).

Mood and Cognition

Mood and Sleep. HT is not indicated as a treatment for mood or sleep disorders. However, overall health-related quality of life is improved for many women taking HT. Data regarding antidepressant effects of HT for the women with and without a diagnosis of depression is mixed. There is some evidence that short-term use of HT may improve mood. However, improvement in vasomotor symptoms may also alleviate depressive symptoms. The progestogen component of HT may worsen symptoms of depression, especially if a woman previously suffered from PMS (NAMS, 2012). A decrease in hot flashes and night sweats that frequently disrupt sleep during the menopause transition is an indirect benefit of HT (Taylor & Manson, 2011). HT is not an antidepressant and depression is not an indication for prescribing HT for a perimenopausal or menopausal woman (NAMS, 2012).

Cognitive Functioning, Dementia, & Alzheimer's Disease. Recent literature suggests a transient, negative effect of the menopause transition on cognition. Long-term effects have not been substantiated. However, data does not support the use of ET or EPT use by peri- or postmenopausal women to reduce the risk of declined cognitive function or Alzheimer's disease based on findings from substudy of the WHI, the WHIMS, and the WHISCA (WHI Study of Cognitive Aging) (Resnick et al., 2006). Small clinical trials support the cognition benefits of women using ET following surgical menopause (NAMS, 2012). Among women older than 65 years, HT does not benefit memory and cognition and EPT has been found to be harmful to memory and associated with a higher risk of dementia (NAMS, 2012; Resnick et al., 2006; Shumaker et al., 2003). In addition, several observational studies have found an association between HT and Alzheimer's disease (NAMS, 2012). It has been hypothesized that, similar to CVD and HT data, the "timing hypothesis" may also relate to HT effects on cognitive functioning. Further study is needed to better understand the complex relationship between hormonal changes during the menopausal transition and cognitive functioning. Based on current evidence, there is no indication that ET or EPT should be prescribed for preventing or treating cognitive conditions associated with aging or chronic health conditions (NAMS, 2012).

Other

Gallbladder Disease. Gallbladder disease is common in postmenopausal women and use of hormone replacement therapy increases the risk. Use of transdermal therapy rather than oral therapy may decrease the risk of developing gallbladder disease associated with HT use (Liu et al., 2008; Santen et al., 2011).

Obstructive Sleep Apnea. It is associated with aging and is more prevalent among postmenopausal women who are not using HT. Androgen excess is also associated with obstructive sleep apnea regardless of BMI (Pierola et al., 2011; Tasali & VanCauter, 2008).

Dry Eye Syndrome. This risk is significantly increased with the use of HT (Jung, Jung, Shin, & Palik, 2010).

Client Education and Counseling Based on WHI and Other Research Findings

When presenting information to women about the WHI study results, it is important to present the absolute excess risk data along with the percentage increases in relative risk. For example, as women make decisions about short-term use of EPT/ET to manage vasomotor symptoms, it is important that they understand that a 26 percent increase in breast cancer risk equals eight more cases of invasive breast cancer per 10,000 woman years. In addition, after the publication of the WHI results, controversy arose about the applicability of the findings to women in their early postmenopausal years. The average age of participants was 63 years, with only 3.5 percent in the 50- to 54-year age range. These early postmenopausal years are when most women will be making decisions about using HT (Santen et al., 2010).

As expected, the results of the WHI and other studies have changed clinical practice related to HT significantly. It is clear that long-term use of 0.625 mg CE with 2.5 mg MPA for women without a uterus must be reevaluated and prescribed based on the individual client's history, needs, and risks. Each woman's situation is different, and treatment for menopause-related conditions must be tailored to the individual, just as are therapies for other conditions, such as hypertension. Are there factors in the woman's history that indicate that hormone therapy use could increase her risks? These factors must be assessed and considered before prescribing any therapy regimen. When women are older and have heart disease, an increased breast cancer risk, or other possible conditions that warrant careful consideration about use of hormones, the provider must evaluate all factors in partnership with the woman, including if hormone therapy or some other therapy would be best, the length of such therapy, and the specific therapy regimen.

The clinician, in close partnership with the client, must consider all the factors in the client's history when counseling women about HT use. Important information to covey to clients includes (1) HT is not indicated to treat/prevent CVD; (2) other measures must be considered, such as lipid-lowering therapies, as well as CV lifestyle changes for CVD prevention/treatment where risk or disease are present; (3) HT is at the lowest possible dosage that is effective in managing menopausal symptoms; (4) use of a progestin/progesterone other than MPA is advised (norethindrone acetate, norgestimate, prometrium); (5) lower doses of both estrogen and progestin are prudent; (6) nonhormonal therapies should be considered and may be better for a client, such as bisphosphonates and SERMS; (7) other more traditional measures for prevention and treatment of osteoporosis must be used (e.g., aerobic and weight-bearing exercises, calcium, vitamin D, no smoking, moderate or no alcohol); (8) annual clinician breast exams and mammography are essential; and (9) local therapies for vaginal atrophy and dyspareunia, including estrogen creams, but not systemic hormone therapy, are advised.

CONCLUSION

The menopausal transition is a normal event in the lives of women across all cultures. As life expectancy increases, a greater proportion of the female population will be in the postmenopausal demographic category. Women may or may not seek health care related to symptoms of the menopausal transition. As health care providers, we have the opportunity to partner with women to optimize their quality of life during this period in their lives. Providing anticipatory guidance and education about the menopausal transition during well woman visits provides women the tools they may need to prepare themselves for the menopausal transition. A healthy lifestyle including nutrition, exercise, stress reduction, and a positive support system can build resilience so that women are able to better manage the menopause transition.

REFERENCES

American College of Obstetricians and Gynecologists (ACOG). (2002). *Guidelines for women's health care* (2nd ed., pp. 130, 171, 314). Washington, DC: American College of Obstetricians and Gynecologists.

ACOG Committee on Gynecologic Practice. (2005). Committee opinion #322: Compounded bioidentical hormones. *Obstetrics and Gynecology, 106,* 1139–1140.

ACOG Committee on Gynecologic Practice. (2011). Committee opinion #483: Primary and preventive care: Periodic assessments. *Obstetrics and Gynecology, 117, 1008–1015.*

Albertazzi, P. (2007). Non-estrogenic approaches for the management of climacteric symptoms. *Climacteric, 10*(Suppl. 2), 115–120.

Anderson, G.I., Limacher, M., Assaf, A.R., Bassfor, T., Beresford, S.A., Black, H., et al. (2004). Effects of conjugated equine estrogen in postmenopausal women with hysterectomy: The women's health initiative randomized controlled trial. *Journal of the American Medical Association, 291,* 1701–1712.

Avis, N.E., Colvin, A., Bromberger, J.T., Hess, R., Matthews, K.A., Ory, M., et al. (2009). Change in health-related quality of life over the menopausal transition in a multiethnic cohort of middle-aged women: Study of women's health across the nation. *Menopause, 16,* 860–869.

Avis, N.E., Ory, M., Matthews, K.A., Schocken, M., Bromberger, J., & Colvin, A. (2003). Health-related quality of life in a multiethnic sample of middle-aged women: Study of women's health across the nation (SWAN). *Medical Care, 41,* 1262–1276.

Ayers, B., Forshaw, M., & Hunter, M.S. (2010). The impact of attitudes towards the menopause on women's symptom experience: A systematic review. *Maturitas, 65,* 28–36.

Beral, V., Reeves, G., Bull, D., & Green, J. (2011). Breast cancer risk in relation to the interval between menopause and starting hormone therapy. *Journal of the National Cancer Institute, 103,* 296–305.

Boston Women's Health Book Collective. (2011). *Our bodies, ourselves* (9th ed.). New York: A Touchstone Book Simon & Schuster

Bray, P.F., Larson, J.C., LaCroix, A.Z., Manson, J.E., Limacher, M.C., Rossouw, J.E., et al. (2008). Women's health initiative investigators. Usefulness of base-line lipids and C-reactive protein in women receiving menopausal hormone therapy as predictors of treatment related coronary events. *American Journal of Cardiology, 101,* 1599–1605.

Burleson, M.H., Todd, M., & Trevathan, W.R. (2010). Daily vasomotor symptoms, sleep problems and mood: Using daily data to evaluate the domino hypothesis in middle-aged women. *Menopause, 17,* 87–95.

Calle, E.E., Feigelson, H.S., Hildebrand, J.S., Teras, L.R., Thun, M.J., & Rodriguez, C. (2009). Postmenopausal hormone use and breast cancer associations differ by hormone regimen and histologic subtype. *Cancer, 115,* 936–945.

Campagnioli, C., Abba, C., Ambroggio, S., Peris, C., Perona, M., & Sanseverino, P. (2005). Polyunsaturated fatty acids (PUFA) might reduce hot flashes: An indication from controlled trials on soy isoflavones alone and with a PUFA supplement. *Maturitias, 51,* 127–134.

Chen, W., Manson, J., Hankinson. S., Rosner, B., Holmes, M.D., Willet, W.C., et al. (2006). Unopposed estrogen therapy and the risk of invasive breast cancer. *Archives of Internal Medicine, 155,* 1027–1032.

Chleblowski, R.T., Anderson, G.I., Gass, M., Lane, D.S., Aragaki, A.K., Kuller, L.H., et al. (2010). Estrogen plus progestin and breast cancer incidence and mortality in postmenopausal women. *Journal of the American Medical Association, 304,* 1684–1692.

Chlebowski, R.T., Anderson, G.I., Manson, J.E., Pettinger, M., Yasmeen, S., Lane, D., et al. (2010). Estrogen alone in postmenopausal women and breast cancer detection by means of mammography and breast biopsy. *Journal of Clinical Oncology, 28,* 2690–2697. (Epub May 3, 2010)

Chlebowski, R.T., Hendrix, S.I., & Langer, R.D. (2003). Influence of estrogen plus progestin on breast cancer and mammography in healthy postmenopausal women: The Women's Health Initiative. *Journal of the American Medical Association, 289,* 3243–3253.

Chlebowski, R.T., Kuller, L.H., Prentice, R.I., Stefacnick, M.I., Manson, J.E., Gass, M., et al. (2009). Breast cancer after use of estrogen plus progestin in postmenopausal women. *New England Journal of Medicine, 360,* 573–587.

Chlebowski, R.T., Schwartz, A.G., Wakelee, H., Anderson, G.L., Stefanick, M.L., Manson, J.E., et al. (2009). Oestrogen plus progestin and lung cancer in postmenopausal women (Women's Health Initiative trial): a post-hoc analysis of a randomised controlled trial. *Lancet, 374,* 1243–1251. (Epub September 18, 2009)

Christiante, D., Pommier, S., Garreau, J., Muller, P., LaFleur, B., & Pommier, R. (2008). Improved breast cancer survival among hormone replacement therapy users is durable after 5 years of additional follow-up. *American Journal of Surgery, 196,* 505–511.

Clayton, A.H. & Ninan, P.T. (2010). Depression or menopause? Presentation and management of major depressive disorder in perimenopausal and postmenopausal women. *Primary Care Companion: Journal of Clinical Psychiatry, 12,* PCC.08r00747.

Col, N.F., Guthrie, J.R., Politi, M., & Dennerstein, I. (2009). Duration of vasomotor symptoms in middle-aged women: A longitudinal study. *Menopause, 16,* 453–457.

Col, N.F., Kim, J.A., & Chlebowski, R.T. (2005). Menopausal hormone therapy after breast cancer: a meta-analysis and critical appraisal of the evidence. *Breast Cancer Research, 7,* R535–R540.

Coon, J.T., Pittler, M.H., & Ernst, E. (2007). Trifolium pratense isoflavones in the treatment of menopausal hot flushes: A systematic review and meta-analysis. *Phytomedicine, 14*(2–3), 153–159.

Davis, S.R., Davison, S.L., & Donath, S. (2005). Circulating androgen levels and self-reported sexual function in women. *Journal of the American Medical Association, 29,* 91–96.

D'Anna, R., Cannata, M.L., Marini, H., Atteritano, M., Cancelleri, F., Corrado, F., et al. (2009). Effects of phytoestrogen genistein on hot flushes, endometrium, and vaginal epithelium in postmenopausal women, double-blind, placebo-controlled study. *Menopause, 16,* 301–306.

Dennehy, C., & Tsourounis, C. (2010). A review of select vitamins and minerals used by postmenopausal women. *Maturitas, 66,* 370–380.

DeValois, B.A., Young, T.E., Robinson, N., McCourt, C., & Maher, E.J. (2010). Using traditional acupuncture for breast cancer-related hot flashes and night sweats. *Journal of Alternative and Complementary Medicine, 16,* 1047–1057.

Espiritu, J.R. (2008). Age-related sleep changes. *Clinical Geriatric Medicine, 24,* 1–14.

Ettinger, B. (2005). Vasomotor symptom relief versus unwanted effects: Role of estrogen dosage. *American Journal of Medicine, 118*(Suppl. 12B), 74–78.

Ettinger, B., Ensrud, K.E., Wallace, R., Johnson, K.C., Cummings, S.R., Yankov, V., et al. (2004). Effects of ultralow-dose transdermal estradiol on bone mineral density: A randomized clinical trial. *Obstetrics and Gynecology, 104,* 443–451.

Evans, M.L., Pritts, E., Vittinghoff, E., McClish, K., Morgan, K.S., & Jaffe, R.B. (2005). Management of postmenopausal hot flushes with venlafaxine hydrochloride: A randomized, controlled trial. *Obstetrics and Gynecology, 105,* 161–166.

Fan, H.G., Mar, N., Houédé-Tchen, N., Chemrynsky, I., Yi, Q.L., Xu, W., et al. (2010). Menopausal symptoms in women undergoing chemotherapy-induced and natural menopause: a prospective controlled study. *Annals of Oncology, 21,* 981–987.

Farague, M., & Maibach, H. (2006). Lifetime changes in the vulva and vagina. *Archives of Gynecology and Obstetrics, 273,* 195–202. (Epub October 6, 2005)

Fournier, A., Berrino, F., & Clave-Chapelon, F. (2008). Unequal risks for breast cancer associated with different hormone replacement therapies: Results from the E3N cohort study. *Breast Cancer Research and Treatment, 107,* 103–111.

Fournier, A., Mesrine, S., Boutron-Ruault, M.C., & Clavel-Chapelon, F. (2009). Estrogen-progestogen menopausal hormone therapy and breast cancer: Does delay from menopause onset to treatment initiation influence risks? *Journal of Clinical Oncology, 27,* 5138–5143.

Geller, S.E., & Studee, L.(2005). Botanical and dietary supplements for menopausal symptoms: what works, what does not. *Journal of Women's Health (Larchmt), 14,* 634–649.

Geller, S.E., Shulman, L.P., van Breemen, R.B., Banuvar, S., Zhou, Y., Epstein, G., et al. (2009). Safety and efficacy of black cohosh and red clover for the management of vasomotor symptoms: A randomized controlled trial. *Menopause. 16,* 1156–1166.

Ghufran, A.J. (2011). Strategies for managing hot flashes. *Journal of Family Practice, 60,* 333–339.

Goldstein, L.B., Bushnell, C.D., Adams, R.J., Appel, L.J., Braun, L.T., Chaturvedi, S., et al. (2011). Guidelines for the primary prevention of stroke: A guideline for healthcare professionals from the American Heart Association/American Stroke Association. *Stroke, 42,* 517–584.

Grady, D., Brown, J.S., Vittinghoff, E., Applegate, W., Varner, E., Snyder, T. (2001). Postmenopausal hormones and incontinence: The Heart and Estrogen/Progestin Replacement Study. *Obstetrics and Gynecology, 97,* 116–120.

Greendale, G.A., Espeland, M., Slone, S., Marcus, R., & Barrett-Connor, E. (2002). Bone mass response to discontinuation of long-term hormone replacement therapy: Results from the postmenopausal estrogen/progestin interventions

(PEPI) safety follow-up study. *Archives of Internal Medicine, 162*(6), 665–672.

Greiser, C.M., Greiser, E.M., & Dören, M. (2010). Menopausal hormone therapy and risk of lung cancer—Systematic review and meta-analysis. *Maturitas, 65,* 198–204.

Grodstein, F., Manson, J.E., Stampfer, M.J., & Rexrode, K. (2008). Postmenopausal hormone therapy and stroke: Role of time since menopause and age at initiation of hormone therapy. *Archives of Internal Medicine, 168,* 861–866.

Hall, L., Callister, L.C., Berry, J.A., & Matsumura, G. (2007). Meanings of menopause: Cultural influence on perception and management of menopause. *Journal of Holistic Nursing, 2,* 106–118.

Harlow, S.D., Gass, M., Hall, J.E., Lobo, R., Maki, P., Rebar, R.W., et al. (2012). Executive summary of the Stages of Reproductive Aging Workshop+10: Addressing the unfinished agenda of staging reproductive aging. *Menopause, 19.* doi:10.1097/gme.0b013e31824d8f40

Harman, S.M., Brinton, E.A., Cedars, M., Lobo, R., Manson, J.E., Merriam, G.R., et al. (2005). KEEPS: The Kronos early estrogen prevention study. *Climacteric, 8,* 3–12.

Heiss, G., Wallace, R., Anderson, G.I., Aragaki, A., Beresford, S.A., Brzyski, R., et al. (2008). Health risks and benefits 3 years after stopping randomized treatment with estrogen and progestin. *Journal of the American Medical Association, 299,* 1036–1045.

Henderson, K.D., Bernstein, L., Henderson, B., Kolonel, L., & Pike, M.C. (2008). Predictors of the timing of natural menopause in the multiethnic cohort study. *American Journal of Epidemiology, 167*(11), 1287–1294.

Hill, D.A., & Hill, S.R. (2010). Counseling patients about hormone therapy and alternatives for menopausal symptoms. *American Family Physician, 82,* 801–807.

Holmberg, L., Iversen, O.E., Rudenstam, C.M., Hammar, M., Kumpulainen, E., Jaskiewicz, J., et al. (2008). Increased risk of recurrence after hormone replacement therapy in breast cancer survivors. *Journal of the National Cancer Institute, 68,* 95–98.

Hulley, S., Grady, D., Bush, T., Furberg, C., Herrington, D., Riggs, B., et al. (1998). Randomized trial of estrogen plus progestin for secondary prevention of coronary heart disease in postmenopausal women. Heart and Estrogen/Progestin Replacement Study (HERS) research group. *Journal of the American Medical Association, 280,* 605–613.

Innes, K.E., Selfe, T.K., & Vishnu, A. (2010). Mind-body therapies for menopausal symptoms: A systematic review. *Maturitas, 66,* 136–149.

International Menopause Society. (2007). IMS updated recommendations on postmenopausal hormone therapy. *Climacteric, 10,* 181–194.

Jin, Y., Hayes, D.F., Li, L., Robarge, J.D., Skaar, T.C., Philips, S., et al. (2008). Estrogen receptor genotypes influence hot flash prevalence and composite score before and after tamoxifen therapy. *Annals of Oncology, 21,* 983–987.

Jung, H.M., Jung, W.J., Shin, K.H., & Paik, H.J. (2010). Effect of hormone replacement therapy on dry eye syndrome in postmenopausal women: A prospective study. *Journal of Korean Ophthalmology Society, 51,* 175–179. Retrieved February 22, 2010, from http://dx.doi.org/10.3341/jkos.2010.51.2.175

Kalish, G.M., Barrett-Connor, E., Laughlin, G.A., & Gulanski, B.I. (2003, April 1). Association of endogenous sex hormones and insulin resistance among postmenopausal women: Results from the postmenopausal estrogen/progestin intervention trial. *Journal of Clinical Endocrinology and Metabolism, 88*(4), 1646–1652.

Labrie, F., Archer, D., Bouchard, C., Fortier, M., Cusan, L., Gomez, J.L., et al. (2010). Vaginal Atrophy: High internal consistency and efficacy of intravaginal DHEA for vaginal atrophy. *Gynecological Endocrinology, 26,* 524–532.

LaCroix, A.Z., Chlebowski, R.T., Manson, J.E., Aragaki, A.K., Johnson, K.C., Martin, L., et al. (2011). Health outcomes after stopping conjugated equine estrogens among postmenopausal women with prior hysterectomy: A randomized controlled trial. *Journal of the American Medical Association, 305*(13), 1305–1314.

Lee, M.S., Shin, B.C., & Ernst, E. (2009). Acupuncture for treating menopausal hot flushes: A systematic review. *Climacteric, 12,* 16–25.

Lethaby, A.E., Brown, J., Marjoribanks, J., Kronenberg, F., Roberts, H., & Eden, J. (2007). Phytoestrogens for vasomotor menopausal symptoms. *Cochrane Database of Systematic Reviews,* (4), CD001395.

Liu, B., Beral, V., Balkwill, A., Green, J., Sweetland, S., Reeves, G., et al. (2008). Gallbladder disease and use of transdermal versus oral hormone replacement therapy in postmenopausal women: Prospective cohort study. *British Medical Journal, 337,* 1–9.

Loibl, S., Lintermans, A., Dieudonné, A.S., & Neven, P. (2011). Management of menopausal symptoms in breast cancer patients. *Maturitas, 68,* 148–154.

Lucas, M., Asselin, G., Mérette, C., Poulin, M.-J., Dodin, S. (2009). Effects of ethyl-eicosapentaenoic acid omega-3 fatty acid supplementation on hot flashes and quality of life among middle-aged women: a double-blind, placebo-controlled, randomized clinical trial. *Menopause, 16,* 357–366.

Lyytinen, H., Pukkala, E., & Ylikorkala, O. (2009). Breast cancer risk in postmenopausal women using estradiol-progestogen therapy. *Obstetrics and Gynecology, 113,* 56–73.

Manson, J.E., Hsia, J., Johnson, K.C., Roussouw, J.E., Assaf, A., Lasser N.L., et al. (2003). Estrogen plus progestin and the risk of coronary heart disease. *New England Journal of Medicine, 349,* 523–534.

Melby, M.K., & Lampl, M. (2011). Menopause: A biocultural perspective. *Annual Review of Anthropology, 40,* 53–70.

Mitchell, J.L., Walsh, J., Wang-Cheng, R., & Hardman, J.L. (2003). Postmenopausal hormone therapy: A concise guide to therapeutic uses, formulations, risks, and alternatives. *Primary Care: Clinics in Office Practice, 30,* 671–696.

Mosca, L., Benjamin, E.J., Berra, K., Bezanson, J.L., Dolor, R.J., Lloyd-Jones, D.M., et al. (2011). Effectiveness based guidelines for the prevention of cardiovascular disease in women–2011 update: A guideline from the American heart association. *Circulation, 123,* 1243–1262. Retrieved from http://circ.ahajournals.org/content/123/11/1243

National Cancer Institute. (2011). *Breast changes during your lifetime that are not cancer.* Retrieved September 15, 2011, from http://www.cancer.gov/cancertopics/screening/understanding-breast-changes/page4

National Institutes of Health (NIH), National Center for Complementary, & Alternative Medicine. (2011). Retrieved from NIH, National Center for Complementary and Alternative Medicine web site: http://nccam.nih.gov/

National Institutes of Health (NIH), Office of Dietary Supplements. (2008a). *Dietary supplement fact sheet: Black Cohosh.* Retrieved from http://ods.od.nih.gov/factsheets/black-cohosh

National Institutes of Health (NIH), Office of Dietary Supplements. (2008b). *Dietary supplement fact sheet: Valerian.* Retrieved from http://ods.od.nih.gov/pdf/factsheets/valerian.pdf

Nelson, H.D. (2004). Commonly used types of postmenopausal estrogen for treatment of hot flashes: Scientific review. *Journal of the American Medical Association, 291,* 1610–1620.

Nelson, H.D., Vesco, K.K., Haney, E., Rongwe, F., Nedrow, A., Miller, J., et al. (2006). Nonhormonal therapies for menopausal hot flashes: systematic review and meta-analysis. *Journal of the American Medical Association, 295,* 2057–2071.

Newton, K.M., Reed, S.D., LaCroix, A.Z., Grothaus, L.C., Erlich, K., & Guiltinan, J. (2006). Treatment of vasomotor symptoms of menopause with black cohosh, multibotanicals, soy, hormone therapy, or placebo. *Annals of Internal Medicine, 145,* 869–879.

NIH, Office of Dietary Supplements. (2008). *Dietary supplement fact sheet: Black cohosh.* Retrieved from http://ods.od.nih.gov/factsheets/blackcohosh

North American Menopause Society (NAMS). (2007). The role of local vaginal estrogen for treatment of vaginal atrophy in postmenopausal women: 2007 position statement of the North American Menopause Society, *Menopause, 14,* 357–369.

North American Menopause Society (NAMS). (2010). *Menopause practice: A clinician's guide* (4th ed.). Mayfield Heights, OH: Author.

North American Menopause Society (NAMS). (2011). *Hormone products for postmenopausal use in the United States and Canada.* Retrieved September 15, 2011, from http://www.menopause.gor/htcharts.pdf

North American Menopause Society (NAMS). (2012). The 2012 hormone therapy position statement of the North American Menopause Society. *Menopause, 19,* 257–271.

Oh, S.W., Myung, S.K., Park, J.Y., Lym, Y.I., & Ju, W. (2010). Hormone therapy and risk of lung cancer: a meta-analysis. *Journal of Women's Health (Larchmant), 19,* 279–288.

Painovich, J.M., Shufelt, C.L., Azziz, R., Yang, Y., Goodarzi, M.O., Braunstein, G.D., et al. (2012). A pilot randomized, single-blind, placebo-controlled trial of traditional acupuncture for vasomotor symptoms and mechanistic pathways of menopause. *Menopause, 19,* 54–61.

Parker, S. (2004). Follicle stimulating hormone: facts and fallacies. *Journal of the British Menopause Society, 10,* 166–168.

Pentti, K., Tuppurainen, M.T., Honkanen, R., Sandini, L., Kröger, H., Alhava, E., et al. (2009). Hormone therapy protects from diabetes: The Kuopio osteoporosis risk factor and prevention study. *European Journal of Endocrinology, 160*(6), 979–983. (Epub March 25, 2009)

Petitti, D.B. (2002). Hormone replacement therapy for prevention: More evidence, more pessimism. *Journal of the American Medical Association, 288*(1), 99–101.

Pierola, J., Nunez, B., Castillo, A.G.F., delaPena, M., Barcelo, A., Alonso-Fernandez, A., et al. (2011). *Menopause is not a risk factor for sleep apnea.* Poster Session, A74 Laboratory and Management Issues for Sleep Disorders, Colorado Convention Center. Retrieved May 15, 2011, from http://ajrccm.atsjournals.org/cgi/reprint/183/1_MeetingAbstracts/A2231.pdf

Prentice, R.I., Chlebowski, R.T., Stefanick, M.I., Manson, J.E., Langer, R.D., Pettinger, M., et al. (2008). Conjugated equine estrogens and breast cancer risk in the Women's Health Initiative clinical trial and observational study. *American Journal of Epidemiology, 167,* 1407–1415.

Ravdin, P.M., Cronin, K.A., Howlader, N., Berg, C.D., Chlebowski, R.T., Feuer, E.J., et al. (2007). The decrease in breast cancer incidence in 2003 in the United States. *New England Journal of Medicine, 356,* 1670–1674.

Resnick, S.M., Maki, P.M., Rapp, S.R., Espeland, M.A., Brunner, R., Coker, L.H., et al. (2006). Effects of combination estrogen plus progestin hormone treatment on cognition and affect. *Journal of Clinical Endocrinology and Metabolism, 91,* 1802–1810. (Epub March 7, 2006)

Rossing, M.A., Cushing-Haugen, K.I., Wicklund, K.G., Doherty, J.A., & Weiss, N.S. (2007). Menopausal hormone therapy and risk of epithelial ovarian cancer. *Cancer Epidemiology, Biomarkers and Prevention, 16,* 2548–2556.

Rossouw, J.E., Anderson, G.L., Prentice, R.L., LaCroix, A.Z., Kooperberg, C., Stefanick, M.L., et al. (2002). Risks and benefits of estrogen plus progestin in healthy postmenopausal women: Principal results from the Women's Health Initiative randomized controlled trial. *Journal of the American Medical Association, 288(3),* 321–333.

Rossouw, J.E., Prentice, R.L., Manson, J.E., Wu, L., Barad, D., Barnabei, V.M., et al. (2007). Post menopausal hormone therapy and risk of cardiovascular disease by age and years since menopause. *Journal of the American Medical Association, 297,* 1465–1477.

Salpeter, S.R., Cheng, J., Thabane, L., Buckley, N.S., & Salpeter, E.E. (2009). Bayesian meta-analysis of hormone therapy and mortality in younger post-menopausal women. *American Journal of Medicine, 122,* 1016–1022.

Santen, R.J., Allred, D.C., Ardoin, S.P., Archer, D.F., Boyd, N., Braunstein, G.D., et al. (2010). Executive summary: Postmenopausal hormone therapy: An endocrine society scientific statement. *Journal of Clinical Endocrinology and Metabolism, 95*(Suppl. 1), S1–S66. Retrieved from http://www.endo-society.org/journals/scientificstatements/upload/jc-2009-2509v1.pdf

Shifren, J., & Schiff, I. (2010). Role of hormone therapy in the management of menopause. *Obstetrics and Gynecology, 115*(4), 839–855.

Shams, T., Setia, M.S., Hemmings, R., McCusker, J., Sewitch, M., & Ciampi, A. (2010). Efficacy of black cohosh containing preparations on menopausal symptoms: A meta-analysis. *Alternative Therapies in Health and Medicine, 16,* 36–44.

Shufelt, C.I., & Braunstein, G.D. (2009). Safety of testosterone use in women. *Maturitas, 63,* 63–66.

Shumaker, S., Legault, C., Rapp, S., Thal, L., Wallace, R.B., Ockene, J.K., Hendrix, S.L., et al. (2003). Estrogen plus progestin and the incidence of dementia and mild cognitive impairment in postmenopausal women: The Women's Health Initiative Memory Study: A randomized controlled trial. *Journal of the American Medical Association, 289,* 2651–2662.

Smith, C.A., & Carmady, B. (2010). Acupuncture to treat common reproductive health complaints: An overview of evidence. *Autonomic Neuroscience: Basic and Clinical, 157,* 52–56.

Somboonparn, W., Davis, S., Seif, M.W., & Bell, R. (2005). Testosterone for peri- and postmenopausal women. *Cochrane Database Systematic Review,* (4), CDC004509.

Sood, R., Shuster, L., Smith, R., Vincent, A., & Jatoi, A. (2011). Counseling postmenopausal women about bioidentical hormones: Ten discussion points for practicing physicians. *Journal of American Board of Family Medicine, 24,* 202–210.

Soules, M.R., Sherman, S., Parrott, E., Rebar, R., Santoro, N., Utian, W., et al. (2001). Executive summary: Stages of reproductive aging workshop (STRAW), Park City, Utah, July 2001. *Menopause, 8*(6), 402–407.

Stefanick, M.I., Anderson, G.I., Margolis, K.I., Hendrix, S.I., Radabough, R.J., Paskett, E.D., et al. (2006). Effects of conjugated equine estrogens on breast cancer and mammography screening in postmenopausal women with hysterectomy. *Journal of the American Medical Association, 295,* 1647–1657.

Suffoletto, J.-A., & Hess, R. (2009). Tapering vs. cold turkey: Symptoms vs. successful discontinuation of menopausal hormone therapy. *Menopause, 16,* 436–437.

Tan, O., Bradshaw, K., & Carr, B.R. (2012). Management of vulvovaginal atrophy-related sexual dysfunction in postmenopausal women: an up-to-date review. *Menopause, 19,* 109–117.

Tasali, E., & VanCauter, E. (2008). Polycystic ovary syndrome and obstructive sleep apnea. *Sleep Medicine Clinic, 3,* 37–46.

Taylor, H.S., & Manson, J.E. (2011). Update in hormone therapy use in menopause. *Journal of Clinical Endocrinology and Metabolism, 96,* 255–264.

Tehrani, F.R., Shakeri, N., Solaymani-Dodaran, M., & Azizi, F. (2011). Predicting age at menopause from serum antimüllerian hormone concentration. *Menopause, 18*(7), 766–770.

Tice, J.A., Ettinger, B., Ensrud, K., Wallace, R., Blackwell, T., & Cummings, S.R. (2003, July 9). Phytoestrogen supplements for the treatment of hot flashes: The Isoflavone Clover Extract (ICE) study: A randomized controlled trial. *Journal of the American Medical Association, 290*(2), 207–214.

Tinelli, A., Malvasi, A., Rahimi, S., Negro, R., Vergara, D., Martignago, R., et al. (2010). Age-related pelvic floor modifications and prolapse risk factors in postmenopausal women. *Menopause, 17,* 204–212.

Toulis, K.A., Tzellos, T., Kouvelas, D., & Goulis, D.G. (2009). Gabapentin for the treatment of hot flashes in women with natural or tamoxifen-induced menopause: A systematic review and meta-analysis. *Clinical Therapeutics, 31,* 221–235.

Trinkhaus, M., Chin, S., Wolfman, W., Simmons, C., & Clemons, M. (2008). Should urogenital atrophy in breast cancer survivors be treated with topical estrogens? *Oncologist, 13*(3), 222–231. Retrieved from http://theoncologist.alphamedpress.org/content/13/3/222.full

Tsai, S.A., Stafanick, M.L., & Stafford, R.S. (2011). Trends in menopausal hormone therapy use of US office-based physicians, 2000-2009, *Menopause, 18,* 385–392.

Vitolins, M.Z., Case, L.D., Morgan, T.M., Miller, M.A., & Burke, G.L. (2010). Soy use and vasomotor symptoms: soy estrogen alternative follow-up study. *International Journal of Women's Health, 2,* 381–386. Retrieved from http://www.ncbi.nlm.nih.gov/pmc/articles/PMC2990907/

Warnecke, E. (2011). What works? Evidence for lifestyle and nonprescription therapies in menopause. *Australian Family Physician, 40,* 286–289.

Wierman, M.F., Basson, R., Davis, S.R., Khosla, S., Miller, K.K., Rosner, W., et al. (2006). Androgen therapy in women: An endocrine society clinical practice guideline. *Journal of Clinical Endocrinology and Metabolism, 91,* 3697–3710.

Williams, R.E., Levine, K.B., Kalilani, L., Lewis, J., & Clark, R.V. (2009). Menopause-specific questionnaire assessment in US population-based study shows negative impact on health-related quality of life. *Maturitas, 62,* 153–159.

Wilson, R. (1966). *Feminine forever.* New York: M. Evans & Company.

Wu, P., Fuller, C., Liu, X., Lee, H.C., Fan, B., Hoven, C.W., et al. (2007). Use of complementary and alternative medicine among women with depression: results of a national survey. *Psychiatric Survey, 58,* 349–356.

Writing Group for the PEPI Trial. (1995). Effects of estrogen or estrogen/progestin regimens on heart disease risk factors in postmenopausal women: The postmenopausal estrogen/progestin interventions (PEPI) trial. *Journal of the American Medical Association, 273*(3), 199–208.

Yates, J., Barrett-Connor, E., Barlas, S., Chen, Y.-T., Miller, P., & Siris, E. (2004). Rapid loss of hip fracture protection after estrogen cessation: Evidence from the national osteoporosis risk assessment. *Obstetrics and Gynecology, 104,* 440–446.

Ziaei, S., Kazemnejad, A., & Zareai, M. (2007). The effect of Vitamin E on hot flashes in menopausal women. *Gynecologic and Obstetric Investigation, 64,* 204–207.

IV ❖ Promotion of Women's Health Care During Pregnancy

CHAPTER ❖ 19

HEALTH PROMOTION AND ASSESSMENT DURING PREGNANCY

Jennifer M. Demma ◆ Karen Trister Grace

The nation's approach to women's health care may well be at the tipping point of redefining the perinatal period to include women's wellness across the reproductive life span. (Freda, Moos, & Curtis, 2006, pp. S43–S44)

Highlights

- Planning for a Healthy Pregnancy
- Immunizations
- Assessment During Pregnancy
- Diagnostic Tests and Methods
- The Developmental Stages of Pregnancy
- Common Complaints
- Adolescent Pregnancy
- Delayed Pregnancy
- Nontraditional Families
- Anticipatory Guidance During Pregnancy
- Danger Signs and Symptoms
- Recognizing Signs and Symptoms of Labor

❖ INTRODUCTION

The ultimate goal of pregnancy is the birth of a healthy infant into a healthy and nurturing family who can provide for his or her physical, psychological, emotional, and spiritual needs. Prenatal care encompasses risk assessment, social services, client education, and medical care. Ideally, this care should begin prior to conception. During pregnancy, many normal physiological changes lead to discomfort or concern for the mother. Health care providers must differentiate between normal and pathological changes, educate clients about changes, and help them to recognize and respond appropriately to signs of pathology and labor. In addition, health care providers need to individualize client education about a multitude of topics, geared toward empowering the pregnant woman and her family, and maximizing the potential for a positive outcome.

Despite advances in prenatal care, several barriers to initiating care exist.

Barriers to Prenatal Care

- *Unrecognized pregnancy:* Pregnancy may go unrecognized because of lack of knowledge about the signs and symptoms of pregnancy, limited body awareness, a history of irregular menses, or obesity.
- *Denied pregnancy:* Pregnancy may be denied, particularly if unplanned, because of the woman's ambivalence regarding motherhood.
- *Limited finances:* Financial constraints, limited health insurance, or unstable housing may discourage or prevent a woman from accessing prenatal care (American College of Obstetricians and Gynecologists [ACOG], 2006b).
- *Inaccessibility of the health care system:* An inconvenient location of the health care facility, lack of transportation, lack of provider availability, or fear of the health care system may make it difficult for a woman to obtain prenatal care.
- *Safety concerns:* A woman may be prevented from accessing prenatal care by a violent or controlling partner, or by concern about the safety of traveling within or outside of her community (ACOG, 2006b).
- *Language barriers:* Limitations in English proficiency have been shown to be a significant barrier in accessing health care services (Timmins, 2002). Women with limited English proficiency may be unaware of available resources for obtaining prenatal care, or may be concerned that their needs will not be met or that they will suffer poor treatment, as a result of their inability to communicate.
- *Cultural barriers:* Some pregnant women may have recently emigrated from countries where prenatal care is not placed in the same context or structure of visits as is found in the United States. Or they come from a culture within the United States that does not value prenatal care provided within the medical community as pregnancy is seen as a wellness state, not a sickness state that requires medicine. This cultural difference and misunderstanding of the norms and expectations may result in clients not initiating or complying with the recommended regimen of prenatal care.

Today, many women have jobs outside the home both for financial reasons and for professional accomplishment. In two-income families, partners often share childrearing responsibilities, and both parents are expected to be active in the care and nurturing of offspring. The concept of *family* has expanded to include nontraditional households, such as same-sex relationships, single-parent families, blended families, and cohabitation.

Clients as consumers desire an optimal outcome in pregnancy, and preconception counseling has gained increasing importance. Throughout pregnancy, women may question the safety of various activities and the effects of substances on the developing fetus. Women and their partners should be included in the decision-making process whenever possible, and encouraged to participate in community prenatal classes, to empower their participation and decision-making ability. When women feel they are in a partnership with their prenatal care providers, they are increasingly able to take responsibility for their health and health care decisions, and better prepared for the life-changing event that is pregnancy and childbirth (Freeman & Griew, 2007).

PLANNING FOR A HEALTHY PREGNANCY

PRECONCEPTION COUNSELING

Awareness and recognition is growing that the ability of prenatal care alone to significantly improve maternal-child health outcomes is limited, and that waiting until pregnancy to provide interventions may be too late for expectant parents to correct unhealthy habits. Since the 1980s, this recognition motivated organizations such as the U.S. Public Health Service, the National Institutes of Health and Human Services (NIH), and the Centers for Disease Control and Prevention (CDC) to recommend that preventive care related to pregnancy begin prior to conception (Freda, Moos, & Curtis, 2006).

Preconception care that once was thought of as a distinct visit, separate from other types of visits, has been reconceptualized into recommendations for incorporating risk assessment, health promotion, and disease prevention strategies into routine visits for women (and men) across the life span (Atrash et al., 2008). The CDC, in 2006, established 10 recommendations for improving preconception health. The recommendations are the following:

Individual responsibility across the life span: Encouraging each individual (female and male) and each couple to have a reproductive life plan.

Consumer awareness: Increasing the public awareness of healthy preconception behaviors.

Preventive visits: Integrating elements of preconception assessment, education, and health promotion interventions into every visit.

Interventions for identified risks: Addressing the risks of women with chronic health problems and infectious diseases that are known to harm pregnancy or are associated with adverse perinatal outcomes.

Interconception care: Targeting interventions for women who have experienced an adverse perinatal outcome.

Prepregnancy checkup: Providing the opportunity for women and their partners to have a prepregnancy visit before conception for risk assessment and health promotion.

Health insurance coverage for women with low incomes: Increasing coverage to improve access to care.

Public health programs and strategies: Integrating preconception health promotion interventions into existing public health programs and initiatives.

Research: Increasing the existing evidence for effective interventions that improve preconception health.

Monitoring improvements: Maximizing the systematic surveillance of existing databases and systems to monitor trends related to improving preconception health.

Part of the motivation for the change to a new understanding of preconception care is the recognition that almost half of all pregnancies in the United States continue to be unplanned, unwanted, or mistimed, despite advances in contraception (Finer & Henshaw, 2006). Women with unintended pregnancies are often more at risk for behaviors that can negatively affect pregnancy and fetal or infant health such as inadequate consumption of folic acid, smoking, late initiation of prenatal care, and limited breastfeeding (Cheng, Schwarz, Douglas, & Horon, 2009). Even with planned pregnancies, many women report being unaware of effects of behaviors or chronic disease states on pregnancy outcomes (Elsinga et al., 2008) and many providers do not incorporate preconception care recommendations into routine care (Atrash et al., 2008).

Regardless of intent to conceive, the principles related to preconception care are an extension of primary care principles but with the added perspective of how factors related to each individual's history, health status, and behaviors could impact a potential pregnancy (Atrash et al., 2008). Prior to conception, prospective parents have an opportunity to make informed decisions and ultimately to make lifestyle adjustments to maximize their chances of a successful outcome in pregnancy (CDC, 2006).

PRECONCEPTION ASSESSMENT

Preconception care and counseling are valuable in identifying risks in the client's medical history and current health status, and their potential impact on a pregnancy. Assessment includes history taking and a physical examination, often augmented by laboratory and/or diagnostic testing (Jack et al., 2008; Moos et al., 2008).

Subjective Data

During the evaluation, obtain detailed information related to medication and supplement use, allergies, immunizations, and medical, surgical, social, reproductive, genetic, and family histories. By identifying problems early, it is sometimes possible to resolve them prior to conception and ultimately improve perinatal outcome (Jack et al., 2008; Moos et al., 2008). Risk factors related to medication usage (i.e., isotretinoins, antiepileptics, anticoagulants), folic acid deficiency, smoking, alcohol use, drug use, health habits (i.e., nutrition, exercise, safety), medical conditions (i.e., diabetes, obesity, hypothyroidism), immunization status, and sexually transmitted infections (STIs) (especially HIV) are all identified as areas for assessment specific to preconception care (CDC, 2006; Moos et al., 2008). This type of comprehensive appraisal is not significantly different than the routine history required at most preventive visits and is intended to assess the health status of the potential mother (or father). The amount of data gathered and the level of counseling or intervention provided will vary depending on each individual at each stage of the reproductive life cycle (Atrash et al., 2008).

Objective Data

Physical Examination. A complete physical examination is often indicated, with special emphasis on the systems identified during the risk appraisal. A thorough pelvic examination should be performed, with consideration of a Papanicolaou (Pap) smear, chlamydia and gonorrhea testing, and/or a wet smear evaluation per screening guidelines (CDC, 2010c).

Diagnostic Tests and Methods. Ordering of testing should be individualized and based on identified risk factors and any current medical conditions. For example, complete blood count (CBC), HIV screening, diabetes screening, thyroid screening, or hemoglobin electrophoresis may be performed if risk factors are identified. Rubella, varicella, and hepatitis B immune status may be verified. Additional genetic screenings may be recommended such as cystic fibrosis (CF) carrier status screening or referral for genetic counseling (Solomon, Jack, & Feero, 2008).

Client Education and Counseling

Preconception counseling and intervention for the client and her partner should focus on the following areas:

- *Menstrual cycles:* Advise the client to keep an accurate record of her menstrual cycles in order to help establish gestational dating.
- *Adequate nutrition and exercise:* Assess nutritional status and habits and provide information on components of a healthy diet. Many women do not follow a healthy diet and are often lacking in essential nutrients. Evaluate intake and quality of dietary fat, protein, and carbohydrates in addition to intake of vitamins A, C, B_6, B_{12}, D, and E, folic acid, calcium, iron, zinc, and magnesium as well as omega-3 fatty acids (American Dietetic Association [ADA], 2008; Gardiner et al., 2008). Advise supplementation as indicated by dietary deficiencies and avoid megavitamin/mineral supplements.

  A vitamin/mineral supplement containing at least 0.4 mg of folic acid per day for the purpose of reducing the risk of a neural tube defect (NTD)–affected pregnancy is recommended for all women, regardless of intent to conceive. Women with a history of an NTD-affected pregnancy are at particular risk in each subsequent pregnancy, and it is recommended that they should take 4 mg of folic acid daily. Folic acid supplementation is recommended at least 1 month prior to attempting conception and through the first 3 months of pregnancy and can be continued throughout pregnancy and postpartum (ADA, 2008; Cunningham et al., 2010). Food sources of folate include leafy green vegetables, legumes, citrus fruits and juices, and fortified breads and cereals (Gardiner et al., 2008).

  Encourage overweight or underweight clients to attain an ideal weight prior to conception. Obesity increases the risk of perinatal morbidity and mortality (Gunatilake & Perlow, 2011). Low pregravid weight increases the risk of premature birth, low birth weight, and intrauterine growth restriction (IUGR) (Moos et al., 2008). Assess level of exercise and activity and encourage weight bearing and cardiovascular exercise according to each individual's needs for fitness and/or weight loss.

  If the client has special dietary needs (e.g., vegetarian/vegan, cultural food restrictions, overweight, underweight), refer her to a dietician. Pay particular attention to recognizing eating disorders or other nutritional risks such as pica and refer as indicated.
- *Avoidance of teratogens and potentially harmful substances:* Warn the client that potential teratogens can be related to diet and lifestyle (e.g., alcohol, mercury in fish), medications (tetracycline, warfarin), environmental exposures (lead, unregulated drinking water/well water), and workplace exposures (chemotherapy, aromatic hydrocarbons [AHC]) (Cunningham et al., 2010; McDiarmid, Gardiner, & Jack, 2008). See Table 19–1 for a selected list of medications and substances that can be teratogenic.
- *Readiness for parenthood:* Assist the family in an assessment of their social, financial, and psychological readiness for pregnancy and commitment to parenthood.
- *Identification of unhealthy behaviors:* Assist individuals and families to identify and alter unhealthy behaviors, such as smoking, alcohol consumption,

TABLE 19–1. Selected Drugs or Substances Suspected or Proven to Be Human Teratogens

Drugs	Substances
Angiotensin-converting enzyme inhibitors Angiotensin-receptor blockers	Alcohol
Aminopterin	Carbon
Androgens	Tetrachloride
Bexarotene	Chlorbiphenyls (PCBs)
Bosentan	Methyl mercury
Carbamazepine	Tobacco
Chloramphenicol	Toluene
Clorimipramine	
Cocaine	
Corticosteroids	
Cyclophosphamide	
Danazol	
Diazepam	
Diethylstilbestrol (DES)	
Efavirenz	
Etretinate	
Isotretinoin	
Leflunomide	
Lithium (may be safe)[a]	
Methimazole	
Methotrexate	
Misoprostol	
Mycophenolate	
NSAIDs	
Paroxetine	
Penicillamine	
Phenobarbital	
Phenytoin	
Radioactive iodine	
Ribavirin	
Statins	
Streptomycin	
Tamoxifen	
Tetracycline	
Thalidomide	
Tretinoin	
Valproate	
Warfarin	

Sources: Buhimschi & Weiner, 2009; Cunningham et al., 2010, Table 14-1; Gentile, 2011; Morrical-Kline, Walton, & Guildenbecher, 2011; Red, Richards, Torres, & Adair, 2011; Tomson & Battino, 2009; Ward & Kugelmas, 2005.

and drug use (i.e., prescription, over-the-counter, and illegal drugs).

- *Infectious diseases:* Screen clients for STIs, tuberculosis, and other infections, as indicated. Provide treatment, counseling, and/or referral appropriate to individual risks (e.g., herpes, HIV) (Coonrod et al., 2008).
- *Treatment of medical conditions:* Ensure that medical conditions that may jeopardize the pregnancy outcome are evaluated. Careful evaluation and counseling should be considered for women with diabetes, hypertension, cardiovascular disease, thyroid disease, phenylketonuria, seizure disorders, renal disease, lupus, asthma, thrombophilias, obesity, and psychiatric disorders (CDC, 2006; Jack et al., 2008). Refer women and their partners to a specialist as needed.
- *Identify genetic risk:* Obtain a three-generation family medical history including information related to genetic abnormalities (Solomon et al., 2008). When risks are identified, refer the couple for genetic counseling and laboratory testing, as indicated (see Figure 19–1).

Name ______________________ Patient # ______________________ Date ______________

1. Have you, the baby's father, or anyone in either of your families ever had any of the following disorders?
   - Down syndrome Yes ___ No ___
   - Other chromosomal abnormality Yes ___ No ___
   - Neural tube defect, spina bifida (meningomyelocele or open spine), anencephaly Yes ___ No ___
   - Hemophilia Yes ___ No ___
   - Muscular dystrophy Yes ___ No ___
   - Cystic fibrosis Yes ___ No ___

   If yes, indicate the relationship of the affected person to you or to the baby's father: ______________
2. Do you or the baby's father have a birth defect? Yes ___ No ___
   If yes, who has the defect and what is it? ______________
3. In any previous marriages, have you or the baby's father had a child, born dead or alive with a birth defect not listed in question 2 above? Yes ___ No ___
   If yes, what was the defect and who had it? ______________
4. Do you or the baby's father have any close relatives with mental retardation or fragile X syndrome? Yes ___ No ___
   If yes, indicate the relationship of the affected person to you or to the baby's father: ______________
   Indicate the cause, if known: ______________
5. Do you, the baby's father, or a close relative in either of your families have a birth defect, any familial disorder, or a chromosomal abnormality not listed above? Yes ___ No ___
   If yes, indicate the condition and the relationship of the affected person to you or to the baby's father: ______________
6. In any previous marriages, have you or the baby's father had a stillborn child or three or more first trimester spontaneous pregnancy losses? Yes ___ No ___
   Have either of you had a chromosomal study? Yes ___ No ___
   If yes, indicate who and the results: ______________
7. If you or the baby's father is of Ashkenazic Jewish, French Canadian or Cajun ancestry, have either of you been screened for Tay-Sachs disease? Yes ___ No ___
   If yes, indicate who and the results: ______________
8. If you or the baby's father is of Ashkenazic Jewish ancestry, have either of you been screened for Canavan disease or familial dysautonomia? Yes ___ No ___
   If yes, indicate who and the results: ______________
9. If you or the baby's father is African American, have either of you been screened for sickle cell trait? Yes ___ No ___
   If yes, indicate who and the results: ______________
10. If you or the baby's father is of Mediterranean, Southeast Asian or African American ancestry, have either of you been tested for ß-thalassemia? Yes ___ No ___
    If yes, indicate who and the results: ______________
11. If you or the baby's father is of Mediterranean, African American or Southeast Asian ancestry, have either of you been tested for α-thalassemia? Yes ___ No ___
    If yes, indicate who and the results: ______________
12. Excluding iron and vitamins, have you taken any medications or recreational drugs since being pregnant or since your last menstrual period? (Include nonprescription drugs.) Yes ___ No ___
    If yes, give name of medication and time taken during pregnancy: ______________

Note: Any patient replying "YES" to questions should be offered appropriate counseling. If the patient declines further counseling or testing, this should be noted in the chart. Given that genetics is a field in a state of flux, alterations or updates to this form will be required periodically.

FIGURE 19–1. Sample Prenatal Genetic Screen. *Sources: AAP & ACOG, 2007; ACOG, 2007e.*

- *Laboratory tests:* Order all appropriate laboratory tests, evaluate the results, and discuss the findings and their implications with the client.
- *Appropriate Vaccinations:* Obtain information related to each client's immunization history and provide for initial or booster vaccines as indicated by recommended immunization schedules for age. If the client is not immune to certain infections, administer the appropriate vaccine. Clients should have all childhood immunizations before conception to protect the fetus from an illness that could produce congenital anomalies and from the theoretical risk of exposure to immunizations (see Immunizations section). Particular attention is given to immune status related to rubella, varicella, and hepatitis B. Advise the client to wait 1 month before attempting conception after administration of any live vaccines (CDC, 2001).
- *Access to care and coverage:* Access to care is an increasingly important public health issue. In addition, many individuals and families are uninsured or underinsured. Refer clients to social workers as indicated for access to information regarding eligibility for federal or state programs such as Medicaid.
- *Effective professional relationship*: To encourage the client's early entry into prenatal care, initiate and nurture a positive professional relationship.

IMMUNIZATIONS

There are a select few vaccinations that may be given during pregnancy, and one that is specifically recommended during pregnancy. Immunity and vaccination status of several illnesses are of particular interest to the prenatal care provider, and are discussed here.

HEPATITIS B VIRUS

Infection with hepatitis B virus carries significant sequelae if the client becomes a chronic carrier. Infection can lead to chronic hepatitis, cirrhosis, or primary hepatocellular carcinoma. A positive test for hepatitis B surface antigen (HBsAg) indicates a high degree of infectivity, and significant risk for the newborn.

All clients should be screened for HBsAg prenatally or, if not then, when they are admitted to the hospital. If HBsAg is positive, further testing of the client, her children, and her sexual partner is advised. The pediatrician should be advised of the mother's positive status and is responsible for appropriate care of the infant (ACOG, 2007g).

If a client is HBsAg and HBsAb (antibody to HBsAg) negative and at risk for infection, immunization is encouraged as pregnancy is not a contraindication. Women considered to be at high risk include health care workers, hemodialysis clients, intravenous drug users, women with multiple sexual partners or a recent STI, women who work or live in institutions for the mentally disabled, and anyone planning travel to a high-incidence country (ACOG, 2007g).

HUMAN PAPILLOMAVIRUS

Human papillomavirus (HPV) is identified as the causative organism in the development of anogenital warts (condylomata acuminata) as well as cervical and other reproductive tract cancers. Transmission of HPV can be reduced with condom use. Two HPV vaccinations are currently available in the United States under the trade names Gardasil® and Cervarix®. Both vaccines are highly effective at preventing HPV infection, but do not treat existing infection. Because both are relatively new, there remain some unanswered questions, such as how long immunity lasts, and the impact of switching from one vaccine to the other midcourse (the vaccination regimen consists of a series of three injections over a 6-month period). Data is also limited on the effect of HPV vaccination on a developing fetus, so for this reason pregnancy is a contraindication to vaccination. If the series has begun prior to pregnancy, it may be continued after the completion of pregnancy. Inadvertent vaccination during pregnancy has not thus far been identified to cause harmful effects, so termination of pregnancy in this event is not recommended. Vaccination should ideally be given prior to coitarche, but is recommended for all unvaccinated women up to the age of 26 (ACOG, 2005a; CDC, 2011a).

INFLUENZA VACCINE

Pregnancy significantly increases the morbidity of influenza infection. The inactivated form of influenza vaccine is generally considered safe at any point in pregnancy, and provides the added benefit of transmission of influenza antibodies to the newborn, for whom vaccination is contraindicated until 6 months of age. The CDC and the ACOG recommend that the flu vaccine be offered to all pregnant clients at the start of or at any point during flu season, regardless of stage of gestation. Those trying to conceive should also be immunized. The live attenuated form of the influenza vaccine is contraindicated in pregnancy (ACOG, 2010a; CDC, 2011a).

RUBELLA

Causing only a mild febrile illness in children and adults, rubella is most significant when it infects pregnant women. Rubella can cause spontaneous abortion or congenital rubella syndrome when contracted in the first trimester of pregnancy. As many as 85 percent of fetuses exposed to maternal infection in early pregnancy develop the significant birth defects associated with congenital rubella syndrome. Congenital rubella syndrome is rare, however, when infection occurs after 20 weeks of pregnancy (CDC, 2011a).

The incidence of rubella in the United States has declined dramatically since the advent of rubella vaccination in 1969, with the majority of cases being among Hispanic adults who were born in countries that do not routinely vaccinate against rubella. In 2004, the CDC declared rubella to be essentially eradicated from the United States (CDC, 2011a).

If the client has a positive serological test, then there is virtually no risk to the fetus if she is exposed to rubella, although isolated cases of congenital rubella syndrome in infants whose mothers had documented immunity have been reported (CDC, 2011a). All prenatal clients should be tested. If seronegative, they should be cautioned to avoid anyone with a rash or viral illness.

All nonimmune clients should be immunized postpartum (see Chapter 22).

ASSESSMENT DURING PREGNANCY

Women's health care during pregnancy begins with a complete history and thorough physical examination during the initial visit. The initial visit is the ideal time to screen for particular risk factors suggesting preterm delivery or other poor outcomes (see Risk Assessment, later in this chapter), and to begin anticipatory guidance on a variety of topics likely to be important to the client.

The health care provider and the client establish the foundation of a trusting relationship by jointly developing a plan of care for the pregnancy. This plan is tailored to the client's lifestyle preferences as much as possible and focuses primarily on education for overall wellness during pregnancy. The ultimate goal is early detection and prevention of potential problems in the pregnancy and support and empowerment of the pregnant woman and her family.

Return office visits include physical evaluation of the client and fetus, client education, and the continuation of a holistic approach to pregnancy care.

DIAGNOSIS OF PREGNANCY

Signs and Symptoms

Signs and symptoms that may be reported by the pregnant client are traditionally categorized into three groups, defined as follows and summarized in Table 19–2.

- *Presumptive:* Signs or symptoms frequently reported with pregnancy, although not conclusive for pregnancy.
- *Probable:* Signs or symptoms that are more reliable indicators of pregnancy, often noted on the physical examination or with laboratory testing.
- *Positive:* Signs or symptoms that provide absolute confirmation of pregnancy, when noted.

Although these signs and symptoms assist in confirming pregnancy, they *cannot* necessarily enable the health care provider to differentiate an intrauterine pregnancy from an ectopic pregnancy.

TABLE 19–2. Signs and Symptoms of Pregnancy

Presumptive	Probable	Positive
Amenorrhea	Abdominal enlargement	Auscultation of fetal heart sounds
Breast tenderness and enlargement	Ballottement	Palpation of fetal movements
Chadwick's sign	Braxton-Hicks contractions	Radiological and/or ultrasonic verification of gestation
Fatigue	Goodell's sign	
Hyperpigmentation	Hegar's sign	
Chloasma	Palpation of fetal contours	
Linea nigra	Positive pregnancy test	
Fetal movements (quickening)	Uterine enlargement	
Urinary frequency		
Nausea/vomiting		

Sources: Davidson et al., 2012; Varney et al., 2004.

Pregnancy Tests

It is important to diagnose pregnancy as early as possible to maximize the benefits from health care and minimize risks to the developing fetus.

Human chorionic gonadotropin (hCG) is detected in pregnancy at about the time of implantation. Levels in normal pregnancy usually double every 1.4 to 2.0 days. Levels peak at approximately 60 to 90 days postfertilization, and then decrease to plateau at 16 weeks of pregnancy (Blackburn, 2007; Cunningham et al., 2010). Tests vary in sensitivity, specificity, and accuracy—influenced by the length of gestation, concentration of specimen, proteins or blood present, and some medical conditions (Davidson, London, & Ladewig, 2012). Serum tests are generally more sensitive than urine tests.

Quantitative, serial measurements of serum beta-subunit hCG (β-hCG) can be valuable in certain situations to help determine the viability of the pregnancy. Serum and urine tests specific for β-hCG have accuracy rates of 99 percent, with few false positives. With urine testing, early gestational age and decreased specimen concentration may yield false negatives (Davidson et al., 2012).

OVERVIEW OF INITIAL PRENATAL VISIT

During the initial visit, the health care provider performs a complete assessment and counsels the client about risk factors and prenatal care. Several components are included.

- *Confirmation of pregnancy:* Perform a β-hCG urine test, auscultate fetal heart tones (FHTs), or perform ultrasound; if all three are negative but pregnancy is still suspected, retest using a radioimmunoassay β-hCG serum test.
- *History:* Obtain a complete medical, surgical, psychosocial, family, and reproductive history (see Chapter 5). Several areas require more in-depth evaluation during pregnancy. Information obtained may help date the pregnancy and identify potential risk factors.
    - Menstrual history—last normal menses, menstrual pattern
    - Contraceptive history—last time used, dates of unprotected intercourse
    - Obstetric history—dates and types of previous deliveries, weights of newborns, lengths of labors, any complications with pregnancies, labors, or deliveries
    - Gynecologic history—STIs, abnormal cervical cytology and treatment, if any
    - Sexual history—number of partners, high-risk behavior
    - Surgical history—especially surgical procedures affecting the uterus
- *Physical examination:* (See Chapter 5). Assess the client's vital signs and perform a complete head-to-toe examination with particular attention to the pelvic evaluation. Establish the client's baseline cervical status. The normal pregnant cervix is usually 3 to 4 cm long, closed, firm in texture, and mid to posterior in position. Testing the adequacy of the pelvis (pelvimetry), if unproven by previous vaginal delivery, may be part of the practice protocol in some settings. Pelvimetry is typically not recommended for routine screening as it has been found to not be predictive of ability to deliver vaginally. It includes measurement of the diagonal conjugate from the posterior inferior edge of the symphysis pubis to the sacral promontory (normally 11.5 cm or greater), which estimates the inlet; the transverse diameter of the midpelvis includes evaluation of the ischial spines (sharp or blunt and degree of prominence) and of the anteroposterior diameter by the shape of the sacrum (curved or flat). The ischial tuberosities should be 8 cm or more apart, and the pubic arch should be 90° or greater (Varney, Kriebs, & Gegor, 2004).
- *Expected date of delivery (EDD):* EDD is calculated using the first day of the last menstrual period (LMP), and Naegele's rule (add 7 days to the date of LMP, subtract 3 months from that date). EDD is confirmed or changed, based on history, physical exam, and ultrasonography, if performed. Clients should be informed that their EDD marks the completion of 40 weeks of pregnancy, which is 10 lunar months, or 9 calendar months.
- *Laboratory tests:* Perform routine laboratory tests (Table 19–3) and additional testing as needed (Table 19–4).
- *Risk assessment:* Refer the client for management of high-risk findings, as indicated.
- *Prenatal educational materials:* Provide and review information about prenatal classes, nutrition, exercise, teratogens, sexuality, and options for infant feeding.
- *Anticipatory guidance and teaching:* May cover a range of topics including physiologic changes of pregnancy, discomforts of pregnancy, psychosocial issues, sibling rivalry, preparation for parenting, and so on.

TABLE 19–3. Routine Tests to Be Performed on All Prenatal Clients

ABO blood group/Rh factor identification/antibody screen
Complete blood cell count with indices (Hb, Hct, MCV, MCH, MCHC)
Rubella titer
Syphilis screening/VDRL, RPR
Hepatitis B surface antigen
Urinalysis and urine culture
Chlamydia screening
Cervical cytology (if indicated by routine screening guidelines)
HIV antibody screening

Hb—hemoglobin
Hct—hematocrit
HIV—human immunodeficiency virus
MCHC—mean corpuscular hemoglobin concentration
MCH—mean corpuscular hemoglobin
MCV—mean corpuscular volume
RPR—rapid plasma reagin
VDRL—Venereal Disease Research Laboratories test

Values may vary according to the laboratory used.
Source: AAP & ACOG, 2007.

TABLE 19–4. Additional Tests Performed on the Basis of the Prenatal Client's History

Blood chemistry
Cystic fibrosis screen
Cytomegalovirus titer
Diabetes screening
Genetic risk screening and/or testing, such as quad screen, amniocentesis, or chorionic villus sampling
Glucose tolerance tests
Group B streptococcus culture
Hemoglobin electrophoresis
Herpes culture
Lead level
Quantitative beta-hCG
Serum iron studies
Thyroid studies
Tuberculin skin test (PPD)
Urine culture
Ultrasonography to evaluate gestational age, fetal anatomy, and/or placental location
Varicella titer

Values may vary according to the laboratory used.

- *Schedule follow-up visits:* Discuss the importance of continued prenatal care and work out a schedule for follow-up visits. The standard schedule for a normal pregnancy is every 4 weeks until 28 weeks, every 2 weeks between 28 and 36 weeks, every week from 36 weeks until delivery, and often biweekly after 40 weeks. Fewer visits or more frequent visits may be determined based on each individual and the health of the woman and pregnancy.

SUBSEQUENT PRENATAL VISITS

At each subsequent prenatal visit, review the chart, patient history, and details of previous visits; measure the client's weight and blood pressure; assess for quickening/fetal movement; determine fundal height; assess FHTs; and, if indicated, evaluate the client's urine for blood, protein, ketones, nitrites, and/or glucose. Also at each visit, evaluate any client complaints, inquire about any danger signs or symptoms, and answer questions appropriately. Leopold's maneuvers should be performed weekly after 35 weeks to determine fetal presentation and position. Counseling on topics such as nutrition, weight gain, exercise, and/or breastfeeding can occur at most visits. Likewise, the clinician should always be attentive to observe or screen for complications such as depression, poor coping, and any signs of potential obstetric complications.

Leopold's maneuvers are performed in the following manner. The first three maneuvers are to be performed while facing the client's head. For the final maneuver, face the client's feet (Davidson et al., 2012):

- Outline the uterus and determine what part of the fetus is at the uterine fundus. The fetal breech feels bumpy, is somewhat soft, and is mostly nonmovable; the fetal head feels firm, is round, and is somewhat more movable.
- Next, using the palms of your hands, gently but firmly palpate the sides of her abdomen. The fetal back will feel firm and almost as a flat, smooth structure; the opposite palm will feel bumpiness of the arms and legs (knees or elbows). It will be harder to determine the position of a fetus not in a side-lying position.
- Now, gently capture the lower portion of the maternal abdomen just above the symphysis pubis between the thumb and fingers of your dominant hand or you can use the pads of the first three fingers of both hands. Check for mobility. If the presenting part is mobile, it is not engaged in the pelvis yet.
- Finally, use the pads of the first three fingers of each hand, gently but firmly palpate toward the axis of the pelvic inlet. For vertex presentations (head down), the cephalic prominence will be initially noted with the fingers of one hand; the fingers of the other hand will proceed further into the pelvis.

For a vertex presentation, if the cephalic prominence is on the same side as the arms and legs, the head is considered flexed. If the vertex and the cephalic prominence are on the same side as the back, the examiner needs to consider either the head is in extension or the possibility that a face presentation exists. Information about descent or station of the presenting part is related to how easy it is to palpate the cephalic prominence. An easily palpable cephalic prominence is above the level of the ischial spines. Placental position and body habitus of the client impacts the ability to gather information with these maneuvers (Cunningham et al., 2010).

Include the partner and family when possible in auscultation of FHTs and palpation of fundal height changes. Share positive aspects of the exam (e.g., normal heart tones, normal growth). Commend the woman and her partner on their efforts toward healthy behaviors. Review the common discomforts of pregnancy and how they may influence elements such as ability to care for other children or sexuality. Encourage the partner's or support person's participation in the pregnancy and labor and delivery process to enhance support systems for the woman and family.

Weeks 4 to 12

Pregnancy confirmation visits are not typically needed if the patient has taken a positive pregnancy test at home. However, it may be indicated to see a woman early in pregnancy especially if she has significant risk factors. The risk for miscarriage is highest in the first trimester, so it is not unusual to see women during early pregnancy to try to establish viability, especially if they have experienced a previous loss. In addition, many women have significant early pregnancy discomforts such as nausea and vomiting, fatigue, and cramping and may need evaluation, reassurance, and education. It is common to have women schedule a first OB visit between 8 and 10 weeks, and sometimes earlier if they are planning genetic testing (i.e., chorionic villus sampling [CVS]).

Weeks 12 to 16

Review laboratory findings with the client and her partner. Offer and order appropriate genetic testing as indicated. Follow-up on and address any medical or pregnancy risk factors. Provide anticipatory guidance related to fetal development and changes to expect as the pregnancy progresses. Counsel the client on lifestyle factors such as healthy nutrition, weight gain, and exercise.

Weeks 16 to 20

Assess for fetal movements (quickening), which typically occur between 16 and 20 weeks of gestation. Offer and order appropriate genetic screening tests. Ultrasound evaluation may be performed to confirm gestational age and assess fetal anatomy. Encourage the woman and her partner or support person(s) to enroll in prenatal childbirth education classes. Continue to provide anticipatory guidance and screen for risk factors.

Weeks 24 to 28

If Rh negative, reevaluate the antibody screen titer. Perform glucose screening for gestational diabetes. Administer RhoGAM (Rh immune globulin) as indicated. Retest hemoglobin and hematocrit. Evaluate the client for risk of preterm labor and consider a cervical assessment including cervical position, consistency, length, and dilation, if indicated.

Clients should be instructed to begin performing fetal movement counts (FMCs) daily starting around 28 weeks' gestation. Inform the client regarding the significance of decreased fetal movement and the need to inform the health care provider promptly of any perceived decrease in fetal movement. The client may be instructed to perform daily FMCs as follows:

- Note the start time, the client may lie in the left lateral position; however, a seated or standing position may also be used.
- Place a hand over the abdomen to palpate movement.
- Remain in this position until you have counted 10 fetal movements.
- Record the end time.

If 10 movements are not obtained within 2 hours, then biophysical fetal assessment is indicated (American Academy of Pediatrics [AAP] & ACOG, 2007). The client should notify her health care provider and further evaluation initiated. See Chapter 21, Assessing Fetal Well-Being, for description of biophysical fetal assessment techniques.

Weeks 28 to 35

Encourage the client to begin the process of finding a health care provider for the infant. Assess the client's breasts and discuss preparation for breastfeeding. Discuss the importance of daily fetal movement as an indicator of fetal well-being. Reassess the client for risk of preterm labor; assess the cervix as indicated. May begin assessing fetal presentation and position with Leopold's maneuvers.

Weeks 35 to 37

Review with the client the signs and symptoms of labor; provide a handout listing them. Obtain a vaginal/anorectal culture for group B streptococcus (CDC, 2010b). Assess for active herpes simplex virus outbreak, in those with positive history. For women at or beyond 36 weeks who are at risk for recurrent genital herpes infection, suppressive antiviral therapy may be considered. Suppressive therapy can include acyclovir 400 mg twice a day or valacyclovir 500 mg twice daily until delivery (ACOG, 2007d). Retest for chlamydia, gonorrhea, syphilis, and/or HIV in those with infections earlier in pregnancy or those at high risk for STIs.

Weeks 37 to 40

Assess fetal position and presentation. Review and negotiate the client's birth expectations. Forward a copy of the client's prenatal records to the hospital labor area, as indicated. Document the client's choice of a pediatrician. Initiate fetal surveillance as indicated. A cervical examination may be performed per the protocol of the institution. Review client plans for postpartum contraception, and reinforce preparation for breastfeeding. Ensure that client has made plans for infant car seat. Review signs of postpartum depression and discuss available resources should client need them.

Week 40 and Beyond

Prepare the client for postdate pregnancy protocol. Perform a cervical assessment and consider membrane sweeping if no contraindications exist, such as cervicitis, low-lying placenta or placenta previa, unknown fetal lie, and vaginal bleeding (de Miranda, van der Bom, Bonsel, Bleker, & Rosendaal, 2006; Varney et al., 2004). Institute fetal surveillance, such as ultrasound, to evaluate amniotic fluid volume; nonstress testing; and semiweekly office visits, according to practice protocol.

GROUP PRENATAL CARE

A model of providing group prenatal care called Centering Pregnancy was developed out of work in the 1970s (Rising, 1998) and has been growing in popularity among providers and clinics involved in caring for pregnant women. Centering Pregnancy involves group prenatal visits of 8 to 12 women lasting approximately 90 minutes at regular intervals throughout most of the pregnancy and postpartum. The model incorporates the elements of risk assessment and all the screening and testing of traditional prenatal care with education and support provided in group sessions (Rising, 1998). The Centering Pregnancy model has demonstrated significant improvements in prenatal care, client and provider satisfaction, and breastfeeding, with ongoing research evaluating outcomes (Manant & Dodgson, 2011).

PROGRESSIVE PHYSICAL CHANGES

The zygotic and embryonic phases of development begin at fertilization, which takes place 2 weeks after the LMP. When considering fetal development, it is important to be clear about whether the time period considered is from LMP or from fertilization, which will be approximately 2 weeks different. The physiology of fetal development is beyond the scope of this text, but it is important to note that the majority of organogenesis occurs in the first trimester, making this the most vulnerable time for the damaging effects of teratogens. Major milestones during the first trimester include the beginning of fetal heart movements at 6 weeks' gestation, closure of the neural tube at 7 weeks' gestation, and rapid head and brain growth beginning in the 7th week. Fetal growth and development continues throughout pregnancy, but critical periods of brain growth occur as late as 38 weeks' gestation, and into early childhood (Blackburn, 2007).

Several physical changes commonly occur during pregnancy (Blackburn, 2007; Varney et al., 2004).

- *Skin:* Increased vascularity; increased pigmentation of face (chloasma), areola, abdomen (linea nigra), and genitalia; striae of breasts and abdomen.
- *Head:* Mild changes in scalp; excessive oiliness or dryness.
- *Eyes:* Mild corneal edema and thickening.
- *Mouth:* Edematous gums; increased gingivitis.
- *Respiration/cardiovascular:* Physiologic dyspnea of pregnancy; progressive elevation of the diaphragm; hand/pedal edema; leg and vulvar varicosities and hemorrhoids. Exaggerated heart sounds, particularly functional systolic murmurs.
- *Breasts:* Increased fullness, tenderness, enlargement, and excretion of colostrum are common by the third trimester.
- *Abdomen:* Distention secondary to flatus and increased uterine size; diminished bowel sounds as peristaltic movements are slowed; enlarging uterus, which displaces abdominal organs.
- *Genitalia/reproduction*
  - *External:* Increased pigmentation; pubic hair may lengthen. Near term, pelvic congestion and overall

swelling of labia majora are common; vulvar varicosities may be noted.
- *Vagina:* Rugation of vaginal mucosa is prominent.
- *Cervix:* Chadwick's (bluish/purple color) and Goodell's (softening with growth of cervical glands) signs are noted. May soften, dilate, and efface close to term.
- *Uterus:* Hegar's (softening of the lower uterine segment) sign often present by 6 weeks' gestation. At 12 weeks' gestation, the fundus is noted at the symphysis pubis; at 16 weeks' gestation, the fundus is midway between the symphysis and the umbilicus. Uterine enlargement occurs in linear fashion (1 cm per week). The uterine fundus can be palpated at the umbilicus at approximately 20 weeks and measures 20 cm. By the 36th week, the fundus is just below the xiphoid process and measures approximately 36 cm; the fundal height may decrease slightly or plateau near term (lightening). Measurement may then no longer correspond with week of gestation. The uterus maintains a globular/ovoid shape throughout pregnancy.
- *Adnexa:* Discomfort may be noted with exam due to stretching of the round ligaments throughout pregnancy. The ovaries are not palpable once the uterus fills the pelvic cavity at 12 to 14 weeks' gestation.
- *Urinary:* The bladder may be palpable; frequency and incontinence are common, particularly with multiparity.
- *Rectal:* Increased vascular congestion with resulting hemorrhoids is often noted.

- *Musculoskeletal:* Increased relaxation of pelvic structures, lordosis, sciatica, and discomfort at the symphysis pubis are common. Pain from round ligament syndrome often noted.
- *Endocrine:* May have mildly enlarged thyroid; however, diffusely enlarged thyroid nodularity or increased firmness is abnormal.

DIAGNOSTIC TESTS AND METHODS

To assess the development of the fetus and the well-being of the mother, the health care provider may use a variety of invasive and noninvasive tests. Commonly recommended tests are described in Tables 19–3, 19–4, 19–5, and 19–6.

ULTRASOUND

Technological advances in *ultrasonic imaging* (see Chapter 21) can enable accurate evaluation or monitoring of several aspects of pregnancy:

- Early first trimester identification of intrauterine pregnancy, ectopic pregnancy, multiple pregnancy, or molar pregnancy
- Demonstration of growth and viability of the embryo
- Identification and evaluation of uterine, fetal, and/or placental anomalies
- Screening for aneuploidy
- Cervical evaluation
- Assisting during procedures such as cerclage placement, cephalic version, CVS, or amniocentesis
- Serial measurements to evaluate fetal growth
- Evaluation of amniotic fluid levels
- Biophysical profile to evaluate fetal well-being in later stages of pregnancy (ACOG, 2009b; Cunningham et al., 2010)

PSYCHOSOCIAL ASSESSMENT AND INTERVENTIONS

An estimated half of all pregnancies in the United States are unintended (Finer & Henshaw, 2006). Therefore, it is reasonable to expect that women may have some initial feelings of ambivalence about the pregnancy when first diagnosed, and may need a period of time for adjustment, evaluation, decision making, and acceptance. Provide options counseling at the initial diagnosis of pregnancy, and referrals and follow-up appointments as necessary. During the first trimester, assess the meaning of pregnancy to the client and the positive, negative, or ambivalent feelings she may have. Explore her feelings about this pregnancy, her economic concerns, and her level of anxiety. Help the client to identify her support systems; suggest childbirth education classes; begin anticipatory guidance counseling as appropriate.

During the second trimester, assess the client's adaptation to pregnancy and to the body changes she has experienced. Explain how fetal growth/development and the client's own body/emotional changes will facilitate adaptation.

During the third trimester, determine how well the client is prepared for birth, delivery, and the physical needs of a newborn including infant feeding and childcare needs. Explore her expectations about labor, birth, and the newborn—and her fears concerning motherhood, pain of labor, loss of control, and harm to herself or the fetus.

TABLE 19–5. Selected Laboratory and Diagnostic Tests Nonpregnant Values, Pregnant Values, and Implications

Test	Nonpregnant Values	Pregnant Values	Implications for Mother/Fetus
Hematology			
Red blood cell count	3.6–5.0/mm^3	Relative decrease	Body fluid increases and normal number of erythrocytes become diluted. Stable during pregnancy.
White blood cell count	4.5–11/mm^3	5–12/mm^3; may increase	
Hematocrit	36–48%	28.6–38.4%	Decreased values reflect overall 50% increase in plasma volume—physiological anemia.
Hemoglobin	12–16 g/dL	11–16 g/dL	Increased oxygen carrying capacity of red blood cells compensates for volume expansion.
Platelets	140,000–400,000/mm^3		May decrease with severe preeclampsia. Rule out immune thrombocytopenic purpura.
Blood chemistry			
Alkaline phosphatase (total)	25–100 IU/L	May double	Elevated in liver conditions; increases due to placental involvement; in diseases involving connective tissue.
Blood urea nitrogen	6–20 mg/dL	8–10 mg/dL	Pregnant values are lower due to physiologic hydremia. In preeclampsia, values can increase to nonpregnant levels due to pathological arterial spasm and vasoconstriction.
Cholesterol (total)	130–200 mg/dL	243–305 mg/dL	Accurate levels not reflected in pregnancy. Do not assess in pregnancy or during lactation as abnormally elevated.
Creatinine	0.4–1.0 mg/dL	0.5–0.7 mg/dL	Pregnant values are lower due to increased glomerular filtration rate. In preeclampsia, values can increase to nonpregnant levels due to pathological arterial spasm and vasoconstriction.
Iron—serum	50–170 mcg/dL	Decrease	Iron demands increase during pregnancy.
Serum alanine aminotransferase	7–35 IU/L		Used primarily to monitor the liver; may increase in severe preeclampsia.
Serum aspartate aminotransferase	10–36 IU/L	May decrease due to abnormal metabolism of pyridoxine	Elevated in conditions where cardiac or hepatic damage occurs; also elevated post intramuscular injections; may also be depressed in diabetic ketoacidosis and beriberi.
Thyroid panel: triiodothyronine (T_3) uptake	25–35%	Decrease	Due to increase of thyroid-binding globulins by estrogen.
Thyroxine (T_4) total	5.4–11.5 mcg/dL	Increase	Basal metabolic rate increases by 25%; increased thyroid-binding globulins. Free T_4 is a more reliable indicator of thyroid function in pregnancy that total T_4.
Thyrotropin	0.4–4.2 mcU/mL		Most sensitive indicator for hypothyroid/hyperthyroid states in pregnancy. May have transient decrease in first trimester from effects of hCG.
Total iron-binding capacity	250–450 mcg/dL	Increase (late pregnancy)	Estrogen increases ability for iron to bind to transferrin, which regulates transport in the body.
Uric acid	2.4–6.0 mg/dL		Pregnant values are lower due to increased glomerular filtration rate. In preeclampsia, values can increase due to pathological arterial spasm and vasoconstriction.
Urinalysis			
Albumin	Negative	Less than 100	Elevations seen in preeclampsia and urinary tract infections.
Creatinine	11–20 mg/kg/24 h	Slight increase	Due to increased glomerular filtration rate.
Glucose	< 0.5g/24 h	Elevated	Due to decrease renal threshold and increased glomerular filtration rate.
Ketones	Negative	Same	Presence may indicate dehydration; starvation states; ketoacidosis in insulin-dependent diabetes mellitus; strenuous exercise.

Values may vary according to the laboratory used.

Sources: Cunningham et al., 2010; Fischbach & Dunning, 2009.

TABLE 19–6. Additional Tests Often Performed During Pregnancy

Test	Values	Significance	Implications
Cystic fibrosis (CF) carrier testing profile	Tests for 34 of the most common CF mutations	Risk for CF carrier status	An abnormal value is followed by screening of the father of the baby. If the father of the baby is tested positive, chorionic villus sampling or amniocentesis can be performed to determine if the fetus is affected.
Nuchal translucency (NT) ultrasound	Specialized ultrasound measurement of NT thickness Calculated multiples of the median (MoM) risk when used with serum markers	Performed between 11 and 136/7 weeks Increased NT measurement associated with risk for trisomy 21, fetal heart defects, skeletal dysplasias, and other genetic syndromes	Increased sensitivity with additional use of serum markers: plasma protein A and free beta-hCG. Can be done as part of integrated, sequential, or contingent screening. Genetic counseling and additional testing recommended with abnormal results.
Maternal serum Alpha fetoprotein (MS-AFP)	Based on MoM Cutoff values are lab dependent	Screening for open neural tube defects (ONTD/NTD). Can detect 75–90% of ONTD and 95% or greater of anencephaly and 85% of ventral wall defects	Relative to maternal weight, age, race, gestational dating, diabetic status, singleton vs. multiple gestation. Genetic counseling, ultrasound, and the option of invasive testing recommended with elevated MS-AFP. Abnormal levels have been associated with risk for preterm birth, fetal growth restriction, and fetal demise.
Multiple-marker screen Triple Screen (AFP, hCG, and unconjugated estriol) Quad screen (AFP, hCG, unconjugated estriol, and dimeric inhibin-A)	Risk calculation	Screening for risk of trisomies 18 and 21 Low AFP and unconjugated estriol levels with elevated hCG and dimeric inhibin-A levels present in most cases of trisomy 21 Low AFP and unconjugated estriol levels and hCG present in most cases of trisomy 18	Calculation of maternal age and three or four biochemical markers to determine risk. Not diagnostic. Can be used independently or in conjunction with first trimester screenings. Genetic counseling, ultrasound, and the option of invasive testing recommended with positive risk screenings.
Fasting blood sugar (FBS)	Fasting values typically not used as independent screening test in normal pregnancy	≥ 105 mg/dL elevated	Abnormal values suspicious for diagnosis of gestational diabetes.
1-hour 50 g glucose challenge test		130–140 mg/dL elevated	Screening done at 24–28 weeks' gestation; consider screen earlier and again at 24–28 weeks if history of 4,000 g infant, history of gestational diabetes, advanced maternal age, obesity, previous fetal death, or other risk factors associated with gestational diabetes.
3-hour 100 g glucose tolerance test			Elevated fasting alone can be diagnostic of gestational diabetes.
FBS		92-95 mg/dL elevated	Requires fasting 8–14 hours prior to testing. Elevated FBS is indicator of probable need for insulin therapy.
1 hour		≥ 180 mg/dL elevated	Criterion: Diagnostic of gestational diabetes if 2 of the 4 values are elevated.
2 hours		≥ 155 mg/dL elevated	Criterion: Diagnostic of gestational diabetes if 2 of the 4 values are elevated.
3 hours		≥ 140 mg/dL elevated	Criterion: Diagnostic of gestational diabetes if 2 of the 4 values are elevated.

Source: Cunningham et al., 2010.

Intimate Partner Violence

Health care providers who care for pregnant women are in a unique position to assess and provide intervention for intimate partner violence. Providers can more easily request that the client be seen alone, without the presence of her partner and other family, due to the intimate nature of the exam to be performed. Providers also examine the entire physical body of their clients, ensuring that they don't miss injuries inflicted in places thought to be unseen. Pregnancy is a particularly vulnerable time for many women, as violence is more likely to begin or intensify (Chambliss, 2008; Jeanjot, Barlow, & Rozenberg, 2008). Violence also predisposes women to complications during their pregnancy, related to stress, delayed start of prenatal care and lack of compliance with prenatal care, higher rates of substance abuse and smoking, and direct complications of violence, such as preterm labor and fetal injury or death (Brown, McDonald, & Krastev, 2008; Chambliss, 2008; Jeanjot et al., 2008).

In the United States, it is estimated that over a half a million sexual or physical assaults against women are perpetrated by intimate partners each year. This rate has declined significantly over the past 20 years, but it remains a significant deadly threat (Catalano, Smith, Snyder, & Rand, 2009). Throughout pregnancy, assess for subtle and overt signs of physical, sexual, and emotional abuse. Because of the prevalence of intimate partner violence, and because it may take time to build enough trust with an abused woman for her to disclose her situation, it is recommended to universally screen *all* pregnant women for intimate partner violence once each trimester (Chambliss, 2008; Salber, 2006). The five-question Abuse Assessment Screen (Figure 19–2) may help to identify abused clients. Also see Appendix B, Selected Screening Tools for Women's Health.

RISK ASSESSMENT

Assessment of a maternity client for risk factors encompasses physical, historical, and psychosocial aspects. The client at risk is identified, evaluated, and observed, with special consideration given to the course and outcome of pregnancy. Screening is done to detect elements such as genetic defects; the risk of preterm labor and delivery; parental-fetal attachment; and hazards in the environment and workplace. Screening should ideally be done at the initial visit, during each remaining trimester, and whenever necessary.

Genetic Screening

The purpose of genetic screening is to identify those at risk for an inherited or acquired defect and to identify unrecognized defects in healthy individuals. It is estimated that 50 percent of spontaneous abortions and 6 to 11 percent of intrauterine fetal deaths and neonatal deaths involve fetuses with aneuploidy (ACOG, 2007c). In addition, approximately 2 to 3 percent of infants have recognizable defects present at birth and an estimated one fourth of children admitted to pediatric hospitals are treated for conditions that have a genetic component (Cunningham et al., 2010; Gabbe, Niebyl, & Simpson, 2007). Clients with potential risks (Figure 19–1) should receive further counseling, testing, education, and guidance in decision making.

Tools for the Detection and Diagnosis of Genetic Defects

- *Family genogram:* A graphic record of family history that emphasizes medical, genetic, and/or other disorders may reveal an inheritance pattern and help to identify whether further laboratory testing and clinical evaluation are needed. Traditionally, a three-generation history is taken and standardized symbols and formatting provide guidance for developing a genogram (Wright & Leahey, 2009) (see Figure 19–3).
- *Noninvasive genetic screening*

  First trimester screening (combined screening): Noninvasive genetic screening tests for fetal aneuploidy focus primarily on detection of risk for trisomies 18 and 21. In the first trimester, measurement of the sonolucent space behind the fetal neck, nuchal translucency (NT) ultrasound, can be performed between 11 and 136/7 weeks (see Chapter 21 for detailed description of testing).

  Second trimester screening

  Quad screening: This multiple-marker screening can be a useful screening test in situations where women initiate prenatal care later in the pregnancy or when access to specialized NT ultrasound is not readily available (see Chapter 21 for detailed description of testing).

  Integrated screening: In an effort to improve detection rates, different screening patterns have been made available. The integrated screening approach can use the first trimester screenings of NT and plasma protein A (PAPP-A) in addition to the quad screen to develop a risk assessment for aneuploidy. The detection rate for Down syndrome

ABUSE ASSESSMENT SCREEN

1. Have you **ever** been emotionally or physically abused by your partner or someone important to you?
YES ☐ NO ☐

2. **WITHIN THE LAST YEAR,**
have you been hit, slapped, kicked, or otherwise physically hurt by someone? YES ☐ NO ☐
If YES, by whom?__________ Total number of times_____

3. Since you've been pregnant, were you hit, slapped, kicked, or otherwise physically hurt by someone? YES ☐ NO ☐
If YES, by whom?__________ Total number of times_____

MARK THE AREA OF INJURY ON THE BODY MAP. SCORE EACH INCIDENT ACCORDING TO THE FOLLOWING SCALE:

SCORE

1= Threats of abuse including use of a weapon _____

2= Slapping, pushing; no injuries and/or lasting pain _____

3= Punching, kicking, bruises, cuts and/or continuing pain _____

4= Beating up, severe contusions, burns, broken bones _____

5= Head injury, internal injury, permanent injury _____

6= Use of weapon; wound from weapon _____

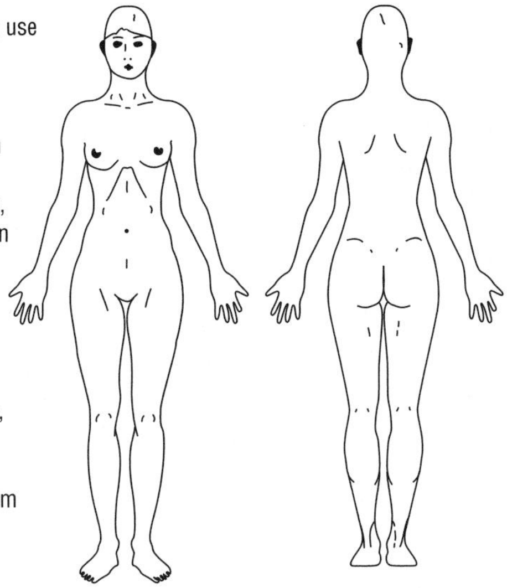

If any of the descriptions for the higher number apply, use the higher number.

4. **WITHIN THE LAST YEAR,**
has anyone forced you to have sexual activities? YES ☐ NO ☐
If YES, who? __________ Total number of times _____

5. Are you afraid of your partner or anyone you listed above? YES ☐ NO ☐

Developed by the Nursing Research Consortium on Violence and Abuse. Readers are encouraged to reproduce and use this assessment tool.

FIGURE 19–2. Abuse Assessment Screen. *Reprinted with permission from author Barbara Parker, RN, PhD, Professor University of Virginia, School of Nursing, Charlottesville, Virginia. Available for use at http://www.nnvawi.org.*

with this method is approximately 93 to 96 percent (ACOG, 2007e; Driscoll & Gross, 2009). The enhanced detection rate must be balanced by the fact that results of the first trimester testing are not provided to the patient and she must wait until the second trimester for the integrated screening result. Similar testing can be done in this integrated approach using serum testing of PAPP-A and the quad screen; however, the detection rate is only approximately 85 to 88 percent (ACOG, 2007e).

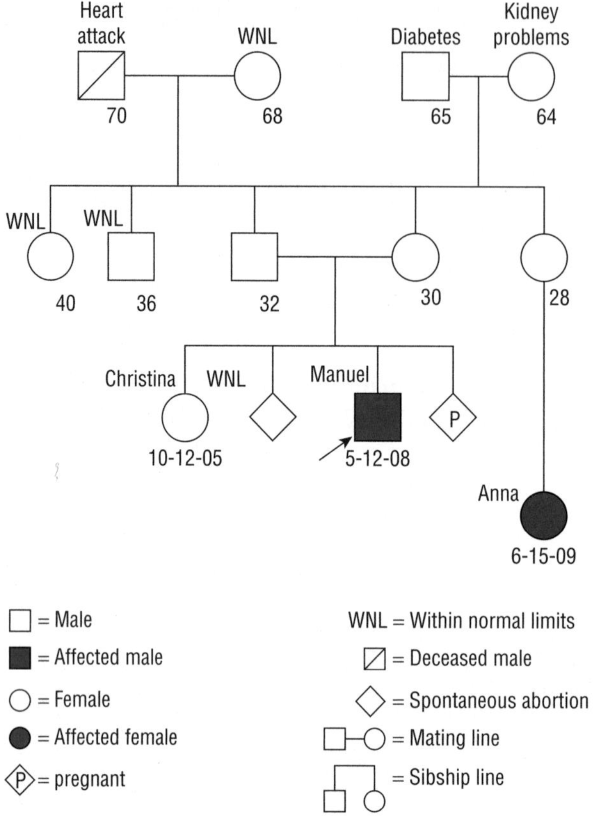

FIGURE 19–3. Screening Pedigree. *Source: Davidson et al., 2012.*

This rate is higher than with quad screen alone and may be a desirable option when NT ultrasound is not available (Driscoll & Gross, 2009).

Sequential screening: This approach can be done in a stepwise or contingent method. In the stepwise sequential screening, the woman receives the results of the first trimester screening tests, and if the testing indicates a high risk for fetal aneuploidy, then diagnostic testing (i.e., CVS) is offered. If the first trimester testing indicates a low or moderate risk, then the second trimester quad screen test is performed and the final result is calculated with both first and second trimester screening results (ACOG, 2007e; Driscoll & Gross, 2009).

With the contingent sequential approach, the woman receives the first trimester screening results, and if the risk for fetal aneuploidy is high, then diagnostic testing would be offered. However, if the first trimester screening is low, then no further serum screening testing is done. If the first trimester screening is intermediate, then second trimester quad screen testing is offered and the final result is calculated with both first and second trimester screening results (ACOG, 2007e; Driscoll & Gross, 2009).

The advantages of the sequential approaches are that the woman receives the first trimester results and does not have to wait until the second trimester to receive them. Another advantage of the sequential approach is a high detection rate of 90 percent with a false-positive rate of 2 to 3 percent (Driscoll & Gross, 2009). Whether the integrated or sequential approach is chosen, a woman must return for her second trimester testing (if indicated), which can be a limitation of these approaches.

- *Invasive genetic testing:* Whereas the first and second trimester screening tests can provide calculated risks for genetic abnormalities, invasive genetic testing is the only way to diagnose fetal aneuploidy during pregnancy at this time. CVS and amniocentesis are two available options for invasive diagnostic genetic testing. These tests can be done after a high-risk screening test result or as the first line of testing. All women, regardless of age, should be offered the option of invasive genetic testing in pregnancy (ACOG, 2007c). This ACOG recommendation represents a change from past practice that limited offering invasive testing as a first line only to women 35 or older at delivery.

CVS is performed by aspirating chorionic villi via a transvaginal or transabdominal approach. Due to the concern of potential risk for limb defects, CVS is typically not recommended before 9 weeks (ACOG, 2007g). Amniocentesis is performed by transabdominal aspiration of amniotic fluid. This diagnostic procedure is typically performed between 15 and 20 weeks and has a fetal loss risk as low as 1 in 300 to 500 based on recent data (ACOG, 2007c).

- *NTD screening:* Detection of NTDs can be done independent of screening testing for fetal aneuploidy or in addition to that testing. A maternal serum alpha-fetoprotein (MS-AFP) test is done by measuring levels of AFP circulating in MS in relation to gestational age, maternal age, weight, race, presence of diabetes, or previous history of NTDs. MS-AFP testing can detect open NTDs, anencephaly, and ventral wall defects with a false-positive rate of 5 percent (Driscoll & Gross, 2009).

  Standard ultrasound or level 2 ultrasound can provide additional screening for markers of genetic abnormalities and indirect visualization of fetal structures to identify structural anomalies. Because of the low sensitivity and specificity of ultrasound alone to screen for fetal aneuploidy, it is not typically recommended as an independent genetic screening test (Driscoll & Gross, 2009). (See Chapter 21 for more information on ultrasound.)
- *CF carrier screening:* CF is an autosomal recessive, life-threatening condition that is most common in non-Hispanic white and Ashkenazi Jewish populations. Regardless of ethnicity, CF carrier testing should be offered and available to any woman desiring screening (ACOG, 2011a). If a woman chooses to have CF carrier testing performed, it can be done at any time before or during pregnancy. Ideally, it should be performed in the preconception period. If a woman is a carrier, then it is recommended to test the male partner or sperm donor (if possible) to determine carrier status. If both individuals are carriers, then an amniocentesis and genetic counseling are offered for diagnosis and interpretation of the CF status of the fetus. Results of CF screening and subsequent testing can take up to 2 weeks; therefore, early screening is important.

Preterm Labor Screening

Preterm labor is traditionally defined as the presence of regular uterine contractions causing cervical dilation and effacement before 37 completed weeks' gestation and after 20 completed weeks. The etiology of preterm labor is unknown. Recent estimates are that approximately 12.8 percent of infants are born premature and the incidence of preterm birth has increased since the mid-1980s. Great disparities exist in the incidence of preterm birth and infant mortality for women of color, especially non-Hispanic black women (Mathews & MacDorman, 2010). Even with the most advanced technology, outcomes are poor for gestations of fewer than 26 weeks. In addition to increased risks of mortality, premature infants are at increased risk for long-term sequelae such as mental retardation, cerebral palsy, chronic lung disease, and vision and hearing loss (March of Dimes, 2010). Significant parental emotional and financial strain may also be experienced after preterm birth.

The demographic, historical, and psychosocial factors associated with increased incidence of preterm labor and delivery are assessed with preterm screening. Early identification of risk factors, continuous assessment of physical changes, education, and treatment that reduces controllable risk factors may help to decrease incidence of preterm birth. Risk factors for preterm birth are multifactorial and can include elements of maternal health that can occur before and during pregnancy. Some factors associated with increased risk of preterm birth are history of cervical loop electrosurgical excision or conization procedures, history of preterm birth, maternal smoking, uterine abnormalities, low prepregnancy BMI, multiple gestation, genitourinary infections, polyhydramnios, and recurrent bleeding during pregnancy (Creasy, Resnik, Iams, Lockwood, & Moore, 2009). (For further information on diagnosis and treatment, see Chapter 20.)

Substance Abuse in Pregnancy

Substance abuse during pregnancy is known to occur across age, race, and class divisions. For this reason, it is useful to practice universal screening of all pregnant women for substance abuse. Additionally, many women are motivated by pregnancy to effect positive change in their lives, making prenatal care providers in an optimal position to reach substance-abusing women. Because of the fear of child custody, criminal, or employment ramifications, however, many women are reluctant to reveal substance abuse histories (Gabbe et al., 2007). Screening is done to detect the use or abuse of any substance known or suspected to exert a deleterious effect on the client or her fetus.

The effects of specific drugs are difficult to assign, because often multiple drugs are used and nutritional status may be poor. Substance use in pregnancy is associated with IUGR, fetal alcohol spectrum disorders, miscarriage, preterm birth, placental abruptions, neurologic impairment and cognitive delay, and congenital malformations (Gabbe et al., 2007). Factors that may impact a drug's fetal effects are duration of use, dosage, timing in gestation, and use of other drugs (Briggs, Freeman, & Yaffe, 2008). Ideally, counseling a client concerning substance abuse begins prior to conception. Open discussions may make a client more aware of the need to prevent pregnancy and to obtain counseling or professional detoxification and rehabilitation services, if necessary. Clients who use substances only occasionally need to be aware of the potential teratogenic effect of even one exposure.

During pregnancy, ascertain whether the mother and fetus have been exposed to harmful substances, assess the mother's need for counseling, and design intervention that targets and eliminates the abuse and decreases potential harm to mother and fetus. Being nonjudgmental is a key to success; a client is more apt to trust and reveal patterns of abuse if the health provider maintains impartial professionalism, without criticism or judgment, at all times.

Initially, the goal of the health care provider is to prevent complications of pregnancy and in utero exposure, thereby minimizing permanent sequelae. Behavioral problems, learning disabilities, and other long-term physical, cognitive, and neurodevelopmental delays and anomalies may be present in the drug-exposed newborn and child. If multigenerational drug use is to be prevented, a link in the chain of addiction must be broken. Getting the client into treatment may help to identify her needs as an individual, teach her how to cope with the stresses that lead to drug use, and perhaps introduce skills for coping and potential parenting. In turn, these measures may enhance parent–child bonding and reduce the incidence of emotional, physical, or sexual abuse and neglect, which are often experienced by children of substance abusers (AAP & ACOG, 2007).

Physical Examination. The physical examination of a woman abusing a chemical substance may reveal fresh needle or track marks, a dazed appearance, inappropriate behavior or affect, extreme agitation or stupor, frequent conjunctivitis, tremors, flecks of paint around the mouth and nose, fetal/maternal tachycardia, or poor maternal weight gain (or weight loss) not attributed to underlying maternal disease.

Plan. Client counseling must continue into the postpartum period. Behaviors that are common among drug-exposed infants, such as feeding difficulties, sleeping only for short intervals, crying shrilly, being difficult to console, and avoiding eye contact, may act as a trigger to a substance-abusing woman without a strong support system or who is not actively involved in a recovery program (Varney et al., 2004).

All women should be screened for substance use and abuse as part of a complete history at the initial visit. Various screening tools exist. In addition to screening as part of a history, the provider may consider using more diagnostic laboratory tests, such as a urine toxicology test. This test detects a variety of drugs of abuse, each one having a range of time since last use when they may be detected. The provider should be aware, however, that the results of this test can have far-reaching implications for the client. Pregnant women who abuse drugs in certain states face criminal prosecution and/or involuntary commitment to treatment facilities. A complete informed consent should be provided to the client, emphasizing the benefits (improvement in our ability to provide good care for her and her baby), the risks (if positive, she may be reported to a local agency according to the requirements of her locality, and custody of her baby may be in jeopardy after delivery), and the client's right to refuse the test altogether. It is essential for the provider to familiarize himself or herself with the regulations, requirements, and implications regarding drug screening and reporting in his or her practice area (ACOG, 2011b).

Assist the substance-abusing client to enroll in a drug rehabilitation program that offers her ease of accessibility and provides optimum social support. (Be aware that resources for treating pregnant substance abusers are often limited and have long waiting lists.) Management includes dietary counseling, ideally by a nutritionist. The client should be seen perhaps every 1 to 2 weeks and begin a regimen of close fetal surveillance to assess fetal well-being, growth patterns, and placental health.

Constant encouragement and motivation are required to reinforce the need for compliance. Be honest about drug effects, but do not humiliate the client. Be open and direct with questions while being supportive of her efforts. Women who are abusing substances may struggle with the ability to appreciate long-term consequences or implications of their actions, and may benefit more from counseling on the immediate effects of substance use on both mother and baby. Most importantly, clients need to understand and value consistent prenatal care, and it should be clear that this will be available to them without judgment, regardless of whether they are able to stop using drugs during their pregnancy.

Nutrition and Weight Gain in Pregnancy

Good nutrition before and during pregnancy decreases the risks of significant health problems for the client and her infant. Studies have shown that the influence of maternal nutrition can impact the health of the infant in adulthood (ADA, 2008; Cunningham et al., 2010; Gunatilake & Perlow, 2011). Women who are underweight or who gain little weight during pregnancy are more likely to have small-for-gestational-age infants. Of greater concern, however, are women who are overweight or obese and become pregnant. It is estimated that over 40 percent of women initiating pregnancy are overweight or obese and that obesity complicates up to 28 percent of pregnancies (Gunatilake & Perlow, 2011). Women who are obese or whose weight gain is excessive are at risk for issues such as spontaneous abortion, gestational diabetes, preeclampsia, gestational hypertension, macrosomia, NTDs, and cesarean birth (ACOG, 2005b; Gunatilake & Perlow, 2011; Smith, Hulsey, & Goodnight, 2008). In addition, obese women are more likely to have preexisting chronic medical problems that may complicate a pregnancy such as cardiovascular disease, depression, chronic hypertension, metabolic syndrome, diabetes, or sleep apnea (ACOG, 2005b; Graves, 2010). Ideally, issues of nutrition and weight should be addressed before conception. Because many women are highly motivated to eat properly during pregnancy (Clark & Ogden, 1999), the nutrition instruction that they receive during pregnancy could result in positive and sustained dietary changes for the entire family.

Subjective Data. Several points are assessed during the first prenatal interview and reassessed as necessary at subsequent visits.

- Nutrition knowledge and any special dietary practices (e.g., vegetarian, vegan)
- A recall of the client's diet, ideally 7-day, though 24-hour is often more attainable
- Food storage and preparation capabilities
- Portion of income spent for food
- Enrollment in Women, Infants, and Children (WIC) program, if needed
- Food-buying practices
- Cultural and religious preferences
- Food aversions or allergies (e.g., lactose intolerance)
- Meanings attached to eating (e.g., celebration)
- Prepregnancy weight and body mass index (see Figure 19–4)
- Activity level and any change since pregnancy
- Lactation during or just prior to pregnancy and plans to breast-feed
- Herbal or vitamin supplement use
- Nicotine, alcohol, medication, or drug abuse
- Psychological disorders (e.g., depression, eating disorders)
- Medical risk factors (e.g., past bariatric surgery, diabetes, hypertension, endocrine disorders)
- Discomforts of pregnancy (e.g., dyspepsia, nausea/vomiting, smell/taste changes)
- Current or past obstetric risk factors (e.g., closely spaced pregnancy, inadequate or excessive weight gain, anemia, fetal growth abnormalities, congenital anomalies, preterm delivery, perinatal loss, gestational diabetes, hypertensive disorders)

Objective Data

Physical Examination. Establish prepregnancy BMI at the initial visit and review recommended weight gain guidelines in order to help the pregnant woman set goals and expectations for pregnancy. At each subsequent prenatal visit, assess adequacy of weight gain.

Diagnostic Tests and Methods

- Height, weight, and BMI at initial visit. Subsequent visits measure weight and evaluate weight gain since last visit as well as total weight gain in pregnancy.
- CBC to screen for anemia.
- One-hour 50 g Glucola to rule out gestational diabetes.
- Urine dipstick, when applicable, to detect proteinuria, glucosuria, and/or ketonuria.
- Serum 25-hydroxyvitamin D levels, when applicable, to detect vitamin D deficiency.

Differential Medical Diagnoses. Normal nutrition in pregnancy ruling out overweight or underweight; anemia; gestational diabetes; drug, alcohol, or nicotine abuse; eating disorders; problems affecting nutrition (e.g., cultural, economic, psychosocial); and complications of pregnancy and medical conditions requiring dietary intervention.

Plan

Psychosocial Interventions. Encourage the client to verbalize any physical and psychosocial problems and explore

Body Mass Index Table

	Normal						Overweight					Obese										Extreme Obesity														
BMI	**19**	**20**	**21**	**22**	**23**	**24**	**25**	**26**	**27**	**28**	**29**	**30**	**31**	**32**	**33**	**34**	**35**	**36**	**37**	**38**	**39**	**40**	**41**	**42**	**43**	**44**	**45**	**46**	**47**	**48**	**49**	**50**	**51**	**52**	**53**	**54**
Height (inches)																	**Body Weight (pounds)**																			
58	91	96	100	105	110	115	119	124	129	134	138	143	148	153	158	162	167	172	177	181	186	191	196	201	205	210	215	220	224	229	234	239	244	248	253	258
59	94	99	104	109	114	119	124	128	133	138	143	148	153	158	163	168	173	178	183	188	193	198	203	208	212	217	222	227	232	237	242	247	252	257	262	267
60	97	102	107	112	118	123	128	133	138	143	148	153	158	163	168	174	179	184	189	194	199	204	209	215	220	225	230	235	240	245	250	255	261	266	271	276
61	100	106	111	116	122	127	132	137	143	148	153	158	164	169	174	180	185	190	195	201	206	211	217	222	227	232	238	243	248	254	259	264	269	275	280	285
62	104	109	115	120	126	131	136	142	147	153	158	164	169	175	180	186	191	196	202	207	213	218	224	229	235	240	246	251	256	262	267	273	278	284	289	295
63	107	113	118	124	130	135	141	146	152	158	163	169	175	180	186	191	197	203	208	214	220	225	231	237	242	248	254	259	265	270	278	282	287	293	299	304
64	110	116	122	128	134	140	145	151	157	163	169	174	180	186	192	197	204	209	215	221	227	232	238	244	250	256	262	267	273	279	285	291	296	302	308	314
65	114	120	126	132	138	144	150	156	162	168	174	180	186	192	198	204	210	216	222	228	234	240	246	252	258	264	270	276	282	288	294	300	306	312	318	324
66	118	124	130	136	142	148	155	161	167	173	179	186	192	198	204	210	216	223	229	235	241	247	253	260	266	272	278	284	291	297	303	309	315	322	328	334
67	121	127	134	140	146	153	159	166	172	178	185	191	198	204	211	217	223	230	236	242	249	255	261	268	274	280	287	293	299	306	312	319	325	331	338	344
68	125	131	138	144	151	158	164	171	177	184	190	197	203	210	216	223	230	236	243	249	256	262	269	276	282	289	295	302	308	315	322	328	335	341	348	354
69	128	135	142	149	155	162	169	176	182	189	196	203	209	216	223	230	236	243	250	257	263	270	277	284	291	297	304	311	318	324	331	338	345	351	358	365
70	132	139	146	153	160	167	174	181	188	195	202	209	216	222	229	236	243	250	257	264	271	278	285	292	299	306	313	320	327	334	341	348	355	362	369	376
71	136	143	150	157	165	172	179	186	193	200	208	215	222	229	236	243	250	257	265	272	279	286	293	301	308	315	322	329	338	343	351	358	365	372	379	386
72	140	147	154	162	169	177	184	191	199	206	213	221	228	235	242	250	258	265	272	279	287	294	302	309	316	324	331	338	346	353	361	368	375	383	390	397
73	144	151	159	166	174	182	189	197	204	212	219	227	235	242	250	257	265	272	280	288	295	302	310	318	325	333	340	348	355	363	371	378	386	393	401	408
74	148	155	163	171	179	186	194	202	210	218	225	233	241	249	256	264	272	280	287	295	303	311	319	326	334	342	350	358	365	373	381	389	396	404	412	420
75	152	160	168	176	184	192	200	208	216	224	232	240	248	256	264	272	279	287	295	303	311	319	327	335	343	351	359	367	375	383	391	399	407	415	423	431
76	156	164	172	180	189	197	205	213	221	230	238	246	254	263	271	279	287	295	304	312	320	328	336	344	353	361	369	377	385	394	402	410	418	426	435	443

FIGURE 19–4. Body Mass Index Table. *Source: http://www.nhlbi.nih.gov/guidelines/obesity/bmi_tbl.pdf.*

interventions with her. Interventions for the normal physiological changes that may interfere with a woman's ability to eat an adequate diet are described later in this chapter (see Common Complaints).

Dietary Interventions. Assuming the client's dietary intake was adequate before conception and her weight is within a normal range, caloric intake (kcal) should increase by approximately 100 to 300 in the last two trimesters for a singleton pregnancy (Cunningham et al., 2010). Educate the client about the dietary adjustments needed to supply nutrients, taking into account the client's cultural, religious, and personal preferences, as well as lifestyle, food preferences, intolerances, and aversions.

High or low activity levels require adjustment of calorie intake. The goal is appropriate weight gain patterns. Variable energy needs of pregnant clients make advising total calorie needs difficult. The client with very low prepregnant weight may need more than 300 kcal/day added to her diet. In addition, little is known about the specific caloric needs of women with multiple gestation pregnancies. Nutritional counseling and recommendations should be individualized to each woman based on her circumstances (e.g., age, activity level, prepregnant BMI, gestation) (ADA, 2008).

Recently, the Institute of Medicine (IOM) (2009) updated the weight gain recommendations for pregnancy. One primary change from the 1990 guidelines relates to obese women (BMI ≥ 30) and the recommended weight gain of 11 to 20 lb (5–9 kg) in pregnancy, compared to the previously recommended 15 lb (7 kg). The BMI categories were also changed to reflect the categories established by the International Obesity Task Force. Weight gain recommendations are no longer different for adolescents, women of short stature, or women of color. The IOM guidelines also provide for weight gain recommendations in women with twin gestation according to prepregnant BMI. The challenge for providers remains in trying to help women achieve weight gain within these guidelines given that most women gain in excess of the recommendations (Siega-Riz, Deierlein, & Stuebe, 2010) (see Table 19–7).

Independent of weight gain, recommended daily allowances of vitamins and minerals are established for pregnant and lactating women (ADA, 2008; Barger, 2010; Cunningham et al., 2010). Most nutrients can be obtained with a healthy diet based on adequate consumption of vegetables, fruits, whole grains, legumes, lean proteins, and calcium-rich foods and avoidance of unhealthy or processed foods and sugar-sweetened beverages (ADA, 2008; Widen & Siega-Riz, 2010). Emphasis is placed on certain micronutrients and minerals in pregnancy such as iron and folic acid, as well as vitamin B_{12} for certain populations (see Table 19–8).

The recommended daily intake of iron in pregnancy is 27 mg (ADA, 2008). All pregnant women are advised to add supplemental iron during pregnancy, especially after the first trimester when the iron needs are greatest (Cunningham et al., 2010). Most prenatal vitamins contain adequate amounts of iron for supplementation. Women with iron-deficiency anemia may need up to 60 mg or more of daily iron supplementation (ADA, 2008; Cunningham et al., 2010). Encourage a diet that includes foods high in iron (e.g., kale, spinach, lentils, beans, lean meats, fortified breads and cereals, and blackstrap molasses). Calcium and magnesium, if given with iron, decrease absorption, while vitamin C enhances absorption.

An estimated 50 percent of NTDs can be prevented with 400 μg of folic acid daily starting before conception and continuing in early pregnancy. Consumption of fortified foods in addition to supplementation with folic acid or with a prenatal vitamin typically provides adequate

TABLE 19–7. Recommendations for Total Weight Gain During Pregnancy

'Prepregnancy BMI	BMI (kg/m^2)	Total weight galn (LBS)	Rates of weight gain in 2nd and 3rd trimester (LBS/week)
Underweight	< 18.5	28–40	1 (1–1.3)
Normal weight	18.5–24.9	25–35	1 (0.8–1)
Overweight	25.0–29.9	15–25	0.6 (0.5–0.7)
Obese	> 30	11–20	0.5 (0.4–0.6)

Source: Institute of Medicine. (2009). *Weight Gain During Pregnancy: Reexamining the Guide.* Reprinted with permission from the National Academies Press, Copyright ©2009, National Academy of Sciences.

TABLE 19–8. Daily Food Plan for Pregnancy and Lactation

Food group	Nutrients provided	Food source	Recommended daily amount during pregnancy	Recommended daily amount during lactation
Dairy products	*Protein, riboflavin,* vitamins A, D, and others, calcium, phosphorus; zinc, magnesium	Milk—whole, 2%, low-fat, *skim,* dry, buttermilk Cheeses—hard, semisoft, cottage Yogurt—plain, low-fat Soybean milk—canned, dry	Four (8 oz) cups (five for teenagers) used plain or with flavoring, in shakes, soups, puddings, custards, cocoa Calcium in 1 cup milk equivalent *to* 11/2 cups *cottage* cheese, 11/2 oz hard or semisoft cheese, 1 cup yogurt, 1 1/2 cups ice cream (high in fat and sugar)	Four(8 oz)cups(fireforll teenagers); equivalent *(M* amount of cheese, yogurt! and so forth *'M*
Meat and meat alternatives	Protein; iron, thiamine, niacin, and other vitamins, minerals	Seef, pork, *veal, iamb, poultry,* animal organ meats, fish, tofu, eggs, legumes, nuts, seeds, peanut butter, grains in proper vegetarian combination (vitamin $B_{1?}$ supplement needed)	Three servings (one serving = 2 oz), combination in amounts necessary for same nutrient equivalent (varies greatly)	Two servings
Gram products, whole grain or enriched	B vitamins, iron; whole gram also has zinc, magnesium, and other trace elements; provides fiber	Breads and bread products such as cornbread, muffins, waffles, hotcakes, biscuits, dumplings, cereals, pastas, rice	Six to 11 servings daily: one serving = one slice bread, 3/4 cup or 1 oz dry cereal, 1/2 cup rice or pasta	Same as for pregnancy
Fruits and fruit juices	Vitamins A and C; minerals, raw fruits for roughage	Citrus fruits and juices, melons, berries, all other fruits and juices	Two to four servings (one seiving for vitamin C). one serving = one medium fruit, 1/2-1 cup fruit, 4 oz orange or grapefruit juice	Same as for pregnancy
Vegetables and vegetable juices	Vitamins A and C; minerals; provides roughage	Leafy green vegetables; deep yellow or orange vegetables such as *carrots,* sweet potatoes, squash, tomatoes, green vegetables such as peas, green beans, broccoli; other vegetables such as beets, cabbage, potatoes, com, lima beans	Three to five servings (one serving of dark green or deep yellow vegetable for vitamin A) one serving = 1/2-1 cup vegetable, two tomatoes, one medium potato	Same as for pregnancy
Fats	Vitamins A and D, linoleic acid	Butter, cream cheese, fortified table spreads; cream, whipped cream, whipped toppings; avocado, mayonnaise, oil, nuts	As desired in moderation (high in calories): one serving = 1 tbsp butter or enriched margarine	Same as for pregnancy
Sugar and sweets		Sugar, brown sugar, honey, molasses	Occasionally, if desired	Same as for pregnancy
Desserts		Nutritious desserts such as puddings, custards, fruit whips, and crisps; other rich, sweet desserts and pastries	Occasionally, if desired	Same as for pregnancy
Beverages		Coffee, decaffeinated beverages, tea, bouillon, carbonated drinks	As desired, in moderation	Same as for pregnancy
Miscellaneous		lodized salt, herbs, spices, condiments	As desired	Same as for pregnancy

Note: The pregnant woman should eat regularly, three meals a day, with nutritious snacks of fruit, cheese, milk, or other foods between meals if desired. (More frequent but smaller meals are also recommended). Four to 6 (8 oz) glasses of water and a total of 8 to 10 (8 oz) cups total fluid intake should be consumed daily. Water is an essential nutrient

recommended daily intake. Women with a history of a child with NTDs are recommended to increase their folic acid intake to 4 mg daily starting 1 month prior to conception and continuing through the first trimester (Cunningham et al., 2010). Smoking and alcohol use decrease folate levels.

Women may choose to follow a vegetarian, vegan, or macrobiotic diet for health, personal, philosophical, ethical, and/or religious reasons. For most of these women, a prenatal or multivitamin supplement is recommended that contains adequate amounts of vitamin B_{12} (ADA, 2008; Widen & Siega-Riz, 2010).

Research is increasing regarding the prevalence of vitamin D deficiency and the importance of adequate levels of vitamin D (and calcium) for bone development and health (Kaludjerovic & Vieth, 2010). Optimal levels of serum 25-hydroxyvitamin D during pregnancy have not been established and routine screening is not recommended. Screening can be considered in women at risk for deficiency such as vegetarians, women in climates with limited sun exposure, or ethnic minorities (ACOG, 2011c). The recommended dietary allowance for pregnant women is 600 international units (IU) of vitamin D daily (ACOG, 2011c) and most prenatal vitamins contain at least 400 IU (Kaludjerovic & Vieth, 2010). Consensus is lacking regarding levels of vitamin D supplementation during pregnancy for women who are deficient. Careful attention needs to be directed to avoiding levels high enough to become toxic; however, supplementation with 1,000 to 2,000 IU of vitamin D daily is considered safe in pregnancy for women with vitamin D deficiency (ACOG, 2011c). Vitamin D can also be obtained through limited sun exposure and consumption of certain fish (e.g., salmon, tuna) or fish oils, fortified milk, cheese, and egg yolks (Kaludjerovic & Vieth, 2010).

Research is also ongoing related to the role of essential fatty acids, especially omega-3 docosahexaenoic acid (DHA) and eicosapentaenoic acid (EPA), in perinatal outcomes. Fatty acids are a vital component of cell membranes, they cannot be synthesized by the body, and DHA and EPA are especially vital for fetal growth and development and subsequent visual and cognitive function (Jordan, 2010). Associations of inadequate levels of essential fatty acids with preeclampsia, preterm birth, and low birth weight have been noted; however, there are not enough data yet to demonstrate a consistently significant relationship. Although omega-6 fatty acids are plentiful in most American diets, omega-3 fatty acids are often lacking. Recommendations for consumption in pregnancy is 200 to 300 mg of DHA plus EPA, which can be found in fish, purified fish oils, or algal oil supplements (Jordan, 2010). Care should be taken to avoid those fish highest in mercury content (e.g., shark, swordfish, tilefish, king mackerel) and to limit consumption to two 6-oz servings a week of fish lower in mercury content (e.g., salmon, canned light tuna, shrimp) (Environmental Protection Agency, 2011).

Vitamin A deficiency is a global health issue in underdeveloped countries. Supplementation is typically not recommended in the United States, and high intake of vitamin A (10,000–50,000 IU) as retinol, not beta-carotene, should be avoided to reduce risk of birth defects (Cunningham et al., 2010). Prevention of foodborne illnesses such as listeriosis and toxoplasmosis is of special importance in pregnancy. All pregnant women should be advised to avoid soft cheeses; unpasteurized dairy products; cold deli meats; and raw, uncooked, or undercooked eggs or meat (ADA, 2008).

Follow-Up. Weight gain should be assessed at each visit. Abnormal weight gains should be evaluated by ruling out obstetric complications (e.g., hyperemesis, edema, infection, gestational diabetes, abnormal fetal growth) and by assessing diet quality, activity levels, food preferences and intolerance, and socioeconomic and psychologic factors (Siega-Riz et al., 2010). Consider referral to a nutritionist or dietician for any client at nutritional risk, with a drug or alcohol abuse problem, with a chronic medical problem that requires a therapeutic diet, with gestational diabetes, or with a vegetarian diet. Additionally, if an eating disorder is identified or psychosocial problems are affecting the client's diet or appetite, refer her to a mental health care provider. If the client has inadequate financial resources, refer her to a social worker for advice about government and private programs such as WIC.

Assessment of Prenatal Attachment

Since the 1980s, maternal-fetal, paternal-fetal, or prenatal attachment has been described and studied in order to define and measure the phenomenon of connection between the parent(s) and the developing fetus (Alhusen, 2008; Ustunsoz, Guvenc, Akyuz, & Oflaz, 2010). Positive correlations have been observed between prenatal attachment and subsequent parent–child attachment in early infancy and childhood. In addition, factors such as social support, gestational age, and prenatal ultrasound testing have demonstrated significant relationships with increased prenatal attachment. Assessing levels of family support, offering ultrasound testing, and evaluating prenatal attachment (especially in the third trimester when it is typically strongest) may help to identify a family at risk for future disruptions with parent–child attachment (Alhusen, 2008; Yarcheski, Mahon, Yarcheski, Hanks, & Cannella, 2008).

THE DEVELOPMENTAL STAGES OF PREGNANCY

Maternal role attainment is not an inevitable, instinctive event initiated by the act of birth; instead, it is an active process requiring personal motivation. It is believed that the roots of this role develop during childhood. During pregnancy, a woman actively works on assuming the behaviors she believes encompass the ideal mother (Attrill, 2002; Gay, Edgil, & Douglas, 1988; Rubin, 1984).

MAJOR THEORIES OF MATERNAL ROLE DEVELOPMENT

Three leading theorists in maternal role development are Reva Rubin, Ramona Mercer, and Regina Lederman.

Reva Rubin's contributions to maternity nursing provide valuable insights into the biopsychosocial experience of childbearing. Rubin developed a framework for the process of maternal role assumption in 1967, although she published from 1961 to 1984. Her early publications *Basic Maternal Behaviors* and *Maternal Touch* are considered classics in maternity nursing (Gay et al., 1988).

Rubin's writings include concepts about body image, self-esteem, and thought process during pregnancy, as well as assumption of the maternal role prior to and after delivery (Gay et al., 1988). Without the desire for children, there is no active motivation to assume a maternal role. Rubin identified maternal tasks and behaviors normally seen during the antepartum and postpartum periods. Assessment of those behaviors can be used to evaluate the mother's progress toward assumption of a maternal role (see Table 19–9) (Gay et al., 1988; Rubin, 1984). Rubin concluded that if the mother perceived a threat to her pregnancy, such as HIV infection or miscarriage, then she was less likely to bond with her infant and, therefore, was at risk for poor attachment.

When Rubin made her initial observations of maternal behaviors, strong consumer participation in childbirth education and health care was in its infancy. Today, childbearing couples have the option of knowing the gender of their fetus, see their fetus through the technology of ultrasound, and are more knowledgeable and less passive than parents of previous generations. Ultimately, some of Rubin's observations may have less relevance for contemporary women, but they are a timeless framework for family-centered maternity care. Using Rubin's three postpartum developmental phases, a mother's progress during the postpartum period may be assessed (Gay et al., 1988; Rubin, 1984) (see Chapter 22). More recently, Ramona Mercer (2004) built upon Rubin's earlier work to describe the concept of "becoming a mother," which more completely defines the process of maternal role development, giving fuller expression to the transformational experience of motherhood. Mercer suggests this transformational experience begins with preparation during pregnancy, followed by learning about and becoming acquainted with her newborn. Over the first few months of the postpartum period she adjusts to her "new normal," ultimately achieving her identity as a mother.

Regina Lederman (1996) views maternal role assumption as identification with motherhood, namely as part of the larger process of psychosocial development in pregnancy that includes taking the developmental step from being a woman without child to being a woman with child. This process is a progressive change in thinking for the mother, away from concerns about self and more toward concern for the mother–infant unit. Two important factors come into play to achieve this goal: motivation and the degree of preparation for the mothering role.

According to Lederman, motivation for motherhood is reflected by the degree to which one expresses the interest and the ability to nurture and empathize with a child. This encompasses the perception of motherhood as a life-fulfilling event. The woman's motivation for pregnancy is questioned if her thoughts toward the child (fetus) are infrequent, aversive, avoided, or denied, or if the woman desires the pregnancy but not the child.

Preparation for motherhood involves acquiring the ability to see oneself as a mother. This is accomplished through *fantasizing/dreaming*, which is an arena for rehearsing motherhood skills. The woman relies on her life experiences of being nurtured and on her ability to identify with other women in their positive role as mothers. According to Lederman, all women bring conflicts to

TABLE 19–9. Reva Rubin Theory: The Antepartum Phase

Trimester	Maternal Task/Behavior	Nursing Significance
First	"Who me?" "Pregnant?" "Now?"	Question of identity—conception thought to be a surprise—resulting ambivalence related to the reality of pregnancy. Incorporation of concept of fetus into self. Acceptance of pregnancy/fetus by self and significant others.
Second	Seeking safe passage for self and child. Ensuring the acceptance of the child fetus. Protective behaviors by the mother for the child.	Acceptance of growing fetus by self, others. Willingness to "house" fetus even with body/role/ego changes. Passage of socially accepted values, behaviors, attitudes, skills from mother to child.
Third	Mother's binding-in to her unknown child. Learning to give of self.	Binding-in developed from initial maternal-fetal bonds to adult–child companionship. These bonds include fetal movements, maternal anatomic changes. Nurturant behaviors given from mother to child.

Sources: Gay et al., 1988; Rubin, 1984.

a pregnancy. But if the conflicts are not resolved through preparation and bargaining during pregnancy, then the woman may find the motherhood role unrewarding, thereby increasing her feelings of inadequacy.

Lederman describes a woman's relationship with her own mother as the final aspect of maternal role development. The availability of the client's own mother, her acceptance of that pregnancy, her respect for the daughter's autonomy, and her willingness to share her previous childbearing/childrearing experiences all impact the outcome of preparation.

Rubin's and Lederman's frameworks are generally considered compatible, although they use different names for similar concepts. Absence of these processes or inability to pass through them satisfactorily may impede the progress of maternal role development (Lederman, 1996; Rubin, 1984). This recognition is fundamental for nursing assessment during pregnancy and the postpartum period.

Implications of Rubin's, Mercer's, and Lederman's Theories

- Identify whether the client is at higher risk for maladaptation at initial and ongoing prenatal visits.
- Monitor the client's progress by observing for expected role behaviors.
- Refer the client for appropriate counseling when maladaptive behaviors are identified.

COMMON COMPLAINTS

Many symptoms that are frequently reported to health care providers are most often attributable to pregnancy but must be evaluated to rule out other pathology.

FIRST TRIMESTER

Breast Pain, Enlargement, and Changes in Pigmentation

Etiology. Physiologic changes that underlie these complaints are the increased levels of estrogen, progesterone, hCG, prolactin, and human placental lactogen, which cause the fat layer of breasts to thicken and the numbers and development of milk ducts and glands to increase. As a result, the breasts, especially the area around the areola, increase in size, weight, and tenderness. The nipples become erect, the areolae darken, the Montgomery's tubercles enlarge, and a slight colostrum discharge may be present (Blackburn, 2007).

Subjective Data. The client may report increasing tenderness, weight, and size of the breasts, darkening of the areolae, and leakage of colostrum from the nipples. The history should not include pain and redness localized in one area of the breast, fever, flu-like symptoms, injury, masses, dimples, bloody discharge, changes in skin texture, or changes in breast or nipple size, shape, symmetry, as these symptoms/signs may indicate other conditions requiring medical follow-up. Some medications are known to cause galactorrhea.

Objective Data. No diagnostic tests are necessary. Physical examination and vital signs are within normal limits. Areas of induration, inflammation, or heat; masses; skin dimpling; skin changes; enlarged nodes; or unilateral or bloody nipple discharge should not be present.

Differential Medical Diagnosis. Breast tenderness, enlargement, and pigment changes due to pregnancy; ruling out mastitis, fibrocystic breast tissue, breast injury, and breast cancer.

Plan

Psychosocial Interventions. Educate the client about the physiology behind breast changes. Inform her that pain often improves in the second trimester but the other changes will remain until after lactation ends. Advise the client to notify the health care provider if any symptoms ruled out during the history taking occur in the future.

Lifestyle Changes. Advise the client to examine her breasts in the same way as before pregnancy, except that no special time of month is indicated. If instruction is necessary, provide it (see Chapter 17).

In addition, the client may need to constantly wear a supportive bra. Correct fit is important as breast size changes in pregnancy. She may find wearing a bra while sleeping more comfortable.

Dietary Interventions. Advise the client to avoid the use of caffeine.

Follow-Up. Clients with symptoms of mastitis must be treated appropriately (see Chapters 17 and 22). Refer the client with symptoms of pathology to a physician.

Constipation

Etiology. Large amounts of circulating progesterone cause decreased motility of the gastrointestinal (GI) tract, resulting in increased water reabsorption from the bowel. The large bowel is also mechanically compressed by the enlarging uterus. The client may have changed her food and fluid intake or exercise level in response to nausea and vomiting, fatigue, culturally prescribed expectations of pregnant women, or medically prescribed treatment (Blackburn, 2007). Prenatal vitamins with iron or calcium can also be constipating.

Subjective Data. The client may report abdominal cramping, flatulence, or increasing difficulty with bowel movements or intervals between them. Stools may be small, hard, round, and dark. Often the client has a history of constipation before pregnancy. Her diet may be high in refined carbohydrates and low in bulk and fluids, and she may rarely exercise. The client may have taken antacids, calcium, iron supplements, anticholinergics, tricyclic antidepressants, or codeine medications, causing constipation. The history should *not* include change in stool (i.e., color, shape, or pattern), diarrhea, abdominal pain, fever, weight loss, anorexia, periumbilical pain, rectal bleeding, pus or mucus in bowels, emotional distress, or excessive laxative use, because these symptoms/signs may indicate other conditions requiring medical or other appropriate follow-up.

Objective Data. Physical examination and vital signs are within normal limits, although hyperactive bowel sounds, constipated stool in the rectum, a palpable mass in the lower left quadrant that disappears after bowel movements, hemorrhoids, or hemorrhoidal tags may be noted.

Differential Medical Diagnosis. Constipation related to pregnancy ruling out preterm labor, pica, GI disease (e.g., irritable bowel syndrome, appendicitis), chronic laxative use, use of medications known to cause constipation (e.g., codeine), or anal pain.

Plan

Psychosocial Interventions. Explain to the client how pregnancy exacerbates the symptoms of constipation and that symptoms should improve after delivery. Advise her to notify the health care provider if any symptoms ruled out during history taking occur in the future.

Medication. Advise the client to avoid mineral oil, as it will decrease the absorption of fat-soluble vitamins. Cathartics are contraindicated in pregnancy.

Review with client what other medication (e.g., calcium supplements, iron) she is taking to determine whether constipation is a side effect—then help her to reduce their use if possible.

- Bulk-forming, nonnutritive laxatives (e.g., Metamucil, FiberCon) (Deglin, Vallerand, & Sanoski, 2011)
  - *Indications:* Occasional constipation.
  - *Administration:* Available in tablets or granules. Take per package instructions.
  - *Side effects and adverse reactions:* If taken without adequate fluids, may swell in throat or esophagus, causing choking.
  - *Contraindications:* Fecal impaction or intestinal obstruction.
  - *Anticipated outcome on evaluation:* Softer stools with decreased constipation.
  - *Client teaching and counseling:* Instruct the client to drink 8 oz of water or more with each dose. Do not use if having difficulty breathing or swallowing, chest pain, or vomiting. If these occur, advise to seek immediate medical attention. She may need to continue treatment for 2 to 3 days before maximum effect is noted.
  - *FDA pregnancy category:* B.
- Docusate sodium (Colace) (Botehlo, Emeis, & Brucker, 2011; Deglin et al., 2011; Manns-James, 2011)
  - *Indications:* Prevention of constipation
  - *Administration:* 50 to 100 mg PO qd bid
  - *Side effects and adverse reactions:* Not significant
  - *Contraindications:* Nausea and vomiting, acute abdominal pain
  - *Anticipated outcome on evaluation:* Soft bowel movement within 24 to 48 hours
  - *Client teaching and counseling:* Use short-term only, make dietary changes in addition to medication use
  - *FDA pregnancy category:* C

Lifestyle Changes. Encourage the client to exercise regularly (according to ACOG guidelines), establish a time of day to defecate, avoid prolonged attempts to defecate, and elevate her feet on a stool while defecating to avoid straining.

Dietary Interventions. Advise the client to eat foods high in bulk (e.g., fresh fruits and vegetables, whole-grain breads and cereals), drink fluids (6 to 8 glasses of water per day), decrease refined carbohydrates, and drink warm fluids on arising to stimulate bowel motility. Explain that if she takes her vitamin/mineral supplement every second or third day or changes to a supplement without iron and calcium temporarily, constipation may be less of a problem. If any foods or juices (e.g., bran, prune juice) have helped the client in the past, encourage their use.

Follow-Up. If prenatal vitamins or iron are discontinued, monitor the client for anemia. Folic acid should be supplemented in the first trimester. If purging or psychosocial stress is causing constipation, refer the client to a mental health care provider. If symptoms of a pathological condition develop, refer the client to a physician.

Excessive Salivation (Ptyalism) and Bad Taste in Mouth

Etiology. The etiology of oral changes is not known. It is theorized that eating starchy foods may stimulate the salivary glands, or that nausea causes a decreased ability to swallow saliva (Blackburn, 2007; Cunningham et al., 2010).

Subjective Data. The client reports increased salivation or a bitter taste in her mouth. History should *not* include a sore throat, fever, flu-like symptoms, heat, pain or lesions in the mouth, bad breath, upper abdominal pain, bloating, lethargy, dental problems, or pica. In addition, assess that the client practices good dental hygiene and does not have symptoms of a psychiatric disorder.

Objective Data. No diagnostic tests are necessary. Physical examination and vital signs, particularly the condition of the mouth and teeth, are within normal limits. Occasionally, perioral irritation, red-coated tongue, swollen glands, drooling, or salivation interfering with speech may occur.

Differential Medical Diagnoses. Excessive salivation related to pregnancy ruling out dental problems, upper GI problems (e.g., stomatitis), upper respiratory disease (e.g., pharyngitis), and pica.

Plan

Psychosocial Interventions. Reassure the client that the complaint is related to pregnancy and that the condition should resolve after the pregnancy. Advise the client to notify the health care provider if any symptoms ruled out during the history taking occur in the future.

Lifestyle Changes. Advise the client to maintain good oral hygiene.

Dietary Interventions. Advise the client to avoid excessive starch intake and to maintain a good diet and adequate hydration. Inform her that sucking hard candy or breath mints or chewing gum may provide relief.

Follow-Up. Refer a client with symptoms of pathology to a physician. Refer a client with symptoms of dental disease to a dentist.

Fatigue

Etiology. Fatigue during pregnancy occurs primarily during the first and third trimesters (the highest energy levels often occur during the second trimester). First-trimester fatigue may be caused by physical changes (e.g., increased oxygen consumption, progesterone and relaxin levels, and fetal demands) and psychosocial changes (e.g., reexamination of roles). Third-trimester fatigue is usually caused by sleep disturbances that result from increased weight, physical discomforts, and decreased exercise.

Subjective Data. The client may report fatigue despite normal amounts of sleep or related to insomnia. Her family or work situation may not allow her to rest during the day. The history should *not* include depression, anxiety, difficulty with concentration, anorexia, anemia, use of medications known to cause drowsiness, exercise intolerance, chest pain or discomfort, change in bowel habits, flu-like symptoms, sore throat, coughing, or dyspnea, or other symptoms/signs indicating other conditions requiring medical or other appropriate follow-up.

Objective Data. The physical examination and vital signs are within normal limits.

A CBC is used to evaluate the client for signs of anemia, infection, or blood dyscrasias.

Differential Medical Diagnosis. Fatigue due to pregnancy ruling out other pathological states.

Plan

Psychosocial Interventions. Explain to the client that increased fatigue is expected in the first and third trimesters. Encourage her to contact the health care provider if she develops other symptoms.

Encourage verbalization of psychosocial problems and explore appropriate interventions. Encourage the client to accept offers of help. Advise the client to avoid, if possible, major life stresses (e.g., moving) during pregnancy.

Medication. Supplemental iron may be appropriate if anemic. No sleeping medications are prescribed.

Lifestyle Changes. Encourage adequate sleep and rest periods; recommend that the client arrange work, childcare, and other activities to permit additional rest. Mild exercise may help lessen symptoms of fatigue (Varney et al., 2004).

Dietary Interventions. Correct nutritional inadequacies, paying attention to total nutrient intake and distribution of those nutrients throughout the day (see Nutrition, later in this chapter, and Table 19–7).

Follow-Up. Refer the client to a physician if symptoms of pathology are evident. When severe psychosocial stress, anxiety, or depression is noted, referral to a mental health care provider is appropriate.

Flatulence

Etiology. The physiological changes that result in constipation also may result in increased flatulence.

Subjective Data. A client may report increased passage of rectal gas, abdominal bloating, constipation, or belching, but not abdominal pain, epigastric pain, use of food or medications that cause gas, change in bowels, greasy bowel movements, anxiety, or depression.

Objective Data. Often, hyperactive bowel sounds or abdominal distention is detected on physical exam.

Differential Medical Diagnoses. Flatulence; rule out irritable bowel syndrome, lactose or food intolerance, medication side effects, hyperventilation, or other GI disease (e.g., malabsorption syndromes).

Plan

Psychosocial Interventions. Reassure the client that increased flatulence is related to pregnancy and should resolve afterward.

Lifestyle Changes. Teach the client measures to avoid constipation. Avoiding gum chewing, large meals, and smoking also will reduce flatulence. The knee-chest position may help expel gas that is causing discomfort (Varney et al., 2004).

Dietary Interventions. Advise the client to limit gas-forming foods (e.g., carbonated beverages, cruciferous vegetables, baking soda, cheese, beans, bananas, peanuts, calcium carbonate supplements). Pasta, corn, and whole grains when cooked, refrigerated, or frozen and then reheated form gas-producing substances. Each cooling and reheating makes them more potent. Mint can increase abdominal gas.

Follow-Up. Refer her to a mental health care provider if symptoms of psychosocial stress are evident.

Headache

Etiology. Headaches during pregnancy are most often of the tension type, and are caused by increased circulatory volume, the effects of estrogen on cerebral blood flow, stress, fatigue, sinus congestion, and eye strain related to ocular changes. Headaches not caused by pathology are very common in pregnancy. Nevertheless, headache, particularly new onset, can be a symptom of serious illness, which must be ruled out. New onset of migraine headache is very rare in pregnancy, and women with preexisting migraines may find that after an initial exacerbation of symptoms in the first trimester, symptoms often decrease or cease altogether as pregnancy progresses (Blackburn, 2007; Manns-James, 2011).

Subjective Data. Focus on the nature, frequency, intensity, location, description of the pain; factors that trigger, worsen, or alleviate it; and changes that have occurred during pregnancy in the quality of the headaches. The client may report a past or family history of headaches or increased stress. The history should *not* include injury to the head, neck, or back; nausea, vomiting, diarrhea; fever; migraine aura; occupational exposure to chemicals; consumption of alcohol, chocolate, or aged cheese; unbalanced intake of calories; fatigue, as these symptoms/signs may indicate other conditions requiring medical or other appropriate follow-up. Pathology may also be present if there is a history of increasing intensity and frequency of headaches, increase with coughing or straining, worse in morning, disrupts sleep; facial edema; changes in the level of consciousness; memory changes; depression; anxiety; motor, visual, or sensory changes; nausea; vomiting; stiff neck; fever; ear or eye pain; rhinitis; flu-like symptoms; injury; or prodomata (i.e., visual, auditory, or sensory changes preceding a headache).

Objective Data. Physical examination and vital signs, particularly blood pressure, weight gain pattern, ophthalmoscopic examination, and ear, nose, throat, neurological, musculoskeletal, and upper respiratory exams, are within normal limits.

A *urine dipstick test* that is negative for protein and ketones reduces the possibility of preeclampsia and dehydration from vomiting.

A CBC is another diagnostic test used (see Fatigue).

Differential Medical Diagnosis. Benign vascular headache of pregnancy ruling out preeclampsia, gestational hypertension, HELLP syndrome, infectious process (e.g., sinus infections), cardiovascular diseases, musculoskeletal disease (e.g., muscle tension headache), neurological disease (e.g., cluster or vascular headache), hypoglycemia, caffeine withdrawal. Chapter 24 has additional discussion about headaches. Caution is advised with the use of the medications described because several are not recommended in pregnancy.

Plan

Psychosocial Interventions. Explain to the client the physiologic changes that are causing the headache and that it may improve in the second trimester. Advise the client to notify the health care provider if any symptoms ruled out during the history taking occur in the future.

Ask the client to keep a diary of activities, foods, and environmental stimuli that occur around the time of the headache. This may reveal triggering factors.

Teach the client symptoms of preeclampsia (headache that is different in nature, visual changes, photophobia, confusion, swelling in the face or hands, severe swelling in the feet, epigastric pain) and encourage immediate contact with the provider.

Medication. Acetaminophen is indicated for headache and other pain (Deglin et al., 2011).

- *Administration:* 325 to 650 mg every 4 hours as needed for pain.
- *Side effects and adverse reactions:* Not significant.
- *Contraindication:* Sensitivity to acetaminophen, chronic alcohol use, liver damage.
- *Anticipated outcome on evaluation:* Reduced headache pain.
- *Client counseling:* Instruct the client to notify the health care provider if headache pain continues. Overdose of acetaminophen requires prompt attention. It has been associated with liver damage. Advise against chronic use.
- *FDA pregnancy category:* B.

Lifestyle Changes. Advise the client to avoid activities and situations that may trigger headaches (stress, smoking, smoke-filled rooms, blinking lights, sleeping late). Advise her to reduce stress as much as possible, get adequate sleep, have her neck and shoulders massaged with heat or cold applied.

Encourage the client to practice relaxation techniques.

Dietary Interventions. Advise the client to eat a regular, balanced diet, to avoid intake of food that triggers headaches (e.g., caffeine, chocolate, nitrites, hard aged cheese, alcohol—especially red wine), and to stay well hydrated.

Consult with or refer to a physician if the headache is severe, does not respond to interventions, requires strong pain killers, or demonstrates other signs of preeclampsia, gestational hypertension, pathology, or eye strain. If caffeine withdrawal is causing headache, advise weaning off caffeine gradually. If signs of severe psychosocial stress are present, refer the client to a mental health care provider. Referral to a pain center may help severe headache that is not due to pathology.

Hemorrhoids

Etiology. Hemorrhoids occur when the vascular submucosa in the rectoanal canal bulges and becomes congested with varicosities. They become significant only when symptomatic. Hemorrhoids are exacerbated during pregnancy by increased intravascular pressure in veins below the uterus, constipation, and straining at stool (Varney et al., 2004).

Subjective Data. The client may report a history of constipation, hemorrhoids before pregnancy, multiparity, increased age, or a family history of hemorrhoids. She may notice swelling, fullness, or a lump at her anus; bright red, painless bleeding on the stool surface during defecation; or increased mucus with defecation. If an anal fissure develops, defecation is often painful.

Objective Data. Physical examination and vital signs may be within normal limits, or hemorrhoids may be visible externally or palpated internally. Anal fissures or hemorrhoidal tags may be noted. Thrombosed hemorrhoids are a painful, shiny, bluish or purple clot-containing mass near the anus.

Diagnostic tests and methods include evaluation of the *hemoglobin level* in the blood. The hemoglobin level may be decreased if bleeding is extensive or prolonged.

Differential Medical Diagnosis. Hemorrhoids exacerbated by pregnancy; rule out abscessed or thrombosed hemorrhoids, rectal lesions (e.g., condyloma acuminata cancerous lesions), all of which may require more extensive medical referral and intervention.

Plan

Psychosocial Interventions. Explain to the client the underlying changes that created or exacerbated the hemorrhoids and assure her that the condition will improve or resolve after pregnancy. Encourage her to contact a health care provider if any symptoms occur in the future.

Medication. Over-the-counter topical anesthetics (e.g., Preparation H, Anusol) may shrink swelling and reduce itching.

Lifestyle Changes. Advise the client to try to avoid constipation by following the measures described in the preceding section (see Constipation). Encourage her to use warm or cool sitz baths (Epsom salts may be added), witch hazel pads (e.g., Tucks®), and ice packs or cold compresses to reduce the size of the hemorrhoids. Furthermore, advise her to avoid straining by elevating her feet on a stool while attempting to defecate. Applying petroleum jelly around the anus before defecating will help reduce pain and bleeding. Resting with feet and hips elevated plus avoiding prolonged sitting or standing can be helpful (Varney et al., 2004).

Kegel exercises will improve circulation. To learn the feel of tightening the pubococcygeal (Kegel) muscles, first have the client sit on the commode and start and stop her urine flow. To do the exercise, squeeze and tighten for 5 to 10 seconds each, anywhere from 30 to 100 times per day (Amir & Bent, 2008). Gentle self-digital replacement of hemorrhoids if possible and careful perineal cleansing habits are also helpful.

Sitz baths may decrease discomfort and also improve circulation (Varney et al., 2004).

Refer the client to a physician if she has symptoms of thrombosed hemorrhoids, does not respond to interventions, or has symptoms of other pathology.

Nausea and Vomiting

Etiology. Physiological changes that cause nausea and vomiting during pregnancy are unknown; however, unusually high levels of estrogen and hCG as well as psychosocial, cultural, and genetic theories have been proposed. Multiple gestation and molar pregnancies are associated with higher incidences of nausea and vomiting. Fifty to 80 percent of pregnant women experience nausea and vomiting. Symptoms often last until the second trimester of pregnancy and are generally considered to be a reassuring sign, in terms of pregnancy outcome (King & Murphy, 2009).

Subjective Data. Nausea and/or vomiting are reported by the client between the 5th and 16th weeks of pregnancy. It may or may not be limited to certain times of the day (King & Murphy, 2009). The history should *not* include fever, lethargy, muscle aches, abdominal pain, cramping, diarrhea, jaundice, back pain, dark urine, changes in the shape or color of bowel movements, vaginal bleeding, head injury, headache, projectile vomiting, vomiting blood, excessive thirst, neurological signs, ataxia, chest pain, ear pain or ringing, or psychosocial distress, as these symptoms/signs indicate other conditions that may require medical or other appropriate follow-up.

Objective Data. Physical examination and vital signs are within normal limits. Significant negatives include the absence of signs of dehydration and vaginal bleeding. A hydatidiform gestation may present with hyperemesis and possible prolonged vaginal spotting. Multiple pregnancies often cause severe nausea and/or vomiting.

Uterine size should be appropriate for dates. FHTs should be audible at 12 weeks' gestation.

Weight loss, dehydration, ketonuria, and hypokalemia suggest hyperemesis gravidarum (King & Murphy, 2009).

Urine ketone and specific gravity tests are used to rule out dehydration. Tests specific to disease suggested by physical and history should be obtained.

Differential Medical Diagnoses. Nausea and vomiting related to pregnancy ruling out hyperemesis gravidarum, multiple gestation, hydatidiform gestation, GI disease (e.g., appendicitis, gastroenteritis), endocrine disease (e.g., hyperthyroidism), neurological disease (e.g., migraines), cardiorespiratory disease, nutritional disease (e.g., pica, vitamin deficiencies, food poisoning), medication overdose, emotional disease (e.g., eating disorders, depression).

Plan

Psychosocial Interventions. Reassure the client that nausea and vomiting usually are limited to the first trimester and are usually related to positive pregnancy outcomes. Advise her to notify the health care provider if any symptoms ruled out during history taking occur in the future.

Medication

- Diphenhydramine (Benadryl) (Deglin et al., 2011; Manns-James, 2011)
  - *Administration:* 50 to 100 mg PO q 4 to 6 hours
  - *Side effects and adverse reactions:* Drowsiness, anorexia, dry mouth
  - *Contraindications:* Hypersensitivity, acute asthma attack, lactation
  - *Anticipated outcomes on evaluation:* Decreased nausea/vomiting
  - *Client teaching and counseling:* May cause drowsiness and dry mouth, practice good oral hygiene, and do not drive while taking
  - *FDA pregnancy category:* B
- Dimenhydrinate (Dramamine) (Deglin et al., 2011; Manns-James, 2011)
  - *Administration:* 50 to 100 mg PO/PR q 4 to 6 hours
  - *Side effects and adverse reactions:* Drowsiness, anorexia

- *Contraindications:* Hypersensitivity
- *Anticipated outcomes on evaluation:* Decreased nausea/vomiting
- *Client teaching and counseling:* May cause drowsiness, avoid driving
- *FDA pregnancy category:* B

◆ Prochlorperazine (Compazine) (Deglin et al., 2011; Manns-James, 2011)

- *Administration:* 5 to 10 mg PO q 4–6 hours; 25 mg rectal suppository twice a day; maximum dose is 40 mg/day
- *Side effects and adverse reactions:* Sedation, anticholinergic effects; maximum dose is 40 mg/day
- *Contraindications:* Hypersensitivity, glaucoma, severe liver, or cardiovascular disease
- *Anticipated outcomes on evaluation:* Decreased nausea/vomiting
- *Client teaching and counseling:* Extrapyramidal symptoms (EPS) and tardive dyskinesia are possible—report to provider if they occur; may cause drowsiness, constipation, and sensitivity to sun; practice good oral hygiene
- *FDA pregnancy category:* C

◆ Promethazine (Phenergan) (Deglin et al., 2011; Manns-James, 2011)

- *Administration:* 12.5 to 25 mg PO/PR q 4–6 hours
- *Side effects and adverse reactions:* Sedation, anticholinergic effects
- *Contraindications:* Hypersensitivity, glaucoma
- *Anticipated outcomes on evaluation:* Decreased nausea/vomiting
- *Client teaching and counseling:* May cause drowsiness, sensitivity to sun; practice good oral hygiene
- *FDA pregnancy category:* C

◆ Metoclopramide (Reglan) (Deglin et al., 2011; Manns-James, 2011)

- *Administration:* 5 to 10 mg PO q 8 hours
- *Side effects and adverse reactions:* EPS, agitation, anxiety, acute dystonic reactions
- *Contraindications:* Hypersensitivity, possible GI obstruction or hemorrhage, seizure disorder
- *Anticipated outcomes on evaluation:* Decreased nausea/vomiting
- *Client teaching and counseling:* May cause drowsiness; notify provider if EPS occur
- *FDA pregnancy category:* B

◆ Ondansetron (Zofran) (Deglin et al., 2011; Manns-James, 2011)

- *Administration:* 4 to 8 mg PO three to four times per day
- *Side effects and adverse reactions:* Headache, constipation, diarrhea
- *Contraindications:* Hypersensitivity
- *Anticipated outcomes on evaluation:* Decreased nausea/vomiting
- *Client teaching and counseling:* EPS are possible—report to provider if they occur
- *FDA pregnancy category:* B

Lifestyle Changes

◆ Ask the client to keep a diary listing when and for how long nausea and vomiting occur and what activities, associated factors, or foods trigger or improve symptoms. Interventions suggested by this diary are most likely to succeed.

◆ Advise the client to rest when the nausea occurs, avoid stress, avoid sights and smells that trigger nausea, refrain from wearing clothing that is tight and constricting about the abdomen, and reduce workloads. Support and assistance from the client's partner may also improve symptoms.

◆ Suggest hypnosis, acupuncture, or acupressure (e.g., Sea-Bands®) (King & Murphy, 2009).

◆ Describe relaxation techniques that may help: progressive relaxation (systematic tensing and relaxing of muscle groups), autogenic training (using suggestions such as "My right arm is heavy"), meditation (repeating a sound or gazing at an object while clearing the mind of all distractions), visual imagery (visualizing self in a relaxing place), and touching/massage.

Dietary Interventions

◆ Symptoms may be relieved by eating small, frequent meals that do not allow the stomach to become too empty or full, including high-carbohydrate or high-protein, easily digested meals and snacks; sipping carbonated drinks, including foods that tend to neutralize stomach acid (e.g., apples, milk, bread, potatoes, calcium carbonate tablets); eating crackers on arising; drinking fluids between meals instead of with meals; and avoiding foods that may irritate the stomach (e.g., spicy or fatty foods). Lemonade and potato chips have more nutrients and may be more effective than soda and crackers.

◆ Sit upright after eating.

◆ If a vitamin/mineral supplement is causing nausea, it may be discontinued until the client is less nauseated, often after about 14 to 16 weeks of pregnancy. Folic acid supplementation is advised.

- Remind the client of the need for adequate hydration (six to eight glasses per day). Sipping lukewarm fluids every 5 minutes is tolerated better than drinking an entire glass of fluid at one time.
- Vitamin B_6 (pyridoxine) has been shown in studies to be safe and effective at reducing nausea, at doses up to 40 mg per day (King & Murphy, 2009).
- Ginger has been shown to be as effective a treatment for nausea and vomiting as vitamin B_6 (King & Murphy, 2009). Ginger may be taken as fresh grated or crystallized rhizome, tea, liquid extract, syrup, or capsules, in divided doses totally 1 g per day (King & Murphy, 2009).

Follow-Up. Consult with a physician regarding any client who is unable to hold down liquids for more than 12 hours, who loses 5 lb or more, who has ketonuria or any symptoms of dehydration or pathology.

Urinary Frequency and Incontinence

Etiology. Urinary frequency and incontinence are experienced by as many as 60 percent of pregnant women, and can begin as early as the first trimester of pregnancy. Contrary to popular understanding that the pressure of the enlarging uterus causes these changes, this appears to account for frequency and incontinence experienced only in the final weeks of pregnancy. The actual etiology appears to be a combination of hormonal changes, increased circulating blood volume, and changes in renal physiology (Blackburn, 2007).

Subjective Data. The client may report increased urination, nocturia, or involuntary loss of urine. The history should *not* include back pain, fever, flu-like symptoms, hematuria, dysuria, urgency, dark, cloudy or blood urine, dribbling, suprapubic pain, polyuria, polydipsia, polyphagia, history of perineal or abdominal trauma, as these symptoms/signs indicate other conditions requiring more thorough follow-up and possible medical referral. She may report use of alcohol or caffeine.

To differentiate urine loss from rupture of membranes (ROM), know that ROM may be described as fluid from the client's vagina that cannot be controlled with Kegel exercises or as fluid that does not smell of urine and that may increase while she is lying down, gush at first when she stands, and then decrease after standing.

Objective Data. Physical examination and vital signs are within normal limits. The costal vertebral angle and suprapubic area are not tender. Vaginal exam does not reveal pooling of amniotic fluid but may reveal a cystocele.

Collect a clean catch urine specimen. (See Chapter 3 for test description and specimen collection information.) The urine can be poured over a urine dipstick. Presence of nitrites, or three to four plus protein, suggests a urinary tract infection (UTI), and presence of glucose suggests need to rule out diabetes (see Chapters 20 and 23).

The *nitrazine test* may help discriminate between vaginal discharge and amniotic fluid. Use of a sterile technique reduces the possibility of introducing infection if the membranes have ruptured. If possible ROM is suspected, a sterile speculum is inserted vaginally and a sterile cotton-tipped applicator is used to remove discharge from the vaginal pool. It is placed on nitrazine paper and the color change is compared with the chart. If the pH is 3.5 to 5, the fluid is normal vaginal discharge. If the pH is 7, the discharge may be amniotic fluid. Note that blood and vaginal discharge associated with certain vaginal infections (e.g., bacterial vaginosis and trichomonas vaginitis) may give a higher than normal pH reading.

The *fern test* also discriminates between vaginal discharge and amniotic fluid. Again, a sterile speculum is used. The sample of vaginal discharge is placed on a clean slide and allowed to dry. Amniotic fluid forms a fernlike pattern under microscopic examination. Inform the client that the nitrazine and fern tests are the best way to discriminate between vaginal discharge and amniotic fluid. Differentiation is important because premature ROM can cause amnionitis or preterm labor. During the speculum exam, the practitioner should also look for fluid leaking from the cervix.

Differential Medical Diagnosis. Urinary frequency/incontinence due to pregnancy ruling out UTI, pyelonephritis, kidney stone, stress urinary incontinence, gestational diabetes, preexisting diabetes mellitus, hypokalemia, and spontaneous ROM.

Plan

Psychosocial Interventions. Review diagrams of female anatomy with the client, to assist her in understanding the anatomical changes that occur during pregnancy that may lead to urinary frequency and incontinence. Reassure her that these symptoms should improve after delivery. Advise the client to notify the health care provider if any symptoms ruled out during history taking occur in the future.

Lifestyle Changes. Resting and sleeping in the lateral recumbent position enhance kidney function. Kegel exercises improve muscle tone.

Dietary Interventions. Advise the client to maintain an adequate fluid intake (six to eight glasses of water) to decrease the incidence of UTIs. Water intake should decrease 2 to 3 hours before bedtime. In addition, advise the client to discontinue drinking beverages that contain alcohol or caffeine.

Follow-Up. A client with UTI must be treated appropriately (see Chapter 24). Refer clients with symptoms of pathology, such as frequently repeated UTIs, to a urologist.

Varicosities of Vulva and Legs

Etiology. Physiologic changes during pregnancy that exacerbate varicosities include increased pressure of the gravid uterus, increased venous pressure, and the effects of estrogen on tissue elasticity. Factors that may contribute to the development of varicosities include genetic predisposition, prolonged standing or sitting, and wearing constrictive clothing (Blackburn, 2007; Varney et al., 2004).

Subjective Data. The client may report aching, throbbing, swelling, or heaviness in the legs or vulvar area, often worse at night. The client may also report multiparity, prolonged standing or sitting, or decreased activity. She may note increased symptoms as she becomes older. A family history of varicosities may be reported. The history should *not* include calf pain, clotting, swelling, redness, tenderness, or a white, cold, numb leg, as these symptoms/signs indicate other conditions requiring immediate medical follow-up.

Objective Data. Diagnostic tests are not necessary. Physical examination and vital signs are within normal limits. Knotted, twisted, and swollen veins, however, are visible in the legs or vulva with possible edema below the varicosities. Peripheral pulses are normal. Significant negatives include no inflammation over the varicosities, equal pedal, and femoral pulses; no firm, cordlike feel; no dependent cyanosis; no positive Homan's sign; no deep pain on palpation; no distention of veins on the dorsal side of the foot after it is elevated 45°; and no restlessness, fever, or tachycardia.

Differential Medical Diagnosis. Varicosities of legs and/or vulva exacerbated by pregnancy ruling out vascular disease (e.g., deep vein thrombosis), edema associated with gestational hypertension, physiologic edema of pregnancy, or other musculoskeletal disease.

Plan

Psychological Interventions. Explain to the client the reasons for the varicosities and inform her that the varicosities are not likely to resolve until after delivery. Advise the client to notify the health care provider if any symptoms ruled out during the history taking occur in the future.

Consider referral to a surgeon for evaluation after delivery or, optimally, after childbearing is complete.

Lifestyle Changes. Some lifestyle changes may help to relieve discomfort. Teach the client proper application of support hose and compression stockings. Have her lie flat and raise her legs to drain the veins. While her legs are elevated, have her roll the stockings on. Advise the client to do this before she rises in the morning and to leave the stockings on until she goes to bed at night.

Instruct the client to avoid crossing her legs and not to wear knee-high stockings or a constrictive band around the legs.

Explain the importance of elevating the legs as often as possible, throughout the day. Advise the client to wear comfortable shoes and to avoid prolonged standing or sitting, altering position frequently. Instruct the client in the use of perineal pads with a sanitary belt or maternity girdle to compress vulvar varicosities.

Encourage Kegel exercises, other mild exercise, and warm tub baths.

Explain to the client the need to avoid leg or vulvar injury, as hemorrhage may result.

Follow-Up. Refer a client with symptoms of pathology to a physician.

SECOND TRIMESTER

Backache

Etiology. The enlarging uterus creates a lordosis of the spine and this shift in the musculoskeletal alignment can cause back discomfort or pain. The high levels of circulating progesterone soften cartilage and cause relaxation of joints and ligaments, which can create or increase discomfort (Bickley, 2009). Increasing breast size may also contribute to upper back discomfort and nighttime backache may result from pressure on the lower back from the gravid uterus.

Subjective Data. The client reports dull, aching pain in the upper or lower back that increases as the day goes on. Ask the client to describe the location, nature, and duration of the pain, exacerbating and relieving factors, the changes in pain that occur with movement, and any radiation of pain. She may be wearing improperly fitting or high-heeled shoes. The client may have gained excessive weight, report being obese before pregnancy, have to stand or sit for long time periods, or be fatigued. She may have large breasts and/or wear an improperly fitting or poorly supporting bra. Many clients lift heavy objects (or their other children) by bending from the waist rather than bending the knees; low back muscles are strained as a result of this movement. There should be *no* history of back injury, surgery, or symptoms of UTI, GI symptoms, vaginal infection, ruptured membranes, uterine contractions, pain or numbness in buttocks, legs, or hips, or neurologic deficit.

Objective Data. No diagnostic tests are done. Physical examination and vital signs are within normal limits; however, lordosis, abnormal gait, or tenderness along paraspinous muscles may be revealed. Significant negatives include no costal vertebral angle tenderness; no pain with straight-leg raises; normal patellar, deep tendon, and plantar reflexes; and a normal neurologic exam. No urinary tract or GI symptoms (see Urinary Frequency and Incontinence), no abnormal vaginal discharge (see Leukorrhea), and no uterine contractions are detected.

Differential Medical Diagnoses. Backache ruling out uterine contractions, genital infections, UTIs, GI disease, kidney stone, pancreatitis, ulcer, musculoskeletal back disorders, including muscle sprain or strain.

Plan

Psychosocial Interventions. Explain to the client the changes underlying the backache, and inform her that it should decrease or resolve after pregnancy. Advise the client to notify the health care provider if any symptoms ruled out during the history taking occur in the future.

Medication. Acetaminophen (see Headache).

Lifestyle Changes. Encourage good posture, wearing of low-heeled shoes, and pelvic tilt exercises to ease backaches. Pelvic tilt exercises help to relieve back pain by relieving muscles often tired from the excessive lordosis of pregnancy. One such exercise can be taught to the client by having her stand against a wall, with knees slightly bent, and insert her hand behind the small of her back. Move the pelvis to roll her uterus up toward her chest and push her buttocks toward the floor. This should push her hand against the wall. Encourage her to do this while standing, walking, and sitting.

Proper body mechanics, particularly when lifting, require her to keep her back straight when lifting and to bend her knees, keeping the object close to her body; if she must hold her breath to lift an object, it is too heavy. Advise her to avoid excessive twisting, bending, and stretching. Inform the client that an exercise program encourages general fitness. Advise the client, when standing for long periods, to rest one foot on a low stool, and when sitting for long periods, to rest her feet on a low stool, to raise her knees above the hips and to sit with her back firmly against the back of the chair. While driving, she should sit straight and position the seat so that her knees are slightly bent when using the pedals. Advise the client to avoid excessive or uninterrupted walking or standing.

Uterine support with a maternity girdle or belt may offer some relief. Inform the client that a firm, supportive mattress may be helpful. Advise her to assume a lateral recumbent position while sleeping, with pillows supporting the back and legs. Sleeping in this position promotes comfort. Advise the client with upper back pain to wear a good, supportive bra. Inform the client that massage and relaxation techniques, as well as use of a heating pad (do not sleep with it), warm tub baths, or cold applications for short periods, may promote comfort.

Dietary Interventions. Advise the client to avoid gaining excessive weight.

Follow-Up. If pain does not respond to intervention, refer the client to a physical therapist. Refer any client who requires strong pain medication or who has symptoms of pathology to a physician.

Dyspnea

Etiology. As many as 70 percent of pregnant women report symptoms of dyspnea during pregnancy, beginning as early as the first or second trimester. Physiologic dyspnea of pregnancy may occur at rest or with exertion, and is thought to be caused by respiratory changes of pregnancy, such as increased respiratory drive and load, oxygenation changes, and increased sensitivity to carbon dioxide and hypoxia (Blackburn, 2007).

Subjective Data. The client reports shortness of breath, dizziness, or lightheadedness. There should be *no* history of headache, sore throat, coughing, flu-like symptoms, perioral numbness, fever, night sweats, wheezing, chest pain, palpitations, indigestion, exercise intolerance, vomiting, sweating, hyperventilation, or anxiety. Neither does the client smoke nor has a history of respiratory or cardiac problems.

Objective Data. Physical examination, particularly of the upper respiratory tract, heart, and lungs, and vital signs are within normal limits.

Differential Medical Diagnosis. Dyspnea related to pregnancy ruling out upper respiratory infection, pulmonary embolism or other pulmonary or cardiac problems, and anemia.

Plan

Psychosocial Interventions. Explain to the client that her dyspnea is related to normal physiologic changes of pregnancy and that it may improve when the fetus drops into the pelvis. Reassure her that it is not an indication that she or the fetus is receiving insufficient air. Advise the client to notify the health care provider if any symptoms ruled out during history taking occur in the future.

Lifestyle Changes. Advise the client not to wear constrictive clothing. Inform the client that sitting up very straight, raising her arms over her head while taking a breath, or elevating her head with pillows may help relieve dyspnea. Lying in the lateral recumbent position displaces the uterus off the vena cava and improves breathing efforts.

Follow-Up. Refer a client with symptoms of pathology to a physician.

Epistaxis

Etiology. The physiologic change underlying nosebleeds (epistaxis) is the high level of circulating estrogen and increases in blood volume. Elevated progesterone levels also cause the capillaries in the respiratory tract become engorged; nasal mucosa becomes hypertrophic and hyperemic and, as a result, bleeds more easily (Blackburn, 2007).

Subjective Data. The client reports that her nose bleeds easily, but she is able to control a nosebleed within 15 minutes. Nosebleeds are usually preceded by blowing the nose, picking at the nose, or overexertion. She has no history of hypertension, bleeding problems, menorrhagia, sinus symptoms, upper respiratory infection, swollen glands, fever, trauma, cocaine or chronic nasal spray use. She may report a history of nasal stuffiness, postnasal drip, or hay fever.

Objective Data. Physical examination and vital signs, particularly blood pressure, are within normal limits. The nasal mucosa may be swollen and dull red or pink, and clotted blood may be observed. Increased vascularization may be evident as may postnasal drip. Nasal polyps, growths, and evidence of cocaine use should not be observed. A CBC may be indicated as a diagnostic test (see Fatigue).

Differential Medical Diagnoses. Epistaxis of pregnancy ruling out upper respiratory infection or disorder (e.g., sinusitis, nasal polyps), hypertension, anemia, bleeding disorders, cocaine or chronic nasal spray use.

Plan

Psychosocial Interventions. Explain to the client the underlying physiologic changes that cause the problem and inform her that the condition should resolve after pregnancy. Advise the client to notify the health care provider if any symptoms ruled out during the history taking occur in the future.

Lifestyle Changes Advise the client, when nosebleeds occur, to loosen clothing around the neck, sit with her head tilted forward, pinch her nostrils for 10 to 15 minutes, and apply ice packs to her nose. Light packing of the nose with sterile gauze may help. Advise the client to avoid overheated air, excessive exertion, and nasal sprays. A cool mist vaporizer may help humidify the air. Do not use if allergic to molds or mildew.

Inform the client that the reduced air pressure at high altitudes may precipitate nosebleeds. Instruct the client to blow her nose gently, one nostril at a time and not to pick at her nose.

Follow-Up. Clients whose nosebleeds cannot be controlled within 15 minutes or who have high blood pressure or symptoms of pathology should be referred to a physician.

Leukorrhea

Etiology. Hyperplasia of vaginal glandular tissue and mucosa result in leukorrhea in the second trimester. The discharge is white or yellow, thin, and more acidic than normal vaginal discharge (Blackburn, 2007; Davidson et al., 2012).

Subjective Data. The client reports increased vaginal discharge. History should *not* include green, watery, bloody, or irritating discharge that smells foul or fishy; vaginal itching or discomfort; fever; flu-like symptoms; abdominal pain; bleeding after intercourse; dysuria or dyspareunia. Ask the client if she has multiple or new sexual partners, recently resumed sexual activity, performed douching, uses any hygiene products, had abnormal cervical cytology in the past, or recently used antibiotics.

Objective Data. Physical examination and vital signs are within normal limits; however, the pelvic exam may show increased but normal-appearing vaginal discharge. Evaluation of the increased discharge can be done using a wet mount test along with pH of the vaginal discharge to rule out candidiasis, trichomoniasis, or bacterial vaginosis as the cause of the discharge. The presence of hyphae, trichomonads, clue cells, and abnormal numbers of coccal bacteria, red cells, and white blood cells may indicate a vaginal infection (CDC, 2010c). The nitrazine and fern tests may also be used (see Urinary Frequency and Incontinence) if there is concern about possible ROM. If indicated by abnormal cervical appearance on exam, or patient history, cervical cytology may be obtained (if not already done at the first obstetrical visit) and testing for chlamydia and gonorrhea may also be indicated. Signs of vaginal infection or herpes simplex may also be noted on exam.

Differential Medical Diagnoses. Physiologic leukorrhea of pregnancy ruling out ruptured membranes, vaginitis, cervicitis, UTI, sexually transmitted diseases (STDs), and cervical dysplasia or neoplasia.

Plan

Psychosocial Interventions. Reassure the client that increased leukorrhea is normal and will decrease postpartum. Advise the client to notify the health care provider if any symptoms ruled out during the history taking occur in the future.

Lifestyle Changes. Advise the client to keep the vulva clean and dry; to avoid pantyhose and other tight or layered clothing; to wear cotton underwear and remove underwear while sleeping at night; and, if using panty liners, to use unscented/nondeodorant brands and to change them frequently. Also, advise her to avoid douching and tampon use unless otherwise instructed by the health care provider. Feminine sprays, powders, and the like should not be used.

Dietary Interventions. Some clients have recurrent candidiasis during pregnancy. Instruct these clients to avoid large amounts of carbohydrates in their diets. If an antibiotic has been prescribed, advise the client to take acidophilus (may be obtained over the counter) or consume a sugar-free yogurt or kefir-containing active cultures or other recommended probiotics.

Follow-Up. Refer all clients with abnormal Pap smears or symptoms of pathology for appropriate follow-up. Clients with symptoms of vaginitis require appropriate treatment (see Chapter 11).

Ligament Pain

Etiology. The physiologic change underlying ligament pain is the growth of the uterus, which causes ligaments in the pelvis to stretch (Davidson et al., 2012). The round ligaments attach to the uterus at the top of the fundus, extend anteriorly and inferiorly to the oviducts, through the inguinal canal, and attach at the labia majora. Other ligaments attach at the upper fundus, extend bilaterally to the upper labia majora and from the posterior cervix to the sacrum (Cunningham et al., 2010).

Subjective Data. Usually in the second trimester, the client reports sharp or dull pain on either or both sides of the uterus. The pain often starts or worsens with moving from sitting to standing, twisting, stretching, or quick movements. The history, however, does *not* include contractions, constipation, diarrhea, vomiting, vomiting blood, changes in stools, low-grade fever, anorexia, periumbilical pain, right lower abdominal or flank pain, UTI symptoms, a tender lump in the groin that tends to worsen the longer she stands, or one-sided constant pain that increases (if the pregnancy is less than 14–16 weeks). These symptoms may indicate problems other than ligament pain, and require further evaluation.

Objective Data. Physical examination and vital signs are within normal limits. Tenderness at the supravaginal insertion site or laterally to the uterus may occur on pelvic exam. Significant negatives include no contractions, cervical dilatation, effacement or softening, ROM, adnexal or abdominal masses, hernias, hyperactive or underactive bowel sounds, rebound tenderness, jaundice, or tenderness on abdominal palpation other than along the affected ligament.

Differential Medical Diagnoses. Stretching of ligaments ruling out preterm labor, ectopic pregnancy, rupture of an ovarian cyst, GI disease (e.g., appendicitis), urinary tract disease (e.g., kidney stone, infection), and inguinal hernia.

Plan

Psychosocial Interventions. Explain to the client the underlying physiologic change causing the pain and inform her that the pain will resolve after pregnancy. Advise the client to notify the health care provider if any symptoms ruled out during history taking occur in the future.

Lifestyle Changes. Advise the client to avoid sudden twisting or stretching movements. Inform her that getting out of bed by turning onto her side and pushing up with her arm will reduce abdominal muscle and back strain.

Leaning toward the affected side while standing may provide relief as well.

Fingertip massage, warm bath, or heat to the affected area may provide relief. Heating pads should not be used over 15 minutes. Advise her to avoid excessive exercise, standing, or walking. Frequent, short rest periods during the day may help.

Medication. Acetaminophen (see Headache) may provide relief when pain is severe.

Follow-Up. Refer clients with symptoms of pathology to a physician.

Muscle Cramps in the Calf, Thigh, or Buttocks

Etiology. The physiologic change underlying muscle cramps is related to changes in serum calcium and phosphate levels, and the mild respiratory alkalosis experienced during pregnancy (Blackburn, 2007).

Subjective Data. The client reports calf, thigh, or buttocks cramps that occur mostly at night or in the early morning, usually beginning in the second half of pregnancy. She may report a similar history with previous pregnancies, excessive exercise or walking, or wearing of high-heeled or poorly supporting shoes. There should be *no* history of deep vein thromboembolic disease, recent trauma or surgery, swelling, lower back pain, muscle strain, neurologic symptoms, arthritis, increased pain or limping with walking.

Objective Data. Physical examination and vital signs, particularly Homan's sign, and pulses are within normal limits. No redness, tenderness, heat, swelling, coldness, numbness, or whiteness appears in a calf or leg.

Diagnostic tests are not done unless pathology is suspected.

Differential Medical Diagnoses. Calf, thigh, or buttocks cramps ruling out thromboembolic disease, varicosities, dehydration, musculoskeletal disease (e.g., sciatica, arthritis).

Plan

Psychosocial Interventions. Explain to the client the physiologic changes that could possibly cause muscle cramping and inform her that the condition should improve after delivery. Advise the client to notify the health care provider if any symptoms ruled out during the history taking occur in the future.

Lifestyle Changes. Advise the client to avoid stretching her legs, pointing toes, walking excessively, and lying on her back and to wear low-heeled shoes.

Instruct the client in calf stretching. Have the client stand 3 feet from a wall and lean toward it to rest the lower arms against the wall, keeping her heels on the floor. Advise her that performing this exercise 10 to 12 times before going to bed may reduce cramping.

Instruct clients to flex the foot of the affected leg to relieve muscle cramping during an acute episode. Massage and warm compresses may help as well.

Dietary Interventions. Assure adequate hydration. Decreasing milk intake may be of benefit, as milk contains high levels of phosphate. Magnesium lactate or citrate supplements may be of benefit as well (Blackburn, 2007).

Follow-Up. Refer a client with symptoms of pathology to a physician.

Pica

Etiology. The physiologic change underlying pica (i.e., eating nonnutritive substances) is unknown. Pica has been ameliorated with correction of anemia in some clients (Cunningham et al., 2010).

Subjective Data. The client may report cravings for nonfood items such as ice, cornstarch, laundry starch, toothpaste, paint chips, dirt, or clay.

Pica may lead to constipation, bowel obstruction or perforation, parotid gland obstruction, anemia, lead poisoning, poor weight gain, parasitic infection, or preterm birth (Cunningham et al., 2010).

Objective Data. Physical examination, particularly of the abdomen and mouth, and vital signs are within normal limits.

Diagnostic tests include the urine dipstick, which if negative for ketones rules out ketonuria, and a CBC to rule out anemia.

Differential Medical Diagnoses. Pica is diagnosed; rule out anemia, ketonuria, obstruction, parasitic intestinal problems, poor nutrition, poor weight gain, and lead poisoning.

Plan

Psychosocial Interventions. Clients may be embarrassed by pica and reluctant to reveal their cravings to health care providers. While respecting cultural variations and remaining nonjudgmental in attitude, explain that eating nonfood items (e.g., starch) may be damaging to the mother and fetus. Advise the client to notify the health care provider if any symptoms ruled out during the history taking occur in the future.

Dietary Interventions. Evaluate the client's diet to determine its adequacy. A high iron diet with iron supplements may be needed with anemia. If pica is diagnosed, explain the need to maintain a healthy diet and that problems could occur if the craved substance either is substituting for nutritious food, blocking nutrient absorption, or is harmful to the mother or fetus.

Follow-Up. Refer a client with symptoms of pathology to a physician or a client eating an inadequate diet to a dietitian. A client without adequate financial resources may be referred to a social worker.

Syncope

Etiology. The physiologic changes underlying syncope (feeling dizzy or faint) are related to expansion of blood volume and pooling of blood in the lower extremities causing postural hypotension (Davidson et al., 2012).

Subjective Data. The client reports lightheadedness or dizziness that lasts a minute or less when she is standing, lying on her back, or changing position. She may report low or sporadic intake of calories. There should be *no* history of loss of consciousness; use of medications; exposure to toxic agents; substance abuse; sinus, hearing, or ear problems; numbness or tingling in the digits or around the mouth; nausea or vomiting; melena; heart palpitations; shortness of breath; neurological symptoms; or anxiety or depression, as these symptoms/signs may indicate other conditions that may require medical or other appropriate follow-up.

Objective Data. Physical examination and vital signs are within normal limits. *Hemoglobin* tests may reveal anemia. Blood sugar level is in normal limits.

Differential Medical Diagnosis. Syncope related to the hemodynamic changes in pregnancy ruling out orthostatic hypotension, compression of vena cava, hyperventilation, anemia, hypoglycemia, dehydration, substance abuse, exposure to a toxic agent, psychosocial stress, or central nervous system, cardiac, respiratory, endocrine, eye, ear, or sinus pathology.

Plan

Psychosocial Interventions. Explain to the client the physiologic changes causing syncope. Advise the client to notify the health care provider if any symptoms ruled out during the history taking occur in the future.

Advise the client to avoid stressful situations. Teach her to recognize hyperventilation. Encourage her to verbalize problems and explore appropriate responses.

Lifestyle Changes. Advise the client to rest in the lateral recumbent position; to change position gradually, holding on to something when rising; or to lower her head below the level of the heart if feeling faint.

To reduce blood pooling in the extremities, instruct the client to apply compression stockings before getting out of bed and to perform leg pumping exercises (flexing and extending the ankle several times).

If being in a crowd induces symptoms, advise the client to move to an open window or go outside and loosen or remove layers of clothing.

Dietary Interventions. Advise the client to eat frequent small meals throughout the day and to maintain adequate protein intake. Assess her diet for adequate calorie and fluid intake and distribution.

Follow-Up. Refer a client with symptoms of pathology to a physician.

THIRD TRIMESTER

Braxton-Hicks Contractions

Etiology. As early as 6 weeks' gestation, the uterus begins painless, irregular contractions known as Braxton-Hicks contractions. The contractions are not strong enough to effect dilation of the cervix, but may be mistaken for labor by the client (Varney et al., 2004).

Subjective Data. The client may report a sudden tightening or pressure in the uterus, without the sensation of building, which lasts from 30 seconds to 2 minutes. The contractions may decrease with position change or emptying of the bladder. History does *not* include regular contractions, vaginal bleeding, bloody show, leaking or ROM, symptoms of UTI, constipation, diarrhea, fever, flu-like symptoms, or cramping, as these symptoms/signs may indicate other conditions requiring medical follow-up. Increased vaginal discharge may signal cervical dilation.

Objective Data. Physical examination and vital signs are within normal limits. The pelvic exam, particularly cervical dilation, effacement, and station, does not demonstrate change over the course of a 1- to 2-hour period. No bleeding from the cervical os or pooling of amniotic fluid is evident. Vaginal discharge is negative for ferning and nitrazine demonstrates a pH of 3 to 3.5. The abdominal exam does not reveal regular contractions, rigid, tender uterus, or suprapubic tenderness. Bowel sounds are normal. The fetus should be normally active.

Differential Medical Diagnoses. Braxton-Hicks contractions ruling out preterm labor, premature ROM, UTI, pyelonephritis, gastroenteritis, constipation, and normal fetal activity.

Plan

Psychosocial Interventions. Reassure the client that Braxton-Hicks contractions are normal. Teach the client to differentiate between Braxton-Hicks and labor contractions. Labor contractions grow longer, stronger, and closer together and occur at regular intervals. Often, activity strengthens labor contractions, but decreases Braxton-Hicks contractions. Labor is differentiated from Braxton-Hicks contractions by the presence of cervical changes.

Advise the client to notify the health care provider if any symptoms ruled out during the history taking occur in the future.

Lifestyle Changes. Advise the client to empty her bladder frequently, though she must stay well hydrated. Inform her that resting in a lateral recumbent position, walking, or exercising lightly may relieve contractions.

Lamaze breathing may ease the discomfort of contractions. Teach the client to breathe slowly and deeply at about half her normal rate. Advise the client to contact the health care provider if contractions become strong or different in character from previous contractions.

Follow-Up. Refer a client with possible preterm labor, premature ROM, or symptoms of pathology to a physician.

Discomfort in the Upper Extremities

Etiology. Postural changes caused by the enlarging breasts may cause a flexion of the neck and slumping shoulders. This plus the retention of fluids can cause aching, numbness, and weakness of the upper extremities. Carpal tunnel syndrome results from swelling in the wrists, causing numbness, tingling, weakness, and pain in the first through third digits (Blackburn, 2007; Davidson et al., 2012).

Subjective Data. The client may report pain, numbness, weakness, or tingling in the upper arms or hands. History does not include cardiac symptoms; symptoms of hyperventilation (numbness around mouth with nausea or sweating); loss of sensation in the extremities; loss of ability to grip; history of trauma to neck, shoulder, arm, or wrist; recent chest trauma or surgery; or arthritis. She may report a past history of carpal tunnel syndrome.

Objective Data. The fingers may exhibit decreased sensation during neurological testing. The hands may be edematous. Pain produced by forced flexion at wrist or tapping on the carpal tunnel indicates carpal tunnel syndrome. Otherwise, the physical examination and vital signs are within normal limits.

Differential Medical Diagnoses. Pain, numbness, tingling, or weakness in the upper extremities ruling out carpal tunnel syndrome, musculoskeletal disease (e.g., arthritis), cardiac problems, or psychosocial problems causing hyperventilation.

Plan

Psychosocial Interventions. Assure the client that the discomfort is related to pregnancy and will resolve after the pregnancy is over.

Lifestyle Changes. Wearing a wrist splint especially to bed at night to prevent sleeping on flexed wrists. During the day, if the hands are affected, raise hands above the head and pump the fists. At night, put the hands over the side of the bed and shake. Avoid aggravating movements, especially fine motor movements (e.g., typing, writing).

Advise wearing a well-supporting bra. Avoid slumping.

Dietary Interventions. See Edema for interventions to reduce swelling.

Follow-Up. Refer any client with symptoms of pathology to a physician. Any client with recurrent hyperventilation should be referred for counseling.

Edema

Etiology. The physiologic change underlying edema is increased capillary permeability caused by elevated hormone levels, as well as decreased plasma colloid osmotic pressure and increased femoral venous pressure. Sodium and water are retained. Thirst increases. Plasma osmolarity is lowered and the osmoreceptors for vasopressin are suppressed. Edema occurs most often in dependent areas. Moreover, the pressure of the gravid uterus slows down venous return to the heart. Consequently, more fluid passes into intracellular spaces (Blackburn, 2007; Cunningham et al., 2010).

Subjective Data. The client reports mild edema in her hands and feet that may worsen as the day progresses. Warm weather or prolonged sitting or standing may increase edema. It should improve by morning. Advise the client not to wear constrictive bands on her legs.

The history does *not* include numbness, loss of sensation or muscle strength in the fingers of either or both hands. Edema is dependent and improves after a night's sleep. There is *no* report or evidence of facial edema, edema in one extremity, especially one leg, confusion, headache, visual changes, fatigue, nausea, vomiting, dyspnea, hives, upper abdominal pain, decreased fetal movement, decreased urine output, or rapid weight gain (i.e., more than 2 lb per week).

Objective Data. Physical examination, particularly of the heart, lungs, extremities, and abdomen, and vital signs are within normal limits. Physiologic edema in pregnancy is not associated with significant proteinuria, nor with blood pressure elevation or quick or significant weight gain. Physiologic edema of the extremities is 0 (no swelling) to +1 (after pressing skin for 5 seconds, the indentation is slight and the contour normal). Deep tendon reflexes are also normal. Jaundice, upper abdominal pain, or headache are not noted.

The urine dipstick for protein should be no greater than a trace.

Differential Medical Diagnoses. Physiologic edema of pregnancy ruling out gestational hypertension; preeclampsia, renal, liver, cardiac, or vascular disease; local trauma or infection to extremities; allergic reaction; carpal tunnel syndrome.

Plan

Psychosocial Interventions. Reassure the client that edema in pregnancy is normal and will resolve after pregnancy. Advise the client to notify the health care provider if any symptoms ruled out during the history taking occur in the future.

Lifestyle Changes. Advise the client to lie in a lateral recumbent position for 1 to 2 hours twice a day and to sleep in that position at night. Also advise her to avoid long periods of sitting or standing. If a client must sit for extended periods, she should also stand—preferably walk—10 minutes every 1 to 2 hours. Regular aerobic exercise may improve blood flow to legs.

Instruct the client not to wear constrictive bands on the legs and arms; however, she should wear maternity support pantyhose.

Inform the client that raising arms and legs above the level of the heart for short periods and pumping hands and feet may decrease edema. Advise her not to curl her hands under her head or pillow at night if they are swollen or numb. Use of wrist supports may decrease swelling and numbness.

Dietary Interventions. Food should be salted to taste; there is no need to restrict salt, though excessive amounts should be avoided. Advise the client to drink 8 to 10 glasses of fluid a day, 4 to 6 of which should be water (reducing fluids does not reduce edema) (Blackburn, 2007; Davidson et al., 2012).

Follow-Up. Consult with a physician regarding a client with symptoms of preeclampsia or with symptoms of pathology. A dietitian may assist with special dietary needs.

Heartburn

Etiology. The physiologic changes underlying heartburn are pressure on the stomach and diaphragm from the growing uterus, decreased GI tone, and esophageal sphincter relaxation (Blackburn, 2007).

Subjective Data. The client reports heartburn and bloating. The client may be under stress, depressed, swallowing air, or overweight. History does *not* include chest pain; shortness of breath; exercise intolerance; palpitations; sweating; anxiety; upper abdominal pain, especially after heavy, fatty, or spicy meals; fatty, foul-smelling stools; anorexia; nausea, diarrhea, constipation, or vomiting; pain in right shoulder, fever, or flu-like symptoms, as these symptoms/signs may indicate other conditions requiring medical follow-up.

Objective Data. No diagnostic tests are necessary. Physical examination, particularly of the heart and abdomen, and vital signs are within normal limits.

Differential Medical Diagnoses. Heartburn related to pregnancy ruling out cardiac problems, GI disease (e.g., cholelithiasis, irritable bowel syndrome), and preeclampsia or HELLP syndrome.

Plan

Psychosocial Interventions. Reassure the client that heartburn is common in pregnancy and should improve or disappear after delivery. Advise the client to notify the health care provider if any symptoms ruled out during history taking occur in the future.

Medication. Calcium carbonate is indicated for hyperacidity. One to two tablets are recommended every hour, as needed (see Nutrition). Abdominal bloating may occur in some clients. Inform the client that calcium carbonate is an additional source of calcium.

- Histamine 2-receptor agonists—cimetidine (Tagamet), famotidine (Pepcid), nizatidine (Axid), ranitidine (Zantac) (Deglin et al., 2011; Manns-James, 2011)
  - *Administration:* Take one tablet orally up to twice daily (according to directions on package) (200 mg cimetidine, 40 mg famotidine, 300 mg nizatidine, or 75 mg of rantidine).
  - *Side effects and adverse reactions:* Famotidine, nizatidine, and ranitidine may cause confusion.
  - *Contraindications:* Hypersensitivity.
  - *Anticipated outcomes on evaluation:* Relief of heartburn.
  - *Client teaching and counseling:* Contact the health care provider with persistent abdominal pain, hemoptysis, or difficulty swallowing. Do not take for longer than 2 weeks without contacting health care provider. May cause drowsiness.
  - *FDA pregnancy category:* B.

Lifestyle Changes. Advise the client not to lie down, bend, or stoop for 2 hours after eating. Inform her that for sleeping, the head of the bed can be elevated 6 inches. Instruct the client not to wear restrictive clothing around the abdomen or waist.

Teach the client to avoid hyperventilation and swallowing of air, which may aggravate dyspepsia.

Advise the client to stop smoking.

Dietary Interventions. Advise the client to avoid hot, spicy, fatty, gas-forming, and acidic foods such as tomatoes and citrus; caffeine; chocolate; and alcohol. Instruct her to eat small, frequent meals and to chew slowly and thoroughly, avoiding lying down for 1 to 3 hours after eating. Inform her that sipping water, milk, hot tea, or a tablespoonful of heavy cream, yogurt, or half-and-half, or chewing gum may help heartburn (Blackburn, 2007).

Follow-Up. Refer any client with symptoms of pathology to a physician.

Insomnia

Etiology. Insomnia in pregnancy may be caused by stress and anxiety or by discomfort in pregnancy or fetal movement (Varney et al., 2004).

Subjective Data. The client may report difficulty sleeping due to generalized discomfort, fetal movements, urinary frequency, vivid dreams, increased stress, or emotional problems.

Objective Data. Physical examination and vital signs are within normal limits with a normal affect and normal neurological exam.

Differential Medical Diagnoses. Insomnia related to pregnancy ruling out physical or emotional disorders (e.g., depression, abuse).

Plan

Psychosocial Interventions. Suggest ways to increase comfort and reduce insomnia (e.g., placing pillows behind her back, raising the head of the bed up on blocks).

- Establishing a regular sleep time and routine may induce sleep.
- Demonstrate exercises that consume less energy (isometric instead of aerobic exercises). Have the client avoid exercise during the 2 hours prior to sleep.
- Recommend exercise for sedentary clients (see Exercise, later in this chapter).
- Relaxation techniques may help.
- Measures to reduce leg cramps may decrease their occurrence (see Muscle Cramps in the Calf, Thigh, or Buttocks).

Dietary Interventions. Advise client to avoid caffeine after midday and heavy meals at the end of the day. Suggest that warm milk may induce sleep. Encourage higher fluid intake earlier in the day, decreasing in the evening. Avoiding high-sugar diets may be helpful.

Follow-Up. Refer the client to a physician if symptoms of pathology are evident. When severe psychosocial stress, anxiety, or depression is noted, referral to a mental health care provider is appropriate.

Joint Pain/Ache

Etiology. The physiologic changes underlying joint discomfort are hormonal. Increased levels of estrogen and relaxin affect collagen synthesis and collagen fibers, resulting in increased mobility of joints, and also increasing the risk for pain and injury to muscles and ligaments. Joint pain may also result from increasing maternal weight, especially in weight bearing areas such as the hip and knee (Blackburn, 2007).

Subjective Data. The client reports pain in the pelvis or hip joints. Sciatic nerve pain is felt in the buttocks and down the back or side of the affected leg. It can be excruciating. Pain often increases after fetal engagement. The history does *not* include contractions; symptoms of UTI; swelling, stiffness, or redness in the joints; pain radiating down legs; intermittent claudication; or fever, abnormally cold and/or white digits, and other flu-like symptoms, as these symptoms/signs indicate other conditions requiring medical follow-up. There is no history of tick bites or being in a wooded area where ticks could bite.

Objective Data. Physical examination, pulses, and vital signs, particularly the joints and musculoskeletal system, are within normal limits; however, tenderness may be noted when palpating the symphysis pubis. There are no signs of labor.

Differential Medical Diagnoses. Joint pain ruling out UTI, contractions, Lyme disease, or other rheumatic, vascular, or joint diseases.

Plan

Psychosocial Interventions. Reassure the client that the discomfort is limited to pregnancy. Advise her to notify the health care provider if any symptoms ruled out during the history taking occur in the future.

Medication. Acetaminophen may be taken (see Headache).

Lifestyle Changes. Advise the client to avoid excessive walking, high-heeled shoes, jarring movements, high-impact activities, or other movements that are found to cause pain. Comfort measures may include applying a heating pad, warm moist heat, or cold packs to the painful area, reclining on the opposite side, and maintaining good posture. Instruct the client that she may place pillows between the thighs and underneath her abdomen to support and align the back while sleeping.

Follow-Up. Refer any client with symptoms of pathology to a physician.

ADOLESCENT PREGNANCY

Adolescent pregnancy is defined as pregnancy occurring between the age of menarche and 19 years of age, but it also can be viewed in relation to emotional maturity and financial independence. Adolescents have among the highest rates of unintended pregnancy, though overall national trends show the rates of adolescent pregnancy, birth, and abortion are all declining (Finer & Henshaw, 2006; Kost, Henshaw, & Carlin, 2010). Despite this decline, the rate of adolescent pregnancy in the United States remains high, and the implications for adolescent mothers and for the long-term impacts and challenges on society are significant (CDC, 2011c). Perinatal morbidity and mortality are significantly higher in adolescent pregnancy, when compared with pregnancies of adult women. Adolescent parenting has devastating effects on long-term educational achievement, earnings, reliance on public assistance, adolescent parenting rates, and incarceration rates for the offspring of these pregnancies (ACOG, 2007f; CDC, 2011c). Consistent with normal adolescent development is a lack of impulse control, fantastic thinking, feelings of invincibility, and limited appreciation for long-term implications of her actions, all of which contribute to the incidence of unintended adolescent pregnancy (Davidson et al., 2012). Many strategies exist in efforts to reduce rates of adolescent sexual experimentation, increase use of contraception by sexually active teens, and reduce the impact of adolescent pregnancy on long-term outcomes (ACOG, 2007f).

OBJECTIVE DATA

A physical exam will reveal changes similar to those seen during an adult physical exam, particularly during the breast, abdominal, and pelvic evaluations. However, the provider should be mindful that this exam may be the client's first experience having a pelvic exam and breast exam, and sensitivity, explanation, and adequate time should be provided accordingly. Evaluate Tanner staging (see Chapter 4), as young adolescents may be physically immature, which would significantly impact growth and development in pregnancy. Evaluate for psychosocial concerns more common in pregnant adolescents, such as eating disorders, substance use, and intimate partner violence or histories of child maltreatment and abuse (Klein & The Committee on Adolescence, 2005). Current guidelines for beginning cervical cytology screening should be followed (see Chapter 5), but screening for STIs is an essential component of the physical exam.

PLAN

Pregnant adolescents are at increased risk of having low birth weight infants and preterm births, as well as inadequate weight gain, preeclampsia, anemia, and STIs (CDC, 2011c; Klein & The Committee on Adolescence, 2005). Moreover, they are at increased risk for cesarean births. Cephalopelvic disproportion may result from immature skeletal development of the pelvis, especially in pregnant teens under the age of 16 (Rasheed, Abdelmonem, & Amin, 2011). It remains the primary goal of the health care provider to promote the best possible pregnancy outcome through client evaluation and education. Therefore, focus education on general health maintenance and how pregnancy needs will change health status. The cognitive abilities of adolescents vary, however, as do their abilities to assimilate information. Foster behaviors that will promote independence in adolescent development.

Encourage the client to maintain peer interactions and continue to work toward educational goals. Help her to clarify the father's role, make use of family support systems, and set realistic goals. Assess the client's cognitive abilities (e.g., concrete versus abstract). Encourage behaviors that foster parenting skills such as attending parenting classes, and demonstration of what has been learned. Be aware of the increased rate of suicide among adolescents, the risk of substance abuse, and the need to promote a nonjudgmental atmosphere in which the client may express views about the pregnancy (CDC, 2010d).

Health care providers need to assess their own value system, particularly to avoid stereotyping. The foundation for a trusting relationship is based on mutual acceptance, caring, and a nonjudgmental approach. Assisting the client to achieve the developmental tasks of adolescence, such as financial, emotional, and physical independence, is the underlying task for the health provider.

ANTICIPATORY GUIDANCE

Medication

Stress the importance of not using medication without first discussing with a health care provider. Stress the importance of not consuming chemical substances during pregnancy without knowledge or direction of a health care provider.

Diet and Exercise

The adolescent diet is notoriously inadequate (CDC, 2010d). The greatest nutritional risk is to adolescents within 4 years of menarche, due to physiologic immaturity (Davidson et al., 2012). Because of the increased risk for inadequate nutrition, it is imperative to stress normal, adequate nutrition and the value of daily prenatal vitamins and iron supplementation. Educate the client on what constitutes appropriate nutritional choices. The physical changes of pregnancy and the growing fetus place the adolescent at risk for altered body image and eating disorders. Careful periodic assessment during prenatal care will aid the health care provider in early detection of inadequate nutrition.

Older adolescents may follow the adult recommendation of an additional 300 kcal per day of dietary intake, but those aged 14 and younger will require an additional 500 kcal per day. Pregnant adolescents will universally require iron supplementation due to the increased needs of pregnancy and the typically iron-poor nature of the adolescent diet. The recommendation for calcium intake for adolescents does not increase above the 1,300 mg per day recommended for all (nonpregnant) adolescents. Careful attention to dietary intake is indicated, but a supplement may be required to achieve this level of intake (Bloom & Escuro, 2008; Davidson et al., 2012). Weight gain recommendations are the same as for pregnant adults, unless the adolescent is under age 16 or within 2 years of menarche, in which case they are recommended to gain at the upper limits of the weight gain recommendations for their BMI category (see Nutrition, later in this chapter) (Rasmussen & Yaktine, 2009). Encourage a balanced diet from the food pyramid and limiting nonnutritious foods and snacks. Instruction in good nutrition is related to maternal/fetal growth needs and should reinforce the need for adherence on the part of the adolescent mother. Advise the client to avoid contact sports but maintain physical activity by walking, swimming, and participating in prenatal exercise classes.

Smoking

Although the harmful effects of smoking cigarettes are well documented, adolescents continue to smoke at alarming rates (CDC, 2010d). Cigarette smoking is highly correlated to early sexual activity; it is often seen as a display of adult behavior, rebellion, or peer pressure (Hansen et al., 2010). (See Tobacco, later in this chapter, for specific suggestions on counseling pregnant women who smoke.)

Education

Assist the client in assessing options for continuing education during pregnancy. Alternatives to traditional schooling may include general equivalency diploma, home tutoring, and schools with special programs for pregnant adolescents. Be aware that with some of these options, peer interaction may be decreased.

Finances

Financial concerns are heightened if education is interrupted as a result of pregnancy. Assist clients with negotiating the complexities of health insurance coverage and job benefits, if applicable. Refer for public assistance programs such as WIC or Aid to Dependent Children, if eligible.

Family Planning

Frequent conception is common with adolescent mothers; between 28 and 63 percent conceive again within 18 months, and 20 to 37 percent give birth again within 24 months (Raneri & Wiemann, 2007). Short- and long-term disadvantages and risks associated with adolescent pregnancy are increased with repeat pregnancy (Raneri & Wiemann, 2007). Strongly encourage the client to choose a reliable method prior to completion of pregnancy, emphasizing options and repeating counseling at various times throughout prenatal care. Explore the client's options for contraception, sexual responsibility, and risk behaviors for STD.

FOLLOW-UP

Adolescent mothers are at higher risk for a wide array of physical, psychosocial, obstetric, parental, and socioeconomic disadvantages and complications. Vigilance and close surveillance and support throughout pregnancy are warranted. In addition, adolescent clients may benefit from referrals to a nutritionist and social services provider, as appropriate and available at a given institution. A follow-up STI screen in the third trimester is recommended as well.

DELAYED PREGNANCY

Increasing numbers of women in the United States are delaying or extending their childbearing years through their late 30s and into their 40s. Advances in contraceptive techniques have enabled greater freedom to time the birth of the first child. An additional reason for delayed childbearing may be the steady increase in late or second marriages. Moreover, for women who previously suffered from infertility, the prospect of bearing a child has improved with advances in reproductive technology.

Women age 35 or older at the time of delivery are considered women of advanced maternal age (AMA). Extensive literature in medicine and genetics has debated whether any significant risks are associated with childbearing after age 35. In general, older gravidas are more likely to experience complications with pregnancy and these complications appear to increase with advancing age—especially after 40 years old. AMA is associated with risks such as infertility, spontaneous abortion, fetal aneuploidy, multiple gestation, preterm birth, low birth weight, intrauterine fetal demise, gestational diabetes, preeclampsia, placenta previa, cesarean delivery, and neonatal intensive care unit admissions (Cunningham et al., 2010; Fretts & Duru, 2008; Shrim et al., 2010; Yogev et al., 2010). However, many of these risks are also related to other factors such as preexisting medical conditions like hypertension and diabetes. With proper control of underlying medical conditions and optimal prenatal care, most women of AMA can have successful pregnancy outcomes.

HISTORY AND PHYSICAL EXAMINATION

For women whose pregnancy occurs later in life, the history and physical examination are the same as for other pregnant clients. Devote particular attention to nutritional and immunization status; reproductive, medical, occupational, and social histories; chemical substance use; and genetic concerns. Offer the client referral for genetic counseling and a review of available genetic testing. Identify any occupational hazards.

DIAGNOSTIC TESTS AND METHODS

The minimum standard tests are recommended; medical conditions may require additional individual assessment. The ACOG (2007e) recommends that all pregnant women, regardless of age, be offered the option of noninvasive or invasive genetic testing.

PLAN

There is no conclusive agreement or definitive recommendations regarding antenatal surveillance based solely on the risk factor of maternal age. Furthermore, antenatal testing has not demonstrated the ability to consistently and significantly predict or prevent those risks related to AMA (Fretts & Duru, 2008). Therefore, prenatal care, anticipatory guidance, and guidelines for caring for older pregnant women are not necessarily different than the routine, individualized care offered to all adult pregnant women. Decision making related to screenings, testing, or interventions is determined by the totality of the clinical picture.

Clinicians are responsible for helping put medical risks into perspective for all pregnant women. Fair, balanced, and evidenced-based counseling is key to helping women of AMA navigate through the information related to age-related risks and making decisions related to testing and antenatal surveillance (Fretts & Duru, 2008; Jordan & Murphy, 2009). Make referrals where appropriate and encourage the client to explore educational resources within the community (e.g., prenatal classes). Tailor follow-up visits to pertinent medical findings and individual needs.

NONTRADITIONAL FAMILIES

The American family has made several remarkable changes in the past 25 years. Today's families include the typical nuclear family and nontraditional families including one-parent households, same-sex parents, single-by-choice parents, unmarried heterosexual couples living together, and those choosing to remain childfree. These patterns are the result of profound social and demographic changes in the United States and are becoming increasingly accepted. The contraceptive revolution of the 1960s greatly influenced family structure by changing the role of women. Selective fertility has played a fundamental role in economic shifts within households. Providers have a responsibility in providing individualized care to adapt to these changes and offer all families a welcoming and nonjudgmental atmosphere where the unique needs and situation of each woman and her family are addressed.

ANTICIPATORY GUIDANCE DURING PREGNANCY

The issues of concern to pregnant women involve safety, comfort, and uncertainty about what to expect during pregnancy, labor, and delivery.

ACCIDENTS OR BLOWS TO THE ABDOMEN

Reassure the client that the amniotic fluid and abdominal structure protect the fetus, although a very serious blow to the abdomen could cause injury (e.g., hitting the steering wheel during an auto accident). Recommend that she contact a health care provider if an abdominal blow should occur. Danger signs include vaginal bleeding; leaking fluid; new, persistent, or severe abdominal pain; uterine contractions; or decreased or no fetal movements. Abusive relationships may intensify during pregnancy. If a woman is in a potentially abusive relationship, abuse may begin once she is pregnant. Refer her to a mental health care provider if abuse is suspected (see Chapter 23).

BATHING

Advise the client that she may take warm (not hot) tub baths if ruptured membranes are not suspected and if she takes safety precautions of keeping the temperature below 100°F and is careful to watch for syncope, overheating, and dehydration. Late in pregnancy, a woman may need help rising out of a low tub.

CHEMICAL USE AND SAFETY

Tobacco

Smoking increases the risk of infertility, spontaneous abortion, preterm labor and delivery, IUGR, premature ROM, placenta previa, placental abruption, low birth weight infant, and perinatal death (ACOG, Committee of Obstetric Practice, 2010; CDC, 2011b). In addition, the risk for sudden infant death syndrome (SIDS) is increased, as is the incidence of childhood respiratory infections (CDC, 2011b). Although the exact mechanisms for the negative effects associated with smoking are unclear, impaired fetal gas exchange, decreased placental blood flow, and the potentially toxic effects of nicotine and other substances all likely play a role in impairing fetal growth and effecting pregnancy outcomes (Cunningham et al., 2010). Smoking cessation at any point in pregnancy is beneficial, but cessation prior to the start of the third trimester demonstrates greatest benefit in neonatal outcomes. Careful attention is needed in women who have quit smoking during pregnancy to help them continue their commitment to abstinence after delivery (Fiore et al., 2008).

Targeted psychosocial smoking cessation interventions and motivational interviewing techniques have demonstrated effectiveness in pregnant women. One intervention includes using the 5 As of *a*sking about smoking status; *a*dvising women who smoke to stop; *a*ssessing each woman's willingness to quit in the next month; *a*ssisting those individuals who express a willingness to quit by providing materials and referrals for cessation; and *a*rranging follow-up visits to help women stop smoking (ACOG, Committee of Obstetric Practice, 2010; Fiore et al., 2008).

Because of either lack of evidence or conflicting evidence related to the safety and efficacy of use of nicotine replacement products or other medications (such as bupropion or varenicline) during pregnancy, these medications should be used only if other methods have failed, the woman is extremely motivated to quit smoking, and the risks of smoking outweigh the risk of medications (ACOG, Committee of Obstetric Practice, 2010; Fiore et al., 2008).

Alcohol

Currently, the best advice for a pregnant woman is complete abstinence from alcohol from preconception throughout pregnancy (CDC, 2010a). This recommendation is based in large part on the fact that there is no known safe level of alcohol use in pregnancy and that even as little as one drink per week during pregnancy has been associated with neurodevelopmental effects in children (March of Dimes, 2008). Of greatest concern is fetal alcohol syndrome (FAS), which is part of a range of disorders associated with alcohol use in pregnancy termed fetal alcohol spectrum disorders. As one of the most common causes of mental retardation, FAS is an entirely preventable birth defect (Cunningham et al., 2010).

Characteristics of FAS include craniofacial dysmorphia, IUGR, microcephaly, and congenital anomalies such as limb abnormalities and cardiac defects. Long-term sequelae include postnatal growth restriction, attention deficits, behavioral disorders, delayed reaction time, and poor scholastic performance. Other adverse outcomes of alcohol usage in pregnancy include intrauterine fetal demise and alcohol-related birth defects involving the heart, liver, kidneys, musculoskeletal system, and/or face and alcohol-related neurodevelopmental disorders involving learning disabilities, memory problems, attention deficits, speech/language delays, and/or psychological disorders (Cunningham et al., 2010; March of Dimes, 2008).

Although most women are often able to quit alcohol use in pregnancy, research indicates that many women use alcohol before they know they are pregnant and are often more likely to continue drinking in pregnancy when they have heavy use pre-pregnancy or are also smoking (Harrison & Sidebottom, 2009). This emphasizes the need for regular screening related to alcohol, smoking, and drug use as a part of routine care and providing interventions to promote cessation in order to maximize preconception health.

Artificial Sweeteners

Moderate consumption of foods or drinks containing sweeteners such as acesulfame potassium, aspartame, saccharin, sucralose, neotame, and stevia that are classified by the FDA as "generally recognized as safe" are considered safe in pregnancy (ADA, 2008; Widen & Siega-Riz, 2010). Women with phenylketonuria should be cautioned to avoid aspartame use (Gabbe et al., 2007).

Caffeine

Though caffeine has not been shown to be teratogenic, high consumption of caffeine may increase risk of spontaneous abortion (Weng, Odouli, & Li, 2008). The ADA (2008) recommends limitation of caffeine to no greater than 300 mg daily during pregnancy. Inform the client of caffeine sources: coffee, tea, chocolate, some sodas, energy drinks, and some over-the-counter pain and cold medications. Explain the physical effects of caffeine withdrawal (e.g., lethargy, irritability, headache) and their usual duration (3–4 days). Mixing decaffeinated and caffeinated products in increasing ratios to wean from caffeine use may reduce these effects.

Illegal Drugs

The risks of using illegal drugs include fetal addiction, prematurity, low birth weight, placental abruption, stillbirth, and hepatitis B and HIV infection. Advise clients to stop using drugs. Refer clients using illegal drugs to a drug detoxification center specializing in the needs of pregnant women or to a mental health care provider whose expertise is drug abuse see Chapter 20. Effects of specific drugs are covered here.

Cocaine. Like many illicit drugs, determining the fetal effects associated with cocaine is difficult due to multiple confounding variables present with women who use cocaine in pregnancy (i.e., smoking, alcohol use, other drug use, and multiple psychosocial and socioeconomic stressors). However, cocaine use in pregnancy has been associated with increased risk for spontaneous abortion, placental abruption, intrauterine fetal demise, preterm labor and birth, IUGR, congenital anomalies, and complications of the neonatal course (Creasy et al., 2009; Gabbe et al., 2007).

Lysergic Acid Diethylamide (LSD). Usage of LSD in pregnancy is not known to be a teratogen or to increase perinatal morbidity or mortality. Long-term effects on development, however, are not known (Cunningham et al., 2010).

Opiates/Narcotics. Though not teratogenic alone, opiates such as heroin may induce intense addiction in both mother and neonate. Neonatal withdrawal symptoms can occur and an increased incidence of SIDS has been found among these infants. Methadone substitution has been successful during pregnancy but must be used in a closely supervised treatment program. Infants of mothers using methadone in pregnancy also frequently experience withdrawal symptoms that can last up to 3 weeks (Cunningham et al., 2010). Narcotic antagonists, such as Narcan® (naloxone), Nubaine® (nalbuphine), and Stadol® (butorphanol) (frequently given in labor) can precipitate withdrawal symptoms in women with a history of opiate use in pregnancy.

Methamphetamines. Methamphetamine use has significantly increased in the United States over the last 30 years. Although the teratogenicity of methamphetamines is not well established, the risk for teratogenic effects of methamphetamines can depend on the substances used to manufacture the product. Effects such as small for gestational age and low birth weight are consistently reported in infants exposed to methamphetamine in utero (ACOG, Committee of Obstetric Practice, 2011).

Marijuana. Marijuana is the most commonly used illicit drug in pregnancy, and it is recommended that women abstain from using it. However, marijuana is not known to be teratogenic (Cunningham et al., 2010). Usage of marijuana during pregnancy has been associated with signs of neurologic impairment in neonates such as tremors, high pitched cries, and exaggerated startle responses, as well as behavioral and developmental delays in children (Gabbe et al., 2007).

Organic Solvents/AHC. These are present in paints, glue, enamel, varnish, lacquer, and resins. They are easily absorbed through the skin, lungs, and GI tract, and easily cross the placenta. Exposure may occur in the workplace or be recreational ("huffing" or "sniffing"). Toluene is the most popular AHC for this purpose. Usage during pregnancy may lead to IUGR, microcephaly, hydrocephaly, limb anomalies, and craniofacial dysmorphia similar to FAS (Cunningham et al., 2010).

Over-the-Counter Medications/ Vitamins/Herbs

Health care providers do recommend specific over-the-counter medications for minor complaints, such as headaches. Some medications are not advised during pregnancy and not all herbs have been well studied. Advise the client not to take any medication/vitamin/herb without first consulting a health care provider. Also advise her that megadoses of vitamins (e.g., vitamins A and D) could harm both her and the fetus; she should take only a vitamin/mineral supplement advised by a health care provider.

Prescription Drugs

Some prescription drugs are harmful to the fetus. Advise the client to report all medications she is taking to her health care provider for evaluation prior to use (see Table 19–10).

Environmental Exposure

Women of childbearing age comprise a significant proportion of the U.S. workforce. Women are exposed to chemicals and infectious agents, demanding labor, and often less than ideal working conditions. *Teratogens* are substances or disorders with the potential to alter the fetus permanently in form or function. Often the effect is dose related; the effect is greatest during fetal organogenesis. In order to be teratogenic, a substance must cross the placenta in high enough doses to expose the fetus at a critical stage of development (Cunningham et al., 2010). The best advice is to avoid chemical exposure before and during pregnancy, particularly in the first trimester when organogenesis is occurring.

The client can be exposed to various chemicals in her work setting, home, or other environments. To reduce exposure when using chemicals (e.g., household cleaning items), the client should ensure that work areas are well ventilated and wear protective gloves. Advise the client to avoid inhaling chemical fumes, particularly from paint or turpentine, and to wash off any chemicals on the skin immediately. Also advise her if she is in doubt about the toxicity of a chemical to which she has been exposed, she should notify a health care provider, call a poison control center, or go to an emergency room.

Knowledge about teratogens is growing. To obtain the most current information, several hotlines are available.

- Reproductive Toxicology Center is a subscription service available to professionals (http://www.reprotox.org)
- National Pesticide Information Center (http://npic.orst.edu/)
- Occupational Safety and Health Administration (http://www.osha.gov/SLTC/reproductivehazards)
- Material Safety Data Sheets (MSDSs) are required to be available whenever chemicals are used in the workplace. Pregnancy issues are addressed.

Lead Poisoning

Elevated lead levels in pregnancy can have significant repercussions for the developing fetus. Research continues into exact levels of critical concern, and specific health effects, but indications are that effects may include poor fetal growth and developmental delays, and potential impacts on sexual maturation and future fertility on female fetuses. Potential sources of exposure include renovation on homes built before 1978, working in construction or other industrial occupations where exposure to lead may occur, traditional lead glazed pottery, and certain alternative remedies and imported foods and cosmetics (Ettinger, Wengrovitz, Portier, & Brown, 2010). Pregnant women who practice pica, and who are recent immigrants to the United States are also considered to be at elevated risk for lead exposure. Advise the client to avoid all potential sources of lead exposure and to discuss with her health care provider her concerns.

CHILDBIRTH EDUCATION METHODS

Pregnant women may be confronted with many alternatives for childbirth preparation classes. Many classes adapt parts of various childbirth education philosophies and often differ in specific or unique techniques to facilitate relaxation during labor and birth (i.e., Lamaze, hypnobirthing). Classes usually comprise five to six pairs, employ varied media to present materials, permit discussion, and ultimately prepare the client and her partner or support person for many different experiences during labor and delivery, including natural childbirth, use of pain medication, vaginal and surgical modes of delivery, and so on (Walker & Worrell, 2008). In counseling the client regarding the many approaches to childbirth education, it is paramount to consider her readiness to learn, knowledge base, attitudes and fears about pregnancy, and the support systems available to her. The organization International Childbirth Education Association (http://www.icea.org) can help women find childbirth educators and classes in their area.

CIRCUMCISION

AAP (1999) states that although there is some evidence of health benefits of circumcision, the evidence is not strong enough to recommend the procedure routinely. Risks of circumcision include bleeding, infection, and isolated reports of rare but serious procedural complications. Potential benefits include decreased incidence of UTI, penile cancer, and a possible association with reduction of risk for HIV and syphilis. Parents are encouraged to consider religious, cultural, and ethnic traditions in their decision. Informed consent is essential.

CONCERN FOR BABY

Reassure the client that her concern about whether the baby will be normal is not unusual. The many tests that are available to diagnose problems prenatally may be discussed, if appropriate. If her concern seems excessive, refer the client for counseling.

CONTACT WITH DISEASES

Ideally, clients should avoid persons with disease, and immunizations should be up-to-date prior to pregnancy. The client should also be assessed for susceptibility to hepatitis B, rubella, and varicella zoster before pregnancy or early in the prenatal period.

Cytomegalovirus

Fifty to 85 percent of pregnant women have been infected with cytomegalovirus (CMV) at some point in their lives, and are seropositive for the IgG antibody. Antibodies do not protect from reinfection, but primary infection during the first half of pregnancy carries the greatest risk to the fetus. Between 0.2 and 2 percent of all neonates show evidence of fetal infection with CMV, but of those, only 5 to 6 percent are affected with congenital CMV syndrome, consisting of growth restriction, microcephaly, intracranial calcifications, chorioretinitis, cognitive, motor and sensorineural delays, hepatosplenomegaly, jaundice, hemolytic anemia, and thrombocytopenic purpura. Because of the frequency of CMV illness among children, pregnant women who work in daycare settings or who have older children who attend day care should avoid contact with saliva, respiratory secretions, urine, and feces, with hand washing and cleaning of toys and cooking, eating, and drinking utensils (AAP & ACOG, 2007; Cunningham et al., 2010) .

Fifth's Disease (Parvovirus B19)

Over half of all pregnant women are immune to parvovirus B19, but fetal death, miscarriage, or fetal hydrops can rarely occur with infection during pregnancy. The most significant time for infection to affect the fetus seems to be between the 10th- and 20th-week gestation, but poor outcomes have been reported with third trimester infection. Clients are advised to avoid exposure to children with undiagnosed rashes, although contagion is reduced after the onset of a visible rash, so daycare workers need not be restricted from work and infected children do not require isolation. Hand washing and standard infection control practices can reduce the chance of maternal infection (AAP & ACOG, 2007; Cunningham et al., 2010).

Listeriosis

Listeriosis is infection with the foodborne bacteria *Listeria monocytogenes*, which is found in unpasteurized dairy products, undercooked poultry, deli meats and hotdogs, raw unwashed produce, and seafood. If contracted during pregnancy, listeriosis can cause stillbirth or miscarriage, preterm delivery, and other complications. Newborns can contract the illness during delivery, and may develop severe infection. Maternal infection should be treated promptly with antibiotics, which may help prevent fetal and neonatal effects. The symptoms are flu-like. To avoid listeriosis, clients should not eat unpasteurized dairy products; soft cheeses, undercooked meat, poultry, fish, or eggs; raw or cold meat, eggs, or seafood (AAP & ACOG, 2007; Cunningham et al., 2010; Gabbe et al., 2007). Advise clients to contact their health care provider if flu-like symptoms occur.

Lyme Disease

Lyme disease can be transmitted to the fetus through the placenta, though no congenital effects have been identified. Antibiotics will cure the client with early stage Lyme disease (Cunningham et al., 2010). Advise avoiding tick bites by wearing long pants tucked into boots and long sleeves in grassy or wooded areas. Insect repellant can be applied to the clothes but not directly to the skin. A skin check for ticks is recommended after potential exposure. Clients should contact a health care provider with suspected exposure.

Measles

Rubeola (or measles) is not linked to fetal defects but may cause miscarriage, preterm labor, or low birth weight. Infection close to term could result in the fetus's developing severe infection without sufficient antibodies to protect it. Avoidance of exposure is advised and contacting the health care provider immediately upon exposure is recommended because an immune serum globulin is available. Vaccination preconception or postpartum for nonimmune women is recommended (Cunningham et al., 2010).

Mumps

Mumps in pregnancy is not associated with congenital anomalies, but can cause miscarriage or fetal death (Ornoy & Tenenbaum, 2006). If not immune or vaccinated, the client should avoid exposure and receive vaccination postpartum. Mumps vaccine is contraindicated during pregnancy, and clients should wait 1 month after vaccination before conceiving (CDC, 2011a).

Rubella

Rubella, also known as German measles, can cause significant harm to the fetus if the client contracts it in the first half of her pregnancy. All clients should be tested prenatally and, ideally, preconceptionally. If nonimmune, advise the client to avoid exposure to anyone with an undiagnosed rash. Advise vaccination preconception and then wait 1 month to conceive. If exposed, contact the health care provider immediately. Nonimmune clients should be vaccinated immediately postpartum (see Chapter 22) (CDC, 2011a).

Sexually Transmitted Diseases

STDs can pose a health threat to the fetus. Assess the client for a history of STDs; ask about the number of sexual partners she has and her use of condoms. Advise her to use condoms if she has multiple partners or a new partner, if she is unsure of her partner's sexual or drug use history, or if her partner has multiple sexual partners.

Educate clients to recognize symptoms of infection and if exposed to high-risk sexual partners to contact a health care provider as soon as possible (see Chapter 14).

Toxoplasmosis

Advise clients to avoid toxoplasmosis infection by not handling raw meat or gardening without gloves and avoiding outdoor sandboxes and cat litter boxes. If the client must change a cat's litter, it should be changed frequently to avoid the development of infectious *Toxoplasma gondii* in the feces, which takes approximately 48 hours to form, and she should wear gloves. Afterward, hands are washed well (Davidson et al., 2012).

Tuberculosis

The incidence of tuberculosis has risen in the United States. If a client is exposed or determined to be at high risk for latent tuberculosis infection, a Mantoux skin test with purified protein derivative (PPD) is advised. In the event of a positive PPD test, a chest x-ray is indicated to determine the presence or absence of active disease. A negative chest x-ray with a positive PPD indicates latent tuberculosis infection, and prophylaxis against active disease may be started during pregnancy if the client is determined to be at high risk for its development. Referral to a physician is indicated for active tuberculosis infection, and consultation or referral may be warranted for a latent infection. Active tuberculosis infection poses significant risk to the pregnant woman, her household contacts, and especially the newborn. In this event, a report to the public health department should be made, and the mother and newborn may need to be separated temporarily after delivery. Advise clients to contact the health care provider if exposure is suspected (AAP & ACOG, 2007).

Varicella Zoster

Varicella zoster virus (chicken pox) can occasionally cause congenital varicella syndrome in the fetus, if the client becomes infected during the first half of the pregnancy. Adults, particularly if pregnant, are at much greater risk than children of developing severe complications from varicella virus. If infected between 5 days prior and 2 days after delivery, the greatest risk is to a newborn that develops the disease before the mother has developed antibodies and transferred them to the fetus transplacentally. Any client without a history of varicella illness or vaccination is advised to avoid contact with infected persons, and contact her health care provider immediately in the event of suspected exposure. Varicella zoster immunoglobulin has not been available in the United States since 2006, but an investigational product called VariZIG is available to select groups, including susceptible exposed pregnant women (CDC, 2011a).

DENTAL CARE

Dental and periodontal problems are associated with poor pregnancy outcomes, including preterm birth. For this reason, clients should be strongly encouraged to follow up with regular dental care during pregnancy, and a regimen of homecare including brushing and flossing should be encouraged and reinforced. Reassure and educate clients who are under the mistaken impression that dental care is contraindicated in pregnancy. The dentist must be told of the pregnancy, and may request a letter of clearance from the prenatal care provider. The letter should note that local anesthesia may be used, specific antibiotics and narcotics may be prescribed, and x-rays may be performed with an abdominal shield (AAP & ACOG, 2007).

EXERCISE

Regular exercise during pregnancy increases a client's sense of well-being, improves sleep, contributes to the prevention of some complications of pregnancy, helps to control weight gain and tone muscles, and, after delivery, hastens recovery. A client who was physically active before conception should be able to engage in the same activities throughout pregnancy (Penney, 2008). You may need to advise clients not to take up new activities or sports if this activity requires balance because their sense of balance is decreased and their joints are looser, which increases the risk of injury. Many exercise programs for pregnant women exist but because exercise specialists are not regulated, advise clients to consult their health care provider and to check the credentials of the instructor.

As a general guideline, clients should avoid sports with high risk for impact, falling, and abdominal trauma (e.g., hockey, soccer, gymnastics, horseback riding, downhill skiing). Likewise, scuba diving and high altitude activities should also be avoided. The client should exercise 30 minutes per day, doing activity of moderate intensity (such as brisk walking) (Penney, 2008). Drinking water before, during, and after exercise to replace what is lost and eating a light snack before exercising are recommended. The clients should take care to ensure that calorie intake takes into account exercise expenditure. After the first trimester, the client should not lie on her back for more than a few minutes at a time. The client should stop exercising and contact a health care provider if any of the following occur: decreased fetal movement, contractions, chest or calf pain, bleeding, suspected membrane rupture, dizziness, shortness of breath (unable to talk comfortably), palpitations, faintness, tachycardia, back pain, pelvic pain or pressure, or difficulty walking (AAP & ACOG, 2007; ACOG, Committee of Obstetric Practice, 2002).

Absolute Contraindications to Exercise in Pregnancy

Several complications of pregnancy may prohibit exercise. These include preterm labor hypertensive disorders of pregnancy, ruptured membranes, incompetent cervix, multiple fetuses, persistent second or third trimester bleeding, placenta previa after 26 weeks' gestation, and significant cardiac or respiratory disease. Clients with other medical comorbidities or high-risk pregnancies should discuss the benefits and risks of exercise with their provider prior to beginning or continuing an exercise regimen (ACOG, Committee of Obstetric Practice, 2002).

FAMILY PLANNING

Encourage the client to begin thinking about family-planning methods before delivery. Ideally, women should space births at least 12 months apart to allow their bodies to recover and replace nutritional reserves, and in order to ensure the best outcomes in the subsequent pregnancy. Individualized counseling should be provided to each breastfeeding woman regarding risks and benefits of immediate initiation of progestin-only pills (POPs). When combined with breastfeeding, the effectiveness of POPs is close to 100 percent, but women and their partners should be advised that taking the POP as little as 3 hours late can decrease the effectiveness (Schuiling & Likis, 2006). If a client has previously used a diaphragm, it must be refitted postpartum. If a client desires sterilization, the procedure may be done on the first postpartum day, during a cesarean birth, or after her postpartum visit. General anesthetic agents, if used, may sedate the infant temporarily if nursing. If the woman's partner decides to have a vasectomy, the procedure can be done at any time. Both partners, however, must be aware that a man is not sterile until his sperm count is zero. Sperm can take 21 days to travel from the testes to the epididymis, so it can take a month or more to reach a sperm count of zero. A second sperm count to confirm is recommended. Chapter 22 provides in-depth information on postpartum use of various contraceptive methods.

FEEDING METHOD

Women have the choice of breastfeeding or feeding their newborns formula from a bottle. Breast milk is the ideal infant food, and should be strongly encouraged by prenatal providers. Health care providers are in a unique position not only to educate women on the benefits of breastfeeding and hopefully influence their decision of feeding method, but also to effect and influence institutional and societal change, to support and encourage breastfeeding mothers in the hospital, in the workplace, and in their daily lives in their communities (ACOG, 2007a, 2007b). It is the recommendation of the AAP (2005) that breastfeeding be the exclusive method of infant feeding for a duration of 6 months, and should be continued after complementary foods are introduced, for at least 6 additional months (a total of 1 year). See Chapter 22 for more discussion of breastfeeding.

Preparation for Breastfeeding

Education about breastfeeding should begin in the prenatal period, ideally in childbirth education classes, in a supportive atmosphere, facilitated by a knowledgeable instructor, and with ample time for questions and discussion. When local childbirth education classes are not available, La Leche League may be a good resource for finding free support groups and educational materials online. Other resources include books about breastfeeding and supportive friends or family members, who have had successful breastfeeding experiences (Riordan & Hoover, 2010). Nipple preparation is unnecessary, even in the case of inverted nipples, for which special exercises and the wearing of nipple shields during pregnancy were once recommended (Riordan & Wambach, 2010).

Formula Feeding

See Chapter 22 for discussion of formula feeding.

FETAL HICCUPS

Hiccups, often described by the mother as a tapping or jumping sensation usually in the lower abdomen, are common and do not harm the fetus.

GRANDPARENTING

The grandparents of the newborn must go through developmental changes, which can either result in a closer, supportive relationship with their children or widen the communication gap. Assess the communication skills, role expectations, and support skills of the parents and grandparents. Encourage the grandparents to learn about new parenting, feeding, and childrearing skills their children may use. Teach good communication skills. Encourage attendance at grandparenting classes if available.

INFANT SAFETY SEATS

By state law in many cases, most hospitals do not discharge infants unless the parents' car is equipped with an infant safety seat. These seats can be rented or purchased and sometimes are available from charitable organizations and government social service offices. Often, local police and fire stations offer services to check that a safety seat is correctly fastened in a vehicle.

RADIATION EXPOSURE

Ionizing Radiation (X-Ray, Radiation Therapy)

At very high levels, ionizing radiation has the potential to cause miscarriage, growth restriction, congenital defects, childhood cancers, and other complications. Dosage of ionizing radiation less than 5 rad is considered harmless to the fetus, though some studies have found associations with childhood cancers at dosages of 1 to 2 rad. Total exposure during a standard two-view chest x-ray is 0.00007 rad. The greatest risk of fetal harm is between 8 and 15 weeks of gestation, and risk is virtually eliminated before 8 weeks and after 25 weeks (ACOG, 2004; Cunningham et al., 2010). Several guidelines are suggested that pertain to exposure to diagnostic x-rays.

- Avoid unnecessary x-rays or wait until after 15 weeks, or use ultrasound or magnetic resonance imaging (MRI). If indicated and approved by an attending radiologist, MRI without contrast may be performed regardless of gestational age (ACOG, 2004; Cunningham et al., 2010). With all testing, weigh risk versus benefits, waiting if possible.
- Advise the client to inform anyone ordering or taking an x-ray that she is pregnant, and to insist on lead shielding of the abdomen.
- Advise the client to follow exactly the directions of the technician to avoid having to retake x-rays.
- Advise a regularly inspected facility staffed with certified technicians and supervised by a radiologist.

Ultrasound

The use of ultrasound, high-frequency sound waves, has not demonstrated fetal or maternal harm in over 35 years of use (Cunningham et al., 2010). Nonetheless, ultrasound should be limited to use for medical indications only.

Nuclear Medicine

Fetal exposure to radiation during nuclear medicine studies can be calculated. Consultation with a specialist is advised (Cunningham et al., 2010).

SAUNAS, HOT TUBS, WHIRLPOOLS, TANNING BEDS, SPA TREATMENTS

As a precaution, advise clients to avoid these activities. Reliable evidence that hyperthermia in pregnancy is teratogenic is lacking, but the theoretical risk of congenital malformations remains. Clients who choose partake in these activities may be recommended to spend no more than 15 minutes in a sauna, and no more than 10 minutes in a hot tub, and to submerge the body from the chest down only, to reduce heat absorption (AAP & ACOG, 2007). Tanning is not advised due to risk of serious sunburn, dehydration, and skin cancer, as well as the possibility of worsening chloasma.

SEXUAL ACTIVITY

Table 19–10 gives a summary of physiological changes that may enhance pleasure or diminish a woman's sexual response during pregnancy. Second trimester changes, such as increased pelvic congestion and vaginal lubrication, may enhance sexual enjoyment. Some couples experience increased intimacy and closeness from the bond pregnancy creates. For other couples, however, pregnancy is often a time of profound emotional and developmental upheaval and can present a developmental crisis for both partners. Sexuality during pregnancy can be affected directly. The health care provider's role involves providing anticipatory guidance through sexuality education and assessment, both at the initial prenatal evaluation and during subsequent visits.

Sexual activity is not contraindicated in a healthy pregnancy. Assure the couple that the fetus will not be injured by sexual activity, including intercourse/penetration, nor is the fetus able to understand what is happening. Encourage the couple to experiment with positions that may be more comfortable (e.g., woman on top, side lying).

Cunnilingus is safe if the partner does not blow air into the vagina. Air embolisms may be fatal (Cunningham et al., 2010). Condoms are advised with anal sex. Advise changing the condom if vaginal intercourse is then desired. If intercourse is prohibited, specify what is meant:

TABLE 19–10. Physiological Changes in Pregnancy That May Influence Sexuality

First Trimester	Second Trimester	Third Trimester
Fatigue and lethargy	Increased pelvic congestion	Physical discomfort, backache
Nausea and vomiting	Increased vaginal moisture	Increasing uterine irritability
Breast tenderness		Excessive pelvic congestion
Abdominal bloating		Vulvar/femoral varicosities
Increased urination		

Sources: Adapted from Cunningham et al., 2010 and Davidson et al., 2012.

orgasm, vaginal penetration, or unprotected penetration. Other forms of sexual expression (e.g., cuddling, kissing, masturbation) may be advised.

Communication

A couple may require help adjusting to changes brought about by pregnancy. Some women or their partners have increased sexual desire, some less. The woman, though, often has an increased need for closeness during pregnancy. She should communicate all of these concerns to her partner. Emphasize to the couple that closeness and cuddling need not always culminate in intercourse. A mental health care provider may be consulted if necessary.

Contraindications to Sexual Intercourse

The following conditions may preclude sexual relations during a portion of the pregnancy (Cunningham et al., 2010).

- History of repeated miscarriage
- History of cervical incompetence, without cerclage
- Current possibility of threatened abortion
- Placenta previa
- Undiagnosed vaginal bleeding
- Premature ROM or preterm labor
- Severe vulvar varicosities

As appropriate, offer the woman and her partner suggestions about sexual frequency, foreplay, and alternate forms of intimacy.

SIBLING RIVALRY

Many parents need reassurance that sibling rivalry is normal.

Techniques to Minimize Rivalry

Parents can use the following techniques to minimize rivalry.

- Enroll the older child(ren) in sibling classes.
- Encourage the older child(ren) to verbalize emotions and acknowledge those emotions.
- Use a doll to role-play safe handling of a newborn.
- Expect and tolerate some regression.
- If the older child(ren) is to be moved from a crib to a bed or into another room to accommodate the newborn, do so before the baby is born, preferably 2 to 3 months before.
- If the older child(ren) desires, buy a gift that she or he can give to the new infant. Be sure that the gift is safe for an infant and request that it be placed in the bassinette (purchase an item that can be cleaned or sterilized). The older child(ren) can then identify the infant in the nursery.
- The first time the child(ren) comes to visit, have the infant in the bassinette. Give the older child(ren) individual attention until he or she expresses an interest in the infant.
- It may also help to have a gift from the infant to the older child(ren).
- Encourage grandparents and visitors to pay attention first to the older child(ren) and to have her or him introduce the baby.
- Find time every day to be alone with the older child(ren).

PREPARATION FOR SURGICAL INTERVENTION

There are several types of surgical intervention that may be indicated for a pregnant woman. These are, primarily, cesarean section, vacuum or forceps delivery, and episiotomy. Providing in-depth education concerning surgical intervention to clients not at risk may erroneously convey to clients that labor and delivery are fraught with danger, adding to their anxiety level and altering their ability to trust in their body's health and strength, and the normalcy of birth. However, clients should be educated about the surgical options that may be suggested to them, to enable them to make informed decisions in partnership with their delivery providers.

Cesarean Birth

Greater than 30 percent of deliveries in the United States are currently completed by cesarean section. Indications for cesarean delivery can include various types of labor dystocia, fetal distress, abnormal presentation such as breech and transverse, and having multiple prior cesarean deliveries. The rate of cesarean section has risen dramatically since 1970, when the rate was 4.5 percent (Cunningham et al., 2010). Several factors may explain the increase that has occurred.

- More advanced-age pregnancies, and greater numbers of nulliparous women, who are thought to be at greater risk for cesarean delivery.
- Greater use of continuous electronic fetal monitoring, which leads to more diagnoses of fetal distress.
- Fewer forcep, vacuum, and vaginal breech deliveries being performed.
- Higher rates of labor induction.

- Higher rates of obesity.
- Increases in elective cesarean delivery.
- Decreases in the availability of vaginal birth after cesarean (VBAC), for women with prior cesarean delivery.
- Greater threat and incidence of legal malpractice suits (Cunningham et al., 2010).

Risks of cesarean section include maternal mortality, damage to proximal organs, wound infection, and risk of complications in future labor and delivery (Cunningham et al., 2010). Surgery is done under regional or general anesthesia with a combination cold-knife and electrocautery techniques. Rates of VBAC have fluctuated from 5 percent in 1985, to 28 percent in 1996, and again to 8.5 percent in 2006, primarily due to concerns about uterine rupture during labor (ACOG, 2010b). The ACOG recommends that VBAC be offered only in hospitals with staff and facilities immediately available for emergency management. Another current controversy with regard to cesarean delivery is the availability of elective, patient-choice cesarean section. Clients may request this option for a variety of reasons, but it is incumbent on the prenatal provider to offer comprehensive, unbiased information, so the client may make the most informed decision possible.

Forceps Delivery and Vacuum Extraction

Forceps and vacuum extractors are instruments that provide added traction and rotation, in order to facilitate vaginal delivery with greater speed, when needed. Indications for these types of operative vaginal delivery include worsening maternal medical conditions or exhaustion, prolonged second stage of labor, or compromised fetal status. Risks may include large vaginal lacerations, possibly extending into the rectum, long-term urinary and fecal incontinence, uterine infection, and trauma and morbidity to the fetus (Cunningham et al., 2010).

Episiotomy

Episiotomy is a surgical incision into the vaginal mucosa and musculature, intended to widen the vaginal opening and hasten delivery. The incision is usually made under local or regional anesthesia. Although once performed routinely in the United States, episiotomies are now used in 30 to 35 percent of vaginal deliveries. Incidence, however, will vary by type of provider. Indications for episiotomy include fetal distress, shoulder dystocia, operative vaginal delivery, and cases where the perineum is noted to be abnormally short, increasing the likelihood of a significant, spontaneous laceration. Complications from episiotomy include bleeding, hematoma, infection, and postpartum discomfort and dyspareunia (ACOG, 2006a).

TRAVEL

General Guidelines

Generally, a client without medical or obstetrical complications can travel until approximately 36 weeks. The client should check with her health care provider prior to traveling. Travel may be contraindicated with complicated or high-risk pregnancies.

- If planning to fly, the client should check with the airline about restrictions.
- Measures to prevent edema in the legs and feet and the risk of thromboembolism can be taken while flying or driving. Specifically, women should be informed to ambulate frequently or perform lower extremity exercises while seated.
- The client should drink adequate fluids and urinate every 2 hours to increase comfort. Light snacks may help reduce nausea.
- The client should not take medication for motion sickness or constipation without first consulting a health care provider.
- Seat belt should be worn over the pelvis at all times while flying.
- The client should be provided with names of obstetricians in the area to which she will be traveling and given a copy of her prenatal record in case of unexpected complications.
- Travelers to high altitudes or where additional immunization is required should consult their health care provider for individual risk assessment (ACOG, 2009a).

Foreign Travel Guidelines

- Immunizations required for travel should be received at least 3 months before conception (see Immunizations). Consultation with an expert advisor at a travel clinic is advisable before traveling to foreign countries during pregnancy.
- Use of chloroquine during pregnancy (to prevent malaria) is safe as is use of insect repellants containing DEET (McGovern, Boyce, & Fischer, 2007). Covering exposed skin, mosquito netting, and spraying bug repellents on clothing reduce the chance of being bitten. In some areas, the strains of malaria

are resistant to chloroquine. Mefloquine is typically not recommended in the first trimester of pregnancy. Because malaria during pregnancy carries increased risk to the mother and fetus, travel to destinations where there is significant risk of malaria should be postponed until after delivery.

- In areas where water has been known to be contaminated, clients should avoid drinking it, as well as eating raw fruits and vegetables and using ice made from contaminated water or glasses washed in it. Water purification tablets containing iodine are not safe for pregnant women. The pregnant woman should drink only boiled or bottled water, soft drinks, or bottled fruit juices and avoid unpasteurized products or milk products (McGovern et al., 2007). Advise the client which medications and antibiotics to use if she should develop nausea, vomiting, or diarrhea and prescribe them for her if necessary.
- All meat should be thoroughly cooked.

Seat Belts

Advise the client to use shoulder and lap belts when traveling in a car. Correct positioning of a seat belt requires that the lap portion be placed below the abdomen, across the upper thighs. The shoulder belt should rest between the breasts. Both belts should be worn snugly.

VIVID DREAMS AND FANTASIES

Vivid dreams and fantasies are common, healthy, and normal during pregnancy. Recurrent themes may indicate an area of concern for the client. Assess the need for intervention. Reassurance of the normalcy of vivid dreams is often all the client requires.

THE WORKPLACE

In general, women may continue to work until labor if their pregnancy is uncomplicated and the jobs present no special hazards (AAP & ACOG, 2007). Physically intense labor, significant fatigue from work, prolonged standing, prolonged work shifts and night shift work, and heavy lifting can increase the likelihood of low birth weight, preterm labor and delivery, or preeclampsia (AAP & ACOG, 2007; Bonzini, Coggon, & Palmer, 2007; Cunningham et al., 2010). The physical setting needs to be assessed for risk of physical harm, exposure to temperature extremes, and exposure to potential teratogens such as radiation, chemicals, indoor air pollution, or infectious agents (Davidson et al., 2012). Ideally, pregnant women would be provided paid maternity leave in order to adequately protect their health and safety during pregnancy and postpartum, but the financial reality is that many women cannot afford to take unpaid leave from work, and so may continue to work in unsafe conditions.

Modifications

Some modifications may be needed in employment.

- Ideally, the client should not work longer than 8 hours per day, 48 hours per week, avoiding shift and night hours. However, no restriction in hours or shift work is specifically recommended by studies of work in pregnancy (Bonzini et al., 2007).
- The client should take at least two 10-minute rest periods and one nutrition break per shift, with adequate rest and restroom facilities available.
- Jobs should be modified if safety may be compromised by dizziness, loss of balance, nausea, and vomiting, strenuous workloads, extreme temperatures, indoor air pollution, ionizing radiation, chemicals, and infectious disease.
- Daycare providers, animal care providers, and meat handlers should be protected from diseases known to cause fetal defects (see Contact With Diseases).
- Be aware that substances permissible by state codes for a nonpregnant individual may be *unsafe* for a pregnant woman and a developing fetus. The Occupational Safety and Health Administration can answer questions about specific substances and situations.
- Each pregnancy should be evaluated to assess the risk of continued working. Factors to assess include past pregnancy complications and outcomes, medical complications of the current pregnancy, obstetrical complications, and the characteristics of the work environment.
- Clients have certain rights that are protected by law. The Pregnancy Discrimination Act requires the employer to treat pregnancy as any other disability would be treated. The Occupational Safety and Health Administration ensures that employers either provide a workplace free of hazards likely to cause death or serious harm or provide information about dangerous chemicals or substances. The Family and Medical Leave Act requires employers of more than 50 persons to give 12 weeks of unpaid leave with birth; with adoption or foster care of a child; with care of a spouse, child, or parent with a serious health

condition; or if unable to perform the job because of any disability including pregnancy. Vacation and sick pay must be given if earned, and health benefits cannot be changed. The same or equal job must be available upon return to work.

DANGER SIGNS AND SYMPTOMS

Potential problems in pregnancy may be indicated by the development of particular signs or symptoms. Should she recognize such a sign, the client should contact her health care provider as soon as possible.

FIRST TRIMESTER

Signs and symptoms of concern in the first trimester may include spotting or bleeding; cramping; painful urination; severe vomiting and/or diarrhea; fever higher than 100.4°F; symptoms of vaginal infection or STIs; persistent or severe low abdominal pain (unilateral, bilateral, or midline); and lightheadedness or dizziness (particularly if accompanied by shoulder pain). If a woman experiences any abdominal trauma, this should be reported to her health care provider. Additionally, women and their partners should be counseled to report any new onset or exacerbations of depression and/or anxiety symptoms.

SECOND TRIMESTER

Signs and symptoms in the second trimester include all those noted for the first trimester plus regular uterine contractions (six or more per hour); unilateral leg or calf pain—especially if accompanied by edema, pain with movement, redness, heat, and tenderness, or coldness, numbness, and whiteness; sudden gush or consistent leaking of fluid; absence of fetal movement for more than 24 hours after quickening; sudden weight gain; significant edema of the face and/or hands; severe upper abdominal pain; or headache with visual changes and/or photophobia.

THIRD TRIMESTER

Signs and symptoms in the third trimester (after 26–28 weeks) include all those noted for the first and second trimesters plus a decrease in daily fetal movement (see Chapter 19). If movement is insufficient, the woman should contact her health care provider immediately. After 37 weeks' gestation, when contractions are 3 to 5 apart minutes if a primipara, or 5 to 8 minutes apart if a multipara, lasting 45 to 60 seconds, and strong in intensity or with the characteristics of true labor, the client should notify her provider. Each woman, though, should be individually counseled based on her pregnancy risk and the distance the client lives from the birthing location. Also, if the client was scheduled for a cesarean birth, has a history of precipitous labor, or has a high-risk pregnancy, she may need to contact her provider earlier.

Signs indicating a client should be evaluated by a provider as soon as possible include a significant decrease in fetal movement; menstrual-like bleeding; constant, severe contractions; or abdominal pain without relief. Rupture or suspected ROM may fall into this category as well, depending on practice protocol.

RECOGNIZING SIGNS AND SYMPTOMS OF LABOR

PRELABOR

The prelabor, or "false" labor, stage can begin 1 month to 1 hour before labor begins. It is a period of cervical softening, effacement, and descent of the presenting part into the pelvis. Dilation of the cervix can also occur during this time.

Subjective Data

Lightening, dropping, or engagement occurs when the presenting part descends into the pelvis. The client notes easier breathing but increased pelvic pressure, cramping, low back pain, and more frequent urination. Among primiparas, lightening can occur 2 to 4 weeks before labor, and among multiparas, it may be as late as during labor. Either increasing (nesting) or decreasing energy levels are noted. Vaginal discharge may increase and thicken. The client may notice loss of the mucous plug (a thick red or brown plug) and/or bloody show (a pink-tinged mucous discharge). Braxton-Hicks contractions may increase and become more intense. They are irregular, feel high and in front, occur suddenly without buildup, and decrease after urinating or changing position.

Objective Data

Physical examination may reveal a weight loss of 1 to 2 lb since the last visit. Softening of the cervix, effacement, and possibly some dilation occur; dilation is occasionally as much as 4 cm. The cervix moves more anterior. With descent of the presenting part into the pelvis, the fundal measurement may decrease and presenting part may palpate vaginally.

ACTIVE LABOR

Subjective Data

In contrast to prelabor, true labor contractions (which effect regular cervical change over a set period of time) are felt in the back, legs, or lower abdomen, and frequently are accompanied by menstrual-like or GI cramping sensations. With walking or over time, they grow longer, stronger, regular, and close together. Essential questions to ask in the immediate triage of a patient in labor (assuming the fundamentals of prenatal and other significant history have been obtained) include whether fetal movement is felt, whether membranes have ruptured, and whether any vaginal bleeding has been noted.

Objective Data

Initial assessment of a client in labor includes fetal assessment with a fetal monitor or handheld Doppler, depending on practice setting, assessment of contraction pattern, either with an electronic tocometer or by palpation and timing, and a physical assessment of the woman. Essential components of the physical exam include vital signs, sterile speculum exam (if ROM is suspected), and possibly a sterile vaginal exam if indicated. A client is said to be in latent labor from the time regular contractions begin, until she is dilated 3 to 4 cm. Active labor is diagnosed when the cervix is dilated 3 to 4 cm or greater, and regular, painful contractions are present, which cause progressive cervical change.

Palpation of the umbilical cord during a pelvic exam signals a life-threatening emergency. The health care provider should attempt to push the presenting part back into the uterus while the physician is contacted immediately (see Chapter 20).

REFERENCES

Alhusen, J.L. (2008). A literature update on maternal-fetal attachment. *Journal of Obstetric, Gynecologic, and Neonatal Nursing, 37,* 315–328. doi:10.1111/j.1552-6909.2008.00241.x

American Academy of Pediatrics (AAP) & The American College of Obstetricians and Gynecologists (ACOG). (2007). *Guidelines for perinatal care* (6th ed.). Elk Grove Village/Washington, IL/DC: American Academy of Pediatrics/The American College of Obstetricians and Gynecologists.

American Academy of Pediatrics (AAP), Section on Breastfeeding. (2005). Policy statement: Breastfeeding and the use of human milk. *Pediatrics, 115,* 496–506.

American Academy of Pediatrics (AAP), Taskforce on Circumcision. (1999). Circumcision policy statement. *Pediatrics, 103,* 686–693.

American College of Obstetricians and Gynecologists (ACOG). (2004). Guidelines for diagnostic imaging during pregnancy (ACOG Committee Opinion No. 299). *Obstetrics and Gynecology, 104,* 647–651.

American College of Obstetricians and Gynecologists (ACOG). (2005a). Human papillomavirus (ACOG Practice Bulletin No. 61).*Obstetrics and Gynecology, 105,* 905–918.

American College of Obstetricians and Gynecologists (ACOG). (2005b). Obesity in pregnancy (ACOG Committee Opinion No. 315).*Obstetrics and Gynecology, 106*(3), 671–675.

American College of Obstetricians and Gynecologists (ACOG). (2006a). Episiotomy (ACOG Practice Bulletin No. 71). *Obstetrics and Gynecology, 107,* 957–962.

American College of Obstetricians and Gynecologists (ACOG). (2006b). Psychosocial risk factors: Perinatal screening and intervention (ACOG Committee Opinion No. 343). *Obstetrics and Gynecology, 108,* 469–477.

American College of Obstetricians and Gynecologists (ACOG). (2007a). Breastfeeding: Maternal and infant aspects (ACOG Committee Opinion No. 361). *Obstetrics and Gynecology, 109,* 479–480.

American College of Obstetricians and Gynecologists (ACOG). (2007b). Breastfeeding: Maternal and infant aspects (Special Report from ACOG). *ACOG Clinical Review, 12*(1), 1S–16S.

American College of Obstetricians and Gynecologists (ACOG). (2007c). Invasive prenatal testing for aneuploidy (ACOG Practice Bulletin No. 88). *Obstetrics and Gynecology, 110*(6), 1459–1467.

American College of Obstetricians and Gynecologists (ACOG). (2007d). Management of herpes in pregnancy (ACOG Practice Bulletin No. 82). *Obstetrics and Gynecology, 109,* 1489–1498.

American College of Obstetricians and Gynecologists (ACOG). (2007e). Screening for fetal chromosomal abnormalities (ACOG Practice Bulletin No. 77). *Obstetrics and Gynecology, 109,* 217–227.

American College of Obstetricians and Gynecologists (ACOG). (2007f). *Strategies for adolescent pregnancy prevention.* Washington, DC: Author.

American College of Obstetricians and Gynecologists (ACOG). (2007g). Viral hepatitis in pregnancy (ACOG Practice Bulletin No. 86). *Obstetrics and Gynecology, 110,* 941–955.

American College of Obstetricians and Gynecologists (ACOG). (2009a). Air travel during pregnancy (ACOG Committee Opinion No. 443). *Obstetrics and Gynecology, 114,* 254–255.

American College of Obstetricians and Gynecologists (ACOG). (2009b). Ultrasonography in pregnancy (ACOG Practice Bulletin No. 101). *Obstetrics and Gynecology, 113*(2), 451–461.

American College of Obstetricians and Gynecologists (ACOG). (2010a). Influenza vaccination during pregnancy (ACOG Committee Opinion No. 468). *Obstetrics and Gynecology, 116,* 1006–1007.

American College of Obstetricians and Gynecologists (ACOG). (2010b). Vaginal birth after previous cesarean delivery (ACOG Practice Bulletin No. 115). *Obstetrics and Gynecology, 116,* 450–463.

American College of Obstetricians and Gynecologists (ACOG). (2011a). Update on carrier screening for cystic fibrosis (ACOG Committee Opinion No. 486). *Obstetrics and Gynecology, 117,* 1028–1031.

American College of Obstetricians and Gynecologists (ACOG). (2011b). Substance abuse reporting and pregnancy: The role of the obstetrician-gynecologist (ACOG Committee Opinion No. 473). *Obstetrics and Gynecology, 117,* 200–201.

American College of Obstetricians and Gynecologists (ACOG). (2011c). Vitamin D: Screening and supplementation during pregnancy (ACOG Committee Opinion No. 495). *Obstetrics and Gynecology, 118*(1), 197–198.

American College of Obstetricians and Gynecologists (ACOG), Committee of Obstetric Practice. (2002). Exercise during pregnancy and the postpartum period (ACOG Committee Opinion No. 267). *Obstetrics and Gynecology, 99,* 171–173.

American College of Obstetricians and Gynecologists (ACOG), Committee of Obstetric Practice. (2010). Smoking cessation during pregnancy (ACOG Committee Opinion No. 471). *Obstetrics and Gynecology, 116*(5), 1241–1244.

American College of Obstetricians and Gynecologists (ACOG), Committee of Obstetric Practice. (2011). Methamphetamine abuse in women of reproductive age (ACOG Committee Opinion No. 479). *Obstetrics and Gynecology, 117*(3), 751–755.

American Dietetic Association (ADA). (2008). Position of the American Dietetic Association: Nutrition and lifestyle for a healthy pregnancy outcome. *Journal of the American Dietetic Association, 108,* 553–551. doi:10/1016/j.jada.2008.01.030

Amir, B., & Bent, A.E. (2008). Nonsurgical management of urinary incontinence and overactive bladder. In R.S. Gibbs, B.Y. Karlan, A.F. Haney, & I.E. Nygaard (Eds.), *Danforth's obstetrics and gynecology* (9th ed., pp. 890–899). Philadelphia: Lippincott Williams & Wilkins.

Atrash, H., Jack, B.W., Johnson, K., Coonrod, D., Moos, M.K., Stubblefield, P.G., et al. (2008). Where is the "W"oman in MCH?*American Journal of Obstetrics & Gynecology, 199*(6), S259–S265. doi:10.1016/j.ajog.2008.08.059

Attrill, B. (2002). The assumption of the maternal role: A developmental process. *Australian Journal of Midwifery, 15*(1), 21–25.

Barger, M.K. (2010). Maternal nutrition and perinatal outcomes. *Journal of Midwifery and Women's Health, 55*(6), 502–511.

Bickley, L.S. (2009). *Bates' guide to physical examination and history taking* (10th ed.). Philadelphia: Lippincott Williams & Wilkins.

Blackburn, S.T. (2007). *Maternal, fetal, and neonatal physiology: A clinical perspective* (3rd ed.). Philadelphia: W.B. Saunders Company.

Bloom, L., & Escuro, A. (2008). Adolescent pregnancy: Where do we start? In C.J. Lammi-Keefe, S.C. Couch, & E.H. Philipson (Eds.), *Handbook of nutrition and pregnancy* (pp. 101–113). Totowa, NJ: Humana Press.

Bonzini, M., Coggon, D., & Palmer, K.T. (2007). Risk of prematurity, low birthweight and pre-eclampsia in relation to working hours and physical activities: A systematic review. *Occupational and Environmental Medicine, 64*(4), 228–243.

Botehlo, N., Emeis, C.L., & Brucker, M.C. (2011). Gastrointestinal conditions. In T.L. King & M.C. Brucker (Eds.), *Pharmacology for women's health* (pp. 605–642). Sudbury, MA: Jones and Bartlett Publishers.

Briggs, G.G., Freeman, R.K., & Yaffe, S.J. (2008). *Drugs in pregnancy and lactation: A reference guide to fetal and neonatal risk.* Philadelphia: Lippincott Williams and Wilkins.

Brown, S.J., McDonald, E.A., & Krastev, A.H. (2008). Fear of an intimate partner and women's health in early pregnancy: Findings from the maternal health study. *Birth, 35*(4), 293–302.

Buhimschi, C.S., & Weiner, C.P. (2009). Medication in pregnancy and lactation: Part 1. Teratology. *Obstetrics and Gynecology, 113*(1), 166–188.

Catalano, S., Smith, E., Snyder, H., & Rand, M. (2009, September). *Female victims of violence.* Bureau of Justice Statistics: Selected Findings (Revised 10/23/09). Retrieved June 14, 2011, from http://bjs.ojp.usdoj.gov/content/pub/pdf/fvv.pdf

Centers for Disease Control and Prevention (CDC). (2001). Notice to readers: Revised ACIP recommendation for avoiding pregnancy after receiving a rubella-containing vaccine. *Morbidity and Mortality Weekly Report, 50*(49), 1117.

Centers for Disease Control and Prevention (CDC). (2006). Recommendations to improve preconception health and health care—United States. A report of the CDC/ATSDR preconception care work group and the select panel on preconception care. *Morbidity and Mortality Weekly Report, 55*(RR-06), 1–23. Retrieved May 7, 2011, from http://www.cdc.gov/mmwr/preview/mmwrhtml/rr5506a1.htm

Centers for Disease Control and Prevention (CDC). (2010a). *Alcohol use in pregnancy.* Retrieved June 21, 2011, from http://www.cdc.gov/ncbddd/fasd/alcohol-use.html

Centers for Disease Control and Prevention (CDC). (2010b). Prevention of perinatal group B streptococcal disease: Revised guidelines from CDC. *Recommendations and Reports: Morbidity and Mortality Weekly Report, 59*(RR-10), 1–32.

Centers for Disease Control and Prevention (CDC). (2010c). Sexually transmitted diseases treatment guidelines, 2010. *Recommendations and Reports: Morbidity and Mortality Weekly Report, 59*(RR-12), 1–114.

Centers for Disease Control and Prevention (CDC). (2010d). US medical eligibility criteria for contraceptive use, 2010. *Recommendations and Reports: Morbidity and Mortality Weekly Report, 59,* 1–88.

Centers for Disease Control and Prevention (CDC). (2010e). Youth risk behavior surveillance—United States, 2009. *Surveillance Summaries: Morbidity and Mortality Weekly Report, 59*(SS-5), 1–148.

Centers for Disease Control and Prevention (CDC). (2011a). *Epidemiology and prevention of vaccine-preventable diseases* (12th ed.). Washington, DC: Public Health Foundation.

Centers for Disease Control and Prevention (CDC). (2011b). *Tobacco use and pregnancy.* Retrieved June 21, 2011, from http://www.cdc.gov/reproductivehealth/TobaccoUsePregnancy/

Centers for Disease Control and Prevention (CDC). (2011c). Vital signs: Teen pregnancy—United States, 1991–2009. *Recommendations and Reports: Morbidity and Mortality Weekly Report, 60*(13), 414–420.

Chambliss, L.R. (2008). Intimate partner violence and its implications for pregnancy. *Clinical Obstetrics and Gynecology, 51*(2), 385–397.

Cheng, D., Schwarz, E.B., Douglas, E., & Horon, I. (2009). Unintended pregnancy and associated maternal preconception, prenatal and postpartum behaviors. *Contraception, 79,* 194–198. doi:10.1016/j.contraception.2008.09.009

Clark, M., & Ogden, J. (1999). The impact of pregnancy on eating behaviors and aspects of weight concern. *International Journal of Obesity and Related Metabolic Disorders, 23*(1), 18–24.

Coonrod, D.V., Jack, B.W., Stubblefield, P.G., Hollier, L.M., Boggess, K.A., Cefalo, R., et al. (2008). The clinical content of preconception care: Infectious diseases in preconception care. *American Journal of Obstetrics & Gynecology, 199*(6), S296–S309. doi:10.1016/j.ajog.2008.08.062

Creasy, R.K., Resnik, R., Iams, J.D., Lockwood, C.J., & Moore, T.R. (2009). *Creasy & Resnik's maternal-fetal medicine.* (6th ed.). Philadelphia: Saunders Elsevier.

Cunningham, F., Leveno, K., Bloom, S., Hauth, J., Rouse, D., & Spong, C. (2010). *Williams obstetrics* (23rd ed.). New York: McGraw-Hill.

Davidson, M., London, M., & Ladewig, P. (2012). *Olds' maternal-newborn nursing & women's health across the lifespan* (9th ed.). Boston: Pearson.

Deglin, J.H., Vallerand, A.H., & Sanoski, C.A. (2011). *Davis's drug guide for nurses* (12th ed.). Philadelphia: F. A. Davis.

Driscoll, D., & Gross, S.J. (2009). Screening for fetal aneuploidy and neural tube defects. *Genetics in Medicine, 11*(11), 818–821.

Elsinga, J., de Jong-Potjer, L.C., van der pal-de Bruin, K.M., le Cessie, S., Assendelft, W.J.J., & Buitendijk, S.E. (2008). The effect of preconception counseling on lifestyle and other behaviour before and during pregnancy. *Women's Health Issues, 18S,* S117–S125. doi:10.1016/j.whi.2008.09.00

Environmental Protection Agency. (2011). *What you need to know about mercury in fish and shellfish.* Retrieved June 29, 2011, from http://water.epa.gov/scitech/swguidance/fishshellfish/outreach/advice_index.cfm

Ettinger, A.S., Wengrovitz, A.G., Portier, C., & Brown, M.J. (2010). *Guidelines for the identification and management of lead exposure in pregnant and lactating women.* Atlanta, GA: US Department of Health and Human Services.

Finer, L.B., & Henshaw, S.K. (2006). Disparities in rates of unintended pregnancy in the United States, 1994 and 2001. *Perspectives on Sexual Reproductive Health, 38,* 90–96.

Fiore, M.C., Jaen, C.R., Baker, T.B., Bailey, W.C., Benowitz, N.L., Curry, S.J., et al. (2008). *Treating tobacco use and dependence: 2008 update.* Rockville, MD: US Department of Health and Human Services.

Fischbach, F.T., & Dunning, M.B. (2009). *A manual of laboratory and diagnostic tests* (8th ed.). Philadelphia: Wolters Kluwer/Lippincott Williams & Wilkins.

Freda, M.C., Moos, M.-K., & Curtis, M. (2006). The history of preconception care: Evolving guidelines and standards. *Maternal Child Health Journal, 10,* S43–S52.

Freeman, L., & Griew, K. (2007). Enhancing the midwife-woman relationship through shared decision-making and clinical guidelines. *Women and Birth, 20,* 11–15.

Fretts, R.C., & Duru, U.A. (2008). New indications for antepartum testing: Making the case for antepartum surveillance or timed delivery for women of advanced maternal age. *Seminars in Perinatology, 32,* 312–317. doi:10.1053/j.semperi.2008.04.016

Gabbe, S.G., Niebyl, J.R., & Simpson, J.L. (2007). *Obstetrics: Normal and problem pregnancies* (5th ed.). Philadelphia: Churchill, Livingston, Elsevier.

Gardiner, P.M., Nelson, L., Shellhaas, C.S., Dunlop, A.L., Long, R., Andrist, S., et al. (2008). The clinical content of preconception care: Nutrition and dietary supplements. *American Journal of Obstetrics & Gynecology, 199*(6), S345–S356.

Gay, J., Edgil, A., & Douglas, A. (1988). Reva Rubin revisited. *Journal of Obstetric Gynecologic and Neonatal Nursing, 17,* 394–399.

Gentile, S. (2011). Drug treatment for mood disorders in pregnancy. *Current Opinion in Psychiatry, 24*, 34–40.

Graves, B.W. (2010). The obesity epidemic: Scope of the problem and management strategies. *Journal of Midwifery and Women's Health, 55*(6), 568–578.

Gunatilake, R.P., & Perlow, J.H. (2011). Obesity and pregnancy: Clinical management of the obese gravida. *American Journal of Obstetrics & Gynecology, 204*(2), 106–119.

Hansen, B.T., Kjaer, S.K., Munk, C., Tryggvadottir, L., Sparén, P., Hagerup-Jenssen, M., et al. (2010). Early smoking initiation, sexual behavior and reproductive health—A large population-based study of Nordic women. *Preventive Medicine, 51*, 68–72.

Harrison, P.A., & Sidebottom, A.C. (2009). Alcohol and drug use before and during pregnancy: An examination of use patterns and predictors of cessation. *Maternal Child Health Journal, 13*, 386–394. doi:10.1007/s10995-008-0355-z

Institute of Medicine (IOM). (2009). *Weight gain during pregnancy: Reexamining the guidelines*. Washington, DC: The National Academies Press.

Jack, B.W., Atrash, H., Coonrod, D.V., Moos, M.K., O'Donnell, J., & Johnson, K. (2008). The clinical content of preconception care: An overview and preparation of this supplement. *American Journal of Obstetrics & Gynecology, 199*(6), S266–S279. doi:10.1016/j.ajog.2008.07.067

Jeanjot, I., Barlow, P., & Rozenberg, S. (2008). Domestic violence during pregnancy: Survey of patients and healthcare providers.*Journal of Women's Health, 17*, 557–567.

Jordan, R.G. (2010). Prenatal omega-3 fatty acids: Review and recommendations. *Journal of Midwifery and Women's Health, 55*(6), 520–528.

Jordan, R.G., & Murphy, P.A. (2009). Risk assessment and risk distortion: Finding the balance. *Journal of Midwifery and Women's Health, 54*, 191–200. doi:10.1016/j.jmwh.2009.02.001

Kaludjerovic, J., & Vieth, R. (2010). Relationship between vitamin D during perinatal development and health. *Journal of Midwifery and Women's Health, 55*(6), 550–560.

King, T.L., & Murphy, P.A. (2009). Evidence-based approaches to managing nausea and vomiting in early pregnancy. *Journal of Midwifery and Women's Health, 54*, 430–444.

Klein, J.D., & The Committee on Adolescence. (2005). Adolescent pregnancy: Current trends and issues. *Pediatrics, 116*, 281–286.

Kost, K., Henshaw, S., & Carlin, L. (2010). *U.S. teenage pregnancies, births and abortions: National and state trends and trends by race and ethnicity*. Washington, DC: Guttmacher Institute. Retrieved April 13, 2011, from http://www.guttmacher.org/pubs/USTPtrends.pdf

Lederman, R. (1996). *Psychosocial adaptation in pregnancy* (2nd ed.). Englewood Cliffs, NJ: Prentice Hall.

Manant, A., & Dodgson, J.E. (2011). Centering pregnancy: An integrative literature review. *Journal of Midwifery and Women's Health, 56*, 94–102.

Manns-James, L. (2011). Pregnancy. In T.L. King & M.C. Brucker (Eds.), *Pharmacology for women's health* (pp. 1045–1085). Sudbury, MA: Jones and Bartlett Publishers.

March of Dimes. (2008). *Drinking alcohol during pregnancy*. Retrieved June 21, 2011, from http://www.marchofdimes.com/Pregnancy/alcohol_indepth.html

March of Dimes. (2010). *Premature birth*. Retrieved June 21, 2011, from http://www.marchofdimes.com/baby/premature_indepth.html

Mathews, T.J., & MacDorman, M.F. (2010). Infant mortality statistics from the 2006 period linked birth/infant death data set.*National Vital Statistics Reports, 58*(17), 1–32.

McDiarmid, M.A., Gardiner, P.M., & Jack, B.W. (2008). The clinical content of preconception care: Environmental exposures.*American Journal of Obstetrics & Gynecology, 199*(6), S357–S361. doi:10.1016/j/ajog.2008.10.044

McGovern, L.M., Boyce, T.G., & Fischer, P.R. (2007). Congenital infections associated with international travel during pregnancy.*Journal of Travel Medicine, 14*(2), 117–128. doi:10.1111/j.1708-8305.2006.00093.x

Mercer, R.T. (2004). Becoming a mother versus maternal role attainment. *Journal of Nursing Scholarship, 36*(3), 226–232.

de Miranda, E., van der Bom, J.G., Bonsel, G.J., Bleker, O.P., & Rosendaal, F.R. (2006). Membrane sweeping and prevention of post-term pregnancy in low-risk pregnancies: A randomised controlled trial. *BJOG: An International Journal of Obstetrics and Gynaecology, 113*(4), 402–408.

Morrical-Kline, K.A., Walton, A.M., & Guildenbecher, T.M. (2011). Teratogen use in women of childbearing potential: An intervention study. *Journal of the American Board of Family Medicine, 24*(3), 262–271.

Moos, M.K., Dunlop, A.L., Jack, B.W., Nelson, L., Coonrod, D.V., Long, R., et al. (2008). Healthier women, healthier reproductive outcomes: Recommendations for the routine care of all women of reproductive age. *American Journal of Obstetrics & Gynecology, 199*(6), S280–S289. doi:10.1016/j.ajog.2008.08.060

Ornoy, A., & Tenenbaum, A. (2006). Pregnancy outcome following infections by coxsackie, echo, measles, mumps, hepatitis, polio and encephalitis viruses. *Reproductive Toxicology, 21*, 446–457.

Penney, D.S. (2008). The effect of vigorous exercise on pregnancy. *Journal of Midwifery and Women's Health, 53*, 155–159.

Raneri, L.G., & Wiemann, C.M. (2007). Social ecological predictors of repeat adolescent pregnancy. *Perspectives on Sexual and Reproductive Health, 39*(1), 39–47.

Rasheed, S., Abdelmonem, A., & Amin, M. (2011). Adolescent pregnancy in Upper Egypt. *International Journal of Gynecology and Obstetrics, 112,* 21–24.

Rasmussen, K.M., & Yaktine, A.L. (Eds.). (2009). *Weight gain during pregnancy: Reexamining the guidelines.* Washington, DC: National Academies Press.

Red, R.T., Richards, S.M., Torres, C., & Adair, C.D. (2011). Environmental toxicant exposure during pregnancy.*Obstetrical and Gynecological Survey, 66*(3), 159–169.

Riordan, J., & Hoover, K. (2010). Perinatal and intrapartum care. In J. Riordan & K. Wambach (Eds.), *Breastfeeding and human lactation* (pp. 215–251). Sudbury, MA: Jones and Bartlett Publishers.

Riordan, J., & Wambach, K. (2010). Breast-related problems. In J. Riordan & K. Wambach (Eds.), *Breastfeeding and human lactation* (pp. 291–324). Sudbury, MA: Jones and Bartlett Publishers.

Rising, S.S. (1998). Centering pregnancy: An interdisciplinary model of empowerment. *Journal of Nurse-Midwifery, 43*(1), 46–54.

Rubin, R. (1984). *Maternal identity and the maternal experience.* New York: Springer.

Salber, P. (2006). Routine screening to increase recognition of intimate partner violence and abuse. In P.R. Salber & E. Taliaferro (Eds.), *The physician's guide to intimate partner violence and abuse* (pp. 34–40). Volcano, CA: Volcano Press.

Schuiling, K., & Likis, F. (2006). *Women's gynecologic health.* Sudbury, MA: Jones & Bartlett.

Shrim, A., Levin, I., Mallozzi, A., Brown, R., Salama, K., Gamzu, R., et al. (2010). Does very advanced maternal age, with or without egg donation, really increase obstetric risk in a large tertiary center. *Journal of Perinatal Medicine, 38,* 645–650. doi:10.1515/JPM.2010.084

Siega-Riz, A.M., Deierlein, A., & Stuebe, A. (2010). Implementation of the new Institute of Medicine gestational weight gain guidelines. *Journal of Midwifery and Women's Health, 55*(6), 512–519.

Smith, S.A., Hulsey, T., & Goodnight, W. (2008). Effects of obesity on pregnancy. *Journal of Obstetric, Gynecologic, and Neonatal Nursing, 37,* 176–184. doi:10.1111/j.1552-6909.2008.00222.x

Solomon, B.D., Jack, B.W., & Feero, G. (2008). The clinical content of preconception care: Genetics and genomics. *American Journal of Obstetrics & Gynecology, 199*(6), S340–S344. doi:10.1016/j.ajog.2008.09.870

Timmins, C.L. (2002). The impact of language barriers on the health care of Latinos in the United States: A review of the literature and guidelines for practice. *Journal of Midwifery and Women's Health, 47,* 80–96.

Tomson, T., & Battino, D. (2009). Teratogenic effects of antiepileptic medications. *Neurologic Clinics, 27,* 993–1002.

Ustunsoz, A., Guvenc, G., Akyuz, A., & Oflaz, F. (2010). Comparison of maternal-and paternal-fetal attachment in Turkish couples.*Midwifery, 26,* e1–e9. doi:10.1016/j.midw.2009.12.006

Varney, H., Kriebs, J.M., & Gegor, C.L. (2004). *Varney's midwifery* (4th ed.). Sudbury, MA: Jones and Bartlett Publishers.

Walker, D.S., & Worrell, R. (2008). Promoting healthy pregnancies through perinatal groups: A comparison of centering pregnancy group prenatal care and childbirth education classes. *Journal of Perinatal Education, 17*(1), 27–34. doi:10.1624/105812408X267934

Ward, R.P., & Kugelmas, M. (2005). Using pegylated interferon and ribavirin to treat patients with chronic hepatitis C. *American Family Physician, 72*(4), 655–662.

Weng, X., Odouli, R., & Li, D.K. (2008). Maternal caffeine consumption during pregnancy and the risk of miscarriage: A prospective cohort study. *American Journal of Obstetrics & Gynecology, 198,* 279.e1–279.e8. doi:10.1016/j.ajog.2007.10.803

Widen, E., & Siega-Riz, A.M. (2010). Prenatal nutrition: A practical guide for assessment and counseling. *Journal of Midwifery and Women's Health, 55*(6), 540–549.

Wright, L.M., & Leahey, M. (2009). *Nurses and families: A guide to family assessment and intervention* (5th ed.). Philadelphia: F.A. Davis.

Yarcheski, A., Mahon, N.E., Yarcheski, T.J., Hanks, M.M., & Cannella, B.L. (2008). A meta-analytic study of predictors of maternal-fetal attachment. *International Journal of Nursing Studies, 46,* 708–715. doi:10.1016/j.ijnurstu.2008.10.013

Yogev, Y., Melamed, N., Bardin, R., Tenenbaum-Gavish, K., Ben-Shitrit, G., & Ben-Haroush, A. (2010). Pregnancy outcome at extremely advanced maternal age. *American Journal of Obstetrics & Gynecology, 203,* 558.e1–558.e7. doi:10/1016/j.ajog.2010.07.039

CHAPTER ❖ **20**

MATERNAL CONDITIONS IMPACTING RISK IN PREGNANCY

Melissa Frisvold ◆ *Debbie Ringdahl*

Highlights

- Infections
- Bleeding
- Anemias
- Hyperemesis Gravidarum
- Hypertension
- Obesity
- Diabetes
- Preterm Labor and Birth
- Multifetal Gestation

❖ INTRODUCTION

A high-risk pregnancy is one in which a condition exists that potentially jeopardizes the health of the mother, her fetus, or both. The condition may be preexisting or occur solely because of the pregnancy. According to the Centers for Disease Control and Prevention (CDC) (Hamilton, Martin, & Ventura, 2009), there were 4,317,110 million live births in the United States in 2007, and an estimated 548 maternal deaths. The maternal mortality rate was 12.7 deaths per 100,000 live births for white women and 26.5 deaths per 100,000 live births for black women. Clearly, black women in the United States have a significantly higher risk of maternal death than white women (Xu, Kochanek, Murphy, & Tejada-Vera, 2010). Women of high parity (Aliyu, Jolly, Ehiri, & Salihu, 2005) and older women (Luke & Brown, 2007) are also at increased risk.

Prenatal care can influence perinatal outcome because it allows timely and appropriate intervention to prevent or lessen the impact of untoward occurrences. In 2007, only 70.79 percent of women in the United States received prenatal care (CDC, 2011d). The early receipt of prenatal care varies substantially among racial and ethnic groups. Lack of or late prenatal care is associated with low birth weight (LBW) infants who are at increased risk of neonatal mortality. The reasons that women frequently give for not seeking prenatal care are lack of money, no transportation, and not being aware of their pregnancy. Also, increased stress levels and inadequate support systems have been associated with complications of pregnancy.

Infant mortality is frequently used as a benchmark of the health status of nations and/or communities. In the United States, the infant mortality has gradually declined in the past 20 years, mostly due to increased technology of caring for the sick neonate. However, the black infant mortality rate was 2.4 times the white infant mortality rate in 2006, a ratio that has persisted for several years (MacDorman & Mathews, 2011). Addressing these disparities in health is one of the goals for *Healthy People 2020*.

High-risk care includes several functions. The clinician assesses the physical and emotional health of the woman; assists the family to activate its own strengths and develop strategies to deal with stressors of high-risk pregnancy; anticipates the needs and concerns the family may have and assists family members to make appropriate plans to meet their needs; educates the woman and her family about all aspects of the treatment and care so that they can actively participate in the management; advocates for the woman and assists her to communicate and interact with the health care system; and counsels the client throughout her pregnancy.

Even with comprehensive, high-quality prenatal care, many of the conditions discussed in this chapter will continue to occur with less than optimal outcome. The goal of care at all times is the best possible outcome for the woman and her family; the ultimate goal is a healthy mother with a healthy infant.

INFECTIONS

HEPATITIS

Hepatitis is an acute, systemic, viral infection and the most frequent cause of jaundice during pregnancy. There are five main types of hepatitis. It occurs as hepatitis A (HAV); hepatitis B (HBV); hepatitis C (HCV), hepatitis D (HDV), and hepatitis E (HEV); and hepatitis D (delta hepatitis). Hepatitis A is an RNA virus that causes an acute, mild, self-limiting hepatitis without major risk to health. Liver enzymes are temporarily affected and the woman does not become a carrier. Hepatitis B is a DNA virus that causes an acute, more severe infection. Among its sequelae are chronic hepatitis, cirrhosis, and hepatocellular cancer. Pregnancy does not affect the severity or outcome of the disease. There are at least six hepatitis C virus (HCV) genotypes with a wide range of prognoses for both progression and treatment response. The principle risk factors for transmission are transfusion of blood products and intravenous (IV) drug use. Hepatitis D is an incomplete viral particle that causes disease only in the presence of HBV. Chronic hepatits D produces more severe disease more often than other forms of chronic hepatitis. Hepatitis E is a virus that is rare in the United States and self-limiting (ACOG Practice Bulletin, 2007d).

Epidemiology

Hepatitis A: Hepatitis A virus (HAV) infection is acquired primarily by the fecal-oral route by either person-to-person contact or ingestion of contaminated food, particularly milk and shellfish, or polluted water. High-risk populations are American Indians, Alaskan Natives, and those living in western states. The rates are highest in children and employees in daycare centers (Fiore, Wasley, & Bell, 2006).

Hepatitis B: Hepatitis B virus (HBV) is transmitted through contaminated blood and blood products and through sexual intercourse. Skin punctures with contaminated needles, syringes, or medical instruments can also transmit the virus. Perinatal transmission does occur. The fetus is not at risk for the disease until it comes in contact with contaminated blood at delivery (CDC, 2005a).

Hepatitis C: Risk factors for obstetric population include women with sexually transmitted diseases such as human immunodeficiency virus (HIV) and hepatitis B, multiple sexual partners, history of blood transfusions, and history of IV drug use (ACOG Practice Bulletin, 2007d).

Hepatitis D: Occurring as coinfection with hepatitis B, it has the same transmission and risks (ACOG Practice Bulletin, 2007d). Perinatal transmission has been reported, but immunoprophylaxis for hepatitis B has been effective in preventing neonatal infection.

Hepatitis E: Although rare in the United States, hepatitis E is endemic in developing countries and is transmitted by fecal-oral route (ACOG Practice Bulletin, 2007d). Risk to obstetric population involves women who travel to developing countries. Once the pregnant woman recovers from the acute phase of infection, perinatal transmission does not occur.

Subjective Data

Viral hepatitis produces flu-like symptoms with malaise, fatigue, anorexia, nausea, pruritus, fever, and right upper quadrant pain. The typical physical presentations are jaundice, hepatomegaly, and upper abdominal tenderness. The stool is usually darkened (ACOG Practice Bulletin, 2007d). The older the woman is, the more severe her symptoms. Infection may be not apparent to the woman or the provider.

Objective Data

Physical examination may reveal a normal general appearance. Jaundice of the skin, sclera, or nail beds may be present.

Hepatitis A: Serological testing to detect the presence of IgM antibody to HAV is diagnostic of acute HAV infection (CDC, 2010b)

Hepatitis B: The diagnosis of chronic or acute HBV infection requires serologic testing. The presence of IgM antibodies to the hepatitis B core antigen is diagnostic of acute HBV infection. The presence of the antibody to hepatitis B surface antigen (HBsAg) is produced after either a resolved infection or vaccination (CDC, 2010b).

Testing for HBsAg should be included in the initial prenatal assessment for all clients (ACOG Practice Bulletin, 2007d) (see Chapter 19). Prepare the client for repeat testing, as HBV screening tests may also be used to monitor the progression of infection.

Serum levels of cellular enzymes found in the liver are evaluated to determine liver damage. When liver damage occurs, increased amounts of these enzymes are released into the bloodstream. As these enzymes are evaluated as part of a complete panel of blood work, usually following a positive screening for HBV or clinical signs of illness, inform the client that enzyme levels will be retested to monitor the severity and progression of disease.

Hepatitis C: Confirmed by the identification of antibody to HCV by performing a second- or third-generation enzyme-linked immunosorbent assay (ELISA) (Scott & Gretch, 2007).

Hepatitis D: For acute infection, serologic test will have positive antigen and positive IgM antibody (Duff, 1998).

Hepatitis E: Confirmation done through electron microscopy of stool sample; fluorescent antibody blocking assay and Western blot assay are also available (Duff, 1998).

Hepatitis G: It can be identified in serum by polymerase chain reaction (Duff, 1998).

Differential Medical Diagnoses

Fatty liver disease, pregnancy-induced hypertension with HELLP (hemolysis, elevated liver enzymes, and low platelets) syndrome, secondary syphilis, drug-induced hepatitis.

Plan

Psychosocial Interventions. Reassure the client that the fetus is at minimal risk if other risk factors are absent. Family members should be encouraged to assist with household and childcare duties to allow the client to rest.

Medication. *Hepatitis A:* Immune globulin (gamma globulin) or immune-specific globulin is indicated for any pregnant woman exposed to HAV to provide passive immunity through injected antibodies. All household contacts should also receive gamma globulin. Gamma globulin is given intramuscularly (IM). Immune globulin intravenous is available to provide passive immunity.

Hepatitis B: Hepatitis B immune globulin (HBIG) contains a high titer of HBsAg, which provides passive immunity to hepatitis B. Pregnant women with definite exposure to HBV should receive HBIG as soon as possible after contact and again 30 days later. Any household or sexual contact should be tested and, if negative, receive immunoprophylaxis with HBIG. Those individuals should also receive the vaccination series. The newborn of a woman positive for HBV should be given HBIG and the hepatitis B vaccine within 12 hours of delivery (ACOG Practice Bulletin, 2007d). Close contacts of women with HBV should also receive HBIG, if not already immunized.

Hepatitis B vaccine is indicated for the newborn of a woman who has tested positive for HBsAg to stimulate the newborn's active immunity. It should be given as soon as possible after birth up to 7 days of life, and again at 30 and 60 days. The CDC (2005a) recommends routine vaccination of all newborns. Dosage recommendations depend upon the status of the mother. The vaccination is not contraindicated during pregnancy.

Hepatitis C, D, and E: No current licensed vaccine for use with hepatitis C or D infection is available. The provision of optimal obstetrical care for women with HCV is limited by the lack of pharmacologic or immunologic measures to decrease the risk of vertical transmission (ACOG Practice Bulletin, 2007d).

Hygienic Measures. All caregivers, whether health care providers or family members, should use universal precautions at all times. Stress to the client and her family that hepatitis A, C, D, and E are highly contagious. Explain the mode of transmission in the instruction and advise family and friends concerning good hand washing and hygiene.

Diet. Recommend a bland diet with additional fluids, depending on the extent of a client's nausea and vomiting. IV fluid hydration may become necessary.

Breastfeeding. Infants who have received prophylaxis at birth and are currently on the immunization schedule should continue breastfeeding.

Follow-Up

Frankly discuss and assess possible drug use, as hepatitis is frequently associated with substance abuse. In addition, as many forms of hepatitis are sexually transmitted, recommend the use of condoms throughout the remainder of the pregnancy, and arrange to repeat screening tests for sexually transmitted diseases, especially HIV infection.

RUBELLA

Commonly called German measles or 3-day measles, rubella is an acute, mild, contagious disease caused by the rubella virus.

Epidemiology

Infection early in pregnancy with rubella, especially during the first 16 weeks, can result in fetal death, miscarriage, or an infant born with birth defects (Plotkin & Reef, 2008).

Transmission occurs by direct contact with urine, stool, or nasopharyngeal secretions with an incubation period of 2 to 3 weeks. Infected individuals can transmit the infection for several days without experiencing the characteristic symptoms or rash. The disease is transmitted to the fetus through transplacental infestation.

The low incidence of rubella and related congenital anomalies is attributed to the availability of rubella vaccine since 1969. It is estimated that 5 to 15 percent of women of childbearing age are susceptible to rubella.

Subjective Data

The client reports a nonpruritic rash, fever, and a feeling of general malaise. She has no history of the disease or vaccination.

Objective Data

Postauricular and occipital lymphadenopathy is present early in process. Fever may range from 99.5 to 101.7°F, and conjunctival erythema (mild conjunctivitis) may be noted. The characteristic maculopapular rash starts on the face, spreads to the trunk, and disappears by the third day.

The diagnostic test used is hemagglutination inhibition (HI). A serum sample is obtained and sent for laboratory evaluation. Antibodies are usually not present in the serum until after the rash has developed. When confirmation of rubella infection is important, as it is in pregnancy, an HI antibody titer is drawn immediately after exposure to the virus and repeated in 2 to 3 weeks. An initial titer of 1:8 or less indicates absence of previous rubella infection. A fourfold rise in antibody titer in 2 to 3 weeks indicates infection. Prepare the client for repeat testing.

When rubella affects the fetus, it is termed *rubella syndrome*; defects of the eyes (cataracts, retinopathy, glaucoma), ears (degenerative changes in inner ear, hearing loss), and heart (patent ductus arteriosus, pulmonary artery stenosis) may result. Also associated with the syndrome are decreased head circumference, mental retardation, and poor childhood growth and language and motor development. Seizures related to encephalitis from central nervous system damage also may occur (Gershon, 2009).

Differential Medical Diagnoses

Rubeola, scarlet fever, drug reaction.

Plan

Ideally, all women have been vaccinated and have adequate immunity; however, it is recommended that all women be screened during the initial prenatal visit. Assessment of rubella status should be included in a preconception visit. If negative, vaccination should be done a minimum of 3 months prior to conception. Counsel clients who do not have adequate immunity to avoid situations in which they may come in contact with infected persons (CDC, 2010a). Vaccination is recommended during the immediate postpartum period. Breastfeeding is not a contraindication to vaccination (CDC, 2008).

If active disease occurs during the first trimester, counsel the client concerning the risks to her fetus. Support her decision to continue or terminate the pregnancy.

VARICELLA ZOSTER (CHICKEN POX)

Varicella zoster is usually acquired during childhood and 95 percent of adults have immunity (Plourd & Austin, 2005). Varicella is a member of the herpes virus family and, like herpes, varicella can lay dormant in the dorsal root ganglia and reactivate later. Less than 10 percent of occurrences are in individuals over 10 years of age. It is a common benign childhood disease that can be more serious in adulthood. In pregnant women, the severity of the disease may be further increased, particularly if there is pulmonary involvement. Once an individual is infected, immunity is usually lifelong. Therefore, varicella is rare in pregnancy; 95 percent of pregnant women have antibodies to varicella-zoster virus (VZV). Immunization is available and may be used prior to conception if indicated.

Epidemiology

Pregnant women are at risk for developing varicella when they come in close physical contact with children who have active infection. The virus is transmitted through direct contact with respiratory tract secretions with an incubation period of 10 to 15 days. Individuals are infectious the 24 hours prior to the rash until all cutaneous lesions have crusted (Daley, Thorpe, & Garland, 2008). According to the CDC (2011f), although complications with varicella are rare, they include skin infections, swelling of the brain, and pneumonia. Maternal pneumonia complicates approximately 10 to 20 percent of cases of varicella, with resulting higher morbidity/mortality than nonpregnant women (Gardella & Brown, 2007).

The incidence of congenital varicella syndrome varies according to the gestational age when the acquisition of varicella occurs. No cases of congenital varicella syndrome have been reported after 28 weeks' gestation (Tan & Koren, 2006). Varicella infection in the first two trimesters of pregnancy results in intrauterine infection in 25 percent of the reported cases and congenital anomalies are seen in 12 percent of infected fetuses (Lamont et al., 2011).

Subjective Data

The client reports fever, malaise, and a generalized pruritic rash predominantly on the trunk. Usually, her history reveals exposure during the previous 2 weeks.

Objective Data

Physical examination of the client reveals a characteristic rash. Fluid from the vesicles may be examined for diagnosis and several antibody tests performed.

Initially, nonspecific symptoms such as headache, malaise, and fever may be present. This phase is followed by a pruritic maculopapular rash that becomes vesicular and then crusts over (Lamont et al., 2011). Prenatal infection can lead to varicella embryopathy or varicella in the newborn. Congenital anomalies associated with varicella are limb atrophy, microencephaly, cortical atrophy, motor and sensory manifestations, and eye problems such as cataracts, chorioretinitis, microphthalmia, and Horner's syndrome.

Diagnostic methods include clinical evaluation of the virus isolated from vesicular fluid. Serologic tests may help document an acute infection. Several antibody tests are also used to detect infection: latex agglutination, ELISA, fluorescent antibody against membrane antigen (UpToDate, 2011c).

Medical Differential Diagnoses

Rubella, rubeola.

Plan

Psychosocial Interventions. Focus on identifying women who are at risk prior to or shortly after exposure to the virus. Counsel any woman who has been exposed and has not previously had the infection to be tested for VZV antibody.

The primary care provider must educate all pregnant women to avoid situations in which they may come in contact with varicella. When infection does occur, women require instructions on how to avoid spread of infection and how to relieve the discomforts of skin eruptions.

Medication. Medication is given for symptomatic relief of pruritic; acetaminophen is given to control fever. For severe varicella infection in pregnancy involving pneumonia and high fever, IV acyclovir may be recommended. Acyclovir has demonstrated safety and can be used in all trimesters of pregnancy.

Pregnant women who are at risk for severe disease or have been exposed to varicella may receive VariZIG, after receiving informed consent (CDC, 2007). VariZIG is a purified human immune globulin and must be administered within 96 hours of exposure.

Immunization. Women of reproductive age should be assessed for varicella immunity prior to pregnancy and offered the vaccine, Varivax (a live attenuated vaccine given in two doses 4 to 8 weeks apart). Pregnancy should be avoided for a minimum of 1 month following the last vaccination. Effects of the varicella virus on the fetus are unknown; therefore, pregnant women should not be vaccinated (CDC, 2007).

Other Interventions. Institute measures to prevent the spread of infection. Isolate the client until the rash has disappeared, which is usually about 7 days. Take respiratory and skin precautions if the client is in labor and in the hospital. Following delivery, she should be isolated with her neonate in a private room.

CYTOMEGALOVIRUS

Cytomegalovirus (CMV) is a DNA virus that is widely spread throughout the human population and can be transmitted to others during primary infection, reinfection, or reactivation (Griffiths, 2009). Congenital infection is different from perinatal infection. Congenital CMV infection is the most common intrauterine infection and the leading infectious cause of mental retardation and sensorineural hearing loss (Yinon, Farine, & Yudin, 2010). Acute congential effects of the neonate include hepatosplenomegaly, thrombocytopenia, hepatitis with jaundice, and/or anemia.

Epidemiology

The etiology of congenital disease involves in utero infection. Congenital CMV infection results from hepatogenous dissemination of virus across the placenta secondary to primary maternal CMV infection. In women, the likelihood of seropositivity has been correlated with low socioeconomic status, older age, multigravidity, large number of sexual partners, and a first pregnancy before age 15. Women who fit these criteria are at most risk for primary CMV infection. Perinatal CMV is acquired through intrapartum exposure to secretions or postpartum exposure to CMV in breast milk or blood transfusions.

Pregnant women acquire active disease mostly from sexual contact, blood transfusions, and contact with children in daycare centers. Reactivation of previous infection can also occur and cause congenital CMV. The estimates of prevalence in the developed world of congenital CMV range between 0.6 and 0.7 percent of all infants (Lombardi, Garofoli, & Stronati, 2010). In women who acquire primary disease during pregnancy, 40 percent of those infants will be affected (Revello & Gerna, 2004).

Subjective Data

Most women with primary infections are asymptomatic. Women may, however, report flu-like symptoms, including myalgia, chills, and malaise (CDC, 2011a).

Objective Data

Lymphadenopathy and hepatosplenomegaly may be present. Blood work demonstrates leukocytosis and lymphocytosis; liver function tests are elevated. Diagnosis is most often made by means of antibody tests, including HI, ELISA, and fluorescent antibody. Serologic testing is key in determining maternal infection. Primary infection is confirmed when seroconversion is documented through the appearance of virus-specific IgG in the serum of pregnant women who previously tested negative. When CMV status prior to pregnancy is unknown, the determination of primary infection is made with the detection of specific IgM antibodies. In order to distinguish between primary and reincurrent infection, the IgG avidity assay may be useful. A high avidity IgG antibody is detected only in recurrent or remote infection (Yinon et al., 2010).

Differential Medical Diagnoses

Mononucleosis, HIV disease.

Plan

No therapy prevents or treats CMV infection. Screening for CMV using cervical cultures or blood tests is not recommended. Women with documented active infection during pregnancy may elect termination of their pregnancy, depending on the gestational age. Discuss the risks and be sensitive to the client's concerns and anxiety. A live attenuated vaccine has been developed, but concerns exist about the ability of the virus to reactivate when shed through the cervix or during breastfeeding. The vaccine is yet to be recommended (ACOG Practice Bulletin, 2001a, reaffirmed 2009).

Teaching all pregnant women about good hygiene and hand washing helps decrease the spread of disease. Advise pregnant women to avoid exposure to individuals with CMV infection (e.g., persons with AIDS). Explain that CMV may be sexually transmitted and advise the use of condoms and limiting sexual partners as strategies that reduce the transmission of the infection.

PARVOVIRUS B19 OR ERYTHEMA INFECTIOSUM (FIFTH DISEASE)

Human parvovirus B19 may display as erythema infectiosum or fifth's disease or "slapped face syndrome" (Lamont et al., 2010). When acute infection occurs during pregnancy, particularly before 18 weeks of gestation, fetal infection and stillbirth are possible.

Epidemiology

The prevalence of infection among pregnant women and fetuses is not known. What is known is that in North America, approximately 65 percent of pregnant women have evidence of past infection. During pregnancy, infection with parvovirus B19 is mostly asymptomatic and causes no harm to the fetus (Lamont et al., 2010). Infection is spread transplacentally, by oropharyngeal route in casual contact, and through infected blood components.

The most significant effect of human parvovirus on the fetus is the occurrence of fetal hydrops. The hydrops develops as a result of aplastic anemia secondary to the viral infection and subsequent congestive heart failure (Markenson & Yancey, 1998). The incidence of hydrops varies from 0 to 38 percent, with most researchers reporting 15 to 27 percent (ACOG Practice Bulletin, 2001a, reaffirmed 2009; Markenson & Yancey, 1998).

Schoolteachers, daycare workers, and women living with school-age children are at highest risk for being seropositive for parvovirus B19, especially if a recent outbreak has occurred in those settings. These women may benefit from a baseline serologic test to determine their susceptibility to infection. There is no antiviral therapy for parvovirus B19 infection (Staroselsky, Klieger-Grossmann, Garcia-Bournissen, & Koren, 2009). Prevention is the best strategy and includes routine hand washing when handling children, cleaning of toys and hard surfaces in contact with infected children, and avoiding the sharing of food or drinks (McCarter-Spaulding, 2002).

Subjective Data

A client may report a facial rash and sometimes arthritic pain of the hands, wrists, and knees.

Objective Data

The most characteristic sign of parvovirus B19 infection is the slapped-face rash, a macular rash that may also be found on the trunk. The rash may have a lacelike pattern on the trunk. The rash may subside only to return in response to stress, exercise, sunlight, or bathing.

Maternal viremia peaks 1 week after infection when infection occurs. Mild fever, athralgia, and headache may occur 10 to 14 days after exposure in approximately 50 percent of the women who have parvovirus B19 infection. If the IgM is positive, indicating maternal infection, the fetus should be monitored weekly by ultrasound examination for the development of hydrops fetalis until 20 weeks' postexposure (de Jong, Walther, Kroes, & Oepkes, 2011).

Medical Differential Diagnoses

Rubella, rubeola, roseola, scarlet fever.

Plan

Sonography. A level II sonogram should be done in any woman with suspicion of parvovirus infection. Serial sonograms should be ordered after acute infection to monitor for the occurrence of hydrops. The health care provider should share what information is available and be sensitive to the client's concerns.

TOXOPLASMOSIS

Toxoplasmosis is a common infectious disease caused by the intracellular protozoan parasite *Toxoplasma gondii*. Primary infection during pregnancy is associated with stillbirth or congenital infection. Symptoms usually appear at birth. About 10 percent of infected infants manifest severe disease characterized by chorioretinitis, cyanosis, pneumonia, hepatosplenomegaly, jaundice, and thrombocytopenia purpura. Infants who survive sustain some permanent neurological damage.

Epidemiology

Risk factors for maternal infection include eating raw or undercooked meats and living in rural areas.

Usual transmission is through ingestion of tissue cysts in contaminated meat or through contact with oocytes in feces of infected cats or farm animals, or eating unwashed fruit, berries, or vegetables with contagious oocytes on their surface. Chances of transplacental transmission to the fetus increases depending upon when the acute maternal infection occurs. The risk of transmission greatly increases with gestational age and is estimated to be as high as 71 percent at 36 weeks (SYROCOT, Thiebaut, Leproust, Chêne, & Gilbert, 2007). Any history of maternal infection affords permanent immunity. Spontaneous abortion, stillbirth, or severe congenital infection occurs in 10 to 15 percent of pregnancies complicated with toxoplasmosis. Serious congenital infection is more likely to occur when maternal infection occurs in the third trimester.

Women who are positive for HIV or who are on immunosuppressive therapy following transplantation will be more susceptible to toxoplasmosis.

The overall incidence is 0.25 to 1.0 per 1,000 live births. In the United States, it is estimated that 22.5 percent of the population, 12 years of age or older, has been infected with *T. gondii* (CDC, 2011c).

Subjective Data

Although most women are asymptomatic, the client may report fatigue, fever, rash, depression, malaise, headache, and sore throat. Infection occurs 1 to 2 weeks after exposure, and the client may remain symptomatic for as long as several months.

Objective Data

Physical examination reveals lymph node enlargement, particularly in the posterior cervical chain.

Diagnosis is made by means of serial toxoplasma antibody tests (two or more) done 3 weeks apart. The second sample shows significantly higher levels of antibodies if active infection is present. An indirect fluorescent antibody test of 1:512 or greater correlates with active infection. Recently, testing for toxoplasma DNA in amniotic fluid has been used to determine presence of fetal infection. Ultrasound is also used to detect findings such as intracranial calcifications, intrauterine growth retardation, microcephaly, neonatal ascites, hepatosplenomegaly, and cardiomegaly, which can all be associated with toxoplasmosis infection (ACOG Practice Bulletin, 2001a, reaffirmed 2009).

Some countries screen all pregnant women for toxoplasmosis during the initial prenatal visit. That is not currently an acceptable approach in the United States.

Differential Medical Diagnosis

Infectious mononucleosis.

Plan

Psychosocial Interventions. Educate prenatal clients about the risk of toxoplasmosis and discuss prevention. Advise pregnant women to avoid handling cat litter, to wear gloves when gardening, to always wash their hands well after handling cats, and to avoid eating undercooked or raw meats. Prevention of disease is the key to management.

Medications. Pregnant women diagnosed with toxoplasmosis during the first 18 weeks should be treated with spiramycin (Montoya & Remington, 2008). The effectiveness of treatment, however, remains controversial. If fetal infection is confirmed after 18 weeks, sulfadiazine, pyrimethamine, and folinic acid are given together to treat the fetus (ACOG Practice Bulletin, 2001a, reaffirmed 2010; Montoya & Remington, 2008). Pyrimethamine should be avoided in the first trimester as it is teratogenic in animals when given in large doses. Azithromycin or clarithromycin may be an alternative to spiramycin to prevent in utero infection, but large clinical trials are necessary to study this potential treatment option (Montoya & Remington, 2008). Treatment of infection in the fetus has shown to improve clinical outcomes (ACOG Practice Bulletin, 2001a, reaffirmed 2010; Montoya & Remington, 2008).

A newborn whose mother was treated antenatally for toxoplasmosis should be treated prophylactically with a combination of pyrimethamine and sulfadiazine (antimalarial drug). An infant with symptoms or an asymptomatic infant with positive cerebrospinal fluid should also be treated.

HUMAN IMMUNODEFICIENCY VIRUS*

HIV is the virus that can lead to acquired immunodeficiency syndrome (AIDS), which is a severe immune-suppressed state. The CDC (2011b) estimates that about 56,000 people in the United States contracted HIV in 2006. HIV destroys specific red blood cells (RBCs), called CD4+ T cells, which are critical to helping the body fight disease. Pregnancy does not appear to accelerate the progression of HIV to AIDS and/or death. In an observational cohort study, where a group of HIV-positive pregnant women were given a highly active antiretroviral therapy during pregnancy, it appeared that the progression of the disease actually slowed. More research is needed to determine the potential underlying biologic mechanisms (Tai et al., 2007). The CDC definition of AIDS is an HIV-infected person with a specific opportunistic infection or a CD4 count less than 200 mm.

Epidemiology

Historically, HIV/AIDS was a disease of homosexual males. Now, the incidence of HIV/AIDS has increased in women. In 2009, there were an estimated 11,200 new HIV infections among women in the United States (CDC, 2011b). Women comprised 51 percent of the U.S. population and 23 percent of those newly infected with HIV, that year. Of the total number of new HIV infections in U.S. women, 57 percent were in blacks, 21 percent were in whites, and 16 percent were in Hispanics/Latinas. The rate of new HIV infections among black women was 15 times that of white women, and over 3 times the rate among Hispanic/Latina women in 2009. Most HIV infections in the United States are HIV-1, but HIV-2 is endemic in other countries such as Africa.

An estimated 7,000 infants are born to HIV-infected women in the United States each year. Most cases of infant HIV infection are due to perinatal transmission. The chances of a woman having an infant who has HIV infection varies from 5 to 60 percent with an average of 20 to 30 percent. The large variance reported in transmission statistics relates to advances in treatment being developed over the short time that women are beginning to be represented in the HIV-positive population. Using prenatal drug treatment has been able to decrease vertical transmission from 25 percent to less than 2 percent (CDC, 2011b). Vertical transmission is affected by the viral load of the mother, status of the maternal immune system, route of delivery, general health of the fetus, presence of maternal infection, and exposure to genital secretions. Usually, the greater the viral load of the mother, the more likely that vertical transmission of the virus will occur (Public Health Service Task Force [PHSTF], 2002). Women with AIDS and a suppressed immune system are more likely to transmit the virus to the fetus. A first twin during vaginal delivery also has increased risk to contract the virus because of its longer exposure to cervical/vaginal secretions. Any delivery complication such as forceps delivery, lacerations, or episiotomy adds to fetal risk for the same reason. Placental vasculitis (chorioamnionitis) facilitates the spread of the virus.

HIV infection is acquired by sexual contact, exposure to blood or bodily fluids, vertical transmission to the fetus, perinatal exposure at delivery, and breastfeeding. Most women with AIDS have acquired the disease through heterosexual contact, and a majority of those women are mothers. Pregnancy rates among women infected with HIV remain high. The implications to discuss this disease in women's and infants' health are obvious.

The relationship between pregnancy and HIV infection is difficult to separate because so many of the women with HIV/AIDs have other risks associated with complications of pregnancy. Many of these women affected by HIV also have problems with drug addiction, lack of access to prenatal care, inadequate nutrition, poverty, and increased incidence of sexually transmitted diseases. Considering these factors, women affected by HIV also have increased risk for preterm delivery, premature rupture of membranes, intrauterine growth retardation, postpartum endometritis, and increased perinatal mortality (PHSTF, 2002).

The risk of acquiring HIV through heterosexual contact is greater for women because semen has high concentration of the virus, and coitus causes more breaks in the vaginal lining as compared to the penile skin. The presence of other genital infections also increases those chances.

Subjective Data

Most people remain asymptomatic after exposure to the virus. Within the first few months of being infected, many persons experience an acute viral infection similar

*Refer to Chapter 15 for a more complete discussion of HIV/AIDS.

to mononucleosis with complaints such as weight loss, fever, night sweats, pharyngitis, rash, and lymphadenopathy. These symptoms resolve within a few weeks and are frequently not perceived by the client as significant.

The woman may experience several episodes of discrete illnesses such as weight loss or an infection with a definitive beginning and end. Once the symptoms subside, the woman returns to a prediagnosis level of function. At some point, these illnesses become chronic and, even though controlled, are not cured. Usually, at this time the woman is on prophylaxis drug therapy. The symptoms experienced at this point are varied and reflect which organ systems are most affected by the virus. Common symptoms include dyspnea and fatigue, decreased muscle strength, cramping pain in the extremities, nausea and vomiting, and recurrent vaginal yeast infections (Holzemer, 2002). Because these are also common complaints associated with pregnancy, identifying onset of illness may be difficult.

Objective Data

HIV infection can be diagnosed by serologic tests that detect antibodies against HIV. See Chapters 3, 15, and 19 for more information about testing and screening. Refer to Chapter 15 for more detailed information on monitoring status of HIV.

Differential Medical Diagnosis

Refer to Chapter 15.

Plan

Prevention. In February 1994, the National Institutes of Health (NIH) announced findings of a study sponsored by the Pediatric AIDS Clinical Trials Group (PACTG), which found that administering zidovudine (AZT) during pregnancy, labor, and delivery and during the neonatal period reduced perinatal transmission of HIV by two thirds. Epidemiological studies have confirmed this finding (PHSTF, 2002). Women with advanced HIV disease or previous antiretroviral therapy were not included in this study. The PACTG recommended the development of national policies and protocols for the counseling and screening of all pregnant women (PHSTF, 2002). Since then, much effort by governmental agencies, professional groups, and concerned citizens has occurred to educate women about this potential preventive strategy. Currently, the NIH has a HIV/AIDS Guidelines Portal that provides guidelines on a multitude of issues related to HIV/AIDS to offer up-to-date and evidence-based information. These guidelines are available at http://www.aidsinfo.nih.gov/default.aspx.

Prenatal Screening. It is the recommendation of the USPSTF (2011) that all pregnant women be screened for HIV. However, screening is optional and not mandatory. It may be either opt-in or opt-out. Opt-out testing is where HIV testing is automatically a part of routine prenatal testing. The client must ask to not be tested and sign a form refusing HIV testing (Branson et al., 2006; U.S. Department of Health and Human Services, 2012). Women who are seropositive for HIV should be counseled about the risk of perinatal transmission and potential for obstetric complications. A discussion of the options on continuing the pregnancy, medication, risks, perinatal outcomes, and treatments is warranted.

Prenatal Care. Women affected by HIV warrant comprehensive prenatal care that can be provided by the local obstetrical care delivery system. Community-based care with appropriate consultation and guidance from the appropriate referral center is preferred. The usual screening tests for normal pregnancy should be done. Screening for gonorrhea; chlamydia; herpes; hepatitis B, C, and D; and syphilis is particularly important. Testing for antibody to CMV and toxoplasmosis is also recommended (CDC, 2006). If not routinely done for the normal pregnant women in the prenatal setting, a tuberculin skin test with follow-up chest x-ray is indicated for the woman who is HIV positive. Vaccinations for hepatitis B, pneumococcal infection, hemophilus B influenza, and viral influenza should be done to offer protection from opportunistic infections. Close scrutiny and follow-up of suspicious Pap smear results are prudent because of the increased risk of cervical changes associated with HPV and HIV (UpToDate, 2011b).

Newborn Screening. It is recommended that HIV testing be done at 14 to 21 days and 1 to 2 months, and again at 4 to 6 months using virologic HIV tests. HIV antibody tests are not used because newborns will carry their mothers' antibodies to HIV for up to 18 months (U.S. Department of Health and Human Services, 2012).

Medication. There is not one best medication regimen that works for everyone. The choice of medications used to treat HIV in pregnancy and postpartum will depend on several factors. These factors include the woman's state of health and stage of HIV infection, CD4 count, other comorbidities such as hepatitis B infection, and personal preference (U.S. Department of Health and Human

Services, 2012). When to start the medication in pregnancy will depend on why the medication is being used. If the pregnant woman needs the medication for her own health, then treatment should begin right away; otherwise, it might be recommended that she wait until the second trimester of pregnancy. See Chapter 15 for more information about current available antiretroviral agents.

It is beyond the scope of this chapter to adequately address the various medication options and which are recommended in pregnancy. Guidelines have been developed by a panel of experts to provide guidance to health care providers on the optimal use of antiretroviral agents in pregnant women. These guidelines developed through the NIH, AIDS*info* (2012) can be accessed online at http://www.aidsinfo.nih.gov/guidelines/html/3/perinatal-guidelines/0/.

Physical Concerns. Fatigue or decreased physical endurance has been identified by HIV-positive clients and their caregivers as a major health care problem. Exercise has been proposed as a strategy to increase endurance and improve mental outlook. Direct positive effect on the immune system has been theorized but as yet has not been demonstrated. Effects of exercise, including prenatal exercises and prepared childbirth, have not been studied for their effects on the HIV-positive pregnant woman.

Psychosocial Issues. Women living with HIV/AIDS have to deal with many challenges (see Chapter 15). When the diagnosis of HIV positive is made, the woman is usually not symptomatic. Therefore, the woman is likely to react with denial. Because of this denial, discussions about planning for the future, accepting preventive treatment for perinatal transmission, and reducing the transmission of HIV to present partners are difficult. Previous experience and general mental health will attribute to the women's ability to cope with the disease and/or the pregnancy. With the emphasis on prenatal screening, many women have to deal with an initial diagnosis of a chronic and potentially fatal disease as well as with stressors of a pregnancy. Those women who abuse drugs are even more difficult to help because of the nature of their lifestyle, which is usually disorganized and without adequate family or community support.

The national AIDS hotline (1-800-342-AIDS) is an excellent source of information for clients and providers. Information for women with HIV/AIDS who need care but can't afford it or need help locating a case manager is available through the Ryan White HIV/AIDS Foundation (2011).

Education/Counseling. The HIV-positive pregnant woman will need education concerning infection control issues at home, safer-sex precautions, stages of the HIV disease, and treatment modalities at these various stages. She will need information about the preventive drug therapies for her unborn child. Much national attention supported with federal funds has been spent to disseminate the prevention of HIV message.

Delivery. Women with unknown HIV status at time of delivery should be offered rapid HIV testing using an opt-out approach (CDC, 2006). The risk of transmission of HIV from mother to child is low for women who take anti-HIV medications during pregnancy and have a viral load near the time of delivery of less than 1,000 copies/mL (U.S. Department of Health and Human Services, 2012). A scheduled cesarean delivery may be the recommended delivery option for women who have not received anti-HIV medications and have a viral load greater than 1,000 copies/mL. It has been shown that the risk of HIV transmission increases when the fetal membranes have been ruptured more than 4 hours before delivery, which may attribute to lower transmission rates in cesarean births. For that reason, fetal membranes should remain intact until delivery. Efforts to reduce instrumentation such as avoiding use of episiotomy, fetal scalp electrodes, and scalp pH assessment are necessary to decrease the newborn's exposure to maternal vaginal secretions and blood.

Newborn. Babies born to women who are HIV positive should receive anti-HIV medication in the nucleoside reverse transcriptase inhibitor class such as AZT (U.S. Department of Health and Human Services, 2012). This medication is started within 6 to 12 hours of birth and continues for 6 weeks.

Breastfeeding. HIV can be transmitted through breast milk. In the United States, infant formula is a safe alternative to breastfeeding. Therefore, it is recommended that HIV-positive mothers in the United States not breastfeed and use formula instead (NIH, AIDS*info*, 2012) (see Chapter 22).

Postpartum Contraception. In some groups, rates of pregnancy in HIV-affected women are high. Reasons women continue to be at risk for pregnancy are complex and multifactorial. Reasons include denial of illness and its meaning, positive secondary gains related to the pregnancy, perception of the low risk of transmission to the child, ethical and cultural beliefs about contraception and conception, lack of access to health care including family planning services, or the inability to negotiate with partner for safer-sex practices including pregnancy prevention practices. For the woman who is also abusing drugs, pregnancy may be a low priority issue for her. Intrauterine devices (IUDs) are usually not advised in these women because of the risk of pelvic infection. All other contraceptive methods are viable options with emphasis that latex condoms should be used in addition to reduce transmission to the partner. Surgical sterilization may be desired and should be discussed. Contraceptive services including sterilization should be available and affordable. Important to any discussion of contraception regarding HIV-affected women is sensitivity to the woman's choice. The provider's responsibility is to ensure that the client makes an informed decision based upon current knowledge. Even though effective contraception seems to be logical for the provider, directive counseling on contraception, especially sterilization, is inappropriate.

Legal Issues. Because of the previous documented discrimination that has occurred in HIV-positive persons, maintaining confidentiality is critical to the woman and her family. Legal issues regarding a positive HIV include insurance coverage, job security, documentation policies, state testing and reporting protocols, and guardianship of surviving children. The provider must maintain current knowledge of local laws and policies that affect the health care of the HIV-affected woman and her newborn. Referral to community legal services is appropriate.

SEXUALLY TRANSMITTED DISEASES AFFECTING PREGNANCY

Many sexually transmitted infections, including HIV, are known to have fatal or severely debilitating effects on the fetus.Table 20–1 summarizes the infections most commonly faced by providers in prenatal care. For early treatment and prevention of vertical transmission, screening for many sexually transmitted diseases is done at the initial prenatal visit. Refer to Chapter 14 for a more detailed discussion of these diseases and their impact on women's health.

PYELONEPHRITIS

Acute pyelonephritis in pregnancy is a common renal disorder defined as the presence of actively multiplying bacteria in the upper urinary tract. It usually, although not always, follows a previous asymptomatic bacteriuria (ASB). *Escherichia coli* is the most common organism for ASB.

Epidemiology

There are many physiologic changes of pregnancy that contribute to an increase in urinary tract infections. In normal pregnancy, there is ureteral and renal calyceal dilatation thought to be due to the relaxation properties of progesterone. The enlarging uterus compresses the ureters and ureteral peristalsis slows. There is incomplete emptying of the bladder due to compression from the uterus and decreased detrusor tone. In addition, due to increases in glomerular filtration, there are elevations in urinary glucose and an alkalization of the urine that facilitates bacterial growth. All of these factors contribute to the increased incidence of urinary tract infections in pregnancy (Jolly & Wing, 2010).

Acute pyelonephritis is the most common nonobstetrical reason for antepartum admissions (Jolly & Wing, 2010). Ascension of bacteria to the kidney will lead to pyelonephritis. Effects on the mother include bacterial endotoxemia leading to endotoxin shock and acute renal dysfunction leading to acute renal failure. Pyelonephritis in pregnancy has been reported to be associated with small-for-gestational age babies and preterm delivery, but recent studies have not corroborated that finding. Transient renal dysfunction, pulmonary insufficiency, septicemia, and anemia are all associated with pyelonephritis in pregnancy (Hill, Sheffield, McIntire, & Wendel, 2005).

Subjective Data

Maternal symptoms include fever, shaking chills, malaise, flank pain, nausea and vomiting, headache, increased urinary frequency, and dysuria. Symptoms of mild cough to severe respiratory distress syndrome are present when severe cases lead to pulmonary dysfunction.

Objective Data

Traditionally, all pregnant women are screened by urine culture on the initial prenatal visit and monitored throughout pregnancy with a dipstick method for presence of nitrites.

For the symptomatic woman, a urine culture is necessary. Bacteriuria, with pyuria and white blood cell casts, will be present in urine examination. A count of 1 to 2 bacteria per high power field in spun urine or more than 20 bacteria in the sediment of a centrifuged specimen of urine collected by bladder catheterization is diagnostic. Hematuria may be present. Urine culture is necessary for diagnosis and determination of causative agent. Determining the causative agent is important in monitoring

TABLE 20–1. Sexually Transmitted Diseases Affecting Pregnancy

Organism	Incidence in Pregnancy	Effect on Pregnancy	Medications	Other Concerns
Herpes simplex virus (HSV)	About 20% of the female population have been diagnosed with HSV and about 2% of women acquire HSV during pregnancy. Infants born to women infected with HSV have a 30–60% chance of acquiring infection. Infants with skin, eye, and mouth infection showed no mortality, but more seriously affected infants with systemic infection have a 60% mortality.	The same painful vesicular lesions appear as in the nonpregnant client. Initial viremia in the first trimester of pregnancy is frequently associated with spontaneous abortion. Not all infants born through an infected birth canal become infected; in fact, most infected infants are not born to women with a history of herpes genitalis. Perinatal transmission is more likely if the initial infection is near the time of delivery. Infants manifest HSV in localized form by lesions on the skin, eyes, or oral cavity. In more severe systemic forms shown by lethargy, poor feeding, fever, irritability, convulsions, jaundice, apnea, shock, and possible death.	Oral and topical acyclovir has been used. Usual regimen is 200 mg orally five times/day for 7–10 days until lesions resolve. Hospitalization for intravenous administration of acyclovir or valacyclovir has been used to decrease chances of infant becoming infected or treat life-threatening maternal infections including encephalitis, pneumonitis, or hepatitis. Some HSV experts recommend prophylactic therapy using acyclovir, valacyclovir, or famciclovir starting at 36 weeks, but definitive evidence as to the risks to the fetus is still inconclusive.	Instructions for the client include symptomatic relief measures as nonpregnant women. Cool perineal compressors, sitz baths, loose-fitting clothes help to alleviate pain. Cesarean delivery is not necessary for every client with a history of herpes: Only recommended when active lesions are present. Infants born through an HSV-infected birth canal should be monitored carefully for neonatal complications. Women need to be instructed to avoid intercourse in the third trimester with partners known or suspected of having HSV. Viral cultures collected during pregnancy are not able to predict viral shedding at delivery. Thus, routine cultures on women with a history of HSV are not recommended. Breastfeeding is allowed if contact with the active lesions is avoided.
Syphilis (*Treponema pallidum*)	40–50% of infants of infected mothers contract congenital syphilis. 20.6 congenital syphilis cases per 100,000 live births in 1998.	Syphilis unaltered by course of pregnancy. Chancre often unnoticed and/or internal and not diagnosed during pregnancy. Treponemas cross placenta as early as 9 weeks of gestation, but fetal involvement rare prior to 18 weeks of gestation. Maternal infection increases risk of endarteritis, stromal hyperplasia, and immature villi. Increased risk of premature labor and birth. Congenital syphilis signs and symptoms: hepatosplenomegaly, osteochondritis, jaundice, rhinitis, anemia, lymphadenopathy, nervous system involvement, periostitis, ocular abnormalities, nonimmune hydrops, IUGR, pseudoparalysis of an extremity.	Benzathine penicillin G. Doseage and length of treatment depend on clinical manifestation and stage of the disease. No known alternative to penicillin treatment in pregnancy. Treat pregnant women with penicillin after desensitization.	All pregnant women should be screened in early pregnancy. Serologic test should be reported in third trimester in populations with high incidence or women at high risk. Infant diagnosed with congenital syphilis should be placed in isolation until treatment administered. All women infected with syphilis should be tested for HIV. Any woman who delivers a stillborn infant after 20 weeks' gestation should be tested for sypilis. No infant should leave the hospital without documentation of results of maternal syphilis test.
Gonorrhea (*Neissaeria gonorrhea*)	Estimated 700,000 cases a year in the United States	85% of infected women have no symptoms. Ophthalium neonatorum results from delivery through infected birth canal. Pelvic inflammatory disease is complication of gonorrhea infection.	Ceftriaxone, 125 mg IM in a single dose, *or* cefixime, 400 mg po in a single dose followed by presumptive treatment for chlamydia. Erythromycin base or stearate 500 mg po qid 3–7 days or erythromycin ethyisuccinate 800 mg po qid 3–7 days. Pregnant women who cannot tolerate a cephalosporin should receive spectinomycin 2 g IM (single dose).	Gonorrhea screening should be done at initial prenatal visit and repeated in the third trimester. Test of cure not recommended when using drug of choice and woman asymptomatic. Test for syphilis with positive gonorrhea. All states have mandated prophylaxis in the first hour of life. Newborn prophylaxis: Tetracycline or erythromycin ointments, silver nitrade ophthalmic drops, and penicillin GM have all been used as prophylaxis. Partners must be treated. Avoid coitus until both partners are cured.

(*Continued*)

TABLE 20–1. (Continued)

Organism	Incidence in Pregnancy	Effect on Pregnancy	Medications	Other Concerns
C Trachomatic (*Chlamydial cervicitis*)	Most common STD. Occurs in 5% of pregnant women with a range of 3–37%. More prevalent in adolescents and young women.	Frequently the woman is asymptomatic. It is a common cause of mucopurulent cervicitis. Chlamydial infection during pregnancy is associated with prematurity and stillbirth. Urinary tract infection caused by chlamydia untreated may progress to pyelonephritis. Infants born vaginally to infected women have a 10–20% chance of acquiring conjunctivitis. The newborn may also develop a pneumonia type of infection with congestion, wheezing, and cough up to 12 weeks of age. It may also cause a middle ear infection in the infant.	Tetracycline, doxycycline, ofloxann are contraindicated in pregnancy. Erythromycin 500 mg qid for 7 days (see Gonorrhea). Azithromycin 1g orally. Amoxicillin 500 mg tid for 7 days.	Fluoroquinolone resistance to *N. gonorrhea* is spreading in parts of Asia, the Pacific, and the U.S. west coast. If women, who have previously been diagnosed and treated with a recommended regimen, have recurrent symptoms; culture and sensitivity are necessary prior to further treatment. Treatment is essential for the sexual partner. Encouragement of abstinence during treatment is important to prevent reinfection. Treatment prior to delivery will eradicate maternal cervical chlamydial infection and prevent vertical transmission to the newborn. Many states mandate the use of erythromycin topical eye ointment within the first 1 hour of birth to prevent both gonorrhea and chlamydial infection. All women positive for chlamydia need to be screened for other STDs.
Trichomonas	Occurs in 20–30% of all pregnant women.	Women may experience diffuse, malodorous, yellow-green discharge or may be asymptomatic. Associated with premature rupture of membranes, preterm delivery, and low birth weight. Recent reports suggest association between any prenatal vaginal infections and preterm delivery.	Metronidazole 2 g initial treatment. Metronidazole 500 mg bid × 7 days. The treatment of asymptomatic trichomonas has not lessened poor outcomes. Avoidance of using metronidazole in the first trimester has been a common practice because of concern of teratogenicity. Recent multiple studies have not demonstrated that association.	Partners need treatment. Instruct the client to avoid sexual intercourse until she and her partner have completed therapy. Screening for trichomonas during pregnancy is not recommended but treatment of symptomatic women recommended.

Sources: ACOG Practice Bulletin, 2007a, 2007b, 2007c, 2007d; CDC, 2010b.

recurring episodes. Also, if the causative organism is group B streptococcus (GBS), intrapartum chemoprophylaxis is recommended to reduce neonatal group B streptococcal disease.

Differential Medical Diagnoses

Acute cystitis, urinary calculi, glomerulonephritis, labor, chorioamnionitis, appendicitis, abruptio placentae.

Plan

Prevention. The incidence of pyelonephritis can be significantly reduced by screening and treating ASB during prenatal visits. Acute pyelonephritis will occur in 25 percent of those women untreated for bacteriuria. Clean-catch urine cultures are recommended at the initial prenatal visit for all pregnant women. If on the client's initial prenatal visit, urine culture reveals > 100,000 organisms per millimeter, the client should be treated regardless of the presence of symptoms. It is important to do a repeat urine culture following treatment because 25 percent of women treated for bacteriuria will experience recurrence and 34 percent will develop acute pyelonephritits (Gilstrap & Ramin, 2001). For those women treated for bacteriuria during pregnancy, prophylaxis antibiotic maintenance may be ordered by some providers throughout the remainder of the pregnancy. Close monitoring and urine screening for all pregnant women at each routine prenatal visit are recommended.

Medication. The choice of antibiotics should be based on microbiology and susceptibility data. For the initial episode of pyelonephritis, a third-generation cephalosporin is the drug of choice (UpToDate, 2011d). In pregnancy, fluoroquinolones should be avoided. Antibiotic suppression is continued throughout the remainder of the pregnancy after an episode of pyelonephritis. Nitrofurantoin 100 mg once or twice daily is a common suppression regimen (Gilstrap & Ramin, 2001). Sulfa drugs need to be avoided in late pregnancy because of the increased risk of neonatal hyperbilirubinemia. Antipyretic agents are used as necessary for fever.

Hospitalization. Historically, all pregnant women with a diagnosis of pyelonephritis were admitted to the hospital for antibiotics and hydration. IV antibiotic therapy continued for 24 to 48 hours after the woman becomes afebrile, and costovertebral angle tenderness subsided. The complications, even though uncommon, are severe and can be life-threatening. Recently, outpatient protocols have been developed in an attempt to provide safe and effective outpatient care of these women. The outpatient model includes IV hydration, IV antibiotics, observation for 24 hours, and discharge once the woman is afebrile. Women with high-risk factors such as signs of sepsis, allergies, respiratory compromise, preterm labor (PTL), gestation greater than 37 weeks, history of substance abuse, or known fetal malformations are not recommended to be managed outside of the hospital (Wing, Hendershott, Debuque, & Millar, 1999). Most providers are continuing to manage pregnant women with initial hospitalization.

Postpartum. About 2 to 4 percent of women develop a lower urinary tract infection postdelivery secondary to factors such as birth trauma, expected bladder hypotonia, residual urine, catheterization, anesthesia, and vaginal examinations. Pyelonephritis can be a likely sequelae to these infections if not treated adequately. Antibiotic therapy for these infections continues for up to 10 days. Education of the new mother should include the importance of completing all medication to decrease incidence of recurrence. Because *E. coli* is the causative organism in most cases, sulfonamides, nitrofurantoin, ampicillin, or cephalosporins are used. Breastfeeding while taking sulfonamides is controversial; however, the risk of an adverse reaction is low in healthy full-term infants (see Chapter 22).

Women who experienced recurrent urinary tract infections or pyelonephritis during pregnancy need radiographic evaluation of the upper urinary tract 3 months postpartum to assess for structural abnormality. Urine for culture and sensitivity should be obtained at the routine postpartum visit.

INTRA-AMNIOTIC INFECTION

Intra-amniotic infection (IAI) is any infection within the intrauterine structures. Although in the past, the terms *chorioamnionitis* and *amnionitis* were used interchangeably, each is a specific diagnosis dependent on the structures affected. The conditions are frequently not detected until after delivery.

The organisms most often isolated from the amniotic fluid of infected women are gential mycoplasmas, anaerobes (including *Gardnerella vaginallis*), enteric gram-negative bacilli, and GBS (UpToDate, 2011a). How these organisms may affect PTL and neonatal sepsis is not clear. GBSs are currently the most common cause of sepsis and meningitis in neonates and young infants.

Perinatal Group B Streptococcal Disease

GBS is a leading cause of neonatal infection in the United States and a significant cause of maternal illness. GBS is a gram-positive bacterium that colonizes in the vagina and when present during pregnancy attributes to maternal and/or neonatal infection (Verani, McGee, & Schrag, 2010).

Epidemiology In most populations studied, from 10 to 30 percent of pregnant women were colonized with GBS in the vaginal or rectal areas. Colonization rates can differ among ethnic groups, geographic areas, and by age; however, rates are similar between pregnant and nonpregnant women. The incidence of GBS is higher in African American women and women under 20 years of age. The amniotic cavity usually protects the fetus from ascending pathogens; however, with rupture of the membranes and onset of labor, ascending infection from the lower genital tract can occur. Infants born to women who have positive GBS cultures prenatally have a significant increase in early onset disease compared to infants born to women whose prenatal cultures were negative (Verani et al., 2010).

The incidence of neonatal sepsis is only 1 to 2 percent; however, infection can be fatal or lead to permanent neurodevelopmental defect (Chandran et al., 2001; McKenna & Iams, 1998; Mitchell, Steffenson, Hogan, & Brooks, 1997). The origin of GBSs in the genital tract is unclear, but the gastrointestinal tract seems the likely source. Reinfection is common through either autoinfection or sexual intercourse.

Subjective Data Women with colonies of GBSs in the genital tract are asymptomatic. With IAI, however, the client may report vague symptoms of fever and malaise, usually in the third trimester after membranes have ruptured.

Objective Data Early diagnosis is difficult because symptoms do not occur until infection has progressed substantially and caused amniotis.

The earliest sign of infection is most likely fever. Uterine tenderness, foul-smelling amniotic fluid, maternal leukocytosis, and tachycardia are detected late in the infectious process.

Cultures can be done to isolate GBSs, but a minimum of 24 hours is needed for test results. Gram stains can provide immediate results but are not specific or reliable for GBSs (McKenna & Iams, 1998).

Differential Medical Diagnoses Pyelonephritis, bacterial vaginosis, gonorrhea.

Plan

Prevention. Research has focused on either inducing protective immunity in the neonate or eradicating colonization from the mother and/or neonate (chemoprophylaxis). Several vaccines to induce antibodies against GBS are being developed but currently no licensed vaccine is available (Verani et al., 2010).

Psychosocial Interventions. All pregnant women need education, especially in the third trimester, on the potential for GBS infection. They also need to be aware of risk factors and screening recommendations. It is unclear whether a woman who has had a child with neonatal sepsis is truly at risk during a subsequent pregnancy, but emotionally she is clearly at risk. Any history of neonatal sepsis can cause apprehension. The provider must recognize this and be sensitive to the client's concerns and questions.

Screening. In May 1996, the CDC in collaboration with the American College of Obstetricians and Gynecologists (ACOG) and the American Academy of Pediatrics released recommendations on the prevention of perinatal group B streptococcal disease. Both a screening-based and a risk factor–based approach have been appropriate. Studies over the past years have demonstrated a reduction in the incidence of neonatal group B streptococcal infection due to the more widespread usage of routine testing and prophylactic treatment (CDC, 2000a, 2000b; Schrag et al., 2000). A revision of the guidelines, which was released in 2002, recommended universal culture-based screening for all pregnant women at 35 to 37 weeks (CDC, 2002). The screening protocol is to obtain one or two swabs from the vaginal introitus and anorectum without using a speculum. Cervical cultures are not acceptable. Appropriate nonnutritive moist swab transport systems (e.g., Amies) are commercially available. Those women positive for GBS should be offered intrapartum penicillin. The other approach is to provide intrapartum chemoprophylaxis for women with risk factors without screening (Verani et al., 2010).

Medication. Antibiotic treatment of women who are colonized during prenatal screening is not effective in eliminating the organism or preventing neonatal disease. Antibiotic treatment prenatally is not recommended. IV penicillin or ampicillin is the drug of choice for intrapartum chemoprophylaxis in women with a documented positive culture for GBS (Verani et al., 2010). Women who are treated based upon risk factors include those who (1) had a previous infant with invasive GBS disease, (2) had GBS bacteriuria during current pregnancy, (3) are less than 37 weeks' gestation and GBS status is unknown, or (4) have temperature equal to or greater than 38°C (100.4°F) (ACOG Practice Bulletin, 2007c).

Delivery. Critical to the implementation of the CDC guidelines is the notification of staff caring for the woman during the intrapartum period. A positive prenatal screening for GBS needs to be clearly documented on the chart. The woman needs to be counseled to the importance of knowing her GBS status and, if positive, needs to know to communicate that to staff in the intrapartum unit. Neonatal colonization usually occurs at the time of delivery, but cesarean birth does not reduce the vertical transmission or infection rates. Presence or suspicion of GBS is not an indicator for surgical delivery.

Neonatal Follow-Up. Routine use of prophylactic antibiotic agents for infants born to mothers who received intrapartum prophylaxis is not recommended. For infants symptomatic of sepsis, several management approaches are being used. Close observation and assessment for sepsis is critical (Verani et al., 2010).

Implications for Providers. Clear documentation of any screening results and management plans is critical. Table 20–2 summarizes risks associated with GBS disease. Systems for communicating prenatal culture results to intrapartum providers and nursing staff must be established. Brochures have been developed by numerous

TABLE 20–2. Risks Associated With Delivering an Infant With Perinatal Group B Streptococcal Disease

Prenatal
< 20 years of age
African American ethnicity
Positive 35- to 37-week GBS culture
Previous delivery of GBS-infected neonate (early onset)
Treatment of GBS bacteriuria in current pregnancy
Intrapartal
Membrane rupture ≥ 18 hours
Fever ≥ 38°C (100.4°F)
< 37 weeks' gestation

Sources: Adapted from Verani et al., 2010, and Ungerer, Lincetto, McGuire, Saloojee, & Gulmezoglu, 2004.

public and private organizations to assist the provider to counsel and educate women and their families.

Implications for Parents. Women and their families need to be aware of the strategies for the early detection, treatment, and prevention of GBS transmission to the neonate. One volunteer organization, Group B Strep Association, has been formed to educate expectant parents about the implications of GBS on neonatal outcome.

BLEEDING

Bleeding during pregnancy is common and can be life-threatening. The March of Dimes (2011a) estimates that bleeding in early pregnancy occurs in 20 to 30 percent of all pregnancies. The amount of bleeding and the time it occurs determine the urgency and management plan.

SPONTANEOUS ABORTION

Spontaneous abortion is the termination of pregnancy before the point of fetal viability. Gestation should not be more than 20 weeks and conceptus should not weigh more than 500 g or be longer than 16.5 cm, crown to rump. *Miscarriage* is the lay term for spontaneous abortion.

Types of abortion are categorized according to signs and symptoms.

- A *threatened abortion* is possible pregnancy loss; however, pregnancy may continue without further problems. Slight bleeding usually occurs, and some uterine contractions are felt as abdominal cramping. Uterine size is compatible with dates, the cervical os is closed, and no products of conception are passed. Prognosis is unpredictable.
- An *inevitable abortion* is a pregnancy that cannot be salvaged. Moderate bleeding and moderate to severe uterine cramping occur, and the cervical os is dilated. Uterine size is compatible with dates. The products of conception are not passed. Prognosis is poor.
- In an *incomplete abortion*, some products of conception are passed. Moderate to severe uterine cramping and heavy bleeding occur. Uterine size is compatible with dates; the cervical os is dilated. Prognosis is poor.
- In a *complete abortion*, all products of conception are expelled. Bleeding may be minimal and uterine contractions have subsided. The uterus is normal prepregnancy size; the cervical os may be opened or closed.
- A *missed abortion* occurs when the embryo is not viable but is retained in utero for at least 6 weeks. Uterine contractions are absent. Bleeding may initially be absent, but spotting begins and later becomes heavier.
- *Habitual abortion* is the experience of three or more consecutive spontaneous abortions.

Epidemiology

A precise etiology of spontaneous abortion does not exist, but varied maternal and fetal factors are attributed to its incidence. There are many causes for spontaneous abortion and include endocrinologic, genetic, microbiologic, and anatomic aspects (Friebe & Arch, 2008).

Anatomic abnormalities of the reproductive tract are usually associated with abortion in the second trimester. Some chronic diseases, such as diabetes, nutritional deficiencies, renal diseases, and lupus erythematosus, also affect a woman's ability to maintain her pregnancy. Moreover, lifestyle practices, such as smoking, substance abuse, and exposure to environmental hazards, are related to early pregnancy loss. Incidence reports reveal that about 20 percent of all pregnant women experience some cramping and bleeding in early pregnancy. About one half of those women continue through an uneventful pregnancy; the other half suffer pregnancy loss.

Subjective Data

Varying degrees of vaginal bleeding, low back pain, abdominal cramping, and passage of products of conception are reported. Usually the severity of cramping progresses and a change is seen in the type of blood lost.

Many women in early pregnancy report spotting, a brown-red vaginal discharge that stains underwear or toilet tissue. Vaginal bleeding that becomes bright red is usually significant. The amount of bleeding is ascertained by the saturation of sanitary napkins and the frequency with which the napkins must be changed. Saturation of one sanitary napkin every hour is significant.

Objective Data

Data is established using categorizations based on the client's signs and symptoms and diagnostic test results.

Uterine size is less than the expected gestational size.

Fetal heart tones are reassuring and dictate a conservative management plan; their absence beyond the 10th week of gestation may indicate a missed abortion.

Cervix may be dilated and soft or products of conception noted at the os; bleeding may be seen.

Real-time sonography will determine the presence of an embryonic sac and detect fetal cardiac motion, which is reassuring and dictates a wait-and-see management approach. If the beta-subunit human chorionic gonadotropin (β-hCG) is greater than 1,000 mIU/mL and if the pregnancy is intrauterine, the gestational sac should be visualized by transvaginal ultrasound (Morin & Van den Hof, 2005). Transabdominal ultrasound of the gestational sac may not be visualized until the β-hCG reaches 6,000 mIU/mL. Absence of the embryonic sac in the uterus may indicate ectopic pregnancy and must be investigated further.

Serial β-hCG measurements scheduled at least 2 days apart correlate with appropriate rise in β-hCG. Blood is collected for each measurement and sent to the laboratory. Beta-hCG levels should double every 2 days in early pregnancy, peak at about 10 weeks, and then gradually decrease during the remainder of pregnancy. Doubling of levels every 2 days indicates viability and favorable prognosis (Cunningham et al., 2010). Failure of the β-hCG level to double is suspicious of ectopic pregnancy or abortion. Although the client requires no specific instructions for this test, waiting the 2 days between specimens may be distressing to her.

Differential Medical Diagnoses

Malignancy, cervicitis, ectopic pregnancy, gestational trophoblastic disease (hydatidiform mole).

Plan

Psychosocial Interventions. Provide information for the client and her partner throughout all phases of threatened or eventual abortion. Reasons for blood tests and sonograms should be openly discussed. Explain to the client that precautions of bed rest and/or pelvic rest will continue until an asymptomatic period of at least 48 hours has elapsed.

The health care provider should understand the many different responses to pregnancy loss. A response may be influenced by the value of the pregnancy to the client or couple, the desire for pregnancy, the length of gestation, history of other pregnancy losses, the couple's relationship, their social network and support, and religious beliefs. Expressions of anger directed toward the care provider are common. Sensitive listening, counseling, and anticipatory guidance are important to assist the woman and her family adjust to the pregnancy loss (refer to Chapter 13, Infertility).

Medication. In some cases, progesterone supplementation via vaginal suppositories has been used successfully for women with known luteal-phase defect associated with spontaneous abortion defect.

Specific Interventions. Threatened abortion requires conservative wait-and-see management, unless symptoms threaten the life of the mother. Bed rest is not shown to affect outcome in threatened abortion but is commonly prescribed. The client at home on bed rest and/or pelvic rest should be instructed to maintain adequate hydration and report ominous signs or symptoms. The client should be evaluated weekly in the health office to determine complete blood count (CBC), serial β-hCG levels, any signs of infection, or a missed abortion.

- Bed rest requires that the woman be away from her job, have limited or no childcare responsibilities at home, and rest in a horizontal position, except when bathing or using the toilet.
- Pelvic rest means no sexual intercourse; no douching or inserting anything into the vagina.
- Instructions for hydration are to drink a minimum of 32 oz of noncaffeinated fluid every 24 hours.
- Clients are taught the signs and symptoms of infection and how uterine contractions and vaginal bleeding may progress.

Inevitable, incomplete, or missed abortion should be treated more aggressively as soon as a definitive diagnosis is made. To prevent infection and uterine hemorrhage, the uterus should be emptied of all products of conception. Dilatation of the cervix can be achieved through insertion of laminaria and aspiration of the products of conception. Use of prostaglandin vaginal tablets is an effective alternative (Rogers & Worley, 2011). If some products of conception remain in the uterus as evidenced by cramping and bleeding, enlarged and/or soft uterus, or fever, suction curettage is recommended. Removal of necrotic decidua decreases the incidence of postabortion bleeding and shortens the recovery period.

Missed abortion usually progresses to inevitable abortion, but a wait-and-see approach can be emotionally intolerable for some women. In such cases, suction curettage is recommended during the first trimester. In the second trimester, dilatation and evacuation may be performed or labor may be induced with an intravaginal prostaglandin E_2 suppository. Some primary care providers use a laminaria to dilate the cervix overnight prior to the procedure, thereby facilitating a less stressful dilatation procedure. For some women, delaying the definitive diagnosis and treatment plan is necessary to help them accept the situation emotionally.

Follow-Up

Instruct the client about the danger signs of infection or incomplete evacuation of the uterus: fever, foul-smelling lochia, excessive bleeding, back or abdominal pain. The Rh factor should be assessed and immunoglobulin administered to Rh-negative, unsensitized women.

Inform the client that she will need to use contraception for at least 4 to 6 months to allow for complete maternal healing and regeneration of endometrial lining. Advise her to have a gynecological exam within 2 to 3 weeks of the abortion.

If a woman has had repeated pregnancy losses, complete evaluation is recommended to determine possible causes; appropriate treatment may be instituted prior to future pregnancies (refer to Chapter 13, Infertility).

ECTOPIC PREGNANCY

Ectopic pregnancy is the implantation of a fertilized ovum outside the uterine cavity (Krause, Janicke, & Cydulka, 2011). Most ectopic pregnancies occur in a fallopian tube, but may also occur in the cervix, on an ovary, or in the abdominal cavity. Following implantation, the embryo grows, but no decidua is present. The structure of the implantation can sustain some growth; however, rupture is usually inevitable. Early signs of pregnancy, including uterine changes and amenorrhea, are present, secondary to hormonal influence. Ectopic pregnancy is a potentially life-threatening condition and involves pregnancy loss.

Epidemiology

The etiology of extrauterine implanatation originates with an interference in normal ovum transport. Women at risk are those who have used an IUD or who have a history of infertility, pelvic inflammatory disease, tubal surgery (e.g., ligation or reconstruction), ectopic pregnancy, or tubal infection (Cunningham et al., 2010).

Ectopic pregnancy accounts for 5 percent of maternal deaths worldwide (WHO, 2007), but the incidence has declined significantly in the United States since the 1970s (Cunningham et al., 2010). It is more prevalent in poor, less advantaged countries. Although maternal mortality has decreased in the United States, the actual number of ectopic pregnancies has increased. The increased incidence appears to be related to factors associated with infertility, such as chronic salpingitis, earlier detection by ultrasound, and sensitive β-hCG assays.

Subjective Data

Classical and atypical presentations are used in diagnosis. The classical clinical presentation includes many of the early signs of pregnancy: 1 to 2 months of amenorrhea, nausea, breast tenderness. The most common presenting symptoms are abdominal pain and irregular vaginal bleeding. Abdominal pain can be unilateral, and mild vaginal bleeding is possible. The client is motivated to seek emergency care when her pain becomes sharper and she experiences more generalized discomfort. She may report gastrointestinal disturbances and feelings of malaise and syncope. She may faint. Classically, pain is referred to the shoulder as the hemorrhage becomes extensive and irritates the diaphragm.

Atypical clinical presentations are not so clearly evident. Many clients report vague or subacute symptoms. They may report menstrual irregularity. Amenorrhea may not be obvious, as intermittent spotting or mild vaginal bleeding may mimic normal menses. Ectopic pregnancy should be considered in diagnosis when any woman of childbearing age reports mild or severe abdominal symptoms. Symptoms do not necessarily correlate with the severity of the condition; mild signs and symptoms may occur with massive hemorrhage (Hick, Rodgerson, Heegaard, & Sterner, 2001; Mashburn, 1999).

Objective Data

Any sexually active woman with a missed menses is at risk for ectopic pregnancy. Use of current diagnostic methods has provided the early detection of ectopic pregnancy before symptoms occur or become severe. When symptoms do occur, they mimic other problems with similar complaints.

Physical examination may reveal symptoms of shock especially after hemorrhage. The woman in early gestation may appear in little discomfort. General signs of shock include cool, clammy skin and poor skin color and turgor. Late signs are hypotension and tachycardia. Abdominal examination may reveal some unilateral adnexal tenderness. A pelvic exam reveals a normal-appearing cervix, but marked tenderness is noted. The vaginal vault may be bloody, usually brick red to brown in color. There may be vaginal tenderness. A tender adnexal mass may be palpated, and the uterus may be slightly enlarged and soft.

Levels of serial β-hCG are used to diagnose ectopic pregnancy. A small amount of functioning trophoblastic tissue, as is found in ectopic pregnancy, will produce a small amount of β-hCG without the amount of expected doubling increases associated with normal pregnancy. In a normal intrauterine pregnancy, hormone levels should double every 2 to 4 days with a predictable slope of increase. Low β-hCG levels are, therefore, suggestive of an ectopic pregnancy and should be followed by a repeated quantitative radioimmunoassay.

A sonogram is used to determine if the pregnancy is intrauterine, to assess the size of the uterus, and to detect presence of fetal viability. If the β-hCG is greater than 1,000 to 2,000 mIU/mL at 35 days of gestation, and the pregnancy is intrauterine, a gestational sac should be visualized by transvaginal ultrasound (Cunningham et al., 2010). Absence of an intrauterine gestational sac is diagnostic of ectopic pregnancy.

Culdocentesis may be done to detect intraperitoneal blood, which will be present following tubal pregnancy rupture. This procedure is carried out during a pelvic exam. The health care provider inserts a needle through the vaginal wall into the cul-de-sac and withdraws whatever fluid is present. Nonclotted blood indicates hemorrhage. The source of bleeding is then identified by means of laparoscopy or laparotomy, and measures are taken to control bleeding.

Differential Medical Diagnoses

Pelvic inflammatory disease, ovarian cyst, ovarian tumor, intrauterine pregnancy, recent spontaneous abortion, early hydatidiform degeneration, acute appendicitis, and other bowel-related disorders.

Plan

Psychosocial Interventions. Inform the client about procedures and support her as early diagnosis and appropriate medical referral are pursued. Because laparoscopy is frequently necessary for a definitive diagnosis, prepare the woman for safe and timely transfer to a hospital. Information about the procedure and management plan should be clearly stated for the client and her partner, a family member, or friend.

Medical Management. Methotrexate, administered IM, is commonly used in the nonsurgical management of ectopic pregnancy (Barnhart, 2009). The client eligible for medical therapy must be hemodynamically stable and the mass must be unruptured, measuring fewer than 4 cm determined by ultrasound. The severe side effects of bone marrow suppression, hepatotoxicity, stomatitis, pulmonary fibrosis, alopecia, and photosensitivity from methotrexate are uncommon in short-term therapy for ectopic pregnancy, but need to be administered with appropriate caution. Single-dose methotrexate is 50 mg/m^2 of body surface area IM. Another regimen is methotrexate, 1 mg/kg of body weight IM every other day, alternating with leucovorin, 0.1 mg/kg IM every other day, for a total of 8 days (Cunningham et al., 2010). Treatment continues until the β-hCG drops equal to or greater than 15 percent in 48 hours or four doses of methotrexate have been given. Serum β-hCG should be monitored weekly until undetected; blood count, platelet count, and liver enzyme levels should also be monitored weekly (Mashburn, 1999). Colicky pain secondary to the stomatitis can mimic ectopic rupture and must be differentiated by assessment for hypotension, tachycardia, or falling hematocrit indicating hemorrhage. Clients should avoid gas-producing foods such as beans or cabbage, which may also mimic ectopic rupture. Clients should also avoid sun exposure while taking the methotrexate because of the photosensitivity of the drug.

Surgical Evacuation of Conceptus. Surgical treatment may involve either salpingectomy (removal of the affected fallopian tube) or the dissection of the ectopic pregnancy while conserving the tube (salpingostomy). Laparoscopy is the preferred surgical approach. A laparotomy should be indicated only in the case of uncontrolled hemorrhage or hemodynamic instability (Barnhart, 2009). Historically, treatment focused on prevention of death, but with the ability to perform linear salpingostomy, emphasis is now on facilitating rapid recovery, preserving fertility, and reducing costs.

Follow-Up

Postoperatively, all Rh-negative unsensitized clients should be given Rh immunoglobulin. Discuss the normal body changes the client will experience. Instruct her concerning contraception, danger signals (e.g., signs of postsurgical infection or hemorrhage), and any further follow-up testing. The emotional needs of clients will vary. Pregnancy may not have been realized prior to diagnosis, and learning about the pregnancy and pregnancy loss in such a short period can be overwhelming (Minnick-Smith & Cook, 1997). Pregnancy should be acknowledged and its meaning discussed. Explain to a client that having one ectopic pregnancy increases her chances for future ectopic pregnancies; however, the risk is less with the use of methotrexate. Review the signs and symptoms of repeated ectopic pregnancy with her. Advise her to practice contraception for at least 2 months to allow for adequate healing and tissue repair. In 20 percent of cases treated with methotrexate, residual tissue remains and causes hemorrhage and other complications. Weekly blood tests for β-hCG levels should be monitored until β-hCG becomes undetectable. The initial follow-up visit should include discussion of the need for follow-up blood testing, emotional responses to the ectopic pregnancy, risk factors, and need for contraception.

Prevention of ectopic pregnancies through screening and client education is essential. Preventing tubal damage from, for example, sexually transmitted disease can decrease the incidence of the disorder. Encouraging the use of condoms can decrease the incidence of many infections responsible for tubal scarring. Early detection and prompt treatment of gonorrhea and chlamydia, when they occur, can decrease morbidity.

Selection of an appropriate contraceptive method is important. Because IUD use may be associated with infections and tubal pregnancy, women need to be informed of the risk and effect of an IUD on future pregnancies.

GESTATIONAL TROPHOBLASTIC DISEASE

Gestational trophoblastic disease is a group of neoplastic disorders that originate in the human placenta. Gestational tissue is present but pregnancy is nonviable.

- *Hydatidiform mole:* The most common type of gestational trophoblastic disease, hydatidiform mole is a benign neoplasm of the chorion in which chorionic villi degenerate and become transparent vesicles containing clear, viscid fluid. Recently, two types of molar gestations have been distinguished: partial and complete. No fetus or amnion is found in the complete mole, but in the partial mole, a fetus or evidence of an amniotic sac is present.
- *Invasive mole (chorioadenoma destruens):* Invasive mole is a complete molar gestation that has invaded the myometrium, metastasized to other tissues, or both. Karyotyping reveals abnormal genetic material resulting from an empty egg or diploid sperm.
- *Choriocarcinoma:* This rare chorionic malignancy may follow any type of pregnancy, even years later. Half of choriocarcinomas occur following hydatidiform molar pregnancy.

Epidemiology

The etiology may be influenced by nutritional factors, such as protein deficiency. Such deficiencies would explain some of the race and geographical differences associated with gestational trophoblastic disease.

The incidence of molar pregnancy varies markedly around the world. Molar pregnancy is more prevalent in Hispanics and American Indians (Smith et al., 2006). The true incidence of partial mole is unknown, because many are diagnosed as spontaneous abortions and tissue karyotyping is not done. Moles do recur in subsequent pregnancies. Age is also a factor; older women have a greater incidence of molar pregnancy.

Subjective Data

Presenting symptoms are similar to those of spontaneous abortion. The client usually reports signs of early pregnancy (amenorrhea, breast tenderness, morning sickness) and presents with vaginal bleeding around the 12th week of gestation. Bleeding may begin as spotting, usually brownish rather than bright red. Some women experience severe nausea and vomiting and are treated for hyperemesis gravidarum. Preeclampsia that develops before 24 weeks should raise an index of suspicion for a molar pregnancy (Cunningham et al., 2010). Uterine cramping may or may not be present.

Objective Data

Physical examination may reveal what is sometimes a first sign of molar pregnancy: expulsion of grapelike vesicles with or without a history of vaginal bleeding. Vital signs are usually stable; no medical emergency exists. The abdomen is soft and nontender; in the vagina, bloody or clear vesicles may be present. The uterus is usually enlarged beyond the point of expected gestation and has a doughy consistency (Cunningham et al., 2010). Ovaries may be enlarged and tender secondary to theca lutein cysts, which develop from ovarian hyperstimulation of high hCG levels. No fetal heart tones or fetal activity is detected.

The sonogram shows the absence of the gestational sac and characteristic multiple echogenic regions within the uterus (Cunningham et al., 2010).

Human chorionic gonadotropin levels are extremely high in molar pregnancies and continue to rise 100 days after the last menstrual period (LMP). No single value is diagnostic; therefore, serial values must be evaluated and compared with the normal pregnancy curve for β-hCG.

Differential Medical Diagnoses

Normal pregnancy, threatened abortion; error in dates, uterine myomas, polyhydramnios, multiple gestation.

Plan

Prompt identification of gestational trophoblastic disease and appropriate referral are essential to management.

Psychosocial Interventions. Explain the diagnostic procedures and follow-up blood work to the client. Explore the meaning of the client's pregnancy with her and her partner, a family member, or friend. Support them in their grieving. Accounting for religious beliefs and cultural practices is crucial in counseling women during treatment concerning the necessity of contraception. Reassurance about future pregnancies is appropriate, because prognosis is good even for women with invasive molar pregnancies (Berkowitz, Tuncer, Bernstein, & Goldstein, 2000).

Medication. If β-hCG levels either rise or plateau after evacuation, chemotherapy is indicated for potential metastatic disease. For women who wish to protect their fertility, single-agent therapy is used, usually methotrexate administered orally (ACOG Practice Bulletin, 2004a).

Other Interventions. Evacuation of the uterus is necessary as soon as the diagnosis is made. Dilatation and curettage (suction curettage) is the safest, most effective method of emptying the uterus. Labor induction with prostaglandins or oxytocin is not recommended (ACOG Practice Bulletin, 2004a). Hospital admission is necessary for adequate anesthesia and nursing surveillance.

A *chest x-ray* is ordered to establish a baseline if there is any question later of invasive disease.

Serial monitoring of β-hCG levels is done weekly until normal for 3 weeks and then monthly for 6 months after the evacuation procedure. Levels of β-hCG are used to detect residual trophoblastic tissue. If any tissue remains, β-hCG levels will not regress. A rising β-hCG level could indicate the presence of a new gestation and must be investigated prior to any extensive diagnostic imagining or therapeutic intervention.

No further intervention is necessary if β-hCG levels decrease to normal, that is, become nondetectable. The postmolar surveillance period is 1 year. When pregnancy occurs prior to this time, the pregnancy may be continued but requires a discussion of risks and close observation (Aghajanian, 2011). *Reliable contraception* must be used during this time because a positive pregnancy test cannot differentiate normal early pregnancy from beginning invasive disease. Reliable and safe contraceptives such as oral contraceptives, medroxyprogesterone acetate (Depo-Provera), or barrier methods are desirable.

PLACENTA PREVIA

In placenta previa, the placenta becomes implanted in the lower segment of the uterus and obstructs the presenting part prior to or during labor. When the cervix begins to dilate, the placenta is pulled away from the endometrial wall and bleeding can occur. Any significant bleeding that leads to hemorrhage can endanger the mother and, if allowed to persist, can interfere with uteroplacental sufficiency.

The three types of previa (total, incomplete, and marginal) are classified by the amount of cervix involved.

- In *total or complete previa*, the entire internal os is covered with placenta.
- In *incomplete or partial previa*, the internal os is only partially covered by the placenta.
- In *marginal or low-lying previa*, the edge of the placenta is at the cervical os but does not obstruct any part of it.

The amount of cervical dilation can affect the classification system. Other systems are based on the amount of placental encroachment over the os at the point of full dilation.

Epidemiology

The etiology of placenta previa is unknown, but certain women are at greater risk than others. Parity is the most common risk factor; old fundal implantation sites are scarred and not suitable for implantation. Other uterine surgical scars, such as those from cesarean birth or myomectomy, increase the chance of placental malimplantation. Advanced maternal age, maternal smoking, and a history of induced or spontaneous abortion have also been reported to be risk factors for placenta previa (Cunningham et al., 2010). Maternal complications such as hysterectomy, intrapartum and postpartum hemorrhage, septicemia, and thrombophlebitis have been noted in the women diagnosed with placenta previa (Crane et al., 2000)

Incidence seems to vary with gestation, although the condition is reported in 1 of every 200 pregnancies. Better diagnostic techniques have revealed gestational differences. For example, in the second trimester, placenta previa is a prevalent finding on sonogram, but as pregnancy progresses the incidence falls. In the third trimester, the lower uterine segment stretches and develops, making the placenta seem to migrate away from the internal os, and the previa resolves.

Subjective Data

The characteristic symptom of placenta previa is painless bleeding during the third trimester of pregnancy. Bleeding may occur as early as 20 weeks of gestation and without any precipitating event. Previa should be suspected in any bleeding that occurs after 24 weeks of gestation. Blood is usually bright red. A woman may experience symptoms of shock, such as syncope. The first bleed, however, is usually not a significant amount.

Objective Data

Vital signs are stable, fetal heart tones are normal, and fetal activity is present. The uterus is nontender with a normal resting tone. Bright red blood is evident on sanitary napkins.

Diagnosis is best made by sonogram. No pelvic exam is done to avoid dislodging any clot that may have formed at the cervix (Oyelese & Smulian, 2006).

Differential Medical Diagnoses

Abruptio placentae, genital lacerations, excessive show, cervical lesions and/or severe cervicitis, nonvaginal bleeding (urinary or rectal), ectopic pregnancy (Rees & Paradinas, 2001).

Plan

The role of the primary care provider lies primarily in the early detection of placenta previa. Referral for appropriate intervention is necessary.

Medication. Not indicated.

Management. The medical plan depends on the extent of hemorrhage and length of gestation. If gestation is less than 36 weeks, an attempt is made to stabilize the mother, administer transfusions as needed, and maintain the pregnancy. Strict hospital bed rest is employed, and the mother and fetus are closely monitored. If bleeding stops and the hematocrit is greater than 30 percent, then gradual ambulation may be allowed. Some women may be allowed to return home with limited activity until further problems arise or labor begins.

Provide the client with clear instructions about pelvic rest and what to do if signs of impending labor or bleeding begins.

During the wait-and-see period, amniocentesis may be done weekly after 36 weeks to document fetal maturity. In addition, serial sonograms are done to determine placement of the placenta and to note any migration. Later in the pregnancy, placental problems can lead to uteroplacental insufficiency and intrauterine growth retardation.

Sonography. Serial sonograms are also used to monitor fetal growth. If bleeding continues or recurs, then operative delivery may be forced.

Delivery. The amount of bleeding, general fetal condition, fetal presentation, and gestation will affect delivery decisions. Once fetal maturity is accomplished, delivery is planned. When gestation is less than 36 weeks and previa is coexisting with PTL, some clinicians are successfully using an expectant approach using tocolysis. The extent to which the os is covered by the placenta determines if vaginal delivery is considered. Cesarean delivery is usually recommended (Cunningham et al., 2010).

Postpartum Follow-Up. It is the same as for other postpartum women. The amount of blood loss is associated with perinatal outcome, even though the number of bleeding episodes does not increase perinatal mortality or morbidity. A mother usually recovers readily from anemia and fluid loss. During the first month of life, the infant is at increased risk for death, compared with infants of the same gestational age and birth weight. The increased risk is probably related to transient episodes of fetal hypoxia.

ABRUPTIO PLACENTAE

Abruptio placentae is the partial or complete detachment of a normally implanted placenta at any time prior to delivery. Detachment occurs more frequently during the third trimester, but may occur anytime after 20 weeks of gestation. The proposed mechanism is that maternal arterioles become thrombosed and lead to degeneration of decidua and, subsequently, to rupture of one vessel.

The resultant bleeding forms a retroplacental clot, which increases pressure behind the placenta and adds to the separation process.

The classification of abruptio placentae is based on the signs and symptoms of abruption in combination with selected laboratory findings.

Epidemiology

The etiology of abruptio placentae is unknown. Maternal smoking, poor maternal nutrition, chorioamnionitis, and use of cocaine are risk factors for premature separation. It appears that increased maternal age increases the risk of abruption. In one research study, the risk of abruption in a woman older than age 40 was 2.3 times more likely than a woman 35 years of age or younger (Cleary-Goldman et al., 2005). Conditions with underlying vascular involvement, particularly hypertension, can predispose a woman to abruption (Ananth, Getahun, Peltier, & Smulian, 2006). Severe trauma, such as an automobile accident or injury secondary to domestic violence, has also been associated with abruption (Cannada et al., 2008). The incidence of battering of women has grown and the incidence of battering during pregnancy is reported to be higher than other times, even though there is no evidence to support this observation (Ballard, Saltzman, Gazmararian, et al., 1998; Moore, 1999).

The true incidence is unknown because abruption occurs in varying degrees. Incidence is reported to be 1:120 births per year (Witlin, Saade, Mattar, & Sibai, 1999).

Subjective Data

Symptoms of abruptio placentae can vary significantly depending on the extent and location of separation. The client may report labor pains with some continual cramping. With more severe abruption, severe, sudden, knife-like pain may be described. The client may experience no bleeding, a small amount of dark old blood, or profuse bleeding. Depending on the amount of blood lost from the systemic circulation, she may experience symptoms of shock, such as syncope.

Objective Data

Physical Examination. May reveal vaginal bleeding (dark old blood or bright red blood), uterine tenderness (local or generalized), increased uterine tone, occasional boardlike quality with little or no relaxation between contractions, lack of fetal heart tones, or signs of fetal distress (such as tachycardia, loss of beat-to-beat variability, or late decelerations). No vaginal or rectal exam is done until placenta previa is eliminated as a diagnosis (Witlin et al., 1999).

Sonogram. Frequently used to locate a retroplacental clot. A clot may not be seen on the sonogram in an early abruption, but if symptoms are severe, time is critical and diagnosis must be made on presumptive signs.

Differential Medical Diagnoses

Placenta previa, placenta accreta, hematoma of rectus muscle, ovarian cysts, appendicitis, degeneration of fibroids.

Plan

Immediate identification of possibility or suspicion of abruptio placentae dictates prompt referral for appropriate stabilization and treatment.

Psychosocial Interventions. Allay the anxiety of the woman and her family. They need to be informed about impending diagnostic tests, possible hospitalization, and surgery.

Management. Maintain respiratory and cardiovascular support (IV fluid, oxygen), as needed, until the client is transported to the hospital. Because of the potential for hemorrhage, development of a coagulopathy disorder is a risk. Hemorrhage, which if not corrected by delivery of the fetus and the placenta, will lead to depletion of the clotting factors and can be life-threatening (Cunningham et al., 2010). Hemorrhage may occur into the postpartum period.

Delivery. Delivery is necessary if severe symptoms are present and condition is life-threatening for the mother or fetus. Whether the fetus is to be delivered by cesarean or vaginal birth will depend on the assessment of the mother and the fetus. If the mother's condition is stable, but the fetus is not viable, cesarean birth is not indicated. Cesarean delivery is indicated when there are signs of fetal distress, maternal hemorrhage, maternal coagulopathy, or poor progress of labor. Fetal well-being is assessed by electronic fetal monitoring. If both mother and fetus are stable, assessment for fetal maturity is done to assist in decisions of the timing of delivery.

Follow-Up

After delivery, care for women with abruptio placentae is the same as that for other postpartum women. It may be necessary to deal with pregnancy loss, or in some cases, when the infant survives, maternal grieving may occur over loss of a normal pregnancy or delivery. Infants may need care in a newborn intensive care unit, which adds to family stress.

ANEMIAS

Anemia is a reduction in the concentration of erythrocytes or hemoglobin in blood (ACOG Practice Bulletin, 2008). A prevalence rate of 21.55 per 1,000 pregnant women was found in a national study when anemia was defined as a hemoglobin concentration of less than 10 g/dL (Adebisi & Strayhorn, 2005). When this data was examined for prevalence by race and age, prevalence among non-Hispanic black women was twice as high as non-Hispanic white women (35 vs. 18 per 1,000 women) and teenaged mothers had the highest prevalence (Adebisi & Strayhorn, 2005). In a normal pregnancy, concentrations of erythrocytes and hemoglobin fall because of a disproportional increase in the ratio of plasma volume to erythrocyte volume (hypervolemia or physiological anemia of pregnancy). During pregnancy, plasma volume increases as much as 45 to 50 percent, but erythrocyte volume increases only 25 percent. Expansion of blood volume and growth of the fetus, placenta, and other maternal tissues increase the demand for iron threefold in the second and third trimesters. Many women have borderline hemoglobin levels before pregnancy; therefore, they do not have the reserve necessary to support these physiological changes.

Hemoglobin concentration decreases after 8 weeks, drops to its lowest level at midpregnancy, and rises slightly or stabilizes near term. Hemoglobin and hematocrit values are expected to return to prepregnancy level by 6 weeks postdelivery unless there was severe blood loss during the intrapartal or postpartal period. The most common causes of anemia during pregnancy and postpartum are iron deficiency and acute blood loss (ACOG Practice Bulletin, 2008). Most pregnant women who do not take iron supplements are unable to maintain adequate iron stores, especially during the second and third trimesters (CDC, 1998a).

The causation of anemia can be attributed to decreased RBC production, increased RBC destruction, and/or blood loss (ACOG Practice Bulletin, 2008). Even though the majority of anemia during pregnancy is caused by iron deficiency, other blood disorders also may contribute to anemia in pregnancy, and an initial low hemoglobin value requires additional lab work. Identification of causation is especially important when evaluating the effects of anemia on pregnancy outcomes. Some other causes of anemia in pregnancy include folate-deficiency anemia and hemolytic anemia caused by the most frequently encountered hemoglobinopathies, thalassemia, and sickle cell. Consultation is recommended with all these disorders except mild to moderate iron-deficiency anemia.

IRON-DEFICIENCY ANEMIA

The CDC (1998a) definition of anemia in iron-supplemented pregnant women is a hemoglobin concentration of less than 11 g/dL (hematocrit 33%) in the first and second trimester or less than 10.5 g/dL (hematocrit 32%) in the third trimester (CDC, 1998a).

Epidemiology

There is limited prevalence data specific to iron-deficiency anemia during pregnancy (Agency for Healthcare Research and Quality, 2006). One report estimated iron-deficiency rates in a low-income, mostly minority population as 1.8 percent in the first trimester, 8.2 percent in the second trimester, and 24.7 percent in the third trimester (Scholl, 2005).

The cause of iron-deficiency anemia is decreased RBC production due to an inadequate iron supply, usually secondary to poor dietary intake. Teenagers and women of low socioeconomic status are at greatest risk because of the likelihood of inadequate or improperly balanced diets (Cunningham et al., 2010). Risk factors for iron-deficiency anemia include a diet poor in iron-rich foods; a diet poor in iron-absorption enhancers; a diet rich in foods that diminish iron absorption; pica; gastrointestinal disease affecting absorption; heavy menses; short interpregnancy interval; and significant blood loss at delivery.

Iron-deficiency anemia during pregnancy has been associated with an increased risk of LBW, preterm birth (PTB), and perinatal mortality (Kidanto, Mogren, Lindmark, Massawe, & Nystrom, 2009; Ren et al., 2007; Scholl, 2005); the mechanism for this association is unknown. There is also research linking maternal iron-deficiency anemia to postpartum depression, with poor results in mental and psychomotor performance testing in offspring (Corwin, Murray-Kolb, & Beard, 2003; Perez et al., 2005; Tamura et al., 2002).

Subjective Data

A woman may experience fatigue or weakness that may affect her ability to perform activities of daily living.

In the second and third trimesters of pregnancy, she may notice shortness of breath on exertion. Evaluating nutrition through dietary recall is important in assessing risk factors.

Objective Data

A hemoglobin assessment is recommended for all pregnant women at their first prenatal visit (Institute for Clinical Systems Improvement [ICSI], 2010). Physical examination of a pregnant woman may suggest iron-deficiency anemia; blood tests confirm it.

Physical examination may reveal pale conjunctiva and mucous membranes.

Hemoglobin concentration or hematocrit is nonspecific for identifying iron-deficiency anemia. Asymptomatic women who meet the CDC criteria for anemia should be further evaluated. Initial evaluation of mild to moderate anemia should include a medical history, family history, physical examination, and CBC, RBC indices, serum iron levels, and ferritin levels (ACOG Practice Bulletin, 2008). An electrophoresis is recommended in certain ethnic groups.

Ferritin levels have the highest sensitivity and specificity for diagnosing iron-deficiency anemia (ACOG Practice Bulletin, 2008). Results characteristic of iron-deficiency anemia show microcytic and hypochromic mature RBCs, low plasma iron levels, high total iron-binding capacity, low serum ferritin levels (less than 10–15 μg/L), and increased levels of free erythrocyte protoporphyrin (see Table 20–3).

Differential Medical Diagnoses

Folate deficiency, thalassemia, sickle cell disease, aplastic anemia, HELLP syndrome.

Plan

Psychosocial Interventions. Inform the client of need to eat a well-balanced diet, emphasizing foods that are high in iron, foods that enhance iron absorption, and foods that reduce iron absorption. The use of patient education materials listing high iron food sources should accompany a discussion of how iron-rich foods are important during and after pregnancy.

Although iron absorption is enhanced when taken prior to a meal, this timing may lead to gastrointestinal disturbances. For pregnant women, taking iron following meals is less problematic because dietary iron absorption is much more efficient during pregnancy. Advise against taking iron with milk, tea, or antacids as they interfere with absorption. Spacing the doses throughout the day aids in absorption. If clients are unable to tolerate the maximum daily dose, individualize administration and dosage. Instruct the client to drink extra fluids to reduce the likelihood of constipation.

Medication. The typical diet provides 15 mg of elemental iron per day, and the recommended daily dietary allowance of ferrous iron during pregnancy is 27 mg, which is present in most prenatal vitamins (ACOG Practice Bulletin, 2008). The CDC (1998a) recommends universal iron supplementation for all pregnant women except those with certain genetic disorders. A Cochrane review concluded that iron supplementation decreases the prevalence of maternal anemia at delivery, but it is uncertain whether this affects perinatal outcome (Pena-Rosas & Viteri, 2009).

The recommended dosage for deficiency anemia is 180 to 200 mg of elemental iron (equivalent two or three 300-mg tablets of ferrous sulfate) per day in separated doses. Total iron supplementation per day should include iron contained in a prenatal vitamin and not exceed the 200 mg of elemental iron daily (Cunningham et al., 2010). For women who cannot tolerate oral iron, parenteral administration may be necessary (Bayonumeu, Subiran-Buisset, Baka, et al., 2002). Ferrous sucrose is preferred over iron dextran (ACOG Practice Bulletin, 2008). Available iron supplements are listed in Table 20–4.

TABLE 20–3. Normal Iron Indices in Pregnancy

Test	Normal Value
Plasma iron level	40–175 μg/dL
Plasma total iron-binding capacity	216–400 μg/dL
Transferrin saturation	16–60%
Serum ferritin level	More than 10 μg/dL
Free erythrocyte protoporphyrin level	Less than 3 μg/g

Source: ACOG Practice Bulletin, 2008.

TABLE 20–4. Iron Supplements

Preparation	Dose
Ferrous fumarate	106 mg elemental iron per 325 mg tablet
Ferrous sulfate	65 mg elemental iron per 325 mg tablet
Ferrous gluconate	34 mg elemental iron per 300 mg tablet
Iron dextran	50 mg elemental iron per milliliter, intramuscularly or intravenously
Ferric gluconate	12.5 mg iron per milliliter, intravenously only
Iron sucrose	20 mg iron per milliliter, intravenously only

Source: ACOG Practice Bulletin, 2008.

Fetal considerations

The amount of iron diverted to the fetus does not appear to be impacted by maternal iron stores; even the newborn of a severely anemic mother doesn't have iron-deficiency anemia (Cunningham et al., 2010). Severe cases of anemia (maternal hemoglobin levels less than 6 g/dL) have, however, been associated with abnormal fetal oxygenation, presenting clinically with nonreassuring fetal heart rate patterns, reduced amniotic fluid volume, fetal cerebral vasodilation, and fetal death (Carles et al., 2003). In these cases, maternal transfusion should be considered for fetal indications (ACOG Practice Bulletin, 2008).

Follow-Up

The diagnosis of iron-deficiency anemia is often presumptive, and iron therapy may be initiated on the basis of a low hemoglobin level alone. There should be an increase in reticulocyte count 7 to 10 days after initiating iron therapy with increase in hemoglobin levels in subsequent weeks. Common clinical practice is to repeat the hemoglobin level in 2 weeks. Failure to respond to iron therapy should be followed by further investigation of causation.

All anemic women should be monitored for infection and signs of intrauterine growth retardation. Following delivery, these women should remain on iron therapy and monitored for recovery for at least 3 months. More than 2 years may be needed to replenish iron stores from dietary sources. Counseling women about this period is important if other pregnancies are planned.

FOLIC ACID DEFICIENCY

Folic acid is a B-complex vitamin essential for cell growth and division. It promotes the maturation of RBCs. During pregnancy, folic acid requirement increase from 50 to 400 μg (ACOG Practice Bulletin, 2008). Additional folic acid intake is recommended when folate requirements are increased, such as multifetal pregnancy, macrocytic anemia, Crohn's disease, alcoholism, and following gastric bypass surgery (ACOG Practice Bulletin, 2008; CDC, 1998b).

Epidemiology

Folic acid deficiency is the most common cause of macrocytic anemia, previously referred to as pernicious anemia (Cunningham et al., 2010). Folic acid deficiency in the United States is usually diet related and coexists with iron-deficiency anemia. It is associated with diets lacking fresh vegetables, legumes, or animal proteins. Green vegetables, peanuts, and animal proteins, especially liver and red meats, are good sources of folic acid. As of 1996, food sources such as breads and cereals are now being fortified with folic acid (Honein, Paulozzi, Mathews, Erickson, & Wong, 2001). Teenagers and women of low socioeconomic status are at greatest risk for folic acid deficiency because of the likelihood of inadequate or improperly balanced dietary intake. Also at risk are women with hemoglobinopathies, multifetal pregnancies, short intervals between pregnancies, and women with excessive ethanol ingestion (Cunningham et al., 2010).

Since the early 1990s, there has been a great deal of attention directed at the role of folic acid deficiency in the development of neural tube defects, leading to the recommendation that all women of reproductive age consume at least 400 μg of folic acid daily (ACOG Practice Bulletin, 2008). The promotion of adequate folic acid intake should be included in all clinical care for women of reproductive age. There is also evidence that women with a history of infants with neural tube defects have a lower recurrence rate if they consume 4 mg of folic acid prior and during early pregnancy (De-Regil, Fernandez-Gaxiola, Dowswell, & Pena-Rosas, 2010).

Subjective Data

A client with folic acid deficiency may experience nausea, vomiting, and anorexia during pregnancy and symptoms of iron deficiency if it coexists. Evaluating nutrition through dietary recall is important in assessing risk factors.

Objective Data

Physical examination may reveal pale conjunctiva and mucous membranes. Signs of folic acid deficiency cannot be distinguished from those of iron-deficiency anemia.

Diagnostic tests include determination of serum folate and RBC folate levels. Levels normally fall during pregnancy; however, a fasting folate level of less than 3 mg/mL in an anemic woman is a presumptive sign for diagnosis. Hypersegmented neutrophilic leukocytes and macrocytic red cells on peripheral smear are diagnostic, but definitive diagnosis is made by bone marrow examination (although seldom necessary). The reticulocyte count is depressed in the folic acid–deficient client, but reticulocytosis usually occurs within 3 days after administration of a folic acid supplementation.

Differential Medical Diagnoses

Iron-deficiency anemia, thalassemia, sickle cell anemia.

Plan

Psychosocial Interventions. Provide the client with information about foods that are high in folic acid. Explain to the client the importance of eating healthful foods every day to benefit herself and her fetus. The use of handouts with high iron food sources should accompany a discussion of how folic acid–rich foods are important for her health before, during, and after pregnancy.

Treatment in Pregnancy. Treatment with daily intake of 1.0 mg of folic acid is recommended. Women with significant hemoglobinopathies, on anticonvulsants such as phenytoin (Dilantin), or with multiple gestation are also advised to supplement with 1.0 mg daily of folic acid. Women who have had a previous infant affected by neural tube defect should be advised to supplement their diet, as mentioned earlier, with daily folate intake of 4 mg/day 2 to 3 months prior to pregnancy and during pregnancy (De-Regil et al., 2010).

Follow-Up

The measures used for clients with folic acid deficiency are the same as those for women with iron-deficiency anemia. The appropriate screening for iron deficiency should be performed and iron supplementation initiated when indicated.

THALASSEMIA

Thalassemias represent a spectrum of hematologic disorders that are characterized by impaired production of one or more of the normal globin peptide chains, leading to increased RBC destruction and anemia. Classification of thalassemia is made according to the globin chain affected, with the most common types being alpha-thalassemia and beta-thalassemia. Thalassemia is an autosomal recessive genetic disorder that occurs more frequently in certain racial and ethnic groups. Symptoms will depend upon the number and location of the missing proteins on the gene. Diagnosis is made by hemoglobin electrophoresis (ACOG Practice Bulletin, 2007a).

Genetic screening identifies couples at risk for offspring with hemoglobinopathies so informed decisions can be made about reproduction and prenatal diagnosis (Davies et al., 2000). Individuals of African, Southeast Asian, and Mediterranean ancestry are at greater risk for thalassemias and should be offered carrier screening. Lower-risk groups include northern Europeans, Japanese, Native Americans, Inuit (Eskimo), and Koreans. Genetic counseling is recommended for couples at risk for having a child with a hemoglobinopathy in order to review the natural history of these disorders, treatment and cure prospects, their risk, genetic testing options, and reproductive choices. Diagnosis of alpha thalassemia minor and major in the fetus can be done through DNA analysis of chorionic villi or cultured amniotic cells (ACOG Practice Bulletin, 2007a).

A combination of laboratory tests is required to screen for hemoglobinapathies. A CBC should be done on all individuals of non-African descent, and CBC with hemoglobin electrophoresis for those of African descent. Determination of mean corpuscular volume is recommended for patients at risk for alpha- or beta-thalassemia, and those with low values (less than 80 fL) are candidates for electrophoresis. If there is a low hemoglobin value, serum ferritin levels are also recommended (ACOG Practice Bulletin, 2007a).

Homozygous alpha-thalassemia or alpha-thalassemia major (Hemoglobin Barts) requires expert obstetrical management. Women with alpha-thalassemia have signs and symptoms of hemolytic anemia, namely, hemosiderosis, a condition characterized by deposition in organs of the iron-containing pigment hemosiderin, which is derived from hemoglobin degeneration. Symptoms may include chills, fever, hypotension, tachycardia, anxiety, nausea, vomiting, renal failure, and shock. Hydrops fetalis and stillbirth are associated with this condition (ACOG Practice Bulletin, 2007a).

Heterozygous alpha-thalassemia carrier does not require change in obstetric management as a normal outcome is expected for the mother and infant. These conditions are usually benign although mild microcytic anemia is common. Iron supplementation is given for documented iron-deficiency anemia. If Asian, the partner should be screened for hemoglobinopathies due to the possibility of fetus being homozygous for alpha-thalassemia.

Heterozygous beta-thalassemia minor (beta-thalassemia carrier) does not require change in obstetric management as a normal outcome is expected for the mother and infant; it is usually associated with asymptomatic mild iron-deficiency anemia (ACOG Practice Bulletin, 2007a). Parenteral iron is contraindicated because of the possibility of exogenous hemosiderosis. This disorder is more common in individuals of Mediterranean, Asian, Middle Eastern, Hispanic, and West Indian descent. Some forms can produce a child with major disease; therefore, partner should be screened for any hemoglobinopathies.

Beta-thalassemia major (Cooley's anemia), which is homozygous β, is rare, and can be a life-threatening condition. It is characterized by severe anemia that results in extramedullary erythropoesis, delayed sexual development, and poor growth (ACOG Practice Bulletin, 2007a). Previously, these affected young women were not expected to survive into the childbearing years. Other countries are now reporting programs that have been following these young men and women into adulthood and report normal vocational, social, sexual, and reproductive goals. The impact of the disorder on pregnancies occurring in these groups is unknown (Psihogios et al., 2002).

Management

Asymptomatic thalassemia carriers do not require any special testing but should receive serial ultrasounds to monitor fetal growth. Nonstress testing is also suggested to evaluate fetal well-being. A good outcome is expected for both mother and infant. Administration of oral iron supplementation is controversial because hemosiderosis is possible (Cunningham et al., 2010). Further discussion is beyond the scope of this chapter; however, medical referral and genetic counseling are recommended.

SICKLE CELL ANEMIA

Sickle cell disease refers to a group of autosomal recessive inherited disorders that involve abnormal hemoglobin (*Hb S*). *Sickle cell anemia* (*Hb SS*) is the most severe form of the disease and carries the risk of severe anemia, sickle crisis, and increased perinatal mortality. *Hb SC* disease occurs in women who are heterozygous for both the S and C genes, and unless it occurs in combination with other hemoglobin variants, there are no adverse effects during pregnancy (ACOG Practice Bulletin, 2007a). Asymptomatic individuals with heterozygous Hb S genotypes (carriers) have *sickle cell trait* (*Hb AS*), which is associated with increased risk of urinary infection but poses minimal risk to the fetus. This group may go undiagnosed until identified through routine prenatal screening because of the lack of symptoms. All women in high-risk groups should be screened during the initial prenatal visit.

A hemoglobin electrophoresis is done to determine the hemoglobin type. Electrophoresis confirms Hb SS, AS, or SC. During their initial prenatal visit, all women of African American women, Greek, Italian, Middle Eastern, or Asian Indian ancestry should be screened or have documentation of S and C hemoglobin status. Solubility tests (Sickledex) are inadequate for diagnosis of sickle cell disorders because they don't differentiate between heterozygous AS and monozygous SS genotypes (ACOG Practice Bulletin, 2007a).

Pregnant women with sickle cell disease should have regular care by or in consultation with obstetricians who are experienced in the management of sickle cell disease and should receive care in institutions that can manage complications of sickle cell disease and high-risk pregnancies (ACOG Practice Bulletin, 2007a).

Epidemiology

Sickle cell disease occurs most commonly in individuals of African origin. Approximately 1 in every 12 African Americans has sickle cell trait and 1 in 600 African American newborns has sickle cell anemia (ACOG Practice Bulletin, 2007a). Clinically significant Hb SC disease occurs in 1 in 833 African Americans and the trait for Hb SC occurs in 1 in 40 (Koshy, 1999). Sickle cell anemia involves periods of hypoxia that lead to destruction of RBCs, hemolytic anemia, and occlusion of blood vessels by abnormally shaped cells. Pregnancy can predispose to periods of hypoxia and trigger a crisis state. Sickling can occur in the renal medulla, leading to reduced oxygen, necrosis of kidney tissue, and renal tubular dysfunction (Koshy, 1999). These factors predispose to an increased risk for bacteriuria, which, if undiagnosed, can progress to pyelonephritis. Painful crisis is the most common cause of recurrent morbidity in Hb SS disease, and if this occurs during the third trimester, it may not resolve until after delivery (ACOG Practice Bulletin, 2007a). Pneumonia and osteomyelitis also occur more frequently among pregnant women with sickle cell disease. As many as 40 percent of patients with Hb SS disease suffer from pulmonary complications; cardiac dysfunction from ventricular hypertrophy is also common (Cunningham et al., 2010).

Pregnancies in women with sickle cell disease are associated with PTL/PTB, premature rupture of membranes, antepartal hospitalization, LBW infants, intrauterine growth restriction (IUGR), and postpartum infection (Sun, Wilburn, Raynor, & Jamieson, 2001). Chakravarty, Khanna, and Chung (2008) reported that sickle cell disease was associated with increased risk of renal failure, various forms of hypertension, and fetal-growth restriction. Patients with Hb SC disease are also at risk for these complications, but to a lesser degree than those with sickle cell anemia (ACOG Practice Bulletin, 2007a).

Subjective Data

Women with sickle cell trait are usually asymptomatic. Women with Hb SC disease have only mild symptoms and frequently are undiagnosed until they experience more pronounced symptoms in pregnancy.

The client with Hb SS reports multifocal pain, dyspnea, malaise, neurological symptoms, and gastrointestinal upset. The crisis state is characterized by pain, dyspnea, and malaise. Pain can be multifocal, occurring in the extremities, chest, abdomen, or back. It frequently occurs in bones and joints. Neurological symptoms include headache, visual changes, and seizures. Liver and spleen involvement results in gastrointestinal symptoms, including nausea and vomiting or severe abdominal cramping. Cunningham and colleagues (2010) identify the importance of considering all potential sources of pain when a pregnant woman with sickle cell anemia is being evaluated for pain. Ectopic pregnancy, placental abruption, pyelonephritis, or appendicitis should also be considered in the differential diagnosis.

Objective Data

Physical examination of the pregnant woman in sickle cell crisis reveals symptoms in several systems.

- Skin is pale and possibly jaundiced.
- Visual acuity and peripheral vision may decrease.
- Signs of distress are apparent. The client experiences shortness of breath and possibly signs of pulmonary embolus or pneumonia.
- Abdomen may be distended with hepatomegaly and palpable spleen. Fundal height may be equal to or less than expected, depending on the client's general health prior to the episode.
- Kidneys are unable to concentrate urine and signs of kidney failure may be evident.
- Fetal heart tones, if present, may be elevated or lack variability.

With Hb SC disease, a dramatic fall in hematocrit occurs in a crisis secondary to a marked sequestration of a large volume of RBCs in the spleen. During pregnancy, these women may have a mild thrombocytopenia associated with increased splenic activity (Telen, 2001).

Differential Medical Diagnoses

Malabsorption syndromes, alcoholic cirrhosis, hookworm infestation.

Plan

Preconception Counseling. Ideally, those women affected by hemoglobinopathies are screened and are aware—prior to conception—of the risks of sickle cell anemia and Hb SC disease to themselves and to a pregnancy. Determining both her own and the partner's status can assist the couple in making appropriate reproductive decisions.

Genetic Referral. The partner of the woman with sickle cell anemia, sickle cell trait, or Hb SC should be tested and, if both are affected and carriers, prenatal diagnosis of the fetus should be offered. Hb S can be identified through hemoglobin electrophoresis and DNA analysis of fetal blood.

Psychosocial Interventions. Involve the client's family in every aspect of care. Provide information and clarification about the disease and its implication for pregnancy, delivery, and the fetus. The provider must be sensitive to the woman's possible fear of dying or fear of losing her infant. A crisis is painful and may be life-threatening.

Education. Reinforce the importance of avoiding factors that precipitate a crisis, such as cold environments, heavy physical exertion, dehydration, and stress (ACOG Practice Bulletin, 2007a). Also discuss the need to recognize symptoms of crisis or complication as soon as possible and to seek care with first signs. Immediate attention can defer the effect on the fetus and frequently decrease the intensity of symptoms. Teach the client the danger signs of pregnancy-induced hypertension and signs and symptoms of infection. Early treatment of common infections, particularly vaginitis and cystitis, may decrease the incidence of more advanced infections, such as pyelonephritis and osteomyelitis. Dietary education about high sources of folic acid and iron should also be provided. Information to women is provided by several organizations such as the Sickle Cell Disease Association of America (http://sicklecelldisease.org), the Sickle Cell Information Center (scinfo.org), and other local coalitions.

Medication. Pregnant women with sickle cell disease need 4 mg of folic acid supplementation because of the continual turn over of RBCs (ACOG Practice Bulletin, 2007a). The CDC (2011e) recommend pneumoccal, influenza, and meningococcal vaccinations for sickle cell patients. There is no specific medication for sickle cell disease or the crisis state. Antibiotics are used for infection. Analgesics are used for pain during a crisis (Marti-Carvajal, Pena-Marti, Communian-Carrasco, & Marti-Pena, 2009). Iron therapy should be initiated only if anemia is present. Some authorities are concerned about iron overload; therefore, iron supplementation is not given unless indicated by serum iron and ferritin levels.

Sickle Cell Crisis. Sickle cell crisis requires hospitalization, enabling administration of transfusions, oxygen, IV therapy for hydration, and sedation and analgesia. The initial clinical assessment should focus on detection of serious medical complications requiring specific interventions, such as acute chest syndrome, infection, dehydration, severe anemia, cholecystitis, and hypersplenism. Obstetricians, hematologists, and anesthesiologists should be involved in the care of a pregnant woman with sickle cell crisis (ACOG Practice Bulletin, 2007a).

Other Interventions. Prophylactic transfusions have been used throughout pregnancy with some success, but the practice remains controversial. Available evidence suggests that the reduction in morbidity and mortality of sickle cell disease in pregnancy can be attributed to improvement in pregnancy management rather than prophylactic transfusions. Blood samples are taken throughout pregnancy to closely monitor cardiac, renal, and liver function. A urine culture and sensitivity should be performed at least once each trimester for women with sickle cell disease, including sickle cell trait. Fetal surveillance by early sonogram to confirm dates and serial sonograms to assess fetal growth is recommended, as well as a plan of antepartal fetal surveillance (ACOG Practice Bulletin, 2007a).

Labor and Delivery. When delivery occurs depends on the condition of both mother and fetus in relation to gestation and the risks and benefits that are presented. After 36 weeks, delivery should be initiated in women with sickle cell anemia as soon as fetal lung maturity is documented. Vaginal delivery is preferred, if possible. General anesthesia should be avoided because of the risk of hypoxia. During labor, fluid overload must be avoided and the woman should remain in the left lateral recumbent position as much that can be tolerated. Oxygen therapy may be necessary. Women with Hb SC disease need the same program of prenatal care as outlined for the woman with sickle cell anemia.

Follow-Up

After delivery, recommend genetic counseling to assist the client and her family to plan future pregnancies. The newborn is screened within the first few days of life. The woman is observed closely for postpartum hemorrhage. Several contraceptive methods are safe and acceptable options for women of childbearing age with sickle cell disease. Because of the potential adverse vascular and thrombotic effects of estrogen containing birth control methods, many clinicians do not recommend their use for this population (Cunningham et al., 2010). Depo-Provera (medroxyprogesterone) has been shown to be another acceptable alternative, and has been associated with reduced incidence of painful crisis (Manchikanti, Grimes, Lopez, & Schulz, 2007).

HYPEREMESIS GRAVIDARUM

Hyperemesis gravidarum (HG) is characterized by persistent vomiting, a weight loss of more than 5 percent, ketonuria, electrolyte abnormalities, and dehydration (Niebyl, 2010). There is not a standard definition of HG but rather a diagnosis of exclusion based on a typical presentation (ACOG Practice Bulletin, 2004b). The repercussions of this condition include increased maternal morbidity as well as social and economic consequences. Severe HG symptoms are the second most common reason for prenatal hospitalization in the United States, representing 11.4 percent of all nondelivery antepartal admissions (Bacak, Callaghan, Dietz, & Crouse, 2005; Lee & Saha, 2011). Treatments used for HG have included abortion, antiemetics, integrative therapies, dietary restriction, hydration, psychotherapy, psychotropic medication, and parenteral nutrition (King & Murphy, 2009).

It is likely that HG represents an extreme end of the continuum of nausea and vomiting of pregnancy. The normal nausea and vomiting of pregnancy is generally time limited with a predictable course: onset occurs about the 5th week after the LMP, peaks at 8 to 12 weeks, and is generally resolved by 16 to 18 weeks of pregnancy (King & Murphy, 2009). Clinical interventions directed at decreasing nausea and vomiting in early pregnancy are intended to prevent worsening symptoms that result in HG. Once symptoms of nausea and vomiting progress, a vicious cycle is set into motion and treatment can be difficult. Some women who experience nausea and vomiting during pregnancy may not receive timely and effective treatment from health care providers and others don't seek treatment because of concerns about safety of treatment options (ACOG Practice Bulletin, 2004a; Lee & Saha, 2011).

There is no diagnostic test available to determine hyperemesis, but the development of an assessment tool by Canadian clinicians and researchers has proved useful for clinical management of symptoms. The Pregnancy-Unique Quantification of Emesis/Nausea (PUQE) index provides identification of severity (mild, moderate, severe) with a concomitant management plan and evaluation of efficacy after 24 hours (Koren et al., 2002; Lacasse, Rey, Ferreira, Morin, & Bérard, 2008).

ETIOLOGY

Although the cause of nausea and vomiting in pregnancy is unknown, it is most likely triggered by the hormonal changes of pregnancy and further influenced by an interplay of genetic, biologic, and psychological factors (Sanu & Lamont, 2011). The onset of nausea and vomiting in early pregnancy coincides with the rise in hCG levels and/or estrogens (Furneaux, Langley-Evans, & Langley-Evans, 2001; Niebyl, 2010). Women with higher levels of hCG, such as those with multiple gestation and hydatidiform moles, are at higher risk for HG, supporting the hypothesis that it is the placenta rather than the fetus that plays a major role in hyperemesis (Niebly, 2010). The occurrence of hyperemesis is theorized to be related to the pregnant woman's response to these triggers based upon her underlying vestibular, gastrointestinal, olfactory, and emotional status (Goodwin, 2002; Lacasse, Rey, Ferreira, Morin, & Bérard, 2009). Thyroid dysfunction and infectious disease (specifically *Helicobacter pylori*) have also been theorized to play a role in hyperemesis (King & Murphy, 2009). Historically, much discussion described deep-rooted distress of pregnancy, which was being transformed into physical symptoms. There is no scientific evidence to support these discussions, but a woman's stress level and personal situation may contribute to her ability to cope and deal with this condition (Buckwalter & Simpson, 2002).

Epidemiology

Between 50 and 80 percent of all pregnant women experience nausea and vomiting of pregnancy; 50 percent have both nausea and vomiting and 25 percent nausea only. The incidence of HG is 0.5 to 2 percent of pregnancies, depending on diagnostic criteria used and population studied (ACOG Practice Bulletin, 2004b). In a Canadian study, Asian and African women had lower rates of nausea and vomiting in the first trimester compared to Caucasian women, even when sociodemographic factors were controlled, leading the investigators to consider genetic and cultural factors (Lacasse et al., 2009).

The most common maternal complications of HG include weight loss, dehydration, micronutrient deficiency, and muscle weakness (Lee & Saha, 2011). Although uncommon, severe dehydration and trauma from severe vomiting can lead to serious medical problems, including acute renal failure, life-threatening complications of continuous retching including Mallory-Weiss tears, esophageal rupture, pneumothorax, pneumomediastinum, and serious vitamin deficiencies (vitamin B_1 and K) leading to Wernicke's encephalopathy and maternal coagulopathy (Lee & Saha, 2011; Niebyl, 2010).

In addition to these physical outcomes associated with HG, significant quality of life issues emerge for women experiencing HG (Munch, Korst, Hernandez, Romero, & Goodwin, 2011). A variety of adverse psychosocial effects have been reported, including economic and employment concerns, depression, anxiety, and fear about future pregnancies (Poursharif et al., 2008). Women report loss of efficiency at work, requirements for time off, and negative effects on the relationship with their partner and children (Attard et al., 2002; McCormick, Scott-Heyes, & McCusker, 2011). In a recent study, of those women with severe nausea or vomiting or HG, 76 percent changed plans for future pregnancies, 15 percent terminated their pregnancies secondary to HG, and 7 percent reported long-term psychological problems (Poursharif et al., 2007).

Most studies have found nausea and vomiting in pregnancy to be associated with favorable fetal outcome (Lee & Saha, 2011). Nausea in pregnancy is associated with lower rates of spontaneous miscarriage (King & Murphy, 2009). However, some adverse fetal outcomes have been associated with severe nausea and vomiting, including LBW and PTB, with lower birth weights associated with more severe symptoms (ACOG Practice Bulletin, 2004b).

Risk factors associated with HG include clinical hyperthyroid disorders, prepregnancy psychiatric diagnosis, history of HG with previous pregnancy, history of motion sickness or migraine, family history, trophoblastic disease, multiple gestation, fetal abnormalities such as triploidy, trisomy 21, and hydrops fetalis, diabetes, gastrointestinal disorders (ACOG Practice Bulletin, 2004b; Fejzo, MacGibbon, Romero, Goodwin, & Mullin, 2011; Lee & Saha, 2011; Zhang et al., 2011). For women hospitalized for hyperemesis in a previous pregnancy, 20 percent require hospitalization for a subsequent pregnancy (Dodds, Fell, Joseph, Allen, & Butler, 2006). Women over the age of 30 and women who smoke have a lower risk of HG (Fell, Dodds, Joseph, Allen, & Butler, 2006). A recent study in Norway found that starting pregnancy either underweight or overweight increased the risk of HG in nonsmokers (Vikanes et al., 2010).

The only identified prevention strategy for nausea and vomiting of pregnancy is the preconceptual use of multivitamins that contain vitamin B_6 and B complex. Several studies have shown that women who were taking a multivitamin before pregnancy had a reduction in the need for medical intervention related to vomiting (ACOG Practice Bulletin, 2004b; Black, 2002).

Subjective Data

Women with HG typically present with severe nausea and episodes of uncontrolled vomiting and retching. It's important to assess severity of symptoms by asking questions that quantify nausea, vomiting, and retching (see PUQE index, Table 20–5). Some women may also report excess salivation or gastroesophageal reflux symptoms such as retrosternal discomfort and heartburn (King & Murphy, 2009). Severely affected women may have muscle wasting, weakness, and/or mental status changes (Lee & Saha, 2011).

Women who experience nausea and vomiting for the first time after 9 to 10 weeks of gestation need to be evaluated for other medical conditions (ACOG Practice Bulletin, 2004b; Ebrahimi, Maltepe, & Einarson, 2010). Nausea and vomiting of pregnancy is not associated with fever or headache, so if these conditions coexist with nausea and vomiting, infection and/or neurological disorders should be further investigated (ACOG Practice Bulletin, 2004b).

Objective Data

Physical Examination. Women may present with signs of dehydration, such as dry mucous membranes, tachycardia, poor skin turgor, and postural hypotension (Lee & Saha, 2011). The uterine, breast, and skin changes are all within normal limits of pregnancy. An abdominal exam should be performed to rule out abdominal causes of nausea and vomiting.

The PUQE index can be used to provide a more objective assessment of nausea and vomiting symptoms (see Figure 20–1) and guidance in making management decisions. Weight should also be measured at each visit to ascertain weight gain or loss.

Laboratory and Radiologic Evaluation. A pregnancy test should be done if a woman presents with severe nausea/vomiting but she hasn't been evaluated for pregnancy. Electrolyte results will generally indicate dehydration if vomiting persists beyond 24 hours. In spite of an association of *H. pylori* with HG, routine screening for gastric infection in women with HG is not recommended (Lee & Saha, 2011). An ultrasound evaluation is useful in identification of risk factors such as multiple gestation and trophoblastic disease. For women with a history of hyperthyroidism, measurements of free thyroxine and free triiodothyronine concentrations should be obtained (ACOG Practice Bulletin, 2004b). Other serious disorders should be ruled out in conjunction with acute management of HG.

Common laboratory tests performed for a pregnant woman who presents with severe nausea and vomiting include CBC, urinalysis, electrolytes, blood urea nitrogen (BUN), creatinine, liver function, serum amylase or lipase, and thyroid-stimulating hormone (TSH). A woman with HG may have an elevated hematocrit, electrolyte disturbances, ketones, elevated liver enzymes, elevated serum amylase or lipase, and lower TSH levels (ACOG Practice Bulletin, 2004b; Lee & Saha, 2011; Niebyl, 2010).

TABLE 20–5. Modified Pregnancy-Unique Quantification of Emesis/Nausea (PUQE) Index

Circle the answer that best suits your situation from the beginning of your pregnancy.				
1. On an average day, for how long do you feel nauseated or sick to your stomach				
> 6 hrs (5 pts.)	4-6 hrs (4 pts)	2-3 hrs (3 pts)	≤ 1 hr (2 pts)	Not at all (1 pt)
2. On an average day how many times do you vomit or throw up?				
7 or more (5 pts)	5-6 (4 pts)	3-4 (3 pts)	1-2 (2 pts)	None (1 pt)
3. On an average day how many times do you have retching or dry heaves without bringing anything up?				
7 or more (5 pts)	5-6 (4 pts)	3-4 (3 pts)	1-2 (2 pts)	None (1 pt)

Total score (sum of replies to 1, 2, and 3): mild NVP, ≤ 6; moderate NVP, 7-12; severe NVP, ≥ 13.

Sources: Lacasse(2008). Validity of the modified-PUQE. American Journal of Obstetrics and Gynecology 198(1), 71; King & Murphy (2009) Evidence-based approaches to managing nausea and vomiting in early pregnancy. Journal of Midwifery and Women's Health 46(6) 430-444; Saxe, & Collins-Bride (2011). Clinical Guidelines for Advanced Practice Nursing, 2nd ed., p 277. Burlington ,MA: Jones & Bartlett.

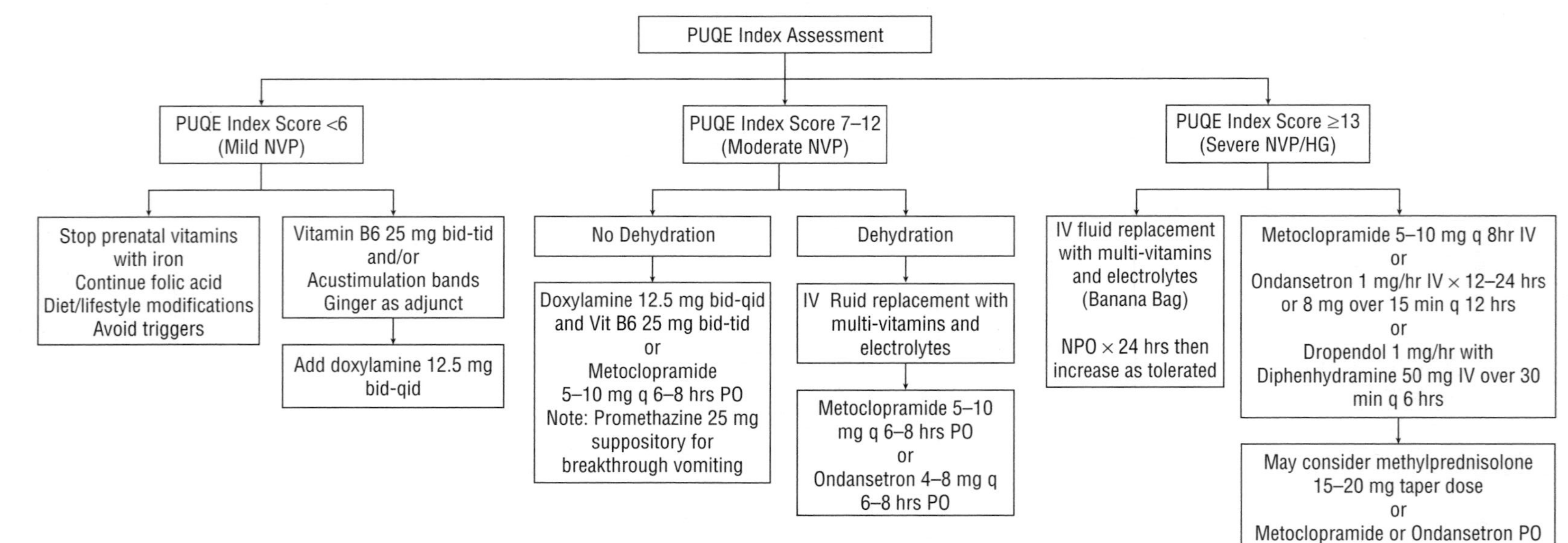

FIGURE 20–1. Protocol for Assessing and Treating Women With Nausea and Vomiting in Pregnancy. *Sources: Adapted from ACOG Practice Bulletin, 2004b; Arsenault et al., 2002; King & Murphy, 2009; and Levichek et al., 2002.*

Differential Medical Diagnosis

Acute thyroidoitis, gastroenteritis, gastroesophageal reflux disease, cholecystitis, pancreatitis, gastric and duodenal peptic disease, irritable bowel disease, viral hepatitis, biliary tract disease, pyelonephritis, appendicitis, and eating disorders.

Plan

A systematic approach to management of nausea and vomiting in pregnancy in combination with more frequent clinic visits (every 4 days to weekly for women with severe symptoms) has been recommended to decrease maternal morbidity and save health care resources (King & Murphy, 2009). Although there are no standard treatment algorithims, the PUQE index, as discussed earlier, can serve as a guide for management decisions based on severity of symptoms (see Figure 20–1).

The general approach to management of nausea and vomiting in pregnancy is to start with dietary and lifestyle modifications, including the use of ginger and vitamin B_6. The treatment pathway for unresolved nausea and vomiting that is more characteristic of HG generally involves the use of IV hydration and pharmacologic therapy. These pathways can typically be managed in an outpatient setting, but hospitalization for ongoing IV hydration, antiemetic medication, and parenteral nutritional support may be required for worsening symptoms and maternal status. These treatment strategies will be reviewed later.

Dietary and lifestyle changes are commonly used as the initial approach to mild nausea and vomiting, although there has been no evidence-based research to substantiate their effectiveness (King & Murphy, 2009; Matthews, Dowswell, Haas, Doyle, & O'Mathuna, 2010). These changes include avoidance of odors, foods, or supplements (iron tablets) that trigger nausea/vomiting; eating small, frequent meals throughout the day (avoiding an empty stomach); avoidance of fatty, rich, or spicy foods; eating crackers before getting out of bed in the morning; and eating a high protein snack before bedtime (ACOG Practice Bulletin, 2004b; King & Murphy, 2009; Niebyl, 2010).

Herbal methods of treating nausea and vomiting in pregnancy include use of ginger, chamomile, peppermint, and red raspberry leaf (King & Murphy, 2009). Of these, ginger is the only one that has research evidence to support its use for management of nausea and vomiting in pregnancy. The use of ginger has been shown to have beneficial effects in several research studies (ACOG Practice Bulletin, 2004b; Ebrahimi et al., 2010). Dosages from 250 to 1,000 per day of ginger root powder, capsule, or extract have been found to reduce the number of episodes of vomiting and the duration and severity of nausea without evidence of any negative pregnancy outcomes (Ebrahimi et al., 2010). Other integrative therapies such as acupuncture, acupressure wristsbands, biofeedback, and hypnosis have also been used by women with some success (ACOG Practice Bulletin, 2004b; Buckwalter & Simpson, 2002; MacCormick, 2010). The majority of studies on the use of pressure or electrical stimulation of P6 (or Negian point) on the inside of the wrist for management of nausea and vomiting have shown positive results (ACOG Practice Bulletin, 2004b; Ebrahimi et al., 2010; King & Murphy, 2009; Lee & Frazier, 2011; Matthews et al., 2010).

Multiple well-designed research studies have demonstrated that vitamin B_6 (10–25 mg every 8 hours) is effective in the treatment of the nausea and vomiting in pregnancy (King & Murphy, 2009; Matthews et al., 2010; Niebyl, 2010). In 1983, a combination of vitamin B_6, antispasmodic dicylcomine hydrochloride, and antihistamine doxylamine (Bendectin) was removed from the U.S. market by the manufacturer due to allegations of teratogenicity, which were later found to be unsubstantiated (Niebyl, 2010). A comparable drug (Diclectin) has been available in Canada since 1979 (Koren et al., 2010) and has been found to reduce the incidence of hospitalization for nausea and vomiting in pregnancy (Niebyl, 2010). The combination of vitamin B_6 and doxylamine has been extensively studied with no evidence of teratogenicity and significant reduction in nausea and vomiting. The ACOG recommends this combination as the first-line therapy for nausea and vomiting (ACOG Practice Bulletin, 2004b; Niebyl, 2010). Oral vitamin B_6 and doxylamine (Unisom SleepTabs®) are available over the counter in the United States.

IV fluid therapy plays a significant role in managing the dehydration and subsequent electrolye imbalance that accompanies HG. IV therapy should be used for women who are unable to tolerate oral liquids for a prolonged period (> 24 hours) or if clinical signs of dehydration are present (ACOG Practice Bulletin, 2004b). Normal saline should be used with the addition of potassium chloride, and optionally, thiamine or a multivitamin solution. IV thiamine should be administered before using dextrose-containing solutions in order to prevent Wernicke's encephalopathy (Lee & Saha, 2011), which can occur when women with a thiamine deficiency receive a large carbohydrate load (King & Murphy, 2009). In some areas, the woman may be able to obtain IV therapy in an office setting, ambulatory care, or emergency room, and in-home IV administration should be considered for women with multiple hospital admissions (Lee & Saha, 2011). Hospitalization for management of HG is generally recommended when there is persistent vomiting and other methods of outpatient treatment have been unsuccessful (ACOG Practice Bulletin, 2004b).

Pharmacologic therapies used for the treatment of HG include vitamin B_6 (see earlier), antihistamines, antiemetics, promotility agents, and other medications such as ondansetron (Zofran) and corticosteroids. Doxylamine and other antihistamines have been found to demonstrate efficacy and safety when used to manage nausea and vomiting during pregnancy. Phenothiazines such as Phenergan and Compazine are also effective in reducing vomiting (Ebrahimi et al., 2010). Metoclopramide (Reglan), an upper gastrointestinal motility stimulant, has been used as a second step when phenothiazines or antihistamines are ineffective or as a first step (administered IV or subcutaneously) when women are admitted to an inpatient setting for treatment of HG (King & Murphy, 2009; Tan & Omar, 2011). Zofran, initially used as an effective treatment for nausea and vomiting associating with chemotherapy, is now also used for treatment of HG (Ebrahimi et al., 2010). Because this drug is expensive, some insurance companies may not approve usage until other methods have proved ineffective (King & Murphy, 2009). Corticosteroids have also been used when women are hospitalized for HG, but research linking usage to a small increase in the risk of oral clefts has resulted in decreased use (King & Murphy, 2009) and ACOG recommends usage only after 10 weeks' gestation (ACOG Practice Bulletin, 2004b).

Dietary counseling is usually added to any medication therapy. The diet can consist of liquids that contain salt, glucose, and potassium such as sports drinks and bouillon. The woman must be able to consume a minimum of 1.0 to 1.5 L of fluid in order to prevent dehydration. Once tolerating liquids, the diet is advanced to brothy soups with noodles or rice. If tolerated, solid starches such as potatoes or pasta are added. Chicken or fish are preferred protein sources. Fatty foods such as creamed soups are avoided because they delay gastric emptying (Koch, 2002).

The primary criterion for use of parenteral or enteral therapy is persistent weight loss and this level of severity requires hospitalization. Enteral (tube) feedings should be initiated first in these circumstances, as sole use of parenteral therapy for women with persistent weight loss is associated with a significant increase in serious complications (ACOG Practice Bulletin, 2004b; Ebrahimi et al., 2010).

HYPERTENSION

The results of a large nationwide study show an increased prevalence of hypertensive disorders among hospitalizations for delivery since 2001, contributing to increased rates of severe maternal morbidity (Kuklina, Ayala, & Callaghan, 2009). The increasing numbers of women entering pregnancy over the age of 40, the rise in multiple births, and the increased incidence of obesity in the United States place more women at risk for the development of hypertensive disorders during pregnancy. From a public health perspective, obesity should be addressed as a primary area of focus in the prevention of hypertensive disorders in pregnancy. There is also growing evidence that women with pregnancies complicated by hypertension have an increased risk of developing hypertension later in life (Lindheimer, Taler, & Cunningham, 2009).

One of the challenges in addressing hypertensive disorders of pregnancy has been changing terminology and diagnostic criteria. The term *toxemia* has been replaced by *preeclampsia* and *pregnancy-induced hypertension* has been replaced by *gestational hypertension*. In 2000, the National High Blood Pressure Education Program (NHBPEP) working group on high blood pressure in pregnancy developed a new classification system with four categories of hypertension in pregnancy: gestational hypertension, preeclampsia/eclampsia, chronic hypertension, and preeclampsia superimposed on chronic hypertension. Preeclampsia is the disorder that is most associated with serious maternal-fetal complications, including fatalities, and remains the focus of most research studies (Lindheimer et al., 2009). The majority of this discussion will be focused on preeclampsia.

CLASSIFICATION OF HYPERTENSIVE DISORDERS OF PREGNANCY

Gestational hypertension is characterized by hypertension (> 140/90) without proteinuria after 20 weeks of gestation and a return of the blood pressure to normal postpartum. Gestational hypertension is a provisional diagnosis: 50 percent of women diagnosed with gestational hypertension between 24 and 35 weeks gestation develop preeclampsia (Barton, O'Brien, Bergauer, Jacques, & Sibai, 2001) and chronic hypertension is diagnosed if there is no resolution by 12 weeks' postpartum.

Preeclampsia is diagnosed in women who have a blood pressure of ≥ 140/90 after the 20th week of pregnancy, confirmed by two readings 4 to 6 hours apart, accompanied by urinary excretion of 0.3 g protein or higher in a 24-hour urine specimen (Report of the NHBPEP working group on high blood pressure in pregnancy, 2000). Previously, if the blood pressure rose 30 mmHg systolic or more than 15 mmHg diastolic above the woman's baseline, she was considered preeclamptic. The NHBPEP working group no longer uses this as a criterion but warns that women experiencing these changes warrant close observation. Edema is also no longer used as diagnostic criteria for preeclampsia, as it is considered too nonspecific (ACOG Practice Bulletin, 2002a).

The ACOG (Practice Bulletin, 2002a) categorizes preeclampsia as mild or severe, with the following clinical features associated with severe preeclampsia: blood pressure higher than 160/110 on two occasions at least 6 hours apart, proteinuria greater than 500 mg in 24-hour urine collection, oliguria (less than 500 mL in 24 hours), pulmonary edema or thrombocytopenia with or without liver damage, and cerebral or visual disturbances, epigastric or right upper quadrant pain, or fetal growth retardation. Other authors note that the potential for rapid fulimation of mild preeclampsia to eclampsia illustrates the need to carefully monitor all patients with a preeclampsia diagnosis (Lindheimer et al., 2009). Eclampsia is defined as the occurrence of new onset of grand mal seizures in a woman diagnosed with preeclampsia (ACOG Practice Bulletin, 2002a), which typically occurs after midpregnancy or postpartum.

Chronic hypertension is diagnosed when a blood pressure of 140/90 or higher develops before pregnancy, is recognized before 20 weeks of gestation, or continues indefinitely postpartum (Report of the NHBPEP working group, 2000). Chronic hypertension is classified as mild (BP > 140/90) or severe (BP ≥ 180/110 mmHg) (ACOG Practice Bulletin, 2001b), with clinical signs that are different from those of gestational hypertension. Due to normal decreases in blood pressure in early pregnancy, chronic hypertension may be masked and incorrectly diagnosed as gestational hypertension when blood pressures are elevated after 20 weeks' gestation.

Preeclampsia superimposed on chronic hypertension is characterized by new onset proteinuria in women with hypertension before 20 weeks' gestation, a sudden increase in proteinuria compared with lesser amounts in earlier gestation, a sudden increase in hypertension, or the development of HELLP syndrome (Report of the NHBPEP working group, 2000). Additionally, women with chronic hypertension who develop headache, scotomata, or epigastric pain may have superimposed preeclampsia (ACOG Practice Bulletin, 2002a).

PATHOPHYSIOLOGY AND ETIOLOGY OF PREECLAMPSIA

Preeclampsia is a multiorgan system disorder of unknown etiology that is characterized by hypertension and proteinuria (Leeman & Fontaine, 2008). The hypertension component is due primarily to vasoconstriction, resulting in an elevation in blood pressure and reduction in blood flow to target organs. In addition to the vascular system, the organs most affected are the kidneys, brain, liver, and placenta. Decreased blood flow to the kidneys results in decreased renal plasma flow and glomerular filtration rates. Decreased blood flow to the brain leads to fluid shift, cerebral edema, and changes in sensorium. Cerebral edema also leads to central nervous system irritability, which can predispose to convulsions. Elevated liver enzymes demonstrate the effect of preeclampsia on the liver. Preeclampsia is also associated with alterations in the coagulation system, most commonly thrombocytopenia. Severe preeclampsia may be accompanied by HELLP syndrome. Symptoms and signs of HELLP syndrome include nausea (with or without vomiting), epigastric pain, upper quadrant tenderness, demonstrable edema, and hyperbilirubinemia.

Although the causation of preeclampsia has not been firmly established, current theories implicate placental and endothelial dysfunction with associated vasospasm as major components of this syndrome (Gibson, 2011). Abnormal placentation is a hallmark of preeclampsia, accompanied by a failure of normal trophoblastic invasion of the spiral arteries (McMaster, Zhou, & Fisher, 2004). Subsequent to abnormal placental implantation, substances are released that activate or injure endothelial cells. The effect of endothelial injury explains the multiorgan system involvement. There are also higher rates of gestational hypertension in pregnancies with excessive placental tissue, as is seen in women with diabetes, gestational trophoblastic disease, and multiple gestation. According to Lindheimer et al. (2009), the most plausible theories focus on the placenta and identify the disorder as a two-stage process. In the first stage, an initiating cause results in placenta-producing factors that enter maternal circulation, including an overproduction of proteins that lead to endothelial dysfunction. The second stage is called maternal and is impacted by these circulating factors and the health of the mother, including preexisting cardiorenal, metabolic, and genetic factors and obesity. These theories demonstrate some congruency between risk factors associated with preeclampsia and pathogenesis.

Epidemiology

Hypertensive disorders of pregnancy occur in 5 to 10 percent of pregnancies and preeclampsia complicates 3 to 5 percent of pregnancies in the United States (Hutcheon, Lisonkova, & Joseph, 2011). Approximately 50 percent of women diagnosed with gestational hypertension will develop preeclampsia and 25 percent of women with chronic hypertension will develop superimposed preeclampsia (Report of the NHBPEP working group, 2000). The prevalence of chronic hypertension varies according to age, race, and body mass index (BMI), occurring in up to 22 percent of childbearing women (Gibson, 2011). Overweight and obese women have an increased risk of entering pregnancy with chronic hypertension (Callaway, O'Callaghan, & McIntrye, 2009). HELLP syndrome occurs in approximately 5 percent of women with preeclampsia (Lindheimer et al., 2009). The incidence of eclampsia in the United States has declined in the past several decades, but serious maternal complications such as coma, stroke, and respiratory distress occur in up to 30 percent of cases (Hutcheon et al., 2011).

Risk factors for preeclampsia include nulliparity, family history of preeclampsia, history of preeclampsia in a previous pregnancy, preexisting hypertension or diabetes, obesity, multiple pregnancy, African American race, and advanced maternal age (> 35) (Report of the NHBPEP working group, 2000). The prevalence of hypertensive disorders in pregnancy is two to three times higher in overweight and obese women compared to normal weight women (Callaway et al., 2009), and a systematic review showed the risk of preeclampsia doubles with each 5 to 7 kg/m^2 increase in prepregnancy BMI (O'Brien, Ray, & Chan, 2003). Women with antiphospholipid syndrome, other thrombophilias, autoimmune disease, kidney disease, and infertility are also at greater risk (Hutcheon et al., 2011). Smoking has been shown to have a protective effect on the development of preeclampsia, reducing its occurrence by 50 percent (England & Zhang, 2007). Risk for recurrence of preeclampsia with a subsequent pregnancy is 7 to 15 percent (Hernandez-Diaz, Toh, & Cnattingius, 2009), and increases to 30 percent if the first two pregnancies were complicated by preeclampsia (Magee, Helewa, & Moutquin, 2008).

Maternal complications associated with preeclampsia are acute renal failure, pulmonary edema, thrombotic complications, and death (Report of the NHBPEP working group, 2000). Women with preeclampsia have a 70 percent greater risk of placental abruption (Hogberg, Rasmussen, & Irgens, 2007). Adverse maternal outcomes are associated with earlier gestational age of onset; maternal mortality rates are significantly higher when preeclampsia occurs before 28 weeks compared to term gestation onset (Hutcheon et al., 2011). Fetal complications of hypertensive disorders of pregnancy include IUGR, prematurity, and stillbirth (Report of the NHBPEP working group, 2000). Additionally, offspring of women with preeclampsia have been found to have long-term adverse health effects, including higher blood pressure in childhood and adolescence (Ferreira, Peeters, & Stehouwer, 2009), increased hospitalization for metabolic disorders (Wu et al., 2009), and increased risk for stroke as adults (Kajantie, Erickson, Osmond, Thornburg, & Barker, 2009).

Screening and Prevention

The traditional method of screening women at risk for preeclampsia is through maternal history. Clinical guidelines issued in the United Kingdom recommend formulation of prenatal visits following preeclampsia risk status determined at the initial prenatal visit (Duckitt & Harrington, 2005). More recently, a variety of markers have been evaluated for use in predicting gestational hypertension and preeclampsia. Researchers in the United Kingdom developed a first trimester screening method to identify women at risk for preeclampsia using a combination of maternal variables, including mean arterial pressure, uterine artery pulsatility index, pregnancy-associated plasma protein A (PAPP-A), and placental growth factor. This algorithim has been especially useful in predicting preeclampsia before 34 weeks (Poon, Kametas, Maiz, Akolekar, & Nicolaides, 2009). In another study, blood pressure measurements combined with maternal risk factors yielded a 76 percent rate of detection for early preeclampsia (Poon, Kametas, Valencia, Chelemen, & Nicolaides, 2011). A systematic review conducted to ascertain the current state of first trimester screening for preeclampsia showed that a combination of five markers yielded the highest detection rates (placental protein 13, placental growth factor, PAPP-A, inhibin A, uterine artery Doppler, maternal characteristics), but detection rates for single markers was low. To date, there isn't a single screening test that can reliably predict preeclampsia (Kuc et al., 2011).

There have been several interventions directed at preeclampsia prevention, including the use of aspirin, calcium supplementation, vitamin C and E supplementation, garlic, nitric oxide, progesterone, exercise, and rest during pregnancy. Systematic reviews through 2011 have only identified two interventions with protective effects for women at higher risk of developing preeclampsia: low-dose aspirin and calcium supplementation. Calcium supplementation (minimum of 1,000 mg/day) was found to halve the risk of preeclampsia, reduce the risk of PTB, and reduce associated death or serious morbidity, with the greatest effect on women with low baseline calcium intake and those considered high risk (Hofmeyr, Lawrie, Atallah, & Duley, 2010). Low-dose aspirin (75–81 mg/day) reduced the incidence of preeclampsia in women with a history of hypertension or preeclampsia (Duley, Henderson-Smart, Meher, & King, 2007) with no evidence of adverse maternal or fetal outcomes (Dastor & Tank, 2010). More research is needed to assess dosage, when treatment should be initiated, and the appropriate high-risk client for this therapy (Duley et al, 2007). Aspirin therapy in normotensive women has not shown to be of benefit and is not recommended by the ACOG Practice Bulletin (2002a). Supplementation with the antioxidant vitamins C and E (Polyzos et al., 2007; Rumbold, Duley, Crowther, & Haslam, 2008), progesterone (Meher & Duley, 2006c), and increased intake of garlic (Meher & Duley, 2006a) have no effect on preeclampsia occurrence. There is also insufficient evidence to evaluate the effect of nitric oxide donors and precursors on preeclampsia (Meher & Duley, 2007). Studies evaluating the effect of exercise and rest during pregnancy in women with normal blood pressure have been inconclusive (Meher & Duley, 2006b, 2006d).

Subjective Data

A thorough review of past medical history, family history, obstetrical history, BMI, and laboratory results should provide the basis of identification of risk for the development of preeclampsia. A woman may report headache; visual disturbances; facial, ankle, and finger edema; or severe heartburn with abdominal pain. Generalized edema may be observed but is not considered a sign of preeclampsia.

Objective Data

Blood pressure must be carefully and consistently measured to be meaningful. Consistent measurements are those obtained in the same arm with the client in the same position, using appropriate size cuff (length 1.5 times the upper arm circumference), and taken at least 6 hours apart (ACOG Practice Bulletin, 2002a). Current antepartal care guidelines recommend blood pressure screening at all prenatal visits throughout the pregnancy (ICSI, 2010). Early detection of an abnormal blood pressure trend over time remains the simplest screening strategy for hypertension in pregnancy.

Weight gain is determined at every visit; although weight gain and edema are not used as diagnostic criteria for preeclampsia, excessive weight gain may signal increased risk, particularly for women who are overweight or obese. The Institute of Medicine (IOM, 2009) weight gain standards (based on BMI) should be used to ascertain excessive gain.

Urine testing is no longer recommended for routine prenatal visits (ICSI, 2010). Conventional urine dipstick measurements are unreliable in quantifying urine protein excretion; they are associated with significant false-positive and false-negative readings (Waugh, Clark, Divakaran, Khan, & Kilby, 2004). In spite of these recommendations, many clinical practices continue to routinely perform urine dipsticks for glucose and protein screening. Urine dipsticks of greater than +2 protein should always be quantified with a 24-hour collection or spot urine protein : creatinine ratio (Gibson, 2011). Spot urine specimens for protein : creatinine ratios have been validated as screening tools, but the 24-hour urine collection remains the gold standard as this provides a high accuracy of total urine protein and creatinine excretion (ICSI, 2010). Two- and 12-hour urine protein testing should also be considered to expedite clinical management of preeclampsia (Abebe, Eigbefoh, Isabu, Eifediyi, & Okusanya, 2008).

Additional laboratory testing is recommended for women at higher risk for developing preeclampsia, particularly those with a history of preeclampsia, chronic hypertension, lupus, preexisting diabetes, antiphospholipid syndrome, and renal disease (ICSI, 2010). It may be useful to obtain baseline blood work for hemoglobin, platelet count, liver function tests, and a 24-hour urine collection during the first trimester should signs and symptoms of preeclampsia occur later in pregnancy (Duckitt & Harrington, 2005). Routine laboratory tests recommended for evaluating a client for preeclampsia include CBC, electrolytes, BUN, creatinine, liver enzymes, bilirubin, and 24-hour urine collection (Gibson, 2011).

Physical examination is essentially normal for a woman presenting with mild preeclampsia. Significant changes can be found as preeclampsia becomes more severe. Worrisome changes can include the following:

Edema. Lower extremity edema is normal in the third trimester of pregnancy. Nondependent edema (face and hands) or rapid weight gain with a generalized edema may warrant further evaluation for preeclampsia.

Neurological. Woman may exhibit a decreased attention span, disorientation, sleepiness, or decreased alertness. Many normal women have hyperactive reflexes and hyperreactive reflexes are common during pregnancy, but clonus reflects neuromuscular irritability associated with severe preeclampsia. Brisk reflexes or clonus may herald an imminent convulsive state. Assessment may thus be helpful in monitoring drug therapy, but it cannot be diagnostic for determining status of gestational hypertension.

Retinal Changes. May include edema and arteriolar spasm.

Lungs. Rales and rhonchi can be heard in affected lobes when pulmonary edema is present.

Liver. Hepatomegaly or upper right quadrant tenderness, or both, may be present.

Fundal Height. A decrease in fundal height (more than 2 cm less than gestational age on two consecutive visits) may indicate IUGR. This finding requires follow-up with serial sonograms (see Chapter 21).

Differential Medical Diagnoses

Diseases that mimic severe preeclampsia or HELLP syndrome including cholecystitis, viral hepatitis, idiopathic thrombocytopenia, hemolytic uremic syndrome, microangiopathic syndrome, fatty liver disease of pregnancy, and peptic ulcer. Appendicitis, kidney stones, pyelonephritis, gastroenteritis, placental abruption, abdominal trauma, migraine headache, stroke, and seizure disorders are other possibilities.

Plan

Early identification of symptoms and subsequent intervention can decrease the severity of disease and improve perinatal outcome. Once preeclampsia is diagnosed, management depends on gestational age and disease severity. Because delivery is the only cure for preeclampsia, the challenging clinical balance is to minimize maternal risk while maximizing fetal maturity. Patients with mild preeclampsia are often induced after 37 weeks and induction with severe preeclampsia is considered after 34 weeks (ACOG Practice Bulletin, 2002a). According to the American Society of Hypertension, "delivery is indicated at any stage of pregnancy if severe hypertension remains uncontrolled for 24 to 48 hours or at the appearance of certain 'omninous signs' such as clotting or liver abnormalities, decreasing renal function, signs of impending convulsions (headache, epigastric pain, and hyperreflexia), or the presence of severe growth retardation or nonreassuring fetal testing" (Lindheimer, Taylor, & Cunningham, 2009, p. 220). Management in an obstetrical practice rather than family practice is indicated for those with preeclampsia. Severe preeclampsia warrants referral to a perinatal specialist, hospitalization, and review of the risks/benefits of delivery.

Education. All clients should be informed of the danger signs of preeclampsia and directed to seek evaluation immediately. The two most significant signs of preeclampsia (proteinuria and hypertension) typically occur without the woman's awareness, and the condition may be serious before overt symptoms occur. The client may need to be taught to take her blood pressure or perform a dipstick urine test.

Expectant Management. More frequent monitoring is recommended for women with mild preeclampsia, including biweekly prenatal visits and weekly laboratory and antepartal testing. According to the NHBPEP working group (2000), ambulatory management of women with mild preeclampsia can be considered in conjunction with frequent maternal/fetal evaluation and health care access, with hospitalization for worsening preeclampsia. Antepartal self-monitoring can also provide valuable information and support client participation and autonomy (see Table 20–6).

Bed rest continues to be recommended in women with preeclampsia, but there is little evidence to support this practice. Intermittent rest in the left lateral position has been promoted to induce diuresis and reduce blood pressure. Sustained bed rest should be avoided as it increases the risk of thromboembolic events and typically results in increased maternal and family stress (Meher, Abalos, & Carroll, 2005).

Hospitalization. Hospitalization is essential in the treatment of severe preeclampsia and chronic hypertension with superimposed preeclampsia. The intrauterine environment becomes increasingly hostile to the fetus, and each day is a delicate balance between the risks and benefits of intrauterine and extrauterine existence. Severe preeclampsia is treated aggressively, as hypertension poses

TABLE 20–6. Antepartal Monitoring of Pregnant Woman With Mild Preeclampsia

Home	Office Visit
Check blood pressure once or twice a day	Check blood pressure twice weekly
Check weight every day	Check weight
Perform urine dipstick twice daily	Assess for proteinuria: screen with urine dipstick or spot protein/creatinine ratio, periodic 24-hour urine collections
Observe symptoms: occipital headaches, blurred vision, irritability or emotional tension, scotoma, epigastric pain, or any signs and symptoms of labor	Assess symptoms: occipital headaches, blurred vision, irritability or emotional tension, scotoma, epigastric pain, or any signs and symptoms of labor
	Obtain baseline serum creatinine, uric acid, creatinine clearance, total urinary protein. Repeat weekly
Record fetal movements daily	Obtain baseline liver enzymes, CBC, platelet count—repeat weekly
	Auscultate fetal heart tones, baseline fundal height, and weekly measurements
	Perform baseline nonstress test (NST) twice weekly
	Measure amniotic fluid index (AFI) one to two times weekly
	Biophysical profile weekly in place of twice weekly NSTs and AFI
	Obtain baseline and serial sonograms every 3–4 weeks

Sources: ACOG Practice Bulletins, 2001b, 2002; Leeman & Fontaine, 2008.

an immediate threat to mother and fetus. Aggressive therapy includes maternal and fetal assessments, medications to prevent seizure activity and stabilize blood pressure, and preparation for delivery. Because of the need for intensive and sometimes invasive monitoring techniques such as invasive hemodynamic monitoring, hospitalization is required with critical obstetrical care provided by appropriate medical and nursing staff (ACOG Practice Bulletin, 2002a).

Medication. For those with preeclampsia, drugs are given to decrease seizure activity and reduce blood pressure. The drug of choice to control or prevent seizure activity is magnesium sulfate (ACOG Practice Bulletin, 2002a), reducing the risk of eclampsia by more than 50 percent (Duley, Gulmezoglu, Henderson-Smart, & Chou, 2010). There is no current recommendation that guides when or who to treat prophylactically, although it is not typically used to treat mild preeclampsia (Lindheimer et al., 2009). Other anticonvulsive medications such as diazepam or phenytoin have been used for control of eclampsia, but magnesium sulfate remains the primary treatment (Duley, Henderson-Smart, & Chou, 2010; Duley, Henderson-Smart, Walker, & Chou, 2010). It is usually given as an initial bolus and subsequently in continuous IV infusion. One fourth of women receiving magnesium sulfate report side effects with flushing being the most common (Duley, Gulmezoglu, et al., 2010). Because magnesium sulfate readily crosses the placenta, the newborn will be affected by the sedative properties of the drug and may exhibit hypotonia, suppressed respiratory effort at delivery, and poor sucking. These effects subside as the newborn excretes the drug over the following 3 to 4 days.

Pharmacological treatment of pregnant women with chronic hypertension remains controversial. The NHBPE working group (2000) recommends antihypertensive therapy for women with mild chronic hypertension when BP exceeds 150 to 160 mmHg systolic or 100 to 110 mmHg diastolic and BP over 180/110 mmHg for women with severe chronic hypertension. If drug therapy is deemed necessary, the use of oral antihypertensives with established fetal safety profiles (e.g., methyldopa, labetalol, hydralazine, long-acting nifedipine) is generally preferred. Angiotensin-converting enzyme inhibitors are contraindicated because they are associated with a characteristic fetopathy (ACOG Practice Bulletin, 2001b). The antihypertensive drug recommended for management of chronic hypertension during pregnancy by the NHBPE working group is methyldopa. Hydralazine is commonly used for acute management of preeclampsia, but requires close observation after administration due to unpredictable hypotensive episodes. The most recent Cochrane review on pharmacologic treatment of high blood pressure during pregnancy recommends that clinician experience and familiarity with drug should also be considered (Duley, Henderson-Smart, & Meher, 2006).

The value of antihypertensive therapy in women with mild to moderate hypertension during pregnancy is not clear (Abalos, Duley, Steyn, & Henderson-Smart, 2007; Podymow & August, 2008). Because not treating women until the diastolic BP reaches 100 mmHg does not appear to increase maternal or fetal risk, and treatment may in fact lower uterine blood flow with no benefit, a policy of close observation is reasonable in mildly hypertensive women, especially when there has been no hypertension before pregnancy and no proteinuria.

Convulsive State. This is an emergency situation and can occur at any time, although the client has usually exhibited signs of severe preeclampsia. Convulsive facial twitching and tonic-clonic contractions of the body occur. Gradually, movements subside, but the client may remain in a coma for an indefinite period. Airway maintenance and oxygen are necessary, and hemodynamic monitoring is useful for appropriate fluid management. Following seizure, the client is hypoxic and acidotic and requires stabilization before delivery. However, rapid dilation and precipitous delivery of the fetus may occur with seizure activity.

Delivery. The only cure for gestational hypertension is delivery of the fetus. Primary goal of management is to allow pregnancy to progress as far as possible without jeopardizing maternal or fetal well-being. Timing and mode of delivery depend on stability of the maternal-fetal unit, gestation, and the cervix. If the cervix is favorable and other factors are controlled, labor is induced with pitocin and magnesium sulfate therapy is administered concurrently to control or prevent seizures. For the woman with eclampsia, delivery should occur as soon as possible after the woman and fetus are stabilized. Cesarean delivery is initiated if immediate delivery is indicated. In the absence of coagulopathy, regional or neuroaxial anesthesia is considered safe and effective (ACOG Practice Bulletin, 2002a).

Follow-Up

Women with hypertensive disorders during pregnancy are at greater risk for developing cardiovascular and metabolic disease later in life; women with preeclampsia have a three- to fourfold increased risk of developing chronic hypertension and nearly two times the risk of ischaemic heart disease, stroke, and venous thromboembolism (Bellamy, Casas, Hingorani, & Williams, 2007). Identifying this risk during the childbearing years provides a screening opportunity to detect women at risk for future heart disease and metabolic syndrome with a focus on primary prevention of cardiovascular disease through lifestyle modifications (Preeclampsia Foundation, 2006). All women with a history of preeclampsia should be advised of this increased risk and interventions for risk reduction should be made available, including lifestyle modifications such as smoking cessation, healthy diet, and regular exercise. Annual screening for hypertension, hyperlipidemia, and type II diabetes should also be considered.

OBESITY

The incidence of obesity has increased in the United States and more women are entering pregnancy with a BMI in the overweight and obese category (Hedley et al., 2004). High prepregnant weight and excessive weight gains during pregnancy have been linked to increased pregnancy complications, higher maternal and infant morbidity/mortality, and long-term health problems for women and offspring. There is a linear relationship between pregnancy outcome and BMI; the higher the BMI of a woman starting a pregnancy, the greater the risk of an adverse pregnancy outcome (Manzanares et al., 2012; Raatikainen, Heiskanen, & Heinonen, 2006). Conversely, women who start pregnancies with a prepregnancy BMI in the normal range are at lower risk for preeclampsia, gestational diabetes, and cesarean delivery (IOM, 2009).

The IOM issued new prenatal weight gain guidelines in 2009, adopting the World Health Organization BMI categories, including overweight and obese categories (see Table 20–7). Linkage between gestational weight gain (GWG) and obesity in children led to the first revision in 2007. Since "Nutrition During Pregnancy" was published in 1990 by the IOM, prepregnancy BMI and excessive GWG have dramatically increased among all population groups.

There is compelling evidence that interventions reducing prepregnant weight among women with BMIs over 30 and limiting GWG favorably impacts perinatal outcomes. Pregnancy is a good time to introduce behavioral and dietary modifications, as pregnant women are typically highly motivated to make changes that will improve pregnancy outcome (Olson & Blackwell, 2011). Phelan (2010) introduced the concept of pregnancy as a "teachable moment" for weight control and obesity prevention. Prenatal care provides a unique opportunity for a pregnant woman to access resources and develop

TABLE 20–7. 2009 Institute of Medicine Recommended Prenatal Weight Gains

Weight Category	Body Mass Index Range	Recommended Pregnancy Weight Gain in lb (kg)
Underweight	< 18.5	28–40 (12.5–18.0)
Normal	18.5–24.9	25–35 (11.5–16.0)
Overweight	25.0–29.9	15–25 (7.0–11.5)
Obese	≥ 30.0	11–20 (5.0–9.1)
Category I	30.0–34.9	
Category II	35.0–39.9	
Category III	≥ 40.0	

Source: Institute of Medicine National Research Council, 2009.

strategies for maintaining a healthy lifestyle. Clinicians who work with pregnant women should develop strategies for teaching women how to make healthy lifestyle and nutritional choices before, during, and after pregnancy.

ETIOLOGY AND RISK

Weight gain during pregnancy is a function of the growing fetus and placenta, as well as the development of fat stores that provide energy reserves for pregnancy and lactation (approximately 7 lb). The majority of this growth occurs in the second and third trimesters. Women who enter pregnancy overweight or obese don't need additional stores of adipose tissue, especially central (around waistline) adiposity that is associated with insulin resistance and a predisposition to developing gestational diabetes (Jevitt, 2009).

All pregnant women have greater nutritional needs during pregnancy, both in caloric and in nutrient intake. Caloric intake increases 300 to 400 kcal during the second and third trimesters; requirements for folic acid, vitamin D, and iron double; and needs for protein, calcium, phosphorus, thiamin, zinc, and pyroxidine increase more than 20 percent (Gabbe, Niebyl, & Simpson, 2007). The challenge for all pregnant women is to consume adequate amounts of nutrients without excessive caloric intake and the concomitant excessive weight gain. Adherence to pregnancy weight gain recommendations is challenging. In a study that predates the 2009 guideline change, approximately 40 percent of normal-weight women, 60 percent of overweight women, and 25 percent of obese women exceeded the IOM recommendations (Chu, Callaghan, Bish, & D'Angelo, 2009). Pregnant women who gain weight within the recommended range have a reduced risk of postpartum weight retention, cesarean delivery, and hypertension (IOM, 2009).

It is clear that poor eating habits and a more sedentary lifestyle contribute to increasing rates of obesity among the general population and pregnant women. Studies examining activity levels of pregnant women show that most pregnant women do not meet the ACOG recommendation for 30 minutes or more per day of moderate activity (Anderson et al., 2008; Lindseth & Vari, 2005). Physical activity in pregnancy has been associated with a lower risk of developing gestational diabetes in pregnancy when compared to sedentary women (Oken et al., 2006).

Obesity causes metabolic changes that can lead to insulin resistance, altered glucose metabolism, and ultimately type 2 diabetes. These metabolic changes are also associated with subfertility. See Chapter 23 for more information on metabolic syndrome.

Epidemiology

Currently, 62 percent of reproductive-aged women in the United States are overweight (BMI > 25 kg/m^2) and 33 percent are considered obese (BMI of 30 kg/m^2 or higher) (Ogden et al., 2006). There is a higher prevalence of obesity among women who are non-Hispanic black (39%) or Hispanic (29%) compared with white women (23%), and among women who have lower levels of education (33% without high school completion compared with 18% college graduates) (CDC, 2005b). It is estimated that 40 percent of pregnant women in the United States are overweight or obese (Kim, Dietz, England, Morrow, & Callaghan, 2007). Additionally, at least 46 percent of pregnant women gain more weight than the IOM recommendations, disproportionately occurring among women who have BMIs > 25 (Jevitt, 2009). Less than 1 percent of women entering pregnancy with a BMI over 30 have a medical condition causing excessive weight gain (Gunatilake & Perlow, 2011).

Pregnant women with excessive GWG are more likely to develop gestational diabetes, preeclampsia, postoperative wound infection, postpartum weight retention, and deliver by cesarean section (Olson & Blackwell, 2011). Independent of GWG, obesity in pregnancy (BMI ≥ 30.0) is associated with increased miscarriage rates, fetal congenital anomaly, thromboembolism, gestational diabetes, preeclampsia, dysfunctional labor, postpartum hemorrhage, wound infections, stillbirth, induced labor, cesarean section, anesthesia complications, and neonatal death (Gauthier et al., 2011; Gawade et al., 2011; Olson & Blackwell, 2011; Waller et al., 2007). There is also linkage between excessive GWG and postpartum weight retention, further connecting GWG and future obesity (Jevitt, 2009; Olson & Blackwell, 2011). Most studies have shown a link between depression and obesity (Jevitt, 2009). LaCoursiere and Varner (2009) identifed higher rates of postpartum depression among obese women, with higher rates correlating with greater degrees of obesity (class I, 22.6%; class II, 32.4%; class III, 40%). There is conflicting data about the risk of PTB in overweight and obese women (Aredas, Qiu, & Gruslin, 2008).

Excessive GWG and high prepregnant BMIs have also been positively associated with increased infant, child, adolescent BMI, and later adult obesity (Ludwig & Currie, 2010; Oken, Rifas-Shima, Field, Frazier, & Gillman, 2008; Oken, Taveras, Kleinman,

Rich-Edwards, & Gillman, 2007; Wrotniak, Shults, Butts, & Stettler, 2008). Research on the offspring of mothers with high BMIs and GWG supports the hypothesis that fetal development may play a role in subsequent obesity and metabolic and cardiovascular disease (Olson & Blackwell, 2011). Fraser et al. (2010) confirmed greater BMI, waist circumference, fat mass, leptin, and systolic blood pressure in offspring of mothers with high prepregnancy weight or excessive GWG before 14 weeks.

Increasing numbers of childbearing women with BMIs > 40 are undergoing bariatric surgery, resulting in more women entering pregnancy with a surgically induced weight loss. The two available bariatric surgical procedures are malabsorbtive (jejunoileal bypass and biliopancreatic diversion) and restrictive (gastric banding and vertical banded gastroplasty), resulting in deficiencies in iron, vitamin B_{12}, folate, and calcium (ACOG Technical Bulletin, 2005). Current research reports generally favorable perinatal outcomes for women who achieve pregnancy after bariatric surgery, with lower rates of gestational diabetes, hypertension, macrosomia, and cesarean delivery compared to pregnancies of obese women who have not undergone bariatric surgery, but higher rates of IUGR (Guelinckx, Devlieger, & Vansant, 2009). Women who have undergone bariatric surgery are advised to delay pregnancy 12 to 18 months after surgery to avoid pregnancy during rapid weight loss (ACOG Practice Bulletin, 2005). They should also be screened for deficiencies and counseled on the need for vitamin supplementation, especially B_{12}, and at least 4 mg of folic acid (Gunatilake & Perlow, 2011).

Subjective Data

Verification of LMP and review of medical, family, social, and past pregnancy history should be conducted, as well as a discussion of pregnancy risks and lifestyle considerations. Developing a positive relationship is important when asking questions about eating habits and physical activity, as this remains a sensitive issue for most women. Jevitt (2009) recommends using the BMI standards for weight gain as the primary vehicle for discussing weight gain rather than the terms *obese* and *morbidly obese*.

Objective Data

Routine prenatal laboratory work and physical examination are conducted. Assessment of uterine size may be difficult due to larger body size, warranting an ultrasound to verify gestational age. BMI should be documented; height and weight obtained.

Differential Diagnosis

Type 2 diabetes and chronic hypertension may be preexisting conditions, warranting additional screening. Women with history of bariatric surgeries may have preexisting vitamin deficiencies, also warranting additional screening.

Plan

Prenatal care for women who have a BMI > 30 or history of bariatric surgery follows the same general schedule as recommended for all pregnant women. However, the increased risk that accompanies high prepregnant weight and excessive weight gain during pregnancy supports the need for a greater clinical focus on lifestyle interventions (diet and exercise), as well as the need for additional laboratory testing, sonographic evaluation, antepartal testing, and strategies to lose weight after giving birth. Women with a BMI > 30 should have a 50 g glucose challenge test at the first prenatal visit and repeated at 26 to 28 weeks. Women with a history of bariatric surgery may also require additional laboratory testing and medical/surgical consultation. The general weight gain recommendations are to gain toward the lower end of the 11 to 20 lb weight gain recommended by IOM, but to avoid weight loss (Gunatilake & Perlow, 2011) (see Table 20–8).

DIABETES

There has been a steady increase in Americans diagnosed with diabetes for the past 20 years, leading to increased numbers of women with pregnancies complicated by diabetes. Type 2 diabetes is often not diagnosed until problems develop, and as many as one fourth of all people in the United States may be undiagnosed (ADA, 2011a). Of particular concern is the increase in type 2 diabetes among young women and diabetes undiagnosed before pregnancy (Lawrence, Contreras, Chen, & Sacks, 2008). The increase in Americans who are classified as overweight or obese, see previous section, has contributed significantly to the increased prevalence of diabetes (IOM, 2009; Nguyen, Nguyen, Lane, & Wang, 2011). The incidence of pregnancies complicated by diabetes has increased 40 percent between 1989 and 2004 (Getahun, Nath, Ananth, Chavez, & Smulian, 2008). Screening and diagnostic testing for diabetes during pregnancy are based on evidence that demonstrates clear linkage between hyperglygemia and adverse perinatal outcomes. Recommended changes in diabetes detection strategies

TABLE 20–8. Clinical Management of Pregnancy Complicated by Obesity

Antepartal Care	Lifestyle Modifications During Pregnancy	Laboratory and Sonographic Evaluation	
1st Visit	1st Visit	1st Visit	Postpartum
Document weight, height, BMI BMI > 30 recorded on problem list Patient education—BMI and weight gain goals—document target weight gain Folic acid 4 mg/day Antepartal screening education	Nutritional counseling tailored for pregnancy, level of BMI, weight gain goals, ethnic preferences Nutrition referral if available Educate and set goals for activity during pregnancy	Routine prenatal labs and 50 g glucose challenge test if BMI > 30 US for dating BMI > 40: baseline evaluation of serum chemistries (uric acid, creatinine, hepatic transaminases, 24 urine for protein)	Watch for s/s infection and/or dehiscence following c/s Compression stockings and early ambulation Postpartum depression education and screening Weight reduction program
FU Visit	FU Visit	FU Visit	
Discuss weight at each visit, review goals, increase frequency of visits if needed to reinforce goals, and repeat nutritional counseling	30 minute/day or more of moderate exercise in absence of medical or obstetrical complications	Antepartal screening for neural tube defects US to monitor fetal growth and infant weight Repeat 50 g GCT at 26–28 weeks	

Sources: ACOG Technical Bulletin, 2005; Jevitt, 2009; Olson & Blackwell, 2011.

for pregnant women will likely result in increased identification of hyperglycemic disorders of pregnancy (International Association of Diabetes and Pregnancy Study Groups [IADPSG] Consensus Panel, 2010).

Diabetes is a group of metabolic diseases characterized by hyperglycemia, resulting from inadequate insulin production, inadequate insulin secretion, or both (ADA, 2011a). There are four main categories of diabetes: type 1, type 2, genetic disorders, and gestational diabetes mellitus (GDM), resulting from interactions among genetics, lifestyle choices, and environmental influences (Avery, 2007). Type 1 diabetes usually occurs during childhood and is characterized by autoimmune destruction of pancreatic beta cells and is managed with insulin and dietary therapy to maintain euglycemia (ADA, 2011a). Type 2 diabetes typically occurs during adulthood among individuals with insulin resistance and relative insulin deficiency and is managed with dietary therapy, exercise, oral hypoglycemic medication, and/or insulin (ADA, 2011b). GDM is defined as "any degree of glucose intolerance with onset or first recognition during pregnancy" (ADA, 2011a, p. S65). New diagnostic standards for both overt and gestational diabetes have recently been introduced by several international and national diabetes organizations (ADA, 2011a). See Chapter 023 for more information on overt diabetes.

Early identification and intensive management of GDM are associated with a decrease in infant morbidity/mortality (Metzger et al., 2007), demonstrating the importance of prevention, early identification, and management of diabetes in women of reproductive age. Women who require insulin during pregnancy to manage gestational diabetes are referred to obstetricians, who may or may not consult with an endocrinologist in order to manage care. Women who have preexisting type 1 or 2 diabetes require immediate referral to specialist care to manage their pregnancy. The majority of the following discussion will focus on GDM.

PATHOPHYSIOLOGY AND ETIOLOGY

In normal pregnancy, profound metabolic alterations occur to support the growth and development of a fetus. Maternal basal metabolism increases as a response to fetal growth. The increase contributes to increased glucose utilization with glucose moving from maternal circulation to the fetus by simple diffusion; insulin does not cross the placental membrane. The increase in glucose to the fetus results in accelerated growth of the fetus. Insulin resistance and maternal reduced sensitivity to insulin action result from hormones produced by the placenta and increase in direct correlation with the growth of placental tissue, rising throughout the last 20 weeks of pregnancy. In most cases, the maternal pancreas is able to increase insulin production to maintain normal glucose levels. However, for women with diminished insulin secretory capacity, decreased suppression of glucose production, and/or impaired insulin sensitivity, a hyperglycemic state resembling type 2 diabetes results in GDM (Bowes et al., 1996). Although the exact causes of insulin insufficiency in GDM are not fully defined, three categories have been identified (1) autoimmune beta-cell dysfunction, (2) genetic abnormalities leading to impaired insulin secretion, and (3) beta-cell dysfunction associated with chronic insulin resistance (Metzger et al., 2007). The increased need for insulin and the tendency toward hyperglycemia emerge most often between 20 and 30 weeks of gestation.

Epidemiology

Approximately 10 percent of pregestational diabetics have type 1 diabetes and 90 percent have type 2 diabetes (Refuerzo, 2011). It is estimated that 7 percent of all pregnant women have GDM, ranging from 1 to 14 percent, varying by population studied and diagnostic tests used (ADA, 2011a). Recent screening recommendations may increase the prevalence of GDM as high as one in five pregnancies (Kim, 2010). Major risk factors for GDM are increasing maternal age, family history of diabetes, history of GDM in a previous pregnancy, history of macrosomic infant, and a prepregnancy BMI in the overweight or obese category. A meta-analysis conducted to estimate the magnitude of association between BMI and GDM risk found that the risk for developing GDM increased substantially as women's BMI increased (Chu et al., 2007). GDM is more common among Asian, Hispanic/Latina, and Native American women (Cheng & Caughey, 2008). Women who have GDM and are overweight have a 50 percent lifetime risk for developing type 2 diabetes (ADA, 2002).

The Hyperglycemia and Adverse Pregnancy Outcome (HAPO) Study, a multicenter epidemiologic study, demonstrated that maternal, fetal, and neonatal risk increased in accordance with maternal glycemia at 24 to 28 weeks, within ranges previously considered normal (ADA, 2011a). This study conclusively showed strong continuous associations between higher maternal glucose levels and increasing frequency of birth weight > 90th percentile, primary cesarean delivery, clinically defined neonatal hypoglycemia, cord C-peptide > 90th percentile, preeclampsia, PTL, shoulder dystocia/birth injury, hyperbilirubinemia, and intensive neonatal care (HAPO Study Cooperative Research Group, 2008). Another large study demonstrated that treatment of mild GDM reduced the risks of fetal overgrowth, shoulder dystocia, cesarean delivery, and hypertensive disorders (Landon et al., 2009). Infants of GDM pregnancies are also at increased risk of hypoglycemia (Ferrara et al., 2007). In addition to the aforementioned risks, women with type 1 and type 2 diabetes are at significantly increased risk of spontaneous abortions, congenital birth defects, and intrauterine fetal death (Refuerzo, 2011). Congenital malformations remain the primary cause of mortality and morbidity in infants of women with overt diabetes (ADA, 2011b).

Screening and Diagnosis

The ACOG recommends that all pregnant women should be screened for GDM by clinical history or laboratory testing (ACOG Practice Bulletin, 2001c). Risk-based screening alone has failed to identify as many as 50 percent of GDM cases (Homko & Reece, 2001). The 1-hour 50 g oral glucose challenge test remains the most common laboratory test for GDM in the United States, offered at 24 to 28 weeks' gestation for low-risk women and during the initial prenatal visit for those at greater risk (Cheng & Caughey, 2008). For women with values between 130 and 140 mg/dL, 3-hour glucose tolerance test (GTT) is undertaken to establish the diagnosis. A glucose screening threshold of 130 mg/mL yields a sensitivity of 99 percent and 22 percent screen positive rate, compared to a sensitivity of 80 percent and 13 percent screen positive rate for 140 mg/mL (ACOG Practice Bulletin, 2001c). Diagnostic criteria for GDM using the 3-hour GTT are listed in Table 20–9, demonstrating variation in diagnostic thresholds. Two elevated values on the 3-hour GTT are diagnostic of gestational diabetes.

There continues to be controversy over universal screening for diabetes during pregnancy, as well as threshhold levels for further diagnostic testing. The U.S. Preventive Services Task Force (2008) has recently recommended that there is insufficient evidence for or against GDM screening. The IADPSG convened in 2008 to review current research and develop recommendations for the diagnosis and classification of hyperglycemia in pregnancy. This group reviewed evidence on hyperglycemia and adverse perinatal outcomes, including a

TABLE 20–9. Diagnosis of Gestational Diabetes Mellitus or Overt Diabetes in Pregnancy

Gestational Diabetes Mellitus
Fasting plasma glucose ≥ 92 mg/dL
1-h plasma glucose ≥ 180 mg/dL
2-h plasma glucose ≥ 153 mg/dL
One or more of these values from a 75 g oral GTT must be equaled or exceeded for a diagnosis of GDM
Overt Diabetes
Fasting plasma glucose ≥ 126 mg/dL
A1C ≥ 6.5%
Random plasma glucose ≥ 200 mg/dL
One of these must be met to identify the patient as having overt diabetes in pregnancy.

Source: IADPSG Consensus Panel, 2010.

comprehensive review of the HAPO Study. It concluded there is a strong linear relationship between degree of hyperglycemia and adverse perinatal outcome, resulting in the development of new GDM diagnostic thresholds for GDM and overt diabetes (see Table 20–9). The overall strategy for detection and diagnosis of hyperglycemic disorders in pregnancy is for universal early testing for overt diabetes in populations with a high prevalence of type 2 diabetes and a 75 g oral GTT (OGTT) at 24 to 28 weeks for women without evidence of overt diabetes or GDM. At this time, there is not a recommendation to routinely perform OGTTs before 24 to 28 weeks' gestation (IADPSG Consensus Panel, 2010).

Women with undiagnosed overt diabetes represent a unique group, as they carry the additional risks of congenital anomalies in offspring, diabetic complications (nephropathy and retinopathy), and the need for treatment and follow-up during and after pregnancy (IADPSG Consensus Panel, 2010). The recommendation made by the IADPSG Consensus Panel was that assessment for overt diabetes should be made at the initial prenatal visit and that fasting plasma glucose, random plasma glucose, or HgbAIC could be used. There remains ongoing discussion and debate about whether there should be universal testing or testing only those classified as high risk for identification of overt diabetes. The ADA recommends screening all women at risk for type 2 diabetes at their initial prenatal visit: women who are overweight and have additional risk factors such as family history of diabetes, history of hypertension, hypercholesterolemia, hyperlipidemia, GDM, or polycystic ovary syndrome (ADA, 2011a). Low-risk women are those who meet all of the following criteria: age < 25 years, normal prepregnant weight, members of ethnic group with a low prevalence of GDM, no known diabetes in first-degree relatives, no history of abnormal glucose intolerance, and no history of poor obstetric outcomes (ADA, 2011b).

Subjective Data

The client with gestational diabetes may be asymptomatic throughout the pregnancy. Psychosocial assessment of women with GDM for depression, eating disorders, stress, and anxiety should also be integrated into each antepartal visit.

Objective Data

The client's history may suggest GDM (see above for risk factors) and warrant screening at the first prenatal visit. For women receiving late prenatal care, glycosuria, excessive prenatal weight gain, and/or fundal height larger than dates warrant testing for gestational diabetes. Urine ketone testing is recommended for GDM patients with severe hyperglycemia and weight loss during pregnancy. Fetal sonograms are performed for detection of anomalies and assessment of fetal growth, with the first ultrasound typically performed at the diagnosis of GDM (Metzger et al., 2007). Daily maternal self-monitoring of blood glucose (SMBG) is the basis for ongoing evaluation of maternal glycemic status. Assessment of fetal growth by ultrasound measurement of fetal abdominal circumference starting in the second and early third trimesters and repeated at 2- to 4-week intervals in conjunction with SMBG can also guide management decisions (Metzger et al., 2007).

For established diabetics, (1) an eye exam is recommended because of the proliferative retinopathy that occurs, (2) early songogram is recommended to confirm dates so that care may be planned and carried out at appropriate intervals, (3) serial sonograms are usually started at 26 to 28 weeks in 4- to 6-week intervals, in order to help in monitoring fetal growth (ACOG Practice Bulletin, 2001c), (4) fetal echocardography is done at 20 to 22 weeks' gestation in women with IDDM to detect presence of cardiac lesions, and (5) serial nonstress testing, biophysical profile (BPP), and/or Doppler umbilical artery velocimetry studies should start at 32 weeks and continue until delivery. All pregnant women should be offered alpha-fetoprotein (AFP) screening for neural tube defects; however, women with preexisting diabetes are at higher risk and, therefore, should be informed of this.

Differential Medical Diagnoses

Pancreatitis, malabsorption syndrome, HG, hyperthyroidism.

Plan

With a diagnosis of GDM, the main goal of treatment is control of blood glucose levels. Glucose levels can be lowered through diet control and insulin administration and/or oral hypoglycemic agents if indicated. The initial management of women with GDM includes education, dietary modifications, light exercise, and close monitoring of blood glucose levels through self-monitoring (Cheng & Caughey, 2008). Regular physical activity lowers fasting and postprandial glucose levels and is considered a useful adjunct to improve maternal glycemia (ADA, 2008). Light exercise after each meal can help reduce postprandial values to a normal range (Cheng & Caughey, 2008). Planned physical activity of 30 minutes per day is recommended for all women with GDM who are able to participate (Metzger et al., 2007). Given the high prevalence of overweight and obesity in women with GDM, weight management usually accompanies the aforementioned strategies (Kim, 2010). Weight gain recommendations follow the most recent IOM guidelines (2009): BMI < 18.5 kg/m^2, 28 to 40 lb; BMI 18.5 to 24.9 kg/m^2, 25 to 35 lb; BMI 25 to 29.9 kg/m^2, 15 to 25 lb; and BMI ≥ 30 kg/m^2, 11 to 20 lb. Medication is utilized when dietary changes don't achieve adequate glycemic control. A recent large clinical trial showed that treatment of GDM with nutrition therapy, blood glucose monitoring, and insulin therapy as needed for glycemic control reduced serious perinatal complications as well as improving maternal health-related quality of life when compared to routine care (Crowther et al., 2005). Educating the client about treatment is critical to the successful management of diabetes. With appropriate counseling and information, the client and her family will be able to deal with all changes in her body as well as in her lifestyle.

The goal of medical nutrition therapy (MNT) for women with GDM is to "promote optimal nutrition for maternal and fetal health with adequate energy for appropriate gestational weight gain, achievement and maintenance of normo-glycemia, and absence of ketosis" (ADA, 2011b, p. S69). All women with GDM should receive MNT at the time of diagnosis, and specific nutrition and food recommendations are based on individual assessment and SMBG (ADA, 2011b). MNT is best managed by a registered dietician or qualified individual with experience in the management of GDM (Metzger et al., 2007). Specific nutrition recommendations are based on individual assessment and SMBG. According to the ADA (2008), the amount and distribution of carbohydrate should be based on clinical outcome measures (hunger, plasma glucose levels, weight gain, ketone levels), with a minimum of 175 g of carbohydrate per day, distributed in three small- to moderate-sized meals and two to four snacks. If insulin therapy is added to MNT, it is especially important to maintain carbohydrate consistency at meals and snacks. Moderate caloric restriction (reduction by 30% of estimated energy needs) in obese women with GDM may improve glycemic control and reduce maternal weight gain without ketonemia. The use of daily food records, weekly weight checks, and ketone checks are recommended to determine individual energy requirements and whether the woman is undereating (ADA, 2008).

The glucose levels should be assessed four times a day (fasting and postprandial), maintaining fasting glycemic levels < 95 mg/100 mL and 1-hour postprandial levels < 140 mg/100 mL or 2-hour postprandiol levels < 120 mg/100 mL (Cheng & Caughey, 2008; Metzger et al., 2007). Many clinicians decrease frequency of blood sugar monitoring once good control is maintained, but there is no data to support duration of good control or appropriate frequency of testing (Metzger et al., 2007). The clinician must be sensitive to the woman's ability to cope with frequent self-monitoring techniques required for glucose management. For some women, acceptance of the diagnosis and perception of the impact of GDM on herself and fetus will affect adherence to treatment regimes.

For a woman with GDM, insulin therapy is initiated if diet and exercise fail to maintain self-monitored glycemia at < 95 mg/100 mL fasting and 140 mg/100 mL 1-hour postprandiol. Because insulin doesn't cross the placenta, there are no fetal risks other than maternal hypoglycemia that may result from accidental insulin overdose (Cheng & Caughey, 2008). There is no data that supports the superiority of one insulin or insulin analog regimen for GDM (Metzger et al., 2007). A common insulin regime includes use of NPH insulin injections two to four times per day, although continuous infusion of a rapid acting insulin analog such as lispro may be used if frequent monitoring is problematic (Kim, 2010). Amounts are adjusted on the basis of daily glucose levels. Insulin dosages frequently are split between the morning and evening to provide around-the-clock coverage. Women who receive insulin should monitor their glucose levels at home daily; this includes a fasting level and at least one 2-hour postprandial level. Women with preexisting diabetes require a larger dose of insulin, and their needs increase throughout pregnancy.

Oral glycemics continue to be investigated for safety; however, current research findings show that glyberide and metformin have a favorable safety profile and the advantage of easier administration (Refuerzo, 2011). A recent systematic review demonstrated that maternal and neonatal outcomes are similar when comparing women with GDM treated with glyberide compared to insulin (Nicholson et al., 2009). The use of metformin for women with polycystic ovary syndrome treated for infertility has also contributed to available research on safety and efficacy during pregnancy, demonstrating no increased risk of congenital anomalies (Glueck, Goldenberg, Streicher, & Wang, 2003; Glueck, Wang, Goldenberg, & Sieve-Smith, 2002) or increase in adverse birth outcomes (Glueck et al., 2002, 2004; Vanky et al., 2004). One study showed a lower rate of developing gestational diabetes later in pregnancy (Glueck et al., 2002).

There is insufficient evidence for specific strategies or timing for antepartal testing for pregnancies complicated by GDM, contributing to a wide range of clinical practices for assessment of fetal status (Kim, 2010) (see Chapter 21). Women with GDM who maintain satisfactory glycemic control on MNT and have no evidence of macrosomia typically begin antepartal testing 37 to 40 weeks with delivery recommended by 40 to 41 weeks (Cheng & Caughey, 2008; Kim, 2010). Management of women with GDM requiring insulin or oral hypoglycemic therapy is managed similar to management of pregestational diabetics: antenatal testing is started at 32 weeks' and induction of labor planned for 39 weeks' gestation (Cheng & Caughey, 2008). Maternal assessment of fetal activity to assess fetal well-being is recommended during the last 8 to 10 weeks of pregnancy for all women with GDM (Kim, 2010).

For women with GDM who do not require insulin or oral hypoglycemic agents, their pregnancies are typically managed expectantly until the due date. Evidence of macrosomia is more likely to result in induction. GDM patients who have not required medical therapy during pregnancy typically don't require insulin during labor and deliver, and those utilizing insulin during pregnancy typically have lower requirements during labor (Cheng & Caughey, 2008). The key to intrapartum management of diabetic women is control of blood sugar within strict parameters. Clients are monitored with fingerstick blood samples every 1 to 2 hours and IV insulin is administered if necessary. An epidural is acceptable analgesia and anesthesia. The management of GDM pregnancies complicated by macrosomia by routine cesarean deliveries remains controversial and no randomized trials currently exist to address this question (Kim, 2010).

Follow-Up

After delivery, insulin needs drastically decrease. The established diabetic may not need to return to insulin therapy for a few days. The client should, however, resume her usual prepregnant glucose-monitoring routine. The gestational diabetic who has been taking insulin will not need to continue. Breastfeeding is recommended for infants of women with preexisting diabetes or GDM, but lactating women have reported fluctuations in blood sugar related to nursing sessions, managed with a carbohydrate snack before or during breastfeeding (Reader & Franz, 2004).

Women with GDM are at increased risk for type 2 diabetes later in life and with future pregnancies. Lifestyle modifications such as weight reduction and increased physical activity are recommended after pregnancy, as this reduces the risk of subsequent diabetes (ADA, 2011b; Lobner et al., 2006). For women who are overweight or obese, information about the increased risks associated with elevated BMI such as metabolic disorders and cardiovascular disease should be provided, as well as future pregnancy risks. Retesting for overt diabetes should occur 6 to 12 weeks postpartum and rescreened at 1- to 3-year intervals based on postpartum blood glucose results (ACOG Committee Opinion, 2009; ADA, 2010) (see Chapter 22). There are no current recommendations for medications to prevent subsequent onset of diabetes among women with a history of GDM (Kim, 2010).

PRETERM LABOR AND BIRTH

A PTB is one that occurs prior to 37 completed weeks of gestation, typically preceded by premature/preterm labor (ACOG Practice Bulletin, 2001a). An important distinction exists in describing neonates that are born too early versus those born too small. Infant weight had traditionally been used as the indicator for gestational age, but this has been replaced by more precise definitions. LBW infants weigh fewer than 2,500 g at birth, regardless of gestational age; very LBW (VLBW) infants weigh fewer than 1,500 g at birth; and extremely LBW infants weigh 500 to 1,000 g. The term *small for gestational age* is used to describe newborns whose birth weight is below the 10th percentile for gestational age. Infants born before 37 completed weeks (preterm) can be small or large for gestational age. With the advent of sensitive pregnancy tests in correlation with accurate menstrual history and improved technology with sonography, gestational age can be accurately determined and differentiated from the premature infant. LBW infants can be the result of prematurity, in some instances a result of a poor intrauterine environment, or a combination of those factors (see Chapter 21).

A premature, or PTB, can occur spontaneously or by medical intervention. The spontaneous delivery includes delivery that spontaneously occurs after PTL, premature rupture of membranes, or premature dilation of the cervix. When a medical or obstetrical disorder is present such as diabetes, gestational hypertension, placenta previa, abruptio placentae, or intrauterine growth retardation, medical intervention may be necessary for the sake of improving the outcome for both mother and fetus, and PTB may occur by choice. This form of indicated PTB is not the focus of this section.

PTB is the one of the leading causes of infant mortality and the leading cause of infant morbidity and remains a challenging area of perinatal health. There is no one test that can accurately predict PTB and little is known how to prevent its occurrence. Clinical practice changes, public health initiatives, and research have done little to change the PTB rate over the past 30 years. This is reflected in the lack of consensus about how to prevent, screen, diagnosis, and treat PTL/PTB. Prevention strategies have primarily focused on developing screening tools to identify those women who are at greatest risk, but this hasn't impacted outcomes. The IOM report *Preterm Birth: Causes, Consequences, and Prevention* (2007) recommends a multidisciplinary approach, acknowledging that PTB is a product of overlapping factors and the most significant gains will occur in prevention.

Clinicians should implement PTL/PTB prevention strategies, including education on nutritional and lifestyle choices such as cigarette smoking, pregnancy spacing, and preconception folic acid supplementation. Following professional guidelines on screening for substance abuse, depression, and domestic violence should be a priority in the provision of health care for women, as all of these have been associated with PTB (Damus, 2008). Screening and diagnosing PTL/PTB is within the scope of practice for any clinician. Intrapartal management of PTL/PTB is generally referred for care by an obstetrician.

FETAL/NEWBORN OUTCOMES

Fetal risk from PTB is associated with the immaturity of the organ systems. Conditions common in the premature infant are respiratory distress syndrome, intraventricular hemorrhage, bronchopulmonary dysplasia, patent ductus arteriosus, necrotizing enterocolitis, sepsis, apnea, and retinopathy of prematurity. Some of the long-term effects are increased risk for neurodevelopmental handicaps such as mental retardation, cerebral palsy (CP), seizure disorder, and visual and hearing impairments (Behrman & Butler, 2007). These births account for 60 to 80 percent of the mortality and nearly 50 percent of the long-term morbidity associated with childbirth (Williamson et al., 2008). Health risks for premature infants persist throughout life with higher rates of chronic health problems, shorter life spans, and generational risks for offspring (Damus, 2008).

Due to many advances in care of premature infants, there has been an increase in survival of VLBW and extremely LBW infants, but morbidity and long-term health problems remain problematic. This is especially true for extremely LBW infants born at the threshold of viability, 25 or fewer completed weeks of gestation. Newborns born at 25 weeks of gestation and/or 701 to 800 g have a 75 percent survival rate, but 50 percent will have multiple long-term health problems (ACOG Practice Bulletin, 2002b). The ACOG Practice Bulletin (2002b) and the American Academy of Pediatrics (2009) have issued reports that address the medical, social, and ethical issues that surface when providing care to this population.

There is a growing body of research literature documenting increased morbidity and mortality among late-preterm infants, those born between 34 (+0) and 36 (+6) weeks. This group represents approximately 70 percent of all PTBs and has been steadily increasing since 1990 (Davidoff et al., 2006). The belief that a fetus is essentially mature by 34 weeks has been shown to be incorrect: compared to term infants, late-preterm infants are at higher risk for developing a variety of medical complications, higher rates of morbidity before initial hospital discharge, higher rates of hospital readmission in the first months of life (ACOG Committee Opinion, 2008a), and higher rates of neonatal and infant mortality (Damus, 2008). For these reasons, the ACOG recommends that preterm delivery should occur only when there is significant maternal or fetal indication for delivery.

ETIOLOGY

The onset of labor involves complex interaction among hormonal/endocrine, structural, and maternal/fetal changes. The release of prostaglandins from the endometrium stimulates uterine activity, leading to cervical ripening, dilatation, and/or membrane rupture. Several theories to explain the onset and maintenance of labor have been proposed, but no one theory by itself has adequately explained the process. Theories proposed to explain the initiation of term labor include (1) progesterone withdrawal, (2) oxytocin initiation, and (3) decidual activation (Goldenberg, Culhane, Iams, & Romero, 2008).

PTL is generally believed to be multifactorial in origin. Initiating factors include infection or inflammation, uteroplacental ischemia or hemorrhage, uterine overdistension, stress, and other immunological processes. Infection has been implicated as a significant risk factor in PTB, including urinary tract infections, pyelonephritis, pneumonia, and sexually transmitted infections such as chlamydia, trichomonas, and bacterial vaginosis (Goldenberg et al., 2008). Screening for and treatment of ASB has been found to reduce the PTB rate (Iams, Romero, Culhane, & Goldenberg, 2008), but antibiotic treatment for genital tract infection has not been shown to reliably reduce risk or the rate of PTB (ACOG Practice Bulletin, 2001a; Iams et al., 2008). The most current Cochrane reviews published on the use of screening and treatment of pregnant women with lower genital tract infection remain inconclusive: There is inadequate evidence to support routine screening and treatment of asymptomatic women (MacDonald, Brocklehurst, & Gordon, 2007), but there is some evidence that screening pregnant women before 20 weeks reduces PTB and LBW (Sangkomkamhang, Lumbiganon, Prasertcharoensook, & Laopaiboon, 2008). From a clinical perspective, screening and treatment of pregnant women who are at higher risk for PTB may be prudent.

The terms *cervical insufficiency* and *cervical incompetence* have been used to describe the inability of the cervix to retain a pregnancy to term. Although both cervical insufficiency and PTL may result in PTB, it is general recognized that cervical changes associated with cervical insufficiency are typically not associated with uterine activity. A diagnosis of cervical insufficiency is typically made based on historical features (ACOG Practice Bulletin, 2003b) and should be managed as a high-risk pregnancy.

Epidemiology

Approximately 30 to 35 percent of PTBs occur for maternal or fetal indications, 40 to 45 percent result from spontaneous labor, and 25 to 30 percent follow preterm premature rupture of membranes (PPROM) (Goldenberg et al., 2008). Chorioamnionitis complicates 10 to 36 percent of PTB with PPROM (Di Renzo et al., 2011). The rates of PTB started to increase in the United States in 1996, with medically indicated PTBs responsible for most of this increase (Goldenberg et al., 2008). Some of this increase can be attributed to the high number of multiple gestations associated with assisted reproduction; since 1990, there has been a 40 percent increase in multiple births and a 400 percent increase in higher-order births (Russell, Petrini, Damus, Mattison, & Schwarz, 2003). Multiple gestations represent 15 to 20 of all PTBs, and 60 percent of twins are born preterm (Goldenberg et al., 2008). Additional factors that have been identified as contributing to a higher PTB rate include an increase in high-risk pregnancies due to advanced maternal age, chronic health problems, obesity, gestational diabetes, preeclampsia, elective inductions and cesarean deliveries driven by consumer and health care provider interests, and litigious environment (Damus, 2008).

In the United States, the PTB rate is 12 to 13 percent, compared to Europe and other developed countries, with rates reported at 5 to 9 percent. Incidence of PTB also varies by gestational age with approximately 5 percent of births occurring at less than 28 weeks, 15 percent at 28 to 31 weeks, 20 percent at 32 to 33 weeks, and 60 to 70 percent at 34 to 36 weeks (Goldenberg et al., 2008). There are significant disparities in PTB rates among different racial and ethnic groups in the United States, with a range of 16 to 18 percent for African American women and 5 to 9 percent for white women. African American women are also more likely to have a very early PTB compared to women from other racial or ethnic groups (Goldenberg, Cliver, et al., 1996; Schempf, Branum, Lukacs, & Schoendorf, 2007). These disparities have not been fully explained by differences in socioeconomic conditions or maternal behaviors (IOM, 2007).

Screening Strategies

Although not proven reliable or sensitive in predicting PTL, risk screening for PTB continues to be used by most primary health care providers to try to identify at risk women and intervene to prevent PTB. There are many socioeconomic, biological, and environmental factors that have been associated with PTB, including maternal demographic characteristics, nutritional status, previous pregnancy history, present pregnancy conditions, existing medical problems, infections, cervical length, and behavioral and environmental risks (see Table 20–10). The most predictive risk factor for preterm delivery is history of previous preterm delivery, with a 15 to 50 percent recurrence rate for women with a previous PTB, depending on the parity and the gestational age of previous births (Goldenberg et al., 2008). Risk increases with each subsequent PTB and as the gestational age of PTB declines (Iams et al., 2008). Additionally, multifetal pregnancy, mid-trimester bleeding, and uterine, cervical, or placental abnormalities better predict PTB (Damus, 2008). Medical risks such as hypertension, preeclampsia, abruptio placentae, diabetes, and congenital malformations are associated with indicated PTB (Ananth & Vintzileos, 2006). As noted earlier, selected bacterial infections are correlated with PTB, but screening for vaginal infections remains controversial. Maternal stress has also been examined, with studies showing an association between depression/anxiety, physical abuse, and strenuous work conditions and PTB (Goldenberg et al., 2008; Littleton, Breitkopf, & Berenson, 2007; Reedy, 2007). Poor nutritional status and a short (< 1 year) interconceptional period are associated

TABLE 20–10. Screening Strategies for Preterm Birth Prevention

- Screening for risk of preterm labor, other than historical risk factors, is not beneficial in the general obstetrical population.
- No current data supports use of home uterine activity monitoring or bacterial vaginosis screening.
- Sonography to determine cervical length and/or fetal fibronectin testing may be useful in determining women at risk for preterm labor. However, their value may rest primarily with their negative-predictive value given the lack of proven treatment options.
- Routine digital cervical exams are not beneficial or harmful.

Sources: ACOG Practice Bulletin, 2001d, 2003a; Alexander et al., 2010; Berghella, Baxter, & Hendrix, 2009; Berghella, Hayes, Visintine, & Baxter, 2008.

with a higher incidence of PTB (Goldenberg et al., 2008). Peridontal disease and obesity have been recently investigated to determine association with PTB, but these studies have been inconclusive (Goldenberg et al., 2008; Iams et al., 2008). One third to one half of women with PTL/PTB have no identifiable risk factors, which prevents early identification and targeted interventions (Iams et al., 2008; Reedy, 2007).

Several other clinical screening strategies have been evaluated for effectiveness in identification of women at risk for PTL/PTB: home uterine monitoring, fetal fibronectin measures, sonographic measurement of the cervix, and digital cervical exams with variable predictive value (see Table 20–10).

Home uterine activity monitoring has been used in an effort to identify PTL for the purpose of diagnosing, monitoring, or adjusting tocolytic therapy. Review of studies fails to demonstrate the effectiveness of uterine monitoring in the reduction of PTB (Iams et al., 2002).

Fetal fibronectin is a glycoprotein that is detected in cervicovaginal secretions taken from the cervical os or posterior vaginal fornix. This test is approved by the FDA for use between 22 and 34 completed weeks' gestation for the assessment of PTL (Goldenberg, Mercer, et al., 1996). A negative result means there is a less than 1 percent chance that PTB will occur in the next 7 to 10 days and a positive result means the risk of PTB during the same time period increases from 3 percent to 14 percent (Honest, Bachmann, Gupta, Kleijnen, & Khan, 2002). Therefore, a positive fetal fibronectin warrants more immediate aggressive treatment and monitoring while a negative fibronectin warrants a wait-and-see approach (ACOG Practice Bulletin, 2001d). A positive fetal fibronectin test increases the predictive value of using sonographic cervical length to further identify women at risk for PTB (Di Renzo et al, 2011). Reedy (2007) developed an algorithm for diagnosis and management of PTL that utilizes fetal fibronectin results as a major component of decision making.

Transvaginal sonogram assessment of the length of the cervix has been used to predict early labor because shortened cervical canal length is associated with preterm delivery (Naim, Haberman, Burgess, Navizedeh, & Minkoff, 2002). This procedure can more precisely measure cervical length and identify funneling, the bulging of membranes into the endocervical canal. Several studies have demonstrated that a pregnant woman with a cervical length of 31 mm or longer had a greater likelihood of having a full-term pregnancy (Iams, 2003) and sonographic cervical length, funneling, and prior history of PTB has correlated with delivery before 35 weeks (de Carvalho, Bittar, Brizot, Bicudo, & Zugaib, 2005). Ultrasound assessment in combination with fetal fibronectin has proven useful in identifying those women who present with signs of PTL who are at greatest risk of delivery (ACOG Practice Bulletin, 2001d, 2003a, 2003b; Goldenberg et al., 2008; Iams et al., 2008). According to Goldenberg and colleagues, "A short cervical length and a raised cervical-vaginal fetal fibronectin concentration are the strongest predictors of spontaneous preterm birth" (2008, p. 75). It is important to note that neither bed rest nor coital abstinence has been studied in women with short cervices (Iams et al., 2008).

Digital cervical exams were once conducted as a standard component of prenatal care in the third trimester in an effort to identify premature cervical dilation. Studies have subsequently shown that detection of those at increased risk (based on cervical effacement and dilation) didn't affect PTB outcome or frequency of interventions for PTL (Alexander, Boulvain, Ceysens, Haelterman, & Zhang, 2010). From a clinical standpoint, there is merit, however, in conducting a thorough and accurate cervical exam for the initial prenatal visit and, whenever signs of PTL emerge, using consistent descriptors and clear documentation (see the following Objective Data).

Prevention

Damus (2008) suggests that PTL/PTB meets the criteria for being a chronic complex disorder and this requires shifting to a preventive approach, similar to heart disease or diabetes. The primary approach to preterm prevention in the United States focuses on strategies to reduce morbidity and mortality of preterm infants (tertiary prevention), as opposed to reducing the risk of PTB before or during pregnancy (primary) or reducing risk in those with known risk factors (secondary prevention) (Iams et al., 2008). PTB prevention requires a multidisciplinary approach with ongoing consideration of the importance of healthy lifestyle for health promotion and disease prevention. Every well woman and/or family planning visit should be conducted with preconception care in mind, "every woman, every time" (Korenbrot, Bender, Steinberg, & Newberry, 2001). Many of the aforementioned risk factors, such as smoking, substance abuse, poor nutrition, and job-related activities, are amenable to change. Educating and counseling women about these issues prior to and during pregnancy could have beneficial effects on the incidence of PTL (Damus, 2008; Heaman, Sprague, & Stewart, 2001; Weiss, Saks, & Harris, 2002). For example, a Cochrane review reported that smoking cessation programs implemented during pregnancy reduced the incidence of PTB (Lumley, Oliver, Chamberlain, & Oakley, 2004). A review of smoking cessation programs found that a 5 to 15-minute pregnancy-specific counseling session significantly reduced smoking rates (Iams et al., 2008). In addition, helping the client to deal with stress, whether it is related to physical exertion from specific physical activities, occupational requirements, or emotional and financial factors, may lower the incidence of PTL (Janke, 1999). Preconceptional interventions designed to control diabetes, hypertension, and asthma can impact the risks of PTB for a future pregnancy (Iams et al., 2008). Health care access issues must also be addressed, so that all pregnant women have access to prenatal care regardless of financial status.

A significant breakthrough in a pharmacologically mediated prevention strategy has been identified in research investigating progesterone supplementation to women who are at higher risk for PTB. Current ACOG recommendations are to offer progesterone to all singleton pregnant women with a documented history of a previous spontaneous PTB (ACOG Committee Opinion, 2008b), typically administered as a weekly IM injection from 16 to 20 weeks' gestation until 37 weeks (Damus, 2008). There still exists the need for further research to evaluate optimal progesterone preparation, dosage, route of administration, and other indications for usage (Dodd, Flenady, Cincotta, & Crowther, 2008).

Client and Staff Education

Client education includes instruction about the signs and symptoms of labor. A client may need to learn strategies to differentiate true uterine contraction from the common cramps or abdominal discomfort associated with pregnancy, as well as instructions on how to time contractions. Recognition of the sensations associated with uterine tightening is important for all pregnant women; ultimately, it is frequency and intensity of uterine activity that alerts them to PTL. Teaching pregnant women to palpate a firm uterus when they have a full bladder, for example, can prove helpful in translating the language of contractions into something more understandable. The term Braxton-Hicks contractions, described as irregular, nonrhythmical, and either painful or painless, has been misleading and created confusion in describing uterine contractions. Women who believe their uterine contractions are Braxton-Hicks contractions because they aren't painful may disregard all uterine activity.

All pregnant women should be instructed to notify the health care provider if leaking of fluid begins, vaginal spotting or bleeding develops, or uterine contractions occur every 10 minutes or more frequently. When a woman perceives regular uterine activity, she should first lie down, preferably on her left side, drink fluids (at least 8 oz), palpate the uterus, and time contractions. The client must be instructed that if contractions do not subside in 30 to 60 minutes, she must be evaluated by a health care provider.

Clinic and hospital staff should be educated to be sensitive to a client's complaints and not to dismiss low backache, cramps, or descriptions of "the baby balling up" as normal discomforts of pregnancy. Emergency room caregivers and answering services should be apprised of the special needs of a PTL client (Weiss et al., 2002).

Subjective Data

A thorough review of health records and an interview that elicits pertinent information about signs and symptoms should be conducted on all women who present with PTL signs and symptoms. Some women fail to recognize the signs and symptoms of PTL perhaps because the symptoms of pelvic pressure increase in vaginal discharge, backache, and menstrual-like cramps mimic symptoms that occur in normal pregnancy (Reedy, 2007). Uterine contractions persistently occur with or without pain or discomfort. Clients may complain of low backache, a sense of lower abdominal pressure, or lower abdominal or thigh pain. Some women experience a change in vaginal discharge from creamy white to more mucoid, blood-tinged, or watery. Asking open-ended questions that allow a woman to describe her subjective experience of abdominal discomfort, pelvic pressure, and/or back pain may result in information about subtle indicators of uterine activity.

Objective Data

Confirmation of estimated date of confinement (EDC) should always be included in the initial assessment of a woman presenting with signs and symptoms of PTL. Ideally, the EDC should be established within the first trimester, but if this has not occurred, then a transabdominal sonogram may be ordered to confirm gestational dates and assist in decisions about delivery. A physical exam should be performed on all women presenting for evaluation of PTL, assessing maternal and fetal health status. Health records should be reviewed to obtain pertinent laboratory results, physical exam findings, and current pregnancy information.

Cervical changes occurring in conjunction with regular uterine contractions are the hallmark of PTL/PTB, but this is often difficult to determine until there are significant cervical changes. Until fairly recently, the following were used as criteria to establish a diagnosis of PTL between 20 and 37 weeks' gestation: four contractions 20 minutes or eight contractions per hour with progressive cervical changes, cervical dilatation greater than 1 cm, and cervical effacement of more than 80 percent. A more common clinical practice is to await cervical change during a period of observation while monitoring uterine contractions. Electronic fetal heart rate monitoring should also be used to assess for signs associated with intrauterine infection, including fetal tachycardia, late decelerations, and decreased baseline variability.

Accurate and consistent documentation of cervical exam findings is important, particularly if sequential exams by the same examiner are not possible. Although the Bishop's score was developed for assessing cervical readiness for induction (Bishop, 1964), it can also be used to assess cervical changes related to PTL/PTB. Cervical exam findings that include information about (1) length of the cervix in centimeters, (2) dilatation in centimeters, (3) cervical consistency, (4) cervical position, and (5) fetal station provide a more precise description of cervical status and documentation of cervical changes (Reedy, 2007).

PPROM is the spontaneous rupture of the amniotic fluid membranes at less than 37 weeks' gestation at least 1 hour before the onset of contractions (Goldenberg et al., 2008). The most common presenting symptom is history of a sudden gushing fluid from the vagina followed by persistent, uncontrolled leakage. Women with suspected PPROM may be evaluated in a clinic or hospital setting and are placed in a recumbent position ("pooling") in order to visualize the pooled aminiotic fluid in the posterior vaginal formix. As with all pregnant women who are being evaluated for ruptured amniotic fluid membranes, vaginal exams should be kept to a minimum to reduce infection. A sterile vaginal exam is done to collect fluid for testing. When applied to a dry slide, amniotic fluid will dry into a microscopic crystallization in a "fern" pattern. It can accurately confirm premature rupture of membranes in 85 to 98 percent of cases. The pH of amniotic fluid if present will be blue-green and range from 6.5 to 7.75. A new product, AmniSure ROM Test (AmniSure International, LLC, Boston, MA), is used for detection of ruptured amniotic fluid membranes, and has been reported to have a better diagnostic accuracy than combined use of nitrazine, fern, and pooling and nitrazine test alone (Lee et al., 2009). A sonogram to determine amniotic fluid volume, fetal presentation, estimated fetal weight, and gestational age is done to prepare for delivery.

Differential Medical Diagnoses

False labor/Braxton-Hicks contractions, urinary tract infection, pyelonephritis, low back pain.

Plan

Developing a treatment plan for this group of women involves consideration of gestational age, risk factors, cervical status, and current clinical practice standards.

Laboratory testing should include urinalysis for culture and sensitivity, urine drug screen, cultures for vaginal infection including GBS, gonorrhea, chlamydia, testing for trichomonas, bacterial vaginosis, fetal fibronectin, and a baseline CBC as a marker for infection (Reedy, 2007).

Any client with suspicion of PTL should have a sterile speculum examination for pH, ferning, and pooled vaginal fluid to rule out PPROM and should have cervical, vaginal, and urinary cultures done. Cultures should be collected from the outer one third of vagina and perineum for GBS, from the cervix for chlamydia and *N. gonorrhoea*, and from the external cervical os and posterior vaginal fornix for fibronectin. Fetal fibronectin should be collected on all women with signs of PTL before the digital cervical exam is performed, and is not reliable if the woman has had intercourse or a cervical exam within the previous 24 hours or has vaginal bleeding. The fetal fibronectin test should be repeated at 2-week intervals when the tests are positive (Reedy, 2007).

The traditional recommendation for women presenting with signs and symptoms of PTL has been bed rest, hydration, and pelvic rest, but none of these have been effective in reducing PTB (Reedy, 2007; Sosa, Althabe,

Belizan, & Bergel, 2004; Yost et al., 2006). These interventions are often implemented in conjunction with tocolytic therapy (Reedy, 2007) and corticosteroid administration. Bed rest remains one of the most widely prescribed medical interventions for PTL, even though it is costly, disruptive to families, produces major side effects in every major organ system, and may either have no effect or have negative effects on fetal outcomes (Maloni, Brezinski-Tomasi, & Johnson, 2001). Prolonged bed rest can lead to higher rates of thromboembolic complications (Kovacevich et al., 2000) and bone loss (Promislow, Hertz-Picciotto, Schramm, Watt-Morse, & Anderson, 2004), in addition to significant psychosocial disruption. In some cases, bed rest may be recommended to authorize reduction in work hours, strenuous physical work, disability, or family medical leave (Reedy, 2007). The effectiveness of hydration in arresting PTL has not been well established, and if tocolytics are used, additional IV fluids may increase the risk of pulmonary edema (Reedy, 2007; Stan, Boulvain, Hirsbrunner-Amagbaly, & Pfister, 2002).

Pharmacologic therapies utilized in the management of PTL/PTB include antibiotic treatment to prevent neonatal infection, steroids for enhancing fetal lung maturity, and tocolytic therapies for halting labor. Antibiotic therapy is recommended for women in PTL to prevent neonatal infection with GBS (Iams et al., 2008). If women at risk for PTB typically present before group B screening (usually performed at 36 weeks), they should be treated presumptively. Additional antibiotic therapy is recommended only if there is a documented infection, such as a urinary tract infection, or there is evidence of chorioamnionitis following PPROM (King, Flenady, & Murray, 2002).

Antenatal administration of corticosteroids to women in PTL is recommended to decrease the incidence of respiratory distress syndrome, intraventricular hemorrhage, neonatal death, necrotizing enterocolitis, infectious morbidity, need for respiratory support, and neonatal intensive care admission (Roberts & Dalziel, 2006). The current recommendation is to give women at risk for preterm delivery within 7 days a single course of corticosteroids between 24 and 34 weeks of gestation with intact membranes and before 32 weeks for premature rupture of membranes (ACOG Committee Opinion, 2011). Either two doses of 12 mg betamethasone (IM) 24 hours apart or four doses of 6 mg dexamethasone (IM) every 12 hours are used. Repeat doses are generally not recommended and use with multiple gestations remains controversial (Roberts & Dalziel, 2006).

Because PPROM is associated with PTL and genital tract infection, decision making with respect to delivery must balance the risk of prematurity with that of maternal/neonatal sepsis. Currently, the conservative approach of delaying delivery is more common, unless infection cannot be controlled with antibiotic therapy. The client is hospitalized, temperature is monitored at 4-hour intervals, and leukocyte count is evaluated every 2 to 3 days. An amniocentesis is considered to rule out subclinical infection. Tocolysis is contraindicated when chorioamnionitis is present.

Tocolytic Medication. The primary role of tocolytic therapy is to delay delivery for women in active PTL for an additional 48 to 72 hours to allow for administration of steroids to promote fetal lung maturity (see earlier) and/or transfer to a facility with skilled personnel (Iams et al., 2008; Reedy, 2007). There is no evidence that tocolytic therapy has reduced the rate of PTB by use during acute episodes or ongoing contraction suppression (Iams et al., 2008). Several types of drugs have been tried to interrupt PTL and prevent premature birth. The following represents findings from the Cochrane review meta-analyses on drugs used to interrupt PTL and/or prevent premature birth: calcium-channel blockers (nifidipine) and an oxytocin antagonist (atosiban) delay delivery by 2 to 7 days with a positive risk–benefit ratio (King, Flenady, Papatsonis, Dekker, & Carbonne, 2003; Papatsonis, Flenady, Cole, & Liley, 2005) but there is limited evidence to support atsiban use as a maintenance therapy (Papatsonis, Flenady, & Liley, 2009); beta agonist drugs (ritodrine or terbutaline) may delay delivery by 48 hours but have more side effects than other agents (Whitworth & Quenby, 2008); magnesium sulfate has a greater neonatal risk profile and is less effective than other agents (Crowther, Hiller, & Doyle, 2002); prostaglandin inhibitor (Indocin) has some evidence to support use for PTL (King, Flenady, Cole, & Thornton, 2005). The mechanism of action for each of these tocolyic drugs is the following:

- Calcium-channel blockers (Nifedipine) acts on calcium channel to promote smooth muscle relaxation.
- Oxytocin antagonists (Atosiban) displaces oxytocin and vasopressin from their receptor sites and thus reduces uterine contractility.
- Beta-mimetics (ritodrine and terbutaline) acts on beta-2 receptors to inhibit muscle activity.
- Magnesium sulfate decreases calcium uptake, resulting in decreased uterine contractility.
- Antiprostaglandins, or prostaglandin synthetase inhibitors (e.g., indomethacin [Indocin]), inhibits the synthesis of prostaglandins, which is a strong stimulant of the uterine myometrium.

In general, tocolytic medications are not indicated when maternal conditions warrant early delivery for the benefit of the woman or the fetus. Tocolytics are contraindicated in women with cardiac disease, significant hypertension related to chronic- or pregnancy-induced hypertension, or the occurrence of antenatal hemorrhage. Tocolysis is not indicated in gestation 37 weeks or greater, cervical dilatation greater than 3 cm, birth weight of 2,500 g or more, fetal distress, intrauterine growth retardation, or maternal infection. Tocolysis is also contradicted in the case of fetal demise or lethal anomaly.

Cerclage. Cerclage seems to be primarily beneficial in cases of structural defect or cervical repair, but identifying appropriate candidates has proven difficult (Iams et al., 2008). Cerclage has only proven beneficial with a diagnosis of cervical incompetence (Di Renzo et al., 2011).

Delivery. PTL is not stopped if severe uterine bleeding or maternal disease or infection is present. If labor is not halted, delivery management is based on fetal size and presentation. Delivery mode should be as atraumatic as possible; cesarean section is frequently performed with breech presentations. Cesarean sections should be performed only for the usual fetal and maternal indications.

MULTIFETAL GESTATION

There has been a dramatic increase in the incidence of multifetal gestation over the past 25 years, primarily due to assisted reproductive technologies (ART) and ovulation drugs to treat infertility (Martin et al., 2009). Of concern is the significant increase in health care problems associated with multiple births, as well as psychosocial and economic consequences (Leonard & Denton, 2006). There is clear consensus that perinatal morbidity and mortality increase with the number of fetuses (ACOG Committee Opinion, 2007). The increased risk of PTBs in multifetal gestations significantly compromises survival and increases risk of long-term disability. Ethical considerations exist when providing care to women who are seeking fertility treatments and those who achieve pregnancy with multiple fetuses. Women who experience infertility may view a multiple pregnancy as a positive outcome, and should be informed of the risks of multifetal pregnancies when undergoing treatment for infertility. The ACOG issued a committee opinion to address its professional responsibility to educate and counsel women about the inherent risks associated with multiple births (ACOG Committee Opinion, 2007) and the American Society for Reproductive Medicine (ASRM, 2009) developed guidelines in an effort to reduce the number of higher-order multiple pregnancies by limiting the number of embryos transferred during in vitro fertilization (see Chapter 13).

It is important for any clinician who cares for women undergoing infertility treatment to understand the range of issues that exist in pregnancies with multiple gestation in order to provide comprehensive care and informed consent. Because of the higher risk associated with multiple gestations, the majority of antepartal and intrapartal care is provided by obstetricians and perinatal specialists. The discussion that follows will be primarily focused on twin pregnancies, as management of triplet and higher-order multiple gestations (more than three fetuses) is outside the scope of primary care. Women with higher-order multiple gestations are best managed in a high-risk perinatal clinic.

ETIOLOGY

Monozygotic twins, also called identical twins, arise from a single fertilized ovum that divides during the early development phase into two embryos with identical genetic material. The time of division determines fetal and placental morphology. The chorion and amnion have already differentiated by approximately 8 days after fertilization, and division results in two embryos within a common amniotic sac (Cunningham et al., 2010). Conjoined twins occur if differentiation occurs after this. Monochorionic twins have a greater risk of spontaneous abortion than dichorionic twins (Sperling et al., 2006). The risk of congenital anomalies in a twin gestation is approximately two times greater than in a single gestation, with higher rates of structural defects in monoamniotic twins (Evans & Andriole, 2010).

Dizygotic twins, also called fraternal twins, arise from multiple ova that are fertilized by multiple sperm. Multiple ovulation results from excessive gonadotropin stimulation. Fraternal twins are not true twins but siblings who share the same intrauterine environment. High-order multiple gestations (more than three fetuses) can result from monozygotic, dizygotic, or mono- and dizygotic division. The increased rates of multiple pregnancies are primarily a consequence of dizygotic twins and higher-order multiples.

MATERNAL ADAPTATION

There is a greater degree of physiologic change that occurs in pregnancies with a multiple gestation compared to single gestations, impacting both maternal and fetal adaptation. Serum β-hCG levels are higher, contributing to higher rates of nausea and vomiting (Little, 2010). Maternal blood volume expansion is 500 mL greater in a twin pregnancy than a single gestation, with a proportionately lower increase in red cell production, contributing to greater rates of maternal anemia (Gyamfi, Stone, & Eddleman, 2005). Compared to singleton pregnancies, women with twin pregnancies have increased cardiac output and arterial blood pressure, placing more stress on the cardiovascular system and contributing to higher rates of gestational hypertension. According to Goodnight and Newman (2009), an increase in resting energy expenditure in twin pregnancies can result in a 40 percent increase in caloric requirements. The increased size of the enlarging uterus also makes respiratory symptoms and musculoskeletal discomforts more problematic in twin pregnancies (Gyamfi et al., 2005). The increased weight and overdistended uterus associated with multifetal pregnancies has also been implicated in the development of varicose veins, sciatica, and difficulty in ambulating (Ayres & Johnson, 2005). The incidence of postpartum hemorrhage from uterine atony is significantly increased secondary to overdistention of the uterus during pregnancy.

Epidemiology

There are currently more than 3 percent of newborns in the United States that are born as multiples, and about 95 percent of these are twins (Martin et al., 2009). As noted earlier, there has been a dramatic increase in multiple gestations with a 70 percent increase in twin births between 1980 and 2004, and a fourfold increase in higher-order multiples (triplets or more) between 1980 and 1998 (Martin et al., 2006). The increased use of fertility treatments in combination with delayed childbearing has contributed significantly to this increase. About one third of the increase in multiple pregnancies is due to the fact that more women over age 30 are having babies (Reddy, Branum, & Klebanoff, 2005), as women in this age group are more likely to conceive multiples. The remainder of the increase is due to the use of ART and ovulation induction. Approximately 65 percent of all twins in the United States are a result of infertility treatments (Evans & Andriole, 2010). In 2005, 1 percent of infants born in the United States were conceived through ART and accounted for 17 percent of multiple births (Wright, Chang, Jeng, & Macaluso, 2008). According to Wright et al. (2008), about 44 percent of ART pregnancies result in twins, and about 5 percent in triplets or more. Similar data is not available for ovulation induction (ACOG Committee Opinion, 2007).

The incidence of multiple gestation varies among countries and races. Nigeria has the highest reported incidence (54 per 1,000 births) and Japan has the lowest incidence (4.3 per 1,000 births) (Cunningham et al., 2010). In spontaneous conceptions, monozygotic twinning is considered a random event, but in pregnancies resulting from exogenous gonadotrophins, the incidence of monozygotic twinning increases two to three times (ACOG Committee Opinion, 2007). Frequency of dizygotic twins is influenced by race, ethnicity, maternal age, heredity, parity, and the use of fertility drugs and other ART (Warner, Kiely, & Donovan, 2000). The greatest risk for conceiving multiples occurs among women who are African Americans, are over 30 years of age, have a personal or family history of fraternal twins, are multiparous, and are undergoing fertility treatment. Reddy et al. (2005) also correlated maternal size with multiple gestations: Taller and/or heavier women were more likely to have twin pregnancies.

As recently as 30 years ago, only half of twin pregnancies were diagnosed before birth (Devoe, 2008). Improved outcomes with early diagnosis of twin pregnancies were noted in a Swedish study; routine ultrasonography identified 90 percent of twin gestations and this was associated with lower infant mortality, LBW rates, and greater gestational age at delivery (Persson, Grennert, Gennser, & Kullander, 1979). Although routine ultrasonography is not professionally endorsed as the standard of prenatal care, the majority of pregnant women in the United States receive one or more prenatal ultrasounds (ACOG Practice Bulletin, 2004c). This practice increases early detection of twin pregnancies, which increases the likelihood of reliable dating and early identification of twin morphology (Devoe, 2008). Early diagnosis by sonography has also documented multiple gestations that resulted in single births (Norwitz, Edusa, & Park, 2005), leading to the term *vanishing twin syndrome* or spontaneous pregnancy reduction. It is believed this occurs in up to 20 to 60 percent of spontaneous twin conceptions, and demonstrates that one or more embryos can be reabsorbed without jeopardizing the remaining embryo (Dickey et al., 2002).

Multifetal pregnancies carry significant increased fetal risk. Spontaneous abortion is three times more likely with twin pregnancies, with the greatest number occurring among monochorionic twin pregnancies (Sperling et al., 2006). Twin gestations represent a disproportionate occurrence of neonatal morbidity related to PTB, LBW, and IUGR. LBW is more common in multifetal gestations due to restricted fetal growth and preterm delivery. Although only 3 percent of births are multiple gestations, they represent 15 percent of PTBs, 20 percent of LBW (less than 2,500 g), and 19 to 24 percent of VLBW (less than 1,500 g) newborns in the United States (Goodnight & Newman, 2009). About 60 percent of twins, more than 90 percent of triplets, and all quadruplets and higher-order multiples are born premature, with the length of pregnancy decreasing with each additional baby. On average, most singleton pregnancies last 39 weeks; twins, 35 weeks; triplets, 32 weeks; and quadruplets, 29 weeks (Martin et al., 2009). Children born from a multifetal pregnancy have a higher risk of CP, learning disabilities, and language/neurobehavioral deficits, with CP as the most significant outcome (Rand, Eddleman, & Stone, 2005; Sutcliff & Derom, 2005).

Monochorionicity is considered another risk factor for twin pregnancies, complicated by twin-to-twin transfusion syndrome (TTTS), IUGR, uteroplacental insufficiency, intraventricular hemorrhage, necrotizing enterocolitis, and death (Little, 2010). TTTS is uncompensated, unidirectional blood flow from one fetus to another (donor to recipient) that occurs in 10 percent of monochorionic twins who share a placenta (Rossi & D'Addario, 2008). The donor twin becomes hypovolemic with suboptimal growth and the recipient becomes anemia, hypervolemic, and hydropic. This is a serious complication of multifetal gestation and requires management by a maternal-fetal specialist.

Women with multiple gestation experience increased risk of other complications such as diabetes, gestational hypertension, HELLP, fatty liver disease, anemia, and urinary tract infections (Little, 2010). The incidence of diabetes occurs in 3 to 6 percent of twin pregnancies and 22 to 39 percent of triplet pregnancies. The incidence of preeclampsia is 2.6 times higher in twin pregnancies (ACOG Practice Bulletin, 2004c), and it also occurs earlier in pregnancy and is more severe (Lynch, McDuffie, Murphy, Faber, & Orleans, 2002). As in singleton pregnancies, severe preeclampsia or gestational diabetes requires delivery to prevent further maternal and fetal problems. The cesarean birth rate is over 80 percent in multifetal pregnancies (Gyamfi et al., 2005), and some authors cite a twofold increase in maternal mortality when comparing women with multifetal pregnancies versus singleton pregnancies (Conde-Agudelo, Belizan, & Lindmark, 2000). Placenta previa and vasa previa are also more common problems in multiple gestations (ASRM, 2006).

Prevention

Optimizing pregnancy outcomes requires consideration of the benefits and risks associated with a multifetal pregnancy. The increase in multiple gestations resulting from infertility treatments with the aforementioned concomitant risks has led to a focus on prevention (see Chapter 13).

Subjective Data

Taking a thorough health history is important to evaluate risk of multifetal pregnancy, with attention to identification of risk factors. During early pregnancy, a woman with multiple gestation may experience more severe nausea and vomiting, which may last well into the second trimester. As the pregnancy progresses, women with a multifetal pregnancy are more likely to present with shortness of breath and musculoskeletal discomforts.

Objective Data

The data used to diagnose the presence of a multiple gestation is collected by physical examination, screening through maternal serum AFP testing, and sonography.

In the first trimester, there may be more rapid weight gain and the uterus is larger than estimated for gestational age. In the second trimester, the most common early sign is a fundal height greater than expected for dates. More than one heartbeat may be heard. Palpation of more than one fetus is not usually possible until the third trimester and even then it may be difficult, especially if there is polyhydramnios or the woman is obese.

An elevated maternal serum alpha protein level between 15 and 18 weeks' gestation is associated with multifetal gestation, but this is only a screening test. Sonography is used for definitive diagnosis and to identify the number of fetuses, as well as documentation of chorionicity (Evans & Andriole, 2010). Early ultrasound improves multifetal detection (Whitworth, Bricker, Neilson, & Dowswell, 2010) and increased opportunity for antepartal surveillance (Devoe, 2008).

Differential Medical Diagnoses

Inaccurate menstrual history, anemia, HG, hyperthyroidism, gestational trophoblastic disease, gestational diabetes, uterine leiomyomas, polyhydramnios, fetal macrosomia, closely attached adnexal mass

Plan

The primary clinical goal in management of a multifetal pregnancy is the same as a singleton pregnancy: to assure a healthy outcome. Given the increased risk for premature birth and fetal growth restriction in twin pregnancies, a focus on prevention of prematurity and early detection of fetal growth restriction must accompany the management of twin pregnancies. One of the clinical challenges is that PTB prevention strategies remain elusive for both singleton and twin births.

The use of progesterone therapy for reduction of PTB in multifetal gestations has not reduced birth rates in multifetal pregnancies (Caritis et al., 2009; Rouse, 2007), and therefore, current evidence doesn't support routine use of progesterone for this group (ACOG Committee Opinion, 2008b). The majority of research studies on use of fibronectin in identifying risk of PTB have been conducted on singleton pregnancies, but there is some evidence that this test may have a negative predictive value for multiple gestations (ACOG Practice Bulletin, 2004c). A systematic review by Lim and colleagues (2011) concluded that second trimester cervical length is a strong predictor of PTB in a multiple pregnancy, but because no prevention strategies are available, they discouraged use of this measure in clinical practice.

There is no current evidence that shows improved outcome in multifetal pregnancies with prophylactic use of cerclage, hospitalization, home uterine active monitoring, or bed rest (ACOG Practice Bulletin, 2004c). Bed rest for women with a multiple gestation has been studied extensively, and although bed rest has not prevented PTB, some evidence suggests that hospitalization with bed rest may improve fetal growth and decrease LBW (Crowther & Han, 2010). Most providers limit a woman's activity based on her lifestyle and general health. When a woman with multiple gestation is placed on bed rest, referral to a support group may assist her in dealing with the many physical and emotional changes she may experience (Ruiz, Brown, Peters, & Johnston, 2001).

Research studies using prophylactic tocolytic therapy in twin gestations showed no consistent effect on PTB, birth weight, or neonatal mortality (ACOG Practice Bulletin, 2004c). Of concern is the increased risk of cardiac stress, pulmonary edema, and gestational diabetes associated with tocolytic use that is amplified in multifetal pregnancies. For this reason, tocolytic therapy should be used cautiously in multifetal pregnancies (ACOG Practice Bulletin, 2004c). Antenatal corticosteroid use for pregnant women between 24 and 34 weeks of gestation who are at risk of PTL within 7 days (including multifetal pregnancies) is recommended by the NIH and ACOG (ACOG Committee Opinion, 2011; NIH Consensus Statement, 2000).

Nutritional Interventions. The physiologic changes and nutritional needs accompanying a twin pregnancy, as well as the increased risk of growth restriction, increase the importance of adequate nutritional intake. According to Luke (2004), women with a twin pregnancy and normal prepregnancy BMI should have a daily intake of 3,500 calories: 175 g protein, 350 g carbohydrates, and 150 g fat. Daily supplementation with 30 mg elemental iron, 1 mg folic acid, 2,000 to 2,500 mg calcium, 14 to 45 mg zinc, and up to 1,000 mg magnesium is recommended by Goodnight and Newman (2009), as well as consideration of additional docosahexaenoic acid and vitamin D supplementation. The 2009 IOM Guidelines for Weight Gain in Twin Pregnancies recommend BMI-specific weight gains: normal weight women, 17–25 kg (37–54 lb); overweight women, 14–23 kg (31–50 lb); obese women, 11–19 kg (25–42 lb).

Education. As discussed earlier, the risks associated with a multifetal pregnancy should accompany infertility counseling and be discussed during antepartal care. All procedures and interventions should be thoroughly explained and the signs of PTL and gestational hypertension should be reviewed. Nutritional education should include a review of the need for a higher intake of protein, minerals, vitamins, essential fatty acids, and calories.

Symptom Management. To address the increased discomfort associated with the physiological changes of multiple gestation, various measures may be implemented. Nausea and vomiting may require IV hydration. Constipation, heartburn, sleeping disturbances, and low back pain interventions should be reviewed. Maternity support hose may be recommended early in pregnancy. A maternity "sling" girdle has been helpful for some women to help support the gravid uterus and alleviate lower backstrain associated with multiple gestation. Exercises, particularly those to stretch and strengthen the lower back muscles, may be suggested. Although excessive fetal movement is reported, it does not warrant intervention. The health care provider can assist women in controlling and coping with changes with anticipatory guidance and education (Ruiz et al., 2001).

Maternal Assessment. Carefully evaluate the usual pregnancy changes with particular attention to signs and symptoms of PTL, anemia, gestational hypertension, and gestational diabetes. Gestational diabetes screening should be conducted after multifetal gestation has been diagnosed and women should be asked about nausea and epigastic pain during the second and third trimester because they are at greater risk for developing HELLP syndrome (ACOG Practice Bulletin, 2004c).

Fetal Surveillance. The same principles for screening and diagnosing fetal abnormalities apply to twin pregnancies, although there are differences in safety and efficacy (Evans & Andriole, 2010). For example, fetuses in multiple pregnancies have a poorer nuchal translucency image score when located further from the abdominal wall (Zohav et al., 2006).

Sonography, BPP, and nonstress test (NST) are among the tests that are commonly used to assess fetal well-being in multifetal pregnancies, with each fetus being evaluated separately. TTTS, monoamniotic twinning, and intrauterine death of a single twin fetus present special challenges to antenatal surveillance (Devoe, 2008) (see Chapter 21).

Sonography is done early in the second trimester to assess fetal structures for anomalies, to determine placental placement, to identify chorionicity and amnionicity, and to assess cervical length. Other findings, such as amniotic fluid volume and fetal presentation, are also useful in assessing fetal risk. TTTS is also diagnosed by sonogram. Although there is no evidence that supports one particular approach to antepartal surveillance of a multifetal pregnancy (ACOG Practice Bulletin, 2004c; Devoe, 2008), sonograms are typically done every 2 to 3 weeks after 28 weeks to assess fetal growth. Fetal growth is usually satisfactory until 30 to 32 weeks of pregnancy, but discordant growth has been observed as early as 22 weeks (Warner et al., 2000). BPP and NST also typically start at 28 weeks and are done weekly. Doppler velocimetry as a measure of fetal well-being for multifetal pregnancy has limited evidence to support its use (Devoe, 2008).

Delivery. Decisions concerning delivery are based on gestational age, estimated fetal weights, presentations in relation to each other, and availability of adequate intrapartum monitoring. Cesarean birth is performed more frequently because of malpresentations and concern for the preterm and LBW fetuses to tolerate a vaginal birth. An intrapartal sonogram is necessary to identify fetal presentations and establish a management plan for delivery.

Follow-Up

Due to the increased energy demands and physical challenges inherent in breastfeeding two newborns, a woman with twins may need additional breastfeeding education and support (see Chapter 22). Neonatal illness and separation can also interfere in parent–child attachment. Most communities have lay groups of parents who have had multiple births, such as Mothers of Twins and Mothers of Multiples. These groups provide supportive counseling, practical suggestions such as how to manage two newborns and where to obtain equipment and supplies, and referrals for financial assistance.

REFERENCES

Abalos, E., Duley, L., Steyn, D.W., & Henderson-Smart, D.J. (2007). Antihypertensive drug therapy for mild to moderate hypertension during pregnancy. *Cochrane Database of Systematic Reviews,* (4), CD002252.

Abebe, J., Eigbefoh, J., Isabu, P., Eifediyi, R., & Okusanya, B. (2008). Accuracy of urine dipsticks, 2-h and 12-h urine collections for protein measurement as compared with the 24-h collection. *Journal of Obstetrics and Gynecology, 28*(5), 496–500.

ACOG Committee Opinion. (2002). *Exercise during pregnancy and the postpartum period* (No. 267). Washington, DC: American College of Obstetricians and Gynecologists.

ACOG Committee Opinion. (2007, June). *Multifetal pregnancy reduction* (No. 369). Washington, DC: American College of Obstetricians and Gynecologists.

ACOG Committee Opinion. (2008a). *Late-preterm infants* (No. 404). Washington, DC: American College of Obstetricians and Gynecologists.

ACOG Committee Opinion. (2008b, October). *Use of progesterone to reduce preterm birth* (No. 419). Washington, DC: American College of Obstetricians and Gynecologists.

ACOG Committee Opinion. (2009, June). *Postpartum screening for abnormal glucose tolerance in women who had gestational diabetes mellitus* (No. 435). Washington, DC: American College of Obstetricians and Gynecologists.

ACOG Committee Opinion. (2011, February). *Antenatal corticosteroid therapy for fetal maturation* (No. 475). Washington, DC: American College of Obstetricians and Gynecologists.

ACOG Practice Bulletin. (2001a, reviewed 2009). *Perinatal viral and parasitic infections* (No. 20). Washington, DC: American College of Obstetricians and Gynecologists.

ACOG Practice Bulletin. (2001b, July). *Chronic hypertension in pregnancy* (No. 29). Washington, DC: American College of Obstetricians and Gynecologists.

ACOG Practice Bulletin. (2001c, September). *Diabetes and pregnancy* (No. 30). Washington, DC: American College of Obstetricians and Gynecologists.

ACOG Practice Bulletin. (2001d, October). *Assessment of risk factors for preterm birth* (No. 31). Washington, DC: American College of Obstetricians and Gynecologists.

ACOG Practice Bulletin. (2002a, January; reaffirmed 2010). *Diagnosis and management of preeclampsia and eclampsia*

(No. 33). Washington, DC: American College of Obstetricians and Gynecologists.

ACOG Practice Bulletin. (2002b, September). *Perinatal care at the threshold of viability* (No. 38). Washington, DC: American College of Obstetricians and Gynecologists.

ACOG Practice Bulletin. (2003a, May). *Management of preterm labor* (No. 43). Washington, DC: American College of Obstetricians and Gynecologists.

ACOG Practice Bulletin. (2003b, November). *Cervical insufficiency* (No. 48). Washington, DC: American College of Obstetricians and Gynecologists.

ACOG Practice Bulletin. (2004a). *Diagnosis and treatment of gestational trophoblastic disease* (No. 53). Washington, DC: American College of Obstetricians and Gynecologists.

ACOG Practice Bulletin. (2004b, April). *Nausea and vomiting of pregnancy* (No. 52). Washington, DC: American College of Obstetricians and Gynecologists.

ACOG Practice Bulletin. (2004c, October). *Multiple gestation: Complicated twin, triplet, and higher-order multifetal pregnancy* (No. 56). Washington, DC: American College of Obstetricians and Gynecologists.

ACOG Practice Bulletin. (2005, March). *Clinical management guidelines for obstetrician-gynecologists: Pregestational diabetes mellitus* (No. 60). Washington, DC: American College of Obstetricians and Gynecologists.

ACOG Practice Bulletin. (2007a, January). *Hemoglobinopathies in pregnancy* (No. 78). Washington, DC: American College of Obstetricians and Gynecologists.

ACOG Practice Bulletin. (2007b). *Management of herpes in pregnancy* (No. 82). Washington, DC: American College of Obstetricians and Gynecologists.

ACOG Practice Bulletin. (2007c). *Premature rupture of membranes* (No. 80). Washington, DC: American College of Obstetricians and Gynecologists.

ACOG Practice Bulletin. (2007d). *Viral hepatitis in pregnancy* (No. 86). Washington, DC: American College of Obstetricians and Gynecologists.

ACOG Practice Bulletin. (2008, July). *Anemia in pregnancy* (No. 95). Washington, DC: American College of Obstetricians and Gynecologists.

ACOG Technical Bulletin. (2005). *Obesity in pregnancy* (No. 315). Washington, DC: American College of Obstetricians and Gynecologists.

Adebisi, O.Y., & Strayhorn, G. (2005). Anemia in pregnancy and race in the United States: Blacks at risk. *Family Medicine, 37,* 655–662.

Agency for Healthcare Research and Quality. (2006). *Screening for iron deficiency anemia in childhood and pregnancy: Update of the 1996 U.S. Preventive task force review* (AHRQ Publication No. 06-0590-EF-1). Rockville, MD: Author.

Aghajanian P. (2011). Gestational trophoblastic diseases. In A.H. DeCherney & L. Nathan (Eds.), *Current diagnosis and treatment obstetrics and gynecology* (10th ed.). Retrieved October 16, 2011, from http://www.accessmedicine.com.ezp1.lib.umn.edu/content.aspx?aID=2392439

Alexander, S., Boulvain, M., Ceysens, G., Haelterman, E., & Zhang, W. (2010). Repeat digital cervical assessment in pregnancy for identifying women at risk of preterm labor. *Cochrane Database of Systematic Reviews,* (6), CD005940.

Aliyu, M.D., Jolly, P.E., Ehiri, J.E., & Salihu, H.M. (2005). High parity and adverse birth outcomes: Exploring the maze.*Birth 32*(1) 45–59.

American Academy of Pediatrics. (2009). Antenatal counseling regarding resuscitation at an extremely low gestational age. *Pediatrics, 124*(1), 422–427.

American Diabetes Association (ADA). (2002). Gestational diabetes mellitus. *Diabetes Care, 33*(Suppl. 1), S62–S69.

American Diabetes Association (ADA). (2008). Nutrition recommendations and interventions for diabetes. *Diabetes Care, 31*(Suppl. 1), S61–S78.

American Diabetes Association (ADA). (2010). Diagnosis and classification of diabetes mellitus (position statement). *Diabetes Care, 33*(Suppl. 1), S62–S69.

American Diabetes Association (ADA). (2011a). Diagnosis and classification of diabetes mellitus (position statement). *Diabetes Care, 34*(Suppl. 1), S62–S69.

American Diabetes Association (ADA). (2011b). Standards of medical care in diabetes—2011. *Diabetes Care, 34*(Suppl. 1), S11–S61.

American Society for Reproductive Medicine (ASRM). (2006). Multiple pregnancies associated with infertility therapy. *Fertility and Sterility, 86*(Suppl. 4), S106–S110.

American Society for Reproductive Medicine (ASRM). (2009). Guidelines on number of embryos transferred. *Fertility and Sterility, 92,* 1518–1519.

Ananth, C.V., Getahun, D., Peltier, M.R., Salihu, H.M., & Vintzileos, A.M. (2006). Recurrence of spontaneous versus medically indicated preterm birth. *American Journal of Obstetrics and Gynecology, 195*(3), 643–650.

Ananth, C.V., Getahun, D., Peltier, M.R., & Smulian, J.C. (2006). Placental abruption in term and preterm gestations: Evidence for heterogeneity in clinical pathways. *Obstetrics and Gynecology, 107,* 785–792.

Ananth, C.V., & Vintzileos, A.M. (2006). Maternal-fetal conditions necessitating a medical intervention resulting in preterm birth. *American Journal of Obstetrics and Gynecology, 195*(6), 1557–1563.

Anderson, K., Karstrom, B., Freden, S., Petersson, H., Ohrvall, M., & Zethelius, B. (2008). A two-year clinical lifestyle intervention program for weight loss in obesity. *Food Nutrition Research, 52.* doi:10:3402/fnr.v52i0.1656

Aredas, K., Qiu, G., & Gruslin, A. (2008). Obesity in pregnancy: Pre-conception to postpartum consequences. *Journal of Obstetrics and Gynaecology Canada, 30*(6), 477–488.

Arsenault, M., Lane, C., MacKinnon, C., Bartellas, E., Cargill, Y., Klein, M., et al. (2002). The management of nausea and vomiting of pregnancy. *Journal of Obstetrics and Gynaecology Canada, 24*(10), 817–831.

Attard, C.L., Kohli, M.A., Coleman, S., Bradley, C., Hux, M., Atanackovic, G., et al. (2002). The burden of illness of severe nausea and vomiting of pregnancy in the United States. *American Journal of Obstetrics and Gynecology, 185*(Suppl.), 220–227.

Avery, M. (2007). Endocrine (Chapter 16). In B. Hackley, J.M. Kriebs, & M.E. Rousseau (Eds.), *Primary care of women: A guide for midwives and women's health providers*. Boston: Jones and Bartlett Learning.

Ayres, A., & Johnson, T. (2005). Management of multiple pregnancies: Prenatal care–Part 1. *Obstetrical and Gynecological Survey, 60*(8), 550–554.

Bacak, S., Callaghan, W., Dietz, P., & Crouse, C. (2005). Pregnancy-associated hospitalizations in the United States, 1999–2000. *American Journal of Obstetrics and Gynecology, 192,* 592–597.

Ballard, T.J., Saltzman, L.E., Gazmararian, J.A., Spitz, A.M., Lazorick, S., & Marks, J.S., (1998). Violence during pregnancy: Measurement issues. *American Journal of Public Health, 88* (2), 274–276.

Barnhart, K.T. (2009). Clinical practice: Ectopic pregnancy. *New England Journal of Medicine, 361*(4), 379–387.

Barton, J.R., O'Brien, J.M., Bergauer, N.K., Jacques, D.L., & Sibai, B.M. (2001). Mild gestational hypertension remote form term: Progression and outcome. *American Journal of Obstetrics and Gynecology, 184*(5), 979–983.

Bayoumeu, F., Subiran-Buisset, C., Baka, N.E., Legagneur, H., Monnier-Barbarino, M., & Laxenaire, M.C. (2002). Iron therapy in iron deficiency anemia in pregnancy: Intravenous route versus oral route. *American Journal of Obstetrics and Gynecology, 186* (3), 518–522.

Bellamy, L., Casas, J.P., Hingorani, A.D., & Williams, D.J. (2007). Pre-eclampsia and risk of cardiovascular disease and cancer in later life: A systematic review and meta-analysis. *British Medical Journal, 335,* 974.

Behrman, R.E., & Butler, A.S. (Eds.) (2007). *Preterm Birth: Causes, Consequences, and Prevention.* Institute of Medicine (US) Committee on Understanding Premature Birth and Assuring Health Outcomes, Washington, DC: National Academies Press.

Berghella, V., Baxer, J., & Hendrix, N. (2009). Cervical assessment by ultrasound for preventing preterm delivery. *Cochrane Database of Systematic Reviews,* (3), CD007235.

Berghella, V., Hayes, E., Visintine, J., & Baxter, J. (2008). Fetal fibronectin testing for reducing the risk of preterm birth.*Cochrane Database of Systematic Reviews,* (4), CD006843.

Berkowitz, R.S., Tuncer, Z.S., Bernstein, M.R., & Goldstein, D.P. (2000). Management of gestational trophoblastic diseases: Subsequent pregnancy experience. *Seminars in Oncology, 6,* 678–685.

Bishop, E.H. (1964). Pelvic scoring for elective induction. *Obstetrics and Gynecology, 24,* 266–268.

Black, F.O. (2002). Maternal susceptibility to nausea and vomiting of pregnancy: Is the vestibular system involved? *American Journal of Obstetrics and Gynecology, 185*(Suppl.), 204–209.

Bowes, S.B., Hennessy, T.R., Umpleby, A.M., Benn, J.J., Jackson, N.C., Boroujerdi, M.A., et al. (1996). Measurement of glucose metabolism and insulin secretion during normal pregnancy and pregnancy complicated by gestational diabetes. *Diabetologia, 39*(8), 976–983.

Branson, B.M., Handsfield, H.H., Lampe, M.A., Janssen, R.S., Taylor, A.W., Lyss, S.B., et al. (2006). Revised recommendations for HIV testing of adults, adolescents, and pregnant women in health care settings. *Morbidity and Mortality Weekly Report, 55*(RR-14), 1–17.

Buckwalter, J.G., & Simpson, S.W. (2002). Psychological factors in the etiology and treatment of severe nausea and vomiting in pregnancy. *American Journal of Obstetrics and Gynecology, 186*(Suppl.), 210–214.

Callaway, L.K., O'Callaghan, M. & McIntyre, H.D. (2009). Obesity and hypertensive disorders of pregnancy. *Hypertension in Pregnancy, 28*(4), 473-493.

Cannada, L.K., Pan, P., Casey, B.M., Hawkins, J.S., Shafi, S., McIntire, D., et al. (2008, October). *Outcomes in pregnant trauma patients with orthopedic injuries.* Submitted for Fall Meeting of American Academy of Orthopaedic Surgeons, Dallas, TX.

Caritis, S.N., Rouse, D.J., Peaceman, A.M., Sciscione, A., Momirova, V., Spong, C.Y., et al. (2009). Prevention of preterm birth in triplets using 17 alpha-hydroxyprogesterone caproate: A randomized controlled trial. *Obstetrics and Gynecology, 113,* 285–292.

Carles, G., Tobal, N., Raynal, P., Herault, S., Beucher, G., Marret, H., et al. (2003). Doppler assessment of the fetal cerebral hemodynamic response to moderate or severe maternal anemia. *American Journal of Obstetrics and Gynecology, 188,* 974–979.

de Carvalho, M.H., Bittar, R.E., Brizot, M.L., Bicudo, C., & Zugaib, M. (2005). Prediction of preterm delivery in the second trimester. *Obstetrics and Gynecology, 105*(3), 532–536.

CDC. (1998a). Recommendations to prevent and control iron deficiency in the United States. *Morbidity and Mortality Weekly Report, 47*(RR-3), 1–29.

CDC. (1998b). Use of folic acid-containing supplements among women of childbearing age—United States, 1997. *Morbidity and Mortality Weekly Report, 47*(47), 131–134.

CDC. (2000a). Early-onset group B streptococcal disease—United States, 1998-1999. *Morbidity and Mortality Weekly Report, 49*(35), 793–797.

CDC. (2000b). Hospital-based policies for prevention of perinatal group B streptococcal disease—United States, 1999. *Morbidity and Mortality Weekly Report, 49*(41), 936–940.

CDC. (2002). Prevention of perinatal group B streptococcal disease: Revised guidelines from CDC. *Morbidity and Mortality Weekly Report, 51*(RR-11), 1–22.

CDC. (2005a). Comprehensive immunization strategy to eliminate transmission of hepatitis B virus infection in the United States.*Morbidity and Mortality Weekly Report, 54,* 1–33. Retrieved from http://cdc.gov/mmwr/PDF/rr/rr5416.pdf

CDC. (2005b). Prevalence of overweight and obesity among adults: United States, 1999-2002. Washington, DC: Author. Retrieved from http://www.cdc.gov/nchs/products/pubs/pubd/hestats/obese/obse99.htm

CDC. (2006). Revised recommendations for HIV testing of adults, adolescents, and pregnant women in health care settings. *Morbidity and Mortality Weekly Report, 55*(RR-14), 1–17.

CDC. (2007). Prevention of varicella: Recommendations of the Advisory Committee on Immunization Practices. *Morbidity and Mortality Weekly Report, 56*(RR-04), 1–40. Retrieved from http://www.cdc.gov/mmwr/preview/mmwrhtml/rr5604a1.htm

CDC. (2008). *Guiding principles for development of ACIP recommendations for vaccination during pregnancy and breastfeeding.* Retrieved from http://www.cdc.gov/vaccines/recs/acip/rec-vac-preg.htm

CDC. (2010a). Control and prevention of rubella: Evaluation and management of suspected outbreaks, rubella in pregnant women, and surveillance for congenital rubella syndrome. *Morbidity and Mortality Weekly Report, 50* (RR-12), 1–23.

CDC. (2010b). Sexually transmitted diseases treatment guidelines. *Morbidity and Mortality Weekly Report, 59,* 1–131.

CDC. (2011a). *Cytomegalovirus and congenital cytomegalovirus infections.* Retrieved from http://www.cdc.gov/cmv/testiing-diagnosis.html

CDC. (2011b). *HIV among women.* Retrieved from http://www.cdc.gov/hiv/topics/women/

CDC. (2011c). *Parasites: Toxoplasmosis.* Retrieved from http://www.cdc.gov/parasites/toxoplasmosis/epi.html

CDC. (2011d). *Prenatal care—Health indicators warehouse.* Retrieved from http://www.healthindicators.gov/Indicators/Prenatalcare_1131/Profile/Data

CDC. (2011e). *Vaccines.* Retrieved June 11, 2011, from http://vaccines/

CDC. (2011f). *Varicella (Chickenpox—in short).* Retrieved from http://www.cdc.gov/vaccines/vpd-vac/varicella/in-short-adult.htm#comp

Chakravarty, E., Khanna, D., & Chung, L. (2008). Pregnancy outcomes in systemic sclerosis, primary pulmonary hypertension, and sickle cell disease. *Obstetrics and Gynecology, 111,* 927.

Chandran, L., Navaie-Waliser, M., Zulqarni, N.J., Batra, S., Bayir, H., Shah, M., & Lincoln, P. (2001). Compliance with group B streptococcal disease prevention guidelines. *American Journal of Maternal/Child Nursing, 26* (6), 313–319.

Cheng, Y.W., & Caughey, A.B. (2008). Gestational diabetes: Diagnosis and management. *Journal of Perinatology, 28,* 657–664.

Chu, S.Y., Callaghan, W.M., Bish, C.L., & D'Angelo, D. (2009). Gestational weight gain by body mass index among US women delivering live birth, 2004-2005: Fueling future obesity. *American Journal of Obstetrics and Gynecology, 200*(3), 271.e1–271.e7.

Chu, S.Y., Callaghan, W.M., Kim, S.Y., Schmid, C.H., Lau, J., England, L.J., et al. (2007). Maternal obesity and risk of gestational diabetes mellitus. *Diabetes Care, 30*(8), 2070–2076.

Cleary-Goldman, J., Malone, F.D., Vidaver, J., Ball, R., Nyberg, D.A., Comstock, C.H., et al. (2005). Impact of maternal age on obstetric outcome. *Obstetrics and Gynecology, 105,* 983–990.

Conde-Agudelo, A., Belizan, J., & Lindmark, G. (2000). Maternal morbidity and mortality associated with multiple gestations.*Obstetrics and Gynecology, 95*(6), 899–904.

Corwin, E.J., Murray-Kolb, L.E., & Beard, J.L. (2003). Low hemoglobin level is a risk factor for postpartum depression. *Journal of Nutrition, 133,* 4139–4142.

Crane, J.M.G., Van den Hof, M.C., Dodds, L., Armson, B.A., & Liston, R. (2000). Maternal complications with placenta previa.*American Journal of Perinatology, 17* (2), 101–105.

Crowther, C.A., & Han, S. (2010). Hospitalization and bed rest for multiple pregnancies. *Cochrane Database of Systematic Reviews*, (7), CD000110.

Crowther, C.A., Hiller, J.E., & Doyle, L.W. (2002). Magnesium sulphate for preventing preterm birth in threatened preterm labour. *Cochrane Database of Systematic Reviews*, (4), CD001060.

Crowther, C.A., Hiller, J.E., Moss, J.R., McPhee, A.J., Jeffries, W.S., Robinson, J.S., et al. (2005). Effect of treatment of gestational diabetes mellitus on pregnancy outcomes. *New England Journal of Medicine, 352,* 2477–2486.

Cunningham, F.G., Leveno, K.J., Bloom, S.L., Hauth, J.C., Rouse, D.J., & Spong, C.Y. (2010). *Williams obstetrics* (23rd ed.). New York: McGraw-Hill.

Daley, A.J., Thorpe, S., & Garland, S.M. (2008). Varicella and the pregnant woman: Prevention and management. *Australian and New Zealand Journal of Obstetrics and Gynaecology, 48,* 26–33.

Damus, K. (2008). Prevention of preterm birth: A renewed national priority. *Current Opinion in Obstetrics and Gynecology, 20*(6), 590–596.

Dastor, A., & Tank, P.D. (2010). The pharmacology of preventing preeclampsia. *Journal of Obstetrics and Gynecology of India, 60*(6), 486–492.

Davidoff, M.J., Dias, T., Damus, K., Russell, R., Bettegowda, R., Dolan, S., et al. (2006). Changes in the gestational age distribution among U.S. singleton births: Impact on rates of preterm birth, 1992 to 2002. *Seminars in Perinatology, 30*(1), 8–15.

Davies, S., Cronin, E., Gill, M., Greengorss, P., Hickman, M., & Normand, C. (2000). Screening for sickle cell disease and thalassemia: A systematic review with supplementary research. *Health Technology Assessment, 4,* 1–9.

De-Regil, L., Fernandez-Gaxiola, A., Dowswell, T., & Pena-Rosas, J. (2010). Effects and safety of periconceptional folate supplementation for preventing birth defects. *Cochrane Database of Systematic Reviews*, (10), CD007950.

Devoe, L. (2008). Antenatal fetal assessment: Multifetal gestation—An overview. *Seminars in Perinatology, 32,* 281–287. doi:10.1053/j.semperi.2008.04.011

Di Renzo, G.C., Roura, L.C., Facchinetti, F., Antsaklis, A., Breborowicz, G., Gratacos, E., et al. (2011). Guidelines for the management of spontaneous preterm labor: Identification of spontaneous preterm labor, diagnosis of preterm rupture of membranes, and preventive tools for preterm birth. *Journal of Maternal Fetal Medicine, 24*(5), 659–667.

Dickey, R.P., Taylor, S.N., Lu, P.Y., Sartor, B.M., Storment, J.M., Rye, P.H., et al. (2002). Spontaneous reduction of multiple pregnancy: Incidence and effect on outcome. *American Journal of Obstetrics and Gynecology, 186*(1), 77–82.

Dodd, J.M., Flenady, V.J., Cincotta, R., & Crowther. (2008). Progesterone for the prevention of preterm birth: A systematic review. *Obstetrics and Gynecology, 112,* 127.

Dodds, L., Fell, D., Joseph, K., Allen, V., & Butler, B. (2006). Outcome of pregnancies complicated by hyperemesis gravidarum.*Obstetrics and Gynecology, 107,* 285–292.

Duckitt, K., & Harrington, D. (2005). Risk factors for pre-eclampsia at antenatal booking: Systematic review of controlled studies. *British Medical Journal, 330,* 565–572.

Duff, P. (1998). Hepatitis in pregnancy. *Seminars in Perinatology, 22* (4), 277–283.

Duley, L., Gulmezoglu, A.M., Henderson-Smart, D.J., & Chou, D. (2010). Magnesium sulphate and other anticonvulsants for women with pre-eclampsia. *Cochrane Database of Systematic Reviews*, (11), CD000025.

Duley, L., Henderson-Smart, D.J., & Chou, D. (2010). Magnesium sulphate versus phenytoin for eclampsia. *Cochrane Database of Systematic Reviews*, (10), CD000128.

Duley, L., Henderson-Smart, D.J., & Meher, S. (2006). Drugs for treatment of very high blood pressure during pregnancy. *Cochrane Database of Systematic Reviews*, (4), CD001449.

Duley, L., Henderson-Smart, D.J., Meher, S., & King, J.F. (2007). Antiplatelet agents for preventing pre-eclampsia and its complications. *Cochrane Database of Systematic Reviews*, (2), CD004659.

Duley, L., Henderson-Smart, D.J., Walker, G., & Chou, D. (2010). Magnesium sulphate versus diazepam for eclampsia. *Cochrane Database of Systematic Reviews*, (12), CD000127.

Ebrahimi, N., Maltepe, C., & Einarson, A. (2010). Optimal management of nausea and vomiting of pregnancy. *International Journal of Women's Health, 2,* 241–248.

England, L., & Zhang, J. (2007). Smoking and risk of pre-eclampsia: A systematic review. *Frontiers in Bioscience, 12,* 2471–2483.

Evans, M.I., & Andriole, S. (2010). Screening and testing in multiples. *Clinical Laboratory Medicine, 30,* 643–654.

Fejzo, M.D., Macgibbon, K.W., Romero, R., Goodwin, T.M., & Mullin, P.M. (2011). Recurrence risk of hyperemesis gravidarum.*Journal of Midwifery & Women's Health, 56*(2), 132–136.

Fell, D., Dodds, L., Joseph, K., Allen, V., & Butler, B. (2006). Risk factors for hyperemesis gravidarum requiring hospital admission during pregnancy. *Obstetrics and Gynecology, 107*(2, Pt. 1), 277–284.

Ferrara, A., Weiss, N.S., Hedderson, M.M., Quesenberry, C.P., Selby, J.V., & Erges, I.J. (2007). Pregnancy plasma glucose levels exceeding the American Diabetes Association thresholds, but below the National Diabetes Data Group thresholds for gestational diabetes mellitus, are related to the risk of neonatal macrosomia, hypoglycaemia, and hyperbiliruninaemia. *Diabetiologia, 50,* 298–306.

Ferreira, I., Peeters, L.L., & Stehouwer, C.D. (2009). Pre-eclampsia and increased blood pressure in the offspring: Meta-analysis and critical review of the evidence. *Journal of Hypertension, 27*(10), 1955–1959.

Fiore, A.E., Wasley, A., & Bell, B.P. (2006). Prevention of hepatitis A through active or passive immunity: Recommendations of the Advisory Committee on Immunization Practices. *Morbidity and Mortality Weekly Report, 55* (RR-07), 1–23.

Fraser, A., Tilling, K., Macdonald-Wallis, C., Sattar, N., Brion, M.J., Benfield, L., et al. (2010). Association of maternal weight gain in pregnancy with offspring obesity and metabolic and vascular traits in childhood. *Circulation, 121*(23), 2557–2564.

Friebe, A.E., & Arch, P. (2008). Causes for spontaneous abortion: What the bugs "gut" to do with it? *International Journal of Biochemistry and Cell Biology, 40*(11), 2348–2352.

Furneaux, E.C., Langley-Evans, A.J., & Langley-Evans, S.C. (2001). Nausea and vomiting of pregnancy: Endocrine basis and contribution to pregnancy outcome. *Obstetrics and Gynecology Survey, 56*(12), 775–782.

Gabbe, S.G., Niebyl, J.R., & Simpson, J.L. (2007). *Obstetrics: Normal and problem pregnancies* (5th ed.). Philadelphia: Churchill Livingstone/Elsevier.

Gardella, C., & Brown, Z.A. (2007). Managing varicella zoster infection in pregnancy. *Cleveland Clinic Journal of Medicine, 74,* 290–2296.

Gauthier, T., Mazeau, S., Dalmay, F., Eyraud, J., Catalan, C., Marin, B., et al. (2011). Obesity and cervical ripening failure risk. *Journal of Maternal, Fetal, and Neonatal Medicine, 25*(3), 304–307.

Gawade, P., Markenson, G., Bsat, F., Healy, A., Pekow, P., & Plevyak, M. (2011). Association of gestational weight gain with cesarean delivery rate after labor induction. *Journal of Reproductive Medicine, 56*(3–4), 95–102.

Gershon, A.A. (2009) Rubella virus (German measles. In G.L. Mandell, J. E. Bennett, & R. Dolin (Eds.). *Mandell, Douglas, and Bennett's principles and practice of infectious diseases, 7th ed.* pp. 2265-2288. [electronic version] Churchill Livingstone.

Getahun, D., Nath, C., Ananth, C.V., Chavez, M.R., & Smulian, J.C. (2008). Gestational diabetes in the United States: Temporal trends 1989 through 2004. *American Journal of Obstetrics and Gynecology, 198*(5), 525.e1–525.e5.

Gibson P. (2011, March 29). *Hypertension and pregnancy, medscape*. Retrieved July 21, 2011, from http://emedicine.medscape.com/article/261435-overview

Gilstrap III, L.C., & Ramin, S.M. (2001). Urinary tract infections during pregnancy. *Obstetrics and Gynecology Clinics of North America, 28* (3), 581–591.

Glueck, C.J., Goldenberg, N., Pranikoff, J., Loftspring, M., Sieve, L., & Wang, P. (2004). Height, weight, motor-social development during the first 18 months of life in 126 infants born to 109 mothers with polycystic ovary syndrome who conceived on and continued metformin through pregnancy. *Human Reproduction, 19*(6), 1323–1330.

Glueck, C.J., Goldenberg, N., Streicher, P., & Wang, P. (2003). Metformin and gestational diabetes. *Current Diabetes Report, 3*(4), 303–312.

Glueck, C.J., Wang, P., Goldenberg, N., & Sieve-Smith, L. (2002). Pregnancy outcomes among women with polycystic ovarian syndrome treated with metformin. *Human Reproduction, 17*(11), 2858–2864.

Goldenberg, R.L., Cliver, S.P., Mulvihill, F.X., Hickey, C.A., Hoffman, H.J., Klerman, L.V., et al. (1996). Medical, psychosocial, and behavioral risk factors do not explain the increased risk for low birth weight among black women. *American Journal of Obstetrics and Gynecology, 175*(5), 1317–1324.

Goldenberg, R.L., Culhane, J., Iams, J., & Romero, R. (2008). Preterm birth 1: Epidemiology and causes of preterm birth. *Lancet, 371*(9606), 75–84.

Goldenberg, R.L., Mercer, B.M., Meis, P.J., Copper, R.L., Das, A., & McNellis, D. (1996). The preterm prediction study: Fetal fibronectin testing and spontaneous preterm birth. *Obstetrics and Gynecology, 87*(5, Pt. 1), 643–648.

Goodnight, W., & Newman, R. (2009). Optimal nutrition for improved twin pregnancy outcome. *Obstetrics and Gynecology, 114*(5), 1121–1134.

Goodwin, T.M. (2002). Nausea and vomiting of pregnancy: An obstetric syndrome. *American Journal of Obstetrics and Gynecology, 185*(Suppl.), 184–189.

Griffiths, P.D. (2009). Cytomegalovirus. In A.J. Zuckerman, J.E. Banatvala, B.D. Schoub, P.D. Griffiths, & P. Mortimer (Eds.),*Principles and practice of clinical virology* (6th ed). West Sussex, UK: John Wiley & Sons. doi:10.1002/9780470741405.ch8

Guelinckx, I., Devlieger, R., & Vansant, G. (2009). Reproductive outcome after bariatric surgery: A critical review. *Human Reproductive Update, 15*(2), 189–201.

Gunatilake, R., & Perlow, J. (2011, February). Obesity and pregnancy: Clinical management of the obese gravida. *American Journal of Obstetrics and Gynecology, 204*(2), 106–119.

Gyamfi, C., Stone, J., & Eddleman, K. (2005). Maternal complications of multifetal pregnancy. *Clinics in Perinatology, 32*(2), 431–442.

Hamiliton, B.E., Martin, J.A., & Ventura, S.J. (2009). Births: Preliminary data for 2007, *National Vital Statistics Reports, 57*(12). Retrieved from: www.cdc.gov/nchs/data/nvsr/nvs/57/nvsr57_12.pdf

HAPO Study Cooperative Research Group. (2008). Hyperglycemia and adverse pregnancy outcomes. *New England Journal of Medicine, 358*(19), 1991–2002.

Heaman, M.I., Sprague, A.E., & Stewart, P.J. (2001). Reducing the preterm rate: A population health strategy. *Journal of Obstetric, Gynecologic, and Neonatal Nursing, 30,* 20–29.

Hedley, A.A., Ogeden, C.L., Johnson, C.L., Carroll, M.D., Curtin, L.R., & Flegal, K.M. (2004). Prevalence of overweight and obesity among U.S. children, adolescents, and adults, 1999-2002. *Journal of the American Medical Association, 291*(23), 2847–2850.

Hernandez-Diaz, S., Toh, S., & Cnattingius, S. (2009). Risk of pre-eclampsia in first and subsequent pregnancies: Prospective cohort study. *British Medical Journal, 338,* b2255.

Hick, J.L., Rodgerson, J.D., Heegaard, W.G., & Sterner, S. (2001). Vital signs fail to correlate with hemoperitoneum from ruptured ectopic pregnancy. *American Journal of Emergency Medicine, 19* (6), 488–491.

Hill, J.B., Sheffield, J.S., McIntire, D.D., & Wendel, G.D. (2005). Acute pyelonephritis in pregnancy. *Obstetrics and Gynecology, 105*(1), 18–23.

Hofmeyr, G.J., Lawrie, T.A., Atallah, A.N., & Duley, L. (2010). Calcium supplementation during pregnancy for preventing hypertensive disorders and related problems. *Cochrane Database of Systematic Reviews*, (8), CD001059.

Hogberg, V., Rasmussen, S., & Irgens, L.M. (2007). The effect of smoking and hypertensive disorders on abruptio placentae in Norway 1999-2002. *Acta Obstetricia et Gynecologica Scandinavica, 86*(3), 304–309.

Holzemer, W.L. (2002). HIV and AIDS: The symptom experience. *American Journal of Nursing, 102*(4), 48–52.

Homko, C.J., & Reese, E.A. (2001). To screen or not to screen for gestational diabetes: The clinical quagmire. *Clinical Perinatology, 28*(2), 407–417.

Honein, M.A., Paulozzi, L.J., Mathews, J.J., Erickson, J.D., & Wong, L.Y.C. (2001). Impact of folic acid fortification of the U.S. food supply on the occurrence of neural tube defects. *Journal of the American Medical Association, 285*(23), 2981–2986.

Honest, H., Bachmann, I.M., Gupta, I.K., Kleijnen, J., & Khan, K.S. (2002). Accuracy of cervicovaginal fetal fibronectin test in predicting risk of spontaneous preterm birth. *British Medical Journal, 235*(7359), 301–304.

Hutcheon, J.A., Lisonkova, S., & Joseph, K.S. (2011). Epidemiology of pre-eclampsia and the other hypertensive disorders of pregnancy. *Best Practices and Research Clinical Obstetrics and Gynaecology, 25*(4), 391–403.

Iams, J.D. (2003). Prediction and early detection of preterm labor. *Obstetrics and Gynecology, 101,* 401–412.

Iams, J.D., Newman, R.B., Thom, E.A., Goldenberg, R.L., Mueller-Heubach, E., Moawad, A., et al. (2002). Frequency of uterine contractions and the risk of spontaneous preterm delivery. *New England Journal of Medicine, 346*(4), 250–255.

Iams, J.D., Romero, R., Culhane, J.F., & Goldenberg, R.L. (2008). Preterm birth 2: Primary, secondary, and tertiary interventions to reduce the morbidity and mortality of preterm birth. *Lancet, 371*(9607), 164–175.

Institute for Clinical Systems Improvement (ICSI). (2010, July). *Routine prenatal care, 14th ed.* Retrieved June 11, 2011, from http://www.icis.org

Institute of Medicine (IOM) (1990). *Nutrition during pregnancy.* Washington, DC: National Academies Press.

Institute of Medicine (IOM) (2007). *Preterm Birth: Causes, Consequences, and Prevention.* Washington, DC: National Academies Press.

Institute of Medicine (IOM). (2009). *Weight gain during pregnancy: Reexamining the guidelines*. Washington, DC: National Academies Press.

International Association of Diabetes and Pregnancy Study Groups (IADPSG) Consensus Panel. (2010). International association of diabetes and pregnancy study groups recommendations on the diagnosis and classification of hyperglycemia in pregnancy. *Diabetes Care, 33*(3), 676–682.

Janke, J. (1999). The effect of relaxation therapy on preterm labor outcomes. *Journal of Obstetric, Gynecologic, and Neonatal Nursing, 28,* 255–263.

Jevitt, C. (2009). Pregnancy complicated by obesity: Midwifery management. *Journal of Midwifery and Women's Health, 54*(6), 445–450.

Jolly, J.A., & Wing, D.A. (2010). Pyelonephritis in pregnancy: An update on treatment options for optimal outcomes. *Drugs, 70*(13), 1643–1655.

de Jong, E.P., Walther, F.J., Kroes, C.M., & Oepkes, D. (2011). Parvovirus B 19 infection in pregnancy: New insights and management.*Prenatal Diagnosis, 31,* 410–425.

Kajantie, E., Erickson, J.G., Osmond, C., Thornburg, K., & Barker, D.J. (2009). Pre-eclampsia is associated with increased risk of stroke in the adult offspring: The Helsinki birth cohort study. *Stroke, 40*(4), 1176–1180.

Kidanto, H.L., Mogren, I., Lindmark, G., Massawe, S., & Nystrom, L. (2009). Risks for preterm delivery and low birth weight are independently increased by severity of maternal anemia. *South African Medical Journal, 99*(2), 98.

Kim, C. (2010). Gestational diabetes: Risks, management, and treatment options. *International Journal of Women's Health, 2,* 339–351.

Kim, S., Dietz, P., England, L., Morrow, B., & Callaghan, W. (2007). Trends in pre-pregnancy obesity in nine states, 1993-2003.*Obesity (Silver Spring), 15*(4), 986–993.

King, J., Flenady, V., Cole, S., & Thornton, S. (2005). Cyclo-oxygenase (COX) inhibitors for treating preterm labour. *Cochrane Database of Systematic Reviews*, (2), CD001992.

King, J., Flenady, V., & Murray, L. (2002). Prophylactic antibiotics for inhibiting preterm labour with intact membranes.*Cochrane Database of Systematic Reviews*, (4), CD000246.

King, J., Flenady, V., Papatsonis, D., Dekker, G., & Carbonne, B. (2003). Calcium channel blockers for inhibiting preterm labour. *Cochrane Database of Systematic Reviews*, (1), CD002255.

King, T., & Murphy, P. (2009). Evidence-based approaches to managing nausea and vomiting in early pregnancy. *Journal of Midwifery and Women's Health, 54*(6), 430–440.

Koch, K.L. (2002). Gastrointestinal factors in nausea and vomiting of pregnancy. *American Journal of Obstetrics and Gynecology, 185*(Suppl.), 198–203.

Koren, G., Boskovic, R., Hard, M., Maltepe, C., Navioz, Y., & Einarson, A. (2002). Motherisk-PUQE (pregnancy-unique quantification of emesis and nausea) scoring system for nausea and vomiting of pregnancy. *American Journal of Obstetrics and Gynecology, 185*(Suppl.), 228–231.

Koren, G., Clark, S., Hankins, G., Caritis, S., Miodovnik, M., Umans, J., et al. (2010). Effectiveness of delayed-release doxylamine and pyridoxine for nausea and vomiting of pregnancy: A randomized placebo controlled trial. *American Journal of Obstetrics and Gynecology, 203*(6), 571.e1–571.e7.

Korenbrot, C., Bender, C., Steinberg, A., & Newberry, S. (2001) *Preconception care: Every woman, every time: Executive summary*. Retrieved from http://www.marchofdimes.com/california/4949_8258.asp

Koshy, M. (1999). Sickle cell disease and pregnancy. *Hematology, American Society of Hematology*, 33–38.

Kovacevich, G., Gaich, S., Lavin, L., Hopkins, M.P., Crane, S.S., Stewart, J., et al. (2000). The prevalence of thromboembolic events among women with extended bed rest prescribed as part of the treatment for premature labor or preterm premature rupture of membranes. *American Journal of Obstetrics and Gynecology, 182*(5), 1089–1092.

Krause, R.S., Janicke, D.M., Cydulka, R.K. (2011). Ectopic pregnancy and emergencies in the first 20 weeks of pregnancy. In J.E. Tintinalli, J.S. Stapczynski, D.M. Cline, O.J. Ma, R.K. Cydulka, G.D. Meckler (Eds.), *Tintinalli's emergency medicine: A Comprehensive study guide* (7th ed.). Retrieved October 9, 2011, from http://www.accessmedicine.com.ezp1.lib.umn.edu

Kuc, S., Wortelboer, E.J., van Rijn, B.B., Franx, A., Visser, G.H., & Schielen, P.C. (2011). Evaluation of 7 serum biomarkers and uterine artery Doppler ultrasound for first-trimester prediction of preeclampsia: A systematic review. *Obstetrics and Gynecologic Survey, 66*(4), 225–239.

Kuklina, E.V., Ayala, C., & Callaghan, W.M. (2009). Hypertensive disorders and severe obstetric morbidity in the United States.*Obstetrics and Gynecology, 113*(6), 1299–1306.

Lacasse, A., Rey, E., Ferreira, E., Morin, C., & Bérard, A. (2008). Validity of a modified pregnancy-unique quantification of emesis and nausea (PUQE) scoring index to assess severity of nausea and vomiting of pregnancy. *American Journal of Obstetrics and Gynecology, 198*(1), 71.e1–71.e7.

Lacasse, A., Rey, E., Ferreira, E., Morin, C., & Bérard, A. (2009). Epidemiology of nausea and vomiting of pregnancy: Prevalence, severity, determinants, and the importance of race/ethnicity. *BioMed Central Pregnancy and Childbirth, 9*, 26. doi:10.1186/1471-2393-9-26

LaCoursiere, Y., & Varner, M. (2009). *The association between prepregnancy obesity and postpartum depression, supported by NIH grant R03-HD-048865* (Abstract No. 92). Presented at the 29th Annual Meeting of the Society for Maternal-Fetal, San Diego, CA.

Lamont, R.F., Sobel, J.D., Carrington, D., Mazaki-Tovi, S., Kusanovic, J.P., Vaisbuch, E, & Romero, R (2011) Varicella-zoster virus (chickenpox) infection in pregnancy. *British Journal of Obstetrics and Gynecology,118(10) 1155–1162.*

Lamont, R.F., Sobel, J.D., Vaisbuch, E., Kusanovic, J.P., Mazaki-Tovi, S., Kim, S.K., et al. (2010). Parvovirus B19 infection in human pregnancy. *British Journal of Obstetrics and Gynecology, 118*, 175–186. doi:10.1111/j.1471-0528.2010.02749.x

Landon, M.B., Spong, C.Y., Thom, E., Carpenter, M.W., Ramin, S.M., Casey, B., et al. (2009). A multicenter, randomized trial of treatment for mild gestational diabetes. *New England Journal of Medicine, 361*(14), 1339–1348.

Lawrence, J.M., Contreras, R., Chen, W., & Sacks, D.A. (2008). Trends in prevalence of preexisting diabetes and gestational diabetes mellitus among a racially/ethnically diverse population of pregnant women, 1999-2005. *Diabetes Care, 31*, 899–904.

Lee, E., & Frazier, S. (2011). The efficacy of acupressure for symptom management: A systematic review. *Journal of Pain Symptom Management, 42*(4), 589–603.

Lee, N., & Saha, S. (2011). Nausea and vomiting of pregnancy. *Gastroenterology Clinics of North America, 40*, 309–334.

Lee, S., Lee, J., Seong, H., Lee, S., Park, J., Romero, R., et al. (2009). The clinical significance of a positive Amnisure test in women with term labor and intact membranes. *Journal of Maternal and Fetal Medicine, 22*, 305–310.

Leeman, L., & Fontaine, P. (2008). Hypertensive disorders of pregnancy. *American Family Physician, 78*(1), 93–100.

Leonard, L., & Denton, J. (2006). Preparation for parenting multiple birth children. *Early Human Development, 82*, 371–378.

Levichek, Z., Atanackovic, G., Oepkes, D., Maltepe, C., Einarson, A., Magee, L., et al. (2002). Nausea and vomiting of pregnancy. Evidence-based treatment algorithm. *Canadian Family Physician, 48*, 267–269.

Lim, A., Hegeman, M., Huis, M., Opmeer, B., Bruinse, H., & Mol, B. (2011). Cervical length measurement for the prediction of preterm birth in multiple pregnancies: A systematic review and bivariate meta-analysis. *Ultrasound Obstetrics and Gynecology, 38*(1), 10–17.

Lindheimer, M., Taler, S., & Cunningham, G. (2009). ASH position paper: Hypertension in pregnancy. *Journal of Clinical Hypertension, 11*(4), 214–225.

Lindseth, G., & Vari, P. (2005). Measuring physical activity during pregnancy. *West Journal of Nursing Research, 27*(6), 722–734.

Little, C. (2010). One consequence of infertility treatment: Multifetal pregnancy. *American Journal of Maternal/Child Nursing, 35*(3), 150–155.

Littleton, H., Breitkopf, C., & Berenson, A. (2007). Correlates of anxiety symptoms during pregnancy and association with perinatal outcomes: A meta-analysis. *American Journal of Obstetrics and Gynecology, 196*(5), 424–432.

Lobner, K., Knopff, A., Baumgartern, A., Mollenhauer, U., Marienfeld, S., Garrido-Franco, M., et al. (2006). Predictors of postpartum diabetes in women with gestational diabetes mellitus. *Diabetes, 55*, 792–797.

Lombardi, G., Garofoli, F., & Stronati, M. (2010). Congenital cytomegalovirus infection: Treatment, sequelae and follow-up. *Journal of Maternal-Fetal and Neonatal Medicine, 23*(S3), 45–48.

Ludwig, D.S., & Currie, J. (2010). The association between pregnancy weight gain and birthweight: A within-family comparison. *Lancet, 376*(9745), 984–990.

Luke, B. (2004). Improving multiple pregnancy outcomes with nutritional interventions. *Clinical Obstetrics and Gynecology, 47,* 146–162.

Luke, B., & Brown, M.B. (2007). Elevated risks of pregnancy complications and adverse outcomes with increasing maternal age. *Human Reproduction, 22*(5), 1264–1272.

Lumley, J., Oliver, S., Chamberlain, C., & Oakley, L. (2004). Interventions for promoting smoking cessation during pregnancy. *Cochrane Database of Systematic Reviews*, (4), CD001055.

Lynch, A., McDuffie, R., Murphy, J., Faber, K., & Orleans, M. (2002). Preeclampsia in multiple gestation: The role of assisted reproductive technologies. *Obstetrics and Gynecology, 99,* 445–451.

MacCormack, D. (2010). Hypnosis for hyperemesis gravidarum. *Journal of Obstetrics & Gynaecology, 30*(7), 647–653.

MacDonald, H., Brocklehurst, P., & Gordon, A. (2007). Antibiotics for treating bacterial vaginosis in pregnancy. *Cochrane Database of Systematic Reviews*, (1), CD000262.

MacDorman, M.F., & Mathews, T.J. (2011). Infants deaths–United States, 2000-2007. *Morbidity and Mortality Weekly Report, 60,* 49–51.

Magee, L.A., Helewa, M., & Moutquin, J.M. (2008, March). Diagnosis, evaluation, and management of hypertensive disorders of pregnancy. *Journal of Obstetrics and Gynecology Canada, 30,* S1–S48.

Maloni, J.A., Brezinski-Tomasi, J.E., & Johnson, L.A. (2001). Antepartum bed rest: Effect upon the family. *Journal of Obstetric, Gynecologic, and Neonatal Nursing, 30*(2), 165–173.

Manchikanti, G., Grimes, D., Lopez, L., & Schulz, K. (2007). Steroid hormones of contraception in women with sickle cell disease.*Cochrane Database of Systematic Reviews*, (2), CD006261.

Manzanares, G., Santalla, H., Vico, I., Criado, L., Pineda, A., & Gallo, J. (2012). Abnormal maternal body mass index and obstetric and neonatal outcome. *Journal of Maternal, Fetal, and Neonatal Medicine, 25*(3), 308–312.

March of Dimes. (2011a). *Pregnancy complications.* Retrieved from http://www.marchofdimes.com/pregnancy/complications_spotting.html

March of Dimes. (2011b). *Preterm labor.* Retrieved from http://www.marchofdimes.com/pregnancy/preterm.html?gclid=CKjWjq3uv6sCFQ0CQAodbVB5uA

Markenson, G.R., & Yancey, M.K. (1998). Parvovirus B19 in pregnancy. *Seminars in Perinatology, 22*(4), 309–317.

Marti-Carvajal, I., Pena-Marti, G., Communian-Carrasco, & Marti-Pena, A. (2009). Interventions for treating painful sickle crisis during pregnancy. *Cochrane Database of Systematic Reviews*, (1), CD006786.

Martin, J., Hamilton, B., Sutton, P., Ventura, S., Menacker, F., Kirmeyer, S. (2006). Births: Final data for 2004. *National Vital Statistics Reports, 55*(1), 1–101.

Martin, J., Hamilton, B., Sutton, P., Ventura, S., Menacker, F., Kirmeyer, S., et al. (2009). Births: Final data for 2006.*National Vital Statistics Reports, 57*(7). Retrieved March 27, 2012, from http://www.cdc.gov/nchs/data/nvsr/nvsr57/nvsr57_07.pdf

Mashburn, J. (1999). Ectopic pregnancy: Triage do's and don'ts. *Journal of Nurse-Midwifery, 44*(6), 549–557.

Matthews, A., Dowswell, T., Haas, D., Doyle, M., & O'Mathuna, D. (2010). Interventions for nausea and vomiting in early pregnancy.*Cochrane Database of Systematic Reviews*, (9), CD007575.

McCarter-Spaulding, D. (2002). Parvovirus B19 in pregnancy. *Journal of Obstetric, Gynecology, and Neonatal Nursing, 31*(1), 107–112.

McCormick, D., Scott-Heyes, G., & McCusker, C. (2011). The impact of hyperemesis gravidarum on maternal health and maternal-fetal attachment. *Journal of Psychosomatic Obstetrics and Gynecology, 32*(2), 79–87.

McKenna, D.S., & Iams, J.D. (1998). Group B streptococcal infections. *Seminars in Perinatology, 22* (4), 267–276.

McMaster, M.T., Zhou, Y., & Fisher, S.J. (2004). Abnormal placentation and the syndrome of preeclampsia. *Seminars in Nephrology, 24*(6), 540–547.

Meher, S., Abalos, E., & Carroll, G. (2005). Bed rest with or without hospitalization for hypertension during pregnancy. *Cochrane Database of Systematic Reviews*, (4), CD003514.

Meher, S., & Duley, L. (2006a). Garlic for preventing pre-eclampsia and its complications. *Cochrane Database of Systematic Reviews*, (3), CD006065.

Meher, S., & Duley, L. (2006b). Exercise or other physical activity for preventing pre-eclampsia and its complications. *Cochrane Database of Systematic Reviews*, (2), CD005942.

Meher, S., & Duley, L. (2006c). Progesterone for preventing pre-eclampsia and its complications. *Cochrane Database of Systematic Reviews*, (4), CD006175.

Meher, S., & Duley, L. (2006d). Rest during pregnancy for preventing pre-eclampsia and its complications in women with normal blood pressure. *Cochrane Database of Systematic Reviews*, (2), CD005939.

Meher, S., & Duley, L. (2007). Nitric oxide for preventing pre-eclampsia and its complications. *Cochrane Database of Systematic Reviews*, (2), CD006490.

Metzger, B.E., Buchanan, T.A., Coustan, D.R., de Leiva, A., Dunger, O.B., Hadden, D.R., et al. (2007). Summary and recommendations of the fifth international workshop-conference on gestational diabetes mellitus. *Diabetes Care, 30*(Suppl. 2), S251–S260.

Minnick-Smith, K., & Cook, F. (1997). Current treatment options for ectopic pregnancy. *American Journal of Maternal/Child Nursing, 22,* 21–25.

Mitchell, A., Steffenson, N., Hogan, H., & Brooks, S. (1997). Neonatal group B streptococcal disease. *American Journal of Maternal/Child Nursing, 22,* 249–253.

Montoya, J.C., & Remington, J.S. (2008). Management of Toxoplasma gondii infection during pregnancy. *Clinical Infectious Diseases, 47,* 554–566. doi:10.1086/590149

Moore, M. (1999). Reproductive health and intimate partner violence. *Family Planning Perspectives, 31* (6), 302–312.

Morin, L.M., & Van den Hof, M.C. (2005). *Ultrasound evaluation of first trimester pregnancy complications.* SOGC Clinical Practice Guidelines, No. 161. Retrieved from http://www.sogc.org/guidelines/public/161e-cpg-june2005.pdf

Munch, S., Korst, L., Hernandez, G., Romero, R., & Goodwin, T. (2011). Health-related quality of life in women with nausea and vomiting of pregnancy: The importance of psychosocial context. *Journal of Perinatology, 31,* 10–20.

Naim, A., Haberman, S., Burgess, T., Navizedeh, N., & Minkoff, H. (2002). Changes in cervical length and the risk of preterm labor. *American Journal of Obstetrics and Gynecology, 186,* 887–889.

National Institutes of Health, AIDS*info*. (2010). *HIV and pregnancy.* Retrieved from http://www.aidsinfo.nih.gov/contentfiles/Perinatal_FS_en.pdf

Neilson, J.P. (2003). Interventions for treating placental abruption. *Cochrane Database of Systematic Reviews,* (1). doi:10.1002/14651858.CD003247

Nguyen, N.T., Nguyen, X.M., Lane, J., & Wang, P. (2011). Relationship between obesity and diabetes in a US adult population: Findings from the national health and nutrition examination survey, 1999-2006. *Obesity and Surgery, 21*(3), 351–355.

Nicholson, W., Bolen, S., Witcop, C.T., Neale, D., Wilson, L., & Bass, E. (2009). Benefits and risks of oral agents compared to insulin in women with gestational diabetes: A systematic review. *Obstetrics and Gynecology, 113*(1), 193–205.

Niebyl, J. (2010). Nausea and vomiting in pregnancy. *New England Journal of Medicine, 363,* 1544–1550.

NIH Consensus Statement. (2000). Antenatal corticosteroids revisited. *Repeat Courses, 17*(2), 1–18.

Norwitz, E.R., Edusa, V., & Park, J.S. (2005). Maternal physiology and complications of multiple pregnancies. *Seminars in Perinatology, 29,* 338–348.

O'Brien, T.E., Ray, J.G., & Chan, W.S. (2003). Maternal body mass index and the risk of preeclampsia: A systematic overview.*Epidemiology, 14,* 368–374.

Ogden, C.L., Carroll, M.D., Curtin, L.R., McDowell, M.A., Tabak, C.J., & Flegal, K.M. (2006). Prevalence of overweight and obesity in the United States. *Journal of the American Medical Association, 295*(13), 1549–1555.

Oken, E., Ning, Y., Rifas-Shiman, S., Radeksy, J., Rich-Edwards, J., & Gillman, M. (2006). Associations of physical activity and inactivity before and during pregnancy with glucose tolerance. *Obstetrics and Gynecology, 108*(5), 1200–1207.

Oken, E., Rifas-Shima, S.L., Field, A.E., Frazier, A.L., & Gillman, M.W. (2008). Maternal gestational weight gain and offspring weight in adolescence. *Obstetrics and Gynecology, 112*(5), 999–1006.

Oken, E., Taveras, E.M., Kleinman, K.P., Rich-Edwards, J.W., & Gillman, M.W. (2007). Gestational weight gain and child adiposity at age 3 years. *American Journal of Obstetrics and Gynecology, 196*(4), 322.e1–322.e8.

Olson, G., & Blackwell, S. (2011). Optimization of gestational weight gain in the obese gravida: A review. *Obstetrical Gynecological Clinics of North America, 38*(2), 397–407.

Oyelese, Y., & Smulian, J.C. (2006). Placenta previa, placenta accreta, and vasa previa. *Obstetrics and Gynecology, 107*(4), 927–941.

Papatsonis, D., Flenady, V., & Liley, H. (2009). Maintenance therapy with oxytocin antagonist for inhibiting preterm birth after threatened preterm labor. *Cochrane Database of Systematic Reviews,* (1), CD005938.

Papatsonis, D., Flenady, V., Cole, S., & Liley, H. (2005). Oxytocin receptor antagonists for inhibiting preterm labour. *Cochrane Database of Systematic Reviews,* (3), CD004452.

Pena-Rosas, J., & Viteri, F. (2009). Effects and safety of preventive oral iron or iron + folic acid supplementation for women during pregnancy. *Cochrane Database of Systematic Reviews,* (4), CD004736.

Perez, E.M., Hendricks, M.K., Beard, J.L., Murray-Kolb, L.E., Berg, A., Tomlnson, M., et al. (2005). Mother-infant interactions and infant development are altered by maternal iron deficiency anemia. *Journal of Nutrition, 135,* 850–855.

Persson, P., Grennert, L., Gennser, G., & Kullander, S. (1979). On improved outcome of twin pregnancies. *Acta Obstetricia et Gynecologica Scandinavica, 58*(1), 3–7.

Phelan, S. (2010). Pregnancy: A "teachable" moment for weight control and obesity prevention. *American Journal of Obstetrics and Gynecology, 202*(2), 135.e1–135.e8.

Plotkin, S.A., & Reef, S.E. (2008). Rubella vaccines. In S.A. Plotkin, W.A. Orenstein, & P.S. Offit (Eds.), *Vaccines* (pp. 735–731). Philadelphia: Saunders.

Plourd, D.M. & Austin, K. (2005). Correlation of a reported history of chickenpox with seropositive immunity in pregnant women, *Journal of Reproductive Medicine 50*(10). 779–783.

Polyzos, N., Mauri, D., Tsappi, M., Tzioras, S., Kamposioras, K., Cortinovis, I., et al. (2007). Combined vitamin C and E supplementation during pregnancy for preeclampsia prevention: A systematic review. *Obstetrical and Gynecological Survey, 62*(3), 202–206.

Podymow, T., & August, P.(2008). Update on the use of antihypertensive drugs in pregnancy.*Hypertension.* 51(4):960-9

Poon, L.C., Kametas, N.A., Maiz, N., Akolekar, R., & Nicolaides, K.H. (2009). First-trimester prediction of hypertensive disorders in pregnancy. *Hypertension, 53*(5), 812.

Poon, L.C., Kametas, N.A., Valencia, C., Chelemen, T., & Nicolaides, K.H. (2011). Hypertensive disorders in pregnancy: Screening by systolic diastolic and mean arterial pressure at 11-13 weeks. *Hypertension in Pregnancy, 30*(1), 93–107.

Poursharif, B., Korst, L., Fejzo, M., MacGibbon, K., Romeros, R., & Goodwin, T. (2007). Elective pregnancy termination in a large cohort of women with hyperemesis gravidarum. *Contraception, 76,* 451–455.

Poursharif, B., Korst, L., Fejzo, M., MacGibbon, K., Romeros, R., & Goodwin, T. (2008). The psychosocial burden of hyperemesis gravidarum. *Journal of Perinatology, 28,* 176–181.

Preeclampsia Foundation. (2006, October 27). Preeclampsia identifies women at risk for cardiovascular disease. *Preeclampsia Foundation Position Statement.* Retrieved March 27, 2012, from http://www.preeclampsia.org/pdf/PositionStmt_LateEffects_Oct06.pdf

Promislow, J., Hertz-Picciotto, I, Schramm, M., Watt-Morse, M. & Anderson, J.J. (2004). Bed rest and other determinants of bone loss during pregnancy. *American Journal of Obstetrics and Gynecology*, 191(14),1077-83.

Psihogios, V., Rodda, C., Reid, E., Clark, M., Clarke, C., & Bowden, D. (2002). Reproductive health in individuals with homozygous beta-thalassemia: Knowledge, attitudes, and behavior. *Fertility and Sterility, 77*(1), 119–127.

Public Health Service Task Force (PHSTF). (2002, February 4). *Recommendations for use of antiretroviral drugs in pregnant HIV—1-infected women for maternal health and interventions to reduce perinatal HIV-1 transmission in the United States.* Washington, DC: Author.

Raatikainen, K., Heiskanen, N., & Heinonen, S. (2006). Transition from overweight to obesity worsens pregnancy outcomes in a BMI dependent manner. *Obesity Research, 14*(1), 165–171.

Rand, L., Eddleman, K., & Stone, J. (2005). Long-term outcomes in multiple gestations. *Clinics in Perinatology, 32,* 495–513.

Reader, D., & Franz, M.J. (2004). Lactation, diabetes, and nutrition recommendations. *Current Diabetes Report, 4,* 370–376.

Reddy, U.M., Branum, A.M., & Klebanoff, M.A. (2005). Relationship of maternal body mass index and height to twinning. *Obstetrics and Gynecology, 105*(3), 593–597.

Reedy, N. (2007). Born too soon: The continuing challenge of preterm labor and birth in the United States. *Journal of Midwifery and Women's Health, 52*(3), 281–290.

Rees, H.C., & Paradinas, F.J. (2001). The diagnosis of hydatiform mole in early tubal ectopic pregnancy. *Histopathology, 38* (5), 409–417.

Refuerzo, J.S. (2011). Oral hypoglycemic agents in pregnancy. *Obstetrics and Gynecology Clinics of North America, 38,* 227–234.

Ren, A., Wang, J., Ye, R.W., Li, S., Liu, J. M., & Li Z. (2007) Low first-trimester hemoglobin and low birth weight, preterm birth and small for gestational age newborns. *International Journal of Gynecology & Obstetrics, 98*(2), 124–128.

Report of the national high blood pressure education program working group on high blood pressure in pregnancy. (2000). *American Journal of Obstetrics and Gynecology, 183*(1), S1–S22.

Revello, M. G. & Gerna, G. (2004). Pathogenesis and prenatal diagnosis of human cytomegalovirus infection. *Journal of Clinical Virology, 29,* 71-83.

Roberts, D., & Dalziel, S.R. (2006). Antenatal corticosteroids for accelerating fetal lung maturation for women at risk of preterm birth. *Cochrane Database of Systematic Reviews*, (3), CD004454.

Rogers, V.L., Worley, K.C. (2011). Obstetrics and obstetric disorders. In S.J. McPhee, M.A. Papadakis, M.W. Rabow (Eds.),*Current medical diagnosis and treatment 2012.* Retrieved October 9, 2011, from http://www.accessmedicine.com.ezp1.lib.umn.edu/content.aspx?ID=9353

Rossi, A., & D'Addario, V. (2008). Laser therapy and serial amnioreduction as treatment for twin-twin transfusion syndrome: A metaanalysis and review of literature. *American Journal of Obstetrics and Gynecology, 198*(2), 147–152.

Rouse, D.J. (2007). A trial of 17 alpha-hydroxyprogesterone caproate to prevent prematurity in twins. *New England Journal of Medicine, 357,* 454–461.

Ruiz, R.J., Brown, C.E., Peters, M.T., & Johnston, A.B. (2001). Specialized care for twin gestations: Improving newborn outcomes and reducing costs. *Journal of Obstetric, Gynecologic, and Neonatal Nursing, 30*(1), 52–60.

Rumbold, A., Duley, L., Crowther, C.A., & Haslam, R.R. (2008). Antioxidants for preventing pre-eclampsia. *Cochrane Database of Systematic Reviews*, (1), CD004227.

Russell, R., Petrini, J., Damus, K., Mattison, D.R., & Schwarz, R.H. (2003). The changing epidemiology of multiple births in the United States. *Obstetrics and Gynecology, 101*(1), 129–135.

Ryan White HIV/AIDS Foundation. (2011). *About the Ryan White HIV/AIDS Program.* Retrieved from http://hab.hrsa.gov/abouthab/aboutprogram.html

Sangkomkamhang, U., Lumbiganon, P., Prasertcharoensook, W.I., & Laopaiboon, M. (2008). Antenatal lower genital tract infection screening and treatment programs for preventing preterm delivery. *Cochrane Database of Systematic Reviews*, (2), CD006178.

Sanu, O., & Lamont, R. (2011). Hyperemesis gravidarum: Pathogenesis and the use of antiemetic agents. *Expert Opinion on Pharmacotherapy, 12*(5), 737–748.

Schempf, A.H., Branum, A.M., Lukacs, S.L., & Schoendorf, K.C. (2007). The contribution of preterm birth to the Black-White infant mortality rate, 1990 and 2000. *American Journal of Public Health, 97*(7), 1255–1260.

Scholl, T. (2005). Iron status during pregnancy: Setting the stage for mother and infant. *American Journal of Clinical Nutrition, 81,* 1218S–1222S.

Schrag, S.J., Zywicki, S., Farley, M.M., Reingold, A.L., Harrison, L.H., Lefkowitz, L.B., et al. (2000). Group B streptococcal disease in the era of intrapartum antibiotic prophylaxis. *New England Journal of Medicine, 342*(1), 15–20.

Scott, J.D., & Gretch, D.R. (2007). Molecular diagnostics of hepatitis C virus infection. *Journal of the American Medical Association, 291,* 724–732.

Smith, H.O., Berwick, M., Verschraegen, C.F., Wiggins, C., Lansing, L., Muller, C.Y., et al. (2006). Incidence and survival rates for female malignant germ cell tumors. *Obstetrics and Gynecology, 107*(5), 1075–1085.

Sosa, C., Althabe, F., Belizan, J., & Bergel, E. (2004). Bed rest in singleton pregnancies for preventing preterm birth. *Cochrane Database of Systematic Reviews*, (1), CD003581.

Sperling, L., Kiil, C., Larsen, L.U., Qvist, I., Schwartz, M., Jørgensen, C., et al. (2006). Naturally conceived twins with monochromic placentation have the highest risk of fetal loss. *Ultrasound Obstetrics and Gynecology, 28,* 644–652.

Stan, C., Boulvain, M., Hirsbrunner-Amagbaly, P., & Pfister, R. (2002). Hydration for treatment of preterm labour. *Cochrane Database of Systematic Reviews*, (2), CD003096.

Staroselsky, A., Klieger-Grossmann, C., Garcia-Bournissen, F., & Koren, G. (2009). Exposure to fifth disease in pregnancy.*Canadian Family Physician, 55,* 1195–1198.

Sun, P., Wilburn, W., Raynor, D., & Jamieson, D. (2001). Sickle cell disease and pregnancy: Twenty years of experience at Grady Memorial Hospital, Atlanta, Georgia. *American Journal of Obstetrics and Gynecology, 184,* 1127.

Sutcliff, A., & Derom, C. (2005). Follow-up of twins: Health, behavior, speech, language outcomes and implications for parents.*Early Human Development, 82*(6), 379–386.

SYROCOT (Systematic Review on Congenital Toxoplasmosis) Study Group, Thiebaut, R., Leproust, S., Chêne, G., & Gilbert, R. (2007). Effectiveness of prenatal treatment for congenital toxoplasmosis: A meta-analysis of individual patients' data. *Lancet, 369,* 115–122.

Tai, J.H., Udoji, M.A., Barkanic, G., Byrne, D.W., Rebeiro, P.F., Byram, B.R., et al. (2007). Pregnancy and HIV disease progression during the era of highly active antiretroviral therapy. *Journal of Infectious Diseases, 196,* 1044–1052.

Tamura, T., Goldenberg, R.L., Hou, J., Johnston, K.E., Cliver S.P., Ramey, S.L., et al. (2002). Cord serum ferritin concentrations and mental and psychomotor development of children at five years of age. *Journal of Pediatrics, 140,* 165–170.

Tan, M.P., & Koren, G. (2006). Chickenpox in pregnancy: Revisited. *Reproductive Toxicology, 21,* 410–420.

Tan, P., & Omar, S. (2011). Contemporary approaches to hyperemesis during pregnancy. *Current Opinions in Obstetrics and Gynecology, 23*(2), 87–93.

Telen, M.J. (2001). Principles and problems of transfusion in sickle cell disease. *Seminars in Hematology, 38*(4), 315–323.

Ungerer, R.L., Lincetto, O., McGuire, W., Saloojee, H., & Gulmezoglu, A.M. (2004). *Prophylactic versus selective antibiotics for term newborn infants of mothers with risk factors for neonatal infection.* Retrieved from http://www.nichd.nih.gov/cochrane/Ungerer/UNGERER.HTM

UpToDate. (2011a). *Intraamniotic infection (chorioamnionitis).* Retrieved from http://www.uptodate.com/contents/intraamniotic-infection-chorioamnionitis

UpToDate. (2011b). *Screening for cervical cancer in HIV infected women.* Retrieved from http://www.uptodate.com/contents/screening-for-cervical-cancer-in-hiv-infected-women

UpToDate. (2011c). *Varicella-zoster virus infection in pregnancy.* Retrieved from http://www.uptodate.com/contents/varicella-zoster-virus-infection-in-pregnancy

UptoDate. (2011d) *Urinary tract infections and asymptomatic bacteriuria in pregnancy.* Retrieved from: http://www.uptodate.com/contents/urinary-tract-infections-and-asymptomatic-bacteriuria-in-pregnancy

USPSTF. (2011). *Screening for HIV.* Retrieved from http://www.uspreventiveservicestaskforce.org/uspstf/uspshivi.htm

U.S. Department of Health and Human Services. (2012). *Recommendations for Use of Antiretroviral Drugs in Pregnant HIV-1-Infected Women for Maternal Health and Interventions to Reduce Perinatal Transmission in the United States.* Retrieved from: http://aidsinfo.nih.gov/guidelines.

U.S. Preventive Task Force. (2008). Screening for gestational diabetes: U.S. preventive services task force recommendation statement. *Annals of Internal Medicine, 148,* 759–765.

Vanky, E., Salvesen, K.A., Heimstad, R., Fougner, K.J., Romundstad, P., & Carlsen, S.M. (2004). Metformin reduces pregnancy complications without affecting androgen levels in pregnancy polycystic ovary syndrome women: Results of a randomized study.*Human Reproduction, 19*(8), 1734–1740.

Verani, J.R., McGee, L., & Schrag, S.J. (2010). Prevention of perinatal group B streptococcal disease: Revised guidelines from CDC, 2010. *Morbidity and Mortality Weekly Report, 59*(RR-10), 1–36.

Vikanes, A., Grjibovski, A., Vangen, S., Gunnes, N., Samuelsen, S., & Magnus, P. (2010). Maternal body composition, smoking, and hyperemesis gravidarum. *Annals of Epidemiology, 20,* 592–598.

Waller, D., Shaw, G., Rasmussen, S., Hobbs, C., Canfield, M., Siega-Riz, A., et al. (2007). Prepregnancy obesity as a risk factor for structural birth defects. *Archives of Pediatrics and Adolescent Medicine, 161*(8), 745–750.

Warner, B.B., Kiely, J.L., & Donovan, E.F. (2000). Multiple births and outcome. *Clinics in Perinatology, 27*(2), 347–361.

Waugh, J.J., Clark, T.J., Divakaran, T.G., Khan, K.S., & Kilby, M.D. (2004). Accuracy of urinalysis dipstick techniques in predicting significant proteinuria in pregnancy. *Obstetrics and Gynecology, 103*(4), 769–777.

Weiss, M.E., Saks, N.P., & Harris, S. (2002). Resolving the uncertainty of preterm symptoms: Women's experiences with the onset of preterm labor. *Journal of Obstetric, Gynecologic, and Neonatal Nursing, 31,* 66–76.

Whitworth, M., Bricker, L., Neilson, J., & Dowswell, T. (2010). Ultrasound for fetal assessment in early pregnancy. *Cochrane Database of Systematic Reviews*, (4), CD007058.

Whitworth, M., & Quenby, S. (2008). Prophylactic oral betamimetics for preventing preterm labour in singleton pregnancies. *Cochrane Database of Systematic Reviews*, (1), CD006395.

Williamson, D.M., Abe, K., Bean, C., Ferre, C., Henderson, Z., & Lackritz, E. (2008). Report from the CDC: Current research in preterm birth. *Journal of Women's Health, 17*(10), 1545–1549.

Wing, D.A., Hendershott, C.M., Debuque, L., & Millar, L.K. (1999). Outpatient treatment of acute pyelonephritis in pregnancy after 24 weeks. *Obstetrics and Gynecology, 94* (5), 683–688.

Witlin, A.G., Saade, G.R., Mattar, F., & Sibai, B.M. (1999). Risk factors for abruptio placentae and eclampsia: Analysis of 445 consecutively managed women with severe preeclampsia and eclampsia. *American Journal of Obstetrics and Gynecology, 180,* 1322–1329.

World Health Organization (WHO). (2007). *WHO: Maternal mortality in 2005: Estimates developed by WHO, UNICEF, UNFPA and The World Bank.* Geneva: Author.

Wright, V.C., Chang, J., Jeng, G., & Macaluso, M. (2008). Assisted reproductive technology surveillance—United States, 2005. *Morbidity and Mortality Weekly Report, 57*(SS-05), 1–23.

Wrotniak, B., Shults, J., Butts, S., & Stettler, N. (2008). Gestational weight gain and risk of overweight in the offspring at age 7 y in a multicenter, multiethnic cohort study. *American Journal of Clinical Nutrition, 87,* 1818–1824.

Wu, C.S., Nohr, E.A., Bech, B.H., Vestergard, M., Catov, J.M., & Olsen, J. (2009). Health of children born to mothers who had preeclampsia: A population-based cohort study. *American Journal of Obstetrics and Gynecology, 201*(3), 269.e1–269.e10.

Xu, J., Kochanek. K.D., Murphy. S.L., & Tejada-Vera, B (2010) Deaths: Final data for 2007, *National Vital Statistics Reports 58*(19). Retrieved from: www.cdc.gov/nchs/data/nvsr/58/nvsr58_19.pdf

Yinon, Y., Farine, D., & Yudin, M.H. (2010). Screening, diagnosis, and management of cytomegalovirus infection in pregnancy.*Obstetrics and Gyncology Survey 65*(11) 736–743.

Yost, N., Owen, J., Berghella, V., Thom, E., Swain, M., Dildy, G.A., et al. (2006). Effect of coitus on recurrent preterm birth. *Obstetrics and Gynecology, 107*(4), 793–797.

Zhang, Y., Cantor, R., MacGibbon, K., Romero, R., Goodwin, T., Mullin, P., et al. (2011). Familial aggregation of hyperemesis gravidarum. *American Journal of Obstetrics and Gynecology, 204*(3), 230.e1–230.e7.

Zohav, E., Segal, O., Rabinson, J., Meltcar, S., Anteby, E., & Orvieto, R. (2006). *Journal of Maternal, Fetal, and Neonatal Medicine, 19*(10), 663–666.

CHAPTER ❖ 21

ASSESSING FETAL WELL-BEING

Michele R. Davidson

It is often a dilemma for the client to make the choices presented by screening and assessment tests.

Highlights

- Psychological Needs of Clients
- Indications for Fetal Assessment
- Nonstress Test and Contraction Stress Test
- Screening for Size/Date Discrepancies
- Alloimmunization
- First Trimester Screening
- Second Trimester Screening
- Ultrasonography
- Biophysical Profile
- Doppler Flow Studies
- Amniocentesis and Chorionic Villus Sampling
- Percutaneous Umbilical Blood Sampling
- Interventions/Treatments for Fetal Conditions
- Preimplantation Genetic Diagnosis
- Evaluation of Fetal DNA in Maternal Blood

❖ INTRODUCTION

The assessment of fetal well-being is both a subjective and an objective task, the success of which depends on open communication between the health care provider and the client. Technological advances in assessing the fetus and improving the chances of delivery of a viable infant not only for older women but also for women with disease have required that the health care provider gain increasing knowledge and skill. Allowing advanced practice nurses to perform antepartum testing not only provides continuity of care by providing education and medical care to the mother and fetus, but also provides access to care in outlying areas where care would otherwise not be available.

On the other hand, technological advances in assessing the fetus may initiate a number of questions, often leaving the health care provider with further questions and a client with new fears and anxieties about her pregnancy. Asking one question always leads to another, as Pandora's box is opened. As extremely preterm infants are now surviving at higher and higher rates, the incidence of disabilities due to extreme prematurity is rising. Infants born at less than 25 weeks have a 51 percent risk of neurodevelopmental disability (Hintz et al., 2011). It will continue to be a struggle to decrease perinatal mortality utilizing technology without increasing morbidity rates.

PSYCHOLOGICAL NEEDS OF CLIENTS

Diagnosis, interpretation, and management or referral are often foremost in providing quality fetal assessment. The advanced practice nurse provides counseling, support, and education for mother and family. These are all critical care elements that help to reduce anxiety about the unknown developing fetus and enable the health care provider to achieve continuity of care.

The widespread use of technology and prenatal testing procedures over the last 30 years has made screening and diagnostic testing a routine part of prenatal care for the pregnant woman and her family. In today's modern society, the number of women who utilize the Internet to obtain pregnancy-related information is approximately 94 percent (Lagan, Sinclair, & Kernohan, 2010). Although the Internet has advantages, such as provision of immediate information, availability of discussion forums to link with other pregnant women, and expansion of availability of alternative methods of care, it also has been associated with increased rates of maternal anxiety. Often this anxiety is unsubstantiated and could be avoided if the information was obtained from their health care provider (De Santis et al., 2010). Many prenatal testing options can now be performed that actually relieve maternal anxiety in that they provide reassurance that having a baby affected with a specific disorder is unlikely or provide definitive diagnostic information that the baby is normal (Jaques et al., 2010). On the other hand, women who have an increased risk identified for their fetus based on first trimester screening will have a longer duration of anxiety to manage, especially if they decide not to undergo more invasive diagnostic testing, such as an amniocentesis (Fisher, 2011). Ultrasonographic scanning often provides greater psychological relief to the patient because immediate visualization of the fetus and positive verbal confirmation of fetal normalcy (within the realm of fetal scanning) often occur. Many women face prenatal testing with great ambivalence because there is initial fear that tests may have unfavorable results, yet many desire to learn the status of their infant (Saff et al., 2009). Therefore, clinicians need to be aware that even the simplest of tests raises concerns and possible anxiety for the patient and her family.

Of utmost importance when counseling clients is to take into account racial-ethnic background, socioeconomic status, education attainment, and language issues. Women in ethnic minority groups, women with lower economic status, and women with lower education levels have been identified as at risk for not making truly informed decisions when being counseled for prenatal testing and screening. Women with language barriers are also at risk (Franson et al., 2009). Cultural differences concerning pregnancy and disability do exist and need to be appreciated in order to provide information that enables the client to make an informed decision about fetal assessment. Variations in knowledge, influences from the care provider and patient family members, and access to prenatal diagnostic services influence a client's decisions as well and need to be assessed with each individual (Bhogal & Brunger, 2010).

The following list of guidelines for emotional support, though by no means complete, does give insight into the time and attention needed for "supportive" care. Because the guidelines listed here apply to most of the tests described in this chapter, they are not repeated with the descriptions of the tests. Although only one or a few specific applications may be given in this list, there are many other situations that are applicable.

EMOTIONAL SUPPORT

- *Counsel the client before and after each test.* Prior to any test, the advanced nurse practitioner ensures that the nature of the test, the information that it will provide, and the possibility of further intervention or testing are explained to the patient. Counseling occurs before optional screening or testing to investigate a perceived risk to the client or fetus. Any risks to the client or fetus also are reviewed. To reinforce discussions and reduce anxiety, provide written information and answer questions thoroughly. Tell the client when test results are expected.

  If maternal or fetal risk is the indication for assessment—for example, in cases of diabetes mellitus—the client needs to understand the particular risk, how it affects her pregnancy, and why various tests are important to assess fetal well-being. Depending on the clinical situation, several testing modalities are used. Often a client may become frustrated when one test cannot provide the necessary information, and it may be difficult for her to appreciate why different tests are required. If the health care provider explains the need for assessment, identifies the benefits for both fetus and patient, and encourages the client to voice her opinions in the decision-making process, the client will see herself as part of the solution, not the problem. Hence, the client is able to positively participate in the plan of care.

  It is often a dilemma for the client to make choices presented by screening and assessment tests. Known as *optimistic bias*, clients tend to perceive their own risks as being less than the risks of others, and abnormal results are often unanticipated by the client (LeRoy, Leach, & Bartels, 2010). Also, if the client is upset over the need for tests or the results of tests, she may not "hear" what is being said. Therefore, include the support person or significant other in the counseling and, if possible, wait until the client is ready to hear available options. A support person can later help the client to recall the plan of care when her anxiety eases.
- *Acknowledge the normalcy of feelings of guilt.* A client may feel guilty if she feels inconvenienced by testing but realizes its importance. Having to put the fetus first for 9 months can be stressful during a healthy pregnancy, much less a complicated one requiring invasive or time-consuming procedures. With preeclampsia, for example, a client may feel guilty about her body not cooperating with the pregnancy process and fear harming the fetus. Allow her to express those feelings. Reinforce the fact that she cannot control the actual preeclampsia process but can work with the health care team to provide the best care possible for her fetus and by doing so is helping her fetus.
- *Provide support when an infant has a chromosomal or structural anomaly.* The parents of a fetus with an abnormality may resent the invasive, lengthy procedures and wonder why they are necessary. The health care provider must be prepared to respond in such situations. The client must be informed of diagnoses and, where appropriate, referred to support groups for additional information. Support groups can be extremely helpful in assisting the client with the transition from being pregnant to caring for an infant who has special challenges. In addition, the client needs to grieve the loss of a perfect child.

  Families who have a lethal anomaly identified during the perinatal period need support as they encounter the grieving process. Mothers often choose to terminate the pregnancy at this point and often feel extreme guilt over this agonizing decision. A minority of women will carry the pregnancy to term and allow nature take its course over time. These women face tremendous psychological challenges as they know their baby will not live, while well-meaning strangers may question them about their baby's future. These women should be referred to support groups along with a professional counselor with experience in perinatal loss issues.
- *Provide support if the client chooses termination.* A client who chooses to terminate her pregnancy for any reason also needs support because, as previously mentioned, this decision is likely to be very difficult. This may be particularly true if termination is performed during the first or second trimester when the client has started "showing," heard the fetal heartbeat, felt movement, seen the fetus with ultrasound, and perhaps confided to friends and family that she is pregnant (LeRoy et al., 2010).
- *Be aware of spiritual distress.* Spiritual distress may be encountered when the patient makes decisions

about pursuing fetal screening, when the patient or fetus requires blood (as with isoimmunization or severe anemia) or blood products (RhoGAM) are indicated. Although it is difficult, the client and health care provider may need to consult with legal sources concerning patient and fetal rights. Spiritual distress may also be encountered with identification of a fetal abnormality, termination of a pregnancy, spontaneous abortion, fetal demise, or neonatal death. Clients who have a fetus with a structural or chromosomal anomaly may feel this is due to punishment for something they have done wrong or as a reflection upon their value as an individual. This can have significant repercussions within the family unit. There may be situations in which the health care provider may not be able to attend to the needs of the client. Further psychological, spiritual, or financial intervention may be necessary. The health care provider can be a valuable mediator in such instances, especially by ensuring that appropriate follow-up for abnormal test results is made available to the client *before* she undergoes various tests (Davidson, Ladewig, & London, 2012).

INDICATIONS FOR FETAL ASSESSMENT

ROUTINE ASSESSMENT

Routine fetal assessment begins at the first prenatal visit and continues with every prenatal visit. A bimanual examination or fundal height measurement is performed as a means to grossly estimate fetal growth. If applicable, the fetal heartbeat is auscultated and the client's perception of fetal movement is determined.

This routine standard of care continues for all pregnancies until birth occurs (see Chapter 19). Some women begin pregnancy with risk factors (e.g., diabetes, hypertension, advanced maternal age) that warrant further fetal surveillance. Additionally, complications of fetal or maternal origin may arise during pregnancy and require fetal testing. In general, surveillance or testing is done to monitor a fetus that may be at risk for poor outcome. But, some tests, such as a first trimester aneuploidy testing, should be offered to all women as a screening method.

ADVANCED ASSESSMENT

Advanced assessment is indicated when there is the risk of uteroplacental insufficiency or a maternal condition exists that puts the mother or fetus at an increased risk of morbidity or mortality. It can also be indicated because of specific, sudden, fetal factors, such as decreased movement. Each clinical situation is individualized for the mother and her fetus. Although some risk factors can be identified at the initial prenatal visit, a significant percentage of problems arise in pregnancies without any risk factors. The following is a list of conditions that may indicate need for advanced fetal assessment. Not all health care providers believe that each of the following conditions warrants testing. Moreover, protocols concerning the onset and frequency of indications that warrant particular tests vary among institutions. As technology progresses and the etiology of fetal compromise is further understood, the list may grow (Davidson et al., 2012).

Fetal Conditions

- Premature rupture of membranes
- Premature labor
- Multiple gestation
- Fetal expose to certain infections (herpes, parvovirus B19, toxoplasmosis, etc.)
- Isoimmunization
- Decreased fetal movement
- Any irregularity of fetal heart rate (FHR)
- Abnormal echocardiogram or presence of cardiac defect or arrhythmia
- History or presence of congenital anomalies
- History or presence of intrauterine growth retardation
- Abnormal amniotic fluid volume (AFV)
- Abnormal screening tests, such as the first trimester screening

Maternal Conditions

- Advanced maternal age (for genetic screening)
- Unexplained vaginal bleeding
- Postdate pregnancy
- Multiple gestation
- Abnormal first or second trimester screening
- Poor obstetric history, history of fetal loss or stillbirth
- Maternal substance abuse
- Nutritional and eating disorders
- Uterine structural anomalies
- Antiphospholipid syndrome
- Placental abnormalities

Maternal and Paternal Conditions

- Biological mother or father of the fetus with a chromosome translocation, carrier of a chromosome inversion, or parental aneuploidy

Significant Maternal Disease

- Chronic hypertension
- Diabetes mellitus, insulin dependent or gestational
- Preeclampsia, eclampsia, gestational hypertension
- Hemoglobinopathies
- Cardiac, renal, pulmonary, or connective tissue disease
- Rheumatic heart disease
- Thyroid disorders
- Systemic lupus erythematosus or autoimmune disease

ADVANCED ASSESSMENT FOR PREGNANCIES AT RISK

The American College of Obstetricians and Gynecologists (ACOG, 2009) endorses antenatal assessment to decrease the incidence of fetal death that occurs as a result of hypoxia and to identify fetuses experiencing anemia. The clinician must take into consideration the type and severity of maternal disease, the risk of adverse fetal outcomes and possible death, and the risk of complications of an unnecessary premature birth due to intervention based upon possible false-positive results.

Disagreement exists about when advanced fetal assessment should begin, but the following guidelines generally can be used.

- *Have an accurate estimation of gestational age for the high-risk pregnancy.* Accurate dating is also important for clients with chronic diseases such as diabetes and hypertension, or a history of an intrauterine-growth-restricted (IUGR) infant.
- *Begin as complications arise.* For example, once intrauterine growth retardation or preeclampsia is diagnosed, fetal surveillance should begin.
- *Anticipate events.* Begin assessment prior to the time the problem arose during the previous pregnancy. ACOG (2009) recommended beginning assessment of at-risk fetuses for women with a previous history of stillbirth at 32 to 34 weeks although it stated ultrasound assessment prior to weekly testing can also be initiated. If the diagnosis occurred at 26 weeks, then fetal surveillance should begin just prior to that time.
- *Begin at 32 to 34 weeks of gestation for at-risk clients.* However, clients with high-risk conditions such as chronic hypertension with IUGR should begin surveillance at 26 to 28 weeks. Weekly assessments are warranted for women with high-risk conditions although some women may warrant more frequent testing (ACOG, 2009). Management should be individualized and based on both fetal and maternal risk factors.
- *Assess the postdate fetus (gestational age greater than 40 weeks).* If the only indication for assessment is postdates, then weekly surveillance is usually acceptable in the presence of a normal AFV measurement. Induction is recommended at 41 weeks to avoid uteroplacental insufficiency that may occur with a deteriorating placenta. Women who refuse induction after 42 weeks should be closely monitored with twice weekly nonstress tests (NST) and weekly ultrasound measurements of AFV (Davidson et al., 2012).
- *Frequency of testing.* This is based on the clinical condition of the mother and fetus. Some diseases dictate frequent testing as fetal compromise could be sudden, as in insulin-dependent diabetes, where testing is usually twice weekly.
- *Assess in the first trimester.* First trimester screening allows for medical therapy to address conditions of the infant. First trimester screening is now routinely offered to all women regardless of age. A nuchal translucency (NT) test via ultrasound is used to determine if there is excess skin on the back of the fetal neck. An increased measurement carries a 33 percent risk of a chromosomal disorder with a 50 percent risk of Down syndrome. The NT alone has a detection rate of 64 to 70 percent. The test specificity increases dramatically, with detection rates of 79 to 87 percent, when NT is combined with serum markers, PAPP-A (pregnancy-associated plasma protein-A), hCG (human chorionic gonadotropin), or free β-hCG (beta-subunit hCG) levels. Newer studies have included other parameters, such as assessing for the presence of the nasal bone. Combined with NT, serum markers, and nasal bone assessment via ultrasound, detection rates are reported to be as high as 93 to 96 percent. Other markers that are commonly used include performing an echocardiogram on fetuses missing the nasal bone because cardiac anomalies commonly coexist with genetic anomalies such as Down syndrome (Nicholaides, 2011).

SEQUENCING ADVANCED FETAL TESTING

Testing can begin for a variety of reasons at any gestational age. Some tests are more appropriate than others. Figure 21–1 provides an algorithm of fetal testing that might be used once problems arise. It is one of many available frameworks to be adjusted within institutional protocols. No single test can be regarded as the exclusive choice for assessing fetal well-being as each test reveals

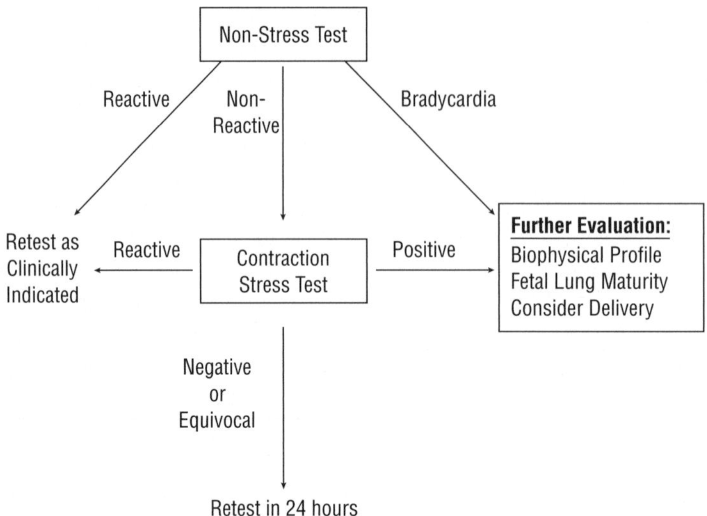

FIGURE 21–1. An Algorithm for Fetal Testing. *Source:* Adapted with permission from Druzin, M., Gabbe, S., & Reed, K. (2002). Antepartum fetal evaluation. In S. Gabbe, J. Niebyl, & J.L. Simpson (Eds.), *Obstetrics: Normal and problem pregnancies* (pp. 313–352). New York: Churchill Livingstone.

different parameters of fetal pathophysiology, often in a complementary manner.

FETAL MOVEMENT

Maternal perception of fetal movement correlates with fetal well-being. Fetal movement is usually perceived by the client at 16 to 20 weeks' gestation. By the use of ultrasound, fetal movement has been noted as early as 7 to 8 weeks (Cunningham et al., 2010). A normal fetus has coordinated movements by 16 to 20 weeks of gestation. Perceived fetal movement is most often related to trunk and limb motion and rollovers, or flips. Generally, during the second half of pregnancy, fetal movement becomes more organized and weaker movements are replaced by stronger movements. Near term, the fetus spends 85 to 95 percent of its time in a quiet or active sleep state, where movement still occurs. Up to 80 percent of gross fetal movement can be perceived by the mother (Creasy, Resnik, Iams, Lockwood, & Moore, 2009). Maternal perception of movement may also diminish, as a result of decreasing AFV, improved fetal coordination, fetal sleep cycles, and increased fetal size, thereby decreasing uterine volume (Cunningham et al., 2010).

Significance of Fetal Movement

Decreased fetal movement may be indicative of asphyxia and intrauterine growth retardation. The compromised fetus decreases oxygen requirements by decreasing activity; documented cessation of activity is a possible indication of impending demise, and a decrease in activity is usually due to chronic, as opposed to acute, nonreassuring fetal status (Creasy et al., 2009). It has been reported that decreased fetal movement may occur prior to fetal death by several days (Cunningham et al., 2010).

Even with a reassuring FHR, decreased fetal movement is a sensitive indicator of fetal distress. It should be a red flag to the clinician when the client reports decreased fetal movement, even in the presence of normal electronic fetal monitoring. Clients with underlying silent problems but no obvious risk factors may be identified only through decreased fetal movement. Approximately 50 percent of fetuses with decreased fetal movement are stillborn, tolerate labor poorly, or require resuscitation at birth (Creasy et al., 2009).

Factors That Decrease Fetal Movement

Maternal use of barbiturates, alcohol, methadone, narcotics, or cigarettes may decrease fetal movement (Cunningham et al., 2010). The drug's effect depends on the amount used, concurrent use of other drugs, and the route by which the drug is taken (i.e., intravenous injection, inhalation, or oral).

Decreased movement, however, may be due to fetal sleep cycles or to inactivity during a particular time of day. Most fetal activity occurs between 9 P.M. and 1 A.M. with periods of inactivity of 20 to 75 minutes in normal pregnancies (Cunningham et al., 2010). Research has shown that fetal activity does not increase after meals; in fact, movement increases with falling maternal glucose levels from 9 P.M. to 1 A.M. (Creasy et al., 2009).

Fetal factors associated with decreased fetal movement or abnormal patterns of fetal movement include hydrocephalus, bilateral renal agenesis, and bilateral hip dislocation. Most fetuses with congenital anomalies may have patterns of movement similar to those of normal fetuses A fetus with severe IUGR (characterized by fetal weight below the 5th percentile for the given gestational age) may have diminished activity. Mild growth restriction, on the other hand, does not appear to reduce the number of fetal movements (Davidson et al., 2012).

FETAL HEART RATE ASSESSMENT

The FHR should be auscultated by 10 to 12 weeks of gestation with a Doppler device although certain maternal factors, such as obesity, may impede the ability to accurately assess the FHR in the first trimester (Davidson et al., 2012). Auscultate the FHR at each prenatal care visit for 1 minute to note rate and rhythm. Take care not to mistake placental flow or maternal heart rate for the FHR. Placental flow or soufflé is a swishing sound different from the actual fetal heartbeat, which is a very distinct, clear beat. To ensure that the maternal heart rate is not confused with the FHR, palpate the client's pulse at the wrist while simultaneously auscultating the FHR through the abdomen with a Doppler device.

Procedure

Place a small amount of ultrasound gel (with a water-soluble base) on the abdomen or directly on a Doppler device. Early in gestation (12–14 weeks), the FHR is best auscultated just above the symphysis with the Doppler. As pregnancy progresses, the FHR is usually heard in the lower abdominal quadrants; however, toward the end of pregnancy if the fetus is not in the vertex position, the FHR is often auscultated near or above the umbilicus. It is easiest to locate the FHR with the client on her back, if she is able to tolerate that position. Most women can tolerate being supine for a few minutes. If the FHR is not found quickly, it may help to locate the fetal back by performing Leopold's maneuvers (see Chapter 19).

Interpretation of FHR

The baseline FHR, beginning at 33 to 34 weeks' gestation, should be 110 to 160 beats per minute (bpm), with allowance for variations in normal accelerations (Davidson et al., 2012; Smith, 2008). As the fetus matures, the parasympathetic and sympathetic nervous systems also mature, thereby decreasing the FHR. A normal heart rate for a term fetus remains at 110 to 160 bpm. However, a fetus of more than 40 weeks may have a heart rate of 110 to 120 bpm due to the greater influence of the parasympathetic system (Smith, 2008). Bradycardia is a baseline heart rate of less than 110 bpm for more than 10 minutes; tachycardia is a baseline heart rate of 160 to 180 bpm for more than 10 minutes (Barclay, 2009). Decelerations or variables may be heard, but they are identified and validated only with external FHR monitoring.

If FHR or rhythm abnormalities are heard, then electronic fetal monitoring is warranted to ascertain the FHR baseline and any periodic patterns. Ultrasound is used to assess cardiac function and note any anomalies. If the FHR is absent, a second Doppler device is used. If the FHR is still not obtained, an ultrasound should be performed immediately to determine fetal viability. Ultrasound is also indicated to document fetal viability if the FHR is not heard by 12 weeks' gestation with a Doppler device or if it is absent after previously being documented (Smith, 2008).

Factors That Influence FHR Detection

The FHR may be heard earlier than 10 to 12 weeks with a Doppler device if the uterus is anteflexed, as opposed to being retroflexed, and if the client has little adipose tissue. Adipose tissue may make it more difficult to hear the FHR early in gestation. The type and age of the Doppler device used may also affect ability to hear the FHR early in gestation.

Advantages and Disadvantages

The procedure is noninvasive, and most clients enjoy hearing the FHR. Listening promotes bonding for mother, father, and siblings and may enable the mother to conceptualize her pregnancy early in gestation, prior to fetal movement. Often fetal movement can also be heard with the doptone device and aids the client in recognizing fetal movement.

On the other hand, the client may be anxious if the FHR is not detected immediately or is not heard at all or if the fetus moves and the FHR is temporarily lost. Because of the immense anxiety that occurs when the practitioner is unable to assess the FHR, additional testing, such as an ultrasound, should be immediately ordered and performed to put the mother at ease and decrease anxiety.

Client Teaching and Counseling

Inform the client of the normal range of heart rate to decrease her anxiety; many women are unaware that the FHR should be 110 to 160 bpm and worry that the fetal heart is beating too fast. Reassurance usually suffices.

NONSTRESS TEST AND CONTRACTION STRESS TEST

The NST and contraction stress test (CST) reflect both the status of fetal cardiac physiology and the fetal status of the central, peripheral, and autonomic nervous systems through heart rate monitoring (Davidson et al., 2012). The tests were developed to assess any indication of uteroplacental insufficiency, thereby predicting the fetus' ability to endure the stress of labor or indicate the need for premature delivery if the fetus is distressed and could be better cared for outside the uterus.

NONSTRESS TEST

Reactivity is present in over 99 percent of fetuses tested using electronic FHR monitoring at 36 to 40 gestational weeks. The NST can be performed after 28 weeks of gestation when the aforementioned fetal systems, particularly the autonomic nervous system, usually reach acceptable maturity and can be assessed; however, there is a 25 percent chance of nonreactivity at this gestational age. The 24- to 28-week fetus is unlikely to have a reactive pattern. Because it is a noninvasive and simple procedure, the NST is appropriate for many clinical indications. In cases of serious fetal or maternal disease, additional tests such as a biophysical profile (BPP) or Doppler flow studies may be performed. The frequency of the testing is determined by maternal and fetal risk and varies depending on practitioner preference (Murray, 2007).

Procedure

Ideally, the client has not been fasting and has not smoked recently as both may affect test results (Murray, 2007). The procedure involves the use of a fetal heart monitor. Two belts are secured around the abdomen. One belt holds the tocodynameter over the fundus, which measures any uterine activity. The other belt holds a transducer over the fetal heart, which measures the FHR. Preferably, the client lies on her left side to avoid supine hypotension. FHR, fetal movement, and uterine contractions (if they occur) are assessed over 20 minutes and recorded on a monitor strip. The client denotes fetal movement by using a handheld "event marker" or by pushing a button on the monitor that marks the strip. Perceived fetal movement is thereby correlated with the FHR. Fetal movement without fetal heart acceleration is atypical, and further workup is warranted.

Interpretation

The NST may be interpreted as reactive or nonreactive. A *reactive NST* is characterized by two FHR accelerations that last 15 seconds and reach 15 beats above baseline FHR in 20 minutes (15-by-15 criterion). If a reactive NST cannot be obtained after 20 minutes, then monitoring is continued another 20 minutes in order to take the fetal sleep-wake cycle into account (Murray, 2007).

Prior to 32 weeks, an acceptable acceleration is 10 beats above baseline lasting 10 seconds or more. However, many fetuses prior to 32 weeks will meet the 15-by-15 criterion, and once this is documented, the fetus should be "held" to this standard in subsequent evaluations (Murray, 2007).

Factors that influence reactivity include maternal sedatives, beta blockers, central nervous system depressants, smoking, maternal fasting, fetal sleep cycles, maternal or fetal disease, and the recent administration of corticosteroids, namely betamethasone. Lengthening the NST another 20 minutes, or choosing another assessment method, may be reasonable to rule out *some* of these variables (Murray, 2007).

When the NST is reactive, it can be repeated at weekly intervals as, in most cases, fetal well-being can be relatively assured for 1 week. Clinical conditions requiring routine weekly NSTs include diet-controlled gestational diabetes, IUGR, preeclampsia, hypertension with normal size fetus, twin gestation without complications, previous history of stillbirth, or being postdates. Type 1 diabetes or gestational diabetes requiring insulin, preeclampsia with IUGR or SGA (small for gestational age), antiphospholipid antibody syndrome, sickle cell disease with crisis during pregnancy, twin gestation with accompanying complications, and maternal Rh alloimmunization all require NST monitoring twice weekly and in some cases more frequently. Frequency of testing is left to the discretion of the clinician, taking into account the clinical aspects of disease that affect maternal and fetal well-being. A woman in an acute sickle cell crisis, for example, warrants continuous monitoring and assessment. The ideal interval for surveillance has not been established; weekly, biweekly, and daily testing are utilized, depending on the clinical situation; however, even with daily testing, fetal demise is encountered on rare occasions (Murray, 2007).

A *nonreactive NST* is characterized by the absence of two FHR accelerations using the 15-by-15 criterion in a 20-minute time frame. Other questionable patterns, such as lack of variability and presence of decelerations, may be noted, however. Additional testing, such as BPP or CST, should be considered in these instances (Murray, 2007).

Periodic FHR patterns that may be viewed during NSTs and CSTs and require evaluation include bradycardia, tachycardia, decelerations, and lack of variability.

Baseline FHR Variability

Interpretation of FHR variability is included in interpretation of any FHR tracing and is considered the most important indicator of fetal well-being.

Baseline FHR variability describes the fluctuation of the FHR observed through irregular changes and fluctuations in the FHR of two cycles per minute or greater with irregular amplitude and inconsistent frequency rather than a smooth continuous line, giving rise to a saw-toothed tracing. Sinusoidal patterns are excluded from this definition (Robinson, 2008). Variability reflects the pathway between the autonomic nervous system and the heart, and is a sensitive indicator of fetal oxygenation (Murray, 2007).

The National Institute of Child and Human Development (NICHD, 2008) no longer distinguishes between *long-term variability* and *short-term variability*, thus these terms should not be used in current practice. Classification of variability is usually evaluated as a unit and excludes the sinusoidal pattern.

Classification of Variability

- *Undetectable:* FHR changes are absent or undetectable.
- *Minimal:* FHR changes are undetectable up to or $\leq$ 5 bpm.
- *Moderate:* FHR changes are 6 to 25 bpm.
- *Marked:* FHR changes are $>$ 25 bpm.

Essentially, FHR changes of 6 to 25 bpm are reassuring; however, minimal or marked variability does not always imply nonreassuring fetal status. Questionable tracings always require a second opinion concerning intervention or further diagnostic testing, such as BPP or CST (NICHD, 2008).

Acceleration

Accelerations are abrupt increases in FHR over baseline, from the time of the onset until the acme is less than 30 seconds. Specifically accelerations are a 15 bpm increase for 15 seconds or more but no longer than 2 minutes. In a preterm fetus less than 32 weeks, a 10 bpm change of 10 seconds or more constitutes acceleration. Prolonged accelerations last longer than 2 minutes but less than 10 minutes. An acceleration lasting longer than 10 minutes is a baseline change (Robinson, 2008).

Deceleration

Decelerations are decreases of FHR below baseline; they can be early, late, or variable. Decelerations are said to be *recurrent decelerations* if they occur in at least 50 percent of the contractions. *Episodic decelerations* are those that occur in less than 50 percent of the contractions appearing infrequently and lacking a regular pattern.

Early decelerations usually occur as a vagal response to increased intracranial pressure with fetal head compression. An early deceleration is uniform in shape with a contraction, beginning and ending with the contraction. It is shallow and symmetrical and usually seen in the active phase of labor, between 4 and 7 cm (Davidson et al., 2012).

Late decelerations are symmetrical decreases in the FHR beginning at or after the peak of the contraction; FHR does not recover until contraction ends. Uteroplacental insufficiency is suspected when late decelerations occur. Markedly compromised fetuses frequently display subtle, shallow decelerations so nurse practitioners should remember that the degree of deceleration has no correlation with the degree of hypoxia or anemia. Late decelerations require immediate intervention and most often warrant immediate delivery (Davidson et al., 2012).

Variable decelerations are usually due to cord compression. Variable decelerations have variable shape, depth, and duration and may occur at any time. Severe decelerations last more than 60 seconds with FHR fewer than 70 bpm. Isolated or recurrent variable decelerations not associated with fetal movement may suggest oligohydramnios or cord compromise or compression and require follow-up with an ultrasound to assess AFV (Robinson, 2008).

Prolonged decelerations are defined as a deceleration in the FHR of at least 15 bpm below baseline for a period of at least 2 minutes but not longer than 10 minutes in duration. A change that occurs longer than 10 minutes is considered a change in baseline (Robinson, 2008).

Use of Vibroacoustic Stimulation

An artificial larynx, or acoustic stimulator, can be used to achieve a reactive tracing and reduce the length of the NST. If fetal movement or accelerations are not noted within 10 minutes during the NST, vibroacoustic stimulation is applied to the woman's abdomen over the fetal head for 1 to 3 seconds. Acceptable accelerations usually result. One or two additional stimuli may be applied at 1- to 2-minute intervals if necessary. Induced accelerations appear to be valid in assuring fetal well-being (Murray, 2007).

Advantages and Disadvantages

The advantages of the NST are that it is easily performed and noninvasive. Furthermore, hearing and seeing the FHR recorded on the tracing may promote maternal-fetal bonding and reduce maternal anxiety, especially for the woman who presents with absent or reduced fetal movement.

The disadvantages of the NST include that it requires someone with expertise to read the results, particularly suspicious patterns. Continuous FHR tracing for the NST may be difficult to obtain if the client is obese or if the fetus is less than 28 weeks, and NSTs are only reactive 50 percent of the time prior to 28 weeks. It can also be a lengthy procedure, particularly if a protocol is not in place for the use of acoustic stimulation. However, use of acoustic stimulation is limited in its utility because the auditory brainstem response in the fetus is not functional until 26 to 28 weeks, so its use is not recommended prior to 28 weeks' gestation (Murray, 2007).

Client Teaching and Counseling

Initially, to avoid client confusion and undue concern, explain the tracings of uterine activity and FHR. The client should also be told what the average FHR is and that variability is normal. Many women are alarmed when the FHR fluctuates (particularly with accelerations), or frightened if the FHR is temporarily lost as a result of a fetal or maternal position change. Explaining the different aspects of FHR monitoring can alleviate many fears. If vibroacoustic stimulation is used, have the client feel and hear the stimulus before applying it to the abdomen.

CONTRACTION STRESS TEST

Although still commonly cited in the literature, the use of CSTs is declining due to the extensive use of ultrasonography and the accuracy of the BPP. The CST is more commonly read or documented when spontaneous contractions are occurring that already meet the criteria for the test itself (Volpe, 2008). This test is performed to note fetal response to uterine contractions, using the principle of induced stress to assess placental insufficiency. It is theorized that if the fetus is hypoxic or has uteroplacental insufficiency, late decelerations will occur with uterine contractions (ACOG, 2009).

Contraindications

Absolute contraindications are history of classical cesarean section, placenta previa or abruptio placentae, premature rupture of membranes, premature labor, multiple gestation, incompetent cervix, previous uterine surgery. Relative contraindications are polyhydramnios or a condition that prohibits adequate uterine monitoring, such as obesity or administration of magnesium sulfate (Murray, 2007).

Procedure

The test procedure is much the same as that for the NST. The client is placed in a semi-Fowler's position to prevent supine hypotension. Attain an initial reading of blood pressure, pulse, and respirations. Blood pressure readings are taken every 10 to 15 minutes; maternal hypotension can decrease uteroplacental perfusion, and therefore, lead to false-positive results (Murray, 2007). The tocodynameter is applied to the fundus, and the transducer placed over the fetal heart. In obese clients, the transducer may have to be handheld to maintain a constant reading of the FHR. A baseline tracing of the fetus is obtained for 15 to 20 minutes. Contractions are achieved by means of nipple stimulation, which causes the release of endogenous oxytocin, or through the use of intravenous oxytocin. Nipple stimulation usually achieves adequate contractions, eliminating the need for intravenous oxytocin and shortening testing time (ACOG, 2009). Spontaneous contractions are acceptable, provided criteria are met. Protocols vary among institutions.

To perform nipple stimulation, the client brushes one nipple with the palmar surface of the fingers, or rolls the nipple between the thumb and index finger through her clothing. Stimulation is stopped after 2 minutes and restarted after 5 minutes if adequate contractions are not obtained. Stimulation is repeated in this cyclic manner for up to four cycles. If this is unsuccessful, one nipple can be stimulated for 10 minutes, stopping when contractions begin and restarting when contractions stop. If needed, both nipples can be stimulated simultaneously for 10 minutes or an electric breast pump can be used to illicit contractions (Murray, 2007).

If no contractions are obtained, or are not sufficient to interpret a CST, an oxytocin infusion is begun. An intravenous line is started with a 21 gauge butterfly needle using half normal saline. The oxytocin infusion is begun at 0.5 to 1.0 milliunits per minute. The rate is doubled every 20 minutes until uterine response is noted. Once adequate contractions are achieved, the infusion is discontinued. Regardless of the method used, the client is monitored until uterine activity returns to baseline and a reactive NST is achieved. If late decelerations are noted, the infusion is immediately stopped and monitoring continues. If the tracing does not become reactive with cessation of oxytocin, emergency birth via cesarean may be warranted.

Interpretation

Interpreting a CST requires three contractions, lasting at least 40 seconds each, within a 10-minute period. Because contractions are recorded through external monitoring, the only criterion they must meet in regard to strength is that they are clearly recorded in order to interpret the tracing. It is also important to note other aspects of the FHR strip, including reactivity (Cunningham et al., 2010).

- *Positive CST:* Late decelerations are present in more than 50 percent of contractions, regardless of contraction frequency. Delivery should be considered or further tests pursued, as the CST has a low positive predictive values and often warrants further evaluation. When birth is indicated, it is typically via cesarean section because the fetus would be unable to tolerate the stress associated with labor (Volpe, 2008).
- *Equivocal CST with hyperstimulation:* FHR decelerations in the presence of hyperstimulation (more than five contractions in 10 minutes or contractions lasting longer than 90 seconds). If hyperstimulation occurs, a BPP can be performed.
- *Equivocal suspicious:* Intermittent late or significant variable decelerations (Cunningham et al., 2010). An unfavorable result warrants BPP testing and possible delivery if additional adverse outcomes are obtained.
- *Negative or normal CST:* No late or variable decelerations. Subsequent testing is based on fetal and maternal conditions and the protocol of the institution (Cunningham et al., 2010).
- *Unsatisfactory CST:* Failure of adequate contractions to occur with nipple stimulation or oxytocin infusion or an uninterpretable tracing (Vogel, 2008). In these circumstances, a BPP is obtained.

Advantages and Disadvantages

Although not as widely used, the CST determines fetal ability to endure labor. If the fetus cannot tolerate the stress of contractions in a controlled testing environment, then it is unlikely the fetus could tolerate labor. Therefore, this screening helps to avoid nonreassuring fetal status.

Nipple stimulation is less costly than oxytocin infusion and does not carry the possible complications associated with venipuncture, such as phlebitis and bruising. Hence, the client may prefer nipple stimulation if she is comfortable touching her breasts in a clinical situation. Providing the client with privacy may reduce feelings of self-consciousness.

Theoretically, the CST carries the potential to induce labor; therefore, it is contraindicated if contractions are to be avoided. In the event that contractions induce nonreassuring fetal status, immediate intervention should be initiated. Another disadvantage is that the CST may take longer than the NST. Clients may become upset with the invasive procedure of oxytocin infusion, if needed.

Client Teaching and Counseling

Review those points included in the discussion of the NST. In addition, inform the client about the possible use of intravenous oxytocin. Clients should be aware that in most cases manufactured contractions do not prompt actual labor, but they may cause slight discomfort. Often contractions are painless.

SCREENING FOR SIZE/DATE DISCREPANCIES

The developing fetus has a genetically predetermined potential for growth but such growth can be influenced by the mother's health, placental function, maternal substance use and abuse, nutrition, fetal anomaly, presence of twins, twin-to-twin transfusion complications, maternal diabetes, polyhydramnios, and perinatal infection. The most common reason for a size/date discrepancy is a dating error (Benson & Bluth, 2008).

Size/date discrepancies are the most common indication for obtaining an obstetrical ultrasound (Benson & Bluth, 2008). When gestational age does not correlate with the apparent size of the uterus or fetus, further evaluation is indicated. The discrepancy may be noted during a bimanual exam or fundal height measurement at a regular prenatal visit, or at delivery when the Dubowitz examination is performed to estimate gestational age of the newborn. If the infant appears smaller or larger than would be expected for the dates, it is very important to determine the actual gestational age of the infant to the best of one's ability. This can impact decisions for interventions if needed. Regardless of when the discrepancy is detected, its cause should be investigated.

PROCEDURES

It is helpful to have good estimates of gestational age by means of pelvic examination or ultrasound in the first trimester. Ultrasound evaluation of gestational age during the first trimester is typically accurate within 3 to 5 days, whereas an ultrasound evaluation to determine dating done in the third trimester can be off by as much as a month (Benson & Bluth, 2008). The last normal menstrual period is recorded and used as the basis for actual gestational age if the client is certain she remembers the first day of her last normal period and if her cycles are about 28 days long. If cycles vary from 28 days, the additional days need to be added or fewer days per cycle need to be subtracted in order to obtain the proper due date.

At each prenatal visit, fundal height is measured or uterine size is assessed to correlate size with gestational age. A measuring tape calibrated in centimeters is used after 20 weeks; the distance between the top of the symphysis pubis and the top of the uterine fundus is measured. The general rule is to consider ultrasound if uterine size is 3 weeks above or below the calculated gestational age, or fundal height is 3 cm above or below the calculated gestational age (Benson & Bluth, 2008). Fundal height is most accurate when the bladder is empty.

Gestational age can be determined and the fetus assessed for abnormalities using ultrasound. A discrepancy in size may simply be the result of incorrect menstrual dates. It is, however, important to rule out other etiologies.

All clients who are at risk for IUGR should have an early ultrasound at 18 to 20 weeks and serial ultrasounds done thereafter, because fundal height measurement alone will miss one third of IUGRs (Davidson et al., 2012). A single ultrasound in late pregnancy cannot detect IUGR (Benson & Bluth, 2008).

DIFFERENTIAL MEDICAL DIAGNOSES

Small for Gestational Age

Small for gestational age is a clinically generic term that describes an infant whose weight is less than 10th percentile without reference to etiology (Cunningham et al., 2010). These fetuses are classified using population-based growth charts. SGA infants have more mortality than their larger-size counterparts; however, some small fetuses are just small and have no risks of morbidity or mortality. Customized growth charts utilize optimal weight as a screening tool and take into account maternal ethnicity, height, weight, and parity at the beginning of pregnancy to calculate ideal and projected weight at the time of birth. These tools seem to be more accurate in predicting fetuses with risk factors than traditional population growth charts (Creasy et al., 2009).

Intrauterine Growth Restriction

Intrauterine growth restriction manifests as a fetal weight below the 10th percentile for age along with clinical evidence of abnormal or dysfunctional growth. There are two types of IUGR. The first type is associated with a normal gestational length but below average birth weight (asymmetrically small). Asymmetrical growth restriction is related to inadequate substrates for fetal metabolism and occurs primarily in the latter part of pregnancy when growth is related to increase in cell size instead of cell number. Musculoskeletal and head dimensions are spared but the abdominal circumference is decreased due to decreasing liver size and subcutaneous fat. Asymmetric IUGR is often due to decreased placental perfusion and maternal vascular disease (Creasy et al., 2009).

The second type is associated with both below average length and weight (symmetrically small). Symmetrical growth restriction occurs with fetal insult during the first trimester, when fetal growth is related to increase in cell number. There is inadequate growth of both the head and the body, all organs are proportionately reduced in size, and the absolute growth rate is decreased. The etiology of the insult may be infection such as cytomegalovirus, maternal drug use or abuse, and chromosomal or congenital anomalies (Creasy et al., 2009).

IUGR fetuses are at risk for perinatal compromise and death, depending on the gestational age, etiology of the IUGR, and severity and progression of maternal disease. Infants born below the 10th percentile for weight and are between 1,500 and 2,500 g have a 5 to 30 times higher mortality rates than those born between the 10th and 90th percentile. When infants are born less than the 10th percentile and weigh less than 1,500 g, the incidence of neonatal mortality is 70 to 100 times greater. Infants below the 6th percentile are at highest risk. Male infants with IUGR experience more deaths than females with similar weights. The incidence of IUGR perinatal deaths related to congenital anomalies is 30 to 60 percent. Symmetric IUGR results in more fetal deaths than asymmetrical IUGR, but this is thought to be related to birth defects and incidence of infection rates; however, in the absence of infection and congenital defects, the rates of death are similar. IUGR infants often have thermoregulatory difficulties and hypoglycemia, not to mention that many IUGR babies are born prematurely, therefore having to cope with the sequelae of preterm birth as well. The perinatal mortality and morbidity are significant. Infants with IUGR are more likely to incur medical problems later in life such as hypertension, type 2 diabetes, and heart and lung disease. These infants also have higher rates of cerebral palsy, lower intelligence scores, and increased mental retardation (Creasy et al., 2009).

The etiology of IUGR can also be divided into three categories (Creasy et al., 2009):

Maternal

- Smoking
- Substance abuse (alcohol, cocaine, heroin)
- Malnutrition
- Medications (phenytoin, trimethadione, warfarin)
- Phenylketonuria
- SGA in mother at birth
- Maternal infection (rubella, cytomegalovirus, HIV, herpes zoster, varicella, toxoplasmosis, *Plasmodium* spp.)
- Maternal hypertensive disease
- Presence of two ascending uterine arteries (instead of one that is typically present)
- Unicornuate uterus
- Excessive maternal exercise in second and third trimester
- Previous pregnancy affected with IUGR

Placental

- Abnormal placenta presentation (circumvallate placenta, placenta previa, abruption placenta)
- Abnormal umbilical cord insertions
- Small placentas
- Failure of the placenta to retain its current weight after 36 gestational weeks
- Placenta hemangiomas

Fetal—adequate substrate from the mother, placenta functioning normally, fetus unable to use the substrate

- Intrauterine infection
- Chromosomal disorders
- Cardiac defects
- Anencephaly
- Hyperinsulinemia

Multiple gestation is also a cause of IUGR, especially in monochorionic-monozygotic twins, with twin-to-twin transfusion occurring as a possible complication. *Twin-to-twin transfusion* occurs when there is an imbalance in the blood supply to the fetuses, which results in overperfusion for one twin and underperfusion for the other. In this scenario, one twin is affected with IUGR and serves as the donor for the other recipient twin. The precise cause of the disorder is not well understood, but it occurs in 15 percent of monochorionic twin pregnancies. The donor twin is typically smaller in size, which results in anemia, cyanosis, and dehydration at the time of birth, while the recipient twin has an excessive amount of blood, redness, and elevated blood pressure readings (Creasy et al., 2009). Treatment may include fetoscopy or fetal laser surgery to interrupt blood flow from one twin to the other. In mild cases, both twins recover; however, in sever cases death of the donor twin is common (National Institutes of Health, 2011).

Large for Gestational Age

An infant may be large for gestational age (LGA), or macrosomic, because of a pathological process, such as diabetes, or because of genetic reasons (e.g., parents of large stature). An LGA infant weighs more than 4,500 g at birth or above the 90th percentile for age (Cunningham et al., 2010).

Risk factors include previous history of macrosomia, maternal obesity, weight gain during pregnancy, gestational or insulin-dependent diabetes, multiparity, male fetus, postdates, ethnicity, maternal birth weight, maternal height, maternal age less than 17 years, and an abnormal 50 g glucose screen with a resulting normal 3-hour oral glucose tolerance test (Cunningham et al., 2010).

The macrosomic infant is at risk for birth trauma, most notably brachial plexus injuries and fractures of the clavicle and humerus associated with shoulder dystocia, as well as asphyxia. Severe asphyxia, while rare, can result in death during a difficult delivery secondary to shoulder dystocia (Cunningham et al., 2010).

Increased uterine size may indicate twins, inaccurate dating, polyhydramnios, or uterine fibroids. Decreased size may indicate fetal demise or oligohydramnios. Both polyhydramnios and oligohydramnios may signify serious fetal anomalies (Creasy et al., 2009).

DIAGNOSIS AND INTERVENTION

Intrauterine Growth Restriction

Diagnosis of IUGR requires ultrasound assessment. The standard indices used are abdominal circumference (AC), head circumference (HC), biparietal diameter (BPD), and femur length (FL). Amniotic fluid volume is assessed as well. These parameters are converted to estimate fetal weight (EFW) using standardized formulas. The diagnosis of IUGR should be based on two ultrasound assessments, 2 to 4 weeks apart (Creasy et al., 2009). An AC that is within normal limits reliably excludes IUGR; a repeat ultrasound is performed in 2 to 4 weeks for confirmation (Cunningham et al., 2010).

When an infant with IUGR is identified in utero, it is essential to determine the etiology of the cause whenever possible. This can be achieved through a history and physical examination. Ultrasound determination of the type of IUGR is of clinical significance as well. Doppler studies are helpful in that fetuses affected with IUGR frequently encounter Doppler arterial velocity abnormalities, which indicate worsening fetal condition that may warrant delivery. Fetal lung maturity studies may be performed to determine optimal timing of delivery. In general, if the fetus is doing well and has normal weekly NST, BPP, and umbilical artery velocimetry results, pregnancy is usually allowed to continue; however, if antenatal testing is unfavorable, then the gestational age and the findings are weighed to determine the best individualized plan of care (Creasy et al., 2009).

Depending on the ultrasound assessment and maternal status, further evaluation of the client and fetus may include fetal karyotyping, maternal serum studies for evidence of viral infection, observation of the client for preeclampsia, and evaluation of the congenital and acquired thrombophylic disorders, particularly if a previous pregnancy was complicated by preeclampsia (Creasy et al., 2009).

Three variables are involved with treatment of IUGR: fetal environment, fetal assessment, and timing of delivery. This is important because IUGR infants have a greater risk of perinatal mortality and morbidity (Creasy et al., 2009).

Improving the fetal environment involves maternal interventions such as consideration of bed rest and stopping work (to increase uterine blood flow), cessation of drug use (alcohol, street drugs, smoking), and aggressive treatment of maternal disease (cardiac and renal conditions, hypertension, malabsorption syndrome). Smoking is the most important risk factor for IUGR and cessation of smoking, even in late pregnancy, provides benefit. Women who quit smoking as late as the 7th month still had infants who weighed more at birth than those women who smoked the entire pregnancy. Tests assessing fetal well-being are fetal movement counts, BPP, Doppler flow studies, AFV assessment, NST, or any combination of these tests. Weekly fetal surveillance is indicated in IUGR, although biweekly assessment is considered with moderate IUGR. Daily surveillance may be indicated, depending on the condition of the mother or fetus (Creasy et al., 2009).

Doppler flow studies have become important in assessing the IUGR fetus and decreasing perinatal death and unnecessary induction of the preterm IUGR fetus. Umbilical arterial velocity monitoring is used to determine adequate blood flow studies to the fetus. Abnormal results in assessment, particularly absent or reverse diastolic flow, should prompt the consideration for delivery, regardless of gestational age (Creasy et al., 2009).

Currently delivery is an optimal treatment for the mature IUGR fetus; the risks and benefits must be weighed for the immature fetus. The use of corticosteroids to decrease neonatal pulmonary and central nervous system morbidity is advised if delivery is likely to occur before 34 weeks of gestation (Creasy et al., 2009; Platz & Neuman, 2008).

Large-for-Gestational-Age Fetus

Diagnosis of *fetal* (as opposed to infant) macrosomia is an estimated weight of greater than 4,500 g (for maternal management, see Chapter 20). Methods to predict birth weight include assessment of maternal risk factors, clinical exam using Leopold's maneuvers, and ultrasound estimation. Single fetal weight estimation via ultrasound has been found to be an unreliable marker for LGA, instead serial ultrasounds in the third trimester are a more accurate diagnostic tool to accurately identify at-risk fetuses (Ben-Haroush, Chen, Hadar, Hod, &Yogev, 2007).

Cesarean delivery is considered if EFW is 5,000 g or greater. It should be noted that infants who are LGA have a higher incidence of birth trauma, operative vaginal delivery, vaginal lacerations with delivery, cephalopelvic disproportion, shoulder dystocia, brachial plexus injuries, clavicle fractures, Bell's palsy, and higher cesarean section rates. They also have a higher incidence of perinatal morbidity and mortality compared to average-size fetuses (Jazayeri, 2010).

Client Teaching and Counseling

Describe to the client the maternal interventions that are to be carried out (see IUGR and Chapter 20). Emphasize that these interventions will increase the chances of a healthy, term infant (if possible) and may heighten her participation with the proposed plan of care.

Many clients believe that a large infant is a sign of good health and that the mother has adequately cared for herself and her infant. The opposite, however, can be true for the mother of a small infant. In some cultures, it may be perceived that a woman who delivers a small infant did not adequately nourish herself or her growing fetus. In the Hispanic culture, large babies are desirable and are believed to be an indicator of good health (Davidson et al., 2012). When counseling clients, it may be difficult to overcome the negative connotations associated with a small infant. Educating the client concerning the underlying processes of abnormal growth patterns may encourage her participation in care.

ALLOIMMUNIZATION

The Centers for Disease Control and Prevention estimate that 1 out of every 1,000 neonates exhibit some sign of alloimmunization. With these decreasing numbers, active management of disease is exceptionally rare. Management begins with the assessment of the maternal blood type, presence or absence of Rh factor, and screening for any atypical antibodies. The identification of alloimmunization constitutes a high-risk pregnancy and appropriate referral should be made to a perinatologist that can obtain phenotyping and monitor titer levels. Antenatal fetal monitoring is begun at 32 weeks to determine fetal well-being. An amniocentesis is performed if delivery is warranted and fetal lung maturity is a determining factor. Some fetuses will require intrauterine transfusions and may need care at a specialized facility (Creasy et al., 2009).

PROCESS OF ALLOIMMUNIZATION

Anti-D IgG antibodies cross the placenta readily, coat fetal cells if they have D antigen, and cause hemolysis. The impact on the fetus of antibodies that are atypical varies according to type (Arora, 2010). The fetus compensates by increasing its production of red blood cells, but if hemolysis is severe, the fetus maximizes red blood cell production in the liver and spleen. The increased demands on the fetal liver result in enlargement, altered function, and decreased albumin production, which lead to leakage of fluid from the fetal vasculature. Ascites and effusions thereby develop. As hemolysis continues, anemia worsens. Ultimately, cardiovascular collapse and fetal death occur. These events describe the process of fetal hemolytic disease, or hydrops fetalis (Cunningham et al., 2010).

Management of an Alloimmunized Pregnancy

In the event of alloimmunization, referral to the appropriate practitioner and health care facility is essential.

FIRST TRIMESTER SCREENING

New testing technologies have introduced early and more effective screening tools to pregnant women. As mentioned in the beginning of this chapter, ACOG (2007a) advocates aneuploidy screening to all pregnant women regardless of maternal age. First trimester screening includes NT testing via ultrasound to screen for the presence of increased nuchal fold measurement in the fetal neck occurring between 11 and 136/7 weeks. Increased measurements indicate the possibility of a chromosomal abnormality such as Down syndrome. NT alone detects 64 to 70 percent of affected fetuses (Cunningham et al., 2010). The addition of serum screening that includes free β-hCG, or β-hCG and PAPP-A, increases detection rates to 79 to 87 percent (Nicholaides, 2011). In the last 10 years, the addition of assessing for the presence of the fetal nasal bone has been established as a means to additionally screen for trisomy 21; however, studies are conflicting and obtaining an accurate assessment can be limited by sonographer skill level. Assessing the nasal bone is a valuable tool in assessing women at risk for Down syndrome and increases accuracy to 93 to 96 percent, whereas NT and serum testing alone yields detection rates of 85 to 95 percent (Nicholaides, 2011). Fetuses with abnormal NT thickness and lacking a nasal bone should also be screened for accompanying heart defects, including tricuspid flow or ductus venosus flow because both can occur in Down syndrome fetuses (Ladewig, London, & Davidson, 2014; Nicholaides, 2011). Most women progress in a sequential process, first having the first trimester screening with ultrasound and serum makers. If abnormal results are obtained, a chorionic villus sampling (CVS) or amniocentesis can be offered to the woman if she desires to pursue definitive testing. Many women will not obtain additional testing, but supportive care should be provided regardless of her decision making. Sequential testing would then offer alpha-fetoprotein (AFP) testing in the second trimester to assess for neural tube defects. For women who do not undergo the first trimester screening with serum markers and NT, a quadruple screen is offered as well.

SECOND TRIMESTER SCREENING

QUADRUPLE SCREENING AND AFP TESTING

The quadruple screening is a combination test that analyzes AFP, hCG, diametric inhibin A, and estriol to screen for neural tube defects and Trisomy's 13, 18, and

21 and is offered during the second trimester for women who have not gotten a NT or NT combination testing with serum markers. Because the first trimester screening with NT and serum markers is considered more reliable, women with those tests performed need only an AFP to screen for neural tube defects in the second trimester. The discussion that follows includes information on AFP testing.

Both the quadruple screen and stand-alone AFP testing may be performed between 15 and 20 weeks, with the greatest accuracy obtained if performed during the 15- to 16-week period (Cunningham et al., 2010). Because neural tube defects occur in 90 percent of women with no risk factors, universal screening should be offered to all women. The MS-AFP (and the only marker if AFP only is being done) is the first marker in the quadruple screening test and detects neural tube defects in 85 percent of cases using this technique alone. The typical cutoff is 2.0 to 2.5 multiples of mean (MoM) of AFP to determine if the test is considered high and yields a 90 percent accuracy rate with a false-positive rate of 3 to 5 percent (Creasy et al., 2009). Other factors that can cause a false-positive result include incorrect calculation of the expected date of delivery, maternal weight, race, and presence of diabetes, twin gestation, fetal anomalies, and fetal death (Cunningham et al., 2010). False elevations may occur if maternal serum was drawn after an invasive procedure such as amniocentesis or CVS (Creasy et al., 2009). Because other factors can produce an abnormal result, clinicians should use caution when revealing abnormal results to expectant parents. The other biochemical markers found only in the quadruple screening test and not done if a first trimester screening was performed are used to predict the incidence of Trisomy's 13, 18, and 21. Abnormal results that define a risk of Down syndrome greater than 1 in 270 are considered suspicious and require further investigation and patient counseling (Davidson et al., 2012).

CLINICAL MANAGEMENT

If an abnormal result is obtained on the quadruple test or AFP, a targeted ultrasound is performed alone or with amniocentesis to assess gestational age and any structural anomalies (Cunningham et al., 2010).

If gestational age is incorrect or if another nonpathological cause of an abnormal value is noted (such as twins), the MoM is recalculated and usually found to be within normal limits. Underestimation of gestational age is the most common reason for an elevated MS-AFP. If a structural anomaly is noted, the fetus should be thoroughly assessed for other anomalies and amniocentesis offered to note genetic aberrations. If no anomaly is apparent and no other cause of an abnormal marker is found, a specialized ultrasound is performed.

Amniocentesis was once the gold standard for detecting neural tube defects and was performed to assess amniotic fluid AFP (AF-AFP) as well as performing a fetal karotype. In amniocentesis, a positive AF-AFP is validated by measuring the amount of acetylcholinesterase (AChE) in the amniotic fluid sample. AChE is present only if there is an open neural tube defect. If the elevated AF-AFP level is due to contamination with fetal blood, AChE will be absent. A low level of AChE or its absence suggests something other than open neural tube defect as the etiology of the elevated AF-AFP. Now it is common to assess for the open NTD by specialized ultrasound if the amniotic fluid is at a normal level; however, because fetuses with an NTD are at a higher risk for a chromosomal abnormality, some women desire an amniocentesis (Cunningham et al., 2010). If an amniocentesis is performed, a detailed ultrasonographic exam should follow the amniocentesis, which is used to detect for structural abnormalities in the fetus (Davidson et al., 2012).

Ninety to 95 percent of clients with abnormal MS-AFP levels have a normal level of AF-AFP. Even though the AF-AFP is normal, the risk for IUGR, premature labor, premature membrane rupture, fetal demise, oligohydramnios, and abruption for clients with abnormal MS-AFP is greater. Elevated levels of β-hCG and low levels of uE3 and PAPP-A have been associated with adverse perinatal outcomes as well. The cause may be due in part to poor placental function. Currently, ACOG does not advise heightened surveillance for abnormal levels of MS-AFP in the absence of an etiology; rather, routine obstetric care is the standard of care until a problem is identified because heightened surveillance has not been proven to improve pregnancy outcome. This advisement is based on the finding that adverse outcomes either are detected with routine obstetric care or remain undetectable despite heightened surveillance (Cunningham et al., 2010).

Amniocentesis should not be narrowly viewed as a test to determine whether to consider termination. Rather, it should be seen as a diagnostic tool. Invasive genetic testing remains the gold standard for fetal diagnosis. Diagnosis of a fetal problem allows the health care provider to supply the client with options for the pregnancy. This may be a referral to a perinatologist for further care or planning of care for the infant at delivery and beyond; termination may be considered as well. By providing information to the health care provider as well as the client, pregnancy outcome and the plan of care can be optimized. In the presence of an open neural tube defect, cesarean delivery appears to retain greater neurologic function and should be considered (Cunningham et al., 2010).

ADVANTAGES AND DISADVANTAGES

Quadruple testing and AFP screening can be done in the office or clinic. If subsequent testing due to abnormal values reveals a fetal problem, treatment (if possible) may be instituted and the client is enabled to prepare and plan care for a child with a chromosomal or structural anomaly. Screening certainly is an advantage for the clinician when planning fetal surveillance, as well as the mode of delivery, and the care that will be needed by the neonate after delivery. Screening and diagnosis in the second trimester also allows the client the option of choosing termination.

There are disadvantages. Maternal serum testing screens for abnormalities; it is not diagnostic. Further intervention is required to assess if an abnormality truly exists; therefore, clients may proceed with amniocentesis unnecessarily (see next section).

CLIENT TEACHING AND COUNSELING

Inform the client of possible test outcomes and clinical sequence of testing that would be advised in the event of abnormal test results prior to drawing the quadruple test or AFP. Many clients can cope with having blood drawn, but the decision to do a chromosomal analysis may pose a cultural or religious dilemma for some. The sequence of events leading to diagnosis after an abnormal test result is often unanticipated. Some clients want to know if the fetus has an abnormality; others prefer not to know until the birth and may decline further diagnostic testing. The health care provider may be caught in the middle in the event of an abnormal result, wherein the fetus will be assumed to be at risk.

ULTRASONOGRAPHY

Ultrasonography uses high-frequency sound waves to produce an image. A transducer directs sound waves toward an object (e.g., the fetus). When the waves interface with solid structures, energy is reflected back to the transducer, which creates electrical voltage. That voltage produces an image on screen. Real-time ultrasound differs from conventional ultrasound. Real-time ultrasound uses a multiple-pulse system of sound waves to note movement, such as fetal breathing; conventional ultrasound uses only a single-pulse system. Most ultrasounds are performed in three or four dimensions. Specialized training is needed to perform and interpret ultrasound. Abdominal ultrasound or a transvaginal probe may be used in assessment.

Ultrasound has no confirmed biologic adverse effects on the fetus (Davidson et al., 2012). This has led many to use ultrasound indiscriminately. Clients often want an ultrasound just to know the sex of the baby. In the early 2000s, shops were even created to provide the parents a memento or keepsake of their baby in the form of an ultrasound DVD. There was concern that this trend would lead to a lack of prenatal care and would fail to identify certain disorders or abnormalities. In 2006, ACOG issued a committee opinion citing opposition to nonmedical use of ultrasound that could provide false reassurance or create false reassurance in the presence of nonreassuring fetal conditions.

Ultrasound technology is widely used in first trimester screening testing and in second trimester to determine structural anomalies and placental placement. Routine ultrasound is now a normal parameter of care in the United States with women with low-risk pregnancies averaging 2.1 and high-risk pregnancies averaging 4.2 ultrasounds. These increases are due to the routine recommendation for first trimester ultrasound screening (NT) and the additional information that can be obtained via ultrasound during pregnancy. Although many insurance companies reimburse for only one ultrasound in an uncomplicated pregnancy, most will cover additional ultrasounds for medical necessity, which may require that the provider write a letter of medical necessity and have it preauthorized with the insurance company. With various changes in health care, the cost-effectiveness of providing routine screening to all women remains an issue. Routine ultrasound examination is now recommended by ACOG (2007b) for all women in the first trimester to undergo aneuploidy screening. Additional ultrasounds are recommended if the AFP or quadruple screen is abnormal as well. In general, ultrasounds are performed based on medical need and clinicians depend on the data to most effectively manage prenatal care (Davidson et al., 2012).

Generally, ultrasonography should provide the information sought (e.g., possible source of bleeding), as well as various parameters depending on gestational age. A

TABLE 21–1. Fetal/Maternal Assessments Possible With Ultrasonography

Ultrasound in the First Trimester Should Obtain the Following Information[a]	Ultrasound in the Second and Third Trimester Should Obtain the Following Information[b]
• Presence or absence of intrauterine gestational sac • Location of gestational sac • Identification of embryo or fetus • Fetal number • Presence or absence of fetal cardiac activity • Crown-to-rump length • Evaluation for ectopic pregnancy • Evaluation of uterus and adnexal structures • Evaluation of fetal growth • Evaluate the cervix • First trimester nuchal translucency testing	• Presence of fetal life, number of fetuses present, and any abnormalities of heart rate or rhythm • Amount of amniotic fluid • Evaluation of cervical insufficiency • Evaluation of vaginal bleeding • Evaluation of fetal position and presentation • Evaluation of abdominal or pelvic pain • Evaluation of suspected uterine mass or abnormality • Size/date discrepancies • Evaluation of premature rupture of membranes • Evaluation of suspected fetal death • Examination of suspected molar pregnancy • Evaluation of suspected amniotic fluid abnormalities • Evaluation of suspected placental abruption • Follow-up on identified anomalies • Evaluation of fetus when a previous sibling born with an anomaly • Location of placenta and its relationship to the cervix • Estimation of the gestational age, using two of the following parameters—biparietal diameter, head circumference, femur length, and abdominal circumference • Attempt to survey fetal anatomy (cerebral ventricles, spine, stomach, urinary bladder, umbilical cord insertion site, and renal regions). Suspected anomalies require a targeted evaluation

[a]Various parameters such as fetal heart activity and the presence of a gestational sac are noted earlier, using vaginal scanning as opposed to abdominal scanning.

[b]Overall, third trimester ultrasounds are not accurate assessment of gestational age and can be off by up to 1 month; dating is most accurate if done before 26 weeks.

Source: Davidson et al., 2012.

distinction is made when a fetus is considered to be at risk for a structural anomaly, or if during a basic scan, there are questionable findings. In this case, the client should be referred for a targeted ultrasound for specialized scanning (Davidson et al., 2012). The health care provider should not assume a lack of responsibility for being knowledgeable and competent when providing even a basic ultrasound, however, as most congenital anomalies occur in the absence of risk factors. The assessments listed in Table 21–1 can be determined during ultrasound examination.

INDICATIONS FOR ULTRASOUND

Gestational Age Determination

Ultrasound is used to establish gestational age throughout pregnancy; however, gestational age is most accurately assessed in the first trimester when there is minimal variation in fetal growth. Gestational age is most accurately estimated by measuring crown-to-rump length (CRL) between 7 and 10 weeks. Based on the CRL, the gestational age can be calculated within 3 days 90 percent of the time (Davidson et al., 2012). Other parameters are used for second and third trimester assessment of gestational age (see previous paragraph). As stated, third trimester ultrasounds are not accurate assessments of gestational age. The margin of error for predicting gestational age is greater as pregnancy advances, particularly in the third trimester. This needs to be taken into account when considering interventions on the behalf of the fetus that may be influenced by gestational age.

Growth Assessment

Ultrasound is indicated when a discrepancy exists between estimated gestational age and uterine size. The ultrasound is done to rule out abnormalities or to correct errors in dating. It is used serially to diagnose IUGR in clients at risk for decreased uteroplacental perfusion, for example, those with hypertension or a history of fetuses with IUGR (Cunningham et al., 2010).

Ratios of various measurements are often given to provide an index for growth. If not, they can be calculated and compared with standardized charts to determine appropriate growth for a particular gestational age.

Detection of Fetal Anomalies

Fetal anomalies can be detected with ultrasound. Assessing fetal structures for anomalies is *fetal scanning*. Ninety-eight percent of fetal structures can be assessed by transvaginal sonography by 14 weeks. The detection rate of fetal malformations being diagnosed on ultrasound is approximately 80 percent (Li et al., 2008). Anomalies related to a polygenic disorder may have the potential to increase detection rates utilizing fetal MRIs; however, the use in fetal diagnosis of genetic disorders typically occurs only in large medical centers and is not currently routine clinical practice (Schmid & Blaicher, 2011). Clients who present with a history of a child with structural anomalies are at an increased risk for reoccurrence in subsequent pregnancies, although the risk is thought to be low. The specific risk factors are based on the type of disorder (Cunningham et al., 2010). Diagnosis of chromosomal abnormalities requires invasive testing, however, and many clients may prefer fetal scanning to assess the fetus and may not wish to obtain more invasive measures because NT carries high screening detection rates. Standard of care dictates referral to highly experienced clinicians when an anomaly is identified (Davidson et al., 2012).

Fetal scans are indicated for women with a family history of disorder or previous anomaly of the abdominal wall or central nervous, renal, brain, gastrointestinal, cardiac, or skeletal system; exposure to any teratogen that produces structural anomalies is also an indication for ultrasound. Sonograms are routine part of prenatal care and serve to identify at-risk fetuses and fetuses that may be affected with a structural or genetic disorder.

Assessment of Amniotic Fluid Volume

Ultrasound assessment of AFV has become a sensitive indicator of fetal well-being, especially when combined with other surveillance methods. The majority of amniotic fluid is produced by the fetal lungs and kidneys; fetal swallowing begins early in the second trimester and subsequently any abnormality with the gastrointestinal or genitourinary tract may be reflected in abnormal AFVs (Blackburn, 2007).

There is a correlation of decreased AFV and placental insufficiency due to the adaptive response the fetus exhibits to hypoxemia. Known as the *brain-sparing effect*, blood is shunted to the vital organs and away from the kidneys. This shunting of blood over a period of time decreases AFV because fetal urine production makes up the majority of amniotic fluid after midgestation. Normal AFV is important for normal fetal growth, fetal movement, and cushioning of the fetus, cord, and placenta (Blackburn, 2007).

Increased AFV has been associated with neural tube defects, gastrointestinal obstruction, immune and nonimmune hydrops, and CNS abnormalities contributing to impaired swallowing. Decreased AFV has been associated with renal abnormalities, gastrointestinal obstruction, and IUGR (Blackburn, 2007).

The method of choice to measure AFV is the amniotic fluid index (AFI). AFI appears to be the most used and the least subjective. The AFI is the sum of the deepest cord-free amniotic fluid pocket in each of the four quadrants of the uterus; at term an AFI of < 5.0 cm is indicative of oligohydramnios and an AFI of > 20 cm indicates polyhydramnios. A table of AFI values based on gestational age has been developed and is widely used to assess AFV measurements (Creasy et al., 2009). Oligohydramnios is defined as an AFI value less than 5th percentile for a given gestational age, and polyhydramnios is an AFI greater than 95th percentile for a given gestational age. Once detected, extremes of amniotic fluid require further evaluation.

Monitoring of a Post-Term Pregnancy

Fetal surveillance is recommended for post-term pregnancies. Perinatal mortality and morbidity is increased for a fetus past 41 weeks (Davidson et al., 2012). Many providers initiate surveillance at 40 weeks and offer induction by 41 gestational weeks. The combination of monitoring AFI, NST, BPP, and fetal movement counts is used to assess the post-term fetus. Gestational age cannot be accurately determined at term (Creasy et al., 2009).

Monitoring an At-Risk Pregnancy

An example of this type of monitoring would be the serial use of ultrasound to monitor a fetus exposed to parvovirus B19. Ultrasound is used to note the development of fetal hydrops, placentomegaly, and growth disturbances. Clients should receive weekly sonographic assessment for up to 10 to 12 weeks after exposure along with Doppler flow studies because the middle artery measurement can be used to demonstrate potential anemia in the fetus (Marino et al., 2010). Ultrasound is also used in a complementary manner to diagnose and monitor the fetus that has been exposed to cytomegalovirus, varicella-zoster virus, and toxoplasmosis (Marino et al., 2010).

Documentation of Fetal Viability

When fetal heart tones are inaudible by Doppler at 12 weeks or if they are absent after previous documentation, ultrasound is indicated to verify cardiac activity. A gestational sac can be seen when β-hCG is 1,000 to 2,000 mIU/mL. Failure to see doubling of β-hCG every 48 hours early in pregnancy may be indicative of an ectopic pregnancy or a nonviable fetus. Cardiac activity should be noted by 7 weeks with transvaginal ultrasound (Davidson et al., 2012).

ADVANTAGES AND DISADVANTAGES

Abdominal ultrasound is noninvasive and may promote bonding, particularly before quickening. Abdominal ultrasound may present a problem for a client experiencing nausea and vomiting during pregnancy, because she must drink approximately 1 quart of water in the hour before examination. Alternatively, the transvaginal probe does not require a full bladder and can be effectively used. Anxiety may be increased if clients are not given information during ultrasound concerning structures seen and the well-being of the fetus. Clients' fears are lessened with positive feedback from the ultrasonographer, but due to the various levels of expertise, information may not be shared with the client until confirmed by a provider with clinical expertise in ultrasonography. Ultrasound must be performed and interpreted by a qualified individual.

Loss of fetus or termination may be more difficult if the client has already viewed the fetus. If ultrasound has promoted bonding, a client may grieve more with demise or termination.

CLIENT TEACHING AND COUNSELING

Explain to the client what ultrasound is. Inform her that no cases of harm to a fetus have been documented. The client needs to be aware that a technician may perform the ultrasound, and, if so, that person can identify structures but cannot interpret findings. Depending on protocol, the radiologist, physician, or practitioner is responsible for discussing the results with the client.

For abdominal ultrasound, the client must drink approximately 1 quart of water 1 hour prior to procedure, and therefore, needs to be aware that there will be pressure on her bladder during ultrasound. For the client undergoing transvaginal ultrasound, explain that a probe will be inserted into the vagina. She can expect some pressure but should not be uncomfortable. Briefly describe the probe and show it to her prior to insertion and reassure the client that the probe will not hurt the fetus or cause miscarriage. A full bladder is not necessary for transvaginal ultrasound. The woman may wish to insert the probe herself.

BIOPHYSICAL PROFILE

Real-time ultrasound allows assessment of various parameters of fetal well-being: fetal tone, breathing, motion, and AFV. These four parameters together with the NST constitute the BPP; however, not all facilities perform NST unless other parameters of the profile are abnormal.

PROCEDURE

Usually the profile is compiled in an outpatient testing center within a hospital or in an outpatient radiology center in the community. Skilled personnel are required to perform the NST as well as to conduct and evaluate the ultrasound. Although the BPP is an advanced surveillance test, nurses with advanced training can perform the ultrasound, score the BPP, and in nonreassuring situations, initiate further assessment.

SCORING

Each component of the BPP is scored as 2 (variable normal) or 0 (variable abnormal). A total score of 10 is possible if the NST is used. Thirty minutes is allotted for testing, although fewer than 8 minutes is usually needed. The following criteria must be met to obtain a score of 2; anything less is 0 (Creasy et al., 2009).

- *Gross body movements:* Three or more discrete body or limb movements.
- *Fetal tone:* One or more full extension and flexion of a limb or trunk, or opening or closing of a hand.
- *Fetal breathing:* One or more breathing movements of at least 30 seconds' duration.
- *Amniotic fluid volume:* One or more pockets of fluid measuring at least 2 cm in two perpendicular planes.
- *Nonstress test:* Performed in the event one of the first four parameters are abnormal; graded as normal (2) or abnormal (0). A normal NST is characterized by two accelerations greater than 15 bpm over baseline, each lasting at least 15 seconds within a 20-minute

TABLE 21–2. Interpretation of Fetal Biophysical Profile Score Results and Recommended Clinical Management

Test Score Result	Interpretation	Perinatal Mortality Within 1 Week Without Intervention	Management
10 of 10 8 of 10 (normal fluid) 8 of 8 (nonstress test not done)	Risk of fetal asphyxia extremely rare	< 1 per 1,000	Intervention only for obstetric and maternal factors; no indication for intervention for fetal disease
8 of 10 (abnormal fluid)	Probable chronic fetal compromise	89 per 1,000	Determine that there is functioning renal tissue and intact membranes; if so, deliver for fetal indications
6 of 10 (normal fluid)	Equivocal test, possible fetal asphyxia	Variable	If the fetus is mature, deliver; in the immature fetus, repeat test within 24 h; if < 6/10, deliver
6 of 10 (abnormal fluid)	Probable fetal asphyxia	89 per 1,000	Deliver for fetal indications
4 of 10	High probability of fetal asphyxia	91 per 1,000	Deliver for fetal indications
2 of 10	Fetal asphyxia almost certain	125 per 1,000	Deliver for fetal indications
0 of 10	Fetal asphyxia certain	600 per 1,000	Deliver for fetal indications

Source: Reprinted with permission from Manning, F. (2001). Intrauterine growth restriction: Diagnosis, prognostication, and management based on ultrasound methods. In A. Fleischer, F. Manning, P. Jeanty, & R. Romero (Eds.), *Sonography in obstetrics and gynecology* (pp. 615–632). New York: McGraw-Hill.

period. An abnormal NST characterized by fewer than two episodes of accelerations or accelerations fewer than 15 bpm above baseline within 20 minutes.

INTERPRETATION

Results of the BPP should be considered in view of the clinical history and the facilities available to care for mother and fetus. The recommendations in Table 21–2 are to be used as guidelines within an existing protocol.

In addition, Doppler flow studies may be utilized to validate clinical decisions.

ADVANTAGES AND DISADVANTAGES

As with ultrasound, the BPP can enhance maternal bonding and help the client recognize fetal movement. The BPP has the sensitivity to predict poor fetal outcome in high-risk pregnancies, as well as to permit assessment of AFV, placental characteristics, and the function of various fetal systems. Expertise is needed to perform and assess the BPP accurately. A modified version of the BPP, which assesses only the NST and AFI, has been utilized as well (Davidson et al., 2012).

CLIENT TEACHING AND COUNSELING

Provide information to the client about ultrasound (see preceding section), as the BPP is usually compiled through the use of abdominal ultrasound. If possible, point out the fetal anatomic structures and indicate the clinical parameters being assessed.

DOPPLER FLOW STUDIES

Doppler ultrasound velocimetry is used to obtain hemodynamic information. By transmitting an ultrasound beam across a blood vessel, the velocity of blood flow can be measured. The umbilical artery has been studied extensively, and its use in monitoring the IUGR fetus has been approved. Umbilical, aortic, cerebral, and uteroplacental circulation can be assessed as well. Skilled practitioners can also measure blood flow in the fetal middle cerebral artery (MCA) to evaluate the fetus for hypoxemia and correlate the MCA value to umbilical artery flow. The brain-sparing effect is seen when comparing the two separate flow studies—umbilical artery flow demonstrates increased flow resistance, while MCA flow resistance is decreased (Cunningham et al., 2010). MCA flow studies are used in conjunction with umbilical arterial Doppler indices.

Because diastolic flow normally increases in relation to systolic peak throughout pregnancy, monitoring a pregnancy at risk for compromise includes noting decreased diastolic flow. Decreased diastolic flow indicates increased placental bed resistance and potential compromise for the fetus due to decreased placental perfusion. Decreased or absent diastolic flow indicates high resistance in the placenta and is often seen in pregnancies complicated by intrauterine growth retardation (Cunningham et al., 2010). These fetuses have higher rates of morbidity and mortality. As placental insufficiency worsens, there is first a decrease in diastolic flow, then an absence, and then reverse diastolic flow is seen (Cunningham et al., 2010). Absence of end-diastolic flow requires more frequent or further testing; the presence of reverse diastolic flow indicates serious fetal compromise and requires further testing and/or intervention (Creasy et al., 2009).

Doppler assessment should be viewed with other clinical data in determining management of a compromised fetus; it should not be the sole parameter in determining fetal well-being, or the basis of clinical decisions. It is not a sensitive screening tool to predict IUGR among unselected populations; rather, it identifies the fetus at risk for adverse perinatal outcome because it is a test of *placental* function as opposed to an assessment of the fetus once IUGR is diagnosed (Cunningham et al., 2010).

Fetal Doppler echocardiography has also been used to study changes in cardiac flow related to disease states such as IUGR, maternal diabetes, fetal anemia, and discordant twins (Cunningham et al., 2010). Maternal uterine artery Doppler flow studies can also detect placental dysfunction.

INDICATIONS

Decreased placental perfusion caused by maternal disease or placental abnormalities is a potential indication for Doppler flow studies. As previously stated, Doppler flow studies can be used once IUGR is diagnosed, but are not used as a screening tool for the general population; MCA flow studies can pinpoint reverse blood flow patterns and are useful in monitoring fetuses affected with severe life-threatening IUGR. Doppler flow studies are used to assess the high-risk fetus at risk for uteroplacental insufficiency and can be used in various fetal or maternal conditions including suspected IUGR; maternal hypertension, collagen vascular disorders, and vascular disease; previous IUGR or demise. Fetal MCA flow studies could be beneficial for suspected IUGR and anemia (Creasy et al., 2009).

Arrhythmias detected with auscultation or electronic fetal monitoring can be identified using M-mode echocardiography (Cunningham et al., 2010; Davidson et al., 2012).

Fetuses diagnosed with cardiac anomalies can benefit from pulsed and color Doppler ultrasonography for accurate diagnosis and cardiac function. Due to the differences in blood flow in the fetus versus the neonate, a congenital cardiac anomaly is not necessarily lethal in utero; care consists of accurate diagnosis of the abnormality, frequency of assessment, possible treatment prior to delivery, and how care will be provided to the neonate after delivery.

PROCEDURE

To evaluate the umbilical artery, the blood flow is assessed during systole and diastole with a Doppler probe, thereby creating a waveform that can be plotted and measured. The systolic/diastolic (S/D) ratio is derived by dividing systolic peak by the end-diastolic component. By measuring the blood flow in the MCA, the peak systolic velocity is measured and is used to monitor fetal anemia of any cause. The use of this measurement has made it possible to assess ongoing fetal alloimmunization and is often used instead of amniocentesis in monitoring affected fetuses (Cunningham et al., 2010). Uterine artery blood flow is helpful in measuring pregnancies at risk for uteroplacental insufficiency such as IUGR and can be useful in preventing stillbirth (Cunningham et al., 2010).

A pulsed wave Doppler probe is used for flow studies. The client lies supine with the uterus slightly tilted, using a wedge or cushion. After transducer gel is placed on the abdomen, the fetus is located with Doppler probe. Flow within the umbilical artery is identified, and the difference between systolic and diastolic flow is displayed. Several readings are taken, and the S/D ratio calculated.

The S/D ratio becomes irrelevant when diastolic flow is absent; therefore, other values are obtained. The pulsatility index (PI), also known as the impedance index, is the S/D ratio divided by the mean velocity; Doppler ultrasound equipment provides these values. The resistance index (RI) is the S/D ratio divided by the systolic value (Cunningham et al., 2010).

INTERPRETATION

The PI, RI, and S/D ratio all normally decrease during pregnancy due to decreased placental resistance (Cunningham et al., 2010). Higher placental resistance is found in the presence of placental insufficiency, detected by a decrease in diastolic velocity. The values for all three indices are calculated and compared with standardized charts for fetuses of the same gestational age. Doppler indices are affected by gestational age, fetal breathing, FHR, and the location on the umbilical cord that is chosen to perform Doppler flow studies; Doppler indices are higher on the fetal end of the cord than the placental end, and this should be taken into consideration when interpreting values.

As previously stated, absence of end-diastolic flow or presence of reverse diastolic flow is correlated with adverse perinatal outcome. Recent research has noted the presence of *reverse diastolic flow* of the umbilical artery in the first trimester to be a possible predictor for poor outcome. However, *end diastolic flow* is often absent in the first trimester and is not necessarily an ominous sign but does require ongoing fetal monitoring.

Reverse diastolic flow, which is caused by increased flow resistance in the placental bed, is an indication for hospitalization and evaluation for delivery. Reverse diastolic flow has been associated with poor perinatal outcome and increased perinatal mortality (Cunningham et al., 2010).

All abnormal results warrant further evaluation, such as FHR monitoring, BPP, ultrasonography to monitor growth, or amniotic fluid indices. Delivery should be considered when other tests indicate imminent fetal danger or when reverse diastolic flow is encountered and extrauterine survival is likely (Cunningham et al., 2010).

ADVANTAGES AND DISADVANTAGES

Doppler has the potential to detect fetal compromise in high-risk pregnancies; it is noninvasive; it has no contraindications. There are also several disadvantages. An experienced individual must perform the test; up to 1 hour is required for a premature fetus. To date, Cunningham et al. (2010) recommend its use in monitoring an IUGR fetus and pregnancies at risk for uteroplacental insufficiencies and not as a screening test for the general obstetric population. Therefore, it should be used in adjunct to other studies. Research continues to determine the indications for Doppler flow studies.

CLIENT TEACHING AND COUNSELING

Provide the same information given for ultrasound testing. The client needs to know why the test is being done, its implications, and how it complements other tests. Be sure to coordinate exams, counseling, and planning sessions; if fetal echocardiography is used due to a cardiac abnormality, be sure to coordinate exams, counseling, and planning sessions with pediatric cardiologists and neonatologists to provide continuity for the client.

AMNIOCENTESIS AND CHORIONIC VILLUS SAMPLING

Both amniocentesis and CVS aid in the diagnosis of chromosomal abnormalities in a fetus. Cytogenetic, biochemical, and molecular testing are utilized in prenatal diagnosis. Cytogenetic testing involves the analysis of chromosomes, which is known as karyotyping. A normal female karyotype is 46,XX. Any change in the normal number of chromosomes is referred to as aneuploidy. Biochemical testing is the assessment of metabolic enzymes, thereby screening for inborn errors of metabolism such as phenylketonuria. Molecular testing involves the use of DNA to diagnose disease (Creasy et al., 2009). Various methods are utilized based upon the diagnosis sought.

Generally, prenatal diagnosis is routinely offered to clients who will be age 35 or older at delivery, because the risk of a chromosomal abnormality is equal to the risk of fetal loss associated with amniocentesis and CVS. Women who have had other affected children or who have abnormal first trimester screening test and, therefore, at risk for aneuploidy are also offered testing.

AMNIOCENTESIS FOR CHROMOSOMAL ANALYSIS

Amniotic fluid is withdrawn from the uterus, and the cells obtained are cultured to identify chromosomal and biochemical abnormalities; amniocentesis is performed at 15 to 20 weeks of gestation (Cunningham et al., 2010). First trimester and early second trimester amniocentesis at 11 to 14 weeks has been investigated. It appears that first trimester amniocentesis carries a higher fetal loss rate and a greater incidence of complications than CVS or traditional amniocentesis; due to increased risk and amniotic fluid culture failures. Therefore, ACOG (2007a) no longer recommends early amniocentesis (Cunningham et al., 2010).

The majority of amniocenteses are performed to rule out chromosomal anomalies. As with CVS, ultrasound must be performed prior to the procedure to confirm gestational age and fetal viability.

Amniocentesis is done with continuous ultrasound guidance and surgical asepsis to avoid infection. A thorough ultrasound exam is performed prior to the amniocentesis to note gestational age, placental location, amount of amniotic fluid, number of fetuses, and any fetal anomalies (Cunningham et al., 2010). After the abdomen is cleansed, a draped sterile ultrasound transducer is used to locate an appropriate pocket of fluid. A 20 to 22 gauge, 3.5-inch-long spinal needle is inserted into the pocket of fluid. Fluid is then aspirated; a 5 mL syringe is used initially and the first 1 to 2 mL of fluid and the syringe are discarded to decrease the risk of contamination of maternal cells collected in the path of the needle. Twenty milliliters of amniotic fluid is then aspirated, transferred to sterile tubes, and taken to the lab for processing. Rh immunoprophylaxis is administered to Rh-negative clients (Davidson et al., 2012).

Indications for Invasive Prenatal Diagnosis

Increased risk of chromosomal anomalies due to advanced maternal age, previous child with chromosomal anomalies, parental balanced translocation or inversion, ultrasound diagnosis of fetal malformations, abnormal first trimester screening, or abnormal maternal serum screening; parents are a carrier of a Mendelian genetic trait; suspected fetal infection or fetal hematologic disorder (Cunningham et al., 2010).

Although ultrasound has become more sophisticated at screening for anatomical landmarks associated with genetic anomalies, and the use of the first trimester screening has enhanced a noninvasive method for screening, amniocentesis remains the gold standard for fetal diagnosis of chromosomal abnormalities (Davidson et al., 2012).

Advantages and Disadvantages

Traditional amniocentesis is associated with a lower risk of complications than CVS, although the risk varies and is related to the experience of the clinician (ACOG, 2007a).

Amniocentesis cannot detect a closed neural tube defect and is associated with some complications. If a fetal anomaly does exist and is not detected until the second trimester with amniocentesis, the client who chooses to terminate her pregnancy is at greater risk for complications than if she had terminated the pregnancy in the first trimester (Cunningham et al., 2010).

Complications

The fetal loss rate is approximately 1 in 300 to 1 in 500 and is influenced by operator experience, presence of already altered placental conditions such as abruption, abnormal placental implantation, fetal anomalies, uterine anomalies, and infection (Cunningham et al., 2010). Minor complications include vaginal spotting, amniotic fluid leakage, and chorioamnionitis. Needle injuries of the fetus have been reported, but are rare (ACOG, 2007a).

Client Teaching and Counseling

Inform the client that she may experience uncomfortable pressure during the procedure, mild cramping up to 48 hours after the procedure, and slight bruising around the insertion site. Reassure the client that fetal heartbeat will be verified after the procedure. Instruct the client to telephone if she notes bleeding, leaking fluid, severe cramping, temperature higher than 100° F, chills, as well as lack of fetal movement if fetal movement has been noted by the client already. Advise the client to avoid strenuous activity or sexual intercourse for 48 hours after the procedure.

Inform the client of the possible risks to herself and the fetus, the significance of abnormal values, and the possible consequences prior to the procedure. Be prepared to counsel the client concerning all possible options.

AMNIOCENTESIS FOR ASSESSING FETAL LUNG MATURITY

Amniocentesis is used in the third trimester to assess fetal lung maturity if delivery is a possibility prior to 37 weeks' gestation. The procedure is performed much in the same way as described for a second trimester amniocentesis. The fluid obtained can be analyzed through a variety of means to assess the risk of respiratory distress in the newborn. Several components are produced as the fetal lung matures, which are secreted in the tracheal fluid, and then released into amniotic fluid. This can then be assessed via amniocentesis. These components can be measured from fluid obtained from a vaginal pool, as in the case of ruptured membranes, but can give false readings on some tests due to vaginal bacteria. Meconium and blood can alter results as well (Davidson et al., 2012).

The following are methods to assess lung maturity: *Lecithin-to-sphingomyelin (L/S) ratio*—Prior to 34 weeks, lecithin and sphingomyelin are found in equal amounts in amniotic fluid. At 35 weeks, the level of lecithin begins to rise. If the L/S ratio is less than 2:1, there is a greater risk of respiratory distress than if the ratio were 2:1 or greater. In the presence of a compromised fetus that could be better cared for outside the uterus, however, an L/S ratio of less than 2:1 may not weigh as significantly if the fetus is expected to deteriorate further if left in utero (Cunningham et al., 2010).

Phosphatidylglycerol (PG)—PG enhances surface-active properties that aid in prevention of alveolar collapse. PG is produced at the end of pregnancy in mature lungs, and the presence of PG is a reliable indication of pulmonary maturity. AmnioStat-FLM is an immunologic semiquantitative agglutination test used to screen for PG; it is reported as either present or absent (Cunningham et al., 2010).

Fluorescence polarization (TDx test for surfactant-to-albumin ratio)—The TDx analyzer is an automated fluorescence polarimeter and is used to assess surfactant content in amniotic fluid. A mature value is 55 mg of surfactant per gram of albumin (Davidson et al., 2012). TDx-FLM II, a second-generation test, has been developed and found to be an excellent indicator of fetal lung maturity.

Foam stability index—Serial dilutions of amniotic fluid are mixed with ethanol. The highest dilution in which foam still persists is read as the foam stability index value. A mature value is 47 or greater (Cunningham et al., 2010).

Lamellar body counts—Lamellar bodies are the storage form of surfactant released by fetal pneumocytes into amniotic fluid; a value of > 32,000 is usually indicative of pulmonary maturity, although some authors suggest a value of 50,000 for maturity, and found lamellar body counts to have the same predictive value as L/S ratios and PG analysis (Cunningham et al., 2010).

Each method has its own level of sensitivity, specificity, and predictive value. Not all of these methods are utilized in every institution. The mean gestational age for lung maturity is 34 to 35 weeks, and 99 percent of fetuses will have lung maturity at 37 weeks. However, the fetus of a diabetic client is the exception, with fetal maturity usually being present by 38.5 weeks (Davidson et al., 2012). In complicated pregnancies, such as those with diabetes, IUGR, and Rh-D alloimmunization, the L/S ratio and presence of PG or the use of the fluorescence polarization test should be used to establish lung maturity.

Corticosteroids were first used in 1972 for women who were anticipated to deliver prematurely to enhance fetal lung maturity; it was found that the incidence of early neonatal death, necrotizing enterocolitis, respiratory distress syndrome, and intraventricular hemorrhage was decreased as well (Davidson et al., 2012). The following clinical scenarios represent women who are candidates for a single course of corticosteroids. Multiple dosages are not recommended (Creasy et al., 2009).

- Clients between 24 and 34 weeks who are at risk for preterm delivery are candidates for corticosteroid therapy unless delivery is imminent or there is evidence the use of corticosteroids will have an adverse effect on the client.
- A client requiring intervention to stop preterm labor is also a candidate for corticosteroids.
- Treatment with corticosteroids for less than 24 hours has been shown to be beneficial; therefore, corticosteroids should be given in the presence of preterm labor unless delivery is imminent.

The use of surfactant, given to the infant through an endotracheal tube at delivery, is decreasing the incidence of neonatal mortality related to respiratory distress syndrome (Cunningham et al., 2010). Surfactant is typically administered via an endotracheal tube but can also be administered via a laryngeal mask airway (Roberts, 2011). The use of corticosteroids antenatally complements surfactant therapy after delivery to reduce mortality in the infant.

CHORIONIC VILLUS SAMPLING

Chorionic villi are of fetal origin, and information concerning chromosome status, enzyme levels, and DNA patterns of the fetus can be obtained through analysis of these cells (Creasy et al., 2009). Chorionic villi divide more rapidly than amniotic fluid cells, providing rapid chromosome analysis with preliminary results within hours and final culture results in 7 to 10 days (Blackburn, 2007). CVS is performed between 10 and 12 weeks, either transcervically or transabdominally; occasionally, a transvaginal route is taken in the presence of retroflexed uterus with a posterior placenta (Cunningham et al., 2010).

After the procedure, fetal cardiac activity is verified with ultrasound, and the fetus is monitored to note any adverse effects. In addition, RhoGAM should be administered to unsensitized Rh-negative clients after the procedure (Davidson et al., 2012).

MS-AFP screening should be offered to all women because CVS cannot detect open neural tube defects. Amniocentesis is the preferred method of diagnosis if testing for open neural tube defects, or if tests require amniotic fluid (ACOG, 2007a).

Indications

Indications for CVS are similar to those for amniocentesis (see previous section). CVS is particularly suitable for the diagnosis of classic genetic disorders with known mutations because the amount of DNA in a few villi is greater than the amount found in 40 mL of amniotic fluid (Cunningham et al., 2010).

Contraindications

CVS is not recommended in the alloimmunized client because CVS may worsen sensitization (Cunningham et al., 2010). Transcervical sampling is preferred with a posterior or low-lying placenta and retroverted uterus.

Transabdominal sampling is preferred with an anterior placenta and is the method of choice in clients who have active vaginal or cervical infection (Creasy et al., 2009).

Advantages and Disadvantages

Compared with amniocentesis, CVS permits quicker diagnosis (7 to 10 days for cell culture, depending on health care facility) and, thereby, earlier recognition of a fetal abnormality. Earlier recognition is helpful if the client must make a decision concerning termination of the pregnancy. Termination during the first trimester presents fewer risks to the client and enhances her privacy because the pregnancy is not yet obvious to others. Moreover, early diagnosis can be essential to recognize various chromosomal anomalies (ACOG, 2007a). Although there is a risk of pregnancy loss (see Complications), very few failures occur in actually retrieving villi and performing chromosomal analysis. In addition, normal findings do reduce parental anxiety at an earlier stage in pregnancy.

One disadvantage of CVS is that currently it is done only in large facilities; not all facilities have the capability or staff with sufficient expertise. Another disadvantage is that CVS tests only for chromosomal anomalies and cannot detect anatomic aberrations, such as open neural tube defects. Also note the complications listed.

Complications

Pregnancy loss varies depending on the center and the expertise of the provider; CVS carries a slightly higher rate of procedure failure and fetal loss than amniocentesis, but the rate has not been found to be statistically significant (Creasy et al., 2009). The risk of fetal loss from CVS is approximately 0.5 percent and is higher than conventional amniocentesis (ACOG, 2007a).

Fetal loss may also be coincidental. Women who are at increased risk for pregnancy loss secondary to their age or having a chromosomally abnormal fetus will have an increased rate of spontaneous abortion despite the risk of CVS or amniocentesis (ACOG, 2007a).

Subsequent limb defects have been associated with CVS; several theories have been proposed (Cunningham et al., 2010). ACOG (2007) recommends that CVS be performed between 10 and 12 weeks to reduce the incidence of limb defects. Limb reduction defects incidence in the general population is 6 in 10,000 births. Limb defects have a higher incidence in CVS testing if performed prior to 10 weeks, so later screening at 10 to 13 weeks is now recommended. Clients should be counseled that when CVS is performed between 10 and 12 weeks, the risk of limb defects is low and probably not greater than the risk to the general population.

Maternal cell contamination and mosaicism (the presence of one or more cell types) are potential sources of diagnostic error; interestingly, confined placental mosaicism has been associated with poor pregnancy outcome, possibly related to abnormal placental function. Amniocentesis is advised for confirmation if mosaicism is assessed in cell culture or direct preparation (Creasy et al., 2009).

Client Teaching and Counseling

Advise the client to call if she experiences moderate vaginal bleeding, severe cramping, leaking fluid, temperature higher than 100° F, or chills. Cramping may continue for up to 48 hours after CVS. The client should avoid strenuous activity and sexual intercourse for 48 hours. Discuss each step of the procedure with the client to help decrease her anxiety.

The client should be aware of the potential risks to herself and the fetus. The consequences of an abnormal result should be discussed prior to the procedure. Be aware of all options available to the client; referrals to perinatologists and pediatricians can help the client to become knowledgeable about her fetus. If the client chooses termination, counsel her appropriately and be knowledgeable about the location of centers for pregnancy termination.

PERCUTANEOUS UMBILICAL BLOOD SAMPLING

The terms *percutaneous umbilical blood sampling* (PUBS) and *cordocentesis* are used interchangeably in reference to the invasive sampling of fetal blood. PUBS was originally done using fetoscopy in the early 1970s. The use of ultrasound has decreased the risks of PUBS, however, and its use for a variety of indications has expanded in the last few years. PUBS not only can be a method to assess fetal well-being but can provide fetal therapy as well. Common procedures performed using PUBS include shunt placement, ablation, and angioplasty (Cunningham et al., 2010).

PROCEDURE

PUBS can be performed at approximately 18 weeks' gestation or later as clinical indications arise (Cunningham et al., 2010). Ultrasound is used to assess fetal viability, position, biometry, location of the placenta, and presence of fetal anomalies. The insertion site of the umbilical cord in the placenta is identified. The maternal abdomen is cleansed and draped, just as for amniocentesis. Under ultrasound guidance, a 20 to 25 gauge needle is inserted into the amniotic cavity and into the umbilical vein; the veins can be distinguished by their size, and the direction of blood flow can be determined by using color Doppler. Confirmation that the blood sample is of fetal origin is imperative; a number of tests are available, including the Kleihauer-Betke test and comparison of mean corpuscular volume (Davidson et al., 2012).

Once the needle has been inserted into the umbilical vein, fetal blood is withdrawn into a syringe (Creasy et al., 2009). Samples can be evaluated for coagulation studies, blood group typing, complete blood count, karyotyping, and blood gas analysis (Cunningham et al., 2010). Due to the risk of transplacental hemorrhage, Rh-negative clients are given RhoGAM (Davidson et al., 2012).

After the age of viability, a course of corticosteroids is advised prior to PUBS (Cunningham et al., 2010). This is to enhance fetal lung maturity due to the risk of preterm labor or for the need for immediate delivery in the event fetal distress occurs during or after PUBS. For this reason, if the fetus is at the age of viability, PUBS should be done only in a hospital setting (as opposed to an outpatient setting) in order to deliver the fetus by cesarean section if needed (Creasy et al., 2009).

INDICATIONS

- Cytogenetic diagnosis: for instance, when rapid karyotype is needed, or if one or more cell types is identified (mosaicism or pseudomosaicism) at amniocentesis or CVS
- Congenital infection: toxoplasmosis, rubella, cytomegalovirus, parvovirus, congenital syphilis
- Congenital immunodeficiency
- Coagulopathies
- Platelet disorders
- Hemoglobinopathies
- Severe IUGR: detect etiology, assess fetal hematologic and acid-base function
- Multiple gestation: twin-to-twin transfusion syndrome
- Fetal therapy: transfusions or pharmacologic agents when transplacental passage of the drug is poor
- Diagnosis and/or treatment: fetal anemia, nonimmune hydrops (Creasy et al., 2009; Cunningham et al., 2010; Davidson et al., 2012)

COMPLICATIONS

Fetal loss varies, depending on indication, operator experience, technique, and gestational age at procedure (Cunningham et al., 2010). Fetal complications can be hemorrhage, hematoma of the cord, placental abruption, and preterm delivery. Maternal complications include amnionitis and transplacental hemorrhage. Risks are higher when the client is obese, when the placenta is posterior, or when PUBS is performed prior to 19 weeks (Creasy et al., 2009).

In general, fetal loss rates due to PUBS range from 1 to 4 percent and higher depending on the indication for PUBS. Fetuses with abnormalities and genetic chromosomal abnormalities have higher loss rates than fetuses with blood disorders that are being treated with the procedure. With such a significant loss rate, only clients with clear indications should be offered this method of assessment. Adequate imaging of the cord is not always possible, and another method of surveillance should be chosen, or PUBS should be postponed. Aseptic technique and limiting the number of puncture sites will reduce complications (Milunsky & Milunsky, 2010). Transversing the placenta may worsen alloimmunization due to intermixing of fetal and maternal blood (Creasy et al., 2009).

ADVANTAGES AND DISADVANTAGES

Fetal karyotype can be obtained from a culture of fetal blood in 24 to 48 hours (ACOG, 2007a). There are a number of indications for PUBS (see previous paragraph) in which the procedure is lifesaving for the fetus; although there is an increased risk of fetal loss with PUBS versus CVS or amniocentesis, fetal loss would be inevitable in some cases. The use of PUBS for fetal transfusion is lifesaving for the fetus with nonimmune hydrops fetalis if the fetus is remote from term (Milunsky & Milunsky, 2010).

The main disadvantage is fetal loss, as well as other complications noted.

CLIENT TEACHING AND COUNSELING

The client needs to be aware of the risks involved, as well as the need for immediate intervention in the event nonreassuring fetal status is noted. Other options, if applicable, should be made available to the client. Counseling and, therefore, fetal loss rates need to be specific in regard to the indication for PUBS. Genetic studies versus transfusion for nonimmune hydrops are completely different indications and require specific counseling based on the status of the client and fetus.

INTERVENTIONS/TREATMENTS FOR FETAL CONDITIONS

Currently, there are several fetal conditions that can be successfully treated in utero through medical management of the mother. These include metabolic and endocrinologic disorders as well as toxoplasmosis and other infectious diseases. Treatment consists of medicating the mother for the specific condition or close monitoring of the fetus if no medications exist for the particular condition. Assessment for therapeutic fetal drug levels can be evaluated through cordocentesis (Cunningham et al., 2010). Fetal surgery is a technique that is rarely used due to the high risk associated with its use. Furthermore, there are few centers in the United States that actually perform fetal surgery and it is limited to very specific abnormalities. Certain abnormalities may necessitate open fetal surgery such as thoracic masses that result in hydrops such as cystic adenomatoid malformation, extralobular pulmonary sequestration, sacrococcygeal teratoma, and spina bifida. Fetal surgery carries considerable risk including fetal death. It is typically attempted when the fetal anomaly present is considered so lethal that without the intervention the fetus will likely die. Other complications can be treated with fetoscopic surgery including twin-to-twin transfusion, diaphragmatic hernia, posterior urethral valves, congenital airway obstruction, and amniotic band release. Cordocentesis is still commonly used for shunt therapy, radiofrequency ablation, and fetal intracardiac catheter procedures. Although less risky than the open fetal surgery or fetoscopy, it still has risks of infection, preterm labor, premature rupture of membranes, fetal injury, and fetal loss (Cunningham et al., 2010). Therefore, with advances in technology, intervention on the behalf of the fetus does not necessarily indicate delivery.

TABLE 21–3. Disorders Currently Being Treated With Fetal Stem Cells

Leukemias, lymphomas, blood cancers
Brain tumors and other cancers
Bone marrow failure disorders
Hemoglobinopathies
Histiocytic disorders
Myelodysplastic/myeloproliferative disorders
Inherited metabolic disorders
Inherited immune system disorders

Source: Adapted from Cord Blood Registry, 2011.

Stem cell transplantation therapy for the fetus is an evolving field. Currently, fetal stem cells are collected via the umbilical cord or placenta and can be used to treat certain malignancies and specific disease processes. They can also be collected from the amniotic fluid although this is in the early stages of being refined. The future use of stem cells for regenerative medicine to treat type 1 diabetes, cerebral palsy, and neonatal brain injury is currently in clinical trials (Cord Blood Registry, 2011). In addition, gene therapy and angiogenesis holds promise. Stem cells are currently being used to treat a variety of diseases and the list continues to grow (Table 21–3). Stem cells can be collected at birth via the umbilical cord and banked for future use. This is known as *cord blood banking*. Cord blood banking is recommended for women with a family history of rare cancers in childhood or for parents who wish to save the cells for future use in the child or a family member. Although the procedure is quite easy to perform, the cost remains high and parents must pay annual fees for cryostorage.

PREIMPLANTATION GENETIC DIAGNOSIS

Preimplantation genetic diagnosis (PGD) is a growing field that aims to assist couples in having a pregnancy free of an identifiable genetic disease. It is the combination of in vitro fertilization and prenatal diagnosis (Davidson et al., 2012). Typically, clients are carriers for an inherited disorder that they do not wish to pass on to their child; a couple may already be raising an affected child or have experienced a miscarriage due to a genetic-related condition. They may have already had previous affected pregnancies that were terminated after prenatal diagnosis and wish to avoid termination in the future for a specific disorder (Davidson et al., 2012).

PGD is performed prior to conception (polar body biopsy) and after in vitro fertilization (blastomere biopsy—6- to 8-cell embryo—and trophectoderm biopsy); if results are negative for the disorder in question, fertilization or implantation can proceed (Davidson et al., 2012). Monogenic disorders are diagnosed using PCR, and FISH is used to diagnose chromosomal abnormalities (Blackburn, 2007). Clients are still advised to undergo prenatal diagnosis to assess for other anomalies.

INDICATIONS

Indications for PGD include many of the same for invasive prenatal diagnosis: increased risk of chromosomal anomalies due to advanced maternal age, previous child with chromosomal anomalies, parental balanced translocation or inversion, and parents are a carrier of a Mendelian genetic trait (Davidson et al., 2012).

Couples who are referred for PGD are usually already aware they are carriers of a genetic disorder or have previously experienced an undesirable pregnancy outcome of genetic origin. Couples may also want to avoid the risk of genetic disease without the dilemma of possible termination that prenatal diagnosis raises.

ADVANTAGES AND DISADVANTAGES

Natural conception and traditional prenatal diagnosis is an acceptable choice for many, particularly when faced with the possible decision to continue or terminate an affected pregnancy that accompanies traditional prenatal diagnosis. For clients who have previously terminated a pregnancy due to anomalies, significant psychological repercussions occur with future pregnancies, one of which is to prepare to terminate a pregnancy again (Cunningham et al., 2010). PGD may be a more desirable option for these clients.

PGD does have potential increased emotional, physical, and financial investment because it is the combination of IVF and prenatal diagnosis. Pregnancy rates vary, but only approximately one third of completed cycles of PGD result in pregnancy. Health insurance carriers will more readily cover the cost of prenatal diagnosis versus PGD, even when the primary reason is to eliminate the transmission of an inherited disorder to a child (Cunningham et al., 2010).

The benefit is detection of specific genetic disorders prior to implantation to avoid the dilemma of possible pregnancy termination of affected fetuses. Ethical considerations have been raised concerning the use of PGD to choose an unaffected embryo to be implanted in order to provide stem cells at birth to treat an affected sibling, as in the case of Fanconi anemia; to provide social sexing for family balancing; and to know which embryos to select or discard based on the definition of what constitutes a serious genetic disorder in the realm of PGD (Cunningham et al., 2010).

EVALUATION OF FETAL DNA IN MATERNAL BLOOD

Fetal DNA is present in maternal blood in small amounts and it is hoped that testing could be offered as early as 8 to 10 weeks to diagnose Down syndrome, Trisomy 21, in high-risk pregnancies. With use of a technique, massively parallel genomic sequencing, sufficient fetal DNA molecules can be obtained to determine if an elevated proportion of cells exist for chromosome 21 (as would be the case in Down syndrome). In one study, this method of testing had a positive predictive value of 91.9 percent and a negative predictive value of 100 percent when using a 2-plex protocol (Chiu et al., 2011).

Research needs to continue in order to develop testing that is affordable, ready to use in the clinic setting, and diagnostic of a variety of fetal abnormalities. At times in the past decade these goals for testing have not seemed feasible. However, recent breakthroughs in genomic testing do hold promise of soon being able to offer women accurate, early, affordable, noninvasive testing for fetal aneuploidies (Hahn, Lapaire, Tercanli, Kolla, & Hösli, 2011).

REFERENCES

American College of Obstetricians and Gynecologists (ACOG). (2006). *Nonmedical use of obstetric ultrasound* (ACOG Committee Opinion No. 297). Washington, DC: Author.

American College of Obstetricians and Gynecologists (ACOG). (2007a). *Invasive prenatal testing for aneuploidy* (ACOG Practice Bulletin No. 88). Washington, DC: Author.

American College of Obstetricians and Gynecologists (ACOG). (2007b). *Screening for fetal chromosomal abnormalities* (ACOG Practice Bulletin No. 77). Washington, DC: Author.

American College of Obstetricians and Gynecologists (ACOG). (2009). *Antepartum fetal surveillance* (ACOG Practice Bulletin No. 9). Washington, DC: Author.

Arora, S. (2010). Alloimmunization to both Rh and Kell system antigens (anti-C and anti-K) in a young thalassemic patient. *Indian Journal of Pathology and Microbiology, 53*(4), 889–890.

Barclay, L. (2009). *Fetal heart rate monitoring guidelines updated.* Retrieved from http://www.medscape.com/viewarticle/705210

Ben-Haroush, A., Chen, R., Hadar, E., Hod, M., & Yogev, Y. (2007). Accuracy of a single fetal weight estimation at 29–34 weeks in diabetic pregnancies: Can it predict large-for-gestational-age infants at term? *American Journal of Obstetrics and Gynecology, 197*(5), 497.e1–497.e6. doi:10.1016/j.ajog.2007.04.023

Benson, C.B., & Bluth, E.I. (2008). *Ultrasonography in obstetrics and gynecology.* (2nd ed.). New York: Thieme Medical Publishers.

Bhogal, A.K., & Brunger, F. (2010). Prenatal genetic counseling in cross-cultural medicine. *Canadian Family Physician, 59*(10), 993–999.

Blackburn, S.T. (2007). *Maternal, fetal, & neonatal physiology: A clinical perspective (maternal fetal and neonatal physiology).* Philadelphia: Saunders.

Chiu, R.W.K., Akolekar, R., Zheng, Y.W.L., Leung, T.Y., Sun, H., Chan, K.C.A., et al. (2011). Non-invasive prenatal assessment of trisomy 21 by multiplexed maternal plasma DNA sequencing: Large scale validity study. *British Medical Journal, 342,* c7401. doi:10.1136/bmjc7401

Cord Blood Registry. (2011). *Diseases treated with stem cells.* Retrieved from http://www.cordblood.com/caregivers/banking/diseases_treated.asp

Creasy, R.K., Resnik, R., Iams, J.D., Lockwood, C.J., & Moore, T.R. (2009). *Creasy & Resnik's maternal-fetal medicine* (6th ed.). Philadelphia: Saunders Elsevier.

Cunningham, F.G., Leveno, K.J., Bloom, S.L., Hauth, J.C., Rouse, D.J., & Spong, C.Y. (2010). *Williams obstetrics* (23 rd ed.). New York: McGraw-Hill Medical.

Davidson, M.R., Ladewig, P.A.W., & London, M.L. (2012). *Old's maternal-newborn nursing & women's health across the lifespan* (9th ed.). Uppers Saddle River, NJ: Pearson.

De Santis, M., De Luca, C., Quattrocchi, T., Visconti, D., Cesari, E., Mappa, I., et al. (2010). Use of the Internet by women seeking information about potentially teratogenic agents. *European Journal of Obstetrics, Gynecology, and Reproductive Biology, 151*(2), 154–157.

Fisher, J. (2011). First trimester screening: The fallout. *Prenatal Diagnosis, 31*(1), 44–49. doi:10.1002/pd.2687

Franson, M.P., Bot, M.L., Vogel, I., Mackenbach, J.P., Steegers, E.A.P., & Wildscut, H.I.J. (2009). Ethnic differences in informed decision-making about prenatal screening for Down's syndrome. *Journal of Epidemiological Community Health, 64,* 262–268. doi:10.1136/jech.2009.088237

Hahn, S., Lapaire, O., Tercanli, S., Kolla, V., & Hösli, I. (2011). Determination of fetal chromosome aberrations from fetal DNA in maternal blood: Has the challenge finally been met? *Expert Reviews in Molecular Medicine, 13,* e16. doi:10.1017/S1462399411001852

Hintz, S.R., Msepia, D.E., Kendrick, M., Wislon-Costello, D.E., Das, A., Bell, E.F., et al. (2011). Early-childhood neurodevelopmental outcomes are not improving for infants born at < 25 weeks' gestational age. *Pediatrics, 127*(1), 62–70. doi:10.1542/peds.2010-1150

Jaques, A.M., Collins, V.R., Muggli, E.E., Amor, D.J., Francis, I., Sheffield, L.J., et al. (2010). Uptake of prenatal diagnostic testing and the effectiveness of prenatal screening for Down syndrome. *Prenatal Diagnosis, 30*(6), 522–530.

Jazayeri, A. (2010). *Fetal macrosomia.* Retrieved from http://emedicine.medscape.com/article/262679-overview

Ladewig, P.A.W., London, M.L., & Davidson, M.R. (2014). *Contemporary maternal-newborn nursing* (8th ed.). Upper Saddle River, NJ: Pearson Education.

Lagan, B.M., Sinclair, M., & Kernohan, G.W. (2010). Internet use in pregnancy informs women's decision making: A web-based survey. *Birth, 37,* 106–115. doi:10.1111/j.1523-536X.2010.00390.x

LeRoy, B.S., Leach, P.M., & Bartels, D.M. (2010). *Genetic counseling practice: Advanced concepts and skills.* Hoboken, NJ: Wiley.

Li, S.L., Chen, X.L., Ouyang, S.Y., Yao, Y., Gong, B., Wen, H.X., et al. (2008). P44.04: Value of level III prenatal ultrasound in prenatal diagnosis. *Ultrasound in Obstetrics and Gynecology, 32,* 459–460. doi:10.1002/uog.6183

Marino, T., Laartz, B., Smith, S.E., Gompf, S.G., Alloboun, K., Martinex, J.E., et al. (2010). *Viral infections in pregnancy.* Retrieved from http://emedicine.medscape.com/article/235213-overview

Milunsky, A., & Milunsky, J. (2010). *Genetic disorders and the fetus* (6th ed.). New York: Wiley-Blackwell.

Murray, M.C. (2007). *Essentials of fetal monitoring* (3rd ed.). New York: Spring Publishing Company.

National Institute of Child and Human Development (NICHD). (2008). *The 2008 National Institute of Child Health and Human Development workshop report on electronic fetal monitoring: Update on definitions, interpretation, and research guidelines.* Retrieved from http://www.ihi.org/IHI/Topics/PerinatalCare/PerinatalCareGeneral/Literature/2008NICHDReportonElectronicFetalMonitoring.htm

National Institutes of Health. (2011). *Twin-to-twin transfusion syndrome.* Retrieved from http://www.ncbi.nlm.nih.gov/pubmedhealth/PMH0002562/

Nicholaides, K.H. (2011, January 5). Screening for fetal aneuploidies at 11 to 13 weeks. *Prenatal Diagnosis, 31*(1), 7–15. doi:10.1002/pd.2637

Platz, E., & Neuman, R. (2008). Diagnosis of IUGR: Traditional biometry. *Seminars in Perinatology, 32*(3), 140–147.

Roberts, K. (2011). *NRP changes: A new game in town.* Retrieved from http://www.aap.org/nrp/pdf/newplayer.pdf

Robinson, B. (2008). A review of NICHD standardized nomenclature for cardiotocography: The importance of speaking a common language when describing electronic fetal monitoring. *Review of Obstetrics and Gynecology, 1*(2), 56–60.

Saff, J.C., Hull, S., Duffer, S., Zornetzer, S., Sutton, E., Marteau, T.M., et al. (2009). Ambivalence toward undergoing invasive prenatal testing: An exploration of its origins. *Prenatal Diagnosis, 30*(1), 77–82. doi:10.1002/pd.2343

Schmid, M., & Blaicher, W. (2011). Genetics of fetal disease: Fetal MRI. *Medical Radiology,* 489–505. doi:10.1007/174_2010_62

Smith, J.F. (2008). Fetal health assessment using prenatal diagnostic techniques. *Current Opinions in Obstetrics and Gynecology, 20*(2), 152–156.

Volpe, J.J. (2008). *Neurology of the newborn* (5th ed.). Philadelphia: Saunders.

CHAPTER ❖ **22**

POSTPARTUM AND LACTATION

Diane Marie Schadewald ◆ Cheri Friedrich

The support and experience previously provided by the extended family are not always easily accessible for today's families.

Highlights

- The Puerperium
- The 4- to 6-Week Postpartum Assessment
- Normal Postpartum Health Assessment
- Assessment of Postoperative Cesarean Birth and Sterilization
- Common Postpartum Complications
- Postpartum Psychiatric Disturbances
- Postpartum Post-Traumatic Stress Disorder
- Early Discharge
- Adjusting to Parenting
- Perinatal Loss
- Breastfeeding
- Bottlefeeding

❖ INTRODUCTION

Knowledge of the normal physiologic changes and complications of the postpartum period, parental roles, perinatal loss, and lactation is essential in managing the care of a client and her family postpartum. The health care provider must be familiar with assessment, diagnosis, management, and follow-up. Knowing when referral is needed for further evaluation and management is also vital.

In the diagnosis and management of complications, it may be necessary to implement emergency measures until definitive care from a consulting medical professional arrives. The postpartum woman may be assessed in a hospital setting, alternative birthing site such as a birthing center, clinic, or home.

The extended family of 40 or 50 years ago has been replaced by nuclear and nontraditional families such as single-parent, same-sex, and blended (two partial families joined to become one). The support and experience previously provided by the extended family are not easily accessible for many families of today. Mandatory early hospital discharge is no longer an issue since legislation passed that makes it illegal to force discharge prior to 48 hours post vaginal delivery or 96 hours post cesarean section. However, for those mothers who choose early discharge the nurturing and infant care skills usually taught by health professionals on the second postpartum day need to be taught in a shortened time frame. This is further complicated because the client's attention is often focused on what awaits her at home. To meet the health needs of today's new mother, some communities provide follow-up telephone calls or home visits.

Many women choosing to breast-feed may be deterred when faced with engorgement, tender nipples, and nonsupportive family and friends. Women who deliver twins may believe that breastfeeding is not possible. The postpartum period provides opportunity to promote a successful experience for the breastfeeding family.

Unfortunately, the postpartum experience is not always joyful. Some women or couples are left to deal with the loss of the fantasized infant as they struggle with the reality of a miscarriage, deformity, or perinatal death. Others experience depression or other psychological problems. Knowing how to help the woman and her family and suggest appropriate referral is imperative. There is a list of support groups at the end of this chapter.

Health care during the postpartum period focuses on evaluation of the physiological and psychological changes that normally occur. Any abnormal findings or dysfunctional behavior detected during the antepartum and postpartum periods should continue to be evaluated.

THE PUERPERIUM

Postpartum, also referred to as the *puerperium*, is the period from delivery of the placenta and membranes to the return of the woman's reproductive organs to their nonpregnant state. It generally lasts about 6 weeks and is divided into three segments. The immediate puerperium is the first 24 hours after delivery; the early puerperium extends from the second postpartum day to the end of the first postpartum week; and the remote puerperium continues to the end of the sixth week.

IMMEDIATE PUERPERIUM

- *Uterine involution:* This process includes shedding of the decidua and endometrium. It is monitored by assessing the amount of lochia and uterine size and tone.
    - Immediately after delivery, the uterus is approximately two thirds to three fourths of the way between the umbilicus and the symphysis pubis; after a few hours, the uterus rises to the level of the umbilicus and remains there or one fingerbreadth below for about 2 days before gradually descending into the true pelvis by 2 weeks postpartum (Cunningham et al., 2010c). Any time the top of the fundus is above the umbilicus, bladder distention or uterine distention from blood or clots is to be suspected.
    - Lochia is the uterine discharge during the puerperium that escapes vaginally. Lochia rubra is the earliest lochia and is red because it contains blood and decidual tissue. It begins immediately after delivery and continues the first 2 to 3 days postpartum.
- *Vagina and perineum:* These structures are quite stretched and edematous following a vaginal delivery. The vagina gapes at the introitus; it is smooth-walled and generally lax. Hematoma should be suspected if the woman reports excruciating pain or is unable to void, or if a tense, fluctuant mass is noted

in the perineal area. Also, inspect the episiotomy for hematoma. Vulvar and rectal hemorrhoids are often present and must be observed for evidence of thrombosis. After delivery, ice bags may be applied to the perineum and hemorrhoids for 30 to 60 minutes; commercial cold pack perineal pads lose their temperature in about 60 minutes and are safe to remain in place. If hand-made ice bags are used, they need to be removed after 60 minutes to prevent a secondary vasodilatory effect.

- *Vital signs:* Blood pressure, pulse, and respirations should be stabilized to within normal limits. Fever is indicative of infection, probably in the genitourinary tract.
- *Bladder:* The bladder is edematous, hypotonic, and congested immediately postpartum. Consequently bladder distention, incomplete emptying, inability to void, and excessive urine residual may develop unless the woman is encouraged to void at least every 4 hours even when she does not feel the need. The risk for bladder distention is also increased because of diuresis that begins almost immediately postpartum.
- *Breasts:* Lactation naturally begins. Colostrum is the first fluid the infant receives from the breast. Engorgement commonly occurs 48 to 72 hours after delivery. An ice bag applied to the breasts and axilla for 15 minutes and then discontinued for 1 hour before being reapplied may give the nonlactating woman some relief from engorgement.
- *Abdominal muscles:* The muscles are flabby, and some degree of diastasis recti is normally present. If the client elected to have tubal sterilization or has a cesarean section, part of the preoperative counseling should include advising the client of a possible increase in pain or discomfort because of the surgery as well as from the postpartum afterpains. If cesarean section was performed, a dressing usually covers the incision, and it should be dry. Staples are generally used in the skin closure and are removed 3 to 4 days postoperatively and often replaced with Steri-strips®.
- *Postpartum blues and grief:* Descriptions are provided in the sections Postpartum Psychiatric Disturbances and Perinatal Loss.

EARLY PUERPERIUM

From the second postpartum day to the end of the first postpartum week additional changes evolve.

- *Uterus:* It decreases to approximately 12 weeks size; barely palpable just above the symphysis pubis.
- *Lochia serosa:* The normal uterine discharge from the vagina that occurs during postpartum days 4 to 10 is lochia serosa. It contains primarily serous fluid, decidual tissue, leukocytes, and erythrocytes. Flow is decreasing. Advise to use pads, not tampons.
- *Vagina and perineum:* The vagina remains smooth, and the perineum may be slightly uncomfortable. If an episiotomy was performed, the sutures will be palpable. Attention should be given for signs of infection or hemorrhoids. Advise against douching as it may alter vaginal pH, wash out protective vaginal organisms, and increase risk for infection. Bathing can soothe and cleanse the perineum. Oils and fragrances should not be used in bath water. If hemorrhoids are present, relief can be obtained with Tucks®, Nupercaine® ointment, Dermaplast® (or similar products), increased fluid and fiber intake, stool softeners as needed, and warm or cool sitz baths. Urinary incontinence may indicate cystocele (see Chapter 16).
- *Breasts:* By this time, the breasts of women who are breastfeeding contain milk. Breast milk usually appears on postpartum days 3 to 5, and is bluish white. A mother may need reassurance that the color is normal and her milk has not become weak (see Breastfeeding section).
- *Abdominal muscles:* These muscles are lax, and a woman needs reassurance that it is normal. Walking may help tone muscles without exerting undue stress.
- *Diuresis and profuse perspiration:* These conditions are normal as long as the woman is afebrile.

REMOTE PUERPERIUM

From the end of the first postpartum week to the end of the sixth week maternal change continues.

- *Uterus:* The uterus returns to its nonpregnant size 4 to 6 weeks following birth.
- *Lochia alba:* The last lochia, lochia alba, begins at about day 10 and continues until approximately day 35 postpartum. It is scant, composed primarily of leukocytes and decidual cells, and is creamy white.
- *Vagina and perineum:* These structures begin to regain tone by 6 weeks postpartum. Rugae are normally present by that time. Atrophy, however, may still be evident in the lactating woman. Of concern are maintaining and strengthening vaginal tone, preventing pelvic relaxation, and promoting nonpainful resumption of intercourse.
- *Breasts:* The breasts begin to adapt to the nutritional needs of the baby; engorgement and mastitis

are primary concerns. Assess the breastfeeding process and family support. The breasts of a nonlactating woman may contain milk for up to 3 months postpartum.

- *Renal system:* Urinary tract infection (UTI) may occur, and continuing assessment is of particular concern for clients with a history of UTI. Women who have had catheterization during the labor and delivery process, especially a Foley catheter, are also at increased risk for UTI postpartum.
- *Abdominal muscles:* Abdominal wall musculature becomes firmer by the end of the sixth postpartum week, but may never regain its prepregnant appearance if the muscles remain weakened and stretched. Diastasis recti resolves or at minimum diminishes.

THE 4- TO 6-WEEK POSTPARTUM ASSESSMENT

SUBJECTIVE DATA

Generally review the woman's systems. Specific determinations also need to be made:

- Number of weeks postpartum.
- General adaptation to motherhood; assess the client's rest and sleep habits, mood, appetite, activity level, exercise program, and nutrition (obtain 24-hour dietary recall to assess nutritional intake).
- Coping ability in caring for baby and making family adjustments or living as single parent.
- Problems with baby (feeding, health concerns, first exam).
- Family adjustments caring for baby.
- Sexual activity (resumption, type of contraceptive used, dyspareunia, and other concerns, including possible lack of desire, fear of discomfort or of becoming pregnant again).
- Family planning method desired; assess previous methods used, length of time used, satisfaction with methods, and reason for discontinuance.
- Financial concerns, plans to return to work and if so plans for pumping and storage of breast milk.
- Safety concerns, experience of any physical or psychological abuse, experience of any desire to hurt herself or the baby.

Ask the client if she has called a health care provider or gone to an emergency room and whether she was admitted or readmitted. In addition, ask if she has had fever, chills, or flu-like symptoms.

- *Breasts:* Assess for engorgement and breastfeeding concerns.
    - Determine when engorgement occurred, how long it lasted, if it has been treated, and how and whether it continues to be a problem or has resolved.
    - If breastfeeding is discontinued, determine the length of breastfeeding and the reason for stopping.
    - If the client is currently breastfeeding, ask her about concerns, frequency, nipple soreness, breast care, and enjoyment of breastfeeding.
- *Lochia:* In the postpartum period, assess the duration of each lochia color in sequence, presence of odor, excessive bleeding, clots, and pain.
- *Return of menses:* Several factors influence the return of menses, such as contraceptive method and breastfeeding. Nonlactating women menstruate 6 to 8 weeks following delivery, and lactating women 2 to 18 months following delivery, depending on whether she is exclusively breastfeeding or if she is supplementing with formula. The first postpartum menstruation is heavier than normal menstruation and often anovulatory. Menses returns sooner in the multipara than the primipara.

OBJECTIVE DATA

Physical Examination

Generally assess the client.

- *General appearance and vital signs:* Compare blood pressure with range before and during pregnancy. Compare weight with prepregnant weight and weight at delivery.
- *Neck:* Determine that the thyroid is nonpalpable. If thyromegaly or nodules are palpated, order thyroid function tests (TFTs) and refer the client for medical evaluation (see Normal Postpartum Health Assessment).
- *Breasts:* Evaluation is influenced by whether the client is lactating.
    - Lactating breasts should be full, without erythema, masses, or lymphadenopathy. Milk should be easily expressed.
    - Nonlactating breasts are soft, without masses or lymphadenopathy. Bilateral galactorrhea may be present in nonlactating women for up to 3 months postpartum; these women should return for evaluation of galactorrhea beyond 3 months. Mechanical stimulation of nonlactating breasts may lead to persistence of milky discharge, but more serious causes should be ruled out.

- *Extremities:* Assess for swelling, varicosities, and phlebitis.
- *Cardiovascular and respiratory systems:* Rate and rhythm should be regular without murmurs or extra heart sounds. Clear, equal breath sounds should be evident bilaterally. Blood volume returns to normal by approximately 1 week postpartum.
- *Abdomen and musculoskeleton:* Assess for costovertebral angle tenderness (CVAT) and tenderness along paraspinous muscles. Inspect for abdominal striae, diastasis, hernias, masses, tenderness, and lymph nodes. If she experienced a tubal ligation or cesarean birth, assess healing of incision. Abdominal musculature involution may require 6 to 8 weeks.
- *Genitalia and reproductive organs:* Evaluation of several structures is performed.
    - External genitalia should be without edema or lesions and nontender. Bartholin's, urethra, and Skene's glands should appear normal.
    - Vagina should appear rugated, except in lactating women when rugae may be decreased secondary to hypoestrogenic state. Episiotomy site should be intact, well healed, and nontender.
    - Cervical internal os should be closed. If it is open, determine whether placental products have been retained. After childbirth, the cervix appears as a transverse slit. It appears stellate if severe lacerations were sustained during childbirth.
    - Uterine corpus at 4 to 6 weeks postpartum is nonpregnant size. If uterine tenderness is detected, consider infection and prepare appropriate cultures (e.g., chlamydia, gonorrhea).
    - Involution of ovaries and fallopian tubes is complete by 6 to 7 weeks postpartum.
    - Inspect rectum for hemorrhoids. Assess sphincter control, especially if third- or fourth-degree laceration was sustained during childbirth.
- *Psychological factors:* Assess affect for mood of mother, and her interaction with infant or other indications of maternal-infant bonding.

Diagnostic Tests

Various tests need to be performed.

- Compare antenatal and postnatal hemoglobin levels and hematocrits.
- Check immunity status for rubella and, if not immune (titer $\leq$ 1:10), confirm that rubella vaccine was given prior to hospital discharge. Check immunity status for varicella and, if not immune, confirm if first dose of vaccine was given prior to hospital discharge. Nursing mothers may be vaccinated.
- If client is Rh-negative, check Rh status of infant and, if clinically indicated, determine whether Rho(D) immune globulin human (RhoGAM) was given to mother postpartum. If RhoGAM was given, seroconversion from rubella or varicella vaccines given prior to discharge should be checked at the postpartum visit, or 6 to 8 weeks after vaccine administration. Theoretically, RhoGAM can block antibody development (Centers for Disease Control and Prevention [CDC], 2011a).
- Check when last Pap smear was done, evaluate results, and determine if repeat Pap is indicated.
- If any sexually transmitted disease was detected during pregnancy, consider repeating tests.

PLAN

- *Psychosocial intervention:* Counseling may be helpful about available social services, public health nursing, and child protective services (see Postpartum Depression Support Groups at the end of this chapter).
- *Family planning:* Ask if the client was satisfied with previously used methods of contraception or if she has concerns regarding the method she wishes to use or is using now. Base your instructions about a method of contraception on the client's level of comprehension. Address safer sex as well as satisfaction with or changes in relationship with sexual partner.
- *Preventive measures:* Encourage health maintenance/health promotion activities, such as breast self-examination, Kegel exercises, annual Pap examination, smoking cessation, weight reduction, and exercise. Reassure mothers that it may take months for them to feel normal again.

FOLLOW-UP

- *Pap smear:* Perform only if indicated (American College of Obstetricians and Gynecologists [ACOG], 2009).
- *Colposcopy:* Perform or refer if indicated.
- *Culture:* Culture for chlamydia or gonorrhea if indicated.
- *Urine testing:* Monitor for urinary tract pathology by performing dipstick. Culture urine if bacteriuria occurred during pregnancy or if physical exam warrants.
- *Blood tests:* Obtain hemoglobin level, hematocrit, or complete blood count (CBC) if indicated.

- *Immunization:* Request rubella immunization and varicella immunization if indicated (Advisory Committee on Immunization Practices [ACIP], 2008).
- *Intravenous pyelogram and urology:* Consider referring the client for intravenous pyelogram and urology consultation if she has a history of pyelonephritis or hematuria of unknown etiology during pregnancy.
- *Glucose testing:* Request 75 g glucola if the client was gestational diabetic (see section Gestational Diabetes). Because glucose tolerance testing in the immediate postpartum period is unreliable, however, there must be a wait of at least 6 weeks postpartum for a reliable testing of carbohydrate intolerance.

NORMAL POSTPARTUM HEALTH ASSESSMENT

Essential aspects of normal postpartum health assessment are pelvic musculature and breast evaluations and contraception counseling. See Chapter 17 for information on breast self-examination. Evaluation of pelvic musculature and contraception counseling are discussed here.

PELVIC MUSCULATURE

Pelvic musculature is assessed following pregnancy to evaluate involution and resumption of nonpregnant function (see Chapter 16). The general function of pelvic musculature is to support pelvic organs and assist urinary continence.

Etiology of Relaxed Pelvic Musculature

Relaxed musculature may be related to childbearing, age, obesity, or lack of exercise.

- Closely spaced pregnancies, vacuum/forcep-assisted vaginal deliveries, or large fetuses can stretch and traumatize pelvic musculature and contribute to relaxation.
- Aging, because of decreased estrogen production, contributes to loss of elasticity.
- Obesity increases intra-abdominal pressure and contributes to relaxation of vaginal muscles.
- Failure to perform Kegel exercises permits continued relaxation.

Subjective Data

A postpartum woman may report sensations of pelvic pressure, urinary incontinence, and lack of perineal support during defecation (Sampselle & Brink, 1990). Specific information needs to be pursued.

Although urinary incontinence has been associated with vaginal delivery, a prevalence of up to 14 percent (MacArthur et al., 2006) in women who have had a cesarean delivery suggests that pregnancy itself may be a risk factor for incontinence (Cunningham et al., 2010c). Therefore, evidence does not support the use of cesarean delivery to decrease incidence of stress urinary incontinence (SUI) in women (Sampselle, Palmer, Boyington, O'Dell, & Wooldridge, 2004). Inquire about

- Involuntary loss of urine during an activity that increases intra-abdominal pressure (e.g., coughing, sneezing)
- Age of onset and circumstances of incontinence
- Increase in severity or number of pelvic symptoms, or both, such as loss of bladder control, incomplete emptying of bladder, a sensation of vaginal pressure, inability to defecate without use of counter pressure.
- Day and night voiding patterns
- Frequency and severity of wetting
- Amount of urine lost (drops, teaspoon, tablespoon, quarter of cup, layer of clothing soaked)
- History of and reasons for previous vaginal or urinary tract surgery
- History of lower back surgery (the pudendal nerve innervates pelvic floor muscles and could have been damaged in surgery)
- Past history of SUI and method of treatment
- Fluid intake
- Medications, including over-the-counter, currently being used
- Use of bladder irritants, such as caffeine, nonnutritive sweeteners
- Number and type of deliveries (vaginal vs. cesarean) and complications (tears, lacerations, etc.)

SUI and detrusor instability should be differentiated (Rosenberg & Dmochowski, 2005). SUI results from an incompetent urethra. Urine is lost immediately with an event that increases intra-abdominal pressure. With detrusor instability (involuntary contraction), the bladder itself is the cause of incontinence. A delay occurs between the precipitating event and urine loss; urine loss may also be sudden and without warning.

Objective Data

The physical exam should be directed toward identifying any physical or neurological conditions that could affect a woman's ability to remain continent. The examination involves abdominal, pelvic, and neurologic assessments.

Assessment of the urine for evidence of infection, glycosuria, hematuria, and proteinuria should be routine, with treatment and further evaluation as indicated. The abdomen is assessed for masses, diastasis recti, organomegaly, peritonitis, and fluid collections. The pelvic examination involves assessing the health of the vulva and vagina, pelvic support, and evidence of urinary leakage. Urethral mobility can be assessed by inserting a lubricated cotton swab into the urethra and assessing for movement > 30° from the horizontal plane with a valsalva maneuver. The neurological evaluation assesses the vaginal strength and integrity of the sacral reflex (Rosenberg & Dmochowski, 2005).

Pelvic Examination. Digital measurement of pelvic muscle strength scale assesses vaginal muscles. Sampselle and Brink (1990) developed scoring criteria for pelvic muscle strength based on pressure, duration of pressure, and alteration in plane of examiner's fingers. The examiner inserts index and middle fingers 6 to 8 cm into the introitus on an anteroposterior plane and ask the client to contract her vaginal muscles around the fingers for as long as possible and as forcefully as possible. Scores range from 1 to 4, with 4 denoting the greatest muscle strength (Table 22–1).

The next step is to assess for cystocele, urethrocele, rectocele, and enterocele. Firmly exert pressure with fingers posterior to the vaginal wall and ask the client to bear down or cough. Observe the vaginal wall to detect an anterior bulge (cystocele or urethrocele). Continue pressing posteriorly with fingers while simultaneously separating them; ask the client to cough or bear down. Observe the posterior wall for a bulge (rectocele or enterocele).

Women should be examined for pelvic organ prolapse in the lithotomy, sitting, and standing positions. Examining the client only in the lithotomy position will obscure some pelvic support defects. Each organ that descends within the vaginal canal should be graded according to the maximum degree of descent. Clinical grading is as follows (ACOG, 2007; Doshani, Teo, Mayne, & Tincello, 2007):

- Grade 0—no descent
- Grade 1—descent between ischial spines and hymen > 1 cm above hymen
- Grade 2—descent between ischial spines and hymen < 1 cm above hymen
- Grade 3—descent within hymen
- Grade 4—descent through hymen

Plan

In a meta-analysis, Hay-Smith, Mørkved, Fairbrother, and Herbison (2008) conclude that women who did pelvic muscle exercises had less urinary incontinence in late pregnancy and 6 months postpartum than women who did not do pelvic muscle exercises. Sampselle and colleagues (1998) found initial pelvic muscle strength had significant effect on pelvic muscle strength at 12 months postpartum, supporting the importance of pelvic muscle exercise.

Pelvic muscle exercises benefit women with cystocele, urethrocele, rectocele, or enterocele that bulges into the vaginal vault but not outside the introitus. They may be done in any position as long as knees are 16 to 18 in. apart. Instruct the client to contract vaginal muscles as tightly as possible for as long as possible; the goal is to hold each contraction for 5 to 10 seconds. Initially, the client should contract her pelvic muscles while slowly counting to 5, hold, and gradually release to the count of 5. Sampselle and Brink (1990) advised a goal of 80 contractions per day (groups of 5 to 20 per session). More recently others have decreased the goal number to 30 contractions per day (Rosenberg & Dmochowski, 2005).

Refer the client to a urologist or gynecologist if she has a "cele" that descends beyond the introitus (a third degree).

CONTRACEPTION COUNSELING

Assessment

Assess a woman's knowledge of and preference for available contraceptive methods (see Chapter 12). She should be instructed in her choice of a temporary or permanent method. Temporary methods include barrier, hormonal, spermicidal devices, and periodic abstinence. Permanent methods are female and male sterilization.

TABLE 22–1. Pelvic Muscle Strength Rating Scale

Characteristic	1	2	3	4
Pressure	None	Weak, feel pressure on fingers, but not all way around	Moderate, feel pressure all around	Strong, fingers compress override
Duration	None	< 1 s	> 1 to < 3 s	> 3 s
Displacement in plane	None	Slight incline, base of fingers move up	Greater incline of fingers along total length	Fingers move up and are drawn in

Source: From Sampselle & Brink, 1990.

Reversible Contraceptive Methods

Combination Oral Contraception. If a breastfeeding mother prefers to use combination oral contraceptive pills (OCPs), advise her not to begin combination oral contraceptives until at least 6 months postpartum. The estrogen in the pill can decrease milk supply even with low-dose pills. If a combination pill is used, the estrogen should be ≤ 35 mcg, it should not be started prior to 8 to 12 weeks postpartum, and the pill should be taken just prior to the greatest interval between feedings (Kennedy & Trussell, 2011).

If not breastfeeding, women may begin combination oral contraception 3 weeks postpartum if they have no increased risk for venous thromboembolic (VTE) disease (CDC, 2011c; Kennedy & Trussell, 2011). Those with risk, such as history of VTE, age > 35, smokers, or delivery by cesarean section, should not start OCPs prior to 6 weeks postpartum. Starting OCPs before 6 weeks postpartum increases the risk of VTE (CDC, 2011c).

Other Combination Contraceptives. Other combination contraceptives include NuvaRing® and ORTHO EVRA® transdermal patch. If any of these methods are chosen, breastfeeding women should not be started on them until at least 8 weeks, but preferably 6 months, postpartum. The same starting guidelines for OCPs should be followed for bottlefeeding mothers when initiating use of these other combination contraceptives postpartum.

Progestin-Only Contraceptives. Progestin-only contraceptives (POCs) such as the minipill, Mirena IUD®, Implanon®, and Depo-Provera® are safe to use in breastfeeding women. They do not interfere with milk production and may even increase milk production. However, they may interfere with initial production of breast milk if given immediately postpartum. Therefore, POCs can be started, Depo-Provera® may be administered and Implanon® or the Mirena IUD® can be inserted, at the time of discharge if not lactating, and 6 weeks postpartum if breastfeeding (Kennedy & Trussell, 2011).

Careful evaluation is needed for women with current depression or with a history of severe postpartum depression if considering use of Depo-Provera as its use has been associated with increased risk for worsening of depression. Counseling related to adequate dietary calcium, vitamin D, and weight bearing exercise are also recommended due to the impact of Depo-Provera on bone density. Additionally, the woman needs to be aware that conception can be delayed up to 9 to 10 months after discontinuation of Depo-Provera (Bartz & Goldberg, 2011).

Barrier Methods. Lubricated condoms may be helpful to decrease discomfort related to vaginal dryness. The client who desires to use the contraceptive sponge should be made aware that it has a higher failure rate for parous women and it should not be used prior to 6 weeks postpartum because of risk for toxic shock. Diaphragms or cervical caps should be fitted at the 6-week postpartum exam, as they cannot be fitted properly before that time because of pelvic changes. Episiotomies are also tender and attempting to fit a diaphragm before 6 weeks would only increase the client's discomfort. Fitting should also be deferred until that time because use while bleeding increases the risk of toxic shock syndrome (Kennedy & Trussell, 2011).

Intrauterine Device. Intrauterine devices (IUDs) can be inserted immediately after the delivery of the placenta, within 48 hours postpartum, or at the 6-week postpartum exam. The copper T380A has been shown to be a safe and effective IUD for postpartum women. Expulsion rates and risk for endometritis are higher in immediate postpartum insertion than at the 6-week exam (Kennedy & Trussell, 2011).

Spermicides. Because breastfeeding can cause a decrease in estrogen, spermicides may add comfort by relieving vaginal dryness during intercourse.

Lactation Amenorrhea Method. It should be stressed that breastfeeding is not considered an effective method of birth control. But, if used solely to supply the infant with food and if the infant is completely breast-fed without any supplements, it may be effective (Kennedy & Trussell, 2011). It is used to space pregnancies in many cultures and can be 98 percent effective during the first 6 months (Kennedy & Trussell, 2011; Mohrbacher & Stock, 2003). Criteria for lactation amenorrhea method include no menses (no vaginal bleeding after the 56th day after birth), *and* no supplementing regularly nor going longer than 4 hours between feedings during the day or longer than 6 hours between feedings at night, *and* the baby is younger than 6 months old (Lawrence & Lawrence, 2011; Mohrbacher & Stock, 2003).

Natural Family Planning. Women who are not exclusively breastfeeding and who do not desire pregnancy should be advised of all available contraceptive options. If the woman doesn't desire medication or contraceptive devices, natural family planning should be discussed with her and her partner. Lawrence and Lawrence (2011) state that most women who are totally breastfeeding are likely to have a first menses that is anovulatory. Unplanned pregnancy rates rise among breastfeeding women after the onset of first menses compared with nonlactating women who use thermal or cervical mucous surveillance methods. Basal body temperature (BBT) cannot be determined unless the woman has had 6 hours of uninterrupted sleep, so thermal surveillance may not be accurate if breastfeeding (Kennedy & Trussell, 2011). Lawrence and Lawrence state that studies showing changes in cervical secretions during lactation are reliable. They recommend the couple note when (1) the infant sleeps through the night, (2) the mother reduces the number of breastfeedings, (3) the infant begins solid food, (4) the infant begins other liquids or a bottle, and (5) illness occurs in either the mother or the infant. They advise abstinence in any of these situations until the situation regarding sign of ovulation is clear.

Cervical mucus changes may be misleading during anovulatory postpartum cycles, as dry mucus is similar to that of preovulatory days during an ovulatory cycle; profuse, thick mucus makes identification of mucous patterns for prediction of ovulation difficult.

- Take BBT if cervical mucus appears or the cervix opens or becomes elevated.
- Infertility of breastfeeding can be reasonably assumed if cervical mucus remains tacky for 3 weeks and does not become clear and stretchy (Davis, 1992). Clear and stretchy cervical mucus is the strongest indicator of return to ovulation and fertility in women who are breastfeeding.
- With intermittent signs of cervical mucus discharge, begin BBT. When mucus lasts 3 or more days and its cessation is accompanied by continued low temperature, breastfeeding infertility can be assumed 2 days after mucus disappears (Davis, 1992; Lawrence & Lawrence, 2011). To better assess mucus, coitus should not be more often than every other day so that the presence of ejaculate and sexual lubrication does not interfere with cervical mucus.

If weaning occurs slowly after 3 to 4 months, daily BBT should be continued and cervical mucus checked for onset of ovulation. Coitus is allowed throughout a 10-day weaning period. The couple should consider themselves fertile on the 11th day until cervical and thermal signs show ovulation has occurred (Davis, 1992). If weaning occurs naturally, the client should monitor for signs of ovulation (Davis, 1992; Lawrence & Lawrence, 2011).

In general, for those planning to use natural family planning, the importance of exclusive breastfeeding, as well as the importance of continuing breastfeeding to maintain postpartum infertility, should be taught to clients and their partners. Refer clients to breastfeeding support groups and local lactation consultants.

ASSESSMENT OF POSTOPERATIVE CESAREAN BIRTH AND STERILIZATION

Following cesarean birth, encourage ambulation to decrease risk of thrombosis and embolism. Assess for thrombophlebitis by checking the lower extremities for edema, positive Homan's sign, muscle pain, tenderness, erythema, or induration along a vein. Give analgesics shortly before ambulation. Monitor intake and urinary output by measurement for 24 hours or institutional policy. Observe wound for infection. Encourage woman's contact with family and infant.

After female sterilization, clients should be aware that mild analgesia, such as nonsteroidal anti-inflammatory drugs (NSAIDs), should provide relief. For women not obtaining relief with NSAIDs, medication such as Tylenol #3® or Percocet® can be used. Observe for infection, hematoma at incision site, including episiotomy (if performed). Encourage contact with infant prior to and after surgery.

THE 2- TO 3-WEEK POSTPARTUM ASSESSMENT

Subjective Data

Several points of information may be gained from the mother or from hospital records at the 2- to 3-week postpartum assessment. Generally review the woman's systems, with specific attention to the following:

- Type of birth (vaginal or cesarean); amount and color of vaginal bleeding; presence of foul odor or clots; length of labor and complications during labor, delivery, and postpartum. Support system during labor and delivery.
- If cesarean birth, determine if staples removed, and inquire about drainage from incision. If vaginal delivery with tubal ligation, ask about umbilical incision. If episiotomy performed, assess for tears, lacerations.
- Assess for amount and frequency of pain with urination; constipation; use of medications (prescription and over-the-counter) and herbs and reason for use; effectiveness of pain medication in obtaining pain relief; hemorrhoids; fever.

- Weight and sex of baby. Inquire regarding problems or concerns with baby (feeding, jaundice, colic, elimination patterns, assistance in caring for baby).
- Number of days in hospital, general well-being of both mother and baby.
- Assess family adjustments: father's role, sibling behavior, extended family. Assess support system.
- Bladder and bowel function. Diet/appetite, sleep patterns/fatigue.

Review the mother's feelings and understandings about delivery. If mother experienced a cesarean birth, explore her understanding of the medical reasons and review type of uterine incision and guidelines for vaginal birth after cesarean. Ask if sexual activity has been resumed. If sexual activity has been resumed, inquire about any pain or discomfort. Inquire about type of contraception being used or whether contraception is desired. Reassure that length of time to reach prepregnant weight may take 1 year.

Objective Data

Physical Examination

General Appearance, Vital Signs, Weight. Does the woman appear rested, fatigued, depressed? Does she appear neat and well groomed or ill-kept? Compare blood pressure to range during pregnancy. Compare weight to prepregnant weight and weight at delivery.

Neck. Thyroid nonpalpable or palpable, but soft and without nodules. If thyromegaly or nodules palpated, evaluate for bruits, obtain TFT, and refer for medical evaluation. (See section Postpartum Thyroiditis for further information.)

Cardiovascular and Respiratory. Regular rate and rhythm without murmurs or extra sounds. Clear, equal breath sounds bilaterally.

Breasts. Lactating: Full, without erythema, masses, or lymphadenopathy. Milk easily expressed. *Nonlactating:* Soft, without masses or lymphadenopathy. Bilateral galactorrhea may be present in nonlactating women for up to 3 months postpartum.

Abdomen and Musculoskeletal. Assess for CVAT and tenderness along paraspinous muscles. Fundus is usually nonpalpable above the symphysis and is nontender to gentle palpation. If cesarean birth or sterilization performed, the incision is well healed without exudate, and nontender. Lower extremities are inspected for redness, warmth, and pain in calves. Assess for Homan's sign (pain elicited with dorsiflexion of foot). (See section Thromboembolism for more information.)

Genitalia/Reproductive. Inspect perineum for swelling, hemorrhoids. If episiotomy noted, assess for edema, erythema, ecchymosis, approximation of edges. Bimanual is generally deferred until 6-week postpartum exam.

Psychological. Assess affect and interactions with infant.

Laboratory Tests. See section Diagnostic Tests, The 4- to 6-Week Postpartum Assessment.

Health Teaching. Review ways to ensure adequate rest (sleep when infant does, avoid late-night television, limit visitations). Advise to change perineal pads frequently and frequent voiding to decrease uterine afterpains. Review perineal cleansing/sitz baths/warm water soaks. Assess whether prenatal vitamins are still being taken. If history of prenatal anemia or postpartum hemorrhage, inquire whether iron supplements are being taken and dosing used. Encourage adequate fluid intake and adequate nutrition to promote tissue healing.

THE 6-WEEK POSTCESAREAN BIRTH ASSESSMENT

The 6-week postpartum evaluation of a woman who had a cesarean birth is the same as that of a woman who delivered vaginally, except that the abdominal incision is assessed following a cesarean birth as well as the perineum and vulva.

COMMON POSTPARTUM COMPLICATIONS

Table 22–2 summarizes the postpartum complications.

GESTATIONAL DIABETES

Gestational diabetes is carbohydrate intolerance that is induced by pregnancy (see Chapter 20).

Epidemiology

Gestational diabetes may persist into the postpartum period. More than 50 percent of women with gestational diabetes develop overt diabetes within 20 years. This likelihood increases if the woman experienced fasting hyperglycemia or the need for use of insulin was present in pregnancy (Cunningham et al., 2010j).

TABLE 22–2. Summary of Postpartum Complications

Complication	Signs and Symptoms	Management
Postpartum hemorrhage (early)	Soft, boggy uterus; cool, clammy skin; fever; tachycardia; vertigo; tachypnea	Maintain patient IV line and begin second line; call physician; type and cross for blood; bimanual uterine massage if boggy uterus; oxytocic agents; elevate right hip; CBC and coagulation studies Meds: Oxytocin 40 units in 1,000 mL of intravenous solution of lactated Ringers at 20–40 mU/min until uterus firm, then continue for 24 hours postpartum or as directed by physician Methylergonovine maleate 0.2 mg intramuscularly Carboprost 250 mcg intramuscularly, repeated as necessary q15–90 minutes for maximum eight doses Misoprostol 400–600 μg oral, sublingual, or rectal
Postpartum hemorrhage (late)	Heavy lochia; foul lochia; fever; opened cervical os; pelvic or back pain; uterine tenderness; prolonged bleeding	Bed rest; physician consultation; breastfeeding if possible Meds: Methylergonovine maleate 0.2–0.4 mg po q6–8h for 2–3 days Antibiotics if infection suspected
Subinvolution	Painless, heavy vaginal bleeding; uterine size larger than expected; uterine tenderness; fever	CBC; endocervical cultures; quantitative beta-HCG Meds: Methergine 0.2 mg q4–6h 3days Augmentin 500 mg qid 7–10 days Azithromycin 500 mg daily for 1–2 days, then 250 mg daily for total of 7 days Doxycycline 100 mg bid × 10 days
Mastitis	Flu-like symptoms; malaise; fever and chills; erythema and swelling of affected breast with possible pitting edema	Milk culture; bed rest; continue breastfeeding; ice packs/warm packs; increased fluid intake Meds: First choice—Dicloxacillin sodium 250–500 mg qid 10–14 days Penicillin allergy: Erythromycin 500 mg qid 10–14 days CA-MRSA: Clindamycin 300 mg qid 10–14 days or trimethoprim/sulfamethoxazole 100 mg bid 10–14 days if infant > 4 weeks of age
Metritis with pelvic cellulitis	Unilateral/bilateral abdominal pain; foul lochia; fever; parametrial tenderness; leukocytosis	Medical consultation; hospitalization; rest Meds: (Intravenous)—Gentamicin and clindamycin are gold standard—give until afebrile for 48 hours Cefotetan 2 g q12h Cefoxitin 1–2 g q6–8h Gentamicin 1.5 mg/kg of body weight in three divided doses q8h with clindamycin 900 mg every 8 hours Single-dose gentamicin: 5 mg/kg Oral: Clindamycin 150–300 mg qid × 10 days Augmentin 500 mg qid × 10 days Cephalosporin 500 mg qid × 10 days
Postpartum thyroiditis (thyrotoxicosis)	Weight loss; increased fatigue; palpitations; heat intolerance; sinus tachycardia	Radioactive iodine uptake; physician referral Propranolol (40–120 mg q8h)
Postpartum thyroiditis (transient hypothyroidism)	Pronounced fatigue; continued weight gain; coarse hair; dry skin; delayed reflexes; psychologic reactions mimicking depression	Elevated TSH; physician consultation Meds: Thyroxine therapy—begin with 0.1 mg/day
Urinary tract infection	Spiking fever; Costovertebral angle tenderness; Dysuria; Urgency; Oliguria.	Urinalysis with culture and sensitivity Meds: Macrobid 100 mg q12h × 3–5 days Sulfamethoxazole/trimethoprim q12h × 3–5 days Cephalexin: 250–500 mg q6h 3–5 days
Appendicitis	RUQ or entire right abdominal tenderness; positive Bryan's sign (pain elicited when enlarged uterus moved to right); positive Alder's test (pain elicited when clinician maintains constant pressure at area of maximal tenderness and woman rolls from supine to left position)	Endocervical and lochial cultures; CBC; UA; medical referral; hospitalization

Sources: ACOG, 1998, 2000, 2002, 2006; Cunningham et al., 2010d, 2010f, 2010g, 2010h, 2010k; French & Smaill, 2009; Lawrence & Lawrence, 2011; Muller et al., 2001; Olson, 2002; Wilson, Shannon, & Shields, 2012.

Subjective Data

The client states she had diabetes during her pregnancy.

Objective Data

The 2-hour oral glucose tolerance test (2hr GTT) was traditionally used to detect diabetes in nonpregnant women (American Diabetes Association [ADA], 2002). Current guidelines advise use of HgbA1C testing for nonpregnant women (Zhang et al., 2010). However, the 2hr GTT continues to be recommended for use postpartum in women previously diagnosed with gestational diabetes, and it is administered at 6 weeks postpartum. The test measures the rate at which a concentrated amount of glucose is removed from the bloodstream (see Chapter 23).

If the test is performed, the procedure requires that for the 3 days preceding the test, the client consumes a diet containing at least 150 g of carbohydrate (300 g preferred) per day. After overnight fasting (12 hours), a sample of blood is taken. The client then drinks a preparation containing 75 g of glucose. She must drink all of the solution. A blood sample is then taken 2 hours later.

Counsel the client regarding the purpose of the test and the need for a high carbohydrate diet during the 3 days prior to the test. Remind the client that overnight fasting is required. In addition, advise her not to drink alcohol and caffeine the evening prior to the test and not to smoke during the 2-hour blood testing.

Differential Medical Diagnosis

Diabetes Mellitus

- *Normal values:* Fasting, < 110 mg/dL; 2-hour plasma glucose, < 140 mg/dL.
- *Impaired glucose tolerance:* Fasting, ≥ 110 and < 126 mg/dL, and 2-hour plasma glucose, ≥ 140 and < 200 mg/dL after 75 g glucose load (ADA, 2002).
- *Diabetic values:* One of the following is needed for a positive diagnosis—unequivocal elevation of plasma glucose ≥ 200 mg/dL and classic symptoms of diabetes, including polydipsia, polyuria, polyphagia, and unexplained weight loss; fasting, ≥ 126 mg/dL on two occasions; 2-hour plasma glucose, ≥ 200 mg/dL after 75 g oral glucose tolerance test (ADA, 2002). Confirming the results by repeated testing on a subsequent day is recommended.

Plan

- *Postpartum care:* In the gestational diabetic not requiring insulin (Class A_1), postpartum care is identical to that of the nondiabetic woman. Insulin requirements fall dramatically postpartum because of the decrease in placental hormones (Cunningham et al., 2010j). Insulin is no longer required postpartally in the woman with gestational diabetes requiring insulin (Class A_2). She should be advised to continue her self-monitoring of blood glucose to be sure she remains euglycemic. In the postpartum woman who had pregestational diabetes, insulin is given at approximately one half of her prepregnancy dose.
- *Psychosocial intervention:* Assess the client's lifestyle and knowledge of diabetes and its management. If lifestyle changes are indicated, counsel the client about the specific change (e.g., diet or exercise). Provide clear, accurate information regarding non-gestational diabetes and its usual signs and symptoms and management. Refer the client to support groups if indicated. Frank diabetes may develop as she ages.
- *Medication:* Medication is not usually needed after 1 to 2 days postpartum.
- *Follow-up:* Refer the client to an endocrinologist if frank diabetes is revealed.

PERSISTENT HYPERTENSION

Gestational hypertension that resolves within 12 weeks postpartum is termed *transient hypertension* (Cunningham et al., 2010e). Chronic hypertension is blood pressure that remains significantly elevated beyond this time frame in the postpartum period. It is usually indicative of chronic vascular disease. (See Chapter 23 for information about hypertension in nonpregnant women.)

Subjective Data

The client may report a family history of hypertension or a diagnosis of gestational hypertension. She may have no specific symptoms.

Objective Data

Physical examination reveals a systolic blood pressure equal to or greater than 140, a diastolic blood pressure equal to or greater than 90, or both. No edema is evident. Reflexes are within normal limits. Other findings are normal.

Diagnostic tests include a urine dipstick for protein, baseline electrolyte, blood urea nitrogen (BUN), and creatinine levels, urinalysis for protein urea, and baseline albumin, calcium, and phosphorus levels. More extensive testing (e.g., electrocardiogram) if indicated by extent of findings.

Differential Medical Diagnoses

Essential hypertension, hyperaldosteronism, hyperthyroidism, pheochromocytoma, renovascular disease.

Plan

- *Psychosocial intervention:* Determine stress levels and sources of stress and counsel the client regarding ways to reduce stress. Referral for support and counseling may be appropriate.
- *Medication:* The safety of medications must be considered if the client is breastfeeding.
- *Lifestyle changes:* Provide dietary counseling to help the client reduce sodium and fat intake. She should maintain adequate complex carbohydrate, protein, and polyunsaturated fats. Counsel regarding exercise for aerobic health. Lactating mothers require information about specific dietary modifications and exercise. Advise mothers to stop smoking; explain cardiovascular changes that occur with smoking. In addition, advise the client not to consume alcohol as it is associated with hypertension in women (Sesso, Cook, Buring, Manson, & Gaziano, 2008).
- *Follow-up:* Postpartum follow-up for those with elevated blood pressure in pregnancy should occur 1 week after hospital discharge; if hypertension persists, consult with a physician or refer the client for management.

POSTPARTUM ECLAMPSIA

Definitions and Pathophysiology

Eclampsia may complicate pregnancies after 20 weeks' gestation and usually occurs closer to term. Eclampsia normally resolves with delivery. Postpartum eclampsia may occur within 48 hours of delivery. Chames, Livingston, Ivester, Barton, and Sibai (2002) did a multicenter analysis of data of women with eclampsia from March 1996 to February 2001 at the University of Cincinnati, the University of Tennessee (Memphis), and Central Baptist Hospital (Lexington). The study focused on women who experienced late postpartum eclampsia. The results showed that 89 women were diagnosed with eclampsia, of which 23 women had late onset (greater than 48 hours). Of these 23 women, only 5 had been previously diagnosed with preeclampsia. More importantly, 91 percent of women with late postpartum eclampsia had at least one symptom suggestive of preeclampsia, but only 33 percent of the women reported the symptom to a health care provider (Chames et al., 2002). This alarming finding underscores the need for health care providers to educate all postpartum women on symptoms of preeclampsia. Printed instructions may be given to all postpartum women at discharge, with instructions to call their health care provider if they experience any of these symptoms. (See Chapter 20 for information about gestational hypertension.)

Subjective Data

The client may report severe and persistent occipital headaches, blurred vision, photophobia, scomata, epigastric or right upper quadrant pain, retrosternal chest pain, shortness of breath, nausea or vomiting, bleeding from mucosal membranes, or jaundice (Cunningham et al., 2010e; Sibai & Stella, 2009).

Objective Data

Physical Examination. Proteinuria and hypertension are present. Edema is no longer included in diagnostic criteria because it is so common in normal pregnancies (National Institutes of Health, 2000). Hypertension is diagnosed when blood pressure is 140/90 mmHg or greater, using Korotkoff phase V to define diastolic blood pressure (ACOG, 2002a, reaffirmed 2010; Cunningham et al., 2010e). Assess for brisk reflexes with clonus.

Diagnostic Tests. Urinalysis, platelet count, BUN, lactate dehydrogenase, alanine aminotransferase, aspartate transaminase, plasma glucose, prothrombin time (PT), partial thromboplastin time (PTT), electrolytes, serum creatinine, fibrinogen. ACOG (2002a, reaffirmed 2010) states that uric acid is only predictive of preeclampsia 33 percent of the time and has not proved useful. Magnetic resonance imaging (MRI) of the brain may be indicated.

Differential Medical Diagnoses

Cerebral venous thrombosis, intracerebral hemorrhage, essential hypertension, encephalopathy, pheochromocytoma, tumors of the central nervous system, metabolic disorders, epilepsy.

Plan

Medical. Refer to the physician for further management and hospitalization; consider neurological consultation. Medication used is identical to management of antepartum client with preeclampsia and consists of anticonvulsant and antihypertensive therapy (see Chapter 23).

Psychosocial. Provide emotional support; address concerns of mother regarding her own safety as well as the care of her newborn.

POSTPARTUM HEMORRHAGE

Traditionally, postpartum hemorrhage has been defined as loss of blood exceeding 500 mL within the first 24 hours after delivery (early postpartum hemorrhage) or after 24 hours but before 12 weeks postpartum (late or secondary postpartum hemorrhage) (ACOG, 2006, reaffirmed 2008; Cunningham et al., 2010c, 2010f; Rath, 2011). In fact, blood loss is about 500 to 600 mL for a vaginal delivery, 1,000 mL for a cesarean delivery, 1,400 mL for elective cesarean hysterectomy, and 3,000 to 3,500 mL for emergency cesarean hysterectomy (Cunningham et al., 2010f; Rath, 2011). Several authors (Cunningham et al., 2010f; Rath, 2011) report inaccuracy of visual measurement of postpartum blood loss, with as much as a 34 to 50 percent underestimation. ACOG (2006, reaffirmed 2008) has defined postpartum hemorrhage as a "10 percent change in hematocrit between admission and the postpartum period or a need for erythrocyte transfusion." However, hematocrit changes do not correlate well with the blood and red blood cell volume deficits that occur with postpartum hemorrhage. Blood pressure may remain normal until 30 to 40 percent of blood volume is lost and may be artificially low if taken by arm cuff. Factors contributing to hemorrhage are uterine atony, coagulopathy, birth canal trauma, and poor general health.

Early Postpartum Hemorrhage

Early hemorrhage refers to that which occurs during the first 24 hours postpartum. Several risk factors have been identified.

- Uterine atony—hypotonic myometrium, interuterine rupture, uterine inversion
- Uterine overdistention (macrosomic infant, multiple fetuses, polyhydramnios)
- Midforceps delivery, forceps rotation, intrauterine manipulation
- Delivery through incompletely dilated cervix
- Prolonged labor, precipitous labor, prolonged third stage (30–60 minutes)
- Use of drugs to induce or augment labor or use of halogenated anesthetics
- History of previous postpartum hemorrhage
- Grand multiparity
- Retained placental tissue, chorioamnionitis
- Distended bladder
- Coagulation defects
- Fibroids
- Placenta previa, placenta accreta, or abruptio placentae
- Obesity

Subjective Data

The client may report vertigo, extreme fatigue, chills, or a history of anemia.

Objective Data

Physical examination reveals cool, clammy skin; fever; rapid, thready pulse; tachypnea; pallor of nail beds; and mucous membranes. Bleeding may not be massive; however, a steady seepage may continue. If uterine atony is the cause of blood loss, the uterus feels boggy and clots are easily expressed with massage.

The CBC provides a reliable measurement of blood loss. CBC and clotting studies (PT, PTT, fibrinogen, and platelet count) are done to determine the nature and extent of any coagulation disorders contributing to the abnormal bleeding. Anticipate blood transfusion and request cross-matching of blood (packed red blood cells). Consult with the physician for management.

Differential Medical Diagnoses

Early postpartum hemorrhage secondary to uterine atony, early postpartum hemorrhage secondary to lacerations, hemorrhage secondary to blood coagulopathies.

Plan

Psychosocial Intervention. Provide emotional support. Inform the client in a calm tone of the procedures that are being instituted. Encouraging the woman to breast-feed will help in the release of oxytocin and, therefore, help facilitate natural uterine contractions.

Other Interventions

- Maintain patent intravenous line and begin second intravenous line.
- Bimanual uterine massage if atonic uterus.

- If bleeding persists and uterus is firm, evaluate vagina, cervix, and uterus for lacerations.
- Elevate right hip (prevent vena cava syndrome).
- Oxygen therapy with face mask at 6 to 8 L per minute; provide positive pressure ventilation if needed.
- Call the physician and inform him or her of client's status and corrective measures already instituted.
- Assess client's response by monitoring vital signs.
- Insert Foley catheter to measure urinary output and to empty an over distended bladder.
- Record intravenous fluids infused.

Medication

First-Line Oxytocin

- *Indication:* Uterine stimulation.
- *Administration:* Diluted in intravenous fluids per hospital or agency protocol; usually 10 to 40 units in 1,000 mL of normal saline or lactated Ringer's solution given at 20 to 40 mU/min (ACOG, 2006, reaffirmed 2008; World Health Organization [WHO], 2009). Oxytocin should never be given as an undiluted IV bolus as it can result in severe hypotension and cardiac arrythmias (Cunningham et al., 2010f).
- *Side effects:* Hypertension, uterine tetany, nausea, vomiting, bradycardia, tachycardia, premature ventricular contractions, water intoxication.
- *Contraindication:* Hypersensitivity to oxytocin.
- *Anticipated outcomes on evaluation:* Decreased uterine bleeding and increased uterine tone.
- *Client teaching:* Inform the client that she will experience increased uterine contractions, which may be quite uncomfortable.

Second-Line Methylergonovine Maleate (Methergine)

- *Indications:* Uterine and vascular smooth muscle constriction.
- *Administration:* Intramuscularly, orally, and, in an emergency, intravenously.
  - *Intramuscular:* 0.2 mg, repeated in 2 to 4 hours (ACOG, 2006, reaffirmed 2008; Cunningham et al., 2010f; WHO, 2009).
  - *Oral:* 0.2 to 0.4 mg every 6 to 8 hours, usually for 2 days.
  - *Intravenous:* Hazardous; should be reserved for emergency control of postpartum hemorrhage. If methylergonovine maleate is given intravenously, 0.2 mg is infused over 60 seconds or longer. Ergot alkaloids can cause profound vasoconstriction.
- *Side effects:* Headache, dizziness, nausea, vomiting, chest pain, palpitation, hypertension (especially when given intravenously).
- *Contraindications:* Hypertension, hypersensitivity to ergot alkaloids, respiratory disease, cardiac disease, peripheral vascular disease.
- *Anticipated outcome on evaluation:* Decreased uterine bleeding.
- *Client teaching:* Inform the client about possible side effects and increased uterine cramping.

Third-Line Prostaglandins

- *Indication:* Uterine contraction.
- *Administration:* Intramuscularly—15-methyl PGF2α (carboprost, Prostin 15M, Hemabate) 250 μg, repeated as necessary every 15 to 90 minutes, up to maximum of eight doses (ACOG, 2006, reaffirmed 2008; Cunningham et al., 2010f; WHO, 2009). Preferable to prostaglandin E_2, which may cause vasodilation or exacerbation of hypotension (ACOG, 2006, reaffirmed 2008). However, Dinoprostin or prostaglandin E_2 (Cervidil, Prepidil, Prostin E_2) is preferable to carboprost for women with heart or lung disease. The dose is 20 mg per rectum every 2 hours.
- *Side effects:* Mild fever, diarrhea, abdominal cramping, vomiting, hypotension, hypertension. Prostaglandins can also cause bronchoconstriction, pulmonary vasoconstriction, hypo- or hypertension, and arterial oxygen desaturation (use with caution in clients with bronchospastic or renal disorders or arterial or pulmonary hypertension).
- *Contraindications:* Hypersensitivity, respiratory disease.
- *Anticipated outcome on evaluation:* Decreased uterine bleeding.
- *Client teaching:* Counsel the client regarding possible side effects, including abdominal cramps, low-grade fever, and diarrhea.

Misoprostel. 400 to 600 μg, orally, sublingually, or rectally. Side effects of fever and shivering are more highly associated with the oral or sublingual route and higher dosages (Mansouri & Alsahly, 2011). It has been found effective for control of postpartum hemorrhage in a randomized controlled trial of 658 patients who received misoprostel by either the oral or the rectal route (Mansouri & Alsahly, 2011).

Anesthesia/Analgesia. Choice of regional or general anesthesia depends upon client's stability, cause of hemorrhage, presence of underlying disease pathology, potential for further blood loss, need for additional surgery, and the expertise of the anesthesiologist.

Follow-Up

Advise the client to eat foods high in protein and iron to aid in tissue healing and build up body iron stores. Iron supplements will be needed for an additional 2 to 3 months postpartum. If blood loss was rapid and severe, monitor for signs and symptoms of Sheehan's syndrome (hypopituitarism).

LATE OR SECONDARY POSTPARTUM HEMORRHAGE

Late hemorrhage occurs after the first 24 hours and up to 12 weeks postpartum. Its usual onset is 6 to 10 days after delivery. Several risk factors have been identified:

- Retained placental tissue
- Uterine subinvolution
- Infection
- von Willebrand disease

Subjective Data

The client may report pelvic or back pain, uterine tenderness, or bleeding for more than 2 weeks.

Objective Data

Physical examination may reveal heavy lochia with a foul odor, fever, an open cervical os after the first week postpartum, and hematoma.

A CBC is ordered (see Early Postpartum Hemorrhage).

Differential Medical Diagnoses

Trauma, blood coagulopathy.

Plan

- *Psychosocial intervention:* Provide emotional support by assisting to calm the client and her family—speaking calmly and giving information about procedures (see Early Postpartum Hemorrhage). She may need help obtaining child or infant care.
- *Medication:* Methylergonovine maleate, oxytocin, or prostaglandin analog as discussed under Early Postpartum Hemorrhage. Antibiotics should be added if endometritis is suspected (see Endometritis).
- *Ultrasound:* Ultrasound examination is done to detect retained placental fragments.

Follow-Up

Consult with a physician to determine need for hospital admission or other management.

SUBINVOLUTION OF THE UTERUS

Subinvolution of the uterus is the arrest or prolongation of the normal involution process that occurs following pregnancy (Cunningham et al., 2010c). Complications of subinvolution include hemorrhage, pelvic peritonitis, salpingitis, and abscess formation.

Epidemiology

Several risk factors are identified in the etiology of subinvolution:

- Distended bladder
- Retained placental fragments
- Endometritis
- Cesarean birth
- Uterine myoma
- Multiparity

Subjective Data

The client may report painless, excessive vaginal bleeding; chills and fever; pelvic or back pain. Obtain sexual history from client—resumption of intercourse, use of sex toys, new partner, contraceptive used and type.

Objective Data

Physical examination of the genitalia and reproductive tract reveals whether the uterus is larger than expected for the period of puerperium and whether fundal height is normal—at the level of the bony pelvis by 2 weeks postpartum. The uterus should return to nonpregnant size at 4 to 6 weeks postpartum (Cunningham et al., 2010c). With subinvolution, the uterus feels boggy and soft and may be tender. Uterine bleeding, excessive lochia, and leukorrhea are possible. Fever may also be present.

Diagnostic tests include serum blood tests, culture of cervical discharge, and ultrasound.

- A CBC is performed to detect anemia and infection.
- An erythrocyte sedimentation rate (ESR) is a diagnostic evaluation for occult infective disease.
- Cervical discharge is cultured to identify a specific infective agent. Before a cervical specimen is obtained, the client should be informed about the use of the speculum, the testing to be done, and the reason for the test.

- Quantitative determination of the beta-subunit human chorionic gonadotropin (β-hCG) assists the health care provider in detecting pregnancy, trophoblastic tumors, and tumors that ectopically secrete hCG. Explain the rationale for requesting the test to the client.
- Pelvic ultrasound is done to evaluate whether placental fragments were retained. As the abdominal probe will be used as part of the exam, instruct the client to drink four glasses of water 1 hour prior to the ultrasound exam.

Differential Medical Diagnosis

Distended bladder, ovarian cyst, pelvic adhesions, malignant uterine tumors, cystitis, gestational trophoblastic disease, anemia, uterine leiomyoma, retained placental fragments.

Plan

Psychosocial Intervention. Inform the client about the diagnosis, suspected etiology, and plan of treatment. Explain that methylergonovine may cause painful uterine contractions. Advise her of the need to rest and avoid overexertion.

Medication. For information on methylergonovine maleate, see Early Postpartum Hemorrhage. If infection is suspected, treat presumptively with antibiotics (Cunningham et al., 2010c, 2010d). Antibiotics that may be used include the following:

Amoxicillin Clavulanate Potassium (Augmentin)

- *Indication:* Broad-spectrum antibiotic. Because augmentin contains a β-lactamase inhibitor, it is effective against bacteria that produce β-lactamase.
- *Administration:* One 500 mg tablet orally every 8 hours for 10 days.
- *Side effects:* Nausea, vomiting, diarrhea, vaginitis, eosinophilia, leukopenia.
- *Contraindication:* History of penicillin allergy.
- *Anticipated outcome on evaluation:* Clinically decreased evidence of infection. Check culture and sensitivity report from earlier cultures to confirm effectiveness of chosen antibiotic.
- *Client teaching:* Instruct the client to complete the 10-day medication regimen. Tell the client to telephone if side effects make compliance difficult or if no improvement in symptoms.

Azithromycin

- *Indication:* Broad-spectrum anti-infective.
- *Administration:* One to two 500 mg doses, then 250 mg daily for a total of 7 days.
- *Side effects:* Diarrhea, nausea, abdominal pain, anorexia, cramping, vomiting.
- *Contraindications:* Hypersensitivity to azithromycin or other macrolides.
- *Anticipated outcome on evaluation:* Decreased clinical evidence of infection. Check culture and sensitivity report to confirm organism's responsiveness.
- *Client teaching:* Explain to the client not to take azithromycin with antacids that contain aluminum or magnesium. May take with or without food and should maintain adequate hydration.

Doxycycline

- *Indication:* Broad-spectrum antibiotic/anti-infective.
- *Administration:* One 100 mg tablet orally every 12 hours for 10 days.
- *Side effects:* Anorexia, nausea, vomiting, diarrhea, esophageal irritation, rashes, photosensitivity.
- *Contraindications:* Hypersensitivity to tetracyclines, pregnancy, lactation. Because elimination is primarily nonrenal, doxycycline, unlike tetracycline, may be used for clients with renal failure.
- *Anticipated outcome on evaluation:* Decreased clinical evidence of infection.
- *Client teaching:* Emphasize the need to complete the 10-day medication regimen. Instruct the client to avoid sun exposure (sunscreen does not seem to decrease photosensitivity) and to take doxycycline with a full glass of water. Do not lie down at least 1 hour after administration to avoid epigastric discomfort. The drug may be taken with meals, as its absorption is not affected by food.

Hospitalization. Hospitalization may be necessary if infection is severe, if pelvic structures in addition to the uterus are involved, or if uterine bleeding is excessive.

Follow-Up

Reassess the uterus in 1 to 2 weeks. Report signs and symptoms of hemorrhage, pelvic peritonitis, salpingitis, or abscess to the physician for further evaluation and management.

ENDOMETRITIS

Postpartum endometritis is inflammation of the decidua following childbirth and is one of the causes of puerperal fever (Chen, Ramin, & Barss, 2010; Cunningham et al., 2010d; French & Smaill, 2009). *Endomyometritis* is the term used to denote that the inflammation also involves the myometrium and parametritis indicates parametrial involvement (Chen et al., 2010). Cunningham et al. (2010d) propose using the term *metritis with pelvic cellulitis*, as most often all three area are involved. Bacteria from an infected surgical incision and/or from a colonized cervix and vagina enter amniotic fluid during labor. Once in amniotic fluid, bacteria invade uterine tissue postpartum. Bacteria invade the remaining uterine decidua up to a few days postpartum. Postpartum endometritis is usually polymicrobial (Chen et al., 2010; French & Smaill, 2009). Anaerobic pathogens are implicated in 40 to 60 percent of endometritis diagnoses following cesarean section, and 25 percent of women will not respond to antibiotic therapy unless an agent giving good anaerobic coverage is also used (ACOG, 1998). Endomyoparametritis is associated with retention of placental or amniotic sac remnants and is potentially life-threatening (Kim, Hayashi, & Gambone, 2010).

Endometritis may have an early onset (within 48 hours after delivery), generally following cesarean birth, or late onset (up to 6 weeks after delivery), usually after vaginal delivery (French & Smaill, 2009).

Epidemiology

Risk factors include cesarean birth, membranes ruptured for longer than 24 hours, prolonged labor, numerous cervical examinations, internal fetal monitoring, meconium stained fluid, cervical lacerations, and bacterial infections from organisms such as *Chlamydia trachomatis*, *Mycoplasma hominis*, *Ureaplasma urealyticum*, *Gardnerella vaginalis*, and *group B streptococcus* (ACOG, 1998; Cunningham et al., 2010d).

Transmission occurs via several routes.

- Lymphatic transmission may be from an infected cervical laceration, uterine incision for cesarean birth, or uterine laceration.
- Direct invasion occurs when cervical laceration extends into connective tissue at the base of broad ligaments, providing direct access to infective organisms.
- Transmission may be secondary to pelvic thrombophlebitis. A thrombus may become purulent, resulting in necrosis of venous walls and pathogenic access to surrounding connective tissue.

Postpartum endometritis occurs in 1 to 3 percent of vaginal deliveries (French & Smaill, 2009). It is 10 times more common with caesarean section (French & Smaill, 2009). The incidence is as high as 90 percent in operative deliveries done for cephalopelvic disproportion without perioperative prophylaxis (Cunningham et al., 2010d).

Subjective Data

A client may report unilateral or bilateral abdominal pain, foul-smelling lochia, malaise, and anorexia. Fever of 38° C or higher on any of two of the first 10 postpartum days or fever of 38.7° C within the first 24 hours postpartum defines puerperal fever morbidity (Adair, 1935).

Objective Data

The client appears wan and lethargic. She also appears to have pain.

- Vital signs show fever; tachycardia may or may not be present.
- Abdominal and musculoskeletal examinations reveal significant lower abdominal pain with tenderness and rebound. Paralytic ileus may cause distention and vomiting (Cunningham et al., 2010d).
- Genitalia and reproductive organs have parametrial tenderness on bimanual exam. The pelvic exam may be normal even with severe endometritis. Uterine subinvolution is possible. Lochial discharge is increased, dark red/brown, and foul smelling. Cervical motion tenderness is also possible.

A CBC is ordered to detect infection or anemia. Leukocytosis (15,000–30,000 cells/mL) may be noted on testing of the serum sample. The client should be counseled regarding the purpose of the test and the method used to obtain the serum sample.

Cunningham and colleagues (2010d) question the appropriateness of obtaining blood or genital tract cultures prior to the initiation of antibiotics. They quote earlier studies that found pathogens in the uterine cavities of healthy postpartum women.

Chest radiography may be used to diagnose pulmonary diseases, to detect mediastinal abnormalities, and to assist in assessment of pulmonary status. Request upright anterior, posterior, and lateral views of chest. Inform the client about the test's purpose. She should be told that the radiology technician will ask her to remove her clothing to the waist, take a deep breath and exhale, and take a second deep breath and hold it while the x-ray is taken. Assure the client that the procedure takes only a few minutes, is painless, and may be safely performed during lactation.

A urine culture and sensitivity may be done to assess for UTI. Urine is collected by sterile catheterization and placed in a sterile container.

Differential Medical Diagnoses

Endometritis, endomyometritis, parametritis, cystitis, pyelonephritis, mastitis, appendicitis, viral disease, septic pelvic thrombophlebitis, paralytic ileus.

Plan

Because of severe, life-threatening complications as noted previously, referral to the physician for consideration of hospital admission is mandatory. Outpatient management for mild cases of late postpartum endometritis, after physician consultation, may be appropriate (Cunningham et al., 2010d). Close follow-up by telephone and returning to the office in 48 hours is mandatory.

Psychosocial Intervention. Inform the client of her diagnosis and treatment plan and inquire about her support systems.

Medication Interventions. Parenteral administration of antibiotics is mandatory in moderate to severe infections and should be continued until the client has been afebrile for 48 hours. Oral antibiotics after parenteral treatment are not necessary and no longer recommended (ACOG, 1998; French & Smaill, 2009).

The gold standard of treatment continues to be gentamicin 1.5 mg/kg and clindamycin 900 mg intravenously every 8 hours (Cunningham et al., 2010d; French & Smaill, 2009). Studies comparing daily with thrice-daily gentamicin found no difference in treatment failure (French & Smaill, 2009).

A higher treatment failure rate occurs when an aminoglycoside and penicillin or ampicillin are used instead of the recommended aminoglycoside and clindamycin. Although second- or third-generation cephalosporins, when compared to clindamycin and gentamicin, appear to be equally effective in treating endometritis, they have a higher incidence of treatment failures (French & Smaill, 2009). The health care provider may choose one of the following as clinically indicated.

Gentamicin. Gentamicin is an aminoglycoside. Onset of action is immediate after IV administration, but unknown if given intramuscularly. Peak serum levels occur in 30 to 90 minutes. Gentamicin toxicity is increased when used for longer than 1 week (ACOG, 1998). Aminoglycocide's bactericidal activity is concentration dependent, and bacterial growth is suppressed for long periods after administration. In addition, there is a phenomenon called *adaptive resistance*, in which bactericidal activity of subsequent doses of an aminoglycoside is decreased by the initial dose. Clinical trials of daily single-dose aminoglycoside therapy apply these principles of aminoglycoside action and have proven to be as effective as conventional multiple-dose regimens with less nephrotoxicity.

- *Administration:* Gentamicin—1.5 mg/kg of body weight in three divided doses IV every 8 hours or for daily single-dose therapy, 5 mg/kg of body weight IV. If serum concentrations are monitored, obtain blood for peak gentamicin level 30 minutes to 1 hour after IV infusion; for trough levels, draw blood just before the next dose. Monitor renal function (output, specific gravity, urinalysis, BUN, creatinine levels, creatinine clearance). Evaluate the client's hearing during therapy.
- *Side effects:* Neuromuscular blockade; ototoxicity (tinnitus, vertigo, hearing loss); nephrotoxicity (cells or casts in the urine; oligouria; proteinuria; decreased creatinine clearance; increased BUN, nonprotein nitrogen, and serum creatinine levels).
- *Interactions:* Numerous, consult drug handbook.

Clindamycin. Clindamycin is an anti-infective.

- *Oral dosage:* 150 to 300 mg every 6 hours.
- *Parenteral:* IM or IV—900 mg every 8 hours (Cunningham et al., 2010d).
- *Side effects:* Nausea, diarrhea, dysphagia, bloody or tarry stools, pain, anaphylaxis; sterile abscess with IM injection.

Augmentin. Augmentin is a broad-spectrum antibiotic (previously discussed under subinvolution) that may used to treat endometritis.

Cephalosporins. The cephalosporins are broad-spectrum antibiotics with β-lactamase activity.

Cefotetan Disodium (Cefotan)

- *Administration:* 2 g every 12 hours until the client is afebrile and asymptomatic for 24 to 48 hours.
- *Side effects:* GI upset, rash, pruritus, local reactions, anaphylaxis, blood dyscrasias, elevated liver enzymes.
- *Precautions:* Penicillin or other allergies, renal impairment, renal or hepatic dysfunction. Monitor PT. Monitor for hemolytic anemia in prolonged use.
- *Contraindication:* Hypersensitivity to cephalosporins and penicillins.

- *Anticipated outcomes on evaluation:* Resolution of symptoms and clinical improvement.
- *Client teaching:* Stress the importance of completing the medication regimen. Instruct the client to report signs of allergy.

Cefoxitin. 1 to 2 g IV every 6 to 8 hours.

- *Side effects:* Maculopapular and erythematous rashes, uriticaria, pseudomembranous colitis, diarrhea, transient neutropenia, hemolytic anemia, hypoprothrombinemia, anaphylaxis, pain induration sterile abscesses at IV site, phlebitis, thrombophlebitis.

Cefotaxime. 1 to 2 g IV every 8 to 12 hours.

- *Side effects:* Fever, maculopapular and erythematous rashes, uriticaria, pseudomembranous colitis, diarrhea, transient elevation of liver enzymes, anaphylaxis, pain induration sterile abscesses at IV site, phlebitis, thrombophlebitis.

Conservative management with antibiotics usually produces a response in 48 hours. A poor response indicates abscess, retention of placental parts, or incorrect diagnosis (ACOG, 1998; Cunningham et al., 2010d).

Fluid Intake. Women with endometritis should increase fluid intake.

Lifestyle Changes. Explain to the client and her partner the client's general need for rest, as well as her need for pelvic rest (including no sexual intercourse).

Follow-Up

Medical consultation is required. In addition, management of candidates for outpatient treatment should include the following: telephone the client daily and schedule a return appointment 48 to 72 hours after treatment begins. Complications of endometritis can be severe and include:

- Septic pelvic thrombophlebitis, pain typically develops after the second or third postpartum day. Fever spikes continue despite antimicrobial treatment. Diagnosis is established using computerized tomography or MRI (Cunningham et al., 2010d). Refer the client for immediate medical treatment.
- Pelvic abscess is usually unilateral. Clinical presentation is 1 to 2 weeks postpartum and surgical drainage is most likely necessary, as rupture can cause peritonitis (Cunningham et al., 2010d). Referral to a physician is indicated.

THROMBOEMBOLISM

Pregnancy is a hypercoagulable state and increased risk for thromboembolism continues into the postpartum period with risk not returning to prepregnancy levels until 42 days after delivery (CDC, 2011c; James, 2010). The postpartum woman needs to be monitored for signs and symptoms of deep vein thrombosis (DVT) including unilateral swelling of an extremity, pain in the calf, redness, and a palpable cord along a vein. The incidence is about 1 per 1,000 being present equally antepartum and postpartum. Pulmonary embolism (PE) with chest pain and shortness of breath is a potential life-threatening complication of DVT. Signs and symptoms of PE can be obvious or subtle. Incidence of PE is around 1 in 7,000 and is also equally present in the antepartum and postpartum period (Cunningham et al., 2010g; O'Connor et al., 2011).

Subjective Data

A woman may complain of abrupt swelling and pain in a leg, shortness of breath, chest pain, cough, syncope, or hemoptysis.

Objective Data

Redness, swelling, and/or warmth in an extremity may be present along with a palpable cord. Homan's sign may be positive, but its predictive value is unclear. The woman with PE may appear short of breath or dypsneic. She may be apprehensive, tachypneic, and tachycardic. A friction rub may be heard (Cunningham et al., 2010g).

Diagnostic testing includes compression ultrasonography as a first-line test with consideration of spiral computerized tomography (CT) as indicated. A ventilation-perfusion scan may be considered in evaluation of PE although it has been widely replaced by spiral CT. D-dimer testing is not reliable in pregnancy or postpartum as levels are normally elevated, however a negative test is reassuring (Cunningham et al., 2010g).

Plan

Consultation with a physician is indicated as hospitalization is necessary. Treatment with intravenous heparin and concurrent start of oral warfarin is indicated for the postpartum woman. Warfarin is contraindicated during pregnancy (James, 2010). Heparin is continued for at least 5 days and until international normalized ratio (INR) is therapeutic. Warfarin starting dose is generally between 5 and 10 mg and then titrated to reach an INR between 2 and 3. Warfarin should be continued for a minimum of 6 months postpartum

(Cunningham et al., 2010g). Warfarin does not readily transfer into breast milk and is considered to pose little risk for breast-fed infants. Higher doses may lead to higher concentrations in breast milk. Infants should be monitored closely for signs of bleeding or bruising (Hale, 2010).

MASTITIS

Mastitis, an inflammation of the breast, may be caused by tight clothing, missed infant feedings, poor drainage of duct and alveolus, or an infecting organism (*Staphylococcus aureus* [consider CA-MRSA], *Escherichia coli*, *Streptococcus*) (Cunningham et al., 2010c; Lawrence & Lawrence, 2011).

Infection may be transmitted from lactiferous ducts to a secreting lobule, from a nipple fissure to periductal lymphatics, or by hematogenic means. Scott, Robertson, Fitzpatrick, Knight, and Mulholland (2008) report an incidence of mastitis of 3 to 20 percent with the majority of instances occurring during the first 4 weeks.

Subjective Data

A woman may report flu-like symptoms, including malaise, fever, and chills. She may also describe a tender, hot, red, painful area or lump in the breast.

Objective Data

Physical examination is usually sufficient to diagnose mastitis. Assess vital signs. Fever is often high; tachycardia is common. Examination of the breasts reveals increased warmth, redness, tenderness, and swelling. The affected lobule is often in the outer quadrant and wedge shaped; the nipple may be cracked or abraded; and the breast distended with milk. Suspect a breast abscess if there is no resolution of symptoms after several days of antibiotic therapy. If an abscess has formed, pitting edema is possible and fluctuation may be felt over the affected area. An abscess usually requires both antibiotics and drainage for resolution (ACOG, 2000); therefore, the client should be referred to a physician for further management.

Diagnostic testing may include a culture and sensitivity, although it was seldom used in the past. With the advent of CA-MRSA as causative organism for mastitis, culture and sensitivity may now be desirable and can be done using an expressed sample of breast milk (Cunningham et al., 2010c). Test results may not be available for 72 hours; however, antibiotic therapy needs to be started immediately.

Differential Medical Diagnoses

Clogged duct, simple breast engorgement, breast abscess, viral syndrome.

Plan

Psychosocial Intervention. Counsel the client regarding the etiology of mastitis. Unless she has been prescribed a sulfa drug (see the following), encourage her to continue breastfeeding, emphasizing that her medication is safe to use during lactation. Inform the client of the signs and symptoms of worsening mastitis and the need to call the health care provider should they develop.

Medication. Dicloxacillin is the first-line treatment choice unless penicillin allergy is present. If that is the case, then erythromycin would be the alternative. Cephalosporins may also be considered. Sulfa drugs (see UTI for discussion of sulfanomides) should not be prescribed if the nursing infant is less than 1 month old (Lawrence & Lawrence, 2011). Therefore, clindamycin is the drug of choice when CA-MRSA is suspected and infant is less than 1 month of age.

Dicloxacillin Sodium (Dynapen, Dycill, Pathocil)

- *Indication:* Treatment of penicillinase-resistant organisms.
- *Administration:* 250 to 500 mg orally every 6 hours for 10 days.
- *Side effects:* Nausea, vomiting, diarrhea, vaginitis.
- *Contraindication:* Hypersensitivity to penicillins.
- *Anticipated outcome on evaluation:* Resolution of mastitis.
- *Client teaching:* Instruct the client to complete the 10-day medication regimen even if she feels better before medication is finished; if medication is not taken for all 10 days, the risk for relapse increases (Cunningham et al., 2010c; Lawrence & Lawrence, 2011). The medication is category B for pregnancy.

Erythromycin

- *Indication:* Treatment if penicillin allergy.
- *Administration:* 500 mg orally every 6 hours for 10 days.
- *Side effects:* Nausea, vomiting, diarrhea, vaginitis.
- *Contraindication:* Hypersensitivity to macrolides.
- *Anticipated outcome on evaluation:* Resolution of mastitis.
- *Client teaching:* Same as for dicloxacillin (Cunningham et al., 2010c; Lawrence & Lawrence, 2011). The medication is category B for pregnancy.

Clindamycin

- *Indication:* Treatment if penicillin allergy and/or treatment if CA-MRSA suspected.
- *Administration:* 300 mg orally every 6 hours for 10 days.
- *Side effects:* Diarrhea, nausea, vomiting, pseudomembranous colitis, leucopenia, rash.
- *Contraindication:* Hypersensitivity to clindamycin or lincomycin. History of colitis, ulcerative or antibiotic induced.
- *Anticipated outcome on evaluation:* Resolution of mastitis.
- *Client teaching:* Same as for dicloxacillin (Cunningham et al., 2010c; Lawrence & Lawrence, 2011). The medication is category B for pregnancy.

Cephalexin (Keflex) or Cephradine (Velosef)

- *Administration:* 500 mg every 6 hours for 10 days; inhibits cell wall synthesis.
- *Side effects:* Nausea, anorexia, diarrhea, maculopapular and erythematous rashes, urticaria, anaphylaxis.
- *Contraindications:* Hypersensitivity to cephalosporins.
- *Anticipated outcome on evaluation:* Resolution of mastitis.
- *Client teaching/counseling:* Finish all medication. If medication not taken for 10 days, there is an increase risk for relapse of infection.

Acetaminophen (Tylenol)

- *Indications:* Antipyretic and analgesic.
- *Administration:* 325 to 650 mg orally every 4 hours as needed, not to exceed 4 g per day.
- *Side effects:* Few, if taken in therapeutic doses. Acetaminophen does not cause gastric bleeding or inhibit platelet aggregation. No relationship to Reye's syndrome has been found. Overdosage can cause hepatic necrosis.
- *Contraindication:* None is known.
- *Anticipated outcomes on evaluation:* Decreased pain and fever.
- *Client teaching:* Inform the client about the effects of overdosage; instruct her to take no more than 4 g per day. She should know the early symptoms of hepatic necrosis: nausea, vomiting, diarrhea, sweating, abdominal discomfort. Tell the client to telephone the health care provider if she experiences symptoms of overdosage.

Candidal invasion, described as incredible pain like "hot cords," is a fungal infection of milk ducts that is becoming more common and is usually a secondary complication from antibiotic treatment of recurrent mastitis. However, it may present as a primary infection. See section Breastfeeding Problems for treatment recommendations.

Breast Care. Ice or warm packs may be applied to the breast, whichever is more comfortable. The client should continue to nurse her infant on both breasts, but begin on the unaffected breast and thus allow the affected breast to let down. Review breastfeeding techniques with the client.

Fluid Intake. The client should increase fluid intake.

Lifestyle Changes. Bed rest, with bathroom privileges, is necessary in the treatment of mastitis to prevent the client from becoming exhausted and thereby worsening the mastitis (Lawrence & Lawrence, 2011).

Follow-Up

Referral to a breastfeeding support group or lactation consultant may be necessary (see Support Groups and Resources).

POSTPARTUM THYROIDITIS

Postpartum thyroiditis is a syndrome of transient or permanent thyroid dysfunction that occurs during the first postpartum year from an autoimmune inflammation of the thyroid (Cunningham et al., 2010g). It may also occur following a pregnancy loss at as early as 5 to 20 weeks' gestation. It results from transient rebound of the autoimmune process following delivery or abortion. The thyroid is unable to regulate both the release of previously synthesized thyroid hormone and the synthesis of new thyroid hormone. It is differentiated from other forms of thyrotoxicosis by the lack of thyroid pain, its transient symptoms with spontaneous remission, and elevated serum antibodies and thyroid hormones (hyperthyroid phase) with concomitant suppression of radioactive thyroid uptake (Abalovich et al., 2007; Cunningham et al., 2010k).

Epidemiology

The incidence of postpartum thyroiditis is 5 to 15 percent; in women who are positive for thyroid peroxidase antibodies (TPO), 30 to 60 percent will develop postpartum thyroiditis (Muller, Drexhage, & Bergout, 2001; Stagnaro-Green et al., 2011). Risk factors for PPT include smoking, type 1 diabetes, and prior history of PPT (Cunningham et al., 2010k). Interestingly, the risk factor of smoking was not found to be significantly associated with PPT in a recent prospective trial of 4,562 women (Stagnaro-Green et al., 2011).

Subjective Data

A client may report symptoms of thyrotoxicosis during the first postpartum month and transient hypothyroidism with symptoms that peak after 3 to 5 months.

Thyrotoxicosis has a rapid onset in the latter half of the first postpartum month and persists for 2 to 4 months, usually resolving by the fourth postpartum month. The client reports weight loss, fatigue that occurs easily, heat intolerance, palpitations, hand tremors, nervousness, or other psychoneurotic reactions (Abalovich et al., 2007; Cunningham et al., 2010k).

In transient hypothyroidism, clinical signs peak between 3 and 5 months postpartum. The client shows progressive and pronounced fatigue, continued weight gain in the latter months of first postpartum year, coarse hair, dry skin, and psychological reactions that mimic depression. Any complaint of fatigue, palpitations, impaired memory, depression, or loss of attention span during the first postpartum year needs to be evaluated for thyroid disease (Abalovich et al., 2007; ACOG, 2002b; Muller et al., 2001).

Objective Data

Physical examination reveals signs unique to both phases of PPT. In the thyrotoxicosis phase, the client exhibits sinus tachycardia, stare or lid lag, brisk reflexes, and a firm, nontender thyroid. Only 50 percent of women have thyroid enlargement (ACOG, 2002b). The transient hypothyroidism phase involves delayed reflexes, psychomotor retardation, and psychological reactions that mimic depression.

The thyroid-stimulating hormone (TSH) test is done to diagnose primary hypothyroidism, differentiating primary from secondary hypothyroidism. If the TSH is normal, repeat it in 4 weeks, because a normal TSH may represent the window phase in which the shift goes from hyperthyroid to hypothyroid (Abalovich et al., 2007). In addition, an elevated level of serum TSH is noted in the hypothyroid phase. The test procedure requires a blood sample. Inform the client of the venipuncture procedure and the rationale for the test and explain test results to her.

The antithyroglobulin antibody test differentiates thyroid diseases such as Hashimoto's thyroiditis and thyroid carcinoma. A blood sample is also used in this test. Inform the client of the purpose of the antithyroglobulin antibody test.

TPO is a diagnostic evaluation for the presence of thyroid microsomal antibodies (ACOG, 2002b; Fischbach, 2009). Tell the client that high antibodies to thyroid peroxidase indicate an increased risk for developing thyroid disease in the first postpartum year (ACOG, 2002b; Cunningham et al., 2010k). A TSH assay should be requested. Women with goiters and a high titer of TPO, but a normal TSH, should have the TSH remeasured in 3 to 6 months.

The radioactive iodine uptake test (contraindicated for pregnant or lactating women) reveals increased uptake in hyperthyroidism of Graves' disease, but decreased uptake in hyperthyroidism of thyroiditis (Abalovich et al., 2007). This diagnostic test evaluates the thyroid's ability to concentrate and retain iodine and is indicated in the diagnosis of thyroid disease.

The test procedure is done in conjunction with a thyroid scan and assessment of thyroid hormone levels. A fasting state is preferred. A liquid form or capsule of radioiodine is administered orally. The radioactivity of the thyroid gland is measured by scanning the gland 2, 6, and 24 hours later (Fischbach, 2009).

Provide the client with information about factors that interfere with, or lower, radioactive iodine uptake: iodized foods and iodine-containing medications (1–3 weeks' duration), vitamin preparations that contain minerals (1–3 weeks' duration), radiographic contrast media (1 week to 1 year, so consult with radiologist), antithyroid medications (2–10 days' duration), thyroid medications (1–2 weeks' duration), antihistamines, corticosteroids, isoniazid, thiocyanate, perchlorate, sulfonamides, tolgutamide, phenylbutazone, adrenocorticotropin, aminosalicylic acid, cobalt, and warfarin sodium anticoagulant (Fischbach, 2009).

Medications and conditions that increase uptake include TSH, pregnancy, cirrhosis, barbiturates, lithium, phenothiazine, iodine-deficient diets, and renal failure (Fischbach, 2009). Tell the client that the test is painless, but requires 24 hours to perform. Restrict iodine intake (e.g., iodized salt, seafood) for at least 1 week prior to the test.

Differential Medical Diagnosis

Graves' disease, postpartum depression, Sheehan's syndrome.

Plan

Psychosocial Intervention. Reassure the client regarding the validity of her symptoms. Explain to her the etiology and management of PPT. Counsel the client regarding spontaneous resolution as well as possible recurrence of the condition with future births. Counsel those who are positive for peroxidase antibodies of the increased risk over time of development of permanent thyroid disease (Cunningham et al., 2010k).

Medication. Levothyroxine (T4) is administered to treat hypothyroidism. Initial doses should be low, beginning with 0.1 mg/day, increasing gradually every 4 weeks until full replacement doses have been achieved. Replacement doses have been achieved when repeat TFTs are within normal limits.

- *Side effects:* Rare when given in therapeutic doses. Excessive doses of levothyroxine may cause thyrotoxicosis; symptoms are anxiety, insomnia, tremors, tachycardia, angina, palpitations, hyperthermia, and sweating.
- *Contraindication:* None is known.
- *Anticipated outcomes on evaluation:* Reversal of signs and symptoms of hypothyroidism and a decline in serum TSH levels.
- *Client teaching:* Instruct the client to take the medication on an empty stomach to enhance absorption; morning administration decreases sleeplessness. Medication should be kept in a light-resistant container. Advise the client to report excitability, irritability, or anxiety. Also advise her not to switch brands of levothyroxine unless approved by the health care provider.

In women with symptoms of thyrotoxicosis, a β-blocker may be used short-term until free thyroxine (FT4) levels are normal (Abalovich et al., 2007). Propranolol (40–120 mg) in divided doses every 8 hours may be used (Abalovich et al., 2007; ACOG, 2002b).

Follow-Up

Referral to a physician is required. Regular checkups are scheduled for laboratory assessment of thyroid function. As the thyroid gland often recovers in 1 year, the health care provider can assess thyroid function and the need for continued thyroid replacement by halving the dose and repeating the TSH 6 to 8 weeks later (Cunningham et al., 2010k). If the TSH continues to be normal, one can assume normal thyroid functioning and the levothyroxine can be discontinued. Yearly assessment of thyroid function is advised (Abalovich et al., 2007).

URINARY TRACT INFECTION

Epidemiology

Risk factors for infection, caused by bacteria in the urinary tract (see Chapter 24), include trauma to the bladder or urethra, such as that resulting from catheterization; history of UTI; sickle cell trait; diabetes mellitus; use of diaphragm, oral contraceptives, or spermicide. Infection can be transmitted in vaginal secretions via sexual intercourse and perineal pads.

In a population-based case-control study, Schwartz, Wang, Eckert, and Critchlow (1999) sought to find risk factors for UTI unique to postpartum women. Anemia, obesity, or diabetes were not risk factors for postpartum UTI, but women with cesarean delivery, tocolytic therapy, induction of labor, renal disease, preeclampsia/eclampsia, unmarried status, and longer hospital stay were at an increased risk. Their data did not identify whether these women had been catheterized, and they recommended prospective, controlled studies to look at continuous versus intermittent catheterization as risk factors for UTI. Cunningham et al. (2010d, 2010h) identify traumatized bladder and bladder distention related to either decreased sensation of fullness or normal postpartum diuresis as risk factors for UTI postpartum.

Subjective Data

A client may report dysuria, oliguria, urinary frequency or urgency, nausea and vomiting, chills, and abdominal pain or cramping.

Objective Data

Physical examination usually reveals that general appearance and vital signs are within normal limits. Fever, however, may be present and is indicative of upper UTI (pyelonephritis). The abdominal exam is done to detect CVAT and suprapubic tenderness.

A urinalysis determines the properties of urine and abnormal products. Pyuria (white blood cells in urine), hematuria (red blood cells in urine), and positive nitrite indicate a UTI and warrant a urine culture. Nitrite test may be falsely negative if bladder bacteria have not had sufficient time to produce nitrite; the client does not eat vegetables, or uses a diuretic. Nitrite testing is also negative with some bacteria, such as staphylococci and streptococci (Fischbach, 2009). The test procedure for urinalysis requires a routine urine sample obtained by voiding. Instruct the client about the purpose of the test and the method of collection.

A urine culture and sensitivity is done to diagnose bacterial infection and identify offending organisms (see Endometritis for a description of the test procedure and client teaching).

Differential Medical Diagnoses

UTI (lower or upper tracts); Chlamydia trachomatis.

Plan

Psychosocial Interventions. Provide the client with information and counsel her regarding the suspected diagnosis and pathophysiology of UTI.

Medication. One of the following drugs is administered. (Amoxicillin is no longer the first choice because many organisms causing UTIs are resistant to ampicillin/amoxicillin.)

Nitrofurantoin (Macrobid)

- *Administration:* One 100 mg tablet orally every 12 hours for 3 to 5 days.
- *Side effects:* Gastrointestinal reactions (nausea, vomiting), headache, vertigo, drowsiness.
- *Contraindications:* Hypersensitivity to the drug, glucose-6-phosphate dehydrogenase (G-6-PD) deficiency, renal disease.
- *Anticipated outcomes on evaluation:* Resolution of the client's symptoms and negative urine culture following treatment.
- *Client teaching:* Advise the client to complete the 3- to 5-day medication regimen even if symptoms disappear before that time. Medication is taken with food or milk. The client should be told to return for a follow-up visit if indicated.

Trimethoprim/Sulfamethoxazole (Bactrim DS, Septra DS, Cotrim DS)

- *Administration:* One tablet orally every 12 hours for 3 to 5 days.
- *Side effects:* Gastrointestinal reactions (nausea and vomiting), rash, blood dyscrasias (hemolytic anemia, leukopenia, thrombocytopenia).
- *Contraindications:* Hypersensitivity to trimethoprim or sulfonamides, G-6-PD deficiency, lactating women with infant less than 4 weeks of age, megaloblastic anemia.
- *Anticipated outcomes on evaluation:* Resolution of the client's symptoms and negative urine culture following treatment.
- *Client teaching:* Instruct the client to complete the 3- to 5-day medication regimen even if symptoms improve or disappear before that time. Medication should be taken with a full glass of water; water intake is increased to decrease crystallization in kidneys. Advise the client to avoid sunlight to prevent burns and to contact the care provider if side effects occur.

Cephalosporins

- *Administration:* Cephalexin—250 to 500 mg orally every 6 hours for 3 to 5 days.
- *Side effects:* Maculopapular rash, urticaria, and gastrointestinal upset. Discontinue medication if allergy symptoms appear (urticaria, rash, hypotension, difficulty breathing).
- *Contraindication:* Hypersensitivity to cephalosporins and penicillins.
- *Anticipated outcomes on evaluation:* Resolution of symptoms and clinical improvement.
- *Client teaching:* Stress the importance of completing the medication regimen. Instruct the client to report signs of allergy.

Quinolones (Ciprofloxacin HC [Cipro])

- *Administration:* One 250 to 500 mg tablet every 12 hours for 3 to 7 days.
- *Side effects:* Headache, tremor, drowsiness, seizures, nausea, diarrhea, dyspepsia, arthralgia, rash, photosensitivity, tendon rupture. This drug is not recommended in lactating women due to the potential for arthropathy and other toxicity (Briggs, Freeman, & Yaffe, 2005). If Cipro is given to a lactating woman, the recommendation is that 48 hours elapse from the last dose of the medication before breastfeeding is resumed (Briggs et al., 2005).
- *Contraindications:* Avoid use with aminoglycosides, beta-lactams because of synergistic effects; antacids that contain aluminum, calcium, or magnesium may interfere with the absorption of Cipro (administer Cipro 2 hours before or 6 hours after antacids); monitor theophylline levels because of an increased risk of toxicity; avoid use with warfarin because of increased PT; iron, vitamins, minerals should be discontinued because they may interfere with ciprofloxacin absorption.
- *Anticipated outcomes on evaluation:* Resolution of the UTI.
- *Client teaching:* Instruct client to finish all medication.

Levofloxacin (Levaquin)

- *Administration:* 250 mg tablet daily for 3 days.
- *Side effects:* Same as for ciprofloxacin.
- *Contraindications:* Same reaction with antacids as with ciprofloxacin; may alter blood glucose levels of people on antidiabetic medication; increased photosensitivity; may alter PT in people on warfarin. The use of levofloxacin, as with ciprofloxacin, is not recommended in breastfeeding mothers.
- *Anticipated outcome on evaluation:* Resolution of the UTI.
- *Client teaching:* Finish all medication.

Follow-Up

Review proper perineal hygiene with the client. In addition, reemphasize her need to increase fluid intake and to void at least every 2 to 4 hours. (Additional follow-up is outlined in Chapter 24.)

ACUTE APPENDICITIS

The appendix may become inflamed as a result of obstruction of the appendiceal lumen by hardened stool, hypertrophy of lymph follicles in the wall of the appendix, or strictures.

Epidemiology

In a pregnancy and the puerperium, the appendix is atypically positioned, as it is in obese individuals. If appendicitis is present and not diagnosed before delivery, there is risk of rupture at the time of delivery related to movement of the uterus. However, development of new-onset appendicitis in the early postpartum period is uncommon (Cunningham et al., 2010i).

Subjective Data

The client may report loss of appetite, abdominal distention, and abdominal pain.

Objective Data

Physical examination may reveal the client to be distressed, obviously in pain. Her vital signs are likely to be within normal limits; temperature may be elevated. Abdominal muscles do not show the classic signs of appendicitis (abdominal guarding and rigidity) in early puerperium, as the appendix does not return to its usual location until involution is completed (6–8 weeks).

- Tenderness is common in the right upper quadrant or entire right abdomen when uterine size is 12 weeks or greater.
- Psoas, obturator, and Rovsing's signs are not predictive of appendicitis in pregnant or postpartum women.
- Bryan's sign is positive if moving the enlarged uterus to the right elicits pain and may be a more reliable indicator of appendiceal pathology.
- Alder's test requires the health care provider to maintain constant pressure at an area of maximum tenderness while the client rolls from the supine position onto her left side. Alder's test assists in differentiating pain of uterine etiology from that of extrauterine origin; pain of uterine origin may be relieved by change in position, whereas pain of extrauterine origin will not be relieved regardless of position.
- Examination of the genitalia and reproductive tract reveals that the lochia is not excessive and has no foul odor, the cervix is closed, and the uterus is nontender.
- Diagnostic tests assess blood, urine, and endocervical samples.
- A CBC and ESR may be obtained. Leukocytosis is nonspecific and does not differentiate appendicitis from other inflammatory causes of abdominal pain. White blood cell counts above 15,000/mm^3 and increased neutrophils should raise suspicion for appendicitis. The ESR is used to monitor an inflammatory or malignant disease. The test also helps to detect and diagnose occult disease. A blood sample must be obtained, and the client counseled regarding the purpose of the test and the method used to obtain the sample.
- Urinalysis and culture. (See Urinary Tract Infection for details of the test procedure and nursing implications.)
- Endocervical cultures are discussed under Endometritis.

Differential Medical Diagnoses

Appendicitis; endometritis; pyelonephritis; tubo-ovarian abscess.

Plan

Counsel the client and her family about the diagnosis and assist the family to arrange for childcare. Immediate referral to a surgeon is mandatory, as complications include death and appendiceal perforation.

POSTPARTUM PSYCHIATRIC DISTURBANCES

Psychiatric disturbances may occur during the puerperium. The disturbances are classified on the basis of their severity:

- *Maternity blues or "baby blues":* Transient, emotional disturbances commonly occurring around the second or fourth postpartum day, lasting from a few hours to 2 weeks.
- *Postpartum depression*:* Characterized by lowered mood, irritability, fatigue, feelings of worthlessness, sleeping and eating changes, and subtle changes of personality.
- *Postpartum psychosis*:* Severely impaired ability to perform daily living tasks.

EPIDEMIOLOGY

Etiology and Risk Factors

The etiology of postpartum psychiatric disorders continues to be unknown. Although theories for the etiology of postpartum psychiatric disorders have included hormonal, neurotransmitter, genetic, epigenetic, and psychological factors, current evidence points to a multifactorial etiology in which the neuroendocrinologic changes of the postpartum period, placed on an individual with a vulnerability to illness, precipitates these disorders (Corwin, Kohen, Jarrett, & Stafford, 2010; Doucet, Dennis, Letourneau, & Blackmore, 2009; Joy & Chelmow, 2011). They exist worldwide with recognition and treatment varying by culture (Beck, 2008a; Callister, Beckstrand, & Corbett, 2010).

Risks of untreated postpartum depression are significant and include tragedies of suicide and infanticide. At minimum, postpartum depression has detrimental effects on both the mother and the infant in terms of parenting and developmental skills. Beck analyzed 19 studies on postpartum depression published between 1983 and 1993. Beck's (1995) meta-analysis found that postpartum depression has a significant adverse effect on mother–infant interaction. Her findings have continued to be validated (Hoffbrand, Howard, & Crawley, 2009). Depressed mothers interact less with their infants and experience anger and guilt over their feelings of loneliness (Joy & Chelmow, 2011). They feel overwhelmed by the responsibility of caring for their infants. Infants of depressed mothers tend to be fussier, vocalize less, and use less positive facial expressions than infants of nondepressed mothers (Beck, 2006, 2008b; Joy & Chelmow, 2011). Long-term effects, including impaired cognitive and emotional development, have also been noted in children over the age of 1 year.

Maternity Blues. Maternity blues are the mildest form of depression and are usually self-limiting. They begin on the second or third postpartum day and last up to 14 days.

Specific risk factors are unknown. Psychological factors may include the conflict caused by cultural expectations to bear children and pursue personal goals and the economic cost of childbearing and childrearing.

Postpartum Depression. Postpartum depression has a slow, insidious onset over several weeks postpartum. It usually begins within 2 or 3 weeks postpartum and may last up to a year (Hoffbrand et al., 2009).

Risk factors for postpartum depression include history of previous depression, history of postpartum depression, prenatal depression, life stress, childcare stress, prenatal anxiety, lack of social support, marital stress, and stressful life events during pregnancy or near term. Depression during pregnancy is one of the most important predictors of postpartum depression (Beck, 2002; Joy & Chelmow, 2011). Women with histories of postpartum depression are at higher risk of recurrent episodes in subsequent pregnancies and are more likely to remain depressed 1 year or longer after delivery. Point prevalence for postpartum depression was found to range from 6.5 to 12.9 percent in the first year in a study sponsored by the Agency for Healthcare Research and Quality (Gaynes et al., 2005). This finding correlates with an earlier analysis by Beck and Gable (2001) in which approximately 13 percent of mothers experienced postpartum depression, but up to 50 percent went undiagnosed. Other studies have indicated that postpartum adolescents may have a higher incidence of postpartum depression. They, as did adult mothers with depression, reported more negative feeding interactions with their infants and reported less confidence in their mothering skills than adolescents without depressive symptoms (Yozwiak, 2009). Therefore, awareness of and screening for postpartum depression is vital.

Postpartum Psychosis. Postpartum psychosis has its onset as soon as 48 to 72 hours after delivery. For others, it will appear within a few weeks or, at most, 3 months postpartum; the affected woman is 16 to 20 times more likely to require hospital admission in the 3 months

*Conditions are prolonged beyond usual period expected for blues.

postpartum than in an equivalent period preconceptionally. Of women who have had a previous episode of postpartum psychosis, 50 to 90 percent will experience another episode in subsequent pregnancy (Cunningham et al., 2010l). Symptoms of postpartum psychosis closely resemble a manic or mixed manic episode and include restlessness, irritability, insomnia, a rapidly shifting mood from depressed to manic, confusion, disorientation, erratic behavior, and delusional thinking often revolving around the infant (Beck, 2006; Joy & Chelmow, 2011).

It is more common in first-time mothers with obstetrical complications (Cunningham et al., 2010l). Psychological factors reflect no definite etiology; the primary risk factor seems to be a history of bipolar disorder (Joy & Chelmow, 2011).

Incidence

Incidence varies among the three classifications. Maternity blues affect 50 to 70 percent of postpartum women (Beck, 2006). During the first 3 months postpartum, 14.5% of women may experience a new onset of depression (Gaynes et al., 2005). Older studies identified that 25 percent of these women are likely to develop chronic, severe depression (Gold, 2002). Postpartum psychosis affects 1 to 2 per 1,000 new mothers (Beck, 2006; Doucet et al., 2009; Joy & Chelmow, 2011).

Subjective Data

Current Symptoms. Symptoms may be similar among the three classifications; however, distinct differences are reported by clients. It is important to identify the major problems causing the client to seek help: severe mood swings, hyperactivity, irritability, depression, obsessional thoughts, insomnia, lack of appetite, difficulty with concentration, hallucinations, delusion, inability to care for herself or child, suicidal or homicidal thoughts.

Maternity Blues. Women with maternity blues report weeping, often alternating with periods of elation; irritability; anxiety; headaches; confusion; forgetfulness; depersonalization; disturbances in sleep pattern; and fatigue (Beck, 2006; Hirst & Moutier, 2010).

Postpartum Depression. Women with postpartum depression report symptoms similar to those of maternity blues but without periods of elation. In addition, these symptoms are more intense and last longer. The client considers herself a failure as a mother; she looks for reasons for the perceived failure and associates it with real or imagined character weaknesses and questions self-worth. She experiences excessive fatigue and excessive weight gain or weight loss. Thinking and speaking may be slow. Suicide is a serious hazard and the method is often well planned (Beck, 2006; Hirst & Moutier, 2010).

Postpartum Psychosis. Women with postpartum psychosis report variable symptoms. Three expressions, or phases, of psychosis are possible: manic phase, delirious state, and psychotic depression (Beck, 2006; Cunningham et al., 2010l; Joy & Chelmow, 2011).

- Manic phase, with symptoms similar to those of the manic phase of bipolar disorder is characterized by racing thoughts, hyperactivity, and mood swings.
- Delirious state symptoms include confusion, dissociative episodes with confusion, dissociative episodes with hostility, and anxiety.
- Psychotic depression symptoms include suicidal tendencies, desire to harm the infant or others, psychomotor retardation, and prominent delusions that are often related to the infant.

History of Present Illness. Ask the client to describe the onset of symptoms. What symptoms were present during pregnancy or after the infant's birth? When were symptoms more severe or less severe, and how long did they last? Have symptoms caused her to make unexpected changes in lifestyle?

Past Psychiatric Condition. Ask the client if she has a history of depression, bipolar disorder, or other psychiatric illness. Were any of the illnesses related to childbearing? Did she receive any psychotropic medication? Did the medication help?

Medical-Surgical-Obstetrical History. Was the pregnancy planned or unplanned? Were there complications with this pregnancy? What happened during labor and delivery? Is there a history of medical illness (thyroid disease, other endocrinological problems)? Did the newborn have any serious health problem?

Family History. Does any family member have psychiatric problems (depression, bipolar disorder, schizophrenia, alcoholism or other substance abuse, anorexia nervosa, bulimia)? What type of help was received? Was medication received and what was the response? What was the client's childhood like? Ask her to describe her relationship with parents and her perceptions of their effectiveness as role models. Is there a history of physical or sexual abuse?

Social History. With whom does the client live? Is there someone with whom she can share the responsibility of caring for the child and house? Are there financial problems? Is she planning to work full- or part-time outside the home or full-time in the home? Is her partner emotionally supportive?

Objective Data

Physical Examination. Excessive weight loss or gain is possible. Affect may be flat; speech and thinking processes may be slow; the woman may be weepy, agitated, or irritable. She may exhibit confusion, hostility, or anxiety. The remainder of the physical examination is most likely within normal limits.

Diagnostics. Consider measurement of TSH in addition to use of a depression screening instrument.

Screening Instruments. Several instruments have been developed to identify those women at risk of postpartum depression. The Edinburgh Postnatal Depression Scale (EPDS) has 10 statements describing depressive symptoms with four possible responses. It is written at the third-grade level. Scores range from 0 to 3 for each item, with higher scores indicating greater severity. A score of 12/13 indicates depression (Doucet et al., 2009; Yozwiak, 2009). It has a positive predictive value of 73 percent. Please see Appendix B for example.

The Postpartum Depression Screening Scale (PDSS) is based on the conceptual definition of postpartum depression, and contains a 35-item Likert response scale, consisting of seven dimensions, with five items in each dimension (Beck & Gable, 2001; Doucet et al., 2009; Yozwiak, 2009). It has a positive predictive value of 90 percent. The woman has a choice of five responses for each question (1 = strongly disagree; 5 = strongly agree). A total score range of 35 to 59 is interpreted as normal adjustment. A total score of 60 to 79 indicates significant symptoms of postpartum depression. A total score of 80 to 175 is a positive screen for major postpartum depression, and the woman should be referred as soon as possible to a mental health team for evaluation (Yozwiak, 2009).

When compared, scores on the EPDS, the PDSS, and the Beck Depression Inventory-II have a strong positive correlation, but none of them have been tested in the adolescent population (Yozwiak, 2009). The EPDS is most widely used of these instruments. There is some evidence that the cutoff point for suspicion of depression for all of these instruments may need to be lowered (Joy & Chelmow, 2011).

Differential Medical Diagnoses

Maternity blues, postpartum depression, postpartum psychosis, postpartum thyroiditis.

Plan

Psychosocial Intervention. During the antepartum period, provide the client with information related to maternal changes, such as mood swings and lifestyle changes that could occur after birth. Suggestions should include coping strategies related to the birth:

- Get plenty of rest.
- Allow family and friends, if available, to help with household tasks and the care for older children.
- Eat a well-balanced diet that is low in salt and sugar and high in complex carbohydrates, protein, and green leafy vegetables.
- Drink plenty of fluids, especially water, and limit caffeine intake.
- Continue prenatal vitamins.
- Perform light exercise daily.
- Ensure some personal time and adult relationships.
- Avail oneself of support groups and other community resources (see Breastfeeding Information/Support Groups at the end of this chapter).

The simplest and most effective means to address postpartum depression would involve early and frequent assessments of postpartum women the first 28 days after discharge and 6 to 8 weeks postpartum. MacArthur and colleagues (2002) randomly assigned 2,064 women in the United Kingdom to a control group receiving routine postpartum care or an intervention group. The control group received the usual six to seven home visits by a midwife during the first 10 to 14 days after birth (extended to 28 days if needed), occasional general practitioner (GP) home visits, health visitor care after 28 days, and a checkup with a GP at 6 to 8 weeks postpartum. The intervention group received an increased number of midwife home visits through 28 days, with an additional visit at 10 to 12 weeks postpartum. At specific home visits, the midwife used symptom checklists and the EPDS to identify and manage health problems. The findings were that women's mental health measures were significantly improved in the intervention group with no difference in the physical health score. Many studies (Doucet et al., 2009) have identified lack of support and life stress as risk factors for postpartum depression. MacArthur and colleagues (2002) demonstrated that mental health can be improved by addressing and managing these problems.

Recently, movement to recognize postpartum psychiatric disorders as a public health issue has occurred. The technique of Health Marketing has been utilized in at least one public health initiative to increase community awareness of these disorders and improve screening (Baisch, Carey, Conway, & Mounts, 2010).

Medication Interventions. It is imperative that postpartum women be screened and treated for postpartum depression so they can function in their role as mother, providing the love so necessary in an infant's and child's life. Risks of untreated postpartum depression are significant as discussed earlier.

Although most authorities agree that the benefits of treating postpartum depression in breastfeeding mothers outweigh any risks (Lawrence & Lawrence, 2011), prudent use of medication during lactation is advisable. A Cochrane Review (Hoffbrand et al., 2009) concluded that antidepressant use for mild to moderate postpartum depression may not be indicated. Individual or group psychotherapy, such as interpersonal therapy (IPT) or cognitive-behavioral therapy (CBT), has been found to be effective for mild to moderate postpartum depression (Beck, 2006, 2008b; Dimidjian & Goodman, 2009; Hirst & Moutier, 2010). However, antidepressant use is indicated for moderate to major postpartum depression; use of antidepressants may be augmented with IPT or CBT in these cases (Hirst & Moutier, 2010; Hoffbrand et al., 2009).

Conditions requiring prompt psychiatric referral include suicidal and/or homicidal ideation, evidence or concern of psychotic symptoms, severe impairment of functional capabilities, avoidance of infant or overconcern of infant's health, failure to respond to therapeutic trial of antidepressants, and comorbid substance abuse (Hirst & Moutier, 2010). Lithium, an antimanic, or carbamazepine, an anticonvulsant, is often used to manage manic episodes. Antipsychotic drugs may be prescribed for women with postpartum psychoses who are experiencing hallucinations or other distortions of reality. For moderate to severe postpartum depression, the treatment of choice is selective serotonin reuptake inhibitors (SSRIs) (Hirst & Moutier, 2010).

Serotonin Reuptake Inhibitors. SSRIs have fewer and less noticeable side effects and a wider margin of safety than tricyclic antidepressants. For bottlefeeding mothers, fluoxetine (Prozac®) 10 mg as starting dose in the morning with dosage increased according to response; it may also be given in divided doses in the morning and at noon. The dosage should not exceed 80 mg per day. Fluoxetine is not recommended for breastfeeding mothers because of case reports of adverse infant response and detectable levels noted in breast milk (Hale, 2010; Hirst & Moutier, 2010). However, if it is the only medication tolerated by the breastfeeding mother, the benefit of its use outweigh the risks. It can also be used safely when the infant is over 4 to 6 months in age (Hale, 2010).

Sertraline (Zoloft) administration begins at 25 mg orally daily for 1 week after which it is increased to 50 mg daily. It is the preferred SSRI for breastfeeding mothers. As the therapeutic response may take 2 to 4 weeks, dosage adjustments can be made after that time frame. The dosage range is 50 to 200 mg daily. Response usually occurs at dosages from 50 to 100 mg daily (Hirst & Moutier, 2010). Levels in breast milk have been undetectable and risk for detectable level is considered remote at dosages up to 150 mg a day (Hale, 2010).

Paroxetine (Paxil) administration begins at 10 mg orally daily. Dosage may be increased in 10 mg increments up to a maximum of 50 mg daily (Hirst & Moutier, 2010). This drug is present in breast milk and has been noted to have adverse effects on infants in utero, but minimal to no effect has been noted in breast-fed infants (Hale, 2010).

Citalopram (Celexa) is not a first choice among the SSRIs for the treatment of depression in lactating women because of possible infant somnolence, weight loss, and decreased breastfeeding (Briggs et al., 2005; Hale, 2010; Hirst & Moutier, 2010). Escitalopram would be preferred over citalopram as a lower dose is transferred to the infant (Kendall-Tackett & Hale, 2010).

- *Side effects:* Nervousness, anxiety, insomnia, headache, somnolence, tremor, nausea, vomiting, dry mouth, arrhythmias, dyspepsia, weight loss, rash pruritus, urticaria. SSRIs may prolong the half-life of diazepam. Use with tryptophan can cause agitation, gastrointestinal distress, and restlessness. Interaction with warfarin or other highly protein-bound drugs can increase serum level. Advise the client of the 2- to 4-week lag before clinical improvement of depression.
- *Contraindications:* Hypersensitivity to any of the SSRIs. In addition, these drugs should not be used within 14 days of cessation of monoamine oxidase inhibitors. Cimetidine may increase the plasma concentration of paroxetine.
- *Anticipated outcome on evaluation:* Remission of symptoms of depression.
- *Client teaching:* Include information about side effects.

Bupropion (Wellbutrin, Zyban) is a mixed serotonin and norepinephrine reuptake inhibitor that has been associated with adverse effects for breast-fed infants in some case reports (Hirst & Moutier, 2010). It is rated as moderately safe for breast-fed infants by Hale (2010).

Tricyclic Antidepressants. Tricyclic antidepressants are not the first choice in treatment of postpartum depression because of their side effects, potential for overdosing, drug interactions, and the need for monitoring therapeutic serum levels. The effects of tricyclics on the nursing infant are unknown, but may be of concern (AAP, 2001; Briggs et al., 2005). However, nortriptyline levels have been undetectable in the plasma of nursing infants; therefore, it may be considered for those who do not tolerate or respond to an SSRI (Hale, 2010; Hirst & Moutier, 2010; Kendall-Tackett & Hale, 2010).

Nursing infants of mothers receiving antidepressant therapy should be monitored for lack of weight gain, irritability that persists, and decreased appetite (Hirst & Moutier, 2010; Kendall-Tackett & Hale, 2010).

Lithium. Lithium is indicated if antidepressant treatment precipitates a manic episode, with symptoms of racing thoughts, hyperactivity, pressured speech, increased energy, and impulsive behavior. Immediate referral to psychiatry is indicated (Hirst & Moutier, 2010). It is also the drug of choice for clients with postpartum psychosis with manic features. Long-term use of lithium can induce goiter and has been associated with degenerative renal changes. Therefore, baseline TFTs (T_3, T_4, TSH) and renal function tests (BUN, creatinine) should be obtained and repeated every 6 months. The American Academy of Pediatrics (AAP) considers lithium to be contraindicated during breastfeeding because of the potential for lithium-induced toxicity in the breastfeeding infant (Briggs et al., 2005).

- *Administration:* Therapeutic range—0.6 to 1.2 mEq/L; higher levels can produce toxicity (nausea, vomiting, diarrhea, shakiness) and extremely high levels can produce death. Serum values should be drawn 8 to 12 hours after the first dose (usually before the morning dose), then weekly to monthly.
- *Side effects:* Nausea, vomiting, diarrhea, thirst, polyuria, lethargy, slurred speech, muscle weakness, fine hand tremor. When administered above the therapeutic range, lithium may cause headache, persistent gastrointestinal upset, confusion, hyperirritability, drowsiness, dizziness, tremors, ataxia, dry mouth, hypotension, rash, and pruritus.
- *Contraindications:* Hepatic disease, renal disease, pregnancy, lactation, severe cardiac disease and if therapy can't be monitored closely.
- *Anticipated outcome on evaluation:* The abatement of manic symptoms.
- *Client teaching:* Include information related to side effects.

Antipsychotic Drugs. Other antipsychotic drugs may also be prescribed for postpartum psychosis. See the current *Physicians' Desk Reference* or a pharmacotherapeutic resource for detailed information. Psychiatric referral is mandatory.

Hospitalization. Because 5 percent of women with postpartum psychosis commit suicide and 4 percent commit infanticide, postpartum psychosis is a true psychiatric emergency warranting hospital admission (Doucet et al., 2009; Hirst & Moutier, 2010).

Follow-Up

Postpartum depression poses serious sequelae for mother, infant, and family during the first postnatal year. Appropriate treatment to alter the mother's mood and enhance her sensitivity to her infant's cues will help strengthen the bond between the mother and infant dyad. Home visits, telephone calls, and psychiatric referral may be part of follow-up care.

Consider telephone calls 3 days after hospital discharge and a home visit 7 days after discharge to assess the client's adaptation to motherhood and family responsibilities. If the mother is adapting well, repeat contact after another 7 to 10 days. On the other hand, if she is experiencing difficulty, refer her to appropriate agencies or support groups (see Breastfeeding Information/Support Groups at the end of this chapter).

- Cognitive and supportive therapies help identify and correct distorted perceptions of reality and encourage the partner or other family member(s) to assist with household and childcare tasks.
- Concurrent marital therapy, in conjoint sessions, is especially helpful if the partner exhibits narcissistic behavior or is a substance abuser.
- Support groups (group therapy) complement individual therapy. They help decrease the sense of isolation.

POSTPARTUM POST-TRAUMATIC STRESS DISORDER

The risk for occurrence of post-traumatic stress disorder (PTSD) in the postpartum period has being recognized (Beck, 2004, 2006; Stone, 2009). Prevalence has been estimated at 5.6 percent (Beck, 2004). A comorbid diagnosis of depression often exists (Stone, 2009). Some other risk factors include an increased fear of the birth process or anxiety related to the birth process, a traumatic or prolonged labor and or delivery, poor communication by labor attendants or other perceived lack of attentiveness, use of medications that alter consciousness during labor or delivery, and poor social support (Beck, 2004, 2006; Stone, 2009).

A woman may complain of nightmares, detachment, irritability, problems with sleep, panic-attack symptoms, flashbacks, or avoidance behaviors. Discussion of the birth experience may be helpful to alleviate any misunderstandings and normalize the woman's reaction. It is recommended that this occurs in the immediate postpartum period. Referral to appropriate psychological care and support systems is indicated for those whose symptoms persist (Beck, 2004; Stone, 2009).

EARLY DISCHARGE

Early discharge follows a hospital stay of 48 hours or fewer and may be chosen by some women. It subjects a woman and her infant to certain risk factors. Physical complications may occur: discomfort at an episiotomy or cesarean incision site, endometritis, mastitis. Physiologic changes may be affected: uterine involution, increased edema and hyperemia of the bladder with possible atony, and diuresis. It became the norm in the late 20th century and childbearing families and health care providers, concerned about the care dictated by managed care companies, influenced the passage of patient-protective legislation at state and federal levels (Martell, 2000). If early discharge is desired, follow-up care in the home or by telephone should be pursued to assess the health needs (physical, psychosocial, and educational) of the mother, the family, and the infant in the early puerperium and to implement nursing plans to meet assessed needs.

The AAP and ACOG (2007) recommend that the length of hospital stay should be individualized for each mother–baby dyad. The decision to discharge should be made in consultation with the family and should not be based on third-party payer policies. When no complications are present, a hospital stay of 48 hours for vaginal birth and 96 hours for cesarean birth, excluding the day of delivery, is appropriate. If a shortened hospital stay of less than 48 hours is desired by the mother, the following criteria should be met:

- Mother is afebrile, with normal rate and quality of pulse and respirations.
- Mother's blood pressure is within the normal range.
- The lochia is appropriate in amount and color for the duration of recovery.
- Pertinent laboratory results are available, including a postpartum hemoglobin or hematocrit.
- The uterine fundus is firm.
- Urinary output is adequate.
- ABO blood groups and RhD type are known, and, if indicated, appropriate amount of anti-D immune globulin has been administered.
- Any surgical wound appears to be healing without complication, with minimal edema and no evidence of infection.
- Mother is able to ambulate without difficulty.
- Mother has no abnormal physical or emotional findings.
- Mother is able to eat and drink without difficulty.
- Arrangements have been made for postpartum follow-up care.
- Mother demonstrates readiness to care for herself and infant, is aware of abnormal deviations, and is able to recognize and respond to danger signs and symptoms.
- Mother had an uncomplicated vaginal delivery following a normal antepartum course and was observed after delivery for a sufficient time to ensure that her condition is stable.
- Family or other support system should be available to the mother for the first few days following discharge.
- The mother should be aware of possible complications and how to notify the practitioner.
- Procedures for readmission of obstetric patients should be consistent with hospital policy, as well as local and state regulations.

For early infant discharge, the AAP and ACOG (2007) recommend the following criteria be met:

- Antepartum, intrapartum, and postpartum course for both mother and infant should be uncomplicated.
- Delivery was vaginal.
- The infant was a single birth at 38 to 42 weeks gestation, and birth weight is appropriate for gestational age according to appropriate intrauterine growth curves.
- The baby's vital signs are documented to be normal and stable for the 12 hours preceding discharge, including respiratory rate of fewer than 60 breaths per minute, a heart rate of 100 to 160 beats per minute, and an axillary temperature of 36.5–37° C (97.7–98.6° F) in an open crib with appropriate clothing.
- The infant has urinated and passed at least one stool.

- The baby has completed at least two successful feedings, and documentation has been made that the baby is able to coordinate sucking, swallowing, and breathing while feeding.
- Physical examination reveals no abnormalities that require continued hospitalization.
- The circumcision site reveals no evidence of excessive bleeding for at least 2 hours.
- Significance of any jaundice present has been evaluated and follow-up plan has been determined.
- The mother's (preferably both parents') knowledge, ability, and confidence to provide adequate care for the baby are documented by the fact that the following training has been received:
    - Breastfeeding or bottlefeeding—The breastfeeding mother–baby dyad should be assessed by trained staff regarding nursing position, latch-on, adequacy of swallowing, and mother's knowledge of urine and stool frequency.
    - Cord, skin, and infant genital care should be reviewed.
    - The mother should be able to recognize signs of illness and common infant problems, particularly jaundice.
    - Instruction of proper infant safety (e.g., proper use of car seat and positioning for sleeping) should be provided.
- Family members or other support persons, including health care providers, such as the family pediatrician or his or her designees, who are familiar with newborn care and are knowledgeable about lactation and the recognition of jaundice and dehydration, are available to the mother and the baby for the first few days after discharge.
- Instructions to follow for emergencies have been communicated.
- Laboratory data is available and has been reviewed, including the following:
    - Maternal syphilis, hepatitis B surface antigen, and HIV status
    - Cord or infant blood type and direct Coombs test result, as clinically indicated.
- Screening tests have been done in accordance with state regulations. If a test was done before 24 hours of milk feeding, a system for repeating the test during the follow-up visit must be in place.
- Initial hepatitis B vaccine has been administered or an appointment scheduled for its administration as indicated by risk status and current immunization schedule.
- A physician-directed source of continuing medical care for both the mother and the baby has been identified. For newborns discharged before 48 hours after delivery, a definitive appointment has been made for the baby to be examined within 48 hours of discharge. The follow-up visit can take place in a home or clinic setting, as long as the personnel examining the neonate are competent in newborn assessment and the results of the follow-up visit are reported to the neonate's physician or designees on the day of the visit.
- Family, environmental, and social risk factors have been assessed. When risk factors are present, the discharge should be delayed until they are resolved or a plan to safeguard the infant is in place. Such factors may include, but are not limited to, the following:
    - Untreated parental substance use or positive urine toxicology results in the mother or newborn.
    - History of child abuse or neglect.
    - Mental illness in a parent who is in the home.
    - Lack of social support, particularly for single, first-time mothers.
    - No fixed home.
    - History of untreated domestic violence, particularly during this pregnancy.
    - Adolescent mother, particularly if other risk factors are present.
    - Barriers to adequate follow-up exist, such as transportation issues, lack of access to telephone, and/or non-English speaking

The AAP and ACOG (2007) recommend any newborn with a shortened hospital stay be examined by an experienced health care provider within 48 hours of discharge. If this visit cannot be assured to take place, they recommend deferment of discharge until a mechanism for follow-up evaluation is identified. The follow-up visit is designed to fulfill the following functions:

- Assess the newborn's general health, weight, hydration, and degree of jaundice and identify any new problems.
- Review feeding pattern and technique, including observation of breastfeeding for adequacy of position, latch-on, and swallowing.
- Collect historical evidence of adequate stool and urine patterns.
- Assess quality of mother–baby interaction and details of infant behavior.
- Reinforce maternal or family education in neonatal care, particularly regarding feeding and sleep position.

- Review results of laboratory tests performed at discharge.
- Perform screening tests in accordance with state regulations and other tests that are clinically indicated.
- Identify a plan for health care maintenance, including a method for obtaining emergency services, preventive care and immunizations, periodic evaluations and physical examinations, and necessary screening.

The AAP and ACOG (2007) recommend that discharge planning for high-risk neonates should begin shortly after admission to ensure a smooth transition from hospital to home. They recommend the following criteria be met before discharge:

- The neonate be given a comprehensive physical examination to identify problems that may require ongoing close surveillance and to provide data on which to base future assessments. If preterm, the neonate was tested for anemia before discharge.
- The neonate is stable physiologically and is able to maintain body temperature without cold stress when the amount of clothing worn and the room temperature are appropriate to what the neonate will experience in the home.
- The neonate is gaining weight steadily on enteral feedings.
- The neonate is able to breast-feed or bottle-feed adequately without cardiorespiratory compromise. If the neonate is unable to feed by nipple, the parents or other care providers are competent in alternative feeding techniques.
- The neonate is free of apnea or can be monitored appropriately at home.
- Family and home environment has been assessed for readiness.
    - Two family members can be identified who are able, available, and committed.
    - Parenting risks and family support system has been evaluated (see above criteria for early discharge).
    - Home environment has been assessed (on-site assessment may be needed). Technology-dependent neonate needs home assessed for 24-hour telephone, electricity, water supply, and adequate heating.
    - Determine if financial support is needed.
- The knowledge, ability, and confidence to provide adequate care for the baby's parents and/or other family members have been assessed by trained staff in the following areas:
    - Preparation, dosing accuracy, and proper storage and administration of medications.
    - Basic neonate care including bathing, cord care, temperature measurement, comforting.
    - Use of oxygen therapy or monitoring equipment, including the ability to set up and monitor oxygen delivery system or monitoring system.
    - Ability to provide appropriate nutrition to the infant, including adequate frequency and volume of feeding and the ability to mix calorically dense formulas.
    - Recognition of signs of illness and acute deterioration.
    - Basic neonatal cardiopulmonary resuscitation.
    - Proper infant safety, including car seat adaptations for infants weighing less than 2,000 g and recommended sleeping positions for premature infants.
- Appropriate immunizations have been given.
- Sensorineural screening, hearing, and fundoscopy have been accomplished as indicated.
- Appropriate metabolic screening has been performed.
- Home community and health care system readiness has been assessed.
    - A physician-directed source of continuing medical care, including periodic assessment of infant development, has been identified.
    - Appropriate follow-up has been arranged with specialty care providers.
    - Plan for neurodevelopmental evaluation is in place.
    - Home nursing visits have been arranged.
    - Emergency plans are in place and emergency services providers are notified.
    - Information from hospital discharge summary is shared as well as home care plans.

HOME VISITS/ FOLLOW-UP TELEPHONE CALLS

A home visit or at minimum a telephone call, when a home visit is not covered by insurance or agreed to by the family, made within the first week of discharge is advised to assess the health and well-being of the mother and infant. These services should be available to any childbearing family. However, the availability may vary from community to community.

MATERNAL ASSESSMENT

Physical inspection, psychological evaluation, and assessment of feeding technique are parts of the maternal exam and can be assessed during home visits.

Physical Examination

Focus on answering the following questions:

General Appearance and Vital Signs

- Does the client appear rested or exhausted?
- Are blood pressure and pulse within her normal limits, based on her baseline vital signs as an inpatient (assuming no gestational hypertension)?
- Does the client complain of chills or fever? If so, determine her temperature.
- In a client with a history of gestational hypertension, how does current blood pressure compare with in-hospital blood pressure?

Breast Health and Care

- Is the client lactating?
- Are the breasts soft, or hard and painful (engorged)?
- Is the client wearing a supportive bra?
- If the client is breastfeeding, how often is the infant nursing?
- Is the client experiencing pain or nipple tenderness when she breast-feeds?
- Does the client feel comfortable with breastfeeding or insecure or worried?

Abdomen and Musculoskeletal System

- Does the client have discomfort or difficulty urinating?
- Is she constipated or does she have hemorrhoids?
- If the client had cesarean birth, how does the incision appear? Are staples present? What is the color of the skin and skin integrity? Is the incision draining? If so, what color is the drainage?
- Is there any back or neck pain or pain in the lower extremities?
- Is there swelling in the lower extremities?

Genitalia and Reproductive Organs

- What is the fundal height?
- Is there uterine tenderness?
- How much lochia is evident and what color is it? Has there been any change in these qualities?
- If an episiotomy was done, is the incision erythematous? Draining? Intact?

Psychological Evaluation

Assess the client's ability to cope: What is her financial status? Did she recently relocate? Are her family and significant other supportive? What is her housing situation? Is she homeless or living in overcrowded conditions?

Provide anticipatory guidance for a client concerning her neonate's behavior. Assess her and her family's knowledge of neonatal and infant development and infant cues. Assess their adjustment to the infant.

Feeding Technique

Assess feeding technique. Who is the primary provider of care for the infant? Does another person in the client's family influence infant feeding, for example, the type of milk given, the frequency of feedings, or the introduction of solids?

Breastfeeding technique may be assessed by asking specific questions. How often does the infant nurse? How is the infant held when breast-fed? Do her breasts feel soft after feeding? Ask the client to describe the infant's suck: Is it strong and vigorous, or does the infant frequently stop sucking and cry? How many wet diapers does the infant have in a day? Infants who are getting enough breast milk have six to eight wet diapers a day. Are supplemental feedings given? If so, ask the client the reason for supplementation.

Consider observing the mother and infant during a feeding session to assess the effectiveness of breastfeeding technique. Bottlefeeding technique may also be assessed by questioning. How often is the infant fed and by whom? What type of milk is given—commercially prepared formula or table milk? How is the infant held during feeding? Is the bottle propped? Is the nipple properly positioned? Are solids given? If so, why and how is infant fed the solid food?

Environment

Assess the home environment for hazards. Smoking increases respiratory infections, invasive meningococcal disease, colic, gastroesophageal reflux, and sudden infant death syndrome (SIDS) (Gaffney, 2001; Moon, Horne, & Hauck, 2007; Peat, Keena, Harakeh, & Marks, 2001). Maternal smoking has also been associated with decreased arousal ability in infants (Richardson, Walker, & Horne, 2009). The risk for SIDS increases threefold for infants exposed to environmental tobacco smoke (Klonoff-Cohen et al., 1995). In a meta-analysis by Peat et al. (2001), a dose-related relationship to adverse outcomes in children was found between both the number of smokers in the home and the amount smoked. In addition, there is an emerging body of information regarding risk from thirdhand smoke, that is, residue from smoking that clings to clothing and furnishings. So, this potential risk should also be assessed (Winickoff et al., 2009).

Infant Care

Assess the client's or caregiver's knowledge of infant cues, infant sleep and wake states, and child developmental stages (see Neonatal Assessment, which follows). Inquire about infant's sleep position (prone, supine, side lying). In healthy infants, the AAP recommends infants no longer be placed in the prone position for sleep. Instead, healthy infants should be placed in the supine or side-lying position. Placing healthy infants in the supine or side-lying position is associated with a lower risk of SIDS. The supine position is also recommended for premature and low birth weight infants (AAP, 2000; AAP & ACOG, 2007).

In addition to the supine position, other recommendations by the AAP and ACOG (2007) to reduce the risk of SIDS include:

- A crib that conforms to the safety standards of the Consumer Product Safety Commission and the ASTM (American Society for Testing and Materials) for sleeping rather than a cradle, bassinet, or adult bed.
- Avoidance of soft surfaces for infant sleep, such as waterbeds, sofas, or soft mattresses; avoidance of soft materials in the infant's sleep environment, such as pillows, comforters, sheepskins, or quilts placed under the infant; loose bedding such as quilts, blankets, or sheets—if used, they should be tucked around the crib mattress to avoid covering the infant's face. Another option would be to use sleep clothing rather than blankets when putting the baby to bed.
- Avoiding bed sharing or co-sleeping. Parents who choose to bed share with their infant should not smoke or use substances such as alcohol or drugs, which may impair their arousal.
- Avoidance of overheating of the infant.
- Some tummy time should be encouraged while the infant is awake and observed to help prevent occipital flat spots and to help with developmental skills.
- Avoidance of devices that have been developed to maintain the supine sleep position, as these devices have not been tested for efficacy or safety.
- Home monitoring, while appropriate for some at-risk infants, has not been shown to decrease the incidence of SIDS.

Health Teaching

Provide the client with information about exercise and rest, nutritional needs, postpartum sexuality and fertility, health care, and the nurturing needs of the infant. (Refer to Readjustment With the Infant's Father for specific information.)

NEONATAL ASSESSMENT

Physical inspection, home safety assessment, and identification of engagement and disengagement cues are parts of the neonatal evaluation, which should be assessed during a home visit.

Physical Examination

The physical examination is important to identify any abnormal findings. It is also important for the health care provider to obtain answers for several questions to make an accurate assessment of the infant.

General Appearance and Vital Signs

- Has the infant gained weight since hospital discharge? Although 5 to 10 percent of birth weight may be lost by both bottle-fed and breast-fed infants, the newborn should return to or exceed birth weight by the second week of life. Weigh the infant if a portable scale is available.
- Does the infant appear healthy?
- When awake, does the infant appear alert, wan, irritable?
- What color is the infant's sclera? If yellow, was bilirubin tested prior to discharge?
- When is the infant's follow-up appointment?
- Is the infant's skin clean, without lesions, bruises, or unexplained markings?

Cardiovascular and respiratory assessments include the infant's apical pulse and respiratory rate. If either is elevated, inquire regarding infant's sucking strength, frequency of feedings, and type of cry (absent, weak, vigorous). If assessment indicates possible infection, refer the client and infant for follow-up.

Abdominal assessment is important to assess abdomen for softness and tenderness. It is also essential to determine the amount and frequency of the infant's voidings and the amount and consistency of stool.

In a male infant, the circumcision site, if present, is assessed for type of discharge and evidence of healing. If circumcision was not done, instruction should be given regarding proper care: Wash external penile skin only, as foreskin of infants and young children cannot be retracted.

Genitalia of a female infant may show a small amount of vaginal blood, which is the result of maternal estrogen in utero.

Home Safety

A hazard-free environment is important. Anticipatory guidance is useful for potential safety problems at different developmental stages of the infant and child. Suggest client not leave infant unattended on bed, table, swing. If client's nails are long, suggest she trim them to keep from scratching or otherwise injuring infant. Suggest to the client, for example, that she tie knots in plastic bags before throwing them away, use child-safety gates, and select toys with no sharp edges or separable, hazardous parts. Keep loose objects from edge of table, sink, or store where a small child could reach up to grab and cause injury.

Child Development

The health care provider should observe nonverbal and verbal cues used by the infant to initiate or stop interaction with the caregiver. An infant's demonstration of disengagement behaviors warrants cessation of caretaking activity and then reassessment of the infant. Evaluate the infant's sleep states (deep or light sleep) and awake states (drowsy, quiet alert, active alert, crying). An infant is most conducive to learning and taking in environmental stimuli when in an active alert state. Point out the infant's engagement and disengagement cues to the mother or care provider.

Engagement Cues

- Verbal cues are feeding sounds (sucking) and crying.
- Nonverbal cues are rooting, alerting signs, facial brightening, smooth cyclic movements of the extremities, mutual gaze, feeding posture, brow raising, and facing gaze (infant looks at parent's or caregiver's face) (Barnard, 1978).

Disengagement Cues

- Verbal cues are spitting, vomiting, hiccoughs, whimpering, crying during caregiving activity, and fussing.
- Nonverbal cues are lip compression, clenching eyes, gaze aversion, yawning, tongue show, increased foot movement, and hand-to-ear movement (Barnard, 1978).

ADJUSTING TO PARENTING

Parenting is a skill that is often learned, to varying degrees of success, by trial and error. Attachment is a process whereby affection develops between infant and parent or caregiver. Reva Rubin's theory of maternal-infant bonding is a classic in maternity nursing. See Table 22–3 for Rubin's description of normal maternal behavior postpartum. Mercer built on Rubin's work and further defined the process of attachment as an emotional or affectional commitment to an individual, facilitated by positive interaction between the two and mutually satisfying experiences (Mercer, 1983, 2004). As discussed in Chapter 19, maternal attachment begins during pregnancy as the result of fetal movement and maternal fantasies about an infant (Davis & Akridge, 1987; Lederman, 1996).

A mother's attitudes about pregnancy may influence her feelings about the infant. Maternal grief over the loss of a fantasized perfect child may result in delayed bonding or attachment if, for example, the infant is born prematurely or with obvious birth defects. The infant's behavior can also affect maternal bonding. The infant's crying, avoidance of eye contact, refusal of breast, or withdrawal of a hand when touched is negative reinforcement for a mother.

Kathryn Barnard developed Nursing Child Assessment Satellite Training (NCAST) tools based on research that she began in the 1970s. These tools enable the health care provider to identify families that need intervention. Current information and training for use of these tools is available at www.ncast.org.

TABLE 22–3. Reva Rubin Theory: The Postpartum Phase

Phase	Behaviors
Taking in	Passive, receptive, dependent infant mode; sleep, food are paramount. Often thought to be a process of regeneration. Mother spends time claiming her infant, bringing the infant into her social fabric. Mother begins with initial touching activities: first fingertips then to whole-hand touching within days 1 to 5 postdelivery.
Taking hold	Increased autonomy, independence usually begin on third day postpartum. Characterized by accomplishing what must be done over the next 2–3 weeks of the postpartum period. Mother demonstrates mastery of her own body's functioning, readiness to master some of her many tasks of motherhood.
Letting go	Starts during second and third weeks postdelivery. Mother begins to separate herself from the symbiotic relationship she and her infant enjoyed during pregnancy/delivery. Prior to this point, guilt was predominate feeling for the mother when separated from her infant.

Sources: Gay, Edgil, & Douglas, 1988; Rubin, 1984.

BARNARD MODEL FOR ATTACHMENT AND PARENTING

Adaptation is a result of caregiver-environment-infant interaction. Kathryn Barnard noted that the infant has the tasks to produce clear clues and to respond to the caregiver. If the infant is unable (due to immaturity, illness, or other physical/neurological problems), the adaptive process is interrupted. The mother/caregiver, in turn, cannot respond to the infant's needs, resulting in feelings of maternal inadequacy. Tasks for the mother/caregiver include being able to respond to the infant's cues, to allay distress, and to provide a growth-stimulating environment. Failure interferes with the infant's ability to adapt. The infant, in turn, becomes frustrated, and learns inappropriate interaction behaviors (Barnard, 1978). The environment is also influential. For example, the family is impacted by the actual birth of the child, social deprivation, or an alternate family style, such as single parenting.

Stress or interference may cause parental insensitivity to an infant's cues, failure of the infant to give reliable cues, and failure of the infant to respond to the parent.

MERCER MODEL FOR ATTACHMENT AND PARENTING

Mercer's (1983) definition of attachment—a process affected by positive feedback through mutually enjoyable experiences—stresses "process" (progressive nature, occurring over time), "positive feedback" (social, verbal, nonverbal, real, or perceived responses of one partner to another), and "mutually satisfying experience" (environment can have positive or negative impact on the mother-infant interaction).

Four stages of attachment are identified:

- *Anticipatory:* Mother seeks out role model.
- *Formal:* This stage begins with the birth of the child and continues for 6 to 8 weeks; the mother's behaviors are affected primarily by the expectations of others.
- *Informal:* Mother begins to develop her own unique role behavior.
- *Personal:* Mother feels comfortable with role and others accept her role performance (Mercer, 1985, 1990).

INHIBITORS OF ATTACHMENT

Maternal Factors

The adverse impact of depression or anxiety on maternal attachment has been studied extensively (Cho, Holdritch-Davis, & Miles, 2008; Zauderer, 2008). Substance abuse has also been noted to have an adverse impact (Alhusen, 2008). Research from the 1990s identified the following factors that influence attachment: Among high- and low-risk women and partners, parental competence is a major predictor of parent-infant attachment (Mercer & Ferketich, 1990). Facilitating parental competence thereby increases parent-infant attachment (Mercer & Ferketich, 1990; Muller, 1996). Parental competence may be defined as the real or perceived ability to care for the physical and psychosocial needs of the infant.

Several factors inhibit attachment and decrease competence.

- Medication, such as narcotics, sedatives, and some forms of anesthesia.
- Physical problems from pregnancy, such as long labor, difficult delivery, or chronic illness.
- Lack of experience in caring for newborns/older infants.
- Learned maternal behaviors that have a negative influence.
- A negative self-concept.
- Lack of a positive support system.
- Grieving a significant loss.
- Anticipatory grieving over an imagined loss of infant, resulting from, for example, complicated pregnancy or postnatal problems.
- Psychological unpreparedness due to premature birth.
- Escape mechanisms, such as alcoholism and drugs.

Infant Factors

Several factors may inhibit attachment.

- Neonatal complications in full-term infants.
- Infant abnormalities.
- Immaturity resulting from premature birth.
- Multiple births.
- Feeding difficulties.

Paternal Factors

A father may exhibit behaviors that inhibit his attachment with the infant.

- Difficulty adjusting to new dependent.
- Failure to relate to newborn.
- Escape mechanisms, such as alcohol and drugs.
- Separation from mother and child because of business or military responsibilities (Mercer, 1983).

Hospital Factors

Hospital procedure may inhibit attachment.

- Separation of infant and mother immediately after birth, at night, and for long periods during day.
- Policies that discourage or inhibit unwrapping and exploring the infant, limiting mother's caretaking.
- Restrictive visiting policies.
- Hospital/intensive care environment.
- Staff behavior not supportive of mother's caretaking attempts and abilities (Baho & Hager, 1998).

PARENTS OF INFANTS WITH MALFORMATIONS

Stages of Adjustment

A wide range of change occurs during adjustment.

- Shock, irrational behavior.
- Denial.
- Grief/anger/anxiety.
- Equilibrium; lessening of anxiety and intense emotional reactions.
- Reorganization (Kennell & Klaus, 1998; Klaus & Kennell, 1983).

Long-Range Impact

Caring for a child with malformation affects all aspects of the parents' lives.

- Financial cost for surgery, medical care for chronic problems, or early stimulation, for example, physical therapy sessions.
- Guilt over time spent with imperfect infant compared with that spent with other child(ren).
- Social support from family and friends having adverse effect on family relationship.

Therapeutic Approach

The health care provider should realize that the infant is not consistent with the parents' fantasized infant and that a therapeutic approach is necessary to address their feelings.

- Parents must mourn the loss of the fantasized child before they can fully attach.
- Guilt accompanies their mourning.
- Resentment and anger are often directed at health care personnel. Allow parents to express their feelings and take the time necessary to experience the full extent of their grief.
- The demands of the imperfect newborn retard mother's attempt to mourn the fantasized child.
- Mourning is asynchronous; that is, progress through the stages of mourning varies for each parent (Kennell & Klaus, 1998; Klaus & Kennell, 1983).
- Parents should not be given conflicting information concerning their infant.
- The health care provider may be a role model for parents by responding to the infant with smiles; the infant's positive features should be pointed out to parents.
- Social services may provide financial assistance, and a support group social, interpersonal, or medical support.
- Arrange for home care visit to ensure after discharge care is being implemented.

Of interest, regarding maternal attachment and children with malformations, is a study by Coy, Speltz, and Jones (2002). Follow-up for infants with cleft lip and palate (CLP) in comparison to infants with cleft palate only and no facial malformation revealed that the maternal-child bond by 24 months was stronger for those with CLP. The researchers hypothesize that this related to a stronger protective response of the mother for the child with the visually obvious malformation. Further study is needed regarding maternal attachment and children with malformations.

FAMILY RELATIONSHIPS

The Secundigravida

The concerns of a woman experiencing her second pregnancy are primarily for her other child and the expectation of caring for two children.

- Concern for first child may cause grieving over the dyadic relationship with the first child and her anticipation of the first child's pain.
- Managing the care of two children may cause a mother to feel overwhelmed. She may have increased expectations of the first child and may doubt her own ability to love two children equally. The temperaments of the new infant and the older sibling may be different.
- Assist the parents in developing confidence in parenting skills through parenting classes that include information about infant and child behavior, home visits, and telephone calls.

- The second pregnancy may not be as exciting or as desired as the first. The mother may not be totally engrossed in mothering her second baby as she was with the first. She may feel sad or guilty.
- Maternal self-perception changes and she sees herself as experienced. She recognizes her needs as separate from those of her role as mother.

Readjustment With the Infant's Father

A negative effect of childbirth may be the breakup of the marriage or relationship. The mother may lack support in childcare and household tasks. Spouse abuse or child abuse may increase. In assessing the couple, focus on their sharing of tasks, sexual relationship, leisure activity, and financial management.

- Sharing of family tasks and responsibilities often occurs following agreement before childbirth on the division of tasks. Equal sharing of child and infant care may be agreed on, or the parents may prefer that the father be primary caregiver for the older child or children. Other parents may prefer that the father assume more household tasks and the mother have the responsibility for infant and children.
- Assess the parenting roles of the mother and father. Assess their self-expectations and their expectations of each other. Parenting behavior can be adaptive (constructive) or maladaptive (nonconstructive, harmful). The health care provider may need to identify normal infant and child behaviors and developmental tasks to the parent or caregiver. Alternative forms of discipline for an older child (e.g., "time out") may need to be discussed. Refer parent or caregiver to parenting classes through, for example, churches or March of Dimes.
- The sexual relationship may be safely resumed 2 weeks postpartum (Cunningham et al., 2010c). Physiological responses in the puerperium may cause a decrease in the intensity of the sexual experience. The decrease is due to thin vaginal walls in the hypoestrogenic state, especially during lactation; delayed congestion of the labia majora and minora until the plateau phase; and decreased strength of orgasmic contractions. Sexual activity is decreased because of fatigue, weakness, vaginal discharge or spotting, perineal pain, tight or lax vaginal muscles, breast discomfort, and decreased vaginal lubrication. Client teaching may include suggestions to enhance sexual comfort and safer-sex behaviors and precautions.
    - Saliva (after postpartum exam) or water-soluble gel (Astroglide®, Replens®, K-Y Jelly®) may be used for lubrication.
    - Lubricated condoms may provide comfort.
    - The female-superior or side-to-side positions may help control the depth of thrusting.
    - Gentle rotation of two fingers around the vagina may aid vaginal relaxation.
    - Other displays of affection (holding, cuddling) are pleasurable if intercourse is not desired.
    - The woman may assist partner to orgasm with masturbation or fellatio. Her partner may help her also achieve orgasm without intercourse.
    - The client should perform Kegel exercises to regain vaginal tone.
    - A nutritious diet will promote healing and a sense of well-being.
- Leisure time for the couple should include time alone. They may enlist the help of family and friends to watch the infant and children. Encourage communication between the couple ("I love you," "You are special to me," "Thanks for your help"). Simple gestures of affection (romantic card or flowers for him or her) provoke loving feelings.
- Management of finances may require referral to a community food bank, social services, or the Women, Infants, and Children (WIC) program.

Single Parent/Working Mother

Address the parent's childrearing difficulties, financial insecurity, role conflict, or social isolation.

- Encourage the parent to verbalize feelings on how absence of one parent may affect parent-infant relationship or child development.
- Identify for the working mother the positive aspects of separation (daily break from infant and childcare while at work).
- Stress the importance of quality rather than quantity of time spent with the infant and children.
- Assist the parent in developing confidence in parenting skills through parenting classes that include information about infant behavior, home visits, and telephone calls.
- Encourage inexpensive activities that are relaxing and enjoyable for parent and infant.
- Financial insecurity may benefit from referral to community food bank, social or legal services, or WIC. In addition, referral for housing or job training may be necessary.

A parent experiencing role conflict and uncertainty concerning responsibilities may benefit from assistance in establishing priorities and assigning appropriate tasks to older children. Referral to appropriate resources may also be necessary to develop essential skills in caretaking and home management.

Social isolation and loneliness may be eased by client's involvement in parental and social groups (apartment complex, church, extended family) and support groups (see list of Support Groups at the end of this chapter).

Same-Sex Families

Same-sex families may include legal guardian relationships, working collectives, roommates, ex-lovers now considered family members, and couples with or without children (Blackwell & Blackwell, 1999). The health care provider should be knowledgeable regarding lesbian, bisexual, and transgender (LBT) issues and health care concerns, comfortable providing health care to the LBT population, and supportive of the LBT family (see Chapter 8).

LBT concerns range from unique to common:

- Fear of custody battles requires referral for legal advice on custody, because a nonbiological lesbian parent may not have a legal right to parent a child if the biological parent, or her partner, dies.
- Fear of HIV infection is possible. An alternative insemination/unscreened donor may have been used for conception or a partner may also have intercourse with men (Addis, Davies, Greene, MacBride-Stewart, & Shepherd, 2009; Institute of Medicine [IOM], 1999). If HIV infection is a concern, counsel LBT women regarding breastfeeding risks, testing, and safer sex (see Chapter 15).
- Battering—physical, emotional, or verbal—is possible. (See Appendix B for assessment tool for abuse.) Refer the woman for counseling, to a shelter, or to a support group.
- Alcoholism affects lesbian relationships and families as it does heterosexual relationships and families.
- Support may be lost from family and friends (Bender, Jorjorian, Lynch, & Cramer, 1998; Weisz, 2009).

A role model should be available to assist with maternal tasks.

- Determine the coparent's involvement in infant care and with partner.
- Encourage the partner's role in parenting.
- Encourage the partner's presence during health care visits.
- Referral to appropriate support groups may be helpful.

Families With Human Immunodeficiency Virus Infection

Human immunodeficiency virus (HIV)-infected families are those families in which one or more persons are infected with the virus. Persons may be asymptomatic carriers or exhibit AIDS, having been diagnosed with opportunistic infections and malignancies. The epidemiology of AIDS is described in Chapter 15.

Women who have tested positive for HIV should be referred to HIV specialists during the postpartum period, so that antiretroviral therapy can be reviewed. Neonatal antiretroviral prophylaxis should begin as soon as possible after delivery, ideally within 6 to 12 hours (Aaron, Abrams, Anderson, & Weinberg, 2010). As HIV treatment and prevention is an evolving field, refer to the AIDS*info* website (http://aidsinfo.nih.gov) for up-to-date guidelines for prevention of perinatal transmission. HIV-infected mothers should be taught how to administer appropriate medications to their infants postpartum, regardless of whether they choose to continue antiretroviral therapy after delivery. Discussion of birth control should include the consistent use of condoms, alone or in addition to any other contraceptive method chosen, to decrease the risk of acquiring other strains of HIV (CDC, 2010b). Oral contraceptives may not be as effective when women are on efavirenz and nevirapine, protease inhibitors, or other medications (rifampin) commonly used for HIV-infected patients (CDC, 2010c). All HIV-infected infants should be referred to a pediatric HIV specialist for antiretroviral therapy. All infants should have serial HIV DNA-PCR testing done at 48 hours, 1 to 2 months and 2 to 4 months. Any positive result should be reconfirmed with a second test sample as soon as possible (AAP & ACOG, 2007).

Teach clients about infection control, such as hand washing, avoiding exchange of body fluids or sharing of razors and toothbrushes, wrapping soiled peripads in sturdy plastic containers, and cleaning soiled surfaces with a dilute bleach solution of 1 part bleach to 10 parts water.

Advise clients to contact the health care provider should they note signs of infection: fever, foul smell of lochia, excessive amount of bleeding, return of bright red bleeding. Clients should also contact the health care provider if there are signs of worsening HIV infection: fatigue, anorexia, weight loss, sore throat, cough, dermatologic disorders, or unusual vaginal discharge. The infant's health care provider should be contacted if the infant exhibits fever, poor feeding, oral thrush, diarrhea, cough, or flu-like symptoms.

Instruct the client on how to avoid other infection (see section Self-Care Strategies in Chapter 15).

Families with HIV may have several areas of concern: personal, health, and family concerns; concern for the needs of the children; financial pressures and concerns; dilemma of disclosure; and the social aspects or challenges of HIV (DeMatteo, Wells, Goldie, & King, 2002). Some of the issues of health and family concerns included a divorce, separation, or abandonment rate of one in five adults, fear of intrafamily transmission through the very acts of intimacy that often bring consolation, fear of transmission through casual contact, increased stress from finances or illness, and the importance of support. Families focused on the children by attempting to maintain normalcy in childhood and by preparing children to become self-sufficient and independent. Parents often fear that disclosure would harm the children, especially in the way others perceive them. Women deal with disclosure in several ways. Some deal with it by bringing the child's medication to the school rather than having it dispensed by the school nurse or by not correcting a child's false assumption for taking antiviral medication (Santacroce, Deatrick, & Ledlie, 2002). Other women with HIV deal with their illness by silencing themselves by denying the importance of their own needs and feelings and put the needs of their families foremost (DeMarco, Lynch, & Board, 2002).

Families With Domestic Violence

It is estimated that every year 4 to 5 million acts of some form of intimate partner violence (IPV) are experienced by women in the United States (CDC, 2011b; McColgan, Dempsey, Davis, & Giardino, 2010). The prevalence of emotional or physical abuse during pregnancy in a sample of 1,519 postpartum women was noted to be 7.4 percent in a recent study (Certain, Mueller, Jagodzinski, & Fleming, 2008). However, others have noted prevalence as high as approximately 20 percent (Shay-Zapien & Bullock, 2010). Older studies identified pregnant women are twice as likely to be assaulted with 40 percent of assaults occurring during the first pregnancy (Humphreys & Neylan, 2001; Shoultz, Phillion, Noone, & Tanner, 2002). The incidence of assaults on women with disabilities ranges from 33 to 83 percent (Kramer, 2002).

Child abuse often coexists or increases with spouse abuse (AAP & ACOG, 2007; Shay-Zapien & Bullock, 2010). It has been estimated that child abuse co-occurs with IPV between 30 and 60 percent of the time (Bair-Merritt & Fein, 2010). The National Coalition for the Homeless (NCH) (2007) includes family violence as a major factor contributing to poverty and homelessness of women on its fact sheet. Screening for domestic violence should be a routine part of history-taking and should be done when the patient is alone. Nonthreatening words and emotionally charged words (e.g., abused woman) should be avoided. Women from different cultures and ethnic backgrounds may respond to violence in different ways, sometimes making it more difficult for them to seek help. Shoultz et al. (2002) did a pilot study using prevention protocols that were tailored to five ethnic groups of women on two rural islands in the state of Hawaii. These women were Caucasian, Hawaiian, Filipino, Japanese, and Hispanic. The women felt that public places (schools, churches, laundromats) would be better places for obtaining information on domestic violence. The women stated that the health care provider should develop a relationship with the client and assure confidentiality. The women believed a broad, open-ended question would be more effective than using a laundry list. The health care provider can begin with a statement such as "Many women are dealing with abuse and violence in their lives, so I routinely ask about it in women" or "I am so concerned about violence that I'm asking all my clients."

Make an assessment for evidence of domestic violence, using either the Abuse Assessment Screen (see Appendix B) or the following questions recommended by the AAP and ACOG (2007, p. 99).

- Within the past year, have you been threatened or actually hit, slapped, kicked, or otherwise physically injured by anyone?
- Since you've been pregnant, have you be threatened or actually hit, slapped, kicked, or otherwise physically injured by anyone?
- Within the past year, has anyone forced you into sexual relations?
- Are you afraid of your partner or anyone you listed earlier? Do you feel safe at home?

It is also imperative to screen for a history of child abuse. Women, who were abused as children, are twice as likely to become victims of IPV, whereas men, who were abused as children, are twice as likely to be perpetrators of IPV (Bloom, 2010). See Appendix B for routine trauma questions for primary care.

Once abuse has been identified, assess the potential for danger for the client. An increase in the severity or frequency of abuse, attempts at choking the woman by her partner, threats or attempts on her part to commit suicide, attempts or threats on his part to commit suicide are some indicators that the client is in danger and consideration for her safety must be undertaken. She should be encouraged to think of a safety plan that may include the following:

- Hiding money
- Hiding extra set of house or car keys
- Set up a code with family/friends
- Ask neighbor to call police if violence begins
- Remove weapons
- Have available social security numbers (his, client's, children's), rent and utility receipts, birth certificates (client's and children's), driver's license, bank account numbers, insurance policies and numbers, marriage license, valuable jewelry, important phone numbers (Anderson, 2002; Kramer, 2002; Mick, 2010).
- Offer information on available shelters, legal and criminal assistance.

When child abuse screenings are positive, it is important to follow up with open-ended questions or statements. Ask the parent how the family might best address the issue. Acknowledge the individual's courage in facing and identifying problems, as well as the family's strengths. Follow-up with the family is essential.

Child or spouse abuse should be considered when a child or adult presents with an injury or symptom that is not consistent with the clinical evidence, when illogical or changing explanations for an injury are given by the parent, or when there is concomitant abuse of the child's mother (AAP Committee on Child Abuse and Neglect, 1998, reaffirmed 2004; Mick, 2010). Individuals should be interviewed separately to provide privacy and convey a sense of respect for the person as an individual.

Empowering strategies to use for the survivor of abuse include acknowledging the abuse, listening, avoiding blame, exploring options, and making referrals (Anderson, 2002; Bloom, 2010; Kramer, 2002).

Homeless Families

The homeless population continues to be a health care and social concern today. Approximately 40 percent of the homeless population are families with children, with the majority most frequently headed by women. Single-parent, female-headed families have a 50 percent greater chance of living below the poverty line than two-parent families. The majority of homeless women cite domestic violence as the prime factor for their being homeless (NCH, 2007).

Health issues for homeless families are staggering.

- Social isolation
- Lack of access to health care
- Physical violence on the streets and in shelters
- Spouse abuse, child abuse, or both
- Substance abuse
- Chronic health problems
- Obesity
- Inadequate diet: insufficient iron, folic acid, calcium; low intake of dairy products, fruits, and vegetables; high intake of total fat, saturated fat, and cholesterol
- Parasites
- Infectious diseases
- Exposure to the elements (Buckner, 1998; Menke, 2000; Oliveira & Goldberg, 2002; Synoground & Bruya, 2000)

Arrange for nursery services so that the client may attend classes in parenting skills and learn about infant behavioral cues. Identify and prevent family violence with counseling or referral. Identify and teach basic foot care: keep feet clean and dry; use proper technique for cutting toenails; use appropriate footwear; wear clean dry socks. Evaluation and care are provided at times and locations convenient to the population to be served. Assist in providing nutritional information to volunteers at soup kitchens. Refer families to community resources for lodging and job training. WIC, substance abuse programs, and domestic violence programs may also be suggested.

Discipline and Parenting Skills in Families

Parenting involves caring for children physically and emotionally in a loving manner so that they are able to become responsible, caring adults. Parenting is not an innate behavior but a learned art. Developing a sense of self-esteem and self-worth in the child is enhanced by discipline, provided that the discipline is supportive and aids in the development of problem-solving skills. Yet many parents attempt to accomplish this task with little knowledge of normal developmental stages of infants and children leading to unrealistic expectations.

Although spanking is not recommended by the AAP, spanking continues to be one of the most common forms of physical punishment (AAP, 1998; Kazdin & Benjet, 2003; Regalado, Sareen, Inkelas, Wissow, & Halfon, 2004; Taylor, Manganello, Lee, & Rice, 2010). As many as 90 percent of U.S. families reported having spanked their children as a form of discipline (Kazdin & Benjet, 2003; Regalado et al., 2004; Taylor et al., 2010). Spanking is an ineffective means of discipline because its effectiveness decreases with subsequent use. Spanking has the following consequences: an increased risk of injury when children under the age of 18 months are spanked; repeated spanking can lead to agitated, aggressive behavior in the child and physical altercation between the child and parent; it models an inappropriate behavior as a solution to conflict and has been associated with increased aggression in preschool and school-age children; spanking alters the relationship between parent and child, making discipline more difficult in adolescence; it is not effective as a long-term approach and makes other strategies (such as time out) more difficult and less effective to use. Also, the pattern of spanking may become sustained or increased, making it more likely for the parent to use as a relief from anger (Kazdin & Benjet, 2003; Taylor et al., 2010).

The AAP suggests alternatives to spanking that would be more positive in changing undesired behavior in children. An effective discipline system has three vital elements: (1) a learning environment characterized by a positive, supportive parent-child relationship; (2) a strategy for teaching and strengthening desirable behaviors; and (3) a strategy for decreasing or eliminating undesirable behaviors (AAP, 1998; Regalado et al., 2004).

A positive, supportive parent-child relationship is fostered through play and warmth and affection for the child by the parent. Parents should be encouraged to provide consistency in daily activities and interactions with the child, paying attention to the child to increase positive behavior and, conversely, ignoring and removing parental attention to decrease frequency or intensity of undesired behaviors. Positive reinforcement can entail special time between parent and child, listening carefully, helping them learn words to describe their feelings, allowing them to make choices whenever appropriate and helping them learn to evaluate the potential consequences, praising behaviors that are desirable, and modeling appropriate behavior and resolution strategies (AAP, 1998; Flaskerud, 2011). Undesirable behavior can be eliminated by making clear what the problem behavior is and what consequence can be expected when this behavior occurs, being consistent in responding to undesirable behavior, being calm and empathetic when correcting behavior, and providing a reason for a consequence for undesired behavior (AAP, 1998).

Many authors define discipline as teaching, not punishment (Brazelton, 1992; Kvols, 1998). Brazelton states that children sense a need for discipline, and toward the end of the second year, they will make this need known by obvious testing. He further states that self-discipline, which is the goal of discipline, comes in three stages: trying out limits, teasing to elicit a response from others as to what is and is not allowed, and internalizing these previously unknown boundaries.

Brazelton (1992) gives the following guidelines for discipline:

- Respect a child's stage of development.
- Fit the discipline to the child's stage of development.
- Discipline must fit the child.
- When your child is with other children, try not to hover.
- Model behaviors for the child.
- After the discipline is over, help your child explain what it's all about.
- Use a time-out, but for a brief period only.
- Ask the child's advice about what might help next time.
- Physical punishment has very real disadvantages.
- Watch out for mixed messages (e.g., telling a child "Don't do that" when you really aren't sure or don't mean it).
- Stop and reevaluate whenever discipline doesn't work.
- Pick up the child to love him or her afterward.
- Remember to reinforce the child when he or she isn't teasing you by commenting on how well he or she is controlling himself or herself.

Additional parenting guidelines identified by Kvols (1998) include:

- Taking care of self
- Encouraging the child
- Give unconditional love
- Offer focused attention to the child, known as genuine encounter moments
- Provide order and routine
- Teach child to make decisions
- Teach child to self-quiet
- Set limits
- Use of natural and logical consequences

PLAN

Effective parenting and discipline can be taught. The primary care visit is an ideal time to teach parents effective discipline strategies (Stein, 2010). The plan to assist families in their adjustment to parenting should offer many alternatives to address the multitude of needs.

- *Practical guidance:* This can include the simple suggestion to lay out clothes at night for the next day to decrease tension in the morning while dressing the infant and older child (children) for day care or school.
- *Child development and behavior:* Teaching a client about child development enables her to better understand older children and the new infant; counseling should address infant's cues and states.
- *Referral:* Individual counseling may be necessary for a client who feels excessively guilty or angry about her first child's reactions to the infant. After counseling the client regarding daily nutritional needs of adults, infants, and children, referral for specific dietary needs may be helpful. Refer the client for legal assistance and domestic violence counseling and assistance if appropriate (see Parenting/Family Support Groups at end of this chapter).

PERINATAL LOSS

Perinatal loss involves miscarriage, ectopic pregnancy, perinatal mortality, both stillbirth and neonatal death. A perinatal loss may also involve a perceived loss, including loss of expectation or giving one's infant up for adoption. Stillbirth or neonatal death (death within the first 28 days of life) is obviously a loss for the mother and the family. Less obvious may be the loss felt by a woman who miscarries or elects to terminate a pregnancy. All of these losses are irrevocable.

Loss of expectation is also a real loss for some women and their families. It may be experienced in the birth of a viable infant who is premature or has congenital anomalies or deformities. Loss of expectation may also be experienced when the birthing act causes losses that precipitate maternity blues even though the infant is healthy. For example, postpartum fatigue may make daily tasks difficult to perform and contribute to postpartum blues or depression.

Also, the woman or couple who give up an infant for adoption experience loss, especially if they bonded with the infant before birth. Giving up the infant does not eliminate these bonds (Callister, 2006; Rubin, 1984).

EPIDEMIOLOGY

In 2009, the United States had an infant mortality rate of 6.8 per 1,000 live births. According to the CDC, the United States slipped to 29th place among world nations as of 2004. Between 2000 and 2005, the preterm birth rate increased from 11.6 to 12.7 percent. Low birth weight infants are five to ten times more likely to die during their first year of life than infants of normal weight. The infant mortality rate for African Americans (13.6 per 1,000 live births) remains at more than twice that of white infants (5.76 per 1,000 live births) (MacDorman & Mathews, 2008).

Out of 4.3 million babies born alive in the United States, 19,000 die during the first 28 days of life from genetic disease and congenital malformations; they constitute 20 percent of total neonatal deaths (Cunningham et al., 2010b). Approximately 35 percent of stillbirths have a congenital defect (Cunningham et al., 2010b). Miscarriages occur in approximately 12 to 26 percent of clinically recognized pregnancies, with 80 percent occurring in the first 12 weeks. Approximately 50 percent of these are caused by chromosomal anomalies (Cunningham et al., 2010a).

Subjective Data

A client may report hopelessness, sadness, loss of appetite, inability to sleep, increased irritability or hostility toward others, preoccupation with the lost infant, social isolation, inability to return to normal activities, and somatic distress (Callister, 2006; Kennell, Slyter, & Klaus, 1970). The client may also have feelings of guilt and preoccupation with her negligence or minor omissions (Callister, 2006; Rubin, 1984). These feelings are also experienced by siblings and grandparents (Callister, 2006).

Objective Data

Data is determined concerning the client and her family's grieving by means of observation and counseling. The primary health care provider can then help them cope with their loss. If the health care provider is to assist the family through its grieving process, he or she must realize mothers and fathers may grieve differently (Callister, 2006). The father may desire sexual activity because he perceives coitus as a way to share and comfort as well as be comforted. The mother may perceive this desire as callousness (Dyregrov & Gjestad, 2011; Swanson, Karmall, Powell, & Pulvermakher, 2003).

Phases of Mourning. Progression through the five stages of mourning varies among individuals and regression may occur (Williams, 2000). Perinatal grieving involves acute grief, which is most intense during the 4- to 6-week period following loss and less intense in the subsequent 4 weeks. The normal grief reaction may last from 6 months to 2 years or may never resolve. The anniversary of the loss may reactivate grief reactions.

- The shock and numbness stage (denial) is expressed as impaired normal functioning. The individual has difficulty making decisions and may be aloof.
- Searching and yearning (anger) constitute the second stage of mourning. Anger and bitterness can be transferred to other people, especially health care professionals. Restlessness and guilt feelings may also be experienced.
- Bargaining, which is usually a brief phase, attempts to delay loss.
- Disorganization (depression) is the phase when the reality of the loss occurs. Depression may occur as the full impact of loss is felt. Guilt feelings remain.
- Resolution may be seen as the individual begins to function better at home and at work. Self-confidence increases. The individual is able to place the loss in perspective with life.

Parental Tasks. Following perinatal loss, parents must work through the loss and make it real. The parents must allow the normal grief reaction to progress. During this time, parents should meet their own needs as well as those of their other children and communicate their feelings to the children.

Multiple Gestation. Parents who experienced a multiple gestation may have an additional or more acute sense of loss from conflicting emotions. Parents need to grieve their deceased infant(s) before relating to the survivor(s). Parents may experience grief from loss of prestige as parents of twins. In addition, they may have a sense of inadequacy, as the death of one child may be perceived as the inability to raise more than one child.

Plan

Psychosocial Interventions. Measures are directed toward helping parents work through loss and make it real. Their coping abilities are assessed and, if indicated, the parents are referred to support groups for counseling.

- Telephone parents (especially important on what had been due date or on the anniversary of death) to reevaluate coping and readjustment. Call during the evening to involve the partner. Provide parents with the phone number of the hospital's maternity floor.
- Advise parents to join support groups (see Parenting/Family Support Groups and Perinatal Loss Support Groups at the end of this chapter).
- Provide anticipatory guidance, counseling parents about the normalcy of grief, its stages, and the varying duration. Warn parents of an emotional roller coaster of good and bad days—days when a sight, smell, or sound may bring back a flood of memories and tears. Most difficult time is 2 to 4 months after death (acute grief).
- Prepare parents to deal with reactions of others, especially well-meaning but insensitive comments.
- Advise couple that it is not uncommon for sexual intimacy to be compromised by avoidance, depression, or disinterest for up to 2 years after the death of a child.
- Facilitate communication and expression of grief with open-ended statements such as "Some fathers have said . . . . Tell me how you feel."
- Ask the father how he's doing—avoid expressing concern for just the mother.
- Recommend postponing pregnancy until both parents have worked through their grief.
- Provide suggestions for dealing with grief.
  - Communicate with partner, family, and friends; talk about the infant or child who died.
  - Eat a well-balanced diet; drink adequate fluids; avoid caffeine and alcoholic beverages. Exercise daily.
  - Avoid tobacco as it depletes the body of vitamins, increases stomach acidity, decreases circulation, and can cause palpitations.
  - Rest daily; rest at night even if unable to sleep.
  - Clarify values; don't be persuaded to act or think as you think you should behave. Ignore shoulds (e.g., "I should be strong and not cry").
  - Ease marital stress. Realize that no two people grieve the same way. Take the time to share thoughts and feelings each day and listen to what your partner is saying. Express affection for each other and other family members throughout the day.
  - Recognize and respect the need for solitary time.
  - Keep mementos of the baby. (Some hospitals provide a picture, a lock of hair, footprints, and/or an ID bracelet and will keep them for a period of time for the family that doesn't take these mementos initially.)
  - Read books, poems, and articles that comfort; avoid scare literature and technical medical bulletins.
  - Keep a diary or journal of thoughts, memories, and mementos. Write poems or letters to the infant.

- Avoid making big decisions or changes for 24 months, and do not let others make decisions for you; put away baby clothes and articles when you are ready.
- Accept help from others; request help from clergy if desired (Callister, 2006; Hutti, 2005).

Medication. Medication is not indicated.

Follow-Up

Follow-up involves continuing observation for resolution of grief. Grief is completed when an individual is able to turn outward and think of others and to formulate plans for the future. The stress related to a perinatal loss diminishes after a future birth but remains present for many (Armstrong, 2007). Give the couple a list of resources they can turn to when they are ready. (See Support Groups and Resources at end of this chapter.) If grief remains unresolved, refer parents to a skilled professional counselor. Unresolved grief may be observed in several behaviors:

- Persistent yearning for recovery of lost objects
- Overidentification with the deceased
- Inability to cry or rage despite desire to do so
- Misdirected anger or ambivalence toward infant
- Lack of support group/person
- Presence of secondary gain (e.g., increased attention to mother)

BREASTFEEDING

Breastfeeding rates continue to rise in the United States. In 2010, 75 percent of new mothers initiated breastfeeding and 43 percent of mothers breast-fed for 6 months, compared to 1996 when only 21.7 percent of mothers were breastfeeding their infants at 6 months (CDC, 2010a; Lawrence & Lawrence, 2011). In Third World countries and in acute poverty-stricken areas in the United States, an infant who is bottle-fed has a greater morbidity and mortality risk within the first year than an infant who is breast-fed (Ip et al., 2007; Lawrence & Lawrence, 2011). Breastfeeding has distinct advantages for both mother and infant and almost no contraindications. Human milk is physiologically compatible with the human infant's digestive tract and provides the exact balance of nutrients, electrolytes, and immunological factors necessary for optimal growth and development. Even the act of suckling employs the use of different muscles and feeding mechanism than bottlefeeding (Lawrence & Lawrence, 2011). Breastfeeding is more convenient for the mother, nothing to heat or spoil, and no extra bottles to transport. A special emotional bond develops between mother and nursing infant.

Evidence continues to support the benefits of breastfeeding (Ip et al., 2007, 2009; Lawrence & Lawrence, 2011) A recent meta-analysis conducted by the Agency for Healthcare Research and Quality indicated that breastfeeding may also lower the risk for breast and uterine cancer (Ip et al., 2007). The relative risk of breast cancer is decreased by almost 5 percent for every 12 months of breastfeeding in addition to a 7 percent decrease for each birth (Beral, 2002). If women breast-fed for 24 months, there would be a two-thirds reduction in breast cancer by age 70 (from an incidence of 6.3 to 2.7 per 100 women) in developed countries (Beral, 2002).

A mother who is breastfeeding for the first time may not have the support of family and friends and needs encouragement, support, and accurate information to become self-assured about breastfeeding. It has been demonstrated that extra breastfeeding support has lead to an increase in duration of breastfeeding (Britton, McCormick, Renfrew, Wade, & King, 2007). Support and teaching should ideally begin during the pregnancy. The health care provider has an opportunity to be the support that many breastfeeding mothers and her infant need to successfully breast-feed.

TYPES OF BREASTFEEDING

Unrestricted Breastfeeding

The infant is put to breast immediately after delivery and then on demand. Breast milk is the major source of nourishment for the first year of life or longer.

The advantages of this type of breastfeeding are that less illness occurs during first year of life (Ip et al., 2007; Lawrence & Lawrence, 2011), the infant has mouth–nipple contact and body contact, and the breast is associated with comfort as well as food. One disadvantage is that unrestricted breastfeeding requires the mother's dedication.

Token Breastfeeding

Restrictions are placed on the duration of breastfeeding and the length of each time at the breast; feedings are scheduled. The mother may pump her breasts and store the milk for others to give (e.g., daycare providers). Weaning often occurs by the third month or earlier.

The main advantage of token breastfeeding is that other family members can participate in feeding the infant. The disadvantages are that the milk supply may decrease, the infant is more susceptible to illnesses, and the infant learns bottle-sucking techniques, which may lead to nipple confusion.

BREAST ANATOMY

Breast tissue comprises glands, supporting connective tissue, and fatty tissue. The primary structures are skin, subcutaneous tissue, and the corpus mammae.

The skin includes the nipple, areola, and general skin. Each nipple contains 23 to 27 milk ducts; each of the tubuloalveolar glands opens separately onto the nipple. The nipple also contains smooth muscle fibers, sensory nerve endings, and sebaceous and apocrine glands. Nipple erection is caused by tactile, sensory, or autonomic sympathetic stimuli. Montgomery's tubercles contain the ductular openings of sebaceous and lactiferous glands. They secrete a substance that protects and lubricates the nipple and areola during pregnancy and lactation.

Subcutaneous tissue lies just below the dermis.

The corpus mammae is divided into the parenchyma and stroma. Parenchyma includes the ductular-lobular-alveolar structures. The lactiferous ductal system connects the alveoli to the nipple. Fifteen to 25 mammary lobi are embedded in fat (Lawrence & Lawrence, 2011). Each lobus divide into lobuli which then divide to alveoli. The stroma comprises connective tissue, fat, blood vessels, nerves, and lymphatics.

PHYSIOLOGY OF LACTATION

Lactation is hormonally controlled. The physiological changes that occur are directed toward mammogenesis, lactogenesis (milk secretion), and galactopoiesis (milk maintenance). Most milk is synthesized in the acini and smaller milk ducts during suckling (Lawrence & Lawrence, 2011).

Mammogenesis

Mammogenesis is the development of the mammary glands to their functional state.

Estrogen stimulates parenchymal proliferation and ductal growth. Luteal and placental hormones increase ductular and lobular formation; prolactin and somatotropin accelerate mammary growth (Lawrence & Lawrence, 2011). Prolactin (from the anterior pituitary gland) stimulates glandular production of colostrum; human placental lactogen stimulates secretion of colostrum by the second trimester (Lawrence & Lawrence, 2011); and progesterone stimulates lobular growth.

Lactogenesis

Milk production by the mammary glands proceeds in two stages.

Stage I of lactogenesis begins 12 weeks before parturition and is preceded by significant increases in lactose, total proteins, and immunoglobulins and decreases in sodium and chloride. Stage II clinically begins postpartum with copious milk secretion that occurs with a drop in progesterone during the first 4 days postpartum; mature milk is established in approximately 10 days (Lawrence & Lawrence, 2011).

Galactopoiesis

Galactopoiesis is the maintenance of established lactation, also known as lactogenesis III. Prolactin stimulates and sustains lactation (milk secretion); oxytocin stimulates milk ejection. An intact hypothalamic-pituitary axis regulates prolactin and oxytocin levels and is essential for the maintenance of milk secretion. Ejection reflex is dependent on receptors in the canalicular system of the breast. Dilation or stretching of the canalicules causes a reflex release of oxytocin: Tactile receptors for both oxytocin and reflex prolactin release are located in the nipple (Lawrence & Lawrence, 2011).

Prolactin secretion is controlled by prolactin inhibitory factor (PIF) produced by the hypothalamus. Suppression of PIF allows the anterior pituitary gland to secrete uninhibited amounts of prolactin. Catecholamine levels in the hypothalamus control PIF. Drugs and events that decrease catecholamines also decrease PIF, thereby causing an increase in prolactin (Lawrence & Lawrence, 2011). Among nonnursing mothers, prolactin levels drop to normal in 2 to 3 weeks, independent of lactation suppression therapy.

Composition of Human Milk

Milk varies with the stage of lactation, time of day, sampling time during a given feeding, maternal nutrition, and the individual. Initially, colostrum is produced. A transitional phase in production leads to secretion of mature milk.

Colostrum. A yellowish, thick fluid produced during the first postpartum week. It contains higher concentrations of sodium, potassium, and chloride than mature milk. Protein, fat-soluble vitamins, and minerals are also in larger concentration than in transitional or mature milk. This high-protein, low-fat milk meets the needs and reserves of the newborn (Lawrence & Lawrence, 2011). The mean energy value is 67 kcal/100 mL of mature milk. Colostrum facilitates the establishment of bifudus flora in the digestive tract and the passage of meconium. It contains abundant antibodies.

Transitional Milk. Secreted beginning 7 to 10 days postpartum and continuing until 2 weeks postpartum. The concentration of immunoglobulins decreases, although lactose, fat, and total caloric content increase. Water-soluble vitamins increase and fat-soluble vitamins decrease to approach the level found in mature milk (Lawrence & Lawrence, 2011).

Mature Milk. The only necessary source of nutrition for an infant's first 4 to 6 months of life and should be the primary source for the first year (AAP, 2005; Lawrence & Lawrence, 2011; Mohrbacher & Stock, 2003).

- Water is the major constituent. A lactating woman requires an increased water intake. If water intake is decreased, sensible and insensible water loss are decreased before water for lactation is decreased.
- Lipids, the second most plentiful constituent, and the most variable, provide the major portion of kilocalories. It is almost completely digestible.
- Proteins constitute 0.9 percent of human milk content (Lawrence & Lawrence, 2011).
- The predominant carbohydrate is lactose. Synthesized by the mammary gland, it is specific for newborn growth and enhances calcium absorption. Lactose appears to be critical for the prevention of rickets, as human milk is relatively low in calcium.
- Minerals essential to the newborn are potassium and iron.
    - Potassium levels are higher than sodium in breast milk (similar to intracellular fluids). Sodium levels in cow's milk are 3.6 times greater than those in human milk (Lawrence & Lawrence, 2011).
    - The concentration of exogenous elemental iron in human milk is 100 mcg/1,100 mL (Lawrence & Lawrence, 2011). Normal infants need 8 to 10 mg per day in the first year of life. Prepared formulas provide 10 to 12 mg per day. Although its concentration in human milk is low, iron is absorbed more readily than iron from other sources. Thus, infants are not at risk for iron-deficiency anemia or depletion of iron stores if they are breast-fed totally during the first 6 months of life (Lawrence & Lawrence, 2011).
    - An adequate supply of vitamins A, E, and C is present in breast milk. The amount of vitamin A in mature human milk is 280 IU and in cow's milk, 180 IU; an infant consuming 200 mL of breast milk every day obtains an adequate amount of vitamin A.
    - Serum levels of vitamin E in breast-fed babies rise quickly at birth and are maintained by approximately 4 weeks postpartum with only breast milk intake (Lawrence & Lawrence, 2011).
    - Vitamin C and other water-soluble vitamins in human milk reflect maternal dietary intake. Human milk is an excellent source of these water-soluble vitamins (Lawrence & Lawrence, 2011).

Resistance Factors and Immunological Significance

Breastfeeding significantly decreases infant morbidity and mortality by protecting against enteropathogens that may contaminate other food or formula. The protective factors contained in breast milk are both cellular and humoral (Lawrence & Lawrence, 2011).

Cellular factors include macrophages, polymorphonuclear leukocytes, and lymphocytes. These cells are phagocytes and they stimulate antibody formation. The humoral factors are immunoglobulins.

- Immunoglobulin A (IgA) is the most important immunoglobulin in terms of biological activity, and it is the most concentrated. IgA also has antitoxin activity against *Escherichia coli* and *Vibrio cholerae* and thereby prevents diarrhea (Lawrence & Lawrence, 2011).
- Bifidus factor is responsible for the growth of *Bifidobacterium bifidum*, the predominant bacteria in the gut of breast-fed infants. The flora of bifid bacteria inhibits pathogenic *Staphylococcus aureus*, *Shigella*, and *Protozoa* and encourages growth of *Lactobacillus bifidus*, which crowds out other bacteria. Lysozyme and lactoferrin act directly to inhibit pathogen growth. The resistance factor protects against *Staphylococcus* infection (Lawrence & Lawrence, 2011).
- Breast milk contains antibodies against poliovirus, coxsackievirus, echovirus, influenza virus, and rhinovirus and thus helps to prevent viral infections (AWHONN, 2000; Lawrence & Lawrence, 2011).
- Breast milk protects against the development of allergies. An infant begins to produce antibodies to cow's milk (which is the basis of formula) within 18 days of ingestion. Syndromes associated with cow's milk allergy include gastric enteropathy, atopic dermatitis, rhinitis, chronic pulmonary disease, eosinophilia, and failure to thrive (Lawrence & Lawrence, 2011).

CONTRAINDICATIONS

Human Immunodeficiency Virus

For women in the United States who test positive for HIV, breastfeeding is contraindicated (AAP, 2005; Lawrence & Lawrence, 2011). Breastfeeding, however, remains the feeding method of choice in countries where the death rate in the first year of life is 50 percent, compared with the 18 percent risk of dying from AIDS when born to an infected mother (Lawrence & Lawrence, 2011).

Untreated Active Tuberculosis

Mothers with untreated active tuberculosis should not breast-feed; however, breastfeeding is permitted if the mother's skin test is positive, and if at the same time there is no radiologic indication of disease and the client has started antituberculin medication. If the mother has a positive tuberculin skin test and positive chest film, she may breast-feed if she is taking antituberculous medication and the sputum culture is negative (Lawrence & Lawrence, 2011). The AAP considers isoniazid, rifampin, ethambutol, and streptomycin compatible with breastfeeding (Briggs et al., 2005). If the sputum culture is positive, breastfeeding may be possible after the mother has taken medication for at least 1 week. Limited isolation from the mother with active disease may be required. The breastfeeding infant may be treated prophylactically by the pediatrician.

Infants With Galactosemia

Infants with galactosemia are unable to digest the simple sugar galactose that is found in breast milk or formula. Galactosemia affects 1 in 60,000 infants. Infants with galactosemia will develop brain, liver, eye, and kidney damage if milk or formula of any kind is ingested (National Center for Biotechnology Information [NCBI], 2009).

Others Contraindications

Breastfeeding is also contraindicated if mothers are receiving diagnostic or therapeutic radioactive isotopes, if mothers are receiving chemotherapeutic agents, or if mothers are using any drugs of abuse (AAP, 2005).

CONDITIONS THAT ARE NOT CONTRADICTORY TO BREASTFEEDING

Hepatitis B Virus

Breastfeeding permitted in protected infants—rapid schedule of immunization (0, 1, and 2 months) of infant would be indicated. Milk donors are screened for this virus (AAP, 2005; Lawrence & Lawrence, 2011; Mohrbacher & Stock, 2003).

Cytomegalovirus

Breast milk also contains appropriate antibodies that protect the infant against cytomegalovirus. There does exist a risk for the infant who is exposed to virus but not a daily dose of antibodies, and risk for severe infection is especially great in premature infant of nonimmune mother (Lawrence & Lawrence, 2011).

Augmentation or Reduction Mammoplasty

Breast augmentation or reduction mammoplasty is not a contraindication to breastfeeding; however, milk production may be impacted. If milk ducts were cut during mammoplasty, breastfeeding may not be possible (Lawrence & Lawrence, 2011). Incisions around the areola usually indicate that some milk ducts were cut and possible nerve damage occurred.

In women who have had implants, the ability to lactate depends on the location of the scars. Periareolar incisions are more apt to disrupt the ducts and the neurological innervation of the nipple. Intact innervation is necessary for the milk ejection reflex. If the periareolar incision is completely circumferential, there will be some patent ducts that will be able to secrete milk to the nipple. Where the ducts have been cut, the breast will be engorged because the milk will not be able to be secreted, and the gland will eventually undergo involution (Chez & Friedmann, 2000).

Pierced nipples are not a contraindication to breastfeeding, but jewelry should be removed before putting the baby to breast.

ELEMENTS OF BREASTFEEDING

Compression of Lactiferous Sinuses

Externally, the infant's mouth should cover the lactiferous sinuses, whereas internally, the correct movement of the infant's tongue provides areolar compression between the infant's tongue and palate. The lactiferous sinuses lie underneath the areola; compression of the lactiferous sinuses removes milk from the breast. Sucking may need to continue for 2 minutes for the full response to oxytocin release.

Number of Feedings per Day

A minimum of eight feedings are necessary in 24 hours, with each feeding providing a minimum of 5 to 10 minutes of swallowing at each breast. During the first 2 weeks, infants may nurse 10 to 12 times in 24 hours.

The milk ejection reflex takes 2 to 3 minutes before it is effective (Lawrence & Lawrence, 2011); limiting nursing to 2 to 3 minutes does not permit the infant to obtain milk. Suck efficiency is critical to breastfeeding success.

Signs that an infant is doing well with breastfeeding include the following:

- Three or more stools every 24 hours, with meconium changing to breast milk stools by day 4.
- Six or more wet diapers every day by day 4.
- Infant is content between feedings.
- Infant awakens easily for feedings about every 3 hours.
- Breasts soften or feel lighter as the baby feeds.
- Nipples are healthy, not cracked or bleeding.
- Breast changes signaling lactogenesis stage II around 72 hours.
- Mother experiences signs of oxytocin and prolactin release—she feels drowsy, gets thirsty, and has uterine contractions/increased flow of lochia while baby is breastfeeding (Lawrence & Lawrence, 2011).

Assessment of Infant at Breast

Assessment of a breastfeeding session requires direct observation. Observe positioning and alignment, areolar grasp, sucking, mother-infant interaction, and maternal perception of infant satiety.

Positioning and Alignment. The infant should be relaxed, in a responsive state, and displaying early hunger cues—rooting and hand-to-mouth activity. Crying is a late hunger cue and it may be difficult for the infant to latch at this stage.

The infant's body should be flexed with the head and trunk aligned so that the head is straight on the breast, not turned laterally or hyperextended (head and body are at breast level). The infant should be brought to the breast, not the breast to the infant. Proper alignment decreases traction on the mother's nipples; the areola and nipple are more easily kept in the infant's mouth; swallowing is facilitated.

The mother's hand should cup her breast, with her fingers supporting the lower portion of the breast and her thumb resting on the upper portion. The infant should be permitted to grasp at least one-half inch of areolar tissue. This position is the "C-hold," and permits the mother to support her breast without distorting the nipple.

Areolar Grasp. The infant must have a correct mouth opening, correct lip flanging, and correct tongue placement. To elicit the grasp gently, tickle the infant's lips with the nipple to stimulate the mouth to open. When the mouth is opened wide, quickly pull the infant close to the breast and center the nipple in infant's mouth. Move the infant's head and trunk as a unit to avoid hyperflexion, hyperextension, or lateral turning of the head. Avoid holding the back of the infant's head to maneuver it onto the breast, because it does not allow the mother to feel rapid arm motion and erodes her confidence if the infant latches on. Placing a hand on the mother's arm and moving it quickly toward her breast allows the mother to feel the quick arm movement.

Breastfeeding Problems. May be determined during systematic assessment of the infant at the breast.

- Problems with grasping the areola may be caused by prissily pursed lips. The infant appears to be drinking through a straw. Only the nipple is grasped, and the mother often experiences nipple pain. The infant receives little milk because the lactiferous sinuses are not compressed. Break the suction by inserting a finger into the corner of infant's mouth and stimulate the mouth to open wide. Alternate sucking of the nipple and the areola through pursed lips will traumatize the nipple and the suck will become inefficient. Friction may abrade the mother's areolar tissue and result in ineffective sucking.
- Another grasping problem is negative pressure in an infant's intraoral cavity, which results in retention of the nipple and areolar tissue in the infant's mouth. This counteracts the naturally retractile nature of nipple tissue, helps to refill the lactiferous sinuses with milk from the lactiferous ducts, and conveys milk to the oropharynx. Negative pressure is achieved when an infant forms an effective seal with the border of his or her mouth.
- Sore nipples cause discomfort, and breastfeeding should not hurt. If the mother has sore, cracked nipples, the cause must be found: review positioning and latch-on of the infant. A variety of measures may be tried to relieve sore nipples.
    - Rule out problems such as monilia. The mother may complain of severe nipple itching or a severe pain when infant nurses. The infant may or may not show signs of thrush. The mother and infant should be treated simultaneously, the mother with Nystatin cream or Mycolog cream rubbed into the nipple after each feeding, and the infant with oral Nystatin (Lawrence & Lawrence, 2011). When recurrent candidiasis is not responding to Nystatin, Lawrence and Lawrence recommend oral fluconazole (Diflucan), with a loading dose of 200 mg, then 100 mg daily for 14 days. Although fluconazole passes through breast milk, it has a safety

profile for newborns and is approved for use at 6 months of age. Lawrence and Lawrence recommend the infant be kept on Nystatin to avoid relapse and either pasteurizing or discarding breast milk of women with candida because freezing does not kill the fungus.
  - Some milk may be expressed before feeding to stimulate the milk ejection reflex, thus allowing for softening of the areola before the infant latches on.
  - Some milk may be expressed onto the nipples after feedings and allowed to air dry.
  - The flaps of the nursing bra may be left open after feedings.
  - Nursing pads with plastic liners should be avoided. Nipple shields might also compound the problem by increasing nipple irritation and confusing the baby so that the baby sucks improperly and further irritates the nipple.
- Change the baby's position
- If artificial nipples (pacifiers, bottles, nipple shields) have been used, discontinuing them would likely be beneficial.

Sucking. Correct sucking requires that the infant's tongue cover the mandibular-alveolar ridge on the lower gum line and curve beneath the areolar tissue.

Evaluate tongue placement by gently pulling infant's lower lip downward. Incorrect tongue placement is indicated by clicking or smacking sounds and drawing in of cheek pads with each suck, or by the loss of large amounts of milk over the infant's chin (Mohrbacher & Stock, 2003). A short tongue or one with a short lingual frenulum may not extend over the lower alveolar ridge.

Evaluate areolar compression by carefully noting the type of sucking and swallowing. A sustained slower mandibular motion indicates nutritive sucking; rapid mandibular motion indicates nonnutritive sucking. Audible swallowing is the most reliable indicator of milk intake. Documentation of an infant's breastfeeding should state: "Breastfed with audible swallowing at each breast."

Breastfeeding Positions

The mother's hand position and how the infant is held are important factors when breastfeeding. The exact position is not as important as long as the latch and the suck are effective. Whichever position the mother uses to nurse her infant, she should be comfortable. Pillows should be used to help support her arm and help her hold the baby close to her breast, relaxed and without muscle strain. The following are four common positions that are taught to breastfeeding mothers.

- *Cradle hold:* The mother sits up, the infant faces her, and the infant's head or arm rests on the mother's forearm or in the crook of her arm. The cradle hold is a good choice for a mother whose infant has low muscle tone; for example, an infant with Down syndrome.
- *Football hold:* The mother sits up, the infant's head faces her breast, and the body is held at the mother's side. Unlike a true football hold, the baby is not tucked under the arm but is held in a more forward position with the mother's arm supporting the infant (Lawrence & Lawrence, 2011). The baby's bottom should be resting on a pillow near the mother's elbow to provide additional support for the mother and avoid muscle strain. The football hold is a good choice for a mother who recently had abdominal surgery, as the position does not put pressure on the incision.
- *Side-lying position:* Both the mother and infant lie on their sides, facing each other, with the infant's feet pulled in close to his or her body. Pillows under the mother's head, behind her back, and under the knee or her upper leg may provide comfort. This position is more restful for mothers and has been found to significantly reduce fatigue among new breastfeeding mothers.
- *Slide-over position:* This position is especially useful with infants who refuse one breast. The mother can begin nursing the infant on the preferred side, then slide the infant over to the less preferred side once the milk ejection reflex has occurred. The infant's body position is not changed; he or she merely slides over.

New research by Colson Meek, and Hawdon (2008) suggest that laid back, semireclining positions might be more effective when breastfeeding. These authors have specifically looked at the relationship between primitive neonatal reflexes and breastfeeding positions, termed *biological nurturing*.

Breast Preparation

To prepare breasts for feeding, first assess them by palpating the tissue and inspecting the nipples and areola; then teach the mother proper care of the breasts. Palpate to detect inelastic breast tissue. Skin that is taut and firm and difficult to pick up is more prone to engorgement. Tissue can be improved by measures to prevent engorgement (Lawrence & Lawrence, 2011).

Assess the nipples and areola by gently compressing each areola between the thumb and forefinger. The normal nipple everts with gentle pressure; the inverted or tied nipple inverts more with gentle pressure. Exercises to evert the nipple are rarely successful and can lead to premature labor (Lawrence & Lawrence, 2011).

Stress the importance of avoiding soap and other drying agents on the nipples. Teach the mother to wash breasts with water only. Routine use of ointments and creams is discouraged, as some have irritants, such as lanolin. Vitamin E or hormone creams or ointments are unsafe on the nipples unless prescribed for a specific problem, and they then should be used only in minute amounts (Lawrence & Lawrence, 2011; Mohrbacher & Stock, 2003). Sebaceous glands and tubercles of Montgomery are easily plugged by repeated application of oily substances.

Extrinsic Factors Contributing to Breastfeeding Problems

Separation at any time, delayed feedings, and introduction of bottlefeedings may interfere with breastfeeding.

Separation of mother and infant interferes with milk ejection reflex; the infant is not able to nurse on demand, causing a delay that contributes to milk stasis and engorgement. If, in the mother's absence, the infant learns to suck on a bottle, then sucking at the breast becomes incorrect, causing pain and trauma.

Delaying first feedings to a healthy infant—an infant is most receptive to nursing in the first 90 minutes after birth—can erode the mother's self-confidence when a sleepy infant is later brought to her to feed. Delay can also decrease the milk ejection reflex.

Limiting the frequency and duration of feedings contributes to breastfeeding problems. The milk ejection reflex occurs 2 to 3 minutes after sucking is initiated (Lawrence & Lawrence, 2011). Limiting nursing interferes with the reflex and the infant's milk supply. The limited feedings contribute to milk stasis and engorgement and sore nipples.

Introducing bottles to an infant interferes with the milk ejection reflex by suggesting to the mother that her milk is insufficient. Bottles cause the infant to become confused as sucking at the breast differs from sucking on a commercial nipple or pacifier. An infant may reject the breast or, on the other hand, suckle frequently and for prolonged periods to be satisfied.

Breastfeeding Infants in Multiple Births

The advantages of breastfeeding infants in a multiple birth are similar to those of breastfeeding a single child: Breastfeeding provides a perfect food that is easily digested and provides immunities; the milk is easily accessible; financial savings are substantial; and a special relationship is promoted between mother and infants. A disadvantage may be that the mother finds breastfeeding multiple infants exhausting. The mother may find a support group helpful (see Support Groups and Resources).

The amount of milk produced is influenced by the size of the infants and the number of breastfeeding sessions. The mother should begin breastfeeding at the earliest possible time. An electric piston-type pump may be needed if infants are unable to suckle. Optimal milk production with minimum pumping will most likely involve eight pumping sessions per day, at least 10 to 15 minutes per breast. A minimum total of 100 minutes pumping over 24 hours is recommended; short, frequent sessions to express milk are more effective and stimulate more milk production than longer sessions with longer intervals (Lawrence & Lawrence, 2011). If only one infant can feed and the other is hospitalized, the mother has two options: (1) Nurse twin A while simultaneously pumping for twin B. Breast milk obtained can be taken to twin B. This schedule is rigorous and may be exhausting for the mother. (2) Begin pumping for twin B a few days prior to the infant's discharge.

Feedings may be simultaneous or individual. Simultaneous feedings are advantageous because both feedings are completed in one session. Simultaneous feedings save time and may take advantage of simultaneous letdowns. A disadvantage is that the mother loses individual time with each infant.

Individual feedings are advantageous because modified scheduling may be employed. For example, the hungrier infant sets the pace, and the second infant is awakened for feedings. A disadvantage of this type of feeding is that it is time consuming.

Simultaneous Feedings

Proper positioning is particularly important for breastfeeding two infants so that the mother does not bear the weight of the infants. Pillows should be firm and support the infants' weight. There are pillows made to assist mothers of twins.

- The double football hold is often used for simultaneous feedings. The head and neck of each infant are supported by the mother's hands, with each infant's body supported by one of the mother's arms and their feet toward her back. The infants' abdomens face up or are rotated in toward the mother's chest or side. An advantage of the double football hold is that the mother can assist with head control; the more difficult to manage infant should be placed on the side easiest for the mother to manage (Fidel-Rimon & Shinwell, 2006; Mohrbacher & Stock, 2003). The mother should not bend over to nurse but, instead, bring the infants close to her.

- In the combination cradle/football position, twin A is held like football and approaches the breast at 12 and 6 o'clock. Twin B is cradled across the mother's chest with her or his abdomen tucked in tightly toward the mother's abdomen and approaches the breast at 9 and 3 o'clock (Fidel-Rimon & Shinwell, 2006; Mohrbacher & Stock, 2003). Two advantages of this position are that it is the most inconspicuous for nursing outside the home, and it is easily mastered if one or both infants have difficulty latching onto the breast.
- In the parallel hold, both infants are angled in the same direction. Twin A is cradled, held with legs behind twin B; the legs simultaneously support twin B's head. The advantage of the parallel hold is that the weight of one twin keeps the second infant attached to the breast. In addition, the mother's arms can rest comfortably on pillows (Mohrbacher & Stock, 2003).
- In the crisscross hold, both infants are in cradle position, with the legs of one crossing over those of the other. The infants are in the crook of the mother's arms and are rotated toward her abdomen. The mother supports the infants by holding their buttocks. A disadvantage is that this position is difficult for infants to maintain; it requires head control (Fidel-Rimon & Shinwell, 2006; Mohrbacher & Stock, 2003).
- "V" position is similar to crisscross. The mother is lying nearly flat on her back with pillows under her head. The infants' heads are at their mother's breasts, forming a "V," with their knees touching her upper abdomen (Mohrbacher & Stock, 2003). This position allows the mother to rest more comfortably; it can be used for night feedings. The disadvantage is that it requires infants to have more head control and assistance in grasping the nipple.

DRUG TRANSMISSION IN BREAST MILK

Transmission of a drug in breast milk from mother to infant depends on several factors:

- Absorption of drug by mother's body: half-life or peak serum time, absorption rate, route of administration.
- Lipid solubility and plasma protein-binding properties of drug.
- Movement of drug from maternal plasma to milk; cell diffusion or active transport.
- Amount of drug ingested by infant.
- Concentration of drug in milk.
- Size and relative metabolic maturity of infant.
- pH of substrate (Briggs et al., 2005; Hale, 2010; Lawrence & Lawrence, 2011).

The effect of the drug can be minimized in several ways:

- Do not use a long-acting form of the drug. Infants have difficulty with excretion and detoxification usually occurs in liver; however, the infant liver is immature.
- Schedule the doses so that the least amount of the drug enters the milk: Have the mother take medication immediately after breastfeeding.
- Choose drug that passes least into milk.
- Advise the mother to take medication as directed, if the medication has been demonstrated to be safe for breastfeeding infants and to watch the infant for unusual signs and symptoms or a change in feeding pattern or activity. She should contact her health care provider if she has any concerns or questions.

The AAP (2001) recommended the following be considered before prescribing medication for the lactating woman: (1) Is the drug really necessary? (2) the safest drug should be chosen; (3) if there is a possibility that a drug may present a risk to the infant, consideration should be given to measurement of blood concentrations in the nursing infant; (4) drug exposure to the nursing infant may be minimized by having the mother take the medication just after she has breast-fed the infant or just before the infant is due to have a lengthy sleep period.

The following list includes drugs both in the contraindicated and in the compatible categories and is not intended to be exhaustive. Be sure to check current sources when prescribing medications to lactating women.

Contraindications

Certain drugs are known to be contraindicated while breastfeeding:

- Alcoholic beverages (interfere with ejection reflex).
- Chronic aspirin use may cause metabolic acidosis in infant and affect platelet function (aspirin or acetaminophen in single dose is not significantly transferred).

- Cocaine intoxication (seizures, irritability, vomiting, diarrhea).
- Chloramphenicol (potential for bone marrow toxicity).
- Cimetidine (unknown effect in nursing infant).
- Doxorubicin (possible immune suppression; unknown effect on growth or carcinogenesis) (AAP, 2001; Briggs et al., 2005; Hale, 2010; Mohrbacher & Stock, 2003).
- Gold salts (rash, kidney and liver inflammation).
- Iodine (preferentially concentrated in milk with concentrations 20 to 30 times those of maternal faserum) (Hale, 2010).
- Methotrexate (possible immune suppression; unknown effect on growth or carcinogenesis) (AAP, 2001; Mohrbacher & Stock, 2003).
- Minor tranquilizers (barbiturates, benzodiazepines).
- Narcotics (methadone for maintenance therapy reported safe).
- Phencyclidine.
- Thiouracil (not, however, propylthiouracil).
- Tobacco (smoking more than 20 cigarettes per day decreases milk supply; passive, inhaled smoke increases risks for allergies, SIDS, pneumonia, and bronchitis). Documented decrease in milk supply and weight gain in infant (possible immune suppression; unknown effect on growth or carcinogenesis) (AAP, 2001; Klonoff-Cohen et al., 1995; Mohrbacher & Stock, 2003).

Drugs requiring temporary interruption are radiopharmaceuticals including indium-111 and gallium-67 (AAP, 2001).

The effects of metoclopramide on nursing infants are unknown. No adverse effects have been reported; however, there is the potential for central nervous system effects (AAP, 2001).

Drugs that have caused significant effects in some nursing infants and should be used with caution include clemastine, phenobarbital, primidone, and sulfasalazine (AAP, 2001).

A mother who uses recreational drugs should not breast-feed.

Amphetamines (crack, speed, ups, uppers) are excreted in breast milk; levels in milk exceed those in maternal serum. Abstinence from amphetamines is recommended until more information is available.

Cocaine (snow, coke, crack, champagne, tool, pearl flake, blow, gold dust, dama blanca) appears to be excreted in breast milk. Cocaine intoxication has been reported in 2-week-old infants. Mothers should not apply cocaine to sore nipples.

Heroin ("H," junk, smack, China white, black tar) crosses into breast milk to cause addiction in breast-fed infants, tremors, restlessness, vomiting, and poor feeding (AAP, 2001).

Hallucinogens are extremely potent and are known to cross the blood brain barrier (Hale, 2010). Although there is limited data on transfer into breast milk, this class of drug is highly contraindicated. Hallucinogens include LSD (lysergic acid diethylamide), mescaline (peyote), psilocybin (found in certain mushrooms), and Ts and blues (combination of pentazocine and tripelennamine).

Marijuana (dope, weed, herb, grass, pot, hashish, hash) has unknown long-term effects on infants; the concentration transferred into breast milk is eight times that in maternal blood (AAP, 2001).

Compatible Drugs

Certain drugs are usually compatible with breastfeeding:

- Acetominophen
- Acylovir
- Amoxicillin
- Azithromycin
- Cefoxitin
- Cimetidine
- Ciprofloxin
- Clindanycin
- Diltiazem
- Erythromycin
- Fluconazole
- Ibuprofen
- Labetalol
- Methyldopa
- Methimazole
- Metoprolol
- Mexilitine
- Minoxidil
- Piroxicam
- Prednisone
- Procainamide
- Progesterone
- Propranolol
- Sumatriptan
- Suprafen
- Terbutaline
- Ticarcillin
- Tolmetin
- Valacyclovir
- Verapamil
- Zolpidem (AAP, 2001; Hale, 2010; Lawrence & Lawrence, 2011)

BREAST PUMPS

Mothers of preterm infants or of newborns hospitalized for other reasons and mothers who work may use breast pumps to build and maintain milk supply. An infant's suckling, however, remains the most efficient pump. Infants suck at approximately –50 to –155 mmHg, with a maximum to –220 (Lawrence & Lawrence, 2011). Pumps that match suckling stimulate the milk ejection reflex and promote milk production most effectively. The vacuum produced by a pump should not exceed the vacuum created by an infant.

Infants nurse in a burst-pause pattern. Suckling has three phases: suction, release, and relaxation. Infants apply suction for less than 1 second each time.

A correctly fitting flange surrounds the areola and allows the nipple to move back and forth during pumping. The flange should engulf and firmly support the breast and allow maximum nipple stretch, yet be small enough to provide gentle nipple friction.

There are different types of pumps. An electric pump obtains more milk and is easier to use than a hand-operated pump or manual expression. The double pump expresses milk most quickly. An intermittent draw pump is less likely to cause trauma and provides better stimulation of the milk ejection reflex.

Manual expression of milk might be necessary in the event a part of the mechanical pump is lost or the pump is left at home. To manually express (pump) milk, the mother first washes her hands. She positions her thumb and first two fingers about 1 to 1½ in. behind her nipple, forming a "C" with her hand. She should then push straight into the chest wall and roll her thumb and fingers forward. The movement is repeated rhythmically; the thumb and fingers are rotated to milk other sinuses. She should express each breast until milk flow decreases, then gently massage the breasts to stimulate milk ejection.

Not recommended for pumping breasts is the traditional bicycle horn pump (Lawrence & Lawrence, 2011). It cannot be sterilized, milk can be easily contaminated, and it has no collection mechanism for milk. It is difficult to clean, it can damage breast tissue, and it expresses milk ineffectively.

Using a Pump

Practicing with pump before actual need for milk will facilitate successful use. A woman should become knowledgeable about the pump several weeks before milk is actually needed; she should practice putting the pump together and using it. Hands should be washed before beginning breast pumping, and manufacturer's instructions followed for cleaning the pump.

The mother moistens the breast with water (to form a seal), centers the nipple in the proper size nipple adapter, and begins pumping at the lowest setting. Using a double pump is the most efficient way to express breast milk. If a single pump is used, the mother should switch breasts when milk flow begins to decrease, which often occurs after 15 minutes.

Storing Milk

If milk is to be used within 48 to 72 hours, refrigeration is sufficient for storage. Milk should be frozen if storage will be longer than 24 hours. Do not freeze in glass containers but in rigid polyprophylene plastic containers to maintain stability of cells and immunoglobulins. Frozen milk can be stored for 1 month in the freezer compartment of a refrigerator or 6 months in a deep freeze. Methods of thawing milk can adversely affect anti-infective factors. Frozen milk should be thawed in the refrigerator and used within 24 hours. Thawing milk in warm water can cause contamination, and subjecting milk to microwave temperatures of 72° to 98° F (medium to high) can result in a marked decrease in anti-infective factors (Lawrence & Lawrence, 2011).

RETURNING TO WORK

Pumping/Expressing Milk

Advise the client to begin freezing milk for later use approximately 14 days before returning to work. She should pump at least three times per day, after breastfeeding the infant. A formula is used to estimate the amount of milk needed per feeding:

$$\frac{\text{infant weight} \times 2.5}{\text{number of feedings}} = \text{ounce per feeding}$$

For example, for a 10-pound infant,

$$\frac{10 \times 2.5}{8} = \frac{25}{8} = \text{approximately 3 oz of milk needed per feeding}$$

A Nuk-type nipple might be used when bottlefeeding, as it most closely resembles breast.

Baby's Refusal of Bottle

Refusing to drink from a bottle can occur among infants approximately 3 months old. Using a bottle along with breastfeeding in the first month of life increases the likelihood of nipple confusion; poor suckling at breast results and establishment of a milk supply that meets the infant's needs is delayed (AWHONN, 2000; Lawrence & Lawrence, 2011). Someone other than mother should use a second feeding skill with the infant, for example, offering milk in a cup or spoon rather than the bottle.

Preparing for Absence

Some guidelines might help the client adapt to the challenges of breastfeeding and spending time away from the infant.

- Suggest to the client that she pack an extra bra and wear a two-piece outfit to facilitate pumping and to camouflage leakage of milk.
- Advise the client to ensure that the infant's caregiver is comfortable with the mother's desire to breast-feed and knows how to handle breast milk.
- Suggest to the client that she pack several diaper bags to obviate the need to return home for forgotten articles.
- Refer the client to a breastfeeding support group (see Breastfeeding Information/Support Groups at the end of this chapter).

BOTTLEFEEDING

Although breast milk is the perfect food for infants, not all mothers choose or are able to breast-feed their infants. Formula feedings should be given to an infant for the first year of life. If the infant is allergic to cow's milk, soy-based formulas may be used.

An amendment was passed in 1980 by Congress to the Food, Drug and Cosmetic Act specifying new regulations for commercially prepared infant formula. This act, the Infant Formula Act of 1980, gave the Food and Drug Administration (FDA) the authority to establish quality-control procedures for infant formula, to establish recall procedures, to establish and revise nutrient levels, and to regulate labeling. Manufacturers were also required to analyze each batch of formula to ensure that all nutrients were present in the correct amounts, to ensure that the formula was stable over the period of recommended shelf life, and to make all records available to the FDA. The year 1986 saw the requirement for standard labeling of nutrition information and directions for preparation become mandatory.

Calories are provided to the infant in the form of carbohydrates, protein, and fat. By the end of the second week in life, full-term infants require 100 to 110 Kcal/kg/day of fluids to maintain cellular growth and function. Preterm infants weighing less than 2,500 g may require 110 to 150 Kcal/kg/day to achieve satisfactory growth. Fluid requirements are higher than in full-term infants because of greater fluid loss. Because of the immature digestive system, premature infants often require different formula than full-term infants.

TEACHING BOTTLEFEEDING

- Point the nipple directly into the mouth and on top of the tongue, rather than toward the palate. The nipple should be full of milk at all times to avoid ingestion of air. The nipple hole should be large enough so that milk flows in drips when inverted; if it is too large, the infant can drink too fast and regurgitate or overeat.
- Stroke, cuddle, and talk to the infant during feedings.
- Never prop bottles or feed infant in totally recumbent (flat) position that can result in positional otitis media.
- Avoid warming bottles in a microwave oven, as milk can become too hot and burn the infant. Formula should be at room temperature.
- Avoid reusing milk from a previous feeding.
- Formula should be prepared as directed and never diluted.

SUPPORT GROUPS AND RESOURCES

BREASTFEEDING INFORMATION/ SUPPORT GROUPS

Ameda Breastfeeding Products
c/o Hollister Incorporated
2000 Hollister Dr.
Libertyville, IL 60048
(877) 992-6332 (USA)
(800) 263-7400 (Canada)
www.ameda.com

International Childbirth Education Association
P.O. Box 20048
Minneapolis, MN 55420
(952) 854-8660
www.icea.org

International Lactation Consultant Association
4101 Lake Boone Trail, Ste 201

Raleigh, NC 27607
(919) 787-5181
www.ilca.org

La Leche League International & Breastfeeding Resource Center
1400 N. Meacham Road
P.O. Box 4079
Schaumburg, IL 60173-4808
(847) 519-7730
www.lalecheleague.org

Medela, Inc.
1101 Corporate Dr.
McHenry, IL 60050
(815) 363-1166
(800) 435-8316
email: customer service@medela.com
www.medela.com
Breast pumps, breast pump rentals (including double pumping system), breastfeeding products.

WOMEN, INFANTS, AND CHILDREN AND FOOD STAMP PROGRAMS

Contact your local health department.

PARENTING/FAMILY SUPPORT GROUPS

Al-Anon Family Groups
World Service Office
1600 Corporate Landing Parkway
Virginia Beach, VA 23454-5617
(757) 563-1600
(888) 425-2666 (Monday through Friday 8 a.m.–6 p.m. EST)
www.al-anon.alateen.org

AYUDA

1707 Kalorama Rd. NW.
Washington, DC 20009
(202) 387-4848
www.ayudainc.org
Resource for immigrant Latina women in the Washington, DC, area.

Birth Defect Research for Children, Inc.
976 Lake Baldwin Lane, Suite 104
Orlando, FL 32814
(407) 895-0802 (Monday through Friday 8 a.m.–5 p.m. EST)
www.birthdefects.org

Custody Action for Lesbian Mothers (CALM)
P.O. Box 281
Narbeth, PA 19702
(215) 667-7508

Knowledge Support & Action (Klinefelter's and other X-related conditions)
P.O. Box 461047
Aurora, CO 80046-1047
(888) 999-9428
www.genetic.org

Little People of America, Inc. (LPA)
250 El Camino Real, Suite 201
Tustin, CA 92780
(888) LPA-2001
www.lpaonline.org

National Association of Developmental Disabilities Council (NADDC)
1660 L Street NW, Suite 700
Washington, DC 20036
(202) 506 5813
www.naddc.org

National Association for Parents of Children With Visual Impairments
P.O. Box 317
Watertown, MA 02471
(800) 562-6265 or
(617) 972-7441
www.spedex.com/napvi/

National Center for Lesbian Rights
870 Market St., Suite 370
San Francisco, CA 94102
(415) 392-6257
www.nclrights.org

National Center on Child Abuse and Neglect/U.S. Department of Health & Human Services
Child Welfare Information Gateway
Children's Bureau/ACYF
1250 Maryland Avenue, SW
Eighth Floor
Washington, DC 20024
(800) 394-3366
Information on programs in individual states, publications, and training manuals.

National Coalition Against Domestic Violence (NCADV)
One Broadway, Suite B210
Denver, CO 80203

(303) 839-1852
Hotline (800) 799-SAFE (7233)
www.ncadv.org/contacthome.httm

National Domestic Violence Hotline
P.O. Box 161810
Austin, TX 78716
(800) 799-SAFE (7233)
(800) 787-3224 (TTY)
www.ndvh.org

National Fragile X Foundation
(800) 688-8765
www.fragilex.org

National Dissemination Center for Children With Disabilities
1825 Connecticut Ave NW, Suite 700
Washington, DC 20009
(202) 884-8200 (Voice, TTY)
(800) 695-0285 (Voice, TTY)
www.nichcy.org

National Organization for Rare Disorders (NORD)
55 Kenosia Avenue
P. O Box 1968
Danbury, CT 06813
(203) 744-0100
(800) 999-6673
www.rarediseases.org/cgi-bin/nord

Neurofibromatosis, Inc.
P. O Box 66884
Chicago, IL 60666
(800) 942-6825
www.nfinc.org

Parents of Down Syndrome Children
c/o The Arc
1660 L Street NW, Suite 301.
Washington, DC 20036
(800) 433-5255
www.thearc.org

Parents Helping Parents
Sobrato Center for Nonprofist-San Jose.
1400 Parkmoor Avenue, Suit 100
San Jose, CA 95126
(408) 727-5775
www.php.com

Pathways Awareness
150 N. Michigan Avenue, Suite 2100
Chicago, IL 606011-800-955-2445
www.pathwaysawareness.org

A not-for-profit organization dedicated to resources for parents on normal growth and development.

Spina Bifida Association
4590 MacArthur Blvd., Ste. 250
Washington, DC 20007-4226
(202) 944-3285
(800) 621-3141
www.sbaa.org

Support Organization for Trisomy 18, 13, and Related Disorders
2982 S. Union St.
Rochester, NY 14624
(800) 716-SOFT (7638)
www.trisomy.org

National Organization of Mothers of Twins Clubs (NOMOTC)
2000 Mallory Lane, Suite 130-600
Franklin, TN 37067-8231
248-231-4480
www.nomotc.org

POSTPARTUM DEPRESSION SUPPORT GROUPS

Postpartum Progress
www.postpartumprogress.com
This site has a list of support groups available listed by state for the United States and by city and province for Canada.

Postpartum Support International
6706 SW 54th Avenue.
Portland, OR 97219
1-800-944-4PPD
www.postpartum.net

PERINATAL LOSS SUPPORT GROUPS

SIDS Alliance
1314 Bedford Ave. Ste 210
Baltimore, MD 21208
(800) 221-SIDS (7437)
www.sidsalliance.org

The Compassionate Friends
P.O. Box 3696O
ak Brook, IL 60522
(630) 990-0010
(877) 969-0010 (Monday through Friday 8 a.m.–5 p.m. CST)
www.compassionatefriends.org

Resolve Through Sharing
1900 South Ave.
La Crosse, WI 54601
(800) 782-7300
www.bereavementservices.org
Educational conferences for health care providers and extensive list of loss and grief support resources.

REFERENCES

Aaron, E., Abrams, E., Anderson, J., & Weinberg, G.A. (2010, May 24). *Panel on treatment of HIV-Infected pregnant women and prevention of perinatal transmission. Recommendations for use of antiretroviral drugs in pregnant HIV-1 infected women for maternal health and interventions to reduce perinatal HIV transmission in the United States* (pp. 1–117). Retrieved July 12, 2011, from http://aidsinfo.nih.gov/contentfiles/PerinatalGL.pdf

Abalovich, M., Amino, N., Barbur, L.A., Cobin, R.H., De Groot, L.J., Glinoer, D., et al. (2007). Clinical practice guideline: Management of thyroid dysfunction during pregnancy and postpartum: An endocrine society clinical practice guideline. *Journal of Clinical Endocrinology and Metabolism, 92*(8), S1–47.

Adair, F.L. (1935). The American Committee of Maternal Welfare, Inc: Chairman's address. *American Journal of Obstetrics & Gynecology, 30*, 868–871.

Addis, S., Davies, M., Greene, G., MacBride-Stewart, S., & Shepherd, M. (2009). The health, social care and housing needs of lesbian, gay, bisexual and transgender older people: A review of the literature. *Health and Social Care in the Community, 17*(6), 647–658.

Advisory Committee on Immunization Practices (ACIP). (2008). *Guidelines for vaccinating pregnant women.* Retrieved June 12, 2011, from http://www.dcd.gov/vaccines/pubs/preg-guide.htm

Alhusen, J.L. (2008). A literature update on maternal-fetal attachment. *Journal of Obstetric, Gynecologic, and Neonatal Nursing, 37*(3), 315–328.

American Academy of Pediatrics (AAP). (1998, April). *Guidance for effective discipline (RE9740).* Retrieved June 16, 2011, from http://www.AAP.org

American Academy of Pediatrics (AAP). (2000, March). *Changing concepts of sudden infant death syndrome: Implications for infant sleeping environment and sleep position (RE9946).* Retrieved May 11, 2002, from http://www.AAP.org

American Academy of Pediatrics (AAP). (2001, September). The transfer of drugs and other chemicals into human milk. *Pediatric, 108*(3), 776–789. Retrieved June 13, 2011, from http://www.AAP.org

American Academy of Pediatrics (AAP). (2005). Breastfeeding and the use of human milk. *Pediatric, 115*(2), 496–506. Retrieved June 13, 2011, from http://www.AAP.org

American Academy of Pediatrics (AAP) Committee on Child Abuse and Neglect. (1998, reaffirmed 2004). The role of the pediatrician in recognizing and intervening on behalf of abused women. *Pediatric, 101,* 1091–1092.

American Academy of Pediatrics & American College of Obstetricians and Gynecologists (AAP & ACOG). (2007). *Guidelines for perinatal care* (6th ed.). Elk Grove Village, IL: Author.

American College of Obstetricians and Gynecologists (ACOG). (1998, March). *Antimicrobial therapy for obstetrical patients* (Educational Bulletin No. 245). Washington, DC: Author.

American College of Obstetricians and Gynecologists (ACOG). (2000, July). *Breastfeeding: Maternal and infant aspects* (Educational Bulletin No. 258). Washington, DC: Author.

American College of Obstetricians and Gynecologists (ACOG). (2002a, January; reaffirmed 2010). *Diagnosis and management of preeclampsia and eclampsia* (Practice Bulletin No. 33). Washington, DC: Author.

American College of Obstetricians and Gynecologists (ACOG). (2002b, August). *Thyroid disease in pregnancy* (Practice Bulletin No. 37). Washington, DC: Author.

American College of Obstetricians and Gynecologists (ACOG). (2006, October; reaffirmed 2008). *Postpartum hemorrhage* (Practice Bulletin No. 76). Washington, DC: Author.

American College of Obstetricians and Gynecologists (ACOG). (2007, September). *Pelvic organ prolapse* (Practice Bulletin No. 85). Washington, DC: Author.

American College of Obstetricians and Gynecologists (ACOG). (2009, November). *Cervical cytology screening* (Practice Bulletin No. 109). Washington, DC: Author.

American Diabetes Association (ADA). (2002). Clinical practice recommendations 2002. *Diabetes Care, 25*(Suppl. 1), s21–s24, s5–s20.

Anderson, C. (2002, April/May). Battered and pregnant: A nursing challenge. *AWHONN Lifelines, 6*(2), 95–99.

Armstrong, D.S. (2007). Perinatal loss and parental distress of the birth of a healthy infant. *Advances in Neonatal Care, 7*(4), 200–206.

Association of Women's Health, Obstetric, and Neonatal Nurses (AWHONN). (2000). *Breastfeeding support: Prenatal care through the first year* (Monograph) (pp. 1–35). Washington, DC: Author.

Baho, K., & Hager, J. (1998, April). Clinical focus: Keeping moms and babies together. *AWHONN Lifelines, 2*(2), 44–48.

Bair-Merritt, M.H., & Fein, J.A. (2010). Intimate partner violence and child abuse. In A.P. Giardino & E.R. Giardino (Eds.), *Intimate partner violence* (Chapter 4, pp. 77–86). St. Louis, MO: STM Learning Inc.

Baisch, M.J., Carey, L.K., Conway, A.E., & Mounts, K.O. (2010). Perinatal depression: A health marketing campaign to improve screening. *Nursing for Women's Health, 14*(1), 20–33.

Barnard, K. (1978). *Learning resource manual.* Seattle: University of Washington, Nursing Child Assessment Satellite Training.

Bartz, D., & Goldberg, A.B. (2011). Injectable contraceptives. In R.A. Hatcher, J. Trussell, A.L. Nelson, W. Cates, D. Kowal, & M.S. Policar (Eds.), *Contraceptive technology* (20th ed., pp. 209–236). New York: Ardent Media.

Beck, C.T. (1995, September/October). The effects of postpartum depression on maternal-infant interaction: A meta-analysis. *Nursing Research, 44*(5), 298–304.

Beck, C.T. (2002). Postpartum depression: A metasynthesis. *Qualitative Health Research, 12,* 453–472.

Beck, C.T. (2004). Post-traumatic stress disorder due to childbirth: The aftermath. *Nursing Research, 53*(4), 216–223.

Beck, C.T. (2006). Postpartum depression: It isn't just the blues. *American Journal of Nursing, 106*(5), 40–50.

Beck, C.T. (2008a). State of the science on postpartum depression: What nurse researchers have contributed, Part I. *Maternal Child Nursing, 33*(2), 121–126.

Beck, C.T. (2008b). State of the science on postpartum depression: What nurse researchers have contributed, Part II. *Maternal Child Nursing, 33*(3), 151–156.

Beck, C.T., & Gable, R.K. (2001, July/August). Comparative analysis of the performance of the postpartum depression screening scale with two other depression instruments. *Nursing Research, 50*(4), 242–249.

Bender, E., Jorjorian, A., Lynch, P., & Cramer, A. (1998). Relationships with women. In Boston Women's Health Book Collective (Ed.), *Our bodies, ourselves for the new century* (pp. 200–228). New York: Simon and Schuster.

Beral, V. (2002, July 20). Breast cancer and breastfeeding: Collaborative reanalysis of individual data from 47 epidemiological studies in 30 countries, including 50,302 women with cancer and 96,973 women without the disease. *Lancet, 360*(9328), 187–195.

Blackwell, D.A., & Blackwell, J.T. (1999, October/November). Building alternative families: Helping lesbian couples find the path to parenthood. *AWHONN Lifelines, 3*(5), 45–48.

Bloom, S.L. (2010). Mental health aspects of intimate partner violence: Survivors, professionals, and systems. In A.P. Giardino & E.R. Giardino (Eds.), *Intimate partner violence* (Chapter 10, pp. 207–250). St. Louis, MO: STM Learning Inc.

Brazelton, T.B. (1992). Discipline. In *Touchpoints: Your child's emotional and behavioral development* (pp. 252–260). New York: Addison-Wesley.

Briggs, G.G., Freeman, R.K., & Yaffe, S.J. (2005). *Drugs in pregnancy and lactation* (7th ed.). Philadelphia: Lippincott Williams & Wilkins.

Britton, C., McCormick, R.M., Renfrew, M.J., Wade, A., & King, S.E. (2007). Support for breastfeeding mothers. *Cochrane Database of Systematic Reviews,* 1. doi:10.1002/14651858.CD001141.pub3

Buckner, J. (1998, June). Displaced children: Meeting the health, mental health, and educational needs of immigrant, migrant, and homeless youth. *Adolescent Medicine, 9*(2), 323–334.

Callister, L.C. (2006). Perinatal loss: A family perspective. *Journal of Perinatal and Neonatal Nursing, 20*(3), 227–236.

Callister, L.C., Beckstrand, R.L., & Corbett, C. (2010). Postpartum depression and culture. *American Journal of Maternal/Child Nursing, 35*(5), 254–261.

Centers for Disease Control and Prevention (CDC). (2010a). *Breastfeeding report card—United States 2010.* Retrieved June 13, 2011, from http://www.cdc.gov/breastfeeding/data/reportcard.htm

Centers for Disease Control and Prevention (CDC). (2010b). Sexually transmitted diseases treatment guidelines 2010. *Morbidity and Mortality Weekly Report, 59*(RR-12), 2–61.

Centers for Disease Control and Prevention (CDC). (2010c). U.S. medical eligibility criteria for contraceptive use, 2010. *Morbidity and Mortality Weekly Report, 59,* 1–88.

Centers for Disease Control and Prevention (CDC). (2011a). *Epidemiology and prevention of vaccine-preventable diseases* (12th ed.). Washington, DC: Public Health Foundation.

Centers for Disease Control and Prevention (CDC). (2011b). Understanding intimate partner violence. *CDC Fact Sheet.* Retrieved July 12, 2011, from http://www.cdc.gov/ViolencePrevention/intimatepartnerviolence/index.html

Centers for Disease Control and Prevention (CDC). (2011c). Update to CDC's U.S. medical eligibility criteria for contraceptive use, 2010, revised recommendations for the use of contraceptive methods during the postpartum period. *Morbidity and Mortality Weekly Report, 60*(26), 878–883.

Certain, H.E., Mueller, M., Jagodzinski, T., & Fleming, M. (2008). Domestic abuse during the previous year in a sample of postpartum women. *Journal of Obstetric, Gynecologic, and Neonatal Nursing, 37,* 35–41.

Chames, M.C., Livingston, J.C., Ivester, T.S., Barton, J.R., & Sibai, B.M. (2002, June). Late postpartum eclampsia: A preventable disease? *American Journal of Obstetrics and Gynecology, 186*(6), 1174–1177.

Chen, K.T., Ramin, S.N., & Barss, V. (2010). *Postpartum endometritis.* Retrieved June 11, 2010, from http://www.uptodate.com/contents/postpartum-endometritis

Chez, R.A., & Friedmann, A.K. (2000, August). Offering effective breastfeeding advice. *Contemporary Obstetrics and Gynecology, 45*(8), 32–33, 37–38, 43–44, 47–48, 50.

Cho, J., Holdritch-Davis, D., & Miles, M. (2008). Effects of maternal depressive symptoms and infant gender on the interactions between mothers and their medically at-risk infants. *Journal of Obstetric, Gynecologic, and Neonatal Nursing, 37,* 58–70.

Colson, S.D., Meek, J.H., & Hawdon, J.M. (2008). Optimal positions for the release of primitive neonatal reflexes stimulating breastfeeding. *Early Human Development, 84*(7), 441–449.

Corwin, E.J., Kohen, R., Jarrett, M., & Stafford, B. (2010). The heritability of postpartum depression. *Biological Research for Nursing, 12*(1), 73–83.

Coy, K., Speltz, M.L., & Jones, K. (2002). Facial appearance and attachment in infants with orofacial clefts: A replication. *Cleft Palate-Craniofacial Journal, 39*(1), 66–72.

Cunningham, F.G., Leveno, K.J., Bloom, S.L., Hauth, J.C., Rouse, D.J., & Spong, C.Y. (2010a). Abortion. In F.G. Cunningham, K.J. Leveno, S.L. Bloom, J.C. Hauth, D.J. Rouse, & C.Y. Spong (Eds.), *Williams obstetrics* (Chapter 9, 23rd ed., pp. 215–237). New York: McGraw-Hill.

Cunningham, F.G., Leveno, K.J., Bloom, S.L., Hauth, J.C., Rouse, D.J., & Spong, C.Y. (2010b). Diseases and injuries of the fetus and newborn. In F.G. Cunningham, K.J. Leveno, S.L. Bloom, J.C. Hauth, D.J. Rouse, & C.Y. Spong (Eds.), *Williams obstetrics* (Chapter 29, 23rd ed., pp. 605–644). New York: McGraw-Hill.

Cunningham, F.G., Leveno, K.J., Bloom, S.L., Hauth, J.C., Rouse, D.J., & Spong, C.Y. (2010c). The puerperium. In F.G. Cunningham, K.J. Leveno, S.L. Bloom, J.C. Hauth, D.J. Rouse, & C.Y. Spong (Eds.), *Williams obstetrics* (Chapter 30, 23rd ed., pp. 646–660). New York: McGraw-Hill.

Cunningham, F.G., Leveno, K.J., Bloom, S.L., Hauth, J.C., Rouse, D.J., & Spong, C.Y. (2010d). Puerperal infection. In F.G. Cunningham, K.J. Leveno, S.L. Bloom, J.C. Hauth, D.J. Rouse, & C.Y. Spong (Eds.), *Williams obstetrics* (Chapter 31, 23rd ed., pp. 661–672). New York: McGraw-Hill.

Cunningham, F.G., Leveno, K.J., Bloom, S.L., Hauth, J.C., Rouse, D.J., & Spong, C.Y. (2010e). Pregnancy hypertension. In F.G. Cunningham, K.J. Leveno, S.L. Bloom, J.C. Hauth, D.J. Rouse, & C.Y. Spong (Eds.), *Williams obstetrics* (Chapter 34, 23rd ed., pp. 706–756). New York: McGraw-Hill.

Cunningham, F.G., Leveno, K.J., Bloom, S.L., Hauth, J.C., Rouse, D.J., & Spong, C.Y. (2010f). Obstetrical hemorrhage. In F.G. Cunningham, K.J. Leveno, S.L. Bloom, J.C. Hauth, D.J. Rouse, & C.Y. Spong (Eds.), *Williams obstetrics* (Chapter 35, 23rd ed., pp. 757–803). New York: McGraw-Hill.

Cunningham, F.G., Leveno, K.J., Bloom, S.L., Hauth, J.C., Rouse, D.J., & Spong, C.Y. (2010g). Thromboembolic disorders. In F.G. Cunningham, K.J. Leveno, S.L. Bloom, J.C. Hauth, D.J. Rouse, & C.Y. Spong (Eds.), *Williams obstetrics* (Chapter 47, 23rd ed., pp. 1013–1032). New York: McGraw-Hill.

Cunningham, F.G., Leveno, K.J., Bloom, S.L., Hauth, J.C., Rouse, D.J., & Spong, C.Y. (2010h). Renal and urinary tract disorders. In F.G. Cunningham, K.J. Leveno, S.L. Bloom, J.C. Hauth, D.J. Rouse, & C.Y. Spong (Eds.), *Williams obstetrics* (Chapter 48, 23rd ed., pp. 1033–1048). New York: McGraw-Hill.

Cunningham, F.G., Leveno, K.J., Bloom, S.L., Hauth, J.C., Rouse, D.J., & Spong, C.Y. (2010i). Gastrointestinal disorders. In F.G. Cunningham, K.J. Leveno, S.L. Bloom, J.C. Hauth, D.J. Rouse, & C.Y. Spong (Eds.), *Williams obstetrics* (Chapter 49, 23rd ed., pp. 1049–1062). New York: McGraw-Hill.

Cunningham, F.G., Leveno, K.J., Bloom, S.L., Hauth, J.C., Rouse, D.J., & Spong, C.Y. (2010j). Diabetes. In F.G. Cunningham, K.J. Leveno, S.L. Bloom, J.C. Hauth, D.J. Rouse, & C.Y. Spong (Eds.), *Williams obstetrics* (Chapter 52, 23rd ed., pp. 1104–1125). New York: McGraw-Hill.

Cunningham, F.G., Leveno, K.J., Bloom, S.L., Hauth, J.C., Rouse, D.J., & Spong, C.Y. (2010k). Thyroid and other endocrine disorders. In F.G. Cunningham, K.J. Leveno, S.L. Bloom, J.C. Hauth, D.J. Rouse, & C.Y. Spong (Eds.), *Williams obstetrics* (Chapter 53, 23rd ed., pp. 1126–1144). New York: McGraw-Hill.

Cunningham, F.G., Leveno, K.J., Bloom, S.L., Hauth, J.C., Rouse, D.J., & Spong, C.Y. (2010l). Neurological and psychiatric disorders. In F.G. Cunningham, K.J. Leveno, S.L. Bloom, J.C. Hauth, D.J. Rouse, & C.Y. Spong (Eds.), *Williams obstetrics* (Chapter 55, 23rd ed., pp. 1164–1184). New York: McGraw-Hill.

Davis, M.S. (1992). Natural family planning. *NAACOG's Clinical Issues in Perinatal and Women's Health Nursing, 3*(2), 280–292.

Davis, M.S., & Akridge, K.M. (1987, November/December). The effect of promoting intrauterine attachment in primiparas on postpartum attachment. *Journal of Obstetric, Gynecologic, and Neonatal Nursing, 16*(6), 430–437.

DeMarco, R., Lynch, M.M., & Board, R. (2002, April). Mothers who silence themselves: A concept with clinical implications for women living with HIV/AIDS and their children. *Journal of Pediatric Nursing, 17*(2), 89–95.

DeMatteo, D., Wells, L.M., Goldie, R.S., & King, S.M. (2002, April). The "family" context of HIV: A need for comprehensive health and social policies. *AIDS Care, 14*(2), 261–278.

Dimidjian, S., & Goodman, S. (2009). Nonpharmacologic intervention and prevention strategies for depression during pregnancy and the postpartum. *Clinical Obstetrics and Gynecology, 52*(3), 498–515.

Doshani, A., Teo, R.E.C., Mayne, C.J., & Tincello, D.G. (2007). Uterine prolapse. *British Medical Journal, 335,* 819–823.

Doucet, S., Dennis, C., Letourneau, N., & Blackmore, E.M. (2009). Differentiation and clinical implications of postpartum depression and postpartum psychosis. *Journal of Obstetric, Gynecologic, and Neonatal Nursing, 38,* 269–279.

Dyregrov, A., & Gjestad, R. (2011). Sexuality following the loss of a child. *Death Studies, 35,* 289–315.

Fidel-Rimon, O., & Shinwell, E. (2006). Breast feeding twins and high multiples. *Archives of Disease in Childhood: Fetal and Neonatal Edition, 91,* F377–F380. doi:10.1136/adc.2005.082305. Retrieved June 15, 2011, from http://www.ncbi.nlm.nih.gov/pmc/articles/PMC2672857/pdf/F377.pdf

Fischbach, F. (2009). *A manual of laboratory and diagnostic tests* (8th ed.). Philadelphia: Lippincott Williams & Wilkins.

Flaskerud, J. (2011). Discipline and effective parenting. *Issues in Mental Health Nursing, 32*. doi:10.3109/01612840.2010.498078

French, L.M., & Smaill, F.M. (2009). Antibiotic regimens for endometritis after delivery (Cochrane review, Issue 2). Oxford: The Cochrane Library, Update Software.

Gaffney, K. (2001, Fourth Quarter). Infant exposure to environmental tobacco smoke. *Journal of Nursing Scholarship, 33*(4), 343–347.

Gay, J., Edgil, A., & Douglas, A. (1988). Reva Rubin revisited. *Journal of Obstetric Gynecologic and Neonatal Nursing, 17*, 394–399.

Gaynes, B.N., Gavin, N., Meltzer-Brody, S., Lohr, K.N., Swinson, T., Gartlehner, G., et al. (2005). *Perinatal depression: Prevalence, screening accuracy, and screening outcome* (Evidence Report/Technology Assessment No. 119) (Prepared by the RTI-University of North Carolina Evidence-based Practice Center, under Contract No. 290-02-0016) (AHRQ Publication No. 05-E006-2). Rockville, MD: Agency for Healthcare Research and Quality.

Gold, L. (2002, March). Postpartum disorders in primary care. *Primary Care: Clinics in Office Practice, 29*(1), 27–41.

Hale, T. (2010). *Medications and mothers' milk* (14th ed.). Amarillo: Hale Publishing.

Hay-Smith, J., Mørkved, S., Fairbrother, K.A., & Herbison, G.P. (2008). Pelvic floor muscle training for prevention and treatment of urinary and faecal incontinence in antenatal and postnatal women. *Cochrane Database of Systematic Reviews*, (4), CD007471. doi:10.1002/14651858.CD007471

Hirst, K.P., & Moutier, C.Y. (2010). Postpartum major depression. *American Family Physician, 82*(8), 926–933.

Hoffbrand, S.E., Howard, L., & Crawley, H. (2009). Antidepressant treatment for post-natal depression. *Cochrane Database of Systematic Reviews 2001*, (2), CD002018. doi:10.1002/14651858.CD002018

Humphreys, J., & Neylan, T. (2001, June). Psychological and physical distress of sheltered battered women. *Health Care for Women International, 22*(4), 401–414.

Hutti, M.H. (2005). Social and professional support needs of families after perinatal loss. *Journal of Obstetric, Gynecologic, and Neonatal Nursing, 34*(5), 630–638.

Institute of Medicine (IOM). (1999). *Lesbian health: Current assessment and directions for the future*. Washington, DC: National Academies Press.

Ip, S., Chung, M., Raman, G., Chew, P., Magula, N., DeVine, D., et al. (2007). *Breastfeeding and maternal and infant health outcomes in developed countries* (Evidence Report/Technology Assessment no. 153) (Prepared by Tufts-New England Medical Center Evidence-based Practice Center, under contract no. 290-02-0022) (AHRQ Publication no. 07-E007). Rockville, MD: Agency for Healthcare Research and Quality. Retrieved June 13, 2011, from http://www.ahrq.gov/downloads/pub/evidence/pdf/brfout/brfout.pdf

Ip, S., Chung, M., Raman, G., Trikalinos, T., & Lau, J. (2009). A summary of the agency for healthcare research and quality's evidence report on breastfeeding in developed countries. *Breastfeeding Medicine, 4*(Suppl. 1), S17–S30.

James, A.H. (2010). Pregnancy and thrombotic risk. *Critical Care Medicine, 38*(2S), S57–S63.

Joy, S., & Chelmow D. (2011). Postpartum depression. *Medscape Reference.* Retrieved June, 13, 2011, from http://emedicine.medscape.com/article/271662-overview

Kazdin, A., & Benjet, C. (2003). Spanking children: Evidence and issues. *Current Directions in Psychological Science, 12*(3), 99–103.

Kendall-Tackett, K., & Hale, T.W. (2010). The use of antidepressants in pregnant and breastfeeding women: A review of recent studies. *Journal of Human Lactation, 26,* 187–195.

Kennedy, K.I., & Trussell, J. (2011). Postpartum contraception and lactation. In R.A. Hatcher, J. Trussell, A.L. Nelson, W. Cates, D. Kowal, & M.S. Policar (Eds.), *Contraceptive technology* (20th ed., pp. 483–512). New York: Ardent Media.

Kennell, J.H., & Klaus, M.H. (1998, January). Bonding: Recent observations that alter perinatal death of a newborn infant. *New England Journal of Medicine, 283*(7), 344–349.

Kennell, J.H., Slyter, H., & Klaus, M.H. (1970, August 13). The mourning responses of parents to the death of a newborn infant. *New England Journal of Medicine, 283*(7), 344–349.

Kim, M., Hayashi, R.H., & Gambone, J.C. (2010). Obstetric hemorrhage and puerperal sepsis. In N.F. Hacker, J.C. Gambone, & C.J. Hobel (Eds.), *Hacker and Moore's essentials of obstetrics and gynecology* (Chapter 10, pp. 128–138). Philadelphia: Saunders Elsevier.

Klaus, M., & Kennell, J. (1983). Adjusting to malformation. In *Bonding: The beginnings of parent-infant attachment* (pp. 140–161). St. Louis, MO: C.V. Mosby.

Klonoff-Cohen, H., Edelstein, S., Lefkowitz, E., Srinivasan, I., Kaegi, D., Chang, J., et al. (1995, March 8). The effect of passive smoking and tobacco exposure through breast milk on sudden infant death syndrome. *Journal of the American Medical Association, 273*(10), 795–798.

Kramer, A. (2002, March). Domestic violence: How to ask and how to listen. *Nursing Clinics of North America, 37*(1), 189–210.

Kvols, K. (1998). *Redirecting children's behavior* (3rd ed.). Seattle, WA: Parenting Press Inc.

Lawrence, R.A., & Lawrence, R.M. (2011). *Breastfeeding: A guide for the medical profession* (7th ed.). St. Louis, MO: Mosby.

Lederman, R. (1996). *Psychosocial adaptation in pregnancy* (2nd ed.). Englewood Cliffs, NJ: Prentice Hall.

MacArthur, C., Glasener, C.M., Wilson, P.D., Lancashire, R.J., Herbison, G.P., & Grant, A.M. (2006). Persistent urinary incontinence and delivery mode history: A six-year longitudinal study. *British Journal of Obstetrics and Gynecology, 113*(2), 281–224.

MacArthur, C., Winter, H., Bick, D., Knowles, H., Lilford, R., Henderson, C., et al. (2002, February 2). Effects of redesigned community postnatal care on womens' health 4 months after birth: A cluster randomised controlled trial. *Lancet, 359*(9304), 378–385.

MacDorman, M.F., & Mathews, T.J. (2008). *Recent trends in infant mortality in the United State* (NCHS Data Brief No. 9). Hyattsville, MD: National Center for Health Statistics.

Mansouri, H.A., & Alsahly, N. (2011). Rectal versus oral misoprostol for active management of third stage of labor: A randomized controlled trial. *Archives of Obstetrics and Gynecology, 283,* 935–939.

Martell, L.K. (2000, January/February). The hospital and the postpartum experience: A historical analysis. *Journal of Obstetric, Gynecologic, and Neonatal Nursing, 29*(1), 65–72.

McColgan, M.D., Dempsey, S., Davis, M., & Giardino, A.P. (2010). Overview of the problem. In A.P. Giardino & E.R. Giardino (Eds.), *Intimate partner violence* (Chapter 1, pp. 1–29). St. Louis, MO: STM Learning Inc.

Menke, E.M. (2000, October/November). Comparison of the stressors and coping behaviors of homeless, previously homeless, and never homeless poor children. *Issues in Mental Health Nursing, 21*(7), 691–710.

Mercer, R.T. (1983). Parent-infant attachment. In L. Sonstegard, K. Kowalski, & B. Jennings (Eds.), *Women's health: Vol. II. Childbearing* (pp. 17–42). New York: Grune & Stratton.

Mercer, R.T. (1985, July/August). Process of maternal role attainment over the first year. *Nursing Research, 34*(4), 198–204.

Mercer, R.T. (1990). *Parents at risk.* New York: Springer Publishing Company.

Mercer, R.T. (2004). Becoming a mother versus maternal role attainment. *Journal of Nursing Scholarship, 36*(3), 226–232.

Mercer, R.T., & Ferketich, S. (1990, March). Predictors of parental attachment during early parenthood. *Journal of Advanced Nursing, 153*(3), 268–280.

Mick, J. (2010). Screening and identification in health care settings. In A.P. Giardino & E.R. Giardino (Eds.), *Intimate partner violence* (Chapter 2, pp. 31–54). St. Louis, MO: STM Learning Inc.

Mohrbacher, N., & Stock, J. (2003). *The breastfeeding answer book* (3rd ed.). Schaumburg, IL: La Leche League International.

Moon, R.Y., Horne, R.S.C., & Hauck, F.R. (2007). Sudden infant death syndrome. *Lancet, 370*(9598), 1578–1587.

Muller, A.F., Drexhage, H.A., & Bergout, A. (2001, October). Postpartum thyroiditis and autoimmune thyroiditis in women of childbearing age: Recent insights and consequences for antenatal and postnatal care. *Endocrine Reviews, 22*(5), 605–630.

Muller, M. (1996, February). Prenatal and postnatal attachment: A modest correlation. *Journal of Obstetric, Gynecologic, and Neonatal Nursing, 25*(2), 161–166.

National Center for Biotechnology Information (NCBI). (2009). *Galactosemia.* PubMed Health. Retrieved June 14, 2011, from http://www.ncbi.nlm.nih.gov/pubmedhealth/PMH0001405/

National Coalition for the Homeless (NCH). (2007). Domestic violence and homelessness. *NCH Fact Sheet # 7.* Retrieved July 12, 2011, from http://www.nationahomeless.org/publications/facts/domestic.pdf

National Institutes of Health. (2000). *Working group report on high blood pressure in pregnancy* (NIH Publication No. 00-3029). Washington, DC: U.S. Government Printing Office.

O'Connor, D.J., Scher, L.A., Gargiulo, N.J., Jang, J., Suggs, W.D., & Lipsitz, E.C. (2011). Incidence and characteristics of venous thromboembolic disease during pregnancy and the postnatal period: A contemporary series. *Annals of Vascular Surgery, 25*(1), 9–14.

Oliveira, N.L., & Goldberg, J.P. (2002, March/April). The nutrition status of women and children who are homeless. *Nutrition Today, 37*(2), 70–77.

Olson, G. (2002, April). Thyroid disease in pregnancy. *Female Patient, 27*(1), 10–16.

Peat, J.K., Keena, V., Harakeh, Z., & Marks, G. (2001, September). Parental smoking and respiratory tract infections in children. *Paediatric Respiratory Reviews, 2*(3), 207–213.

Rath, W.H. (2011). Postpartum hemorrhage: Update on problems of definitions and diagnosis. *ACTA Obstetricia et Gynecologica Scandinavica, 90,* 421–428.

Regalado, M., Sareen, H., Inkelas, M., Wissow, L., & Halfon, N. (2004). Parents' discipline of young children: Results from the national survey of early childhood health. *Pediatrics, 113*(6), 1952–1958.

Richardson, H.L., Walker, A.M., & Horne, R.S.C. (2009). Maternal smoking impairs arousal patterns in sleeping infants. *Sleep, 32*(4), 515–521.

Rosenberg, M.T., & Dmochowski, R.R. (2005). Overactive bladder: Evaluation and management in primary care. *Cleveland Clinic Journal of Medicine, 72*(7), 149–156.

Rubin, R. (1984). *Maternal identity and the maternal experience.* New York: Springer Publishing Company.

Sampselle, C., & Brink, C. (1990, May/June). Pelvic muscle relaxation: Assessment and management. *Journal of Nurse Midwifery, 35*(3), 127–132.

Sampselle, C., Miller, J., Mims, B., DeLaney, J.O.L., Ashton-Miller, J.A., & Antonakas, C.L. (1998, March). Effect of pelvic muscle exercise and transient incontinence during pregnancy and after birth. *Obstetrics and Gynecology, 91*(3), 406–412.

Sampselle, C., Palmer, M.H., Boyington, A.R., O'Dell, K.K., & Wooldridge. (2004). Prevention of urinary incontinence in adults. *Nursing Research, 53*(6S), S61–S67.

Santacroce, S.J., Deatrick, J.A., & Ledlie, S.W. (2002, April). Redefining treatment: How biological mothers manage their children's treatment for perinatally acquired HIV. *AIDS Care, 14*(2), 247–260.

Schwartz, M.A., Wang, C.C., Eckert, L.O., & Critchlow, C.W. (1999, September). Risk factors for urinary tract infection in the postpartum period. *American Journal of Obstetrics and Gynecology, 181*(3), 547–553.

Scott, J.A., Robertson, M., Fitzpatrick, J., Knight, C., & Mulholland, S. (2008). Occurrence of lactational mastitis and medical management: A prospective cohort study in Glasgow. *International Breastfeeding Journal, 3,* 21.

Sesso, H.D., Cook, N.R., Buring, J.E., Manson, J.E., & Gaziano, J.M. (2008). Alcohol consumption and the risk of hypertension in women and men. *Hypertension, 51*(4), 1080–1087.

Shay-Zapien, G., & Bullock, L. (2010). Impact of intimate partner violence on maternal child health. *American Journal of Maternal Child Nursing, 53*(4), 206–212.

Shoultz, J., Phillion, N., Noone, J., & Tanner, B. (2002, July). Listening to women: Culturally tailoring the violence prevention guidelines from the "put prevention into practice" program. *Journal of the American Academy of Nurse Practitioners, 14*(7), 307–315.

Sibai, B.M., & Stella, C.L. (2009). Diagnosis and management of atypical preeclampsia-eclampsia. *American Journal of Obstetrics and Gynecology, 200*(5), 481.e1–481.e7.

Stagnaro-Green, A., Schwartz, A., Gismondi, R., Tinelli, A., Mangieri, T., & Negro, R. (2011, June). High rate of persistent hypothyroidism in a large-scale prospective study of postpartum thyroiditis in southern Italy. *Journal of Clinical Endocrinology and Metabolism, 96,* 652–657.

Stein, M. (2010). Teaching parents effective discipline during a health supervision visit. *Pediatrics, 125*(2), e442–e443. Retrieved June 18, 2011, from http://pediatrics.aappublications.org.ezp2.lib.umn.edu/content/125/2/e442.full

Stone, H.L. (2009). Post-traumatic stress disorder in postpartum patients. *Nursing for Women's Health, 13*(4), 284–291.

Swanson, K.M., Karmall, Z.A., Powell, S.H., & Pulvermakher, F. (2003). Miscarriage effects on couples' interpersonal and sexual relationships during the first year after loss: Women's perceptions. *Psychosomatic Medicine, 65,* 902–910.

Synoground, G., & Bruya, M.A. (2000, May). Meeting the health needs of homeless or low-income persons: Role of the nurse practitioner. *Clinical Excellence for Nurse Practitioners, 4*(3), 138–144.

Taylor, C., Manganello, J., Lee, S., & Rice, J. (2010). Mothers spanking of 3-year-old children and subsequent risk of children's aggressive behavior. *Pediatrics, 125*(5), e1057–e1065. doi:10.1542/peds.2009-2678. Retrieved June 17, 2011, from http://pediatrics.aappublications.org.ezp2.lib.umn.edu/content/125/5/e1057.full.pdf+html

Weisz, V.K. (2009). Social justice considerations for lesbian and bisexual women's health care. *Journal of Obstetric, Gynecologic, and Neonatal Nursing, 38,* 81–87.

Williams, G.B. (2000, April/May). Grief after elective abortion. *AWHONN Lifelines, 4*(2), 37–40.

Wilson, B.A., Shannon, M.A., & Shields, K. (Eds.). (2012). *Pearson nurse's drug guide*. Upper Saddle River, NJ: Pearson Prentice Hall.

Winickoff, J.P., Friebely, J., Tanski, W.E., Sherrod, C., Matt, G.E., Hovell, M.F., et al. (2009). Beliefs about the health effects of "thirdhand" smoke and home smoking bans. *Pediatrics, 123,* e74–e79. doi:10.1542/peds.2008-2184

World Health Organization (WHO). (2009). *WHO guidelines for the management of postpartum haemorrhage and retained placenta*, Geneva, Switzerland: Author.

Yozwiak, J.A. (2009). Postpartum depression and adolescent mothers: A review of assessment and treatment approaches. *Journal of Pediatric and Adolescent Gynecology, 23*(3), 172–178. doi:10.1016/j

Zauderer, C.R. (2008). A case study of postpartum depression & altered maternal-newborn attachment. *American Journal of Maternal Child Nursing, 33*(3), 173–178.

Zhang, X., Gregg, E.W., Williamson, D.F., Barker, L.E., Thomas, W., Bullard, K.M., et al. (2010). A1C level and future risk of diabetes: A systematic review. *Diabetes Care, 33*(7), 1665–1673.

V ❖ Primary Care Conditions Affecting Women's Health

CHAPTER ❖ **23**

COMMON MEDICAL PROBLEMS: CARDIOVASCULAR THROUGH HEMATOLOGICAL DISORDERS

Mary Benbenek ◆ *Mary Dierich*

Coronary artery disease was once considered a male affliction, although women are now recognized to be at equal, and in some circumstances greater, risk. Men and women may differ, however, in onset, distribution, and presentation of this disease.

Highlights

- Cardiovascular Disorders
- Dermatologic Disorders
- Ear, Nose, and Throat Disorders
- Endocrine Disorders
- Gastrointestinal Disorders
- Hematological Disorders

❖ INTRODUCTION

A number of disorders or medical problems are seen in practice that are clinically significant to women or are significant in any general population. It is, of course, beyond the scope of this text to touch on all medical concerns. But an effort has been made in this edition to expand and discuss subjects of interest to primary care providers. For convenience, coverage of these common concerns—listed alphabetically by organ system—has been divided into Chapters 23 and 24. In Chapter 23, cardiovascular disorders; dermatologic disorders; ear, nose, and throat disorders; endocrine disorders; gastrointestinal disorders; and hematological disorders are covered. In Chapter 24, musculoskeletal injuries, neurological disorders, ophthalmologic disorders, pulmonary disorders, and urinary tract disorders are discussed. Chapter references provide guidance in finding more in-depth information, and the index should be consulted for the location of specific problems.

The provider's level of comfort and competence in managing medical problems depends on experience, medical resources, location of practice, access to diagnostic testing, practice protocols, and scope of practice.

CARDIOVASCULAR DISORDERS

Cardiovascular disease remains the number one cause of death for women, approximately one death per minute in American women (Roger et al., 2011). The annual direct cost of cardiovascular disease is over $324 billion (American Heart Association [AHA], 2011b). The cardiovascular disorders considered here are two common risk factors (hyperlipidemia and hypertension) for coronary artery disease (CAD) and mitral valve prolapse (MVP). It should be noted that the AHA (Mosca et al., 2011) recently suggested that a number of lifetime patterns were associated with longevity and ideal cardiovascular health. Markers include the absence of cardiovascular disease *and* cholesterol < 200 mg/dL, blood pressure of 120/80, fasting glucose of 100 mg dL, lean body mass of 25 kg/m^2, no smoking, physical activity at recommended levels, and a diet that prevents hypertension. Those at high risk for the development of cardiovascular events include those with diabetes, chronic renal disease, cerebrovascular disease, peripheral artery disease, or abdominal aortic aneurysm. Women at risk for the development of cardiovascular disease include those who have a first-degree relative with early cardiovascular disease, treated or untreated hypertension, treated or untreated dyslipidemia, central adiposity or metabolic syndrome, subclinical vascular disease (coronary calcification, carotid plaques), poor diet or poor exercise tolerance/physical inactivity, or are smokers. In addition, those with a personal history of systemic autoimmune disease such as lupus or rheumatoid arthritis or a history of preeclampsia, gestational diabetes, or pregnancy-induced hypertension are also at risk for the development of cardiovascular disease (Mosca et al., 2011). It is important to keep in mind that women's risk of cardiovascular disease (especially stroke) outstrips that of men as they age. Therefore, because of their longer life spans, early prevention becomes especially relevant for women.

HYPERLIPIDEMIA

Hyperlipidemia is an increased plasma lipid concentration of cholesterol, triglycerides, or both. Water-insoluble lipids are carried in the bloodstream by lipoproteins, which are complex molecules made up partly of cholesterol and triglycerides. Lipoproteins transport both dietary and endogenous lipids from sites of absorption or synthesis to sites of storage or metabolism.

High levels of low-density lipoprotein (LDL) are injurious to the vascular intima and lead to the deposition of cholesterol. This and other thrombolic events combine to form atherosclerotic plaques within the vessel, narrowing the lumen and eventually reducing blood flow to many tissues. Optimal goals for LDL and indications for treatment are given in Table 23–1.

Classification of Lipoproteins

Four principal classes of lipoproteins have been determined (Braun & Rosenson, 2001).

- Chylomicrons are the major transporters of dietary triglycerides.
- Very low-density lipoproteins (VLDLs) are responsible for the transport of endogenous triglycerides.
- LDLs are the major transporter of cholesterol.
- High-density lipoproteins (HDLs) collect cholesterol from the tissues to return it to the liver, thereby acquiring the pseudonym "good cholesterol."

TABLE 23–1. Low-Density Lipoprotein (LDL) Cholesterol Goals of Therapy

LDL Cholesterol	Level for Drug Treatment Consideration (after therapeutic life changes)	Goals of Therapy
Without coronary heart disease and with fewer than two risk factors	190 mg/dL or higher	Less than 160 mg/dL
Without coronary heart disease and with two or more risk factors	160 mg/dL or higher	Less than 130 mg/dL
With coronary heart disease	130 mg/dL or higher	100 mg/dL or less

Electronic 10-year risk calculators available at http://hp2010.nhlbihin.net/atpiii/calculator.asp.

Source: American Heart Association recommendations for goals of therapy accessed from http://www.nhlbi.nih.gov/guidelines/cholesterol/atglance.htm.

Epidemiology

Hyperlipidemia occurs in 25 percent of the U.S. adult population. Risk factors are a high-fat diet, genetic predisposition, sedentary lifestyle, cigarette smoking, and underlying diseases (diabetes mellitus, hypothyroidism, chronic renal disease, liver or gastrointestinal disorders). These may all contribute to an alteration in lipid values (Fletcher et al., 2005).

Levels of LDLs and HDLs are predictors of risk (see Table 23–2). Although LDL level is a powerful predictor of CAD in men, HDL level appears to be a better predictor of risk for CAD in women. Even with higher average total cholesterol and higher LDL levels, women have fewer cardiovascular events than men, possibly due to their higher HDL levels. A cholesterol to HDL ratio of 4 or less is considered acceptable; a ratio of 6 or above warrants an aggressive treatment approach. Hyperlipidemia can occur in pregnant women and treatment is not indicated. Follow-up at 6 months postpartum or at cessation of breastfeeding is recommended. Research is almost exclusively based on men; until further studies of women are completed, it is considered clinically prudent to apply to women the same recommendations used in the care of men. In recent years, the aggressive treatment of hyperlipidemia is estimated to have brought about a 24 percent reduction in CAD (Ford et al., 2007).

Subjective Data

The client reports a first-degree relative with known hyperlipidemia, a family history of premature CAD, or a medical condition associated with hyperlipidemia such as diabetes. An extensive diet, exercise, and health belief history is key in assessing the client's current status and future teaching needs.

TABLE 23–2. Classification of Total, High-Density Lipoprotein (HDL), and Low-Density Lipoprotein (LDL) Cholesterol (measured in mg/dL)

Total Cholesterol		HDL Cholesterol		LDL Cholesterol	
				< 100	Optimal
< 200	Desirable	< 40	Low	100–129	Near optimal/ above optimal
200–239	Borderline high	> 60	High	130–159	Borderline high
≥ 240	High			160–189	High
				≥ 190	Very high

Source: NCEP, 2001.

Objective Data

Although the physical examination may be entirely normal (see Coronary Artery Disease), physical findings that are consistent with hyperlipidemia are obesity, xanthomas, lipemia retinalis, corneal arcus, and hepatosplenomegaly.

Hyperlipidemia Screening. Although there is no agreed-upon interval for screening, lipid screening for women should start at age 45 unless indicated earlier by risk (U.S. Preventive Services Task Force [USPSTF], 2008). In general screening should occur every 5 years, although that time frame is variable depending on whether repeated screening results are normal or patients have been diagnosed with dyslipidemia. Although lipid levels are less likely to change in people over age 65, the absolute benefit in terms of cardiovascular health for older adults is greater than in younger adults, so no upper age to screening has been established. Every 1 percent decrease in high serum cholesterol reduces risk for CAD by 2 percent. Significantly elevated triglycerides should be treated to prevent pancreatitis.

For screening, it is more important to assess cholesterol and HDL cholesterol (HDL-C) (USPSTF, 2008). A random (nonfasting) total cholesterol can be done as a screening measure in low-risk patients. For fasting assessment, the blood sample is drawn after a minimum of 8 hours of fasting. Values that classify clients as moderate to high risk are based on at least two separate studies by venipuncture, drawn 2 months apart. If the difference is less than 30 mg/dL, the two values are averaged. If the difference is more than 30 mg/dL, another sample is obtained and the three values are averaged. Values less than 100 mg/dL are optimal for LDL cholesterol (LDL-C) control (AHA, 2011a). Inform the client that she may drink water when fasting.

Differential Medical Diagnoses

Differential diagnoses include diabetes mellitus, liver disease (obstructive, hepatocellular, or hepatic storage disorder), hypothyroidism, renal disease (nephrosis and renal failure), hormonal imbalance (estrogens, progestins, and androgens), hyperuricemia, acute intermittent porphyria, and alcoholism.

Plan

A majority of clients with hyperlipidemia are managed by their primary care provider. Treatment must be individualized with respect to age, risk factors, clinical status, and presence or extent of CAD (see Table 23–3). The major prevention strategy is increasing activity and decreasing weight (Institute for Clinical Systems Improvement, 2009).

Psychosocial Interventions. Provide support and encourage clients who are changing their diet and level of physical activity to reduce lipid blood levels. Clients should have realistic expectations and be given objective evidence of their efforts. If medications are indicated, reinforce that nonpharmacological interventions are also essential to lowering lipids. Some individuals may have a genetic predisposition to elevated serum cholesterol and, consequently, have less response to nonpharmacological interventions. Avoid attributing high levels to noncompliance without adequate evaluation.

Medication. Consider discontinuing medications that may adversely influence lipid levels (prednisone, beta blockers, hormones, and diuretics). Medication chosen to lower lipid levels is specific to the client and the desired effect on lipid profile. Adherence to any drug regimen necessitates that the client be informed of the benefits of the drug, its potential side effects, cost, and convenience. This is especially true for older people. Few studies have focused on this age group, but post hoc analyses have shown that they have a greater risk reduction than younger populations (Lloyd-Jones et al., 2010; Williams et al., 2002). However, it must be recognized that it takes 2 years for benefits to accrue from medication management of lipids; therefore, a careful assessment must include potential life span, quality of life, and cost (Lloyd-Jones et al., 2010). A motivational feedback mechanism is provided by repeated serum cholesterol evaluation, which reflects the progress made.

Hydroxymethylglutaryl-Coenzyme A Reductase Inhibitors. The statins (rosuvastatin, atorvastatin, simvastatin, fluvastatin, lovastatin, and pravastatin) reduce cholesterol by inhibiting the enzyme that catalyzes the rate-limiting step in cholesterol synthesis (National Cholesterol Education Program [NCEP], 2002) and are the drug of choice to treat those with LDL-C > 190 mg/dL (Fletcher et al., 2005). A major side effect with this class of medications is muscle myopathy and also liver toxicity. Creatine phosphokinase and liver transaminases should be checked prior to instituting treatment and regularly during treatment.

- *Administration:* These medications are taken once a day with the evening meal or twice daily with meals.
- *Side effects:* Myalgias and elevated liver enzymes are known side effects; however, they are generally well tolerated.

TABLE 23–3. Therapeutic Approaches to Low-Density Lipoprotein (LDL) Cholesterol Lowering in Persons With Coronary Heart Disease (CHD) or CHD Risk Equivalents

Subcategory of LDL Cholesterol Level	LDL Cholesterol Goal	Level at Which to Initiate Dietary Therapy	Level at Which to Initiate LDL-Lowering Drugs
> 160 mg/dL	< 100 mg/dL	≥ 100 mg/dL	Increase statin dose or add second therapeutic agent (ezetimibe, bile acid sequestrant, or nicotinic acid)
≥ 130 mg/dL	< 100 mg/dL	≥ 100 mg/dL	Start drug therapy simultaneously with dietary therapy
100–129 mg/dL	< 100 mg/dL	≥ 100 mg/dL	Consider drug options[a]
< 100 mg/dL	< 100 mg/dL	TLC diet and emphasize weight control and physical activity	LDL-lowering drugs not required

An LDL cholesterol goal of < 70 mg/dL may be desirable for those at very high risk.

[a]Some authorities recommend use of LDL-lowering drugs in this category if an LDL cholesterol < 100 mg/dL cannot be achieved by therapeutic lifestyle changes (TLC) diet. Others prefer use of drugs that primarily modify other lipoprotein fractions (e.g., nicotinic acid and fibrate). Clinical judgment also may call for withholding drug therapy in this category.

Source: NCEP, 2001, 2004.

- *Contraindications:* Consult with a hepatologist when clients have known liver disease. Avoid concomitant use with potentially hepatotoxic drugs (e.g., isoniazid).
- *Anticipated outcome on evaluation:* Cholesterol levels decrease.

The following drug classes should not be offered as primary prevention for prevention of cardiovascular disease. An exception is fibrate therapy, which can be initiated if patients do not tolerate statins. The remaining are offered as secondary prevention for lowering LDL-C levels (Mosca et al., 2007; National Institute for Health and Clinical Excellence [NICE], 2008). However, for primary prevention of severe hypertriglyceridemia, fibrates and nicotinic acid are used to prevent pancreatitis (Grundy et al., 2005).

Gemfibrozil (Lopid), Fenofibrate, and Chlofibrate (Atromid S). These drugs are fibric acid derivative that is indicated primarily to lower plasma triglycerides. They also lower cholesterol, but to a lesser extent, and may raise HDL (NCEP, 2002).

- *Administration:* Give orally 30 minutes prior to a meal.
- *Side effect:* Gastrointestinal distress is known to occur.
- *Contraindication:* Do not administer to clients with impaired renal or hepatic function or to pregnant or breastfeeding women.
- *Anticipated outcome on evaluation:* Total cholesterol decreases, with a greater effect on triglycerides.
- *Client teaching:* Counsel the client to be alert for drug interactions.

Bile Acid Sequestrants (Cholestyramine and Colestipol). These agents reduce cholesterol by binding bile acids in the gut (NCEP, 2002).

- *Administration:* A powder, which is mixed with a liquid, or chewable bars are taken in two to four divided doses.
- *Side effects:* Gastrointestinal complaints are common. Bile acid sequestrants may interact with fat-soluble vitamins. Triglycerides tend to increase.
- *Contraindication:* Do not administer to pregnant women.
- *Anticipated outcome on evaluation:* Both LDL and total cholesterol levels decrease.
- *Client teaching:* Usually lower cost than other anticholesterol agents. Require much cooperation on the client's part. Also advise the client that the preparations have a gritty quality and should be taken several hours apart from other medications.

Nicotinic Acid (Niacin). Nicotinic acid reduces cholesterol by inhibiting its synthesis in the liver (NCEP, 2002).

- *Administration:* Usual drug dosage is in divided doses. Start with the smallest dose and gradually increase as tolerated until the desired effect is achieved.
- *Side effects:* Pruritus, gastrointestinal distress, and severe flushing are known side effects that decrease over time.
- *Contraindication:* Do not administer to clients with liver abnormalities.
- *Anticipated outcome on evaluation:* All lipoprotein levels are normal.
- *Client teaching:* Advise the client that nicotinic acid is the least expensive of the medications. Flushing, a side effect, may be controlled by not drinking alcohol or warm fluids and taking one 325-mg aspirin tablet 30 minutes before the nicotinic acid, if there is no contraindication to the use of aspirin.

Surgical Intervention. None known.

Lifestyle Changes. Physical activity might include 30 minutes of aerobic exercise daily to increase HDL levels and facilitate weight loss. Cigarette smoking increases LDL levels. Encourage your client to discontinue smoking.

Dietary Interventions. Refer to the AHA's progressive dietary plan for hyperlipidemia. Clients may benefit from consultation with a dietitian, especially if the diet becomes more complex with additional restrictions imposed because of other illnesses (Gidding et al., 2009). Dietary measures are safe and cost-effective and may eliminate the need for drugs to lower cholesterol.

All family members should be involved. Meet with them collectively or at least with the primary meal provider. Emphasize the foods that can be eaten rather than those that cannot. The AHA recommends the following daily parameters for a heart healthy diet (Mosca et al., 2011).

- Four to five cups of fruits and vegetables per day.
- 3.5 oz of oily type fish twice per week.
- 30 g/day of fiber.
- Three servings of whole grain per day.
- Less than or equal to five servings per week of sugar, lemonade, or sorbet.

- Greater than or equal to four servings of nuts, legumes, and seeds.
- Decrease saturated fats to less than 7 percent of caloric intake and trans fat to none of the caloric needs.
- Cholesterol is limited to < 150 mg/day.
- Alcohol is limited to one or fewer servings per day.
- Sodium is limited ≤ 1,500 mg/day.
- A *food diary* is recorded to target problem areas and provide feedback for the client and provider.
- A specific *food plan* is described during dietary counseling. For example, recommend mozzarella cheese made with skim milk or any dairy product with less than 1 percent fat. Recommend chicken or fish instead of beef. Offer suggestions on how to cook meat (broil, boil) to reduce fat content.

Follow-Up

Ascertain whether the expectation of a 10 to 20 percent decrease in total cholesterol was reached after approximately 6 weeks of dietary modification. Before considering any change in the treatment plan, individuals who have no additional risk factors should continue dietary interventions for at least 6 months. Most medications reduce total cholesterol an average of 20 to 25 percent and triglycerides 40 to 50 percent within 6 weeks. From post hoc analysis of existing statin studies, it appears that cholesterol reduction is just as beneficial or even more beneficial for those over age 65 than it is for those under age 65 (Kirby, 2011; Williams et al., 2002). Much remains to be learned concerning the management of hyperlipidemia as it relates to age and risk of CAD.

HYPERTENSION

Hypertension is the average of two or more readings on two or more occasions of a systolic blood pressure of 140 mmHg or greater and/or a diastolic blood pressure of 90 mmHg (Joint National Committee: 7th Report [JNC VII], 2003). The prevalence of hypertension is nearly equal between men and women ages 45 to 64, but thereafter, women have a much higher rate of hypertension (Robinson, 2007). One in three Americans over age 18 suffer from hypertension (AHA, 2011b). However, at 43 percent prevalence, African Americans have the highest rate of hypertension in the world (Hertz, Unger, Cornell, & Saunders, 2005). The direct and indirect costs to treat hypertension approach 76.6 billion annually (AHA, 2011c).

Epidemiology

Essential hypertension is idiopathic and most common. Most individuals (90%) will develop hypertension over the course of their lifetimes. It affects approximately 50 million Americans (JNC VII, 2003). More aggressive treatment of elevated systolic blood pressure in recent years has been estimated to have decreased coronary heart disease rates by 20 percent (Ford et al., 2007).

Hypertension affects women in all stages of life. But women have less hypertension before menopause, possibly because of higher levels of estrogen or lower levels of androgen or because of lower blood volume (Packer, 2007). Women who have a history of preeclampsia have double the risk of ischemic heart disease, stroke, or venous thrombosis 5 to 15 years after the pregnancy (Bellamy, Casas, Hingorani, & Williams, 2007). Over 50 percent of women older than age 60 have hypertension. Risk factors are a genetic predisposition, age older than 40, minority status, alcoholism, less educated, and/or lower socioeconomic group (JNC VII, 2003), and after age 65, more women than men are afflicted with hypertension (Roger et al., 2011). Hypertension is the leading risk factor for coronary heart disease, congestive heart failure, stroke, retinopathy, renal disease, and the progression of dementia. Reduction of stroke risk (30–40%), myocardial infarction risk (20–25%), and heart failure risk (50%) have been demonstrated when hypertension is treated (JNC VII, 2003).

Reversible risk factors include medication, alcohol abuse, excessive dietary sodium (> 1,500 mg/day), obesity, and systolic blood pressures (130–139) in prehypertensive patients who don't experience a drop in resting blood pressure at night (JNC VII, 2003). Secondary hypertension, which is uncommon, may be caused by polycystic kidneys, renovascular disease, aortic coarctation, Cushing's syndrome, and pheochromocytoma.

Subjective Data

A client with hypertension is most often asymptomatic but may complain of chest pain, headache, visual, dizziness, or neurological changes. She may report a family or personal medical history of hypertension, diabetes, kidney disease, hypothyroidism, cardiovascular disease, or stroke. Be alert for deviations from usual blood pressure readings or a history of elevated blood pressure. Note results and side effects of previous treatments. Identify risk factors including recent weight gain or loss, changes in exercise or diet, increased sodium, alcohol intake, smoking, or recreational drug use. Obtain a complete psychosocial history including socioeconomic status, emotional stress, coping mechanisms, and cultural habits. List all prescription and nonprescription medications that may contribute to hypertension (JNC VII, 2003).

Objective Data

Physical Examination. May include the following:

- *General:* Obesity (note pattern). Body mass index (BMI) ≥ 25.
- *Fundoscopic:* Arteriovenous compression or nicking, hemorrhages, exudates, or papilledema.
- *Neck:* Thyroid abnormalities, carotid bruits, jugular/venous distention.
- *Lungs:* Wheezes, rales, or rhonchi.
- *Heart:* Murmurs, rubs, gallops, displaced point of maximal impulse, regular rate and rhythm.
- *Abdomen:* Bruits, masses, hepatosplenomegaly, or enlarged kidneys.
- *Vascular:* Absent or diminished pulses.
- *Neurologic:* Absent or diminished sensation.
- *Extremities:* Edema, cyanosis, clubbing.

Blood pressure findings that are abnormal are episodic elevations, discrepancies between blood pressures in contralateral arms, and decreased pressures in the lower extremities. Specific measures may be taken to ensure accurate blood pressure readings.

- Seat the client with her arm supported and positioned at the level of her heart with feet flat on floor (legs uncrossed).
- Cigarettes should not be smoked or caffeine ingested within 30 minutes of the measurement.
- Have the client rest for about 5 minutes before measuring blood pressure.
- Use appropriate cuff size. The rubber bladder should be two-thirds the size of the arm.
- Check readings in both arms. Note any discrepancies.

Diagnostic Tests. Laboratory tests include a complete blood count (CBC), chemistries to evaluate kidney and liver function, lipid profiles, and urinalysis to assess renal function (JNC VII, 2003). These are done to provide baseline values, for the selection and surveillance of medications, and to monitor for sequelae from hypertension.

Differential Medical Diagnoses

Pheochromocytoma, thyroid or parathyroid disease, renal disease, Cushing's syndrome, primary aldosteronism, alcoholism, coarctation of the aorta, sleep apnea, and iatrogenic origin (drug effects).

Plan

The goal of hypertension workup and treatment is to (1) identify and reduce risk factors, (2) determine other causes of high blood pressure (renal disease, thyroid disease, drugs, etc.), and (3) to prevent end organ damage. The target goal for hypertension treatment is a systolic blood pressure of < 140. If this goal is met, it is likely that the diastolic pressure will be under 90. For those patients with a history of diagnosed hypertension, diabetes, or chronic kidney disease, the blood pressure goal is < 130/80 (JNC VII, 2003). Table 23–4 shows the current classification of the stages of hypertension with indications for treatment.

Psychosocial Interventions. Involve the client in decisions concerning treatment. Acknowledge hypertension as a chronic disease that can be controlled but not cured. Contract with the client for follow-up at predetermined intervals.

Lifestyle/Dietary Changes. Dietary modification may be an essential lifestyle change. Ideally, BMI should be kept between 18.5 and 24.9. Encourage the Dietary Approaches to Stop Hypertension diet, which is low fat, low salt, and high in fiber. Avoid caffeine and encourage smoking cessation. Advise the client to limit alcohol intake (JNC VII, 2003).

Physical activity may include a 30-minute aerobic exercise program most days of the week (JNC VII, 2003). The program should be initiated gradually. An overall increase in physical activity is encouraged; the benefits are numerous and include:

- HDL levels increase.
- Arterial blood pressure decreases.
- Glucose intolerance improves.
- Risk of colon cancer decreases.
- Knee, hip, and back pain decreases.
- Progression of dementia slows.
- Stress decreases.

Advise the client to stop smoking. Cessation reduces the risk of CAD. One year after quitting smoking, the risk for CAD is half that of a smoker's (U.S. Department of Health and Human Services [USDHS], 2011). The most successful strategies are likely to involve both pharmacological and behavioral methods (USDHS, US Surgeon General's Report, 2010).

TABLE 23–4. Classification of Blood Pressure for Adults Age 18 and Older

Category	Systolic (mmHg)		Diastolic (mmHg)	Lifestyle Modification	No Compelling Indications	Compelling Indications
Optimal	< 120	AND	< 80	Encourage	No antihypertensive drugs indicated	
Prehypertension	120–139	OR	80–89	Yes	No antihypertensive drugs indicated	Antihypertensives for those with chronic kidney disease or diabetes to keep systolic blood pressure < 130
Hypertension						
Stage 1	140–159	OR	90–99	Yes	Thiazide-type diuretics for most. May consider ACEI, ARB, BB, CCB, or combination	Drug(s) for the compelling indications[a] Other antihypertensive drugs (diuretics, ACEI, ARB, BB, CCB) as needed
Stage 2	≥ 160	OR	≥ 100	Yes	Two-drug combination for most (usually thiazide-type diuretic) and ACEI or ARB or BB or CCB)	Drug(s) for the compelling indications[a] Other antihypertensive drugs (diuretics, ACEI, ARB, BB, CCB) as needed

ACEI—angiotensin-converting enzyme inhibitor

ARB—angiotensin receptor blocker

BB—beta blocker

CCB—calcium channel blocker

[a]Compelling indications include heart failure, post myocardial infarction, diabetes, chronic kidney disease, recurrent stroke prevention, and high coronary disease risk.

Source: JNC VII, 2003.

Biofeedback and relaxation have been demonstrated to have modest results in reducing blood pressure in selected groups and may be the most useful treatment for mild hypertension.

Medication. Medication for moderate or severe hypertension decreases potential cardiovascular mortality and morbidity. Clients with mild hypertension benefit from medication in that it arrests the progression to a more severe condition and reduces the risk of cerebrovascular accidents. For individuals with a diastolic blood pressure persistently higher than 90 mmHg, the benefits of drug therapy outweigh the risks (JNC VII, 2003).

Single-dose therapies are usually a first-line choice to improve compliance and reduce side effects and expense in stage one hypertension in all age groups. However, older people may need lower starting doses due to side effects manifested with polypharmacy and poorer renal function. Medications cleared by the kidneys should be adjusted when glomerular filtration rate is below 60. In particular monitor for orthostasis (drop of ≥ 10 mmHg with associated dizziness or faintness). Patients at risk for orthostasis include those with multiple antihypertensives and diabetics, and those on diuretics, vasodilators, or psychotropes. When choosing a drug, consider concomitant medical problems, for example, beta blockers can mask hypoglycemic problems in diabetes and worsen asthma; some calcium channel blockers (nifedipine) can exacerbate migraines, even though some are used for migraine prophylaxis. Also consider race: African Americans are more likely to respond favorably with dual therapy, for example, when diuretics are used with calcium channel blockers (JNC VII, 2003).

- *Diuretics:* Diuretics reduce blood pressure by decreasing volume and thereby decreasing preload. They are classified by mechanism and site of action.
  - *Thiazides and sulfonamides* (chlorothiazide, hydrochlorothiazide, indapamide, metolazone) should be used as initial therapy for most people with hypertension. These agents are inexpensive and well tolerated. However, in those with sulfa allergies, they are contraindicated. These agents may raise lithium blood levels and serum cholesterol. Concomitant administration of nonsteroidal anti-inflammatory drugs (NSAIDs) may antagonize thiazide or sulfonamide effectiveness or cause electrolyte disturbances and sexual dysfunction. These drugs should be avoided in cases where there is a history of gout or hyponatremia.
  - *Potassium-sparing agents* (amiloride, triamterene) are used with caution with clients who are renal compromised (older people) or are using angiotensin-converting enzyme inhibitors (ACEIs). These agents can also potentiate the effectiveness of ACE and calcium channel blockers.

- *Loop diuretics* (bumetanide, furosemide, torsemide) can cause a powerful diuresis, intervascular volume depletion, and electrolyte disturbances. Older people are particularly prone to dehydration with this class of drugs and may also have difficulty getting to the bathroom predisposing them to falls. Potassium supplementation is often required.

- *ACEIs (benazepril, captopril, enalapril, lisinopril, ramipril):* ACEIs are indicated to suppress the renin-angiotensin-aldosterone system. Structure, absorption, and duration of action differ slightly among these drugs. They are particularly effective for congestive heart failure and are indicated for those with diabetes to preserve renal function. Administer ACEIs once or twice daily. Although they are generally well tolerated, adverse effects may include cough (persistent and nonproductive), angioedema, hypotension, rash (most common with captopril), and hyperkalemia. Monitor renal function. Avoid potassium-containing salt substitutes (JNC VII, 2003). For those with an ACE-induced cough, angiotensin receptor blockers (ARBs) can be used with good results. Drugs in this class include candesartan, irbesartan, losartan, valsartan, and olmesartan.
- *Beta blockers:* Beta blockers (atenolol, metoprolol, propanolol, timolol, and nadolol) and calcium channel blockers (diltiazem, verapamil, amlodipine, felodipine, and nifedipine) are also used for hypertension. Beta blockers have been shown to decrease morbidity and mortality and remain initial drugs of choice after diuretics (JNC VII, 2003).
- *Combination therapy:* For those with acute myocardial infarction or unstable angina, antihypertensive therapy should include a beta blocker and an ACEI. For those with a high recurrent stroke risk, chronic kidney disease, or diabetes, combination therapy with one of the antihypertensives being an ACEI or an ARB has been shown to improve long-term outcomes. In those with renal disease, a rise in serum creatinine up to 35 percent above the baseline is acceptable when on ACEIs (JNC VII, 2003).

Follow-Up

Arrange for periodic evaluation for target organ damage (potassium and serum creatinine one to two times per year) and continue to reinforce the client's lifestyle modifications, educating the client that hypertension is the leading cause of heart disease and stroke. Intervals between office visits vary and depend on the degree and lability of hypertension. Adjust medication after 3 to 4 weeks if the client's response is inadequate. However, once the blood pressure goal is reached, visits every 3 to 6 months are sufficient (JNC VII, 2003).

Address reasons for unresponsiveness to therapies. For clients who are following nonpharmacological therapeutic recommendations in addition to medications, a trial of step-down therapy and drug withdrawal may be considered after blood pressure has been at goal level for 1 year.

CORONARY ARTERY DISEASE

Coronary artery disease is caused by altered blood flow in the coronary arteries related to narrowing of the vessel due to damage to the intima by plaque and chronic inflammation resulting in reduced oxygenation of the myocardium. Myocardial ischemia occurs when oxygen demand exceeds oxygen supply. The supply–demand balance may be disturbed by coronary atherosclerosis, vasospasm, thrombus formation, or cardiomyopathy.

Epidemiology

CAD, also known as atherosclerosis, coronary heart disease, ischemic heart disease, or hardening of the arteries, was once considered a male affliction, although women are now recognized to be at equal and, in some circumstances, greater risk than men. Men and women, however, may differ in the onset, distribution, and presentation of this disease (Biswas & Bastian, 2002; Mosca, Mochari-Greenberger, Dolor, Newby, & Robb, 2010). For those who are free of cardiovascular disease at age 50, the lifetime risk of developing cardiovascular disease (CAD, stroke, heart failure, peripheral vascular disease) is 51.7 percent for men and 39.2 percent for women (Lloyd-Jones et al., 2010). Of the deaths attributed to cardiovascular disease, 51 percent are due to CAD (National Center for Health Statistics [NCHS], 2009a). CAD is the main cause of heart attacks (Centers for Disease Control and Prevention [CDC], 2011a).

CAD is distributed differently than is cardiovascular disease overall, with American Indians (6.6%) and whites (6.5%) having the highest prevalence rates and Hispanics (5.7%) and blacks (5.6%) having nearly equal prevalence. The prevalence of CAD, for those over age 20, in men is 9.1 percent, and in women, it is 7 percent, with black women having a higher prevalence (8.8%) than black men (7.8%) (Pleis, Lucus, & Ward, 2009). Black women not only have the highest CAD rate, they also have the highest death rate from CAD and cardiovascular disease in general (Roger et al., 2011).

CAD is the leading cause of death for both men and women (CDC, 2011a) and causes one in six deaths in the United States (Heron et al., 2009). More than 500,000 Americans die each year of heart attacks. Almost half are women (CDC, 2011a). CAD is the most common cause of cardiovascular disease deaths (Mieres et al., 2005). For women, because CAD is underrecognized and undertreated, the initial cardiac event is fatal in 40 percent of incidents (Mieres et al., 2005). The direct and indirect cost of CAD exceeds $316.4 billion annually (CDC, 2011a). According to the most recent NHIS/NCHS figures available, nearly 64 percent of CAD deaths in women could be avoided by controlling modifiable risk factors and making lifestyle changes (Lloyd-Jones et al., 2010). It is believed that changes due to lifestyle and environment account for 44 percent of the decrease in CAD in recent years (Ford et al., 2007).

Modifiable Risk Factors. Factors that may influence the development of CAD include cigarette smoking, obesity, physical inactivity, hypertension, diet, and hyperlipidemia.

Nearly 18 percent of women over age 18 still smoke (CDC, 2009). Cigarette smoking is a powerful risk for cardiovascular events (Goldenberg et al., 2003; Lloyd-Jones et al., 2010). It increases the risk of CAD two to four times that of a nonsmoker (USDHS, 2010), but the risk is reversible within a year of cessation of smoking (Anthonisen et al., 2005). Stopping smoking is estimated to have provided a 12 percent reduction in CAD in recent years (Ford et al., 2007). Smoking low-tar and low-nicotine cigarettes does not reduce the risk of cardiovascular events. Women who smoke *and* use oral contraceptives are more likely to have a heart attack (Hulley et al., 2002).

Obesity also presents a formidable risk with > 66 percent of adults either obese or overweight (Lloyd-Jones et al., 2010). Clients who are more than 30 percent overweight are more likely to develop heart disease, even if this is their only risk factor (Stampfer, Hu, Manson, Rimm, & Willett, 2000).

Physical inactivity—a sedentary lifestyle—contributes to CAD by unfavorably altering serum lipid ratios. Fifty-nine percent of adults admit to no vigorous activity (NCHS, 2009b).

Nonmodifiable Risk Factors. Nonmodifiable risk factors for CAD are family history, age, gender, and diabetes.

A strong family history of CAD (CAD diagnosed in brother/father before the age of 55, or in mother/sister before the age of 65) is significant. Early sudden cardiac death of a first-degree relative warrants a more aggressive approach in controlling modifiable risk factors, even if the client is asymptomatic (Banerjee et al., 2009; Mosca et al., 2011).

Age and gender differences are difficult to distinguish because research studies on women and cardiovascular disease are inadequate. The average age of onset of CAD among men is between 40 and 44 years. Women tend not to develop heart problems until after menopause (Mieres et al., 2005), most likely because of the cardioprotective effects of estrogen. After menopause, the risk of CAD increases steadily and reaches that of males in the seventh decade of life (Mieres et al., 2005). If menopause is iatrogenic (the uterus and ovaries are surgically removed), the risk of a heart attack rises more sharply than if menopause occurs naturally. Exogenous estrogen may increase the risk of heart disease of older women and is no longer recommended for cardioprotective effects (Mosca et al., 2011). Diabetes mellitus not only increases the risk of CAD (Wilson & Meigs, 2008) but is a major predictor of mortality following a myocardial infarction (Lloyd-Jones et al., 2010).

Subjective Data

Premenopausal women have two times the death rate of men for acute myocardial infarction. Morbidity and mortality associated with myocardial infarction are higher among women, because of the failure to identify CAD earlier in women. Women (especially older women) frequently experience nausea, overwhelming fatigue, dizziness, trouble sleeping, shortness of breath, or anxiety and these anginal symptoms more likely are attributed to noncardiac causes (MedicineNet, 2011).

Women are likely to report chest pain or pressure (angina) as their first symptom of a heart attack described as fullness, squeezing, indigestion, heartburn, or upper body discomfort (NHLBI, 2011a, 2011b). Intensity of pain does not always correlate with severity of disease (Anderson et al., 2007). Angina may be described as a minor ache or crushing chest pain. Pain is often accompanied by nausea, vomiting, lightheadedness, fainting, or a cold sweat. Clients may relate only associated symptoms such as dyspnea and diaphoresis with exertion. Treatment of silent ischemia is based more on objective than on subjective findings.

A thorough history includes the onset, character, location, radiation, frequency, duration, precipitating factors, relieving factors, and associated symptoms. If the client reports a clear relationship between her symptoms and physical exertion, a cardiac origin is highly suspected.

Objective Data

Physical Examination. May reveal nothing abnormal; however, signs of CAD may include the following:

- *General appearance:* Obese, anxious, dyspneic.
- *Vital signs:* High or low blood pressure, tachycardia or bradycardia, fever.
- *Skin:* Cyanosis, diaphoresis.
- *Eyes:* Arcus senilis, xanthomas, hypertensive retinopathy.
- *Neck:* Jugular venous distention, carotid bruits.
- *Lungs:* Rales, rhonchi, wheezes, or diminished breath sounds.
- *Heart:* Murmurs, gallops, rubs, clicks, irregular rhythms, displaced point of maximal impulse, heaves, and thrills.
- *Vascular system:* Absent or diminished peripheral pulses, bruits, edema, mottling.
- *Abdomen:* Hepatomegaly, bruits.

Diagnostic Tests. Laboratory testing includes a CBC and renal basic metabolic panel (BMP), thyroid-stimulating hormone (TSH), C-reactive protein (CRP), and liver function tests to determine underlying disease and identify risk factors. If ischemia is suspected, troponins, total creatine kinase, creatine kinase myocardial band, and brain natriuretic peptide (if dyspneic) should be obtained.

Presently, assessing the risk of CAD is difficult. Many of the tests currently used evaluate the degree of established disease or the damage from existing CAD. However, two tests (evaluation of coronary artery calcification [CAC] and carotid intima-media thickness [IMT]) are proving useful for risk stratification of CAD, and may be covered by insurance in the future. The AHA and other groups currently recommend that CAC and carotid IMT be reserved for those in the intermediate risk group for whom therapy is being considered, but may post undue risk for the individual (Mosca et al., 2011). Detrano et al. (2005) demonstrated that subjects with CAC scores of > 100 were 7 to 10 times more likely to have a coronary event. CAC scores may prove useful in predicting how aggressively both hypertension and cholesterol should be controlled (Lloyd-Jones et al., 2010). Carotid IMT uses ultrasound to assess the degree of narrowing of the carotid vessels and is currently employed after stroke or after the development of carotid bruits (Smith, Greenland, & Grundy, 2000). However, carotid IMT may allow intervention in young adulthood for those with scores above the 75th percentile, as these patients have a two- to three-time greater risk of myocardial infarction or stroke (O'Leary et al., 1999).

Electrocardiogram (ECG) permits myocardial ischemic changes to be seen in ST segment elevation or, more commonly, depression. This noninvasive test is essential to detection of myocardial ischemia and is the test of choice for triaging patients with chest pain (Amsterdam et al., 2010). However, a normal ECG does not rule out diagnosis of infarction or ischemia. Dysrhythmias, such as atrial fibrillation or atrial flutter, may be detected. The procedure lacks specificity and sensitivity in women, particularly younger women, those with atypical chest pain and breast attenuation.

The chest x-ray assists in differential diagnosis and in evaluating the progress of disease. It may reveal increased pulmonary markings or cardiomegaly (Amsterdam et al., 2010).

Exercise tolerance testing (ETT), a stress test, identifies the location of ischemic vessels by recording the changes that occur during exercise on an ECG. ETT remains the initial diagnostic test for symptomatic women who are capable of exercise and are at intermediate risk of CAD (Mieres et al., 2005). It is now recommended that ETT should be done early after presentation in low-risk patients (Amsterdam et al., 2010). Patients recommended for this procedure are those who can exercise, those without ECG readings that preclude interpretation of the ETT, those who are not on digoxin, and those without left ventricular hypertrophy (Anderson et al., 2007). Women ≥ age 50 who have either typical or atypical chest pain or women under age 50 with typical chest pain are recommended to have this test. Those who have multiple-risk factors, symptoms, or diabetes should also be considered candidates for testing. For women, this test has a sensitivity of 61 percent (Mieres et al., 2005).

Echocardiogram is the most sensitive, noninvasive diagnostic test used to measure cardiac size and function. It determines abnormalities in the motion of the myocardium, abnormalities in structure and ventricular function, and hypertrophy. A transthoracic echocardiogram is noninvasive. Dobutamine stress echocardiography has excellent negative predictive value for future obstructive events (Amsterdam et al., 2010) and is significantly more sensitive and accurate than ETT (Mieres et al., 2005).

Nuclear perfusion studies have low false-positive rates and should be used to stratify risk for women at intermediate to high-risk categories prior to a cardiac event (Mieres et al., 2005). Pharmacologic studies are recommended when exercise testing does not yield conclusive information or the client is deconditioned or disabled, prohibiting her from sustaining a level of exertion necessary to complete the testing. A day is usually required to complete the test (Amsterdam et al., 2010). These tests can be inaccurate due to breast tissue attenuation and smaller left ventricles in women (Mieres et al., 2005).

Computed tomography coronary angiogram provides a noninvasive way to determine the anatomy and patency of the cardiac vessels. It does carry the risk of allergy to the IV dye as well as renal function issues. Unlike in cardiac catheterization, narrowed vessels cannot be treated, necessitating a second procedure. Although this procedure has excellent diagnostic value, cardiac catheterization remains the most widely used test of anatomic function (Amsterdam et al., 2010).

Cardiac catheterization is the most definitive test to determine the location and extent of CAD (Agostoni et al., 2006). It is ordered based on the results of the exercise stress test and the level of risk an individual carries and should be performed as the initial diagnostic testing on symptomatic women with a known history of CAD and those with an abnormal resting ECG and suspected CAD (Mieres et al., 2005). In experienced laboratories, it is performed with low mortality (0.2–0.7%) or severe vascular complications (0.7–2.6%). Females are at higher risk of local complications (Agostoni et al., 2006). A catheter is threaded through to the coronary vessels retrograde usually from the femoral arteries and dye is injected in order to determine narrowing or occlusion of the cardiac vessels. The client should anticipate a standard preoperative workup.

Differential Medical Diagnoses

Thoracic outlet syndrome, MVP, anemia, substance abuse, costochondritis, gastroesophageal reflux disorder, esophageal spasm, panic disorder.

Plan

As interventions are employed, continued surveillance of symptoms, medications, and risk factors is required.

Psychosocial Interventions. Provide anticipatory guidance about diagnostic testing and the nature of the disease. Assist clients in gaining a sense of control over the disease through risk reduction. Clients need to know the risks and benefits of all treatment options to make informed decisions about their lives and health.

Medication. Coupled with a reduction in modifiable risk factors, medication is a viable option for up to two thirds of clients with CAD. In weighing medical against surgical intervention, the key factors are the extent and location of coronary artery occlusion. Need to evaluate order of recommendation with particular emphasis on older people.

- *Nitrates:* Nitrates (imdur, isosorbide, nitroglycerin) may be used independently or with other medications. Nitrates are used as an antianginal agent because of their vasodilating effect.
  - *Administration:* Sublingual, topical, transdermal, and oral (long-acting or chewable tablet) forms are available. The sublingual form acts within 15 seconds and has a 15- to 30-minute duration of action. Ointments and transdermal patches may last 12 hours or longer.
  - *Side effects:* Headaches are common. They may be relieved by changing the dosage, route of administration, or if taken with acetaminophen. Other reactions to nitrates are hypotension, dizziness, and palpitations.
  - *Contraindication:* Do not administer to clients with severe hypotension.
  - *Anticipated outcome on evaluation:* Anginal episodes decrease or are eliminated.
  - *Client teaching:* Include information about all possible side effects and indications for intermittent use of nitrates as needed. Remind patient when taking nitrates for the first few times that they can cause lightheadedness and that they should be careful with positional changes.
- *Aspirin:* Aspirin lowers the risk of myocardial infarctions in persons at increased risk for atherosclerosis and thrombogenesis, including persons who have had a myocardial infarction, unstable angina, or postcoronary artery bypass grafting. Aspirin inhibits platelet aggregation and prevents formation of arterial thrombi on atherosclerotic plaques.
  - *Administration:* Daily aspirin therapy (unless contraindicated) of 75 to 325 mg should be used in women who have diagnosed CAD and is reasonable for women with diabetes. If a woman is intolerant of aspirin therapy, clopidogrel should be used. There is less evidence for daily therapy in healthy women for myocardial infarction or stroke

prevention. However, low-dose aspirin (81 mg) may be useful in this situation if there is little risk of gastrointestinal bleeding or hemorrhagic stroke (Mosca et al., 2011).

- *Side effects:* Gastrointestinal upset and bleeding.
- *Contraindication:* Do not administer to clients with gastric ulcerative disease and coagulopathies.
- *Anticipated outcomes on evaluation:* Progression of atherosclerotic disease slows, and the likelihood of thrombolic events decreases.
- *Client teaching:* Include information about side effects. Aspirin needs to be used consistently to be an effective preventive measure. Aspirin used in older people does increase the risk of gastritis and potential for gastrointestinal bleed. Make sure the patient knows to report any untoward side effects or symptoms.

◆ *β-Adrenergic receptor antagonists:* Beta blockers, used for 12 months, are indicated for those with an ischemic heart event and preserved left ventricular function. However, indefinite use of beta blockers should be implemented for those with left ventricular failure unless otherwise contraindicated and may be considered for those with CAD or vascular disease with normal left ventricular function (Mosca et al., 2011). These drugs attenuate increased blood pressure and heart rate during activity, thereby decreasing the workload of the heart. They have been shown to decrease mortality postmyocardial infarction.

- *Administration:* The new β_1 selective agents block myocardial receptors with little effect on bronchial or smooth vascular muscle—a benefit to those with asthma or claudication.
- *Side effects:* Depression, impotence, peripheral vascular ischemia, and palpitations are known to occur. The beta blocker may decrease the effectiveness of other medications such as oral hyperglycemic agents.
- Contraindication:Do not administer to clients with heart failure, sick sinus syndrome with atrioventricular block, bradycardia (fewer than 50 beats per minute), and asthma.
- *Anticipated outcome on evaluation:* Symptoms of angina, heart rate, and blood pressure decrease.
- *Client teaching:* Plan to continue indefinitely. Review and encourage the client to report any side effects at all visits.

◆ *ACEIs/ARBs.* ACEIs are recommended after myocardial infarction, with clinical evidence of heart failure (EF < 40), or in those with diabetes and if intolerant of ACEIs, ARBs should be implemented. In addition, aldosterone blockade should be started in women after a myocardial infarction, assuming that they have been started on therapeutic doses of both a beta blocker and an ACEI and they have clinical symptoms of heart failure with an ejection fraction of less than 40 percent and they do not have hypotension, renal dysfunction, or hyperkalemia (Mosca et al., 2011). See Hypertension section for more details on use of these agents.

Surgical and Other Interventions. In percutaneous transluminal coronary angioplasty, a balloon is introduced into an artery and inflated at the site of an atherosclerotic plaque. In dilating the vessel, the balloon flattens the plaque against the arterial wall, reducing its thickness. Stents are often used to prevent the vessel from restenosing. With the newer drug eluting stents, the restenosis rate is reported at roughly 5 percent (Hamid & Coltart, 2007). Complications include acute restenosis or vessel dissection, with the possibility of open heart surgery or death.

Coronary artery bypass grafting is performed for select groups of clients with multivessel disease, left main CAD, or ventricular aneurysm. Generally, anginal symptoms markedly improve and improvement persists at least 10 years. Surgical risks may be increased or decreased, depending on the extent of disease and the presence of other underlying medical problems at the time of surgery.

Lifestyle/Dietary Changes. Such changes can dramatically reduce morbidity and mortality. Primary prevention focuses on modifying risk factors: hypertension, hyperlipidemia, cigarette smoking, obesity, and physical inactivity (Mosca et al., 2011). Advise the client to follow a low-cholesterol and low-fat diet (see Hyperlipidemia).

Physical activity is tailored to the individual client, considering her overall physical condition and cardiac history. Advise the client to avoid exertional activities during extreme weather conditions or after a heavy meal. The client should always carry nitroglycerin and alert the health care provider to any change in symptoms. Advise the client about cardiac rehabilitation programs, especially if she is having difficulty returning to an acceptable level of physical activity.

Cigarette smoking is a significant risk factor and should be discontinued. Involve the client in a smoking cessation program.

MITRAL VALVE PROLAPSE

Valvular heart disease is caused by one of three factors: (1) high velocity flow through normal or abnormal valves, (2) forward flow through normal or narrowed valves, or (3) backward flow through incompetent valves. Most systolic murmurs are benign, while diastolic or continuous murmurs usually represent pathology and should be further evaluated. MVP is a relatively benign and common disorder. Its distinguishing pathology is billowing of one or both valve leaflets into the left atrium (Bonow et al., 2008).

Epidemiology

MVP can be either a familial or a nonfamilial disorder and, if familial, is a genetic disorder of autosomal dominance; offspring have a 50 percent chance of being affected if one parent has the disorder. MVP occurs in several connective tissue diseases, other cardiovascular processes, and miscellaneous muscular and thyroid abnormalities. The causative factor seems to be characteristic dysgenesis of collagenous valvular tissue (Bonow et al., 2008).

Studies show that MVP is the most common valvular abnormality in the United States, with about 3 to 6 percent of the general population affected (Greene, 2008). Prevalence, using echocardiographic criteria, varies from 1 to 2.5 percent of the population (Bonow et al., 2008). Women tend to be affected more than men, and in general, it is a disease appearing in the fifth decade of life (Greene, 2008).

Complications are mitral regurgitation, infective endocarditis, thromboembolism, ventricular dysfunction leading to cardiac arrhythmias, and pulmonary hypertension. Less than 2 percent of MVP cases have sudden death. The role of MVP in thromboembolic disease is less clear. It is often considered a factor in unexplained cerebral ischemic events especially for those under age 45 (Bonow et al., 2008).

Mitral regurgitation is caused most often by MVP, although only a very small percentage of clients with MVP progress to mitral regurgitation. Moreover, a small number within that group become hemodynamically impaired (Auten, 1996; Bonow et al., 1998). Mortality predictors include moderate to severe mitral regurgitation, left ventricular ejection fraction of less than 50 percent, or thickened valve leaflets, although typically MVP survival rates are similar to nonafflicted individuals (Bonow et al., 2008).

Anxiety is not a causative factor in the development of MVP, but it can be a manifestation. Heart, hormone, and chemical disturbances may account for the symptomatology of panic disorder; however, they are not yet understood.

Subjective Data

A client with MVP is usually asymptomatic; however, she may report chest pain and/or palpitations. The exact etiology of pain is unknown. The chest pain is atypical for angina and usually nonexertional. It may result from mechanical stress on the papillary muscle, from coronary artery spasm or embolism, left ventricular dysfunction, rate-related supply/demand imbalance, independent CAD, or extracardiac conditions. Heart palpitations are also common. Other symptoms include complaints of fast heart rate, skipped beats, lightheadedness, fatigue, weakness, dyspnea, anxiety, and postural phenomena (Bonow et al., 2008).

Objective Data

MVP is identified primarily by means of physical examination, with electrocardiogram, and echocardiogram confirming the diagnosis and extent of the disease and associated complications (Bonow et al., 2008). Laboratory tests are done to rule out other suspected medical problems. See Coronary Artery Disease and Hypertension sections for tests done to rule out medical problems that may be associated with MVP.

Physical Examination. Usually normal unless MVP is associated with other conditions. Cardiac findings include an isolated, high-pitched, mid to late systolic click. The client may have a late systolic murmur (late or pansystolic murmurs indicate mitral regurgitation). Chest auscultation is best done with the diaphragm over the cardiac apex. Examine the client in the supine and left lateral recumbent positions. The click is heard earlier and occupies much of systole when sitting or standing. Valsalva maneuvers will increase the length and often the intensity of MVP. Postural auscultation is the key to diagnosis. Standing will lengthen and intensify the MVP murmur, while brisk squatting or passive leg raising in the supine position will soften the murmur or may make the murmur disappear entirely. If the client is squatting, the click may be closer to S2 (Bonow et al., 2008). Murmur often disappears during pregnancy because of expanding blood volume and the subsequent increase in left ventricular cavity size.

Diagnostic Tests. Chest x-ray can help in the initial screening of these patients yielding information regarding cardiac silhouette, pulmonary findings, and calcifications. Abnormal findings on either chest x-ray or ECG (left ventricular hypertrophy or old myocardial infarction) in the presence of a murmur should lead to further examination with echocardiogram to evaluate the cardiac chambers and blood flow through the valves (Bonow et al., 2008).

The echocardiogram is recommended to confirm MVP, to determine the extent of mitral regurgitation, and to assess the possibility of MVP in asymptomatic patients with significant murmur (diastolic, late systolic, continuous, or grade three plus murmurs, murmurs that radiate to back or neck, or murmurs associated with clicks) or for patients who have murmurs and clinical symptoms such as ischemia, syncope, thromboembolism, infective carditis, or congestive heart failure. It is recommended to determine whether mitral valve leaflets have hypertrophied, which increases the risk of infective endocarditis and progression to mitral regurgitation. It is also used for risk stratification in those with known MVP. However, routine repetition of echocardiogram is not indicated in those with MVP without regurgitation or with minimal regurgitation for whom symptoms have not appeared or changed in intensity (Bonow et al., 2008).

Differential Medical Diagnoses

Marfan's syndrome, rheumatic fever, trauma, hypertrophic cardiomyopathy, atrial septal defect, anorexia nervosa, pectus excavatum, connective tissue disorders, anxiety or depressive disorders.

Plan

Psychosocial Interventions. Educate the client about her common, benign condition. The valve functions properly, and usually no treatment is needed. MVP does not appear to alter the course of pregnancy. Periodic auscultatory examinations are necessary to note any changes. For clients with no complications, activities and exercise are not limited. However, for those with moderate left ventricular enlargement, left ventricular dysfunction, uncontrolled tachyarrhythmias, prolonged QT intervals, syncope, previous resuscitation from cardiac arrest, or aortic root enlargement should be discouraged from participating in competitive sports (Bonow et al., 2008).

Medication. Although not usually required, medications may be prescribed.

Beta-adrenergic or calcium channel blockers are usually effective in controlling palpitation symptoms (Bonow et al., 2008). *Anxiolytic drugs* are recommended *only* if there is an underlying anxiety disorder.

Anticoagulants and antiplatelet medications are a possible therapeutic intervention for those at high risk for thromboembolic disease. Aspirin therapy (75–325 mg daily) is indicated for those (1) at any age who have MVP and transient ischemic attacks (TIAs) or (2) who are under age 65 with atrial fibrillation and MVP and have no history of hypertension, mitral regurgitation, or congestive heart failure. Aspirin therapy is also a reasonable choice for patients with MVP and a stroke history but (1) no history of mitral regurgitation, hypertension, congestive heart failure, or (2) in situations when warfarin therapy is contraindicated. On the other hand, warfarin therapy is indicated in MVP patients with atrial fibrillation if they (1) are over age 65 or (2) have hypertension, mitral regurgitation, or congestive heart failure no matter their age. Those who have MVP with a stroke history as well as mitral regurgitation, atrial fibrillation, or thromboembolism should also be on warfarin. Warfarin therapy could also be considered reasonable in patients with MVP and stroke history if there is echogenic evidence of leaflet thickening or for those who have MVP and continued TIAs despite aspirin therapy (Bonow et al., 2006).

Antimicrobial prophylaxis to prevent endocarditis is reasonable only for those undergoing dental procedures or oral mucosa perforation if the patient has a prosthetic valve or prosthetic material was used in a valve repair; prosthetic materials in the heart or surrounding vessels (stents) have a previous history of endocarditis or have coronary heart disease. In the absence of infection, prophylaxis is no longer recommended for nondental procedures such as transesophageal echocardiogram, esophagogastroduodenoscopy (EGD), or colonoscopy. Bacteremia should be considered if a client experiences unexplained malaise or fever for greater than 48 hours; drawing of at least two sets of blood cultures from different sites prior to starting antibiotics is recommended in this situation (Bonow et al., 2008).

Surgical Interventions. Valve repair or replacement is indicated for symptomatic and hemodynamically significant mitral regurgitation. The procedure depends on the extent and etiology of disease (Bonow et al., 2008).

Follow-Up

Recommend follow-up every 3 to 5 years for asymptomatic clients without regurgitation. Annual follow-up is

TABLE 23–5. Key Dermatologic History Questions

What did the rash look like when it first appeared?
Has the rash spread?
What past or current treatment? Results?
Previous occurrence?
Pruritic? Painful?
Any other household members with similar rash?
Recent history of new medication or cosmetic?
Any other symptom or medical problem?

Source: Whitmore, 2007.

recommended for those who are symptomatic, have a change in their symptoms, or have moderate to severe regurgitation (Bonow, Carabello, Chatterjee, & Shanewise, 2006).

DERMATOLOGIC DISORDERS

Skin problems account for many primary care visits. Rashes or lesions may appear on exposed areas of the body or on the face and may cause the client embarrassment and concern. She is likely to seek attention promptly and may expect rapid resolution. The provider needs to be a "derm detective," taking a thorough history and using observational skills. See Table 23–5 for key dermatologic history questions and Table 23–6 for clinical finding specific to different types of dermatoses.

SCALING MACULES, PATCHES, AND PLAQUES

Superficial Fungal Infections

Superficial mycotic infections of the skin are identified according to the area of the body affected. There are two main classes of organisms: Tinea and Candida. The lesions are varied in appearance, but almost all caused by Tinea have a scaly appearance. These scales may be scraped and examined for hyphae under a microscope using KOH wet mount.

Epidemiology. Tinea and candidal dermatophyte infections are common in adults and children and in hot, humid climates. Women who are diabetic, are obese, and exercise to the point of profuse sweating may be especially prone to recurrent candidal infections. Exposure to infected pets may precede ringworm (Schalock, Hsu, & Arndt, 2011; Winland-Brown, Porter, & Allen, 2011).

Subjective/Objective Data, Associated Findings, and Differential Diagnoses. See Table 23–6.

Diagnostic Tests. *Tinea versicolor*, *Tinea corporis* (ringworm), and *Tinea pedis* are usually diagnosed on the basis of history and characteristic appearance/distribution. Scales on the lesion may be scraped onto a slide, covered with KOH, and examined under the microscope for hyphae if diagnosis in doubt. *Tinea capitis* (scalp ringworm) and *Tinea unguium* (nail fungus) are diagnosed by fungus culture before treatment is begun (Schalock et al., 2011; Winland-Brown et al., 2011).

Plan

Psychosocial. Fungal infections may cause body image disturbance and concern regarding contagion. Nail infections may require months of treatment before resolution. Reassurance about self-limited nature of most common dermatoses is helpful to the client. Be open to these issues.

Medication Administration. Various classes of antifungal medications are available for the treatment of fungal infections. See Table 23–7 for a list categorizing fungal medications and clinical indications. Antifungal medications can be applied topically or administered orally depending on severity, location, and diagnosis. Tinea capitus, tinea unguium, and systemic candidiasis require treatment with oral agents. Before beginning oral antifungal agents, hepatic function and CBC baseline should be obtained. Oral antifungals have numerous drug interactions and should be prescribed carefully. Newer oral antifungals such as terbinafine and itraconazole have fewer side effects than older antifungals. See an up-to-date drug handbook for full prescribing information for antifungal therapy.

Diet/Lifestyle. *Tinea capitus:* Griseofulvin, an oral antifungal often prescribed for tinea capitus, has a slightly metallic taste. Encourage the client to maintain adequate nutrition as sense of taste may be altered. Stress importance of adherence to daily dose of oral antifungal when prescribed to prevent relapse. Advise the client to avoid overexposure to sunlight when taking griseofulvin. Alcohol should be avoided during treatment with oral antifungals. Stress the importance of personal hygiene and scalp care, not sharing combs, brushes, hats, towels.

Tinea capitis can be spread by asymptomatic carriers. All members of the client's household should use selenium sulfide shampoo or 2 percent ketoconazole shampoo three times weekly until the client is cured. The shampoos need to remain on the scalp for 5 minutes prior to rinsing (Aly, Forney, & Bayles, 2001; Elewski, 1999b; Goldstein, Smith, Ives, & Goldstein, 2000; Martin & Elewski, 2002).

TABLE 23–6. Scaling Macules, Patches, and Plaques

Diagnosis	Subjective Data	Objective Data Distribution	Differential DX
Tinea versicolor	Mildly pruritic	Pale macules that do not tan Fine scale when scraped (KOH+) Young adults Mainly on trunk	Vitiligo (no pigmentation) Lyme disease
Tinea corporis (ringworm)	Mildly pruritic May have cat	Annular lesion with scaly border and central clearing or scaly patches with distinct border Exposed areas	Psoriasis (on knees, elbows) Secondary syphilis (on palms, soles) Pityriasis rosea (more lesions)
Tinea capitis (scalp ringworm)	Usually asymptomatic May have asymptomatic carrier in family	Scaly plaque of alopecia or broken hairs Kerion formation may occur (inflamed, boggy nodule) Cervical adenopathy Diagnosis on basis of fungal culture Scalp	Seborrheic dermatitis (oily scales) Impetigo (more inflamed, honey colored crust) Psoriasis
Tinea pedis (athlete's foot)	May have intense itching and burning	Scaling and fissuring of toe webs or scaling, thickening and cracking of skin of heel and sole KOH+ Feet, toes	Contact dermatitis (appears on dorsum of foot) Dyshidrosis (KOH–, vesicles) Eczema, pitted keratolysis
Tinea unguium	Usually asymptomatic Often history of Tinea pedis	Thickened, yellow crumbly nails Keratin and debris under nail Diagnosis by fungal culture Finger and toenails	Psoriasis (pitting of nails) Candidiasis (no debris)
Pityriasis rosea	Occasional pruritus History of larger lesion preceding eruption	Fawn-colored, oval scaly macules or papules in Christmas tree pattern on back Spring and fall Young adult females more than males Trunk distribution	Secondary syphilis (nonpruritic on palms and soles, RPR+) Tinea corporis (fewer lesions)
Eczema and nummular eczema	Pruritic History of atopy (asthma, allergy)	In flare, weepy, inflamed, lichenified skin Often Dennie's lines (infraorbital fold) and nasal crease May have secondary impetiginization Distribution eczema—face, sides of neck, flexural aspects of knees, elbows, wrists Nummular: backs of hands, fingers, extensor aspects of forearms, legs	Contact dermatitis (differentiated by history and distribution) Psoriasis (silvery scales)
Seborrheic dermatitis	Pruritus in hairy areas Chronic	Yellow, grayish greasy scales in irregular patches Dandruff on scalp Seborrheic areas of body: scalp, eyebrows, nasolabial folds, presternal and public regions	Psoriasis (red plaques with silvery scales) Tinea capitis (positive fungal culture)
Psoriasis	May or may not be pruritic Family history First eruption 12–20 years old	Begins as pink macules covered by fine silver scale Enlarges to coalesce to well-demarcated plaques that are raised from the surrounding skin Pinpoint bleeding with removal of large scale (Auspitz's sign) Pitting of nails Characteristic distribution: knees, elbows (extensor surface), scalp, lumbosacral area, and often gluteal folds	Seborrheic dermatitis (see previous) Nummular eczema (see previous)
Cutaneous Lupus Erythematosus	Asymptomatic Onset in 40s	Red, scaly round or oval plaques 5–20 mm diameter with well-defined border Scales are tacklike May result in alopecia and scarring with hypo or hyperpigmentation Characteristic butterfly pattern on face, also on scalp, hairline, ears	Seborrheic dermatitis (scales greasy)

Sources: Goldstein et al., 2000; Hsu, Le, & Khoshevis, 2001; Lee & Simpkins, 2000; Martin & Elewski, 2002; Noble, Forbes, & Stamm, 1998; Schalock, Hsu, & Arndt, 2011; Sontheimer & Kovalchick, 1998; Weinstein & Berman, 2002; Werth, 2001; Whitmore, 2007; Youngquist & Usatine, 2001.

TABLE 23–7. Antifungal Medications

Class	Common Drugs	Indications and Comments
Azoles (imidazoles and triazoles)		Fungal skin infections: tinea pedis, tinea corporis, candidiasis (topical or vaginal formulation)
Imidazoles	Clotrimazole (Lotrimin)	Most common. For tineas and yeast vaginitis (topical)
	Miconazole (Aloe Vesta)	For tineas and yeast vaginitis (topical)
	Econazole (Spectrazole)	Clotrimazole with betamethasone 0.05% (topical)
	Oxiconazole (Oxistat)	Used for tinea corporis, pedis (topical)
	Ketoconazole (Nizoral)	Also used to treat tinea capitus, not curative (topical, oral, shampoo formulations)
Triazoles	Terconazole (Terazol)	Used for yeast vaginitis (covers *C. glabrata*) (topical)
	Fluconazole (Diflucan)	Used for yeast vaginitis and candidiasis (oral tablet)
	Itraconazole (Sporonox)	Treatment of superficial and systemic fungal infections (oral formulation)
Allylamines		Treatment of superficial and systemic fungal infections (oral and topical formulations)
	Terbenafine (Lamisil & Lamisil AT)	Tinea corporis and tinea pedis (oral and topical)
	Naftifine (Naftin)	Tinea corporis and tinea pedis (topical)
	Butenafine (Mentax)	Tinea corporis and tinea pedis (topical)
Polyene antibiotic		Treatment of fungal skin infections, oral candidiasis, yeast vaginitis; primarily effective against Candida species
	Nystatin (Mycostatin)	Tinea corporis, candidiasis, yeast vaginitis (oral, cream, liquid)
Miscellaneous	Tolnaftate (Tinactin)	Tinea corporis, tinea pedis (topical, cream, liquid, powder, spray, gel)
	Griseofulvin	Treatment of tinea capitus and pedis (oral tablet or liquid)
	Gentian Violet	Bactericidal to gram-positive organisms, inhibits candidiasis (topical application, stains skin and clothing)
	Cyclopirox-olamine (Loprox, Penlac)	Tinea unguium, pedis, corporis, candidiasis (topical)

Tinea unguium: Advise the client to file nails daily. In clients who acquired infection from artificial nails, advise them infection may recur if artificial nails are worn again. Toenail onychomycosis usually occurs with tinea pedis. Will need to treat tinea pedis in order to minimize reoccurrence of onychomycosis.

Tinea pedis: Educate the client regarding conditions that lead to pedal infection (e.g., trapped moisture between toes, going barefoot in community showers and bathing places). Advise the client to wear cotton socks, change several times a day if profuse sweating of feet, and dry between toes thoroughly.

Tinea corporis: Educate the client regarding spread of fungal skin infections. Apply topical antifungal products twice daily for up to 3 weeks consistently to eradicate infection. If contact with pets or children, they should also be examined for fungal infections. Exercise equipment such as yoga mats may also harbor fungal organisms. If recurrent infections, consider dietary contributors such as high glucose diet or the possibility of an underlying diabetes mellitus.

Follow-Up. Advise the client to return to clinic if no response after 2 to 3 weeks of topical treatment for tinea corporis, tinea pedis, and tinea versicolor. Prior to initiating another wave of treatment or using an alternative medication, verify continued presence of scales or hyphae using KOH and consider repeat culture (Winland-Brown et al., 2011). Advise the client that it may take months for pigment to return to previous shade.

In the case of tinea versicolor, using selenium sulfide, econazole, or ketoconazole shampoo weekly for a month after initial treatment of 7 days may prevent recurrences. Apply shampoo to the skin for 10 minutes prior to bathing (Winland-Brown et al., 2011). Also instruct her to avoid using products such as bath or massage oils, which can increase the risk of reinfection because of the lipophilic properties of the organism responsible for tinea versicolor (*Malassezia furfur*) (Hort & Mayser, 2011).

For tinea capitus and tinea unguium, the client should be instructed to return for follow-up at 1 month. If there is improvement, but not eradication, therapy may be continued for an additional 2 to 4 weeks for tinea capitus and for up to 6 months for tinea unguium. CBC and liver function should be monitored. Ciclopirox solution 8 percent, a topical nail lacquer, or naftifine gel 1 percent can be used for treatment of mild to moderate onychomycosis. Application is twice daily for 6 to 18 months for toenails and 4 to 6 months for fingernails. This treatment may be preferred if unable to tolerate the oral regimens (Winland-Brown et al., 2011).

Before treating tinea capitus, the organism should be identified by fungal culture. Appropriate oral antifungal therapy can then be started. Topical antifungals will not eradicate infection but twice weekly shampooing with selenium 2.5 percent will decrease shedding of spores.

Refer to a physician or dermatologist if not responding to therapy in expected time frame or if condition worsens.

PITYRIASIS ROSEA

The cause of pityriasis is unknown. Because it is generally a disease of children and young adults, does not recur, and often follows an upper respiratory infection, a viral etiology (HHV-6 or HHV-7) is possible. It could also be a postviral immunological reaction (Schalock et al., 2011; Youngquist & Usatine, 2001).

Epidemiology

Most common in young adults and slightly more common in females. Usually occurs in fall or spring. Previously it has been thought that there may be an association between pityriasis and familial histories of asthma and atopic dermatitis (Hsu, Le, & Khoshevis, 2001; Youngquist & Usatine, 2001).

Subjective/Objective Data, Associated Findings, and Differential Diagnoses

See Table 23–6.

Diagnostic Tests. Pityriasis resembles the rash of secondary syphilis but is usually differentiated by distribution and lack of palm or sole involvement. A rapid plasma reagin (RPR) titer should be drawn if diagnosis is in doubt or if the client is at risk for syphilis.

Plan

Psychosocial Interventions. Reassure the client that this is a self-limited problem and is not thought to be contagious. Lesions may remain hyperpigmented in Asian, Latino, and African American clients for several weeks.

Medication. Pityriasis resolves spontaneously in 1 to 3 months without treatment. Management is mostly symptomatic; if pruritus is present, antihistamines such as diphenhydramine 25 to 50 mg at bedtime may reduce discomfort and promote sleep. Recently, acyclovir 800 mg four times daily for 7 days has been found to be helpful (Schalock et al., 2011). Topical steroid creams may also eliminate the discomfort but will not reduce the duration of the disease. Use low- to mid-potency preparations (e.g., 1% hydrocortisone, triamcinolone 0.1%), depending on degree of inflammation, applied two to three times daily in thin film (see Table 23–8) (Schalock et al., 2011; Youngquist & Usatine, 2001).

Colloidal oatmeal baths (Aveeno) may provide relief from pruritus. Packets may be purchased without prescription for nominal cost. Advise the client to mix with tepid water and soak two to three times per day for 10 to 15 minutes.

- *Adverse effects:* See Table 23–8.
- *Contraindications:* Sensitivity to steroid cream. Use cautiously if possibility of fungal or bacterial skin lesion, if impaired circulation (may increase risk of skin ulceration).
- *Expected outcome on evaluation:* Advise the client rash may take 1 to 3 months to clear.

Follow-Up

Advise the client to call or schedule visit if rash worsens or if persists more than 3 months.

ATOPIC DERMATOSES: ECZEMA AND NUMMULAR ECZEMA

Atopic dermatitis is a chronic disease with exacerbations and remissions throughout the lifetime of the client. It is usually diagnosed in infancy. Its most prominent feature is uncontrolled scratching that seems to arise spontaneously. This is known as the itch–scratch cycle, the more the skin is rubbed or scratched, the more highly pruritic it becomes. Nighttime scratching to the point of excoriation of the skin can occur.

TABLE 23–8. Topical Corticosteroids

Generic Name (brand name)	Potency Class	Indications and Comments
Hydrocortisone[a]	Low	Seborrhea, mild eczema, mild contact dermatitis
0.5 & 1.0% cream and lotion		Available over the counter
Desonide 0.05%[a]	Low	As for hydrocortisone, but more efficacious, especially for lesions on face
(Tridesilon)		By prescription
		Expensive
Triamcinolone acetonide 0.1% ointment, cream and lotion (Kenalog, Aristocort)	Medium	Eczema and nummular eczema, pityriasis rosea, psoriasis, contact/allergic dermatitis, dyshydrosis Use lotion on scalp
Mometasone[a] furoate 0.1% cream and lotion (Elocon)	Medium	Same as triamcinolone
Fluocinolone acetonide 0.025% cream and ointment (Lidex)	Medium	Same as triamcinolone
Betamethasone dipropionate 0.05% cream and lotion (Diprosone, Maxivate)	High	Psoriasis, cutaneous lupus erythematosis Eczema, severe contact/allergic dermatitis
Amcinonide 0.1% ointment, cream and lotion (Cyclocort)	High	Same as betamethasone
Fluocinonide 0.05% gel, ointment, cream, and lotion (Lidex)	High	Same as betamethasone
Clobetasol propionate 0.05% cream and ointment (Temovate)	Ultra	Limit use to 2 continuous weeks Cannot occlude
Halobetasol propionate 0.05% cream and ointment (Ultravate)	Ultra	Slightly more effective in psoriasis than clobetasol Same as clobetasol

[a]Note fluorinated.

NOTE: Vehicle choice depends on distribution, extent, area of body, and cosmetic consideration.

Ointment: Use where additional moisturizing desired
Use if client reports stinging with cream
Can be occlusive, for given strength more efficacious than creams
Can cause maceration, acne
May not be suitable for cosmetic reasons

Lotion: Use for hairy areas or where large areas involved
May be drying to the skin
Short exposure time, may rub off before absorbed

Cream: Usually best vehicle choice
Mild emollient
Can be comedogenic

Gel: Use when drying effect desired, good for scalp

Size of dispenser usually small (15 g) and large (60 g). For an adult of average size, it takes 20 to 30 g to cover body once. One arm is covered by about 3 g in one application. One palm requires about 0.5 g in one application.

Adverse effects: Topical steroids may cause local irritation, overgrowth of bacteria or fungus, acneiform eruption, hypopigmentation, striae, miliaria. Advise the client to use sparingly and never on mucous membranes or in genital area. Can be systemically absorbed if not used carefully. Mid- to high-potency steroids on face can cause hypopigmentation, rosacea-like rash. Striae formation in the genital-groin area can occur with fluorinated topical steroids; therefore, only hydrocortisone should be used in these areas.

Sources: Clark, Queener, & Karb, 2000; Johnson & Nunley, 2000a; Schalock, Hsu, & Arndt, 2011.

Nummular eczema appears most commonly as coin-shaped lesions on the extensor surfaces of forearms and legs. Eczema in adults affects mainly the flexural aspects of elbows, wrists, and knees. The epidemiology and treatment is the same for both.

Epidemiology

Most clients with eczema note flares in times of stress and fatigue. Serum IgE levels are often elevated in individuals with severe disease. They may also have asthma and/or hay fever. Nummular eczema is more common in adults (Whitmore, 2007).

Subjective/Objective Data and Differential Diagnoses

See Table 23–6.

Plan

Psychosocial Interventions. Stress management and helping the client get restful, restorative sleep are important. An exercise and fitness program and courses in meditation, yoga, or biofeedback may be necessary. Because this is more often than not a lifetime problem with unexplained recurrences, the client may experience a feeling of helplessness. She may also have body image concerns. Use of makeup may have to be limited. It is important to be sensitive to these issues and to provide support.

Medications. Steroid creams and/or ointments are the cornerstone of treatment. See Table 23–8 for sample list of low-, mid-, and high-potency steroids. See any drug handbook for full listing of topical corticosteroids. Choice of steroid is determined by severity of presentation. Start with low- to mid-potency steroids if possible but may initially require a high-potency topical steroid for severe eczema or hand eczema for 2 to 3 weeks twice a day, then taper to every other day, then to weekends only. Only low-potency steroids should be used on the face or in the genital area. As soon as inflammation subsides, have the client switch to emollients, such as Eucerin or Aquaphor, or use concurrently with corticosteroid preparations, allowing 30 minutes between applications. Restoring the moisture content to the skin is essential to treatment. Tapering steroid use is important to minimize rebound flares. See Pityriasis Rosea for more information on topical steroids.

Severe or extensive outbreak may require oral prednisone taper. Start with 40 mg, then taper down by 10 mg amounts every 2 days over a period of 10 to 14 days. See any drug handbook for special precautions relative to oral corticosteroid therapy.

Acute weeping lesions may be treated with aluminum subacetate solution (Domeboro soaks) or colloidal oatmeal (Aveeno) in tepid baths or as wet dressings for 10 to 15 minutes two to three times a day. The skin is rinsed, patted dry, and topical steroid is applied after bathing or soaking.

If yellow, honey-colored crusts or pustules appear, secondary impetiginization may have occurred. Antistaphylococcal medications such as dicloxacillin 250 mg qid, cephalexin (Keflex) 500 mg tid to qid, or erythromycin 250 mg qid (if allergic to penicillin) may be prescribed for 7 days.

Adverse effects of both antibiotics include nausea, vomiting, diarrhea. Contraindicated in those clients with known hypersensitivity.

Systemic antihistamines, such as hydroxyzine 25 mg, may help to control pruritus especially at night. It may be taken every 6 hours.

Adverse effects include drowsiness, dry mouth, blurred vision, constipation, and urinary retention (Wilson, Shannon, & Shields, 2012).

See any drug handbook for full prescribing information.

Immunomodulators such as pimecrolimus and tacrolimus are also used to treat eczema. They can be used alone or in conjunction with topical corticosteroids. See any drug handbook for full prescribing information. These agents require Medicaid preauthorization. In 2006, a block-box warning was added because of a possible link to the development of lymphatic cancers and light-induced skin cancers (Elias, 2009).

Lifestyle Modifications. See prior discussion of psychosocial interventions. It may be helpful for the client to keep a symptom diary including cosmetic use, foods eaten, stressful events when she first notes flare-up to increase insight, and sense of control. Modifications in skin care such as use of moisturizers or emollients several times a day and avoidance of prolonged hot water baths and of wool clothing next to the skin are helpful. She should keep her fingernails trimmed and filed. Lowering of the thermostat in winter prevents overheating and perspiring. Prompt showering after workouts helps eliminate irritative properties of perspiration.

Follow-Up

During flare-ups, evaluate client every week for response to therapy. Telephone contact is also helpful to provide support. Have the client call at first signs of flare.

DYSHIDROSIS (DYSHIDROTIC ECZEMA)

Dyshidrosis, sometimes incorrectly called pompholyx, is a very common eczematous dermatitis of the hands and feet characterized by symmetrical, recurrent, chronic small vesicles on the palms, soles, and sides of the fingers. It is intensely pruritic.

Epidemiology

First appearance is usually in young adulthood and in times of stress. Hand eczema is more common in young women, but there is no clear correlation with age or gender. It has been associated with atopy and nickel allergy (Lofgren & Warshaw, 2006).

Subjective/Objective Data and Differential Diagnoses

See Table 23–9.

Diagnostic Tests. Diagnosis is usually made on the basis of history and characteristic appearance. Because of its appearance on palms and soles, an RPR to rule out secondary syphilis is suggested. It may coexist with tinea pedis (athlete's foot) so KOH prep may be indicated. Pompholyx is differentiated from dyshidrosis by larger lesions and more acute, severe disruption (Lofgren & Warshaw, 2006).

Plan

Psychosocial Interventions. Clients who internalize stress to a great degree or who are obsessive-compulsive may need referral for psychological counseling. Fissuring and chapping of the skin may be disfiguring. Advise the client that prevention of flares is key. See lifestyle measures following.

Medication. Mid- to high-potency steroid cream or ointment may be helpful to decrease pruritus and to treat peeling and fissuring, which occur after vesicular stage. If weepy and eczematous, advise application of cool, moist compresses or Burow's soaks (Domeboro) twice a day for 15 minutes to dry, debride, and reduce swelling before application of topical steroid (see Table 23–8). Oral steroids are generally not used because of chronicity of condition.

Advise the client that dyshidrosis may not respond well to topical steroids, except for relief of pruritus and inflammation. Acute flares usually resolve within 2 to 3 weeks.

TABLE 23–9. Vesicular Dermatoses

Diagnosis	Subjective Data	Objective Data Distribution	Differential DX
Contact or allergic dermatitis	Pruritic Burning History of trigger	Weeping, encrusted vesicles, and bullae in acute stage May have linear streaking pattern Distribution: asymmetric and pattern may be diagnostic Look for site of contact	Impetigo (positive culture)
Scabies	Pruritus especially at night History of contagion, overcrowded living	Excoriations and vesiculopapular lesions and burrows Distribution is diagnostic; webs of fingers, toes, heels of palms, buttocks, breasts, elbows, axillae Rarely on face Early in course lesions isolated	Scabies (location, no weeping) Eczema (distribution, scaling, history)
Herpes simplex labialis	Burning, tingling often precedes eruption Recurrent Triggered by stress, sunlight	Small grouped vesicles on erythematous base Blisters fragile and may present as erosion Distribution: vermillion border of lip, rarely in mouth	Aphthous ulcers (ulcers only on oral mucosa or gingiva)
Herpes zoster	Very painful Usually not recurrent	Grouped, tense vesicles in linear pattern Distribution: typically only on face or trunk spreading over 1–2 dermatomes	Poison ivy, oak (vesicles confluent not grouped)
Dyshidrosis	Very pruritic Recurrent Triggered by stress Common in young adults	Tapioca vesicles 1–2 mm that may coalesce to form blisters that dry and become scaly or fissured Distribution is characteristic: palms, fingers, soles of feet	Tinea pedis (between toes) Secondary syphilis (RPR+, not vesicular) Herpes simplex virus if immunocompromised

Sources: Callahan, Adal, & Tomecki, 2000; Elgart, 2002; McCrary, Severson, & Tyring, 1999; Schalock, Hsu, & Arndt, 2011; Schmader, 2001; Stankus, Dlugopolski, & Packer, 2000; Venna, Fleischer, & Feldman, 2001; Whitley & Gnann, 1999; Yeung-Yue, Brentjens, Lee, & Tyring, 2002.

Other

- Antihistamines may help relieve itching.
- Topical immunomodulators such as tacrolimus and pimecrolimus have also shown efficacy.
- Immunosuppressive or anti-inflammatory agents such as azathioprine, methotrexate, and cyclosporine have also been used in severe cases (Lofgren & Warshaw, 2006).

Lifestyle. Avoiding irritants is the key to preventing flares. Advise the client to wear cotton gloves inside latex or plastic gloves when hands are immersed in water. Always use hand cream after washing hands, especially those creams containing emollients, such as Eucerin and Aquaphor.

Follow-Up

Evaluate the client after 7 to 10 days of therapy for response.

SEBORRHEIC DERMATITIS

Seborrheic dermatitis is a more localized form of chronic atopic dermatitis that is usually confined to the scalp. It may spread to the forehead, eyebrows, and nasolabial folds. On the body, it may appear in the groin, axillae, and presternal region. The hallmark of seborrhea is greasy yellow or grayish scales overlying irregular reddish patches of the skin. Blepharitis is a complication of seborrheic dermatitis. (See discussion in Disorders of the Eyelid in Chapter 24.)

Epidemiology

There is a genetic predisposition that begins in infancy, remits and then recurs in adolescence and/or adulthood. It is more common in men. Occurrence has been linked to hormone levels, fungal infections, nutritional deficits, and neurogenic factors. There appears to be a causal link to the Malassezia yeast species found on seborrheic regions of the body (head, trunk, and upper back) (Schwarz, Janusz, & Janniger, 2006). Flares occur in cold weather months, when the air is dry. Clients with Parkinson's disease or HIV infection may be more at risk (Martin & Elewski, 2002; Schalock et al., 2011).

Subjective/Objective Data and Differential Diagnoses

See Table 23–6.

Plan

Psychosocial Interventions. Due to scalp and face involvement, it may be source of great distress to the client. It is highly visible and often gives appearance of poor hygiene. The client will need reassurance and prompt resolution. Like eczema, condition may be exacerbated by emotional stress, food allergies, and fatigue.

Medication. Shampoo two times per week with shampoos containing 2.5 percent selenium sulfide or 1 to 2 percent pyrithione zinc (e.g., Head&Shoulders®) or corticosteroid (fluocinolone) or salicylic acid. Shampoo three times per week with shampoos containing coal tar or ketoconazole.

Shampoo daily with ketoconazole shampoo or tea tree oil. If flakes are difficult to remove, try applying warm olive oil or mineral oil to scalp, allowing it to soak in for several hours, and shampooing with dishwasher liquid or tar shampoo. If the daily use of the selenium or pyrithione shampoos is damaging her hair, advise following these products with a moisturizer (Johnson & Nunley, 2000a). Advise that shampoos may cause pruritus.

Topical calcineurin inhibitors (immunomodulators) such as Elidel and Protopic have also been used. Be advised that the long-term use of these products is not recommended due to a possible association with the development of lymphoma.

Treatment of the scalp may improve affected areas of the face. On intertriginous areas, shampoos may be used but avoid greasy ointments. Advise the client to avoid using ketoconazole shampoo on genital area.

Lid margins may be cleaned with baby shampoo (Johnson&Johnson®) applied undiluted with a cotton swab at night.

Diet/Lifestyle. Once the seborrhea is controlled, the client may reduce the use of medicated shampoos to twice a week or as needed. Advise the client that hygiene and environment play a role in exacerbations. Sweat retention tends to make it worse as well as lapses in daily shampoo routine. Stress reduction, adequate rest, nutrition, and hydration promote healthy skin and scalp.

Follow-Up

Have the client telephone or schedule visit to discuss response to therapy after 1 to 2 weeks, depending on severity of presentation.

PSORIASIS

Psoriasis, like eczema, is a lifelong, chronic disease (with acute flares) whose course is unpredictable. It is characterized by red plaques that are covered with silvery or white scales. Its cause is unknown but there is mounting evidence that at least one gene on chromosome 17 is responsible for familial psoriasis (Linden & Weinstein, 1999). Immunologic factors may also play a role. Clients with psoriasis have an increased incidence of human leukocyte antigens (Schalock et al., 2011).

Epidemiology

Onset is often in young adulthood, but may also appear initially in children or older adults. It is not uncommon, and 2 percent of the U.S. population may be affected. Up to 40 percent of clients with psoriasis may also develop psoriatic arthritis with polyarticular involvement (Winterfield, Menter, Gordon, & Gottlieb, 2005).

Subjective/Objective Data, Associated Findings, and Differential Diagnoses

See Table 23–6.

Plan

Psychosocial Interventions. Because psoriasis typically affects exposed areas of the body, it can have a huge impact psychologically. Early onset appears to have the greatest negative effect on the quality of life, impacting both social and occupational sectors.

Medication. Mid- to high-potency topical steroids are most often used. (See Table 23–8 or any drug handbook for examples.)

- *Administration:* Use twice daily for 2 to 3 weeks. Greater penetration may be achieved by removal of the superficial scale by soaking or by use of a keratolytic agent such as salicylic acid. (See discussion of salicylic acid use in section on warts.) Switch to lower-potency steroid combined with nightly application of tar gel product such as Estar® or Psorigel®. Warn the client that tar is messy to apply and will stain clothes and sheets.

Because topical corticosteroids do not produce long-term remission and may make psoriasis more difficult to treat in the long run, they are usually combined with other agents. One such agent is topical calcipotriene, a vitamin D_3 analog that is available as a cream, ointment, and solution. A multiphasic approach combining calcipotriene and a topical corticosteroid is usually best. First, the client should apply the topical steroid and calcipotriene twice daily until the plaques are flat, about 4 weeks. Calcipotriene is then solely applied to the lesions twice daily, saving the topical steroid for "pulse" therapy: that is, twice daily for only 2 days a week. Once the lesions have progressed from bright red to pink, the calcipotriene is used alone and the topical steroid is discontinued (Pardasani, Feldman, & Clark, 2000).

Calcipotriene cannot be used on the face. Side effects include skin irritation (15% of patients) and hypercalcemia if more than 100 g of it is used weekly. Use cautiously in clients with impaired renal function or a history of kidney stones (Pardasani et al., 2000).

Oral steroids are seldom used by the primary practitioner due to frequent rebound flares and worsening of the condition. Scalp lesions may be treated with tar shampoos (Neutrogena T/Gel) used daily or 2 percent ketoconazole (Nizoral) shampoo by prescription used twice weekly.

If psoriasis affects more than 30 percent of the body, refer to a dermatologist for light therapy with ultraviolet B (UVB) three times a week for PUVA (psoralen plus UVA). PUVA may increase the risk of cataract formation and skin cancer. Other therapies used by dermatologists include methotrexate, cyclosporine, and synthetic retinoids. Refer to pharmacology text for further information on these agents (Lebwohl et al., 2001; Pardasani et al., 2000).

There is increasing emphasis on using new biological agents with potentially fewer side effects to treat psoriasis. Three new agents that have been approved to treat psoriasis include alefacept, efalizumab, and etanercept. Patients with persistent recurrent psoriasis should be referred to dermatology for continued management (Schalock et al., 2011; Winterfield et al., 2005).

Oral antihistamines at bedtime such as hydroxyzine (Atarax) 25 mg may be helpful if pruritus is severe or interferes with rest.

- *Expected outcome on evaluation:* Advise the client psoriasis is a chronic condition with periods of flare and remission.

Diet/Lifestyle. Some clients may find exposure to sunlight is beneficial but warn them about harmful effects of prolonged exposure such as skin cancer and premature aging of the skin. Sunscreen should always be worn. Advise the client to try to avoid trauma to affected areas and to resist rubbing and scratching in order to avoid secondary infection. Arthritis associated with psoriasis often improves with successful skin treatment. Daily use of emollients may help prevent flares. Avoid emollients containing lactic acid or alpha-hydroxy acids because they can be irritating (Pardasani et al., 2000).

Follow-Up

Follow weekly during flares. If the client is referred to a dermatologist, request treatment plan to ensure continuity of care.

CUTANEOUS LUPUS ERYTHEMATOSUS

Cutaneous lupus erythematosus (CLE) is an umbrella term that refers to 15 different clinical manifestations of lupus erythematosus (see Chapter 24). CLE may present as a skin eruption with or without systemic disease. Patients are more likely to have systemic disease when they have more generalized skin eruptions than when they have eruptions confined to the head or neck. Drugs that may act as inducers to CLE include penicillamine, ACEIs, sulfonylureas, calcium channel blockers, antifungals, and thiazide diuretics (Patel & Werth, 2002).

There are three categories of CLE: (1) acute CLE, (2) subacute CLE (SCLE), and (3) chronic CLE. Acute CLE is the "butterfly rash" or malar rash commonly associated with lupus erythematosus, although the macular rashes may appear on sun-exposed areas of the body: V-area of the neck, forearms and calfs, and trunk (Schalock et al., 2011; Sontheimer & Kovalchick, 1998). Most clients with acute CLE have concurrent symptoms of systemic lupus erythematosus and 10 percent go on to develop severe forms of systemic lupus erythematosus, often with kidney and central nervous system involvement (Sontheimer & Kovalchick, 1998). SCLE presents with nonscarring, well-defined, red annular lesions, red scaly plaques, or a papulosquamous rash (Hsu et al., 2001). SCLE is the most photosensitive of the types. Chronic CLE comprises several chronic skin diseases specific to lupus erythematosus. The most commonly seen subcategory of chronic CLE is discoid lupus erythematosus (DLE). Localized discoid lupus erythematosus presents as lesions on the face and scalp that cause scarring. Between 25 and 40 percent of clients experience spontaneous remission and only 5 percent of afflicted persons will develop full-blown systemic lupus erythematosus (Werth, 2001). If the scarring lesions are not limited to the head and scalp, then the woman has generalized discoid lupus erythematosus and her risk of progressing to full-blown systemic erythematosus is greater (Sontheimer & Kovalchick, 1998). Squamous cell carcinoma can also develop in DLE lesions (Patel & Werth, 2002).

Epidemiology

CLE first appears in young adults with equal frequency in men and women. A familial pattern has been observed. It is a lifelong disease with exacerbations occurring after sun exposure (Sontheimer & Kovalchick, 1998; Werth, 2001).

Subjective/Objective Data, Associated Signs, and Differential Diagnosis

See Table 23–6.

Plan

The goals of treatment are to improve appearance and prevent lesion progression. Clients should be referred to a dermatologist for biopsy. The examination should include a substantive history, CBC, sedimentation rate, antinuclear antibody (ANA), and urinalysis.

Psychosocial Interventions. Discoid lupus can cause scarring, patchy alopecia, and loss of pigment (especially in darker complexioned individuals). The cosmetic results can be devastating. Aggressive and early treatment may help avoid scarring and permanent alopecia. Be supportive and alert to the need for psychological counseling. It is identified as the third most common cause of dermatological work disability (Patel & Werth, 2002).

Medications. High-potency topical steroids are the initial treatment (see Table 23–8 or any drug handbook). As the skin lesions improve, titrate the potency of the topical steroids downward until using a low-potency preparation (Werth, 2001). A dermatologist may inject triamcinolone 2.5 to 10 mg/mL once a month into lesions before advancing to systemic medications such as antimalarials.

- *Expected outcome on evaluation:* Lesions usually respond to triamcinolone injection.
- *Client teaching:* The client should be aware of medications that can increase sensitivity to sunlight including doxycycline, thiazides, and piroxicam.
- *Lifestyle:* The client should avoid outdoor activities during times of the day when sunlight is strongest (10 a.m.–3 p.m.). Advise use of sunscreen with high SPF always. Protective clothing should be worn.

Follow-Up

Request visit notes and treatment plan from the dermatologist. Some clients may be managed by primary care provider after initial referral.

VESICULAR DERMATOSES

Contact Dermatoses

Contact dermatoses can be classified into two main types: irritant contact dermatitis (ICD) and allergic contact dermatitis (ACD). Eighty percent are due to exposure to common universal irritants, such as soap, solvents, and detergents. The most common contact allergens include poison ivy, poison oak, nickel, latex, hair dye, topical medications, perfumes, cosmetics, and adhesive tape. Allergy to an antibiotic may cause dermatitis. The presentation of contact dermatoses may be acute as in poison ivy or subacute if repeated exposure has occurred and sensitization has developed over time.

Epidemiology. Older people may be more prone to contact dermatitis due to thinning of the skin and loss of protective moisture. Certain occupations, especially those requiring contact with irritants and allergens cited previously, are at increased risk (Schalock et al., 2011; Whitmore, 2007).

Subjective/Objective Data, Associated Features, and Differential Diagnosis. See Table 23–9.

Plan. The first step in treatment is to remove the offending agent. The client may have to be referred to a dermatologist for patch testing if diagnosis of agent unclear.

Psychosocial Interventions. This is usually a self-limited problem, which is resolved in 2 to 3 weeks once the offending agent is removed. Practitioners should be aware, however, that removal of the offender may cause distress, by necessitating a change in lifestyle, occupation, or grooming.

Medications. Classes of medications to treat contact dermatitis include corticosteroid formulations, immunomodulators, barrier creams, emollients, drying agents, tumor necrosis factor-alpha products, phosphodiesterase inhibitors, and UV light. When prescribing topical corticosteroids, the site, frequency of application, and vehicle should be considered. Topical corticosteroids may be more effective in the treatment of ACD than in ICD (Cohen & Noushin, 2004). Oral antihistamines may be effective to treat pruritus. See Medications section under Atopic Dermatoses for overview of medications.

Other. UV light may be useful in treating chronic ICD or ACD unresponsive to systemic or topical corticosteroids.

If the client is experiencing chronic unresponsive contact dermatitis, oral corticosteroids such as prednisone may be given in a taper over 2 to 3 weeks depending on cause. For extensive poison ivy, a slow taper of 2 to 3 weeks is usually recommended. A steroid dose pack is insufficient in this case (Usatine & Riojas, 2010).

Follow-Up. Evaluate the client after 1 week of treatment for response. Refer to a dermatologist if not responding to treatment or if patch testing indicated.

INFESTATIONS

Scabies

Scabies is an intensely pruritic dermatitis caused by infestation with the mite *Sarcoptes scabiei*. The female mite burrows under the skin and deposits eggs, which hatch and mature over a 3-week incubation period, causing intense pruritus. It can be passed on by person-to-person contact or through bedding and clothes. It spreads on the skin by fingernail contamination.

Epidemiology. All ages affected and all socioeconomic groups. Outbreaks occur in nursing homes and hospitals (Venna, Fleischer, & Feldman, 2001).

Subjective/Objective Data and Differential Diagnoses. See Table 23–9.

Diagnostic Tests. Usually diagnosed on basis of history and appearance of burrows in characteristic locations, webs of fingers, genitalia. Burrows can be opened with scalpel blade at the end or dark point, and mite can be placed on slide and examined under oil immersion for confirmation.

Plan

Medication. Permethrin cream (Elimite) 5 percent. Applied neck to toes, with special care to include webs of fingers and toes, axillary, gluteal folds, under breasts. Advise the client not to wash hands after application, should be left on overnight 8 to 14 hours, and then rinsed. Single application is usually effective. Elimite is pregnancy category B, unknown safety in breastfeeding. See any drug handbook for complete prescribing information.

Bed Bugs

Bed bugs from the insect family, Cimicidae, cause an intensely pruritic dermatitis. Bed bug infestation is characterized by itchy red raised welts often appearing in a linear pattern of three bites, "breakfast, lunch, and dinner" sequential feeding. The face, neck, and limbs are commonly involved. There is no cure for bed bugs as they have become resistant to many chemicals, and treatment targets symptoms such as corticosteroids and antihistamines for itching and antibiotics in the case of secondary infection. Eradication of the infestation through environmental treatment is recommended along with prevention of infestation.

Plan

Psychosocial Interventions. May cause embarrassment to the client due to concern over hygiene. Client education is important concerning mode of transmission, occurrence in all socioeconomic groups. Advise her that partner may be infected (common site is penile shaft and glans for scabies) and should be treated.

Lifestyle Modification. Instruct the client to wash all bedding, clothes, and towels in hot soapy water and dry on hottest dryer setting. Nonwashable items may be placed in airtight plastic bag for 2 weeks or sent to dry cleaner. Advise the client of possibility of reinfection if partner is not treated. Advise her she may spread infestation to others up to 24 hours after completion of treatment. Special attention is needed for furniture or inanimate objects to eradicate bed bugs.

Follow-Up. Advise the client to call to schedule visit if treatment is not effective.

Herpes Simplex

Herpes simplex (cold sore or herpes labialis) is a recurrent infection caused by the virus *Herpesvirus hominis.* It appears as tightly clustered vesicles on the vermillion border of the lips, but may appear on other areas of the face. The blisters are fragile, and most common presentation is a secondary erosion that forms a crust. Following the initial infection, the virus remains dormant in the dorsal root ganglia and reactivates during times of stress, trauma, head colds, fever, and exposure to sunlight. The first episode may be asymptomatic.

Epidemiology. Herpes simplex infection is transmitted by exposure to a clinically infected person, an asymptomatic virus shedder, or reactivation of a latent infection. Appearance of the vesicle occurs 3 to 5 days after exposure and lasts 5 to 10 days. Contagion is possible during the first few days of vesicle appearance. Vesicles usually appear in the same site with recurrent infections. Lesions may not clear in immunocompromised individuals (Schalock et al., 2011; Yeung-Yue, Brentjens, Lee, & Tyring, 2002).

Subjective/Objective Data and Differential Diagnoses. See Table 23–9.

Diagnostic Tests. Usually diagnosed on basis of prior history but can be confirmed by opening vesicle dome with small needle, swabbing fluid exudate with sterile swab, and sending for viral culture.

Plan

Psychosocial Interventions. The client may be concerned about appearance and contagion. Discuss importance of frequent handwashing to prevent autoinoculation and refraining from oral sex. Advise her that lesion usually resolves in a week. Be sensitive to issues of possible sexual transmission and address them accordingly. Client education is very important to clear up misconceptions between type 1 and type 2 herpes. See discussion of herpes simplex virus in Chapter 14.

Medication. Topical treatment of orolabial herpes is available in several formulations. Acyclovir ointment may be applied five times daily for 4 days. Penciclovir cream (Denavir®) 1 percent may be applied every 2 hours while awake for 4 days and Docosanol (Abreva®) may be applied five times per day until healed. Generally, topical formulations are less effective than systemic treatment. Oral antiviral agents such as acyclovir, valacyclovir, and famciclovir may be given episodically at first sign of outbreak to lessen duration of symptoms and reduce viral shedding. Acyclovir (Zovirax®) 200 mg may be given five times daily or 400 mg three times per day for 5 days. Famciclovir (Famvir®) 250 mg may be given twice daily for 5 days or valacyclovir (Valtrex®) 2 g may be given twice for 1 day. Acyclovir 400 mg twice daily or valacyclovir 500 mg daily may also be prescribed for prophylaxis of frequent recurrences (Usatine & Tinitigan, 2010). See an up-to-date drug handbook for complete prescribing information.

Lifestyle. Advise the client to apply sunscreen before exposure to sunlight. May also put warm, moist cloths, but advise the client these cloths may contain virus and should not be handled by other household members. Careful and frequent handwashing is the key to prevent spreading to vulnerable contacts such as older people and infants.

Follow-Up. Advise the client to call to schedule visit if not cleared in 7 to 10 days.

Herpes Zoster

Shingles or herpes zoster is a painful vesicular eruption along a dermatome. It is caused by reactivation of the varicella-zoster virus whose first appearance causes chicken pox.

Epidemiology. In younger adults, thoracic dermatomes are most often affected. In older adults, the area of distribution of the trigeminal nerve is frequently involved. If more than two dermatomes are affected, individual may be immunocompromised.

Postherpetic neuralgia is an excruciatingly painful complication, especially if the trigeminal nerve is involved. The infection may also spread to the eye and cause a dendritic pattern conjunctivitis. Disseminated zoster in immunocompromised individuals may be life threatening (Lee & Simpkins, 2000; Schmader, 2001).

Subjective/Objective Data and Differential Diagnoses. See Table 23–9.

Diagnostic Tests. History and appearance are usually diagnostic, but a viral culture will confirm diagnosis. (See previous discussion on herpes simplex for method of culture.) Confirmation by culture is especially important if vesicles cross several dermatomes. If this is the case and the culture is positive for herpes zoster, the client should be evaluated for immunocompromise.

Plan. Refer immediately to the ophthalmologist if the eye appears to be involved. Refer to a physician if appears to be disseminated, involves more than two dermatomes, or appears on face or scalp.

Psychosocial Interventions. Facial appearance may cause body image disturbance. Reassure the client that infection usually resolves in 2 to 3 weeks and does not recur (unless immunocompromised).

Medication. Oral acyclovir 800 mg five times a day for 7 days if started within the first 72 hours may accelerate clearing and reduce pain. (See discussion of acyclovir in Chapter 14.) Valacyclovir 1 g orally three times daily for 7 days and famciclovir 750 mg once daily or 500 mg twice daily or 250 mg three times daily for 7 days are also effective, but must be started within 72 hours of the appearance of the zoster rash (Usatine & Tinitigan, 2010). Famciclovir 500 mg three times daily for 7 days is also an acceptable dosage regimen (Wilson et al., 2012).

Extending the duration of acyclovir treatment to 10 days may reduce the incidence of postherpetic neuralgia. Evidence suggests Valtrex may be slightly superior to acyclovir in reducing postherpetic pain (Holten, 2006). Clients 60 years old and older and immunocompromised clients are at greatest risk for this painful condition (Lee & Simpkins, 2000).

Colloidal oatmeal soaks (Aveeno) or calamine lotion may be soothing to the skin. Systemic steroids demonstrate no efficacy in reducing postherpetic pain and are not recommended (Usatine & Tinitigan, 2010).

Follow-Up. Evaluate the client in 1 week for response. Refer to a physician immediately if condition does not improve.

PUSTULAR AND NODULAR DERMATOSES

Acne Vulgaris

Acne is a common skin condition under the influence of hormonal and genetic factors. It usually starts with stimulation of the sebaceous glands by androgen; therefore, its appearance coincides with puberty. Sebaceous glands increase in size, and output of sebum rises to a point where plugging of the follicle occurs. Bacteria, mainly *Propionibacterium* acnes, causes breakdown of the sebum, disruption of the follicle wall into the dermis, and subsequent inflammation (Johnson & Nunley, 2000b; Thiboutot, 2000).

Epidemiology. First appears in mid to late adolescence and usually wanes in severity in 20s but can persist in women into their 40s. Begins with oily skin and plugged follicles known as whiteheads (closed comedones) and blackheads (open comedones) over the nose and forehead. The sebum inside the plugged duct may cause irritation to adjacent skin and produce inflammatory lesions, nodules, and pustules. Severe cystic acne is more common in males and is rarely found in women. Women often find acne worsens just before menses and may improve (or become worse) with pregnancy. Its course during a lifetime is unpredictable but appearance of cysts and family history of scarring are bad prognosticators (Johnson & Nunley, 2000b; Thiboutot, 2000).

Subjective/Objective Data and Differential Diagnoses. See Table 23–10.

Diagnostic Tests. Diagnosis is made on basis of history and appearance. Pustular lesions resistant to treatment may have to exudate sent for culture and sensitivity.

TABLE 23–10. Pustular and Nodular Dermatoses

Diagnosis	Subjective Data	Objective Data Distribution	Differential DX
Acne vulgaris	Usually onset at puberty May have mild pain, itching May have history of topical or oral steroid use	Inflammatory, open and closed comedones, papules and pustules nodules, and cysts with scarring but hallmark is comedone Distribution: face, neck, upper back, chest, shoulders	Folliculitis (hairy areas, rare on face)
Rosacea	Middle-aged onset History of flushing, burning, esp. with hot food and drink	Inflammatory papules, flushing, telangiectasia Comedones absent Often associated with seborrhea and blepharitis Distribution: only on face	Acne vulgaris (comedones prominent)
Impetigo	Pruritus	Pustules (may have macules and vesicles also) Honey-colored crust When crust removed, leaves denuded area Distribution: often on face	Contact dermatitis (trigger, linear pattern)
Folliculitis	Itching and burning History of hot tub use, diabetes, excessive sweating	Pustules at base of hair follicle May have erythema of surrounding skin Distribution: hairy areas of body	Acne (see above) Impetigo (see above) Pseudofolliculitis (pustules at side not in follicle, caused by ingrown hair)
Furuncles and carbuncles	Painful Common in diabetics, obese with oily skin, staph carriers	Abscess of hair follicle with enlarging, conical shape May coalesce to form carbuncle Becomes flocculent with purulent discharge Distribution: most common sites are hairy areas exposed to irritation, friction, moisture as face, neck, axillae, buttocks, groin, upper back	Inflamed epidermal cyst (history of cyst, cheesy exudate) Acne (not in follicle)
Warts	No symptoms unless on sole of foot (painful)	Flesh-colored papule or nodule 1–10 mm that may form mosaic Surface is rough, verrucated (sawtoothed), or flat May be pedunculated or have cauliflower-like appearance Plantar warts resemble corns or calluses Distribution: anywhere on body but commonly on hands, face, neck, upper trunk, soles of feet, genital area	Squamous cell cancer (biopsy always if in doubt)

Sources: Elgart, 2002; Higgins & Du Vivier, 1999; Johnson & Nunley, 2000b; O'Dell, 1998; Rhody, 2000; Schalock, Hsu, & Arndt, 2011; Thiboutot, 2000.

Plan

Psychosocial Interventions. Acne is an overwhelming concern to adolescents and young adults. Depending on its severity, it can lead to depression and social isolation. The practitioner must be alert to these concerns and anticipate any need for psychological counseling. Be supportive of appropriate coping mechanisms (Johnson & Nunley, 2000b; Thiboutot, 2000).

Medications. Treatment is directed to predominant type of lesion. Medication options include topical tretinoins, benzoyl peroxide, salicylic acid, azelaic acid, topical antibiotic preparations, oral antibiotics, oral isotretinoin, herbal therapies. The aim is to prevent scarring. Be sure to ask the client about efficacy of past and present treatments. Advise her to avoid astringents unless the skin is very oily and to use only on oily spots.

Choice of vehicle for topical agents depends on appearance of the skin. Creams and lotions moisturize, but creams are heavier and may be more appropriate for very dry or irritated skin. Gels and solutions are alcohol based and tend to dry the skin. Client preference should also be taken into consideration.

For the comedonal stage, over-the-counter products that contain salicylic acid (Stridex®), resorcinol, sulfur (Sulforcin®), and/or benzoyl peroxide (Fostex®, Clearasil Maximum Strength®) are fairly effective if used on a regular basis. Alpha-hydroxy acids loosen follicular plugging. Most topical formulations cause drying and may initially worsen appearance.

The most effective agent is topical tretinoin (Retin-A®) because it unplugs comedones and prevents new ones from forming. It is considered appropriate for almost all acne. It is available in various strengths and formulations including creams and gels. It may be used alone or in combination with oral antibiotics. See any drug handbook for full prescribing information.

- Topical tretinoin should be discontinued prior to attempting conception or as soon as pregnancy is detected as it is teratogenic.

If the client is able to tolerate, benzoyl peroxide can be used in the morning and tretinoin at night. Benzoyl peroxide (concentrations 2.5% gel and lotion; 5 and 10% gel, lotion, and cream) is effective against *Propionibacterium* acnes and inflammation, and tretinoin speeds cell turnover and prevents new comedones. This combination can be a very effective treatment and can result in dramatic clearing after 6 to 8 weeks (Schalock et al., 2011; Thiboutot, 2000).

Topical antibiotics such as clindamycin (Cleocin T®) available 10 mg/mL as gel, lotion, or cream and erythromycin (A/T/S, Erycette®) 2 percent gel, ointment, or solution may be used in combination with tretinoin. See any drug handbook for complete prescribing information.

- In more difficult cases, a benzoyl peroxide–erythromycin gel combination (Erythromycin/BP gel) can be used in the morning with tretinoin at night. Initially, start using each on alternating nights until adjustment to irritating effects.
- Contraindication is known sensitivity to any ingredients.
- Advise the client it may take at least 4 weeks to achieve desirable results.

If papules and pustules predominate and there is scarring, consider adding an oral antibiotic, such as erythromycin 250 mg qid, tetracycline 500 mg po bid, or minocycline 100 mg bid. Minocycline is the least photosensitizing of the tetracyclines, is somewhat more effective than tetracycline, and can be taken with food (Johnson & Nunley, 2000b; Thiboutot, 2000). See any drug handbook for complete prescribing information.

Topical antibiotic preparations such as erythromycin gel or clindamycin (Cleocin T) may be used on their own but be aware that *Propionibacterium* acnes can develop resistance to both these preparations. Use erythromycin gel in combination with benzoyl peroxide as discussed previously (Johnson & Nunley, 2000b; Thiboutot, 2000).

If acne does not respond to any of the aforementioned therapies, the client should be referred to dermatology and may be a candidate for oral isotretinoin. Because of its teratogenicity, extreme care must be taken if used by clients of childbearing age. The client should have a negative pregnancy test on record and begin taking the isotretinoin on the first day of menses. Oral isotretinoin is not prescribed by primary care, and should be prescribed only by a dermatologist who is knowledgeable in prescribing and monitoring this medication (Strauss et al., 2007).

If the client is taking oral contraceptives, switch her to a lower androgen formulation. The U.S. Food and Drug Administration (FDA) labels Ortho Tri-Cyclen®, a triphasic combination of norgestimate and ethinyl estradiol, for the treatment of acne in adolescent girls and women (Johnson & Nunley, 2000b).

Diet/Lifestyle. There is no evidence that chocolate or fatty foods make acne worse. Nor does vigorous scrubbing or sun tanning make it better. Gentle cleansers, such as Dove®, Basis®, Neutrogena®, Purpose®, or Cetaphil®, maybe helpful. Advise the client never to pick or squeeze pimples; this can lead to scarring. Review current cosmetic products. Changing to oil-free makeup can lessen comedone formation. Reassure the client best results come from adherence to agreed-upon treatment plan and patience, and may take 4 to 6 weeks to see improvement.

Follow-Up. Refer clients with severe or cystic acne to the dermatologist. After 1 week of treatment plan, evaluate the client, then again at 1 month.

Rosacea

Rosacea is a chronic skin condition that develops in middle age. It may progress through four stages:

Stage I: Prerosacea—transient flushing and erythema of the face and neck

Stage II: Vascular rosacea—persistent erythema and telangiectasia

Stage III: Inflammatory rosacea—multiple inflammatory papules and pustules

Stage IV: Glandular hyperplastic rosacea—(usually in men) lymphedema and hypertrophy of connective tissue (Higgins & du Vivier, 1999)

May also develop ocular rosacea (Barclay, 2009).

Epidemiology. Rosacea affects women three times more than men. Onset is between ages 30 and 50. Fair-skinned individuals are predisposed to rosacea, which is thought to be a reactionary flush to specific precipitating factors, including alcohol, sunlight, stress, vasodilating drugs, and hot/spicy foods (Higgins & du Vivier, 1999; Schalock et al., 2011).

Subjective/Objective Data and Differential Diagnoses. See Table 23–10.

Diagnostic Tests. Diagnosis is usually made on the basis of history and appearance. If lupus or cutaneous sarcoidosis is suspected, diagnosis is made by biopsy and client should be referred to a dermatologist.

Plan

Psychosocial Interventions. Rosacea is a chronic disease, and treatment is continuous. Reassure the client that early intervention and prevention of flares help. Body image concerns and embarrassment should be addressed. A glandular, hyperplastic stage (usually seen in men) may cause rhinophyma in which the nose appears enlarged and bright red or violaceous. The client may be suspected of being a heavy drinker because of flushed appearance of the skin.

Medications. Metronidazole (MetroGel 0.75%, Metrocreme 1%) is the topical treatment of choice (Barclay, 2009). If rosacea is severe, oral antibiotics such as tetracycline or minocycline may be used concurrently with topical treatment. See any drug handbook for full prescribing information. Isotretinoin oral dosing is under study. Initial trials suggest efficacy in rates of remission and treatment of rhinophyma. Please see discussion of isotretinoin in Acne Vulgaris section.

Diet/Lifestyle. Discuss triggers of flushing and erythema such as excessive cold, wind, heat, alcohol, and spicy foods. There is slight evidence to support the avoidance of skin care products containing witch hazel, alcohol, menthol, eucalyptus oil, peppermint, or sodium lauryl sulfate. Moisturizing and sun protection may also be useful (Barclay, 2009).

Follow-Up. Evaluate the client in 1 week for tolerance of therapy, then again at 1 month. Refer to a dermatologist if condition worsens or rhinophyma (enlarged red nose) (Higgins & du Vivier, 1999; Schalock et al., 2011).

Impetigo

Impetigo is a contagious infection of the skin that is caused by *Staphylococcus aureus* coagulase positive and/or group A beta-hemolytic streptococcus (GABHS). Most cases of impetigo today are due to *Staphylococcus.* The lesions may be vesicles, pustules, and/or bullae, but the diagnostic feature is honey-colored crust (Elgart, 2002; O'Dell, 1998).

Epidemiology. Most common in childhood, especially on the face around the nares, but in adults can occur on any exposed surface. It can spread to others. Secondary impetiginization can occur with eczema or other vesiculobullous dermatoses and is treated as impetigo (Elgart, 2002; O'Dell, 1998).

Subjective/Objective Data and Differential Diagnoses. See Table 23–10.

Diagnostic Tests. Diagnosis is usually based on history and appearance. Treatment is empiric with broad-spectrum antibiotic covering staph and strep, but culture and sensitivity of exudate may be helpful if resistant organisms in community are a concern.

Plan

Psychosocial Interventions. Reassure the client impetigo responds very quickly to oral antibiotics.

Medication. Dicloxacillin 250 mg po qid for 7 days, Keflex 500 mg po qid or tid for 7 days or, if allergic to penicillin, erythromycin 250 mg qid for 7 days. Care should be taken when prescribing erythromycin to older people due to effects on QT and potential interactions with other medications. See any drug handbook for full prescribing information.

If not responsive to therapy, cultures of the lesions should be obtained, and if methicilln-resistant *Staphylococcus* aureus (MRSA) cultured, trimethoprim/sulfamethoxazole, tetracycline, or clindamycin should be added. See a drug reference book for dosing information.

If impetigo is localized to small area, mupirocin 2 percent ointment (Bactroban) may be used topically three times a day for 7 to 10 days. Resistance of *Staphylococcus aureus* and MRSA to mupirocin has emerged at a rate of 5 to 10 percent (Sadegh & Burdick, 2010). A newer topical preparation, retapamulin 1 percent ointment applied twice daily for 5 days has shown clinical efficacy and was approved by the FDA in 2007 for treatment of impetigo (Sadegh & Burdick, 2010).

Lifestyle. Warm, moist compresses may be used to soften and remove crusts. Advise the client to separate washcloths and towels from other household members.

Follow-Up. Advise the client to call or to schedule visit if not resolved in 5 to 7 days.

CELLULITIS

Cellulitis is an infection of the skin and subcutaneous tissue without purulent formation.

Epidemiology

Cellulitis may follow superficial injury to the skin, folliculitis, stasis ulcer. Often the initial insult may be inapparent. It is caused primarily by gram positive cocci, such as *staphylococcus* or *streptococcus.*

Subjective Data

The client complains of pain and tenderness.

Objective Data

Diffuse border of warm, red skin.

Diagnostic Tests. Diagnosed on basis of appearance. Bacterial culture from injection and aspiration of saline rarely yield valuable results and may further spread cellulitis.

Differential Diagnoses

Severe contact dermatitis may resemble cellulitis but is pruritic and not as painful.

Plan

Psychosocial Interventions. Reassure the client that with prompt treatment and adherence to treatment plan, cellulitis resolves promptly.

Medications. See prior discussion of impetigo.

Diet/Lifestyle. Advise the client to apply warm soaks at least three times a day, elevate extremity. If legs or feet affected, limit ambulation as much as possible.

Follow-Up

Mark area affected and evaluate within 1 to 2 days by telephone contact or office visit. Close follow-up needed for frail and/or older client, client with hand or anogenital involvement.

Folliculitis

Folliculitis is an infection or inflammation of the hair follicle caused by *Staphylococcus aureus* (or if arises after use of hot tub, *Pseudomonas aeruginosa folliculitis*), by a fungal dermatophyte, by oils (industrial or cosmetic), or by perspiration. The causative agent can be differentiated on the basis of history, location of the pustules, bacterial culture, KOH preparation and fungal culture, and lack of response to antibacterial therapy.

Epidemiology. Bacterial folliculitis is more prevalent in diabetics. Common sites are the axillae, face, back of the neck, breasts, thighs, and perineum. Folliculitis may appear during the first week of oral steroid therapy (steroid acne) or may flare when dose is tapered. Hot tub folliculitis appears in 1 to 4 days after use of a contaminated tub. The rash is tender and pruritic (Luelmo-Aguilar & Santandreu, 2005).

Fungal folliculitis is characterized by the clustering of the follicular pustules, commonly on the hands, arms, legs, and scalp. In women, infection often occurs when the dermatophyte from tinea pedis is spread to the legs when shaving. The follicles cluster on the lower legs. Fungal folliculitis can also arise from misdiagnosed tinea corporis that is treated with steroids. Pustular follicles then arise on the face and dorsum of the hand (O'Dell, 1998; Rhody, 2000).

Pseudofolliculitis is caused by ingrowing hairs. Pustules and papules are located beside the follicle but not in the follicle.

Subjective/Objective Data and Differential Diagnoses. See previous discussion and Table 23–10.

Diagnostic Tests. Bacterial culture and sensitivity, fungal culture, and/or KOH prep are ordered as appropriate. Often empiric treatment is started based on history and appearance while waiting for culture result.

Plan

Psychosocial Interventions. Because pustules appear on exposed areas, client may have body image concerns.

Medication. If bacterial in origin, dicloxacillin 250 mg qid for 14 days (see discussion under Impetigo). Small areas may be treated with mupirocin 2 percent ointment (see discussion under Impetigo). Other options include Zithromax, first-generation cephalosporins such as cephalexin (see Impetigo section), penicillinase-resistant penicillins, and fluoroquinolones (Stulberg, Penrod, & Blatny, 2002). For CA-MRSA, treat with trimethoprim/sulfamethoxazole, doxycycline, fluoroquinolones, linezolid, or clindamycin (Abrahaiman & Moran, 2007; Daum, 2007). May consider addition of rifampin. Folliculitis due to *Pseudomonas aeruginosa*, sometimes called "hot tub folliculitis," usually resolves spontaneously and there is no treatment that makes the course progress more rapidly.

Acetic acid 5 percent compresses can be applied for 20 minutes twice a day to four times a day for relief of symptoms (Toner & Krivida, 2009). In severe cases, mastitis, or immunocompromised patients, ciprofloxacin 500 to 750 mg po bid is recommended (Toner & Krivida, 2009).

Fungal folliculitis usually responds only to oral antifungals such as griseofulvin (see Tinea Capitus). Confirm by fungal culture before starting therapy.

Folliculitis on the back, which has been diagnosed as acne and does not respond to acne treatment, may be due to *Pityrosporum orbiculare*, which is treated with topical 2.5 percent selenium sulfide applied for 15 minutes daily for 3 weeks.

Medication is not indicated for irritant folliculitis, except for use of drying soaks such as Burow's or benzoyl peroxide. Aluminum subacetate (Burow's) soaks or compresses twice a day for 15 minutes provide soothing relief to skin, especially if exudative.

Lifestyle. Control of blood sugars is helpful in diabetics. Advise women who acquire infection as a result of shaving legs to use depilatory until resolved or use disposable shavers. Treat water in hot tubs with appropriate chemicals. If irritant folliculitis is caused by occupational exposure to oil, suggest the client wear protective clothing and gloves. She may need to switch to oil-free makeup.

If excessive perspiration is the cause, suggest the client shower promptly after exercise, avoid tight, occlusive clothing, and lose weight if indicated.

Follow-Up. Evaluate the client in 7 days for response to therapy. Culture if not responding and consider referral to a dermatologist if immunocompromised.

Furuncles and Carbuncles

A furuncle (abscess or boil) is an infection of the hair follicle. It is more extensive and deep-seated than folliculitis and involves the adjacent tissue. Furuncles develop acutely with sudden onset of pain and tenderness. If the furuncles enlarge and coalesce, they may form a carbuncle (Schalock et al., 2011). Carbuncles are more likely to evolve into cellulitis than furuncles.

Epidemiology. Furuncles are caused by *Staphylococcus aureus*. Heat and moisture favor their development, especially where trauma has occurred. Immunocompromised individuals and patients with diabetes or who are obese are at higher risk for development. At risk for recurrent infections are those who chronically carry *Staphylococcus aureus* in their nose or throat.

Subjective/Objective Data and Differential Diagnoses. See Table 23–10.

Diagnostic Tests. Bacterial culture of exudate after incision and drainage is recommended. Treatment is started immediately and is modified if needed based on sensitivity.

Plan

Psychosocial Interventions. Furuncles often develop in the axillae and the anogenital area causing pain and embarrassment. Be alert also to hygiene and body image concerns.

Medications. Systemic antibiotics are usually unnecessary unless there is surrounding cellulitis. (See previous discussions of these agents in sections Folliculitis and Impetigo.) See previous section for treatment of CA-MRSA (Stevens et al., 2005). If the client is chronic carrier, application of mupirocin 2 percent ointment to the nares, anogenital area, and axillae may help eliminate carrier state (O'Dell, 1998; Stevens et al., 2005).

Local Measures. Warm soaks applied for 20 to 30 minutes three times a day may help immobilize lesions and prevent spread. Advise the client not to manipulate furuncles to minimize risk of much deeper and even systemic infection. Fluctuant lesions should be incised, drained, and packed. Incision and drainage is the best management.

Lifestyle. Because furuncles may develop in moist, warm areas, advise the client to wear loose clothing and fabrics that allow perspiration to evaporate and to avoid use of petroleum, oil-based cosmetics and lotions.

Follow-Up. Evaluate the client in 1 week for response to therapy. If furuncle incised and drained, schedule the client for daily evaluation to change packing, irrigate. Refer to a physician if infection recurs. The client or intimate contacts may be staph carriers.

Warts (Human Papillomavirus)

Warts are benign tumors of the skin caused by the human papillomavirus. There are more than 63 types of human papillomavirus and some have premalignant potential. Cutaneous warts fall into three broad classifications:

Common warts

Plantar warts of the foot

Flat warts

They can occur on any part of the body including the hands, face, and feet. Mucosal warts arise on mucous membranes such as the conjunctiva, oral mucosa, larynx, and anogenital area (Elgart, 2002; Schalock et al., 2011). (See discussion of genital warts in Chapter 14.)

Epidemiology. Warts often arise in childhood and regress spontaneously, usually in 1 to 2 years. In adults, they are less likely to regress. They are caused by a virus and have an incubation period of 2 to 18 months. Warts are contagious by fomites, by autoinoculation from one area to another, and from person to person. Warm, moist environments subjected to trauma or friction favor the growth. A single very small papule may grow to 5 to 10 mm, and new warts may cluster around to form a mosaic of 3 cm (Elgart, 2002). Plantar warts are most difficult to treat.

Subjective/Objective Data and Differential Diagnoses. See Table 23–10.

Diagnostic Tests. Usually diagnosed on basis of appearance. Biopsy indicated if located on sun-damaged skin; if large, chronic wart in older people; if color, border change; if long-standing wart of finger (high potential for squamous cell cancer).

Plan

Psychosocial Interventions. Concern about appearance leads many women to seek treatment. Depending on location, warts may also interfere with work, hobbies, or activities of daily living. Reassure the client that even though common cutaneous warts are benign, you appreciate her concern regarding possible malignancy or skin cancer. Give the client realistic expectations of successful treatment. It may take several visits to eradicate lesions. Give the client option of no treatment by pointing out possibility of spontaneous regression, possibility of skin damage, scarring from treatment.

Treatment. Any suspicion of squamous cell carcinoma must be biopsied. Any mucosal wart should be excised immediately and sent to the pathologist.

There are three mainstays of treatment for cutaneous warts: salicylic acid, cantharidin, and liquid nitrogen cryotherapy. Imiquimod, an immunotherapeutic agent, may also be applied to persistent warts.

Salicylic acid is available over the counter under various trade names (Compound W, Wart-Off, Freezone).

- *Administration:* Apply to the entire area after bathing and soaking the wart for several minutes. Pat dry and use applicator to cover the wart. Adjacent skin should be avoided, may use petrolatum to protect. Use every night and rinse off in morning. For warts on soles of feet (plantar warts), may cover with occlusive dressing or salicylic plaster. Apply daily. Remove dead skin by filing off with pumice stone. Frequency of treatment is dependent on tenderness and results. Alternately warts can be frozen in the office with liquid nitrogen applied with pressure for three to four cycles of 5 seconds until wart whitens. Repeat treatments may be applied every 2 weeks.
- *Adverse effects:* Warn the client about local irritation. Contraindicated to salicylic acid if allergic to aspirin.
- *Client teaching:* May require repeated treatments, less effective than cantharidin but less painful.

Cantharidin (Cantharone) is not available at all pharmacies. It is a blistering agent that must be formulated from its ingredients by the pharmacist and is for office use only.

- *Administration:* Solution is applied to wart with a wooden applicator and left on for 24 hours under an occlusive dressing. Instruct the client to remove with mild soap and water the next day. It is reapplied weekly depending on results.
- *Adverse effects:* Moderate to severe pain may develop 12 to 24 hours after treatment.
- *Contraindications:* Known sensitivity to agent. Use with caution if the client is diabetic, or has impaired circulation.

Other. Duct tape has been shown to be effective in wart treatment. It may be applied to the wart six out of seven nights for 4 weeks, then removed followed by soaking the area and then debriding with a pumice stone (Focht, Spicer, & Fairchok, 2002).

See Chapter 14 for discussion of liquid nitrogen cryotherapy.

Lifestyle. Advise the client that warts are contagious and may be spread to other areas of the body or to other close contacts after a break in the skin or maceration. The virus may also be transmitted from gym mats, edges of swimming pools, and shower floors (Schalock et al., 2011).

Follow-Up. Evaluate response to therapy after 1 week. Advise the client to call if significant pain develops after office treatment. Refer insulin-dependent diabetics, those who do not respond to treatment, to a dermatologist.

ANOGENITAL PRURITUS

Anogenital pruritus is a diagnosis of exclusion after all other causes of pruritus have been ruled, such as viral or bacterial infection, infestation, sensitivity to soaps or chemicals, psoriasis, or atrophic vaginitis. Poor hygiene may be at fault.

Epidemiology

Pruritus vulvae is not uncommon in women. It does not involve the anal area in most cases.

Subjective Data

Intense pruritus, especially at night. The client may report scant white discharge.

Objective Data

Absence of physical findings is the rule. May see excoriations, erythema, and/or fissuring.

Differential Diagnoses

Candidiasis, pediculosis, contact or allergic dermatitis, psoriasis, seborrhea, atrophic vaginitis, human papillomavirus, anal strep.

Plan

Psychosocial Interventions. Condition may be extremely embarrassing to the client and may lead to social isolation in extreme cases.

Medication. A short course of a moderate topical steroid cream applied twice a day for 2 weeks usually resolves. Wash hands after use and avoid contact with eyes (Weichert, 2004).

- *Adverse effects:* May burn or sting.
- *Contraindication:* Known sensitivity.
- *Client teaching:* Scrupulous hygiene.

Other. Sedating oral antihistamines such as Atarax may be used at bedtime to reduce itching and promote sleep.

Diet/Lifestyle. If constipation present, may be exacerbating pruritus. Follow high-fiber diet, drink plenty of fluids. Advise cleaning the skin after every bowel movement with moistened soft cloth. Sitz baths may also relieve discomfort.

Follow-Up

Reevaluate after 7 to 10 days for response to therapy.

DERMATOLOGICAL CONDITIONS NEEDING REFERRAL

Erysipelas

Erysipelas is a superficial cellulitis of the upper dermis found commonly on the legs, feet, and face (Callahan, Adal, & Tomecki, 2000). Over a period of a few days, it spreads rapidly to form a smooth, erythematous hot area. It is caused by beta-hemolytic streptococcus. The client may appear toxic on presentation with chills, fever, and pain. If erysipelas is not treated immediately, it can spread systemically and be fatal (Callahan et al., 2000; Schalock et al., 2011).

Epidemiology. Can occur at any age. Older clients and those who are immunocompromised are at greatest risk. Occurs after break in the skin or trauma (Callahan et al., 2000; Schalock et al., 2011).

Subjective Data. The client may report first appeared as small papule near nose and spread rapidly. May complain of chills, fever, and malaise.

Objective Data. Edematous, sharply marginated hot red area that may have vesicles or bullae on surface. May pit to finger pressure.

Diagnostic Tests. White count and erythrocyte sedimentation rate (ESR) are elevated. Blood culture may be positive for strep.

Differential Diagnoses. Urticaria following insect bite (resolves over next 24 hours). Cellulitis has less definite margin (Callahan et al., 2000).

Plan. Refer to a physician immediately. The client is put on bed rest with affected body part elevated (Callahan et al., 2000). Usually treated with dicloxacillin 250 mg orally four times a day or penicillin with clavulanate potassium 500 to 875 mg orally twice a day. For clients allergic to penicillin, a macrolide antibiotic may be used (Schalock et al., 2011). If the woman is frail or immunocompromised, she may require hospitalization and intravenous antibiotics.

Erythema Nodosum

The lesions of erythema nodosum are large, 4 to 10 cm red, painful slope-shouldered or flat-topped plaques that appear on the anterior lower legs and less commonly on the thigh. The most common causes of this inflammatory vascular reaction include reactions to medications such as sulfa, penicillin, and progestins; infections such as streptococcus, deep mycoses, tuberculosis, hepatitis B, and syphilis; autoimmune disease and malignancies such as sarcoidosis, leukemia, and inflammatory bowel disease (Whitmore, 2007).

Epidemiology. More common in women. May appear in pregnancy.

Subjective Data. The client may report fever, malaise, and joint pain before appearance of nodules.

Objective Data. Usually bilateral distribution on anterior lower leg or around ankle. Warm to touch, 4 to 10 cm in size, tender.

Differential Diagnoses. Cellulitis does not appear as multiple lesions. Erythema multiforme has a more general distribution.

Plan

Psychosocial Interventions. Erythema nodosum may be the presenting sign of a chronic, serious disease. Psychosocial support for such a diagnosis should be anticipated.

Treatment is based on underlying cause. Consult with a physician regarding further workup. Comfort measures include NSAIDs and, in some cases, bed rest.

Palpable Purpura

Purpura arises from the escape of the red blood cells (RBCs) into the skin due to an immune complex mechanism or trauma. It has two forms, petechiae (3 mm or less) and ecchymoses (larger than 3 mm). Purpura does not blanch with pressure. Nonpalpable purpura is caused by platelet abnormalities, actinic purpuras, and use of steroids. The most common cause of nontraumatic palpable purpura is a cutaneous vasculitis secondary to infection, connective tissue disease, or medication sensitivity. Noninflammatory etiologies include subacute bacterial endocarditis, amyloidosis, and embolic disease. Some palpable purpura is idiopathic. Serious causes and any underlying blood dyscrasia must be ruled out (Zieve, 2000).

Epidemiology. Depends on underlying cause.

Subjective Data. A careful history will often lead to diagnosis. Key items are recent onset of pharmacotherapy, fever, history of collagen vascular disease, malignancy, sexually transmitted disease, travel history, and insecticide exposure.

Objective Data. Careful examination of the skin, heart, lungs, abdomen, joints, and genitalia. Laboratory tests may include CBC, ESR, blood cultures, ANA, rheumatoid factor, blood urea nitrogen, creatinine, and urinalysis. Range of tests depends on likely etiology and client's presentation. Skin biopsy may be needed if cause is not self-limited such as drug reaction or infection.

Differential Diagnoses. Cutaneous vasculitis, bacteremia, Rocky Mountain spotted fever, subacute bacterial endocarditis, amyloidosis, trauma, cholesterol emboli, disseminated intravascular coagulation, pseudo-purpura such as Kaposi's sarcoma, Sweet's syndrome (fever, rash on upper body 5–10 days after upper respiratory infection); may be marker of leukemia (Zieve, 2000).

Plan. Consultation with a physician to outline diagnostic tests and possible further referral.

Skin Cancer

Skin cancer is the most common type of cancer in the United States. It is estimated that there are more than 1 million new cases of skin cancer per year in the United States (National Cancer Institute, 2011a, 2011b). The three most common types are basal cell cancer, squamous cell cancer, and malignant melanoma. Basal and squamous cell cancers are more common; however, malignant melanoma accounts for almost all the deaths. Women, because of their sun bathing, are particularly at risk. The U.S. Public Health Service's Healthy People 2020 program (2011) recommends efforts to reduce sunburn and use of artificial sources of UV light for tanning in children and adults in the United States.

Basal Cell Skin Cancer. Basal cell cancer arises from basal keratinocytes. It grows by direct extension and destruction of surrounding tissue. Metastasis is uncommon (Whitmore, 2007).

Epidemiology. Risk factors are similar for all types of skin cancer (Goldstein & Goldstein, 2001; National Cancer Institute, 2011a, 2011b; Sachs, Marghoob, & Halpern, 2001), although the type and pattern of UV light exposure may vary between cancers (National Cancer Institute, 2011a, 2011b) (see Table 23–11).

- Fair skin that burns easily and tans poorly
- Substantial time spent outdoors, particularly occupational, for example, farmers and sailors
- History of childhood sunburns
- Family history of skin cancer
- X-ray, radiation burn sites, UV light therapy, chronic venous stasis ulcers
- Arsenic ingestion (rare)
- Immunosuppression

TABLE 23–11. Skin Cancer Prevention Guidelines

1. *Avoid sun exposure*
   - Skin types I–IV are especially susceptible.
   - Protect infants and children. Children cannot protect themselves and significant increased risk may be associated with exposure in first decade.
   - Use caution with sun-sensitizing medications: tetracycline, tricyclics, antihistamines, antipsychotics, hypoglycemics, diuretics, antieoplastics, retin A.
2. *Avoid tanning salons. Artificial sunlight is no safer than sunlight.*
3. *When you must be in the sun, protect yourself*
   - Avoid peak times for ultraviolet B (UVB): 10 a.m. to 3 p.m.
   - Wear protective clothing: hats, especially broad-brimmed; light-colored clothing.
   - Beware of reflective surfaces: snow and cement.
   - Use sunscreen or sun block whenever going outdoors: Choose strong enough sun protection factor (SPF). Apply adequate amounts of sunscreen; manufacturer's directions are more than most people use. Apply lotion 30 to 60 minutes before expected sun exposure, as it takes time for para-aminobenzoic acid (PABA) to bind in the stratum corneum. Reapply at least every 40 to 80 minutes and more frequently if swimming or perspiring.
4. *Types of sunscreens/sunblocks*
   - Chemical sunscreens
     - PABA and PABA esters are the first choice because they effectively block UVB, which is associated with skin cancers.
     - Non-PABA sunscreens include benzophenones and cinnamates, which weakly block UVB; use if allergic to PABA.
   - Physical sunblocks: zinc oxide and titanium dioxide; opaque and often cosmetically unacceptable.
5. *Skin type and choice of SPF*

Skin Type	Skin Color and Sunburn History	SPF
I	Very fair: always burns, never tans	≥15
II	Fair: burns easily, tans minimally	≥15
III	Light brown: burns moderately, tans gradually and uniformly	10–15
IV	Moderate brown: burns minimally, always tans well	6–15
V	Dark brown: rarely burns, tans profusely	6–15
VI	Deeply pigmented: never burns	Low

Sources: Goldstein & Goldstein, 2001; Jerant, Johnson, Sheridan, & Caffrey, 2000; Schalock, Hsu, & Arndt, 2011.

Fair skin and sun exposure are the key risk factors. More than 90 percent of basal cell cancer occurs on sun-exposed areas of the head and neck but are rare on the back of the hand. The cancer may occur at sites of previous trauma, such as in thermal burns and scars. Basal cell cancer has many clinical forms that vary in appearance and malignant potential.

It is estimated that one in seven Americans will develop basal cell cancer. It is the most common type of skin cancer in the United States. Basal cell cancer is common among Caucasians and rare among African Americans. It may occur at any age. The incidence markedly increases after age 40 but basal cell carcinomas are becoming increasingly common in 20- to 30-year-olds. Thirty percent of individuals who develop basal cell carcinoma are at risk to develop another skin cancer within 5 years (American Academy of Dermatology, 2010).

Subjective Data. Basal cell cancer is primarily asymptomatic; its course is unpredictable. The lesion may remain small with almost no perceptible growth for years or it may grow rapidly. Symptoms such as enlargement, change in color, pain, itching, and bleeding should be investigated. If a client is uncertain about how long a crust lesion has been present, have her return for follow-up in 2 weeks. If the suspicious lesion remains unchanged, refer her for biopsy (Goldstein & Goldstein, 2001; Jerant, Johnson, Sheridan, & Caffrey, 2000).

Objective Data. Because the early stages of skin cancer are primarily asymptomatic, screening is crucial. A complete physical exam reveals more than six times the pathology revealed by exams limited to normally exposed sites. Physical examination should employ a magnifying lens and good lighting to observe suspicious lesions. It is helpful to wet the lesion with oil or an alcohol swab and stretch the lesion between two fingers to check for color patterns. Look for signs of dysplastic nevus syndrome (seeTable 23–12). In addition to good visualizations, careful palpation for lymphadenopathy is necessary.

Basal cell cancer usually begins as a small shiny papule that enlarges over months and develops telangiectasias and a pearly border. After time, it develops a central ulcer that recurrently crusts and bleeds. Less common

TABLE 23–12. Differential Diagnoses of Dysplastic Nevi

Sign	Common Mole	Dysplastic Nevi
Shape	Round or oval	Irregular
Margins	Sharp, well circumscribed	Hazy, indistinct
Color	Light brown to black, uniform pigmentation	Variegated tan, dark brown on pink background
Topography	Flat or smooth dome shape	"Fried egg" shape, papular center with macular periphery or pebble contour
Size	Usually < 6 mm	Usually > 5 mm, up to 12 mm
Number	Usually 12 to 25	One or many, often > 100
Location	Usually face and upper extremities	Mostly on covered areas: buttocks, scalp, and female breasts
Age of onset	Few appear after early adulthood	Continue to appear after age 35

Sources: Kanzler & Mraz-Gernhard, 2001; Schalock, Hsu, & Arndt, 2011.

TABLE 23–13. Differential Diagnosis of Skin Cancer

Benign skin lesions	Nevi, seborrheic keratosis, cysts, skin tags, dermatofibromas, keloids
Dermatoses	Seborrhea, eczema, psoriasis, human papillomavirus, fungi
Lesions with premalignant potential	Actinic keratosis, leukoplakia, dysplastic nevus syndrome
Skin cancers	Basal cell cancer, squamous cell cancer (Bowen's, Paget's), malignant melanoma, mycosis fungoides (rare T-cell lymphoma that originates in skin)
Cutaneous metastasis	3–5% of those with metastatic disease develop secondary skin cancers

Sources: Goldstein & Goldstein, 2001; Jerant et al., 2000; Kanzler & Mraz-Gernhard, 2001; Schalock, Hsu, & Arndt, 2011; Whitmore, 2007.

forms of basal cell cancer appear as flat plaques. Keep in mind that the lesion may take many forms. A basal cell carcinoma of the eyelid may have the appearance of a sty that recurs on the lower lid (Schalock et al., 2011).

Diagnostic tests may be performed by a dermatologist following referral. A suspicious lesion is evaluated and skin biopsy may be necessary.

Differential Medical Diagnoses. See Table 23–13.

Plan

PSYCHOSOCIAL INTERVENTIONS. Help the client to understand the importance of compliance with referrals and treatment regimens. Reassure her that prompt referral and treatment results in a high rate of cure, about 90 to 95 percent.

The following organizations provide materials for client and health care education on skin cancer:

National Cancer Institute: http://www.cancer.gov/cancertopics/types/skin

Skin Cancer Foundation: http://www.skincancer.org/

MEDICATION. 5-Fluorouracil (5-FU) and imiquimod have been FDA approved for treatment of superficial basal cell cancers (Skin Cancer Foundation, 2011a, 2011b)

SURGICAL INTERVENTIONS. Surgical excision, radiotherapy, cryotherapy, curettage and electrodesiccation, and Mohs micrographic surgery may be recommended following skin biopsy (National Cancer Institute, 2011a). Mohs micrographic surgery is the surgery of choice for squamous and basal cell cancers (Skin Cancer Foundation, 2011a, 2011b)

LIFESTYLE CHANGES. There is no safe tan. Sun exposure accelerates photoaging (Schalock et al., 2011). Convincing young women to avoid sun tanning is *very* difficult because of cultural norms and feelings of invulnerability. In prevention education, an emphasis on photoaging may be more effective. All people wrinkle; the question is how much and how soon. Have the woman look at how smooth and soft the skin of her upper inner arm is and compare it with that on the back of her hand. This demonstrates photoaging. Encourage all women to follow the skin cancer prevention guidelines in Table 23–11.

Follow-Up. Referral to a dermatologist is necessary after identification of a suspicious lesion.

Squamous Cell Cancer. Squamous cell cancer arises in the epithelium and is the second most common skin cancer (American Academy of Dermatology, 2010). Like basal cell cancer, squamous cell cancer is most common on areas exposed to the sun; however, distribution is somewhat different. Squamous cell cancer is commonly found on the scalp, the back of the hand, the ear, and the lower lip. It often arises from a precursor lesion called *actinic keratosis*. Actinic keratosis, a premalignant skin condition of older people, may appear as flat tan or brown spots with adherent scales and mild surrounding erythema. These often feel rough. Induration, inflammation, and oozing suggest degeneration into malignancy. Squamous cell cancer arising from actinic keratoses is not aggressive but can eventually metastasize. Squamous cell cancers that arise at thermal burn sites or sites of chronic inflammation have a higher metastatic potential than squamous cell cancers evolving from actinic keratoses (Garner & Rodney, 2000; Sachs et al., 2001).

Epidemiology. The etiology of squamous cell cancer differs somewhat depending on the type; however, all of these cancers usually appear on sun-exposed areas of fair-skinned persons. These types (simplified here) and their locations include Bowen's disease, on the trunk and extremities; Paget's disease, on the areola, nipple, and vulva; and extramammary Paget's disease, on the anogenital region, axilla, external ear canal, and eyelids.

Paget's disease of the areola manifests as a sharply demarcated area of erythema and scaling, often with oozing and crusting. It is associated with breast cancer, but easily confused with eczema. By contrast, eczema is bilateral and resolves with treatment; Paget's lesions are mostly unilateral and progressive.

Squamous cell cancer is common in the oral cavity of women who smoke and drink, often on the posterior lateral borders of the tongue. Leukoplakia, a white opaque patch found on the lips, oral mucosa, and vulva, is a precursor lesion that may degenerate into squamous cell cancer.

Subjective Data. Squamous cell cancer is primarily asymptomatic, but a client may report itching, irritation, bleeding, or a change in skin appearance.

Objective Data. See Objective Data under Basal Cell Cancer.

Physical examination reveals a variable appearance among clients, but the lesions usually begin as a reddish papule or plaque with a scaly or crusted surface. It may mimic dermatitis. Later, the lesion may appear nodular or warty. Eventually, it ulcerates and invades underlying tissue. Lesions on the lower lip may start with a thickened, dry, scaly surface on the vermillion border. Later it may progress to a nodule. Lesions of the lower lip, especially those on the inside mucous membrane, are very aggressive and demand prompt referral for treatment (Garner & Rodney, 2000).

Diagnostic evaluation and management are carried out by a dermatologist.

Differential Medical Diagnoses. See Table 23–13.

Plan

PSYCHOSOCIAL INTERVENTIONS. Emphasize the importance of skin cancer prevention (see Table 23–11). Some actinic keratoses may regress if the client avoids sun exposure. Stress the importance of the treatment regimen outlined by the specialist. Refer her to the resources listed for basal cell cancer.

MEDICATION. 5-FU is being investigated for treatment of superficial squamous cell carcinoma, but is not yet FDA approved. 5-FU is not indicated for treatment of invasive squamous cell carcinoma. Imiquimod may be effective to treat invasive squamous cell carcinoma, but is not FDA approved (Skin Cancer Foundation, 2011a, 2011b).

SURGICAL INTERVENTIONS. Excision, cryosurgery, or electrodesiccation and curettage may be performed depending on the extent of the lesion. Mohs micrographic surgery is the surgery of choice for squamous and basal cell cancers (Skin Cancer Foundation, 2011a, 2011b).

LIFESTYLE CHANGES. See those recommended for clients with basal cell cancer.

Follow-Up. Continue to monitor the client for new lesions every 3 months and teach her how to perform monthly self-examinations of the skin.

Malignant Melanoma. Malignant melanoma arises from melanocytes. It is associated primarily with sun exposure. Because most malignant melanomas arise from pigmented moles, any change in a mole is always of concern. Removal of benign moles does not decrease the risk for malignant melanoma. It may develop anywhere there are melanocytes or pigmented skin, such as mucous membranes, eyes, and the central nervous system. Malignant melanoma may arise de novo, that is, from sites where no mole is visible.

Malignant melanoma is deadly. Early identification and prompt surgical excision offer the only change for cure. The radial growth phase is a "window of opportunity" during the first several months to years of a malignant melanoma. A mole removed while it is less than 0.76 mm deep is associated with a 93 percent cure rate. Excision of vertical growths greater than 4 mm results in only 50 percent survival at 5 years (Padgett & Hendrix, 2001).

Dysplastic nevus syndrome is now known as familial atypical mole and melanoma syndrome. It is a familial syndrome found in 2 to 5 percent of the population. Individuals with dysplastic nevus syndrome have at least 6 percent lifetime risk for malignant melanoma. Clients exhibit large asymmetric and irregularly pigmented nevi. If they have two close family members with malignant melanoma, their lifetime risk for developing malignant melanoma is over 50 percent and may approach 100 percent (Kanzler & Mraz-Gernhard, 2001; Whitmore, 2007).

Epidemiology. About 68,130 new cases of malignant melanoma were diagnosed in 2010 and there were 8,700 deaths due to melanoma in 2010 (National Cancer Institute, 2011a, 2011b). Melanoma in women occurs more commonly on the limbs.

The most important risk factor for melanoma is skin color. It is rare in African Americans. In non-blacks, major risk factors include number of moles, tendency to freckle, tendency to burn in sunlight, past history of sunburns (especially in childhood), family history of atypical nevi, and family history of malignant melanoma. Immune dysfunction may also be a risk factor. Past research indicates that immunocompromise may allow transformation of dysplastic nevi into malignant melanoma (Jerant et al., 2000; Padgett & Hendrix, 2001).

Subjective Data. Four major symptoms are enlargement, color change, pain (sometimes itch), and bleeding. Most clients present with only one symptom; any symptom warrants referral for evaluation. Refer to a dermatologist all women with a family history of dysplastic nevus syndrome, especially if they also have a family history of melanoma.

Objective Data. A physical examination will help identify suspicious changes. The ABCDs (asymmetry, border, color, diameter, surface/sensation) can assist practitioners, as well as clients, in performing skin exams (see Table 23–14).

Physical examination focuses on sun-exposed areas (back, head, and neck) where most malignant melanomas occur. Acrolentiginous melanoma is a rare, but rapidly fatal lesion, occurring most often among African Americans on their palmar, plantar, or nail bed surfaces. Each of the several types of melanoma has its own particular idiosyncrasies and growth patterns. Be suspicious of variegated color, irregular borders and surfaces, and an increase in size.

Small dysplastic nevi may be difficult to differentiate from common moles on physical exam. If the client has a family history of dysplastic nevus syndrome and any questionable lesion, refer her to a dermatologist.

Diagnostic tests are conducted by a dermatologist. Refer any suspicious lesion for evaluation and probable biopsy.

Differential Medical Diagnoses. See Table 23–13.

Plan

PSYCHOSOCIAL INTERVENTIONS. Educate the client about moles and reassure her that not all moles are harmful. In general, people are born without moles. Small, flat, tan "common" moles develop in childhood and increase in size and number after puberty. They may become smooth domes. By early adulthood, individuals average 12 to 25 moles. In individuals who live long lives, the moles recede and disappear before death.

MEDICATION. Refer to a dermatologist.

SURGICAL INTERVENTION. Surgical excision may be performed. Referral to dermatology is recommended as achieving clear margins is important during excision.

LIFESTYLE CHANGES. Encourage the client to follow skin cancer prevention guidelines (see Table 23–11). She should also perform monthly self-exams of the skin and stop smoking.

Follow-Up. Refer a client with any suspicious lesion to a dermatologist. If dysplastic nevus syndrome is suspected, refer the client. With numerous dysplastic nevi, baseline photographs and perhaps serial photodocumentation are needed.

Immunocompromised clients may be seen every 3 to 4 months by the dermatologist. Family members of clients with dysplastic nevus syndrome must be screened; often an early operable melanoma is found in a distant relative. All women should be taught the ABCDs of melanoma (see Table 23–14). A complete skin exam should be conducted at the time of the client's annual physical. Encourage women to examine their skin monthly at home.

TABLE 23–14. ABCDs of Skin Cancer

A	Asymmetry	One half shaped unlike the other
B	Border	Irregular, notched, or scalloped
C	Color	Haphazard shades of brown, red, blue, gray
D	Diameter	Greater than 6 mm (size of the tip of a pencil eraser)
S	Surface or sensation	Surface distortion may be subtle or obvious, assess by focusing light at side of lesion; sensation refers to itch, burn, or pain

EAR, NOSE, AND THROAT DISORDERS

These disorders are frequently encountered in primary care; the most common—the common cold, otitis media, acute sinusitis, and pharyngitis—will be addressed here.

THE COMMON COLD

The common cold is a mild, self-limited condition caused by a viral infection of the upper respiratory mucosa. The nasal mucosa is prominently involved.

Epidemiology

Studies of the common cold demonstrate that age and environmental contacts are the two major factors influencing the extent of illness. Numerous groups and hundreds of viral strains cause cold symptoms. Rhinoviruses are the most common group. Others include coronaviruses, respiratory syncytial virus, adenovirus, echovirus, coxsackievirus, and parainfluenza virus.

Transmission is primarily via direct contact with infected secretions, usually hand-to-hand and subsequent hand-to-face contact. It is evident that good handwashing is crucial in breaking the chain of transmission. Less often, transmission occurs via respiratory droplets from coughs or sneezes. Crowds and poor ventilation promote transmission. The incubation period is usually 48 to 72 hours.

Incidence of the common cold among average adults is two to four colds per year but parents of small children have about six colds per year. The vast majority of these illnesses are benign and self-limited; however, they have a major social and financial impact. They are responsible for more absences from work and school than any other type of illness.

Subjective Data

The client's chief complaints are malaise, rhinorrhea, and a scratchy throat. Nasal secretions are usually clear and copious at onset, changing to mucoid appearance later in the illness. Mucopurulent secretions *do not* necessarily indicate a secondary bacterial infection. Fever is rare in adults. Symptoms peak in 2 to 4 days, then gradually resolve. The total course of the illness is usually 5 to 10 days. When nasal symptoms last longer than 10 to 14 days, the client needs to be evaluated for sinusitis or allergies (Meltzer, 2002).

Objective Data

Physical examination reveals a benign general appearance. Fever is either low grade or absent. Nasal mucosa is often edematous with clear discharge. The pharynx appears to have mild erythema. Lymphoid hyperplasia of the posterior pharynx is more common than tonsillar enlargement. Lymph nodes are usually nonpalpable, but small anterior cervical nodes may be palpable. Lungs are clear.

Differential Medical Diagnoses

Bacterial infections (*Mycoplasma pneumoniae, Chlamydia psittaci,* GABHS); viral syndromes (Epstein-Barr or mononucleosis, cytomegalovirus); allergic rhinitis (seasonal, associated itching and copious clear nasal discharge) (Meltzer, 2002). Colds resolve in a few days; other syndromes are more severe and/or longlasting.

Plan

A large part of intervention is helping the client care for herself.

Psychosocial Interventions. Educate the client on the expected course of her illness and the need for self-care. Empower her to pursue self-care when appropriate. Provide information about viral and bacterial infections.

Medication. See Table 23–15.

TABLE 23–15. Overview of Oral Medication Types Used for the Common Cold

Class	Indications	Side Effects	Contraindications
Decongestants	Shrink swollen nasal mucosa	Neurologic agitation, increased blood pressure	Avoid with hypertension
Antihistamines	Dry up mucous membrane secretions	Drowsiness (no effect on blood pressure)	Avoid with asthma and history of asthma "flair" with use of antihistamines
			Avoid giving with sedating medications or alcohol
Antipyretics/analgesic	Relieve discomfort or fever	Gastrointestinal irritation with nonsteroidal anti-inflammatory drugs	Aspirin is associated with Reye's syndrome; use acetaminophen, especially in clients under age 18

Numerous drugs are included in each class. See specific pharmacotherapeutics texts for details.

Sources: Brunton, 2002; Ebel, 2004.

Lifestyle Changes. Lifestyle changes may help prevent the spread of colds. Advise clients to practice good handwashing and to avoid hand-to-face contact. Increasing fluid intake helps keep secretions loose and moving. Physical activity may be carried out as tolerated. Strongly encourage cessation of smoking, as it increases the risk for secondary bacterial infections affecting ears, sinuses, and lungs.

Follow-Up

Teach clients to look for pain (in ear, face, or chest), fever (higher than 102°F or that recurs after initial few days), and distressing cough that is associated with dyspnea, fever, or localized chest pain, or that is persistent and progressive.

OTITIS MEDIA

Otitis media is an acute infection of the middle ear. The majority of infections are caused by eustachian tube dysfunction, which in adults is caused primarily by edema from viral upper respiratory infections and allergies. Cigarette smoking and exposure to tobacco smoke may also be predisposing factors for the development of otitis media in adults (Murphy & Kyungcheol, 2006). Barotrauma (flying/scuba diving) and cancer can also impair eustachian tube function. Chronic negative pressure in the middle ear leads to serious effusion and overgrowth of respiratory tract bacteria, with subsequent purulent discharge and inflammation (Pichichero, 2000).

Epidemiology

Studies indicate that otitis media is a bacterial disease of the respiratory tract mucosa. The three primary pathogens are *Streptococcus pneumoniae*, *Haemophilus influenzae*, and *Moraxella catarrhalis* (previously *Branhamella catarrhalis*). Resistant strains of *M. catarrhalis* and *H. influenzae* can produce beta-lactamase, which inactivates penicillin and amoxicillin. Incidence reports show at least 4.4 percent of the adult population has one episode per year of otitis media (Tigges, 2000). Otitis media is most often a secondary bacterial infection following a viral upper respiratory tract infection or problems with allergies.

Subjective Data

Usually the client reports a history of viral respiratory infections, allergies, smoking, or barotrauma. She describes unilateral or bilateral ear pain associated with decreased hearing. Systemic symptoms are uncommon in adults. New onset of recurrent otitis media with no preceding history of upper respiratory infections or allergies may be indicative of cancer, especially in women who smoke and drink alcohol.

Objective Data

Data is gathered primarily from physical examination of the ears.

Physical examination reveals a general benign appearance. Vital signs are usually normal; fever is rare. The external canal of the ear should appear normal, with no tragus or mastoid tenderness. Otoscopy is used to evaluate five parameters of tympanic membrane appearance:

Otoscopic Exam

- *Color:* Erythema is consistent with acute infection.
- *Contour:* The membrane may be bulging in acute suppurative otitis media, and retracted in serous otitis.
- *Translucence:* The membrane may be thick and opaque in chronic otitis.
- *Structural changes:* An irregular light reflex or blisters indicate infection.
- *Mobility:* A light reflex should move with insufflation; immobility is consistent with infection.
- *Mastoid:* Should not be tender.
- *Nasal cavity:* Turbinate may be erythematous, gray, and boggy. A clear discharge may be present.
- *Oropharynx:* May be benign or changes are consistent with allergic rhinitis or pharyngitis.
- *Neck:* Nodes may be present.

If the canal is obscured by copious purulent drainage and the possibility of rupture exists, do not instill anything into the ear or attempt to clean it out. Diagnostic tests are not usually indicated. An audiogram may be helpful in assessing hearing, and tympanometry may help assess mobility.

Differential Medical Diagnosis

Several conditions of a serious nature should be considered.

- External otitis is also called "swimmer's ear." The canal is usually swollen with exudate and tender with external manipulation of the ear. Treatment with otic drops, usually an antibiotic ear drop combined with a corticosteroid such as CortisporinOtic® or Ciprodex®, is required.

- Serous otitis media is characterized by a retracted tympanic membrane, possibly an air-fluid level, and often decreased hearing. There is no erythema, and the condition is common with allergies and upper respiratory infections.
- Mastoiditis is a life-threatening condition caused by the spread of infection from the middle ear to the air cells of the mastoid process. Any tenderness over the mastoid should lead to suspicion of mastoiditis. Refer the client immediately for hospitalization.
- Meningitis usually causes the client to appear toxic; severe neck pain occurs with flexion.
- Malignant otitis externa is associated with a 50 percent fatality rate and is seen in diabetics and in those immunocompromised with external otitis. Refer the client to a physician immediately (Tigges, 2000).

Plan

Medication. Use of antibiotics and other medication is debatable. In European countries, such as The Netherlands, antibiotics are not prescribed because improvement is seen in 10 days regardless of treatment. In this country, however, it is felt that the risk of suppurative complications is too great, supporting aggressive treatment with antibiotics (Pichichero, 2000; Tigges, 2000).

In general, the first choice is amoxicillin (Amoxil, Biomox) 250 to 500 mg orally three times daily; the second choice is amoxicillin-clavulanate potassium (Augmentin) 875 mg (amoxicillin component) twice daily for 5 to 7 days; or if non–type I penicillin sensitivity reaction, a second- or third-generation cephalosporin such as cefpodoxime (Vantin) 100 to 200 mg every 12 hours, cefuroxime axetil (Ceftin) 250 to 500 mg every 12 hours, cefprozil (Cefzil) 250 to 500 mg every 12 hours, and cefdinir (Omnicef) 300 mg every 12 hours or 600 mg daily for 5 to 7 days. Antibiotics for patients with type I penicillin sensitivity reaction include azithromycin (Zithromax, Z pack 5-day course), or clarithromycin (Biaxin) 250 to 500 mg every 12 hours can also be used. For analgesia, acetaminophen and NSAIDs usually suffice. Decongestants have never been proven to shorten the course of otitis media and are used symptomatically only for nasal congestion. Refer to a pharmacotherapeutics text for details.

Tympanostomy (myringotomy) is not usually required for adults. Refer the client to an ear, nose, and throat specialist if she does not improve after two or three 10-day treatment regimens.

Lifestyle Changes. Advise the client to avoid vigorous nose blowing and to increase fluid intake. Encourage the client to stop smoking, as smoking increases the risk of otitis media. For fluid behind the ear, teach the client to carry out gentle autoinsufflation: She manipulates the posterior pharynx (swallowing, chewing gum, yawning) to speed drainage of fluid from the middle ear.

Follow-Up

Ask the client to return to the clinic if acute symptoms, such as pain, are not improved in 48 hours or if she is not asymptomatic in 10 days.

ACUTE SINUSITIS

Acute sinusitis is infection of one of the four sinuses: maxillary, frontal, ethmoid, and sphenoid. The mucosal lining becomes swollen and occludes air exchange and mucous drainage, resulting in inflammation, bacterial replication, and purulent discharge.

Epidemiology

Acute sinusitis affects one in seven adults and accounts for roughly 20 percent of antibiotic prescription in adults (Rosenfeld et al., 2007). Studies reveal that numerous conditions can predispose an individual to acute sinusitis. The most common risk factors are viral upper respiratory infections, allergic rhinitis, and dental extraction and abscesses. Barotrauma (flying or diving), foreign bodies, tumors, and polyps are less common but they can block the ostia (or openings) to the sinuses (Chrostowski & Pongracic, 2002). It is important to distinguish acute bacterial rhinosinusitis from viral rhinosinusitis. Acute bacterial rhinosinusitis is characterized by persistence of acute rhinosinusitis 10 days or more after onset of symptoms or bimodal pattern where symptoms recur after initial improvement (Rosenfeld et al, 2007).

The primary organisms causing acute sinusitis are *Streptococcus pneumoniae*, *Haemophilus influenzae*, *Moraxella catarrhalis*, group A streptococci, and staphylococci. Organisms involved in chronic infections include those already listed as well as mixed anaerobes, which are often difficult to treat (Chrostowski & Pongracic, 2002).

Incidence reports show acute sinusitis as a common condition; it complicates about 0.5 percent of all upper respiratory infections.

Subjective Data

Taking a detailed history is imperative, as a physical exam is of limited use in making the diagnosis.

The classic history is a preceding upper respiratory infection lasting 5 days or longer, with subsequent development of copious yellow-green nasal discharge and intense, localized facial pain, worse on forward bending. Discomfort is often intense and constant. Depending on which sinus is infected, the pain may be referred to the teeth or palate (maxillary), the eyebrow area (frontal), or behind the eyes or at the top of the head (ethmoid and sphenoid). Note whether symptoms are unilateral or bilateral. Some infections present with only a history of purulent nasal discharge and fatigue, with no associated face pain. Infection can be acute (up to 3 weeks), subacute (3 weeks to 3 months), or chronic (more than 3 months). The time frame is important to ascertain as chronic infection is more difficult to treat and at times may require surgical intervention (Chrostowski & Pongracic, 2002).

Objective Data

Physical Examination. Reveals a benign general appearance. Vital signs are usually normal; fever is rare. If fever is high, consider referral. (Caution: Clients are in pain and may be taking analgesics that mask fever; ask if they have taken any acetaminophen, aspirin, or NSAIDs in the previous 4 hours.) A purulent nasal discharge and edematous turbinates may be noted, as may a purulent postnasal drip. Sinuses are difficult to assess; percussion for tenderness and transillumination are often unreliable. Abnormal eye movements, facial edema, and erythema around the eyes suggest spreading cellulitis; immediate referral is necessary.

Diagnostic Tests. Because plain films of the sinus offer only low specificity and sensitivity, more clinicians are using computed tomography (CT) scans (without contrast) when such tests are indicated. Sinusitis is typically diagnosed on clinical signs and symptoms and does not require radiographic testing to diagnose. In cases of treatment failure, however, CT scan may be useful. CT scans offer good visualization of the ostiomeatal complex, the openings of the anterior ethmoid, maxillary, and frontal sinuses. Nasal endoscopy allows direct visualization of the anatomic and pathologic features of the nose.

Differential Medical Diagnosis

Viral upper respiratory infections, allergic rhinitis, rebound medicamentosa from topical decongestants, dental extractions and abscesses, nasal polyps, and tumors (Chrostowski & Pongracic, 2002).

Plan

Psychosocial Interventions. Encourage the client to comply with the antibiotic regimen. Educate her about the warning signs and symptoms of complications: facial swelling, visual problems, high fever, increased pain.

Medication. Antibiotics, decongestants, analgesics, and topical corticosteroids may be helpful. A recent meta-analysis of antibiotic versus placebo treatment indicated that antibiotic treatment should be considered on an individual case-by-case basis rather than prescribed universally to treat sinusitis. The benefit of antibiotic therapy was of only moderate clinical significance (Bailey & Chang, 2009). Patients with immunocompromise, recent antimicrobial therapy (2–4 weeks), poor oral dentition, fever greater than 101°F, coincident bacterial infection elsewhere, symptoms greater than 30 days, elevated inflammatory CRP (> 100 mg/L), sinus surgery, or nasal polyp should be treated. Other patients may go through a 7-day watchful waiting period, and if no improvement in symptoms during that time, then start on an antibiotic (Rosenfeld et al., 2007).

The *antibiotic* of first choice is amoxicillin, 500 mg orally three times daily for 10 days, or high-dose amoxicillin, 875 mg twice daily, when there are young children who attend day care in the home or there was previous treatment with an antibiotic in the preceding 4 to 6 months. Alternatives include second- or third-generation cephalosporin such as cefuroxime axetil (Ceftin), cefprozil (Cefzil), cefpodoxime (Vantin), or cefdinir (Omnicef) if not a type 1 penicillin sensitivity or trimethoprim/sulfamethoxazole double strength (Bactrim DS) twice daily for 10 days or azithromycin (Z pack) for 5 days. If macrolide or sulfa-based antibiotic is used, there may be ineffective treatment of *Haemophilus influenzae* or resistant *Streptococcus pneumoniae* (Radojicic, 2006). See drug prescribing guide for complete recommendations on dosing. Chronic sinusitis may require 21 days of therapy or more.

Decongestants may help to shrink tissue and drain infection. Monitor hypertensive clients closely.

Analgesics include NSAIDs, which help to ease the pain and edema.

Antihistamines are usually avoided, as they may dry mucous membranes and impair ciliary movement to clear sinuses.

Topical corticosteroids may shrink tissue and promote drainage reducing symptom burden

Guaifenesin is an expectorant, but there is currently no strong evidence to support recommending it for treatment of sinusitis.

Caution is suggested with topical nasal steroid use in sinusitis as, if there is a viral component, the viral load may be increased with such use (Gerzevitz, Porter, & Dunphy, 2011).

Surgical Interventions. Surgical management may be recommended by an ear, nose, and throat specialist if the client's symptoms do not improve.

Lifestyle Changes. Use of a room humidifier, hot showers, and nasal saline nose drops may keep mucous membranes moist and draining. Saline nasal irrigation may provide symptoms relief and decrease need for medication. Application of warm packs to the affected area may provide comfort. Increasing fluid intake also helps to keep secretions loose. Advise physical activity as tolerated, and discourage smoking.

Follow-Up

Consider the potentially lethal complications of acute sinusitis, including periorbital cellulitis and abscess leading to meningitis, osteomyelitis, or cavernous sinus thrombosis. Refer clients to a physician if they appear toxic, have a high fever, or exhibit redness or swelling around the eyes, difficulty moving the eyes, or double vision.

Symptoms should improve greatly 48 to 72 hours after starting antibiotics. If not, refer the client to a physician. All symptoms should resolve before completion of medications. If not, or if they recur, refer the client to a physician. Rule out tumors and polyps if acute episodes recur or if symptoms persist with treatment. Assess for and treat allergic rhinitis after acute symptoms resolve.

PHARYNGITIS

Pharyngitis, an inflammatory condition of the pharynx, has numerous causes. Three causes discussed here in depth are GABHS, infectious mononucleosis, and *Neisseria gonorrhoeae* (see Table 23–16).

Epidemiology

Identification of GABHS necessitates immediate treatment, because these organisms can cause rheumatic fever if untreated and if associated with local suppurative complications such as tonsillar abscess (Gerzevitz et al., 2011). Infectious mononucleosis is acute infection with the Epstein-Barr virus. Although pharyngitis caused by mononucleosis cannot be treated, it should be identified so that the client can be monitored for potentially lethal complications, such as airway compromise and splenic rupture. Pharyngitis caused by *N. gonorrhoeae* may be confused with pharyngitis caused by GABHS or mononucleosis, but it must be identified so that sexual partners can be treated (Gerzevitz et al., 2011).

Transmission of GABHS (scarlet fever) occurs primarily among children of school age or people living under crowded living conditions, such as college dormitories and military barracks. Mononucleosis is primarily a disease of the young passed through mucous membrane secretions. Gonorrheal pharyngitis is most commonly seen among homosexual males, but should be considered in any sexually active adult with a sore throat who fails to respond to treatment (Gerzevitz et al., 2011).

Incidence reports show that GABHS are responsible for about one third of the sore throats seen in primary care. GABHS causes 5 to 20 percent of sore throats among persons older than 15 (Lang & Towers, 2001). Ninety percent of the population has had mononucleosis by age 40. Most adults are not aware that they had it in childhood. The infection tends to be more severe if contracted as an adult (Gerzevitz et al., 2011). Gonorrhea is responsible for about 1 percent of pharyngitis infections among adults treated in primary care.

Subjective Data

Pharyngitis caused by GABHS is associated with a classic history of sudden onset of malaise, fever (usually higher than 101°F), tender anterior cervical nodes, headache, and a severe sore (not scratchy) throat. Nasal symptoms are infrequent and cough is rare. Often a woman has been exposed to small children. If an abscess is present, the client may experience excruciating unilateral pain and may report drooling or spitting saliva, rather than swallowing it. Ask the client about a history of abscesses, as recurrence is common.

Infectious mononucleosis in adults usually presents with a history of gradual onset of fatigue that becomes severe (sleeping 12–14 hours per day). Appetite decreases. Sore throat begins, and the client complains of aches around the neck caused by prominent neck adenopathy. Fever is variable; temperature may be normal to greater than 103°F. Side tenderness and jaundice may be caused by hepatosplenomegaly. Symptoms are most prominent in the first 2 weeks, and gradual full recovery usually occurs in 6 weeks (Lang & Towers, 2001).

Gonorrheal pharyngitis may be mild or severe. The diagnosis is suspected if a client reports a new sexual partner and oral sex. Chlamydia may also be considered

TABLE 23–16. Differential Diagnosis of Pharyngitis

Bacterial Diseases	Viral Diseases	Other Diseases
Group A beta-hemolytic streptococcus	**Mononucleosis**	**Mycoplasma**
Large tonsils beefy red ± exudate	Large tonsils, palatine petechiae ± exudate	Rarely diagnosed in absence of bronchitis/pneumonia
Fever (> 101° F)	Fever may or may not occur	
Nodes anterior and very tender	Nodes posterior or generalized	**Candida**
Rash, scarlatina, sandpaper-like	Rash, faint, maculopapular	"Thrush," rule out AIDS, cancer, and diabetes
Often headache	Headache may or may not occur	
Often vomit once	Persistent anorexia/fatigue	**Allergies**
No cough	Rare cough	Consider if "cold lasts > 3 weeks," worse in morning and nighttime, postnasal drip
Gonorrhea	30% splenomegaly	
1% of sore throats in adults ± exudate	10% hepatomegaly	**Spirochetes**
History of oral sex	**Common cold**	Syphilis
Diphtheria	Upper respiratory infection caused by rhinovirus, etc., usually nasal symptoms may be hoarse	Acute necrotizing ulcerative gingivitis
Pseudomembrane		Ulcers on gums
Unimmunized population	**Herpes simplex**	"Trench mouth"
Haemophilus influenzae	Ulcers on gums, hard palate tissue and lips	**Dehydration**
Rare in adults	**Coxsackievirus**	**Irritant gases**
Epiglottis in children	Ulcers on soft palate and tonsillar pillars	**Trauma**
Group D and C streptococci	**Cytomegalovirus**	**Foreign body**
Rarely cause suppurative complications, therefore not treated	Mononucleosis-like syndrome may be asymptomatic or quite ill, will shed virus, dangerous to pregnant women with no immunity	**Neoplasm**
Tuberculosis	**Measles, mumps, rubella, varicella**	

Sources: Gerzevitz, Porter, & Dunphy, 2011; Lang & Towers, 2001.

as the causative organism. The diagnosis is primarily suspected if persistent sore throat is not cured by usual management (Gerzevitz et al., 2011).

Objective Data

Because physical examination cannot differentiate between viral and bacterial causes of pharyngitis, specific laboratory tests are required for diagnosis.

Physical Examination. Findings depend on the etiology (see Table 23–16). The client may be flushed, appear sick, and have fever. A fine, red, sandpaper-like rash is consistent with GABHS (scarlet fever). A maculopapular rash is consistent with mononucleosis and hemorrhagic pustules with gonorrhea. Jaundice can occur in mononucleosis. Nasal congestion and a hoarse voice are primarily of viral origin and are rare in pharyngitis caused by GABHS, mononucleosis, or gonorrhea. "Hot potato" voice and drooling are red flags and may indicate an abscess. In pharyngitis caused by GABHS, tonsils are often large and beefy red with a thick white exudate. Suspect an abscess or peritonsillar cellulitis if the soft palate shows unilateral bulging, if the uvula is deviated or edematous, or if the client will not open her mouth because of pain (Lang & Towers, 2001). Never force a client's mouth open; if epiglottis is present, it may cause spasm and occlusion of the airway.

Neck adenopathy is nonspecific. As a rule, however, large, very tender anterior nodes are consistent with pharyngitis caused by GABHS or gonorrhea; posterior cervical nodes and generalized adenopathy are more consistent with pharyngitis caused by mononucleosis. The lungs should be clear. Abdominal examination may reveal side tenderness, indicating hepatosplenomegaly from mononucleosis or the mononucleosis-like cytomegalovirus. Genitalia are examined only if gonorrhea is suspected.

Diagnostic Tests. Specific for bacterial and viral infections. For pharyngitis caused by GABHS, in-office rapid strep tests or cultures are helpful. The white blood cell (WBC) count may be slightly elevated in streptococcal pharyngitis, but may be greater than 15,000 if an abscess exists.

For infectious mononucleosis, the mononucleus spot test (or heterophile antibody test) often does not turn positive for 5 to 12 days or longer after onset of illness. The CBC is usually normal or shows a slightly decreased WBC count with a predominance of lymphocytes and monocytes. The diagnosis may be made with a blood smear showing 20 percent atypical lymphocytes. If the client exhibits the classic clinical picture of mononucleosis but the monospot remains negative, consider ordering a battery of tests to rule out cytomegalovirus, toxoplasmosis, and histoplasmosis.

For gonorrheal pharyngitis, order a throat culture; use calcium alginate swabs, plate on Thayer-Martin medium, and incubate.

Differential Medical Diagnoses

See Table 23–16.

Plan

Psychosocial Interventions. Explain to the client her condition or the differential diagnoses being considered if tests were inconclusive. Inform her about the course of treatment to expect and the red flag symptoms that should prompt her to call the health care provider.

Medication. Refer to a current pharmacotherapeutics text for details.

For pharyngitis caused by GABHS, administer penicillin V (Betapen-VK) 250 to 500 mg orally four times daily for 10 days (administer erythromycin or Zithromax if the client is allergic to penicillin V). If the patient is not tolerating oral intake well, may give Bicillin L-A intramuscularly 1.2 million units in office times once.

Note: Although amoxicillin is effective against GABHS, do not give it when the strep test is negative and mononucleosis cannot be ruled out as cause of exudative pharyngitis. Clients with mononucleosis develop a total body maculopapular rash if given amoxicillin (Lang & Towers, 2001). For pharyngitis caused by infectious mononucleosis, analgesics such as ibuprofen may be given. Steroids may be used if tonsillar enlargement threatens the airway (Gerzevitz et al., 2011).

For gonorrheal pharyngitis, if uncomplicated, inject ceftriaxone sodium (Rocephin) 125 to 250 mg (by weight) intramuscularly (see Chapter 14 for recommendations). Also administer oral doxycycline (Vibramycin) or azithromycin (Zithromax) to treat the possibility of concurrent chlamydial infection.

Surgical Interventions. Surgery may be needed if abscess is present. Refer the client for needle aspiration and possible incision and drainage.

Lifestyle Changes. If pharyngitis-caused mononucleosis is diagnosed, encourage the client to listen to her body and to rest when she feels tired. She should avoid vigorous activity for about 6 weeks and protect her sides because of the risk of rupturing the spleen (Gerzevitz et al., 2011). Otherwise, activity is as tolerated. Warn the client to avoid hepatotoxins, such as alcohol. The client may use warm saline gargles and lozenges if she feels they help.

If gonorrheal pharyngitis is diagnosed, education about safer-sex practices should be discussed and all sex partners should be tested and treated.

If pharyngitis caused by GABHS is diagnosed, decreased activity and alcohol avoidance are recommended. In general, encourage clients to increase fluids and nutrition. Discourage smoking.

Follow-Up

Follow-up is specific to the condition. Pharyngitis caused by GABHS should improve greatly in 48 hours; otherwise have the client return to rule out abscess or other infection. Clients with pharyngitis caused by mononucleosis are sickest on about days 4 to 8 of illness and should be followed on the basis of the clinical picture. Observe for airway obstruction, hepatitis, and splenic enlargement. Instruction to avoid contact sports in the case of splenic enlargement should be given.

Clients with gonorrheal pharyngitis are at risk for numerous complications, such as disseminated gonococcal infection with bacteremia and purulent arthritis. Ensure that all sexual contacts are treated.

ENDOCRINE DISORDERS

The four most commonly occurring endocrine disorders discussed in this chapter are hypothyroidism, hyperthyroidism, thyroid nodules, and diabetes.

HYPOTHYROIDISM

Hypothyroidism is a clinical syndrome associated with subnormal levels of circulating thyroid hormones. A client may be asymptomatic; the condition may be mild to severe.

Myxedema is the advanced form of hypothyroidism characterized by proteinaceous infiltration of the skin and subcutaneous tissues with multiple organ system involvement (Cooper, 2001; Klein & Ojamaa, 2001; Yen, 2007).

Epidemiology

The cause differs among the four types of hypothyroidism: primary, secondary, goitrous, and transient. Recently, a distinction is made for subclinical hypothyroidism as well.

Primary hypothyroidism is characterized by atrophy or destruction of thyroid tissue due to an autoimmune response. Primary hypothyroidism accounts for more than 90 percent of hypothyroid disease. Primary hypothyroidism may also be iatrogenic (following radioiodine therapy or thyroidectomy for hyperthyroidism), idiopathic, or the result of a congenital disorder (cretinism) (Cooper, 2001; Toft, 2001; Yen, 2007).

Secondary hypothyroidism results from insufficient stimulation of an intrinsically normal gland. It may occur in primary disorders of the pituitary or hypothalamus, which result in deficiencies of TSH or thyrotropin-releasing hormone.

Goitrous hypothyroidism is due to defective thyroid hormone synthesis and is characterized by development of a goiter. Goitrous disorders include Hashimoto's thyroiditis; iodine deficiency; acquired hypothyroidism, caused by the use of goitrogens (propylthiouracil [PTU], methimazole, lithium, or iodine); peripheral resistance to thyroid hormone; and infiltrative disorders (amyloidosis, sarcoidosis, lymphoma, or malignancy).

Transient hypothyroidism can occur as the result of pregnancy or significant illness (Yen, 2007). It usually resolves within 6 months of onset, and close monitoring is all that is required (Abalovich et al., 2007; Klein & Ojamaa, 2001).

Subclinical hypothyroidism sometimes referred to as early or mild hypothyroidism is characterized by elevated TSH and normal T3 and T4 values. Progression of overt hypothyroidism occurs in 3 to 18 percent of individuals affected (McDermott & Ridgway, 2001).

Routine screening of asymptomatic adults is not recommended. The USPSTF (2004c) found insufficient evidence for or against screening. It may be clinically prudent, however, to screen those at increased risk, namely, older women, newborns, those with a strong family history of thyroid disorders, postpartum women 4 to 8 weeks after delivery, and clients with autoimmune disease (Cooper, 2001; Toft, 2001; Yen, 2007).

The onset of hypothyroidism is most common in women between 30 and 60 years of age. It develops in both men and women. It is a common disorder of older people. The prevalence of thyroid disease in clients more than 60 years of age is about 4 percent, eight times higher than in the general population (Cooper, 2001; Toft, 2001; Yen, 2007).

Subjective Data

Hypothyroidism is easily misdiagnosed because its presentation is nonspecific and it involves multiple organ systems. Less than one third of older people manifest typical symptoms: cold intolerance; weight gain; dry skin; weakness; fatigue; hoarseness; inattention or difficulty concentrating; dizziness; constipation; arthralgias; muscle cramps; menstrual irregularities, particularly menorrhagia; galactorrhea; and depression.

Objective Data

Physical Presentation. Depends on the progression of disease from a subclinical one to a medical emergency, such as that which often precedes myxedema coma.

Physical Examination

- *General appearance:* Flat affect; low-pitched, slow speech.
- *Vital signs:* Bradycardia, hypertension.
- *Skin:* Thin, brittle nails with transverse grooves; dry, scaly cool skin with a diffuse wavy pallor.
- *Head:* Coarse, dry, brittle hair with alopecia; facial edema; enlarged tongue; thinning or absence of the lateral eyebrows.
- *Neck:* Normal, enlarged, small, or absent thyroid; thyroid nodules; tracheal deviation.
- *Chest:* Exertional dyspnea, pleural effusions.
- *Heart:* Cardiomegaly, arrhythmias.
- *Abdomen:* Gastrointestinal hypomotility, ascites.
- *Neurologic exam:* Cerebellar dysfunction, delayed deep tendon reflexes, parathesias, peripheral neuropathies.
- *Endocrine system:* Galactorrhea.

Diagnostic Laboratory Tests. Reveal levels of circulating thyroid hormones. The active thyroid hormones are tetraiodothyronine (thyroxine or T4) and triiodothyronine (T3). Both T3 and T4 circulate in the serum, bound to three proteins: thyroxine-binding globulin, thyroxine-binding prealbumin, and albumin. The small fractions of T3 and T4 that circulate free (not bound to protein) are the active forms. Alterations in thyroxine-binding globulin (e.g., with pregnancy, estrogen replacement, or the use of oral contraceptives) may change total circulating T3 and T4 levels but do not affect free unbound forms.

Primary hypothyroidism is confirmed by a high level of TSH and a low level of free T4. A serum TSH is the most sensitive test; it is elevated in more than 95 percent of clients with hypothyroidism (Cooper, 2001; Toft, 2001; Yen, 2007).

Secondary hypothyroidism is differentiated from primary hypothyroidism by the thyrotropin-releasing hormone test of pituitary-thyroid regulation. If secondary hypothyroidism is suspected, the client should be referred to an endocrinologist.

Differential Medical Diagnoses

Cardiac disorders, renal disorders, neuromuscular disorders, and depression are common diagnostic considerations.

Plan

Psychosocial Interventions. It may be necessary to address acute anxiety reactions, which are often among the manifestations of this multisystem disorder. Reassure the client that her symptoms will gradually abate with treatment. Depressed clients may benefit from short-term counseling.

Medication. Levothyroxine (Levoxine, Synthroid), a synthetic T4 hormonal replacement, is the medication of choice.

- *Administration:* Usual recommended starting dose is levothyroxine 25 to 50 μg/day. However, in asymptomatic cardiac patients and patients younger than age 60, starting at full dose (1.6 μg/kg, usually 100–125 mcg daily) has not been shown to cause negative outcomes, but has caused earlier resolution in symptoms (Roos, Linn-Rasker, van Domburg, Tijssen, & Berghout, 2005; Vaidya & Pearce, 2008). Dosage may be increased by 25 mcg every 6 weeks according to TSH levels. Dosages need to be adjusted with caution in older people and in clients with cardiac disease. These individuals should be started at low dose at 25 μg/day.
- *Side effects:* Palpitations and dysrhythmias are known to occur, particularly in clients with cardiac disease.
- *Contraindications:* Contraindications are outweighed by the risk of not treating the hypothyroidism. Use caution, however, in clients with cardiac disease and older people.
- *Evaluation of drug action:* To ensure equilibrium, measure serum TSH values no sooner than every 6 weeks after initiating therapy and again 3 to 4 months after a maintenance dose is reached. Annual TSH values are done to monitor therapy, as needs may change with time.
- *Client teaching:* Review with the client signs and symptoms of hypothyroidism and hyperthyroidism, which may indicate the need for medication change.

The decision to treat subclinical hypothyroidism must be evaluated on an individual basis. If the client is symptomatic, a trial of levothyroxine may be indicated; however, there is no evidence to support routine treatment. If the client has coexisting medical problems, a referral to an endocrinologist is indicated (Vaidya & Pearce, 2008).

Lifestyle Changes. The daily medication regimen and chronic condition may cause the client to alter her self-perception. Encourage positive, affirming activities. Diet and exercise are not restricted.

Follow-Up

Once the maintenance dose has been established, annual visits are all that may be required to check the TSH level and reinforce client teaching.

HYPERTHYROIDISM (THYROTOXICOSIS)

Thyrotoxicosis is a hypermetabolic state that results from an excess of circulating thyroid hormone. Excessive thyroid hormone does not always result from thyroid gland hyperactivity; thus thyrotoxicosis, not hyperthyroidism, is the preferred term.

The most common condition is diffuse toxic goiter (Graves' disease), an autoimmune disorder. Thyroid-stimulating immunoglobulin binds to thyroid cell receptors and stimulates overproduction of thyroid hormones T4 and T3. The cause of thyroid-stimulating immunoglobulin production is unknown. Graves' disease is characterized by diffuse thyroid enlargement (goiter), hyperthyroidism, ophthalmopathy, and occasionally pretibial myxedema (Toft, 2001; Yen, 2007).

Other causes of thyrotoxicosis include toxic multinodular goiter, toxic adenoma, subacute thyroiditis, autoimmune thyroiditis, excessive exogenous thyroid hormone, excessive pituitary TSH, or trophoblastic disease (Yen, 2007).

Epidemiology

Graves' disease, which accounts 60 to 80 percent of all cases of thyrotoxicosis, appears to be familial in origin. Family history also shows an increased incidence of other autoimmune disorders. Toxic multinodular goiter (Plummer's disease) accounts for 15 to 20 percent of thyrotoxicosis and usually occurs in areas where there is iodine deficiency. It is usually seen after age 50 in individuals with preexisting nontoxic goiter. Silent thyroiditis occurs fairly frequently in postpartal women.

Graves' disease occurs predominantly among women 20 to 40 years old. Up to 2 percent of women are affected. Either sex at any age may be affected (Toft, 2001).

Subjective Data

Clients may report tremulousness; palpitations; exertional tolerance and dyspnea; heat intolerance; increased perspiration; eye irritation, excessive lacrimation, photophobia, and diplopia; dyspnea; unexplained weight loss despite increased appetite; frequent bowel movements; fatigue; weakness, especially of the proximal muscles; and decreased menstrual flow or amenorrhea.

Objective Data

Symptoms are related to excessive sympathomimetic activity and increased catabolic activity. Older people do not usually present with classic symptoms. Cardiac symptoms, including atrial fibrillation, are more common among older people, whereas goiter and eye symptoms may be absent.

Physical Examination

- *General appearance:* Rapid, rambling, anxious speech.
- *Vital signs:* Tachycardia, systolic hypertension, widened pulse pressure.
- *Skin:* Warm, smooth, moist skin and onycholysis.
- *Eyes:* Exophthalmus, proptosis, upper lid retraction, periorbital swelling.
- *Neck:* Enlarged, soft thyroid gland, nodules, thyroid bruits.
- *Chest:* Tachypnea.
- *Heart:* Atrial fibrillation, hyperdynamic apical impulse, systolic flows murmur.
- *Vascular system:* Bounding peripheral pulses.
- *Abdomen:* Hyperactive bowel sounds.
- *Musculoskeletal system:* Myopathy, especially in the proximal lower extremities.
- *Central nervous system:* Fine tremor, hyperreflexia.

Diagnostic Laboratory Tests. Show an elevated serum free T4 and a low TSH. If results are normal yet suspicion remains high, refer the client to an endocrinologist for further evaluation. Additional studies might include a serum T3 or thyrotropin-releasing hormone test. An enzyme-linked immunoabsorbent assay for anti-thyroid autoantibody might also be done to differentiate between autoimmune thyroiditis and toxic multinodular goiter and toxic adenoma. Expectorants, amiodarone, herbals containing large amounts of seaweed, or ionated contrast dyes may precipitate thyrotoxicosis (Lee & Ananthakrishnan, 2011). Dopamine hydrochloride and corticosteroids can suppress TSH levels (Cooper, 2001; Toft, 2001; Yen, 2007).

If diagnosis is not clear after laboratory testing, radiographic imaging studies, thyroid nuclear scintigraphy iodine 123 may be useful to diagnose.

Differential Medical Diagnoses

Amphetamine or cocaine abuse, anxiety states/panic disorder, chronic obstructive pulmonary disease, pheochromocytoma, myeloproliferative disease, diabetes.

Plan

Treatment must be individualized with consideration to the etiology and severity of disease, client's age, concomitant disease, and risks and benefits of therapeutic modalities (Klein & Ojamaa, 2001; Yen, 2007).

Psychosocial Interventions. Reassure the client that her condition is not a malignant process and can be treated quite effectively.

Medication. Antithyroid drugs, beta blockers, and radioactive iodine are used.

Antithyroid Drugs. Antithyroid drugs are not without significant side effects; in rare cases, potentially fatal reactions can occur. The client should be referred to an endocrinologist for treatment. Methmazole (Tapazole) 5 to 20 mg/day initially; 5 to 20 mg/day maintenance; thought to be the more potent than PTU; may be given in one daily dose. PTU 300 to 600 mg/day initially; 50 to 200 mg/day maintenance; must be given in three equally divided doses because of its shorter half-life; PTU is the drug of choice in pregnancy as it is more highly protein bound and crosses the placenta less readily. Liver function must be monitored carefully in patients receiving PTU as there is increased risk for liver toxicity (Lee & Ananthakrishnan, 2011). The medication may be reduced by half when the client's symptoms have resolved, the goiter has decreased, and the T4 has normalized. It is not useful to check labs more often than every 4 to 8 weeks. Drug therapy is maintained for 1 year. Approximately 50 to 60 percent of clients will experience a relapse (Cooper, 2001; Toft, 2001; Yen, 2007).

- *Side effects:* The most frequent side effects are rash, malaise, fever, urticaria, arthralgia, gastrointestinal disturbances, and loss of taste. Transient leukopenia occurs in approximately 12 percent of adults.
- *Contraindication:* Do not administer antithyroid drugs to clients with cardiac disease.
- *Anticipated outcome on evaluation:* Level of circulating thyroid hormone decreases as evidenced by a return to normal TSH level.
- *Client teaching:* Inform the client that although the duration of therapy is controversial, it is rarely longer than 2 years.

Beta Blockers. Beta blockers are indicated to alleviate symptoms of thyrotoxicosis: tachycardia, palpitations, hypertension, tremor, heat intolerance, and anxiety. Beta blockers are used as an adjunct to radioactive iodine until its therapeutic effect is achieved. Propranolol (Inderal) is the most commonly used beta blocker. The goal is to titrate the dose to maintain a heart rate between 70 and 90 and decrease other symptoms. The usual dose is 160 mg/day in either divided doses or long-acting preparation. See section on hypertension for further discussion of beta blockers. Beta blockers should not be administered to patients with history of asthma. Calcium channel blockers may be prescribed when Beta blocker therapy is contraindicated or not tolerated (Lee & Ananthakrishnan, 2011).

Iodine or iodinated contrast agents are sometimes administered to block conversion to T4 to T3 in patients with Graves' disease. These agents should not be given to patients with toxic multinodular goiter or toxic adenoma.

Radioactive Iodine. Radioactive iodine is the treatment of choice for clients over age 40. The client is referred to an endocrinologist for administration.

- *Administration:* The tracer dose of radioactive iodine in tablet form is administered and followed by irradiation.
- *Side effects:* Within the first year, hypothyroidism occurs in 10 percent of those treated. The likelihood of hypothyroidism developing increases by 5 percent each subsequent year over the next 20 years.
- *Contraindication:* Radioactive iodine is never administered to pregnant women.
- *Anticipated outcome on evaluation:* If an adequate dose of radioactive iodine is given, it will be 100 percent effective. Approximately 20 percent of clients require a second dose. Complete resolution of symptoms occurs within 6 months of treatment.
- *Client teaching:* Inform the client that radioactive iodine is inexpensive and effective. Many clients then exhibit hypothyroidism and require T4 replacement. Periodic testing for hypothyroidism (TSH level) should be done indefinitely. The amount of radiation received is comparable to the amount necessary to perform a barium enema. Clients should not become pregnant for 6 months after treatment.
- *Surgical interventions:* Surgical intervention is limited and controversial. It may be an option for pregnant women or for those who do not respond to antithyroid medications.

Surgical Therapy. Thyroidectomy, partial or complete, is the oldest means of treating thyrotoxicosis, but is most often reserved for special cases currently.

Follow-Up

The treatment will dictate the follow-up. Educate the client about the symptoms of hyper- and hypothyroidism.

THYROID NODULES

A thyroid nodule is a mass that presents as a single palpable nodule or as a part of a multinodular gland. The diagnostic challenge is to distinguish a benign nodule from a malignancy.

Epidemiology

Studies often reveal a history of radiation exposure. The period of latency ranges from 5 to 35 years, with an average of 20 years. A family history of thyroid malignancies or endocrine tumors is common. About 20 to 30 percent of persons exposed to ionizing radiation develop palpable thyroid abnormalities; 50 percent have nodules. Of those nodules, 30 to 50 percent are malignant. Single nodules are more likely to be malignant than is a multinodular gland (Hermus & Huysmans, 1998; Yen, 2007).

Incidence reports reveal that about 4 percent of the adult population has thyroid nodules; the incidence increases to 5 percent among individuals older than 60 years. Nodules are four times more common in women than men; however, malignant nodules are more common in men. At least 95 percent of all palpable nodules are benign (Hermus & Huysmans, 1998; Yen, 2007).

Thyroid cancer is rare, and deaths from thyroid cancer are even rarer.

Subjective Data

A client may report a medical history of thyroid disorders, endocrine tumors, and/or head or neck irradiation. Although most women are asymptomatic, a client may have hoarseness, vocal cord paralysis, and dysphagia.

Objective Data

Physical Examination. May be unremarkable or reveal symptoms of hypo- or hyperthyroidism. Nodules range from barely palpable to visible; their physical characteristics do not secure a diagnosis of benign or malignant. Although nodules may be tender, most are nontender. Thyroid malignancy is suggested by a solitary firm nodule with associated nontender cervical lymphadenopathy.

Diagnostic Methods. These include thyroid function tests, biopsy, and imaging. Laboratory tests usually show normal thyroid function (Cooper et al., 2009).

A fine-needle aspiration biopsy is the most reliable diagnostic method. If the aspirate shows malignancy, the probability is that it is 95 percent correct. If suspicious, a 45 percent chance of malignancy is probable. Biopsy determines which nodules will be surgically excised; biopsy is the only definitive evaluation and surgery the definitive treatment. Ultrasonography determines consistency but does not define benign versus malignant disease. It is used as a guide for fine-needle aspiration. The test procedure requires an experienced cytologist. It is safe, inexpensive, and accurate. A fine-needle aspiration biopsy followed by a thyroid scan for suspicious lesions seems to be the most cost-effective approach.

Radionuclide imaging classifies nodules as hot or cold. A malignant lesion incorporates less iodine than normal thyroid tissue; therefore, it should appear cold. This technique is not sensitive; although a hot nodule reduces the likelihood of malignancy, it does not exclude the possibility (Hermus & Huysmans, 1998; Yen, 2007).

Thyroid suppression is controversial and logistically difficult to interpret because of clinical limitations in sizing nodules.

Differential Medical Diagnoses

Hemorrhagic cysts, Hashimoto's thyroiditis.

Plan

Psychosocial Interventions. Inform the client that although it is rare for a nodule to be malignant, the risk is real.

Surgical Interventions. Surgical management of thyroid cancer is controversial. It is generally agreed that the nodule be removed and suppressive therapy utilized. The amount of thyroid to be removed (one lobe or total thyroidectomy) and the method of follow-up may vary.

Follow-Up

Refer all clients with thyroid nodules to an endocrinologist who will manage treatment.

DIABETES MELLITUS

Diabetes mellitus is a chronic disorder that is characterized by hyperglycemia; associated with major abnormalities in carbohydrate, fat, and protein metabolism; accompanied by a marked propensity to develop relatively specific forms of renal, ocular, neurologic, and premature cardiovascular diseases (American Diabetes Association [ADA], 2011a).

Diabetes often presents with clinical signs and symptoms of polyuria, polydipsia, polyphagia, weight loss, and/or blurred vision with persistent hyperglycemia. Previously, diagnostic criterion was limited to when fasting plasma glucose levels exceed 110 and/or random plasma glucose levels exceed 126 on at least three separate occasions (ADA, 2002a, 2002b). In 2010, the ADA added the option of use of a glycosolated hemoglobin A1c (HgbA1c) result of greater than or equal to 6.5 percent (confirmed by repeat testing in absence of unequivocal hyperglycemia) for diagnosis of diabetes when a laboratory method certified by the National Glycohemoglobin Standardization Program and standardized to the Diabetes Control and Complications Trial is available. They also changed the diagnostic criteria for fasting plasma glucose levels to a level greater than or equal to 126 mg/dL with or without symptoms (confirmed by repeat testing in absence of unequivocal hyperglycemia) and the random plasma glucose level to greater than or equal to 200 mg/dL for those with symptoms (ADA, 2010).

The causes of diabetes are unknown, although current thought includes genetic predisposition, unknown precipitating events, progressive autoimmune destruction of pancreatic beta cells, and obesity (ADA, 2010; Hu et al., 2001).

Epidemiology

The majority of diabetes can be classified into two types: type 1 or insulin-dependent diabetes mellitus (absolute insulin deficiency) and type 2 or non-insulin-dependent diabetes mellitus (NIDDM). (Type 2 diabetes is currently subdivided into insulin resistance with insulin deficiency or insulin secretory defect with insulin resistance.) Some patients will not clearly fit into one category or the other (ADA, 2011a, 2011b). Roughly 90 to 95 percent of diabetes cases are type 2. Roughly 7 percent of all pregnancies are complicated by gestational diabetes (ADA, 2010). Women who experience gestational diabetes may be at higher risk for the development of type 2 diabetes over time. Additionally, hyperglycemia during pregnancy may actually be a manifestation of impaired glucose tolerance prior to pregnancy. The International Association of Pregnancy and Diabetes Study Group recommends that women found to be hyperglycemic at their first prenatal visits should be diagnosed with overt diabetes rather than gestational diabetes (ADA, 2010). Other types of diabetes can be associated with other specific conditions or syndromes (pancreatic, endocrine, medications) and are beyond the scope of this book.

Type 1 (Insulin-Dependent or Absolute Insulin Deficiency) Diabetes. According to the National Diabetes Information Clearinghouse (2011), type 1 diabetes annual incidence rate in the under 20 age group is 19.7 per 100,000 for those under 10 and 18.6 per 100,000 for those between 10 and 20 years of age. Type 1 can develop at any age, although generally most cases are diagnosed when the client is under 30 (ADA, 2011b). Overall, type 1 diabetes comprises only 5 to 10 percent of all diabetes cases. Type 1 diabetes may result from autoimmune destruction or from unknown etiologies,

Clients with type 1 diabetes are insulinopenic. Insulin therapy is essential to prevent rapid and severe dehydration, catabolism, ketoacidosis, and death. They are usually lean and often have experienced significant weight loss, polyuria, and polydipsia before presentation.

Type 2 (Non-Insulin-Dependent or Insulin Resistance and Relative Insulin Deficiency) Diabetes. Type 2 diabetes is characterized by fasting hyperglycemia, insulin secretory defects, and insulin resistance. It is usually diagnosed after age 40 but can occur at any age. It affects an estimated 90 to 95 percent of Americans diagnosed with diabetes. Many individuals with type 2 diabetes are overweight or obese. Because type 2 diabetes is a slowly progressive disease that often is asymptomatic, it may go undiagnosed (ADA, 2011b).

The likelihood of developing type 2 is approximately equal by sex but is greater in African Americans, Hispanics, and Native Americans. Obesity (more than 20% over ideal body weight), a family history of diabetes, age 40 or over, hypertension, hypercholesterolemia, gestational diabetes, or having one or more infants weighing more than 9 lb at birth are major risk factors (ADA, 2011b; Yanovski & Yanovski, 2002).

Type 2 diabetes is characterized by insulin resistance and is present in the majority of all clients with fasting blood sugar greater than 126. Sites of insulin resistance include hepatic and peripheral tissues. Postbinding abnormalities are primarily responsible for insulin resistance. Impaired binding may be secondary to associated obesity and hyperinsulinemia but may also contribute to impaired tissue insulin sensitivity. Diet recall may reveal high fats, sweets, and starches. There is evidence that weight reduction, exercise, and diet change are beneficial in primary and secondary prevention of NIDDM (ADA, 2011a, 2011b).

The ADA recommends screening adults with one or more risk factors every 3 years.

Impaired Glucose Tolerance. Impaired glucose tolerance is characterized by a fasting plasma glucose level of > 110 mg/dL and < 125 mg/dL, a HgbA1c of 5.7 to 6.4 percent, or a 2-hour oral glucose tolerance test result of 140 to 199 mg/dL (ADA, 2011b). These clients may develop type 2 diabetes and should be monitored closely.

Subjective Data

The client may report a history of weight loss, polydipsia, polyuria, polyphagia, blurred vision, endocrine disorders, alcoholism, pancreatitis, gestational diabetes, medications (e.g., steroids, thiazide, diuretic), frequent urinary tract infections, yeast vaginitis, poor healing wounds, or a family history of diabetes.

Objective Data

- *General:* Recent weight gains or losses.
- *Eyes:* Fundoscopic-diabetic retinopathy.
- *Mouth/throat:* Candidiasis.
- *Gastrointestinal:* Diminished bowel sounds. Right upper quadrant (RUQ) tenderness (pancreatitis).
- *Genitourinary:* Vulvovaginal candidiasis.
- *Neurological:* Decreased sensation peripherally, gait disturbances, carpal tunnel syndrome.
- *Extremities:* Decreased pulses, poor healing wounds, temperature, or color changes.
- *Diagnostic:* A random blood sugar over 200 mg/dL at any time. A fasting blood sugar > 126 mg/dL, a HgbA1c greater than 6.5 percent, or a two-hour oral glucose tolerance test over 200 mg/dL (confirmed by repeat testing in absence of unequivocal hyperglycemia) (ADA, 2011b).
- *Other lab:* Elevated amylase (pancreatitis) or lipids (especially triglycerides).

Differential Medical Diagnoses

Medication induced diabetes (steroids, thiazide, diuretics), hypothyroidism, hyperthyroidism, HIV, substance abuse.

Plan

The goals are to achieve normal metabolic control, reduce the potential for development of complications, promote a reasonable body weight, and encourage healthy eating habits. The Diabetes Control and Complications Trial (ADA, 2002b) showed an overall reduction in potential complication when these goals are achieved. Before treating, assess the client's self-care attitudes, abilities, and priorities.

Treatment modalities include dietary modifications, increased physical activity, pharmacologic intervention, and intensive and continued client education (ADA, 2011a).

Psychosocial Interventions. The diagnosis of diabetes is a lifelong, life-altering one. Explore the client's perception of self-image, health beliefs, and perception of diabetes. Consider a referral to a diabetes support group.

Dietary Interventions. The client should be encouraged to follow a low-fat, no-added-salt diet and to avoid sweets. Consider a referral to a nutritionist and the local chapter of the ADA or the local diabetes educators in your community.

Physical Activity. Encourage the client to develop a regular exercise plan based on her current fitness level. Establish fitness goals and follow-up at regular visits.

Pharmacologic Intervention. The type 1 diabetic is essentially insulinopenic and requires exogenous insulin. The type 2 or NIDDM diabetic will require pharmacologic intervention when diet modification and increased physical activity fails to control glucose levels alone. The physiologic abnormalities of NIDDM progress gradually over time and then lose efficacy. Five years of success on a given treatment is what may reasonably be expected.

Oral Agent Therapy. Therapies for insulin deficiency:

- *Sulfonylureas.* All sulfonylureas act by increasing the secretion of endogenous insulin in response to fasting and postprandial blood glucose levels. In choosing a sulfonylurea (or any agent), expense, ease of dosing, comorbid conditions, and efficacy in lowering blood glucose must be considered (see Table 23–17). There is greater risk for hypoglycemia with these agents, particularly among older people. Doses should start low with slow titration. They should be used with caution in patients with impaired renal (serum creatinine > 2.0) or hepatic function. Glyburide is the longest acting agent of the sulfonylureas and may contribute to hypoglycemia more than other agents in the class and, for that reason, is used less often. See any drug handbook for dosing information.
- *Amino acid derivatives (rapeglinide and nateglinide).* These medications lower postprandial and fasting blood sugar with greatest effect on postprandial blood glucoses. They should be administered within 30 minutes of meals. This class should not be prescribed with sulfonylureas due to increased risk of hypoglycemia. See any drug handbook for dosing information.
- *Alphaglucosidase inhibitors (acarbose and miglitol).* This class of medications targets postprandial glucose by blocking enzymes that digest starches in the small intestine resulting in decreased absorption of glucose. They can be used in combination with any other oral agent; however, there is some indication that they may decrease the bioavailability of metformin, while having an additive effect on gastrointestinal side effects. Usage is limited by side effect profile that includes increased flatulence, diarrhea, and abdominal distention. These agents should be taken at the beginning of a meal. See any drug handbook for dosing information.

TABLE 23–17. Non-Insulin Agents for Control of Diabetes

Oral Agent Therapy		
Agent	Dose Range (mg)	Doses/Day
	First-Generation Sulfonylureas	
Tolbultamide	500–3,000	bid or tid
Tolazamide	100–1,000	qd or bid
Chlorproamide	100–500	qd
	Second-Generation Sulfonylureas	
Glipizide	2.5–40	qd or bid
Glyburide	5–20	qd
Micronized glyburide	0.75–12	qd
Gliperamide	1–4	qd
	Other Agents	
Acarbose	25–50	tid with meals
Metformin	500–2,000	bid or tid
Pioglitazone[a]	15–30	qd
Rosiglitazone[a]	2–8	bid
Repaglinide	0.5–4	30 min before meals
Nateglinide	60–120	30 min before meals
Sitagliptan	25–100	Daily

Injectable Agent Therapy				
Agent	Dose Range	Doses/Day	Peak	Half-life
Exenatide	5–10 mcg	bid	2 hours	2.4 hours
Liraglutide	0.6–1.8 mg	Daily	8–12 hours	~13 hours

[a]Use is restricted (FDA, 2011).

Sources: Ahmann & Riddle, 2002; Hsu et al., 2001; Warren-Boulton, Greenberg, Lising, & Gallivan, 1999; Wilson, Shannon, & Shields, 2012.

Therapies for insulin resistance:

- *Biguanide (metformin or glucophage).* Metformin targets fasting blood sugar and should be considered first line for treatment of NIDDM in those who have no contraindications and are able to tolerate it. Metformin is absorbed from the gastrointestinal tract over approximately 6 hours and excreted by the kidneys without being metabolized. It decreases glucose production in the liver and increases glucose uptake but does not cause clinical hypoglycemia. It has no effect on pancreatic insulin secretion and requires the presence of insulin to be effective. It is used to overcome insulin resistance. It can be given alone or with other oral agents, Byetta, or insulin. Metformin has been shown to promote weight loss in some patients.
    - Administration: Metformin is available as 500 and 850 mg tablets. The starting dose is low with once a day dosing initially to offset gastrointestinal side effects with titration over 1 to 2 weeks to twice daily dosing. The extended release form may reduce gastrointestinal side effects. Usual dosing is 1 to 2 g daily dose divided into two doses. There is no clinical benefit to prescribing amounts greater than 2 g/day.
    - Adverse effects: Metformin can cause a metallic taste, diarrhea, nausea, vomiting, and anorexia. Most of these symptoms diminish or disappear with a decreased dose or discontinuance of the drug.
    - Lactic acidosis: All biguanides inhibit lactate metabolism, and increased concentrations of the

drug associated with renal impairment can cause lactic acidosis. Even a temporary reduction in renal function, such as occurs after angiography, can cause lactic acidosis. The drug should be discontinued 2 days before such procedures and restarted only after renal function returns to normal. Increased alcohol intake, conditions associated with hypoxemia (heart failure, shock, hepatic failure), or surgery are indication for stopping metformin (ADA, 2002b). Metformin is contraindicated in females with a serum creatinine ≥1.4.

- *Thiazolidinediones (pioglitazone and rosiglitazone).* These insulin sensitizer agents have been found to have health risks and their use has been discouraged by some. Rosiglitazone has been linked to cardiovascular risks, and pioglitazone to risk for bladder cancer, and another drug in this category, troglitazone, was removed from the market in 2000 because of risk for liver toxicity (AAFP, 2011). They act to decrease insulin resistance by making muscle, fat, and liver cells more sensitive to insulin. They also decrease gluconeogenesis in the liver. They also have effects on lipids, increasing HDL, increasing LDL, and decreasing TG. Pioglitazone has more favorable lipid effects than rosiglitazone (Goldberg et al., 2005). The FDA (2011a) requires that use of rosiglitazone be limited to those patients who are currently using the drug and for whom no other treatment is effective. This may be done through Risk Evaluation and Mitigation Strategy. These agents require monitoring of liver function and should be avoided in patients with history of liver disease. See any drug handbook for dosing information.

Combination Therapy. The combination of *metformin* and *sulfonylurea* was found superior to treatment with either drug alone (ADA, 2002b). This has been shown to lower plasma glucose and glycosylated hemoglobin values in clients with NIDDM who had poor responses to maximal doses of a sulfonylurea. It is recommended to start with either metformin or a sulfonylurea, increase as indicated, and add the second agent when the maximum dosage has been reached. Due to the progressive nature of diabetes in some clients, oral agents will fail and insulin should be started. For most, this will mean a permanent commitment to insulin. There are numerous combination drugs available including metformin/sulfonylurea, metformin/thiazolidinedione, metformin/amino acid derivative, metformin/dipeptidyl peptidase, and sulfonylurea/thiazolidinedione.

Therapies for incretin deficiency:

- *Dipeptidyl peptidase IV inhibitors (sitagliptin and saxagliptin).* These agents inhibit enzymes in the gut that inactivate gastrointestinal hormones (incretins) that stimulate the release of insulin from the pancreas after eating before blood sugar rises. They target postprandial blood glucose levels. These agents can be used as monotherapy or in combination with other agents. They are not likely to cause hypoglycemia when used as monotherapy, but have a limited effect on glycosylated hemoglobin. They may contribute to increased upper respiratory infections and are associated with headaches and gastrointestinal upset. A reduced dosage is required in patients with renal impairment. See any drug handbook for dosing information.
- *Incretin mimetic (Byetta and Victoza).* These agents mimic the action of incretin by enhancing the glucose-dependent insulin release that occurs after eating, inhibiting glucagon production, and delaying gastric emptying. They target postprandial glucose levels. They can be used as monotherapy or adjunct therapy, but are most often used as adjunct therapy. Sulfonylurea dosages should be reduced if these are added to reduce the incidence of hypoglycemia. They should not be used in patients with renal impairment. Victoza carries a black-box warning that it has been linked to the development of thyroid cancer and patients should be carefully screened for family or personal history of thyroid cancers. Both of these medications are injected subcutaneously. They may promote weight loss.
- *Synthetic human amylin analog (pramlintide).* Amylin is a hormone produced in the beta cells of the pancreas along with insulin. This drug is used as an adjunct to postprandial glucose control in type 1 and type 2 diabetic patients who are using premeal insulin. It helps promote control of postprandial blood glucose by slowing intestinal glucose absorption, decreasing glucagon release, and delaying gastric emptying. It may promote weight loss and is effective in reducing premeal insulin needs.

Insulin Therapy

INSULIN-DEPENDENT DIABETES (TYPE I). In these clients, the production of insulin by the beta cell is lost and the client becomes dependent on the use of exogenous insulin. Understanding the actions of the various insulins is crucial to designing an insulin program that will mimic the body's own insulin release.

Intensive insulin therapy in three or more injections a day, with home glucose monitoring, will provide ideal control. The basal dose of insulin is given as either a long-acting or an intermediate-acting insulin. A bolus dose is given premeal to mimic the endogenous release of insulin at mealtimes. Typically, 50 percent of daily insulin is given as basal insulin and 50 percent is given as bolus insulin. Starting dose for type 1 diabetes is 0.3 units of insulin per kilogram per day. Before adjusting doses, confirm diet and exercise patterns, recent illnesses or stressors, any hypoglycemia or hyperglycemia events, or other medication changes (see Table 23–18).

NON-INSULIN-DEPENDENT DIABETES (TYPE 2). These clients may require exogenous insulin to supplement decreased endogenous production or decreased insulin response. The starting dose in NIDDM is 0.4 to 0.5 units of insulin per kilogram per day. It is best to match the peak action of insulin to the rise in glucose that occurs in the early morning hours between 3 and 8 a.m. Therefore, the evening dose could be administered at bedtime (Stoller, 2002).

Follow-Up

Follow-up should be individualized based on the client's current needs. Perform regular screening for microvascular and macrovascular complications (ADA, 2011a). Glycosylated hemoglobin should be monitored quarterly to biannually dependent on control, renal and liver function should be monitored at least annually dependent on medication regimen, and urine microalbumin and urinalysis should be monitored at least annually. Additionally, diabetic patients should have annual eye exams, biannual dental exams, and quarterly foot exams. Additional diagnostic and laboratory testing will be dependent on comorbidities. Regular review of the client's home glucose monitoring diary and technique as well as reinforcement of dietary and exercise recommendations is advised. If diabetes is difficult to control, consider other medications as the cause—thiazide can cause hyperglycemia. Beta blockers can mask the signs and symptoms of hypoglycemia.

TABLE 23–18. Insulin Therapy

	Onset of Action	Peak	Duration
Short Acting			
Regular	30–45 minutes	2–3 hours	5–6 hours
Insulin aspart	30 minutes	1–3 hours	3–5 hours
Insulin lispro	30 minutes	30 minutes to 3 hours	2–6 hours
Intermediate Acting			
NPH	2–3 hours	6–9 hours	12–14 hours
Lente	2–3 hours	6–9 hours	12–14 hours
Long Acting			
Ultralente	4–10 hours	8–20 hours	18–28 hours
Insulin glargine	5 hours	Has no pronounced peak	18–28 hours

Sources: Ahmann & Riddle, 2002; American Pharmaceutical Association, 2001; Warren-Boulton et al., 1999.

METABOLIC SYNDROME

Metabolic syndrome is characterized by a constellation of findings: central obesity, hypertension, cholesterol abnormalities including high triglycerides and low HDL, insulin resistance with elevated fasting blood sugar, and increased risk for clotting. Having three of the five criteria is diagnostic for metabolic syndrome (Grundy et al., 2005). These symptoms are risk factors for the development of CAD, stroke, and diabetes mellitus over time. Metabolic syndrome is sometimes referred to as syndrome X and dysmetabolic syndrome. Metabolic syndrome has been linked to polycystic ovary syndrome, fatty liver, onset of type 2 diabetes mellitus in first-degree relative before the age of 60.

Epidemiology

Metabolic syndrome occurs in males and females. It is estimated that 20 to 30 percent of the adult population in industrialized countries has metabolic syndrome (NHLBI, 2010). Aging, genetic predisposition, lack of exercise, and hormonal changes contribute to the development of metabolic syndrome.

Objective data

The waist-to-hip ratio in female patients with metabolic syndrome is typically greater than 9 and waist circumference is greater than 35 in., which are hallmarks of central or abdominal obesity. Blood pressure is typically greater than 130/85. Total cholesterol is usually elevated and triglycerides are greater or equal to 150 mg/dL and HDL is less than 50 mg/dL in women. Fasting blood sugar is greater than 100 mg/dL or patient is treated with drug therapy for elevated blood glucose.

Differential Medical Diagnoses

Type 2 diabetes mellitus, hyperlipidemia, obesity, hypothyroidism, hypertension, polycystic ovary syndrome.

Plan

Psychosocial Interventions. Involve the client as an active partner in management. She may be distressed by being overweight and may require support to reinforce lifestyle changes aimed at managing symptoms.

Medications. Medications that target accompanying risk factors may be prescribed. Blood pressure may be controlled by the use of ACEI such as lisinopril. Blood sugar is often controlled by prescribing metformin or glucophage, a biguanide, which acts to lower blood sugar, improve insulin resistance, and may promote weight loss as well. Target glycosylated hemoglobin is less than 7.0 percent. There is evidence to suggest that metformin may also help restore fertility in those patients with concurrent polycystic ovary syndrome when blood sugars return to normal. A statin medication or a fibric acid derivative may be started for cholesterol abnormalities provided liver function is within normal limits. Choice of lipid-lowering agent may depend on LDL levels. Patients at high risk for clot formation should be started on low-dose aspirin (81 mg) daily. Patients at lower risk may be started on low-dose aspirin for prophylaxis.

Lifestyle/Dietary Changes. Weight loss and increased activity levels are promoted. Target BMI is less than 25 kg/m^2. Goal is to reduce body weight by 7 to 10 percent during the first year of therapy (Grundy et al., 2005). Thirty to 60 minutes of activity at moderate intensity is recommended 5 days of the week or more.

Follow-Up

Follow-up should be regularly scheduled to obtain blood pressure and blood sugar control as well as to promote and reinforce lifestyle changes.

GASTROINTESTINAL DISORDERS

This section covers the following disorders: gastroesophageal reflux disease, peptic ulcer disease, gallbladder disease, irritable bowel syndrome (IBS), anal fissures, and hepatitis.

GASTROESOPHAGEAL REFLUX DISEASE

The American Gastrointestinal Society uses the Montreal Consensus Conference definition of gastroesophageal reflux disease (GERD) stating that it is a "condition that develops when the reflux of stomach contents causes troublesome symptoms and/or complications" (Vakil et al., 2006). Symptoms worsen with lying down or bending over and antacids alleviate the symptoms of heartburn. In this situation, GERD is the presumptive diagnosis unless proven otherwise (DeVault & Castell, 2005). Etiology reveals that hiatal hernias predispose to GERD, but are not pathognomonic. Contributing factors include gastric hyperacidity, impaired esophageal clearance, increased volume of gastric contents, and altered mucosal resistance (Hubbard, 2002; Ray, Secrest, Chien, & Corey, 2002).

Epidemiology

GERD is common at all ages, but more prevalent among persons 60 to 70 years old. The prevalence of GERD in Americans is estimated at 26 percent, with Hispanics having nearly a 50 percent prevalence rate (Yuen et al., 2010).

Early diagnosis and appropriate treatment can prevent secondary complications, such as esophageal strictures, ulcers, Barrett's esophagus, bleeding, pulmonary disease, and hoarseness.

Subjective Data

The client describes a burning sensation or pain underneath the sternum followed by a bitter taste. It may be related to certain foods. Intensity varies, but the sensation usually increases after eating, with forward bending, when supine, or with vigorous exercise. Less common symptoms that may be reported are odynophagia (painful swallowing), dysphagia, and pulmonary manifestations, such as nocturnal coughing, wheezing, and hoarseness.

Objective Data

Physical examination is usually benign. Two approaches are recommended to diagnosis of GERD in those without alarm symptoms (bleeding, anemia, early satiety, dysphagia, unexplained weight loss of > 10%, persistent vomiting, previous esophageal malignancy or peptic ulcer disease, lymphadenopathy, or epigastric mass) under age 55 (Kahrilas, Shaheen, & Vaezi, 2008; Talley & Vakil, 2005). One approach is testing and treating for *Helicobacter pylori* while simultaneously trialing an acid suppressant medication. A second approach is to treat empirically with a proton pump inhibitor (PPI) for 4 to 8 weeks. If an unsatisfactory response is obtained, the dose should be increased or the drug changed. If no response is still forthcoming than test and treating for *H. pylori* and follow up, EGD is recommended (Kahrilas et al., 2008; Talley & Vakil, 2005). Those who respond to either of these therapies can be presumed to have GERD. For those age 55 and over or for those with alarm signs, prompt EGD is recommended (Talley & Vakil, 2005).

Endoscopy. The most definitive approach to diagnosis (DeVault & Castell, 2005) is recommended for patients with GERD symptoms accompanied by dysphagia (Kahrilas et al., 2008). It allows direct visualization of the esophagus using a scope and biopsy of the mucosa to reliably diagnose Barrett's esophagus. Treatment with PPI is warranted prior to EGD to prevent misdiagnosing inflammatory changes. A normal EGD does not rule out GERD, but the inflammatory changes of Barrett's esophagus or esophagitis always confirms GERD (DeVault & Castell, 2005). Endoscopy is usually performed under conscious sedation. Advise the client of the risks (allergic reaction to sedatives, perforation, discomfort/gagging) and benefits of the procedure. It is associated with increased risks for clients who have cardiopulmonary disease, are older people, or are otherwise debilitated.

Esophageal Manometry. Indicated for clients who are not responding to twice daily dosing of a PPI and have a normal appearing esophagus on endoscopy (Kahrilas et al., 2008). Lower esophageal pressure is measured, and esophageal peristalsis and the competence of the lower esophageal sphincter are assessed.

A 24-Hour pH Monitor (a portable unit). Indicated for those with no abnormalities on endoscopic exam and no abnormalities on manometry (Kahrilas et al., 2008). Useful in determining the total acid exposure and identifying episodes of nocturnal reflux and for those without erosive changes on EGD, but in whom acid suppression therapy fails. It is also used to detect the correct placement of the manometer for esophageal manometry (DeVault & Castell, 2005). The pH probe is manually placed in the esophagus; reflux is defined by a distal esophageal pH less than 4.

Differential Medical Diagnoses

Peptic ulcer disease, esophageal strictures, Barrett's esophagus, angina, pancreatic disease, esophageal candidiasis, Zollinger-Ellison syndrome, respiratory disease (Kahrilas et al., 2008).

Plan

In determining the management of symptoms, consider their severity, the cost of procedures, the risk-benefit of diagnostic testing, the age and health status of the client, and the cost of medications.

Psychosocial Interventions. Involve the client as an active partner in management. She should know that the condition is chronic but manageable.

Medication. Medications are not corrective but protect the mucosa from chronic insult. They suppress and neutralize acid and are cytoprotective. Neither surgical nor medical intervention has been shown to regress Barrett's esophagus (DeVault & Castell, 2005). Empirical therapy with antisecretory drugs is a reasonable initial strategy for treatment (Kahrilas et al., 2008).

The acid PPIs (omeprazole, rabeprazole, esomeprazole, pantoprazole, lansoprazole) inactivate the hydrogen-potassium ATPase enzyme that drives the proton pump of the parietal cell. Currently, the PPIs are the mainstay of GERD therapy both for initial treatment and for long-term maintenance having been shown to be more efficacious at eliminating symptoms and healing erosions than any other class of medications (DeVault & Castell, 2005; Kahn, Santana, Donnellan, Preston, & Moayyedi, 2007). There is no evidence of improved efficacy if these drugs are combined with H2 receptor antagonists. Patients should be given twice daily PPI therapy if not responsive to initial treatment with daily dosing. Side effects include headache, diarrhea, constipation, and abdominal pain (Kahrilas et al., 2008). For those with erosive esophagitis, alternate dosing and weekend therapy have not been proven useful in long-term management of GERD (DeVault & Castell, 2005; Kahrilas et al., 2008). However, it is recommended for those with esophagitis that the lowest effective dose for symptom control be used (Kahrilas et al., 2008). Long-term use of PPI may lead to vitamin B_{12} deficiency (Hendler & Rorvik, 2001), magnesium deficiency (FDA, 2011b), and increased risk of osteoporosis and subsequent fractures (Yang, Lewis, Epstein, & Metz, 2006). PPIs should be used with caution in those taking clopidogrel (Gilard et al., 2008) and a recent study has suggested that PPIs are associated with a fourfold increase in certain arrhythmias (Marcus et al., 2010). PPIs should be taken one-half hour before a meal.

H2 receptor agonists block parietal cell actions and thereby decrease gastric acid formation. They are as effective as antacids but have a longer duration of action. They can be obtained as over-the-counter medications. Few side effects are noted; however, close observation for drug interactions is important particularly in elders due to side effect profile and multiple drug interactions.

Sucralfate (Carafate tablets) binds bile salts and pepsin, aids mucosal regeneration, and enhances prostaglandin synthesis, making it cytoprotective. Timing of this drug is difficult particularly in those with polypharmacy.

Surgical Interventions. Surgery may be indicated for clients who have evidence of reflux and failed or are intolerant of PPI therapy (Kahrilas et al., 2008). Surgery is reserved for those who have not responded to simple therapeutic maneuvers or medications, or have advanced disease or complications, such as esophageal stricture, severe bleeding, and pulmonary aspiration. There is little evidence that surgery is protective against the subsequent development of cancer. Surgery is effective in 90 percent of cases; the Nissen fundoplication procedure restores sphincter competence; however, recent studies show that within 5 years of surgery, up to 30 percent of patients resume medications for symptom control. Postoperatively, patients may experience difficulty belching, increased flatulence and diarrhea, as well as dysphagia (Kahrilas et al., 2008). More surgical repairs are now done endoscopically as data is more favorable for this approach than an open approach (DeVault & Castell, 2005).

Lifestyle/Dietary Changes. Pregnancy and obesity may exacerbate symptoms. Lifestyle and dietary changes may be effective initial and adjunctive therapies (Kahrilas et al., 2008). Controlled studies, however, show their benefits are limited to decreasing esophageal acid exposure (DeVault & Castell, 2005).

The diet should not include offending foods such as spicy foods, high-fat foods, alcohol, citrus juices, chocolate, carbonated beverages, and caffeine. Ideal body weight should be maintained and smoking discouraged (Kahrilas et al., 2008). Advise the client to take the following measures:

- Avoid recumbent positions within 3 hours of a meal.
- Elevate the head of the bed on 4- to 6-in. blocks or on a bed wedge.
- Avoid bending forward.
- Avoid constricting clothing.

Follow-Up

Follow-up to determine response to therapy, to reinforce nonpharmacological measures, and to assess for respiratory symptoms.

GALLBLADDER DISEASE

The gallbladder diseases discussed in this chapter include cholecystitis, cholelithiasis, and choledocholithiasis.

Cholecystitis is acute inflammation of the gallbladder, usually caused by a gallstone blocking the outlet of the gallbladder or cystic duct. Edema, infection, and ulceration result. If this process continues, necrosis, perforation, and peritonitis may result. It is characterized by constant and severe upper quadract pain in acute cases.

Cholelithiasis is the presence or formation of gallstones. Generally, gallstones form whenever cholesterol is oversaturated. Gallstones are classified by composition (Greenberger & Paumgartner, 2008). Cholesterol stones constitute 80 percent of all gallstones in the United States and contain, in addition to cholesterol, bile acids, calcium salts, proteins, and phospholipids. *Choledocholithiasis* are stones in the common bile duct which left untreated may progress to gallstone pancreatitis, biliary cirrhosis, or bacterial infection of the bile duct.

Epidemiology

It is estimated that there are 20.5 million cases of gallbladder disease in the United States, with 14.5 million cases occurring among women (Barnes, 2010). The incidence increases with age (Everhart, 2008). Gallbladder disease occurs primarily among overweight women 40 to 65 years of age. Nearly 50 percent of women will experience gallbladder disease by age 75. Other risk factors include ethnicity (American Indian), diabetes, morbid obesity, rapid weight loss, parenteral nutrition (Barnes, 2010; Thomas, 2011). There is a 50 percent chance of recurrence with a previous history of gallbladder disease (Thomas, 2011).

The incidence of gallstones in the United States is approximately 10 percent. Seventy-five percent of stones are thought to be the cholesterol type (Thomas, 2011). Gallbladder disease results in 750,000 cholecystectomies per year (SSAT, 2006). If left untreated, it may progress to cholangitis or pancreatitis, both medical emergencies.

Subjective Data

Initially, a client reports diffuse, intermittent, and temporary RUQ pain, ache, or pressure that occurs at night or early in the morning and may radiate to the right back or flank. It progresses to a continuous, more severe pain and may radiate to the epigastrium or right shoulder. Onset of pain may be sudden and last from 20 minutes to 5 or 6 hours; it may continue as a dull ache for 24 hours or longer. Intervals between episodes vary considerably, from weeks to years. Pain may be accompanied by nausea, vomiting, constipation, or fever (Thomas, 2011).

Objective Data

Physical examination during the acute phase of disease maybe helpful along with diagnostic tests.

Physical Examination. Not helpful in the nonacute phase. During the acute symptom phase, specific changes may be observed:

- *General:* Restless, fever, jaundice.
- *Eyes:* Icteric.
- *Chest:* Clear to auscultation, splinting with respiration.
- *Abdomen:* RUQ tenderness; Murphy's sign (pain to palpation in RUQ) positive in cholecystitis, negative in biliary colic, choledocholithiasis, or cholangitis; a palpable globular mass may be found behind the lower border of the liver.

Both cholecystitis and choledocholithiasis can progress to cholangitis, which is a medical emergency and characterized by Charcot's triad—RUQ pain, fever, and jaundice.

Diagnostic Laboratory Tests. Cholecystitis: Elevated alkaline phosphatase, bilirubin, WBC, and CRP. Choledocholithiasis: Elevated serum bilirubin, conjugated bilirubin, alkaline phosphatase, AST, and ALT. In gallstone pancreatitis, ALT is elevated, while in acute pancreatitis, amylase and lipase are elevated. Cholangitis: May reveal elevations of serum transaminases, alkaline phosphatase (due to obstructed biliary tract), or serum lipase or amylase (gallstone pancreatitis). An increase in WBCs with a left shift denotes cholecystitis or cholangitis.

Ultrasonography is the diagnostic technique of choice as it is fairly sensitive. Ideally, the patient should be fasting up to 6 hours prior to the procedure. It is a quick and inexpensive way to evaluate the liver, pancreas, and other abdominal organs.

Endoscopic retrograde cholangiopancreatography aids in the diagnosis of common duct calculi, biliary dilatation, cystic duct obstruction, and cancer. Stones in the common bile duct can be removed during the procedure, but there is a high risk of pancreatitis postprocedure.

An *oral cholecystogram* is a diagnostic evaluation for cholelithiasis. The client takes iopanic or tyropanoic acid tablets the night before the exam. The dye concentrates in the gallbladder and permits its visualization the following day. The method is well tolerated. It is 90 to 95 percent accurate in detecting stones.

Cholescintigraphy (gallbladder radionucleotide scan or hepatobiliary iminodiacetic acid [HIDA] scan) is more sensitive than ultrasound, but takes longer to perform. Radioactive dye is injected and taken up by the bile allowing more precise visualization of the level of the blockage.

Differential Medical Diagnoses

Angina, peptic ulcer disease, esophageal spasm, appendicitis, intestinal obstruction, gastroesophageal disease, pancreatitis, myocardial ischemia, pyelonephritis, hiatal hernia, hepatitis, and kidney stones.

Plan

Psychosocial Interventions. Discuss with the client that surveillance of recurrence alone may be suitable management for infrequent symptoms and little disability.

Medication. Medication is limited to comfort measures. A client who has asymptomatic gallstones can be monitored and will not necessarily require intervention.

Surgical Interventions. The laparoscopic approach to cholecystectomy is the treatment method of choice for symptomatic gallstone disease. It reduces postoperative pain as well as hospitalization and at-home recovery time and allows same day discharge much of the time. An open approach is used when there is a high index of suspicion for malignancy, cirrhosis, or late in pregnancy.

Lithotripsy, extracorporeal shock-wave therapy of gallstones, although popular a few years back, has fallen out of favor.

Follow-Up

Refer clients with acute cholecystitis to a collaborating physician, gastrointestinal specialist, or surgeon for evaluation and treatment. Acute cholecystitis can be a life-threatening emergency. Major complications are perforation of the gallbladder with resultant peritonitis and internal biliary fistula. Fever, severe pain, and elevated WBC counts are indications for prompt surgical referral. The size, number, and location of gallstones influence the decision to treat aggressively versus conservatively. A more aggressive approach will likely be based on greater pain and disability from biliary attacks.

FUNCTIONAL BOWEL DISORDERS: IRRITABLE BOWEL SYNDROME AND CHRONIC CONSTIPATION

Functional bowel disorders are a group of syndromes that are identified only by symptoms (Longstreth et al., 2006). Two of the most common syndromes (IBS and chronic constipation not covered by IBS) are discussed here. Both syndromes are characterized by disordered transit of the gut. The Rome III criteria have standardized diagnosis and treatment of these syndromes. The etiology of IBS is probably multifactorial. Contraction of colonic smooth muscle is controlled by cyclic alterations of smooth muscle membrane potential. In IBS, the normally orderly movement of colonic contents is altered. The entire gut, particularly the colon, is affected. It is estimated that 10 to 20 percent of adults and adolescents worldwide are afflicted with this syndrome (Longstreth et al., 2006). IBS is diagnosed by excluding other disease entities (Quigley et al., 2009).

Epidemiology

IBS occurs most often among women with first presentation between the ages of 15 and 65, with first presentation to a physician generally between ages 30 and 50 (Quigley et al., 2009). It is one of the most common reasons for referral to gastrointestinal specialists. About 30 percent of the general population may have symptoms, but only 14 percent seek medical attention. There are roughly 3 million ambulatory care visits per year for IBS. Caucasians are affected at twice the rate of blacks and females four times that of males. It is estimated that 10 to 15 percent of adults in the United States have IBS (Quigley et al., 2009). Chronic constipation affects 42 million Americans and is the second most common diagnosis for gastrointestinal complaints in ambulatory care after GERD. In 2004, 13 million prescriptions were filed for these diseases at over $750 million.

Subjective Data

A careful history is the key to diagnosis of both syndromes. Stress has not been shown to precipitate IBS although stress may aggravate symptoms. Poor dietary habits may also be influential. With IBS, 42 to 87 percent of patients report nausea, heartburn, and dyspeptic symptoms. Colic abdominal pain varies in intensity. It may be precipitated by eating, but is typically relieved by a bowel movement. A client may experience diarrhea, constipation, or both. In addition, she may report abdominal distention, increased amounts of rectal mucus, and a feeling of incomplete evacuation. Associated nongastrointestinal symptoms may include lethargy, muscle/joint pain, headache, urinary symptoms, dyspareunia, insomnia, and medication intolerance. IBS frequently coexists with other syndromes including fibromyalgia (20–50% of patients), temperomadibular joint disorder (64%), chronic pelvic pain (50%), and nonulcer dyspepsia and biliary dyskinesia (Quigley et al., 2009).

Patients who have chronic constipation may report straining at defecation, infrequent, or hard or lumpy stools, or incomplete defecation that do not meet the criteria of IBS. Functional constipation occurs in 27 percent of people and is more common in non-Caucasians and women (Longstreth et al., 2006).

Objective Data

Diagnosis for IBS is often made only after other gastrointestinal disorders have been excluded. Consequently, expensive and unnecessary testing may occur. However, further workup should be considered if any of the following occurs: onset of symptoms after age 50, short (acute) history of symptoms, unintended weight loss, nocturnal symptoms, family history of inflammatory bowel disease or colon cancer, rectal bleeding, anemia, recent antibiotic use, abdominal or rectal masses, elevated inflammatory markers, or fever. A detailed history and patterns of other inflammatory diseases in the population guides the workup. At minimum, the initial workup should include a physical examination with abdominal inspection, auscultation, and palpation, as well as a digital rectal exam (Quigley et al., 2009). Workup and treatment is similar to constipation predominant IBS workup (Longstreth et al., 2006).

Physical Examination. May reveal diffuse abdominal tenderness. A rectal exam is essential. Hemorrhoids and anal fissures are evaluated.

Diagnostic Laboratory Tests. If there is a low suspicion for parasites or celiac disease, CBC, ESR or CRP, thyroid function studies, and stool for occult fecal blood may be all the laboratory workup needed. However, if parasites are suspected, examination of stools for ova and parasites (particularly Giardia) is recommended. Serological studies for celiac disease and the ESR would be done if celiac disease is suspected (Quigley et al., 2009). Negative findings point toward the functional bowel diseases.

A *colonoscopy* is additionally indicated for clients older than 40 years or with a strong family history of colon cancer/polyps or for those with persistent diarrhea (Quigley et al., 2009). This test allows sampling of the intestinal mucosa to rule out Crohn's disease and malignancy. Usually, colonoscopy is performed utilizing conscious sedation.

Diagnostic Criteria. Symptoms should occur during the last 3 months for at least 3 or more days per month, with the onset of symptoms being greater than 6 months prior to diagnosis (Longstreth et al., 2006; Quigley et al., 2009). Patients diagnosed with IBS should have abdominal pain or discomfort along with two of the three following criteria: (1) pain or discomfort is relieved with defecation, (2) onset is associated with change in the frequency of stooling, or (3) there is a change in the form or appearance of the stool (Quigley et al., 2009). Supporting factors that occur at least 25 percent of the time help classify patients into IBS subtypes to direct treatment include (1) fewer than three bowel movements per week, (2) hard or lumpy stools, (3) straining at defecation, (4) more than three bowel movements per day, (5) loose (mushy) or watery stools, (6) urgency, (7) mucous passage with stools, (8) abdominal fullness, bloating, or swelling, or (9) a sense of incomplete defecation. Those with diarrhea predominant IBS have one or more of the features from points 1 through 8 and hard stools less than 25 percent of the time. The diarrhea-type IBS occurs about one third of the time and is more common in men. The constipation predominant subtype features symptoms from points 1 through 3 or symptom 9, with loose stools less than 25 percent of the time and also occurs about one third of the time and is more common in women. IBS may also be of the mixed form that has features from both subtypes or occurs cyclically and is estimated to occur in one third to one half of cases (Quigley et al., 2009).

Like IBS, chronic constipation symptoms must be present at least 6 months prior to diagnosis, and have occurred in the last 3 months. At least two of the following must be present during at least 25 percent of defecations: (1) straining, (2) lumpy or hard stools, (3) sensation of incomplete evacuation, (4) sensation of blockage/obstruction, or (5) manual maneuvers to facilitate defecation. Several other criteria do not have a percentage limit but include fewer than three defecations per week, loose stools rarely being present without laxative use, or insufficient criteria to meet an IBS diagnosis (Longstreth et al., 2006). Conditions or diseases often associated with chronic constipation include diabetes, hypothyroidism, hypercalemia, decreased steroid production during the luteal phase of the menstrual cycle, neurologic disorders such as Parkinson's disease or multiple sclerosis, pelvic surgery that may have damaged the pelvic nerve plexus, drug side effects, and poor dietary habits.

Differential Medical Diagnoses

Laxative abuse, lactose intolerance, celiac sprue/gluten enteropathy, ovarian cancer, diverticulitis, endometriosis, pelvic inflammatory disease, Crohn's disease, ulcerative colitis, colon cancer, parasitic infestation, small intestine bacterial overgrowth, sorbitol intolerance, thyroid disorders, diabetes, eating disorders.

Plan

Psychosocial Interventions. Although symptoms can be stress related, overemphasizing the role of stress can induce confusion and guilt in the client. She should know that IBS is a chronic condition that can be managed. Reassure her that her condition is not cancer and will not progress to inflammatory bowel disease. Symptoms are controllable, although it may take time and a trial-and-error approach to find the right therapeutic management for an individual. A plan should focus on diet and lifestyle. Discuss stress reduction techniques.

Medication. Treatment is based on symptoms control. For constipation predominant IBS, bulking agents, though not supported in the literature, are frequently recommended, osmotic laxatives and stool softeners are used, and agents with anticholinergic properties are avoided. Stimulant laxatives may be added to the above for those with chronic constipation. On the other hand, patients with diarrhea predominant IBS may benefit from regular dosing of loperamide (Quigley et al., 2009). Cholestryramine (Longstreth et al., 2006), tricyclic antidepressants (Quigley et al., 2009), or selective serotonin reuptake inhibitors (Quigley et al., 2009) may also improve the situation. Where pain is the predominant component of IBS, antispasmodics may be used (Longstreth et al., 2006; Quigley et al., 2009), although compliance is difficult due to side effects. A promising agent, tegaserod (Zelnorm), was removed from the market by the FDA because of a risk of increased heart attack and stroke. Currently, there is no evidence to support the use of charcoal-containing agents or simethicone in treating accompanying flatulence or bloating (Quigley et al., 2009).

Psyllium is a bulk laxative that improves regularity and is the main pharmacotherapeutic intervention for either the constipation or the diarrheal subtypes of IBS (Quigley et al., 2009). *Polyethylene glycol (Miralax)* has been shown to improve stool frequency in the constipation subtype of IBS (Graham, 2009).

Loperamide HCl, 2 mg every morning or 2 mg twice daily, will help control diarrhea (Quigley et al., 2009).

Antispasmodic agents such as dicyclomine hydrochloride (Bentyl) are used for abdominal pain and cramping (Quigley et al., 2009).

A tricyclic antidepressant or *selective serotonin reuptake inhibitor* is used when depression, with or without anxiety, is present and may help decrease abdominal pain (Quigley et al., 2009).

Lubiprostone (Amitizia) has been approved by the FDA at 8 mcg twice daily for treatment for the constipation subtype of IBS. Side effects include nausea, diarrhea, abdominal pain, and headache.

Alosetron (Lotronex), although approved by the FDA to treat the diarrheal subtype of IBS, carries a black-box warning regarding ischemic colitis and interacts with many common medications. After introduction, it was removed from the market, but then reallowed into the U.S. market with significant postmarket surveillance. Common side effects include upset stomach and hemorrhoids.

Lifestyle/Dietary Changes. These changes include modifications in diet, exercise, and elimination.

Dietary treatment for functional bowel disease is not well supported in the literature, but frequently recommended. Review the diet of the patient and adjust fiber recommendations (usually lowering fiber requirements). Patients should avoid insoluble fiber (bran) and increase soluble fiber (oats), to eat at regular hours, to chew food thoroughly, and to increase intake of noncaffeinated fluids, especially water. Reducing caffeinated beverages to three cups daily and avoiding alcohol and carbonated beverages may all improve symptoms. For diarrhea predominant IBS, avoidance of lactose, fructose, and sorbitol may be helpful (NICE, 2008). Probiotic trials in IBS treatment have been promising (Longstreth et al., 2006; Quigley et al., 2009). For those with chronic constipation, a high fiber (20–30 g) diet is recommended, along with increasing noncaffeinated beverages of eight to ten 8-oz glasses per day.

Daily exercise is helpful (Longstreth et al., 2006). Also advise the client to avoid straining at bowel movements; the urge to defecate should be promptly followed by elimination and clients should take advantage of the colonic reflex that occurs 20 to 30 minutes after eating a meal to help evacuate a bowel movement.

Follow-Up

A diagnosis of IBS does not require frequent x-rays or colonscopic examinations. In general, no follow-up is needed unless diarrhea persists longer than 2 weeks or symptoms continue to cause persistent inconvenience or dysfunction (Quigley et al., 2009). Encourage the client to return should her symptoms exacerbate or change. IBS is a chronic illness that requires support and reinforcement of the prescribed therapeutic regimen.

HEPATITIS

Hepatitis is an inflammation of the liver caused by any one of several viruses or other factors. Five different viruses—hepatitis A, B, C, D, and E—are responsible for most liver infections. Hepatitis B, C, and D lead to chronic hepatitis, a disease that can lead to cirrhosis, hepatic cancer, and death.

Hepatitis A is the most common form of hepatitis. Hepatitis A is spread through a fecal-oral route and is most contagious in the late incubation period before symptoms develop. People at risk include international travelers, people who travel or come from areas to areas where the hepatitis A vaccine is not routinely dispensed, daycare employees, homosexuals, and illicit drug users. The number of new cases of hepatitis A has decreased each year due to widespread vaccination of children. There are an estimated 36,000 new cases annually in the United States (Wasley, Grytdal, & Gallagher, 2008) with the greatest number of cases in the 20 to 39 age group. Hepatitis A does not produce long-term complications, and recovery is usually complete in 1 to 2 months. Infected individuals do not remain carriers and attacks resolve on their own.

It is estimated that 200,000 to 300,000 persons become infected with hepatitis B virus (HBV) each year in the United States, with the greatest number of cases in males 25 to 44 years old (Wasley et al., 2008). Approximately 730,000 people in the United States have chronic, asymptomatic HBV infection (Wasley et al., 2010). Routine screening for HBV infection in the general population is not recommended; however, routine screening of pregnant women at their first prenatal visit is strongly recommended (USPSTF, 2004a, 2009). Those at risk for hepatitis B include people who had blood transfusions before 1987, health care workers, immigrants, mothers who are infected passing on the virus to their children in the prenatal period, hemodialysis patients, those with multiple sexual partners, homosexuals, and IV drug users. HBV is discussed in more detail in Chapter 14.

Hepatitis C is the most common bloodborne pathogen in the United States and is spread through contaminated needles, blood transfusions (especially prior to 1992), and possibly sexual contact (AHRQ, 2010; USPSTF, 2004b). Symptoms are similar to hepatitis B. Over 3.2 million Americans are chronically infected with HCV (Wasley, Miller, & Finelli, 2007). Fifty to 80 percent or greater of those with acute infection progress to chronic disease, with 20 to 30 percent advancing to cirrhosis (Iosue, 2002; Lauer & Walker, 2001). Hepatitis C is one of the most common reasons for liver transplantation (Wasley et al., 2010). Liver cancer is also possible. No vaccine has been developed for hepatitis C (CDC, 2011b). People at risk for hepatitis C include IV drug users, those with piercings or tattoos, those who have sex with infected people or multiple partners, those who had blood transfusions before July of 1992, health care workers, children born to infected mothers, and hemodialysis patients.

Hepatitis D occurs in conjunction with hepatitis B. Transmission is from contaminated needles; sexual contact is less likely. There is no vaccine for hepatitis D, although vaccination against hepatitis B is protective (CDC, 2011b). People at risk include IV drug users, those who live with or have sex with infected people, or patients who received blood transfusions before 1987.

Hepatitis E is a virus spread similarly to hepatitis A. Hepatitis E is rare in the United States. The FDA has not approved a vaccination for hepatitis E (CDC, 2011b). Those at risk include international travelers or people who live with or have sex with infected people.

Subjective Data

The client may complain of fatigue, lack of appetite, nausea and vomiting, muscle and joint aches, low-grade fever, rash, abdominal pain, diarrhea, headache, and jaundice.

Objective Data

Exam may be normal in acute phase

- *General:* Client may be ill-appearing and/or jaundiced.
- *Eyes:* Icteric in acutely ill.
- *Oropharynx:* Pharyngitis may be present in hepatitis A.
- *Lungs:* Rhonchi and/or wheezing.
- *Heart:* Sinus tachycardia associated with fever.
- *Abdomen:* Striae, decreased bowel sounds, diffuse or RUQ tenderness, hepatomegaly, and possibly splenomegaly.
- *Extremities:* Joint tenderness and possibly joint swelling.

Diagnostic Tests. Most laboratories offer acute and convalescent hepatitis panels that include hepatitis A and B. Polymerase chain reaction is used to detect hepatitis C (Lauer & Walker, 2001; USPSTF, 2004b). High-risk patients should be screened routinely (USPSTF, 2004a, 2004b). In addition, patients with unexplained rises in ALT and AST levels, hemophiliacs, and IV drug users should routinely be screened.

Chemistry panels to assess electrolyte and liver function, CBC to assess for anemia, platelet counts and coagulation screen to assess clotting abilities and liver function.

Differential Medical Diagnoses

Drug-induced hepatitis, gallbladder disease, other viral syndromes, and metastatic cancer.

Plan

Treatment is supportive and aims to prevent complications and death especially in chronic forms of the disease. Encourage small frequent meals earlier in the day. Nausea progresses throughout the day. Clients unable to tolerate PO fluids will require IV fluids and antiemetics. No specific drug therapy is available for uncomplicated hepatitis. Avoid exposure to hepatotoxic drugs.

Psychosocial. Counseling concerning high-risk behaviors and the possibility of transmission. Encourage the client to have sexual partner(s) tested if indicated. If possible, the client should avoid sex as long as HBsAg is in the serum.

Medication

Vaccines. The hepatitis A vaccine has been proven efficacious in children; a two-dose single antigen regimen or a three-dose dual antigen, covering hepatitis A and B (Twinrix), is now recommended for adults who fall into the high-risk categories. If the combined vaccine (Twinrix) is given, it should be at 0, 1, and 6 months. Immunocompromised adults should have lower total doses spread out (CDC, 2011b).

Recombivax HB and Engerix-B are the vaccines licensed for use in the United States for hepatitis B immunization. Both are given in a three-dose series, with the second and third doses administered 1 and 4 months after the first dose. Immunocompromised adults should have lower total doses spread out (CDC, 2011b). Pregnancy and lactation are not contraindications (Alsace & Maradiegue, 2000). Injection into the deltoid muscle or anterolateral thigh is recommended because injection into the buttocks has been associated to damage the neurovascular bundles (CDC, 2011b). Soreness at the injection site is the most common side effect. See Chapter 14 for more information on HBV immunization and postexposure prophylaxis.

Interferons and antivirals are used to treat hepatitis B and C. These medications cause fatigue, headache, fever, rigors, and have psychiatric side effects such as depression, irritability, and insomnia. Liver transplantation may be considered for those who fail medical therapy.

Follow-Up

Follow-up to provide continued support, check for resolution of acute symptoms, and follow liver enzymes and coagulation panels one to two times a week. As symptoms resolve, the interval between visits may be lengthened. Recheck liver function studies, hepatitis convalescent panels, and coagulation studies 6 months after resolution of acute symptoms. Refer clients with evidence of chronic disease to a hematologist. Chronic carriers and their families need to be counseled to avoid transmission risks, anxiety, and/or depression related to the diagnosis.

HEMATOLOGICAL DISORDERS

The last section of this chapter covers most of the common and a few of the rarer disorders of the blood. It begins with an overview of anemia and then differentiates among iron-deficiency anemia (IDA), thalassemia, anemia of chronic diseases, and finally less common anemias: glucose-6-phosphate dehydrogenase deficiency; sickle cell anemia and sickle trait; anemia caused by vitamin B_{12} deficiency; and folate deficiency.

TABLE 23–19. Differential Diagnoses of Anemia by Erythrocyte Morphology

Microcytic Anemia (MCV[a] < 80)	Macrocytic Anemia (MCV > 100)	Normocytic Anemia (MCV 80–100)
Iron deficiency	Vitamin B_{12} deficiency	Anemia of chronic disease[b]
Thalassemia	Folate deficiency	Endocrinopathy
Anemia of chronic disease[a]	Liver disease	Hemolysis
Sideroblastic	Alcoholism	Myeloma
Aluminum toxicity	Myelodysplastic syndromes	Renal disease
	Marked reticulocytosis	Sideroblastic anemia[a]
	Spurious anemia	Bleeding
		Aplastic anemia

[a]Mean corpuscular volume.

[b]Some overlap can occur depending on stage of disease.

Sources: Adamson & Longo, 2008; Astor, Muntner, Levin, Eustace, & Coresh, 2002; Babior & Bunn, 2001; Benz, 2008; Waterbury, 2007.

OVERVIEW OF ANEMIA

Anemia is a *sign* of an *underlying* problem; it is not a diagnosis. Identifying anemia is the beginning of a workup, much as identifying a fever is the start of a diagnostic workup. Correcting the anemia may be of little importance compared with finding its cause.

In general, anemia is defined either as a reduction in RBC volume measured by hematocrit or a decrease in the percent concentration of hemoglobin in the peripheral blood. In women, hemoglobin concentrations below 12 g/100 mL or hematocrit values less than 37 percent are indicative of anemia (Killip, Bennett, & Chambers, 2007). Clinical practice sites and laboratories may vary in their parameters.

Laboratory values may be affected by age, sex, altitude, smoking, and hydration state. Beware of "spurious anemia" caused by hemodilution during pregnancy and congestive heart failure. Look at the individual's clinical picture (Adamson & Longo, 2008; Waterbury, 2007). All blood cell types (RBCs, WBCs, and platelets) are derived from the pluripotent stem cells in the marrow. Pancytopenia, or a decrease in all cell types—WBCs (leukopenia), RBCs (anemia), and platelets (thrombocytopenia)—requires referral to a hematologist.

Three mechanisms cause anemia: blood loss; decreased red cell production, usually as a result of insufficient building supplies such as iron, vitamin B_{12}, and folate; and increased red cell destruction (hemolysis). To determine the mechanism, ask the following three questions:

What is the mean corpuscular volume? Mean corpuscular volume (MCV) is one of three RBC indices and indicates blood cell size. Normal MCV is approximately 80 to 100 fL. According to the MCV, anemias are categorized as microcytic, normocytic, or macrocytic (see Table 23–19).

What is the reticulocyte count? Reticulocytes are immature RBCs that retain nuclear particles for 24 hours after leaving the marrow. Normally, reticulocytes constitute about 1 to 1.5 percent of circulating RBCs. Increased reticulocyte count (> 3%) may be an indication of rapid bleeding or hemolysis as the body attempts to replenish lost RBCs. Reticulocyte counts less than 1 percent may indicate nutritional deficiencies or marrow dysfunction (Adamson & Longo, 2008; Waterbury, 2007).

What is the clinical picture? Based on the client's demographic characteristics and problem list, certain types of anemia would be suspected (see Table 23–20).

Among the many types of anemia (most of them rare), three account for approximately 90 percent of the anemias in the United States. They are IDA, thalassemia, and anemia of chronic diseases (Adamson, 2008; Adamson & Longo, 2008; Benz, 2008).

TABLE 23–20. Differential Diagnosis Suggested by Clinical Picture

Female	Iron Deficiency
Race	
Blacks	G-6-PD, thalassemia, hemoglobinopathies
Mediterranean origin	G-6-PD, thalassemia
Southeast Asians	Hemoglobinopathies (e.g., HgB E)
Infections	G-6-PD, immune hemolysis
Thyroid disease	IDA, pernicious anemia
Alcoholism	Bleeding, folate deficiency, IDA, sideroblastic anemia, hemolysis, hypersplenism
Renal failure	Decreased production, hemolysis, bleeding
Connective tissue disorders	Anemia of chronic diseases, IDA, hemolysis
Cancer	Anemia of chronic diseases, hemolysis
Lead exposure	Sideroblastic anemias, IDA
Drugs	
Sulfa	G-6-PD
Dilantin	Megaloblastic anemia (folate), pure red cell aplasia
Antitubercular drugs	Sideroblastic anemia
Gold	Aplastic anemia

G-6-PD—glucose-6-phosphate dehydrogenase deficiency

IDA—iron-deficiency anemia

Sources: Adamson, 2008; Adamson & Longo, 2008; Astor et al., 2002; Babior & Bunn, 2001; Benz, 2008; Waterbury, 2007.

IRON-DEFICIENCY ANEMIA

Iron-deficiency anemia can be caused by inadequate dietary intake of iron, diminished absorption of iron from the intestine, or loss of iron through bleeding. Because the body aggressively recycles iron, adults with reasonable nutrition do not experience deficits. Nutritional inadequacies occur primarily in infants, children, and pregnant women. It is estimated that toddlers, premenopausal women, and pregnant women obtain only 60 percent of the recommended daily requirement for iron (Bellanger, 2010). Celiac disease may result in malabsorption of iron in the intestine leading to IDA. In a woman who is not pregnant, blood loss is assumed to be the cause of IDA. In premenopausal women, menstruation is the primary cause of blood loss. In postmenopausal women and in men, IDA is presumed to result from occult gastrointestinal blood loss (rule out colon cancer) until proven otherwise (Adamson, 2008; Waterbury, 2007).

Epidemiology

Studies reveal that IDA among pregnant women is caused by nutritional deficits, and among nonpregnant women, primarily by blood loss (Waterbury, 2007). Risk factors for bleeding include frequent heavy menses, miscarriages, abortions, deliveries, and surgeries. On average, women lose about 50 mL of blood per month as a result of menses; women with heavy menses may lose five times this amount. Oral contraceptive use decreases menstrual blood flow 30 to 60 percent and thus protects against IDA. Progestin-containing contraceptive methods may also decrease blood loss. Risk factors for occult bleeding include gastrointestinal disorders (Crohn's diverticulosis) and a family history of colon cancer or hemolytic anemias (Adamson, 2008).

Incidence reports show that IDA is the most common nutritional disorder in the world. It is seen primarily in children; however, it is estimated to occur in 20 percent of adult women, 50 percent of pregnant women, and 3 percent of adult men (Adamson, 2008).

Subjective Data

Subjective data varies for premenopausal and postmenopausal women. Premenopausal women report heavy or frequent menses. Acute loss of large volumes of blood may cause the sudden onset of shortness of breath, faintness, thirst, weakness, and rapid pulse. More commonly, however, blood loss is slow and subtle, especially in postmenopausal women. In that manner, the body is able to adjust to the gradual decrease in RBCs; no symptoms develop until the hemoglobin is 6 to 8 g/dL. In severe chronic cases, symptoms may include fatigue, dysphagia, sore tongue or mouth, and pica.

History taking should focus on sources of blood loss or hemolysis. Ask about blood donations, recent surgeries, epigastric burning or pain, melena (rectal bleeding), family history of colon cancer, medications, diet, smoking, alcohol use, NSAID use, previous anemia, and splenectomy (Adamson, 2008; Waterbury, 2007).

Objective Data

Physical Examination. May reveal nothing abnormal. Occasionally, however, signs of anemia may be detected.

- *General appearance:* Fatigue, tachypnea.
- *Vital signs:* Increased pulse and respirations; may be orthostatic, with decreased blood pressure on standing.
- *Skin:* Pallor, tenting, pale palpebral conjunctiva, nails with spooning, separation, and ridges.
- *Mouth:* Angular stomatitis (sores at corners of mouth), cheilosis (red, sore lips), glossitis (beefy red tongue consistent with vitamin B_{12} deficiency).

- *Chest:* Rapid respiratory rate, rales.
- *Heart:* Flow murmurs, tachycardia.
- *Abdomen:* Splenomegaly (hemolysis), hepatomegaly (liver disease, alcoholism), masses (colon cancer), epigastric tenderness (gastritis).
- *Pelvic exam:* Rule out mass.
- *Rectal exam:* Rule out mass, guaiac stool.
- *Central nervous system:* Altered mental status (rule out lead poisoning and vitamin B_{12} dementia), paresthesia (pernicious anemia) (Adamson, 2008; Waterbury, 2007).

Diagnostic Tests. Performed in stages; avoid the expensive shotgun approach to ordering tests.

Initial laboratory tests include a baseline CBC with indices (MCV, mean corpuscular hemoglobin, mean corpuscular hemoglobin concentration) and reticulocyte count. A fecal test for occult blood (FIT test) is done on the basis of the clinical picture and age of the patient.

Initial findings are evaluated. If data reveals microcytic (MCV < 80), hypochromic anemia with a low reticulocyte count, the diagnosis is most likely IDA. A serum ferritin should be ordered. Ferritin is one of the earliest markers for IDA. A serum ferritin level < 12 to 25 ng/mL is indicative of IDA. Normal range for ferritin is 30 to 300 ng/mL. The diagnosis can be confirmed prior to treatment by ordering an iron panel, which usually comprises a serum iron, total iron-binding capacity, and percent saturation. IDA usually occurs gradually. The continuum of change begins with decreased serum ferritin and progresses to decreased serum iron, increased total iron-binding capacity with decreased percent saturation, and finally to decreased MCV and hemoglobin (indices usually are normal until hemoglobin is 10 g/dL) (Adamson, 2008; Bellanger, 2010; Waterbury, 2007).

Consult a physician if laboratory data is not consistent with the clinical picture or the hematocrit is less than 25 percent/dL. Also plan consultation if the client has a positive stool guaiac, history of bleeding, or a family history of colon cancer.

Follow-up tests are crucial to ensure that the diagnosis is correct and that anemia is resolving with treatment. At 1 week, the reticulocyte count should increase 5 to 10 percent; at 1 month, the hemoglobin should increase 2 points; at 2 to 3 months, all normal levels should be reached. Iron is continued another 3 months or more (Adamson, 2008; Adamson & Longo, 2008; Waterbury, 2007).

Differential Medical Diagnoses

See Tables 23–19 and 23–20.

Plan

Psychosocial Interventions. Reassure the client with IDA secondary to menses or pregnancy that her condition is common. Advise her that it takes at least 6 months to completely refill iron stores. Stress the importance of follow-up laboratory tests to confirm the diagnosis. Encourage compliance with oral iron and dietary measures. If the client is postmenopausal, explain the need for further testing to locate the source of blood loss.

Medication. Ferrous sulfate is given once IDA has been documented, confirmed by laboratory tests, and the underlying cause has been diagnosed and treated.

- *Administration:* A 300 to 325 mg tablet of ferrous sulfate is taken three times a day, with 500 mg vitamin C (to aid absorption), for a minimum of 6 months (Adamson, 2008; Adamson & Longo, 2008; Bellanger, 2010; Waterbury, 2007). Enteric-coated and extended-release formulations are better tolerated, but result in diminished absorption (also see Chapter 11, Menstruation and Related Problems and Concerns).
- *Side effects:* The most frequent side effects are gastrointestinal, nausea, constipation, and black stools. The difficulty tolerating iron may be minimized if the client consumes the dose with food, starting slowly with one tablet per day, increases her fluid intake, and increases her dietary fiber. Increase the dose as tolerated.
- *Contraindications:* Do not administer iron if a deficiency has not been documented by laboratory tests. Iron overload can be fatal and hard to reverse. Mistakenly treating other types of anemia, such as sideroblastic anemia and anemia of chronic diseases, with iron can lead to overload and death (Adamson, 2008; Adamson & Longo, 2008; Waterbury, 2007).
- *Client teaching:* After diagnosis, explain to the client that follow-up and treatment will continue for about 6 months. Stress the importance of obtaining follow-up laboratory tests at 1 and 3 months and continuing medications as ordered. Advise the client to keep iron out of the reach of children.

Dietary Interventions. The diet should include foods high in iron: lean meats, egg yolk, shellfish, leafy greens, raisins, and dried apricots and peaches. Advise the client to avoid taking iron with tea, antacids, or dairy products.

The iron supplement contained in multivitamins (18 mg iron) will not correct IDA but will help prevent recurrences of the problem in menstruating women. The average U.S. diet contains 10 to 15 mg of iron per day; only about 1 to 2 mg per day is absorbed. Dietary measures alone are usually insufficient to correct the iron losses from heavy menstruation. Generic once-daily multivitamins with iron are a reasonable approach to avoiding IDA in otherwise healthy women, but will not correct an anemia (Adamson, 2008; Adamson & Longo, 2008; Waterbury, 2007).

Follow-Up

All clients should be retested to confirm the IDA diagnosis and to determine if the anemia is improving. (As stated earlier, after 1 month with adequate treatment, the hemoglobin should increase 2 points; at 2 to 3 months, the ultimate goal of the hemoglobin within normal range should be reached. Iron supplementation is continued for 3 months thereafter.) If the client is compliant, yet no improvement occurs, reconsider the diagnosis.

THALASSEMIA

Thalassemia encompasses a group of hereditary anemias in which synthesis of one or both chains of the hemoglobin molecule (α and ß) is defective. A low hemoglobin level and a microcytic, hypochromic anemias result. Individuals who are heterozygous for α- or ß-thalassemia have *thalassemia minor*; those who are homozygous have *thalassemia major*. ß-Thalassemia major (Cooley's anemia) is a fatal condition. The most severe form of α-thalassemia major results in hydrops fetalis syndrome.

Epidemiology

In the United States, ß-thalassemia minor occurs primarily among African Americans and persons of Mediterranean descent. α-Thalassemia occurs primarily among Southeast Asians. Its transmission is genetic. ß-Thalassemia minor is a silent carrier state in which the individual fails to produce a ß hemoglobin chain. The body compensates by selectively producing hemoglobin A_2, which does not require a ß chain (Benz, 2008; Waterbury, 2007). α-Thalassemia minor is a more benign state and more difficult to diagnose, as hemoglobin A_2 does not increase and other confirmatory tests are not readily available for adults. ß-Thalassemia affects around 10 to 15 percent of those of Mediterranean and Southeast Asian descent and around 0.8 percent of African Americans. Of those impacted by thalassemia in the United States, only about 1,000 cases are severe (Benz, 2008).

Subjective Data

Thalassemia minor is an asymptomatic condition, diagnosed inadvertently primarily by abnormal laboratory findings.

Objective Data

Physical examination reveals nothing abnormal.

A routine CBC will indicate a combined extremely low MCV (usually less than 65 fL) and only a slightly decreased hemoglobin (usually between 10 and 12 g/dL) (Benz, 2008; Waterbury, 2007).

Hemoglobin electrophoresis can confirm a diagnosis of ß-thalassemia because of the increased level of hemoglobin A_2; the test cannot confirm α-thalassemia. The clinical picture and other laboratory results must be evaluated.

The test for α-thalassemia is not easily available. If, however, a client has a clinical picture consistent with ß-thalassemia trait (very low MCV and mild anemia) yet hemoglobin electrophoresis does not show an increase in hemoglobin A_2, suspect the α-thalassemia trait. Refer the client for genetic counseling.

Differential Medical Diagnoses

See Tables 23–19 and 23–20.

Plan

Psychosocial Interventions. Make the appropriate genetic counseling referral and support the client as she makes decisions regarding childbearing. Reassure her that she is not sick and does not need lifelong treatment for anemia.

Medication. None is required. Caution the client that blindly and constantly supplementing her diet with iron tablets is dangerous and a needless expense (Benz, 2008; Waterbury, 2007).

ANEMIA OF CHRONIC DISEASES

Anemia of chronic diseases is a common but poorly understood condition. It is seen in clients with cancer or chronic inflammatory disorders, such as lupus and rheumatoid arthritis. Despite adequate iron supplies, the body cannot use its stored iron. RBCs may be normocytic or microcytic; no uniform hematologic picture can be outlined (Benz, 2008; Waterbury, 2007).

Epidemiology

The cause of anemia of chronic diseases is unknown, although it is associated with chronic inflammatory conditions.

Subjective Data

The condition is usually asymptomatic. When anemia becomes severe, symptoms relative to the coexisting chronic disease may exacerbate. In addition, symptoms of anemia, such as fatigue and shortness of breath, may be present.

Objective Data

For information on the physical examination, see Iron-Deficiency Anemia.

No specific diagnostic tests are conclusive; the anemia is primarily a diagnosis of exclusion. A CBC may reveal normocytic or microcytic anemia; however, no consistent pattern is found in other tests. The serum ferritin is usually adequate. For diagnosis, refer to a physician.

Differential Medical Diagnoses

See Tables 23–19 and 23–20.

Plan

Psychosocial Interventions. Support the client in dealing with chronic illness.

Medication. In some cases, treatment with erythropoietin may be helpful, but in many cases, no treatment is required (Waterbury, 2007). Caution the client to avoid taking iron unless prescribed: excess intake may cause iron overload (Benz, 2008; Waterbury, 2007). Ask the client if she is taking an NSAID. Gastrointestinal bleeding and subsequent iron deficiency may confuse the clinical picture.

Follow-Up

Consultation with a physician is necessary for all clients with anemia of chronic diseases. If anemia is severe, refer the client to a hematologist.

LESS COMMON ANEMIAS

These rarer but still prevalent anemias are usually caused by dietary deficiencies and/or genetic inheritance.

Glucose-6-Phosphate Dehydrogenase Deficiency

Glucose-6-phosphate dehydrogenase deficiency, which is inherited, causes a hemolytic anemia. The enzyme protects RBCs against breakdown by free oxygen. Until an acute hemolytic episode is triggered, the client remains asymptomatic. Hemolysis can be precipitated by viral or bacterial infections or by certain oxidizing drugs.

Glucose-6-phosphate dehydrogenase deficiency is usually discovered accidentally; for example, a pregnant woman who is followed with serial hematocrits may be diagnosed when a marked anemia develops after treatment with an antibiotic, such as sulfa. If hemolysis is severe, she is referred to a hematologist. The woman is instructed to avoid aspirin, sulfa, nitrofurantoin, primaquine, phenacetin, and some vitamin K derivatives (Luzzato, 2008).

Glucose-6-phosphate dehydrogenase deficiency is seen primarily in African Americans, persons from Southeast Asia, and persons of Mediterranean descent (Luzzato, 2008).

Sickle Cell Anemia

Sickle cell anemia is an inherited disease seen primarily in clients of African descent. People with *sickle cell trait* have erythrocytes containing 20 to 40 percent hemoglobin S, with the remaining hemoglobin appearing as normal adult.

Epidemiology. Sickle cell anemia and sickle cell trait are caused by various genetic defects in hemoglobin chains. Roughly 8 percent of the African American population in the United States carry the sickle cell gene. Occasionally, sickle cell trait occurs in persons of Mediterranean, Arabian, or East Indian descent (Waterbury, 2007).

Subjective Data. Most often persons with sickle cell trait are asymptomatic; occasionally, however, episodes of hematuria, increased bacteriuria, and pyelonephritis during pregnancy are associated with this trait. Clients with sickle cell anemia will report frequent painful crises.

Objective Data. Examination is usually benign in sickle cell trait and between sickle cell disease crises. See Tables 23–19 and 23–20 for differential diagnoses.

Plan. Management consists primarily of documenting the condition, encouraging genetic counseling, and reassuring the client that sickle cell trait is benign. Clients in acute crisis should be referred for emergency management.

Vitamin B_{12} Deficiency

Anemia caused by vitamin B_{12} deficiency is megaloblastic, most often caused by pernicious anemia and occasionally by gastrointestinal disorders that result in gastrectomy. Lack of dietary vitamin B_{12} is rarely a problem, as body stores last 3 to 5 years. Vitamin B_{12} absorption, however, may be affected. It requires the intrinsic factor produced by the stomach lining and an intact ileum, where absorption actually occurs. Pernicious anemia is an autoimmune disorder that usually becomes symptomatic around age 60 when the stomach is unable to produce intrinsic factor; as a result, the small intestine is unable to absorb vitamin B_{12}. The classic triad of vitamin B_{12} deficiency includes weakness, sore tongue, and paresthesias (particularly loss of vibratory sense). The Schilling test is used for diagnosis. Treatment involves monthly vitamin B_{12} injections (Hoffbrand, 2008).

Folate Deficiency

Folate deficiency, related primarily to inadequate nutrition, may cause a megaloblastic anemia. Folate does not accumulate in the body; therefore, the anemia is more common than that caused by vitamin B_{12} deficiency. Folate deficiency most commonly occurs during pregnancy and among alcoholics. Lab work reveals a megaloblastic anemia (MCV > 100) and a decreased folate level. Diagnosis is confirmed by an appropriate clinical response to administration of folic acid, usually 1 mg per day. Management should also address the underlying condition, such as alcoholism. Sources of folic acid (leafy vegetables, fruits, nuts, and liver) should be increased in the diet. Certain drugs, for example, dilantin and trimethoprim, inhibit folate absorption. It is interesting to note that the macrocytic anemias caused by vitamin B_{12} and folate deficiency can cause false-positive Pap smears. Abnormal Pap smears should be repeated after adequate treatment with vitamin B_{12} or folic acid (Hoffbrand, 2008).

REFERENCES

Abalovich, M., Amino, N., Barbur, L.A., Cobin, R.H., De Groot, L.J., Glinoer, D., et al. (2007). Clinical practice guideline: Management of thyroid dysfunction during pregnancy and postpartum: An endocrine society clinical practice guideline. *Journal of Clinical Endocrinology and Metabolism, 92*(8), S1–S47.

Abrahaiman, F., & Moran, G. (2007). Methicillin resistant *Staphylococcus aureus* (MRSA) infections. *New England Journal of Medicine, 357,* 2090.

Adamson, J.W. (2008). Iron deficiency and other hypoproliferative anemias. In A.S. Fauci, E. Braunwald, D.L. Kasper, S.L. Hauser, D.L. Longo, J.L. Jameson, et al. (Eds.), *Harrison's principles of internal medicine* (17th ed., pp. 628–634). New York: McGraw-Hill.

Adamson, J.W., & Longo, D.L. (2008). Anemia and polycythemia. In A.S. Fauci, E. Braunwald, D.L. Kasper, S.L. Hauser, D.L. Longo, J.L. Jameson, & J. Loscalzo (Eds.), *Harrison's principles of internal medicine* (17th ed., pp. 355–362). New York: McGraw-Hill.

Agency for Healthcare Research and Quality (AHRQ). (2010). *The guide to clinical preventative services 2010–2011.* Retrieved May 11, 2011, from http://www.ahrq.gov/clinic/pocketgd1011/pocketgd1011.pdf

Agostoni, P., Anselmi, M., Gasparini, G., Morando, G., Tosi, P., De Benedictis, L., et al. (2006). Safety of percutaneous left heart catheterization directly performed by cardiology fellows: A cohort analysis. *Journal of Invasive Cardiology, 18*(6), 248–252.

Ahmann, A.J., & Riddle, M.C. (2002). Current oral agents for type 2 diabetes. *Postgraduate Medicine, 111,* 32–46.

Alsace, N.H., & Maradiegue, A.H. (2000). Gastrointestinal health. In P.V. Meredith & N.M. Horan (Eds.), *Adult primary care* (pp. 380–430). Philadelphia: Saunders.

Aly, R., Forney, R., & Bayles, C. (2001). Treatments for common superficial fungal infections. *Dermatology Nursing, 13,* 91–94.

American Academy of Dermatology. (2010). Suntelligence: How sun smart is your city? *Fact Sheet.* Retrieved from http://www.aad.org/stories-and-news/news-releases/eb7480d2-ada3-4707-a585-9b703ab45137

American Academy of Family Physicians (AAFP). (2011, June 22). Bladder cancer data prompt labeling update for pioglitazone. *AAFP NEWS NOW.* Retrieved from http://www.aafp.org/online/en/home/publications/news/news-now/health-of-the-public/20110622pioglitazone.html

American Diabetes Association (ADA). (2002a). Position statement: Screening for diabetes. *Diabetes Care, 25,* S21–S24.

American Diabetes Association (ADA). (2002b). Standards of medical care for patients with diabetes mellitus. *Diabetes Care, 25,* S33–S49.

American Diabetes Association (ADA). (2010). Position statement: Diagnosis and classification of diabetes mellitus. *Diabetes Care, 33,* S1, S62–S69.

American Diabetes Association (ADA). (2011a). Position statement: Standards of medical care in diabetes. *Diabetes Care, 34,* S1, S11–S61.

American Diabetes Association (ADA). (2011b). Position statement: Diagnosis and classification of diabetes mellitus. *Diabetes Care, 33,* S1, S62–S61.

American Heart Association (AHA). (2011a). *Cholesterol lowering drugs, goals of therapy*. Retrieved June 10, 2011, from http://www.americanheart.org/presenter.jhtml?identifier=4510

American Heart Association (AHA). (2011b). *Heart disease and stroke statistics: 2010 updates*. Retrieved June 10, 2011, from http://www.american heart.org/presenter.jhtml?identifier=3018163

American Heart Association (AHA). (2011c). *High blood pressure statistics*. Retrieved June 4, 2011, from http://www.americanheart.org/presenter.jhtml?identifier=4621

Amsterdam, E.A., Kirk, J.D., Bluemke, D.A., Diercks, D., Farkouh, M.E., Garvey, J.L., et al. (2010). Testing of low-risk patients presenting to the emergency department with chest pain: A scientific statement from the American Heart Association. *Circulation, 122,* 1756–1776. doi:10.1161/CIR.0b013e3181ec61df

Anderson, J.L., Adams, C.D., Antman, E.M., Bridges, C.R., Califf, R.M., Casey, D.E., et al. (2007). ACC/AHA 2007 guidelines for the management of patients with unstable angina/non–ST-elevation myocardial infarction. *Journal of the American College of Cardiology, 50,* 652–726.

Anthonisen, N.R., Skeans, M.A., Wise, R.A., Manfreda, J., Kanner, R.E., & Connett, J.E. (2005). The effects of a smoking cessation intervention on 14.5-year mortality: A randomized clinical trial. *Annals of Internal Medicine, 142,* 233–239.

Astor, B.C., Muntner, P., Levin, A., Eustace, J.A., & Coresh, J. (2002). Association of kidney function with anemia: The third National Health and Nutritional Examination Survey (1988–1994). *Archives of Internal Medicine, 162,* 1401–1408.

Auten, G. (1996). Endocarditis: Current guidelines on prophylaxis, diagnosis, and treatment. *Consultant,* 973–993.

Babior, B.M., & Bunn, H.F. (2001). Megaloblastic anemias. In E. Braunwald, S.L. Hauser, A.S. Fauci, D.L. Longo, D.L. Kasper, & J.L. Jameson (Eds.), *Harrison's principles of internal medicine* (15th ed., pp. 676–680). New York: McGraw-Hill.

Bailey, J., & Chang, J. (2009). Antibiotics for acute maxillary sinusitis. *American Family Physician, 79*(9), 757–758.

Banerjee, A., Silver, L.E., Heneghan, C., Welch, S.J.V., Bull, L.M., Mehta, Z., et al. (2009). Sex-specific familial clustering of myocardial infarction in patients with acute coronary syndromes. *Circulation: Cardiovascular Genetics, 2,* 98–105.

Barclay, L. (2009). Treatment of acne rosacea reviewed. *Medscape*. Retrieved from http://www.medscape.com/viewarticle/708768

Barnes, D.S. (2010). *Gallbladder and biliary tract disease*. Retrieved from http://www.clevelandclinicmeded.com/medicalpubs/diseasemanagement/hepatology/gallbladder-biliary-tract-disease/

Bellamy, L., Casas, J.P., Hingorani, A.D., & Williams, D.J. (2007). Pre-eclampsia and risk of cardiovascular disease and cancer in later life: Systematic review and meta-analysis. *British Medical Journal, 335*(7627), 974.

Bellanger, R. (2010). Iron deficiency anemia in women. *U.S. Pharmacist, 35,* 50–58.

Benz, E.J. (2008). Disorders of hemoglobin. In A.S. Fauci, E. Braunwald, D.L. Kasper, S.L. Hauser, D.L. Longo, J.L. Jameson, & J. Loscalzo (Eds.), *Harrison's principles of internal medicine* (17th ed., pp. 635–642). New York: McGraw-Hill.

Biswas, M.S., & Bastian, L.A. (2002). Risk factors for heart disease among women: Communicating probabilities of disease. *Journal of Clinical Outcomes Management, 9,* 333–340.

Bonow, R.O., Carabello, B., de Leon, A.C., Jr., Edmunds, L.H., Jr., Fedderly, B.J., Freed, M.D., et al. (1998). Guidelines for the management of patients with valvular heart disease: Executive summary. A report of the American College of Cardiology/American Heart Association Task Force on practice guidelines (Committee on Management of Patients with Valvular Heart Disease). *Circulation, 98,* 1949–1984.

Bonow, R.O., Carabello, B.A., Chatterjee, K., de Leon, A.C., Faxon, D.P., Freed, M.D., et al. (2008). 2008 Focused update incorporated into the ACC/AHA 2006 guidelines for the management of patients with valvular heart disease: Practice guidelines.*Circulation, 118,* e523–e661.

Bonow, R.O., Carabello, B.A., Chatterjee, K., & Shanewise, J.S. (2006). ACC/AHA 2006 guidelines for the management of patients with valvular heart disease: Executive summary. *Circulation, 114,* 450–527.

Braun, L.T., & Rosenson, R.S. (2001). Assessing coronary heart disease risk and managing lipids. *Nurse Practitioner, 26,* 30–37.

Brunton, S. (2002, Spring). Allergy management strategies: An update. *Patient Care*, pp. 16–25.

Callahan, E.F., Adal, K.A., & Tomecki, K.J. (2000). Cutaneous (non-HIV) infections. *Dermatologic Clinics, 18,* 497–508.

Centers for Disease Control and Prevention (CDC). (2009). *Early release of selected estimates based on data from the 1998–2008 National Health Interview Survey*. Retrieved May 24, 2011, from http://www.cdc.gov/nchs/data/nhis/earlyrelease/200906_08.pdf

Centers for Disease Control and Prevention (CDC). (2011a). *Heart disease facts: America's heart disease burden*. Retrieved May 17, 2011, from http://www.cdc.gov/HeartDisease/facts.htm

Centers for Disease Control and Prevention (CDC). (2011b). *Hepatitis C information for the public*. Retrieved May 11, 2011, from http://www.cdc.gov/hepatitis/C/cFAQ.htm#

Chrostowski, D., & Pongracic, J. (2002). Control of chronic nasal symptoms. *Postgraduate Medicine, 111,* 77–95.

Clark, J.B.F., Queener, S.F., & Karb, V.B. (2000). *Pharmacological basis of nursing practice* (6th ed.). St. Louis: Mosby.

Cohen, D.E., & Noushin, H. (2004). Treatment of irritant and allergic contact dermatitis. *Dermatologic Therapy, 17*(4), 334–340.

Cooper, D.S. (2001). Subclinical hypothyroidism. *New England Journal of Medicine, 345,* 260–265.

Cooper, D., Doherty, G., Haugen, B., Kloos, R., Lee, S., Mandel, S., et al. (2009). Revised American Thyroid Association management guidelines for patients with thyroid nodules and differentiated thyroid cancer. *Thyroid, 19,* 1167–1214.

Daum, R. (2007). Skin and soft-tissue infections caused by methicillin-resistant staphylococcus aureus. *New England Journal of Medicine, 357,* 380–390.

Detrano, R.C., Anderson, M., Nelson, J., Wong, N.D., Carr, J.J., McNitt-Gray, M., et al. (2005). Coronary calcium measurements: Effect of CT scanner type and calcium measure on rescan reproducibility-MESA study. *Radiology, 236,* 477–484.

DeVault, K.R., & Castell, D.O. (2005). Updated guidelines for diagnosis and treatment of gastroesophageal reflux disease. *American Journal of Gastroenterology, 100,* 190–200.

Ebel, M.H. (2004). Cochrane for clinicians. Cochrane briefs: Antihistamines for the common cold. *American Family Physician, 70*(3), 486.

Elewski, B.E. (1999a). Tinea capitis: A current perspective. *Journal of the American Academy of Dermatology, 42,* 1–20.

Elgart, M.L. (2002). Skin infections and infestations in geriatric patients. *Clinics in Geriatric Medicine, 18,* 89–101.

Elias, P. (2009). An appropriate response to the black box warning: Corrective barrier repair therapy in atopic dermatitis. *Clinical Medical Dermatology, 2,* 1–3.

Everhart, J.E. (Ed.). (2008). The burden of digestive diseases in the United States (NIH Publication No. 09-6443). In *US Department of Health and Human Services, Public Health Service, National Institutes of Health, National Institute of Diabetes and Digestive and Kidney Diseases* (pp. 1–192). Washington, DC: US Government Printing Office.

FDA. (2011a). *Drug safety communication: Avandia (rosiglitazone) labels now contain updated information about cardiovascular risks and use in certain patients. Safety announcement.* Retrieved August 6, 2011, from http://www.fda.gov/Drugs/DrugSafety/ucm242422.htm#sa

FDA. (2011b). *Drug safety communication: Low magnesium levels can be associated with long-term use of proton pump inhibitor drugs (PPIs) safety announcement.* Retrieved May 29, 2011, from http://www.fda.gov/Drugs/DrugSafety/ucm245011.htm#Data_Summary

Fletcher, B., Berra, K., Ades, P., Braun, L.T., Burke, L.E., Durstine, J.L., et al. (2005). Managing abnormal blood lipids. *Circulation, 112,* 3184–3209.

Focht, D.R., Spicer, C., & Fairchok, M.P. (2002). The efficacy of duct tape vs cryotherapy in the treatment of verruca culgaris (the common wart). *Archives of Pediatric and Adolescent Medicine, 156,* 971–974.

Ford, E.S., Ajani, U.A., Croft, J.B., Critchley, J.A., LaBarthe, D.R., Kottke, T.E., et al. (2007). Explaining the decrease in U.S. deaths from coronary disease, 1980–2000. *New England Journal of Medicine, 356,* 2388–2398.

Garner, K.L., & Rodney, W.M. (2000). Basal and squamous cell carcinoma. *Primary Care: Clinics in Office Practice, 27,* 447–458.

Gerzevitz, D., Porter, B.O., & Dunphy, L.M. (2011). Eyes, ears, nose, and throat. In L.M. Dunphy, J.E. Winland-Brown, B.O. Porter, & D.J. Thomas (Eds.), *Primary care: The art and science of advanced practice nursing* (3rd ed., pp. 245–330). Philadelphia: F. A. Davis Company.

Gidding, S.S., Lichtenstein, A.H., Faith, M.S., Karpyn, A., Mennella, J.A., Poplin, B., et al. (2009). Implementing American Heart Association pediatric and adult nutrition guidelines: A scientific statement from the American Heart Association Nutrition Committee of the Council on Nutrition, Physical Activity and Metabolism, Council on Cardiovascular Disease in the Young, Council on Arteriosclerosis, Thrombosis and Vascular Biology, Council on Cardiovascular Nursing, Council on Epidemiology and Prevention, and Council for High Blood Pressure Research. *Circulation, 19*(8), 1161–1175.

Gilard, M., Arnaud, B., Cornily, J.C., Le Gal, L., Lacut, K., Le Calvez, G., et al. (2008). Influence of omeprazole on the antiplatelet action of clopidogrel associated with aspirin. *Journal of the American College of Cardiology, 51*(3), 256–260. doi:10.1016/j.jacc.2007.06.064

Goldberg, R., Kendall, D., Deeg, M., Buse, J., Zagar, A., Pinaire, J., et al. (2005). GLAI Study Investigators: A comparison of lipid and glycemic effects of pioglitazone and rosiglitazone in patients with type 2 diabetes and dyslipidemia. *Diabetes Care, 28,* 1547–1554.

Goldenberg, I., Jonas, M., Tenenbaum, A., Boyko, V., Matetzky, S., Shotan, A., et al. (2003). Current smoking, smoking cessation, and the risk of sudden cardiac death in patients with coronary artery disease. *Archives of Internal Medicine, 163,* 2301–2305.

Goldstein, A.O., Smith, K.M., Ives, T.J., & Goldstein, B. (2000). Mycotic infections: Effective management of conditions involving the skin, hair, and nails. *Geriatrics, 55,* 40–42.

Goldstein, B.G., & Goldstein, A.O. (2001). Diagnosis and management of malignant melanoma. *American Family Physician, 63,* 1359–1368.

Graham, L. (2009). ACG releases recommendations on the management of irritable bowel syndrome. *American Family Physician, 79,* 1108–1117.

Greenberger, N.J., & Paumgartner, G. (2008). Diseases of the gallbladder and bile ducts. In A.S. Fauci, E. Braunwald, D.L. Kaspe, S.L. Hauser, D.L. Longo, J.L. Jameson, et al. (Eds.), *Harrison's principles of internal medicine* (17th ed., pp. 1991–2000). New York: McGraw-Hill.

Greene, J.B. (2008). *Mitral valve prolapse*. Retrieved on June 26, 2011 from US Pharmacist: http://www.uspharmacist.com/content/t/cardiovascularmitral_valve_prolapse/c/10153/dnnprintmode/true/?skinsrc=[l]skins/usp2008/pageprint&containersrc=[l]containers/usp2008/simple

Grundy, S., Cleeman, J., Daniels, S., Donato, K., Eckel, R., Franklin, B., et al. (2005). Diagnosis and management of the metabolic syndrome: A National Heart, Lung, and Blood Institute scientific statement. *Circulation, 112,* 2735–2752.

Hamid, H., & Coltart, J. (2007). Miracle stents': A future without restenosis. *Mcgill Journal of Medicine, 10*(2), 105–111.

Healthy People 2020 United States Department of Health and Human Services. (2011). *2020: Topics and objectives > Cancer.* Retrieved from http://www.healthypeople.gov/2020/topicsobjectives2020/objectiveslist.aspx?topicid=5

Hendler, S.S., & Rorvik, D.R. (Eds.). (2001). *PDR for nutritional supplements.* Montvale, NJ: Medical Economics Company, Inc.

Hermus, A.R., & Huysmans, D.A. (1998). Treatment of benign nodular thyroid disease. *New England Journal of Medicine, 338,* 1438–1447.

Heron, M.P., Hoyert, D.L., Murphy, S.L., Xu, J., Kochanek, K.D., & Tejada-Vera, B. (2009). Deaths: Final data for 2006. *National Vital Statistics Report, 57,* 1–80.

Hertz, R.P., Unger, A.N., Cornell, J.A., & Saunders, E. (2005). Racial disparities in hypertension prevalence, awareness, and management. *Archives of Internal Medicine, 165*(18), 2098–2104.

Higgins, E., & du Vivier, A. (1999). Alcohol intake and other skin disorders. *Clinics in Dermatology, 17,* 437–441.

Hoffbrand, A.V. (2008). Megaloblastic anemias. In A.S. Fauci, E. Braunwald, D.L. Kasper, S.L. Hauser, D.L. Longo, J.L. Jameson, et al. (Eds.), *Harrison's principles of internal medicine* (17th ed., pp. 643–651). New York: McGraw-Hill.

Holten, K.B. (2006). FPIN's clinical inquires: Treatment of herpes zoster. *American Family Physician, 73*(5), 882–884.

Hort, W., & Mayser, P. (2011). Malassezia virulence determinants. *Current Opinion in Infectious Diseases, 24,* 100–105.

Hsu, S., Le, E.H., & Khoshevis, M.R. (2001). Differential diagnosis of annular lesions. *American Family Physician, 64,* 289–296.

Hu, F.B., Manson, J.E., Stampfer, M.J., Colditz, G., Liu, S., Solomon, C.G., et al. (2001). Diet, lifestyle, and the risk of Type 2 diabetes mellitus in women. *New England Journal of Medicine, 345,* 790–797.

Hubbard, P.M. (2002). Update on gastroesophageal reflux disease. *American Journal for Nurse Practitioners, 3,* 9–18.

Hulley, S., Furberg, C., Barret-Connor, E., Cauley, J., Grady, D., Haskell, W., et al. (2002). Noncardiovascular disease outcomes during 6.8 years of hormone therapy. *Journal of American Medical Association, 288,* 58–65.

Institute for Clinical Systems Improvement. (2009). *Lipid management in adults.* Retrieved May 24, 2011, from http://www.icsi.org/lipid_management_3/lipid_management_in_adults_4.html

Iosue, K. (2002). Chronic hepatitis C: Latest treatment options. *Nurse Practitioner, 27,* 32–49.

Jerant, A.F., Johnson, J.T., Sheridan, C.D., & Caffrey, T.J. (2000). Early detection and treatment of skin cancer. *American Family Physician, 62,* 357–368.

Johnson, B.A., & Nunley, J.R. (2000a). Treatment of seborrheic dermatitis. *American Family Physician, 61,* 2703–2710.

Johnson, B.A., & Nunley, J.R. (2000b). Use of systemic agents in the treatment of acne vulgaris. *American Family Physician, 62,* 1823–1830.

Joint National Committee: 7th Report (JNC VII). (2003). *Prevention, detection, evaluation, and treatment of high blood pressure.* Retrieved on April 30, 2011, from http://www.nhlbi.nih.gov/guidelines/hypertension/jnc7full.htm

Kahn, M., Santana, J., Donnellan, C., Preston, C., Moayyedi, P. (2007). Medical treatments in the short term management of reflux oesophagitis. *Cochrane Database Systematic Review, 2,* CD003244.

Kahrilas, P.J., Shaheen, N.J., & Vaezi, M.F. (2008). American Gastroenterological Association Medical Position Statement on the Management of Gastroesophageal Reflux Disease. *Gastroenterology, 135*(4), 1383–1391.

Kanzler, M.H., & Mraz-Gernhard, S. (2001). Primary cutaneous malignant melanoma and its precursor lesions: Diagnostic and therapeutic overview. *Journal of the American Academy of Dermatology, 45,* 260–276.

Killip, S., Bennett, J., & Chambers, M. (2007). Iron deficiency anemia. *American Family Physician, 75,* 671–678.

Kirby, M. (2011). *Lipid lowering in the ageing population.* Retrieved May 24, 2011, from http://www.gerimed.co.uk/_documents/resources/GM2.1104.06.pdf

Klein, I., & Ojamaa, K. (2001). Thyroid hormone and the cardiovascular system. *New England Journal of Medicine, 344,* 501–509.

Lang, M.M., & Towers, C. (2001). Identifying poststreptococcal glomerulonepthritis. *Nurse Practitioner, 26,* 34–47.

Lauer, G.M., & Walker, B.D. (2001). Hepatitis C virus infection. *New England Journal of Medicine, 345,* 41–52.

Lebwohl, M., Drake, L., Menter, A., Koo, J., Gottlieb, A.B., Zanolli, M., et al. (2001). Consensus conference: Acitretin in combination with UVB or PUVA in the treatment of psoriasis. *Journal of the American Academy of Dermatology, 45,* 544–553.

Lee, S., & Ananthakrishnan, S. (2011). *Hyperthyroidism. Medscape.* http://emedicine.medscape.com/article/121865-overview

Lee, V.K., & Simpkins, L. (2000). Herpes zoster and postherpetic neuralgia in the elderly. *Geriatric Nursing, 21,* 132–135.

Linden, K.G., & Weinstein, G.D. (1999). Psoriasis: Current perspectives with an emphasis on treatment. *American Journal of Medicine, 107,* 595–605.

Lloyd-Jones, D., Adams, R.J., Brown, T.M., Carnethon, M., Dai, S., De Simone, G., et al. (2010). Heart and stroke statistics 2010 update: A report from the American Heart Association. *Circulation, 121,* e46–e215. doi:10.1161/CIRCULATIONAHA.109.192667

Lofgren, S., & Warshaw, E. (2006). Dyshidrosis: Epidemiology, clinical characteristics, and therapy. *Dermatitis, 17,* 165–181.

Longstreth, G.F., Thompson, W.G., Chey, W.D., Houghton, L.A., Mearin, F., & Spiller, R.C. (2006). Functional bowel disorders.*Gastroenterology, 130,* 1480–1491.

Luelmo-Aguilar, J., & Santandreu, M. (2004). Folliculitis: Recognition and management. *Journal of Clinical Dermatology, 5,* 301–310.

Luzzato, L. (2008). Hemolytic anemias and anemia due to acute blood loss. In A.S. Fauci, E. Braunwald, D.L. Kasper, S.L. Hauser, D.L. Longo, J.L. Jameson, et al. (Eds.), *Harrison's principles of internal medicine* (17th ed., pp. 652–662). New York: McGraw-Hill.

Marcus, G.M., Smith, L.M., Scheinman, M.M., Nitish, B., Lee, R.J., Tseng, Z.H., et al. (2010). Proton pump inhibitors are associated with focal arrhythmias. *Innovations in Cardiac Rhythm Management* (Online journal article). Retrieved June 30, 2011, from http://innovationscrm.com/showarticle.aspx?id=79

Martin, E.S., & Elewski, B.E. (2002). Geriatric dermatology, Part II: Cutaneous fungal infections in the elderly. *Clinics in Geriatric Medicine, 18,* 59–75.

McCrary, M.L., Severson, J., & Tyring, S.K. (1999). Varicella zoster virus. *Journal of the American Academy of Dermatology, 41,* 1–14.

McDermott, M.T., & Ridgway, E.C. (2001). Subclinical hypothyroidism is mild thyroid failure and should be treated. *Journal of Clinical Endocrinology and Metabolism, 85*(10), 4585–4590.

MedicineNet. (2011). *What are the symptoms of heart attack in women and how are they diagnosed?* Retrieved June 4, 2011, from http://www.medicinenet.com/heart_attack/page7.htm

Meltzer, E.O. (2002, Spring). Allergic rhinitis: A systemic inflammatory process. *Patient Care,* 7–15.

Mieres, J.H., Shaw, L.J., Arai, A., Budoff, M.J., Flamm, S.D., Hundley, W.G., et al. (2005). Role of noninvasive testing in the clinical evaluation of women with suspected coronary artery disease. *Circulation, 111,* 682–696.

Mosca, L., Banka, C.L., Benjamin, E.J., Berra, K., Bushnell, C., Dolor, R.J., et al. (2007). Evidence-based guidelines for cardiovascular disease prevention in women: 2007 update. *Circulation, 115*(11), 1481–1501.

Mosca, L., Benjamin, E.J., Berra, K., Bezanson, J.L., Dolor, R.J., Lloyd-Jones, D.M., et al. (2011). Effectiveness-based guidelines for the prevention of cardiovascular disease in women—2011 update: A guideline from the American Heart Association. *Circulation, 123*(11), 1243–1262. Doi:10.1161/CIR.0b013e3182009701

Mosca, L., Mochari-Greenberger, H., Dolor, R.J., Newby, L.K., & Robb, K.J. (2010). Twelve-year follow-up of American women's awareness of cardiovascular disease risk and barriers to heart health. *Circulation: Cardiovascular Quality and Outcomes, 3,* 20–127.

Murphy, T.F., & Kyungcheol, Y. (2006). Mechanisms of recurrent otitis media: Importance of the immune response to bacterial surface antigens. *Annals of the New York Academy of Sciences, 830,* 353–360.

National Cancer Institute. (2011a). *Skin cancer.* Retrieved from http://www.cancer.gov/cancertopics/types/skin

National Cancer Institute. (2011b). *Skin cancer screening (PDQ ©).* Retrieved from http://www.cancer.gov/cancertopics/screening/skin/HealthProfession/page2

National Center for Health Statistics (NCHS). (2009a). *Compressed mortality file: Underlying cause of death, 1979 to 2006.* Retrieved June 1, 2011, from http://wonder.cdc.gov/mortSQL.html

National Center for Health Statistics (NCHS). (2009b). *Health, United States, 2008, with special feature on the health of young adults.* Retrieved June 4, 2011, from http://www.cdc.gov/nchs/hus.htm

National Cholesterol Education Program (NCEP). (2001). Executive summary of the third report of the National Cholesterol Education Program (NCEP) Expert Panel on detection, evaluation, and treatment of high blood cholesterol in adults (Adult Treatment Panel III). *Journal of the American Medical Association, 285,* 2486–2497.

National Cholesterol Education Program (NCEP). (2002). *Third report of the National Cholesterol Education Panel (NCEP) expert panel on the detection, evaluation and treatment of high blood cholesterol levels in adults: Final report.* Retrieved May 24, 2011, from http://www.nhlbi.nih.gov/guidelines/cholesterol/atp3full.pdf

National Cholesterol Education Program (NCEP). (2004). *ATP III update 2004: Implications of recent clinical trials for the ATP III guidelines.* Retrieved May 24, 2011, from http://www.nhlbi.nih.gov/guidelines/cholesterol/atp3upd04.htm

National Collaborating Centre for Nursing and Supportive Care. (2008). *Irritable bowel syndrome in adults. Diagnosis and management of irritable bowel syndrome in primary care*

(Clinical Guideline No. 61). London: National Institute for Health and Clinical Excellence.

National Diabetes Information Clearinghouse. (2011). *National diabetes statistics*. Retrieved August 8, 2011, from http://diabetes.niddk.nih.gov/dm/pubs/statistics/#ddY20

National Heart, Lung, and Blood Institute (NHLBI). (2010). Metabolic syndrome. *Diseases and Conditions*. Retrieved on June 4, 2011, from http://www.nhlbi.nih.gov/health/dci/Diseases/ms/ms_whatis.html

National Heart, Lung, and Blood Institute (NHLBI). (2011a). *What is coronary heart disease?* Retrieved June 4, 2011, from http://www.nhlbi.nih.gov/health/dci/Diseases/Cad/CAD_WhatIs.html

National Heart, Lung, and Blood Institute (NHLBI). (2011b). *Women and heart disease*. Retrieved June 4, 2011, from http://www.nhlbi.nih.gov/health/dci/Diseases/hdw/hdw_signsandsymptoms.html

National Institute for Health and Clinical Excellence (NICE). (2008). *Lipid modification. Cardiovascular risk assessment and the modification of blood lipids for the primary and secondary prevention of cardiovascular disease*. Retrieved June 11, 2011, from http://www.guideline.gov/content.aspx?id=14318&search=lipids

Noble, S.L., Forbes, R.C., & Stamm, P.L. (1998). Diagnosis and management of common tinea infections. *American Family Physician, 58,* 163–177.

O'Dell, M.L. (1998). Skin and wound infections: An overview. *American Family Physician, 57,* 2424–2432.

O'Leary, D.H., Polak, J.F., Kronmal, R.A., Manolio, T.A., Burke, G.L., & Wolfson, S.K. (1999). Carotid-artery intima and media thickness as a risk factor for myocardial infarction and stroke in older adults. *New England Journal of Medicine, 340,* 14–22.

Packer, C.S. (2007). Estrogen protection, oxidized LDL, endothelial dysfunction and vasorelaxation in cardiovascular disease: New insights into a complex issue. *Cardiovascular Research, 73,* 6–7.

Padgett, J.K., & Hendrix, J.D., Jr. (2001). Cutaneous malignancies and their management. *Otolaryngologic Clinics of North America, 34,* 523–553.

Pardasani, A.G., Feldman, S.R., & Clark, A.R. (2000). Treatment of psoriasis: An algorithm-based approach for primary care physicians. *American Family Physician, 61,* 725–733.

Patel, P., & Werth, V. (2002). Cutaneous lupus erythematosis: A review. *Dermatologic Clinics, 20,* 373–385.

Pichichero, M.E. (2000). Acute otitis media: Part 1. Improving diagnostic accuracy. *American Family Physician, 61,* 2051–2056.

Pleis, J.R., Lucus, J.W., & Ward, B.W. (2009). Summary health statistics for U.S. adults: National health interview survey, 2008. *Vital Health Statistics, 10,* 242. Retrieved June 4, 2011, from http://www.cdc.gov/nchs/data/series/sr_10/sr10_242.pdf

Quigley, E., Fried, M., Gwee, K.A., Olano, C., Guarner, F., Khalif, I., et al. (2009). *World Gastroenterology Organisation Global Guideline irritable bowel syndrome: A global perspective*. Retrieved on June 24, 2011, from http://www.worldgastroenterology.org/assets/downloads/en/pdf/guidelines/20_irritable_bowel_syndrome.pdf

Radojicic, C. (2006). Sinusitis: Allergies, antibiotics, aspirin, asthma. *Cleveland Clinic Journal of Medicine, 73*(7), 671–678.

Ray, S.W., Secrest, J., Chien, A.P.Y., & Corey, R.S. (2002). Managing gastroesophageal reflux disease. *Nurse Practitioner, 27,* 36–53.

Rhody, C. (2000). Bacterial infections of the skin. *Primary Care: Clinics in Office Practice, 27,* 37–42.

Robinson, K. (2007). *Trends in health status and health care use among older women* (Aging Trends No. 7). Atlanta, GA: U. S. Department of Health and Human Services, Centers for Disease Control and Preventions, National Center for Health Statistics.

Roger, V.L., Go, A.S., Lloyd-Jones, D.M., Adams, R.J., Berry, J.D., Brown, T.M., et al. (2011). Heart disease and stroke statistics—2011 update: A report from the American Heart Association. *Circulation, 123,* e18–e209. Retrieved June 15, 2011, from http://circ.ahajournals.org/cgi/reprint/CIR.0b013e3182009701v1

Roos, A., Linn-Rasker, S., van Domburg, R., Tijssen, J., & Berghout, A. (2005). The starting dose of levothyroxine in primary hypothyroidism treatment. *Archives of Internal Medicine, 165,* 1714–1720.

Rosenfeld, R.M., Andes, D., Bhattacharyya, N., Cheung, D., Eisenberg, S., Ganiats, T.G., et al. (2007). Clinical practice guideline: Adult sinusitis. *Otolaryngology-Head and Neck Surgery, 137,* S1–S31.

Sachs, D.L., Marghoob, A.A., & Halpern, A. (2001). Skin cancer in the elderly. *Clinics in Geriatric Medicine, 17,* 715–738.

Sadegh, A., & Burdick, A. (2010). Dermatologic manifestations of impetigo: Treatment and medication. *Medscape*. Retrieved from http://emedicine.medscape.com/article/1052709-treatment

Schalock, P.C., Hsu, J.T.S., & Arndt, K.A. (2011). *Lippincott's primary care dermatology*. Philadelphia: Wolter Kluwer/Lippincott Williams & Wilkins.

Schmader, K. (2001). Herpes zoster in older adults. *Clinical Infectious Diseases, 32,* 1481–1486.

Schwarz, R., Janusz, C., & Janniger, C. (2006). Seborrheic dermatitis: An overview. *American Family Physician, 74,* 125–132.

Skin Cancer Foundation. (2011a). *Moh's micrographic surgery*. Retrieved from http://www.skincancer.org/mohs-micrographic-surgery.html

Skin Cancer Foundation. (2011b). *Squamous cell carcinoma*. Retrieved from http://www.skincancer.org/scc-treatment-options.html

Smith, S.C., Greenland, P., & Grundy, S.M. (2000). Prevention Conference V: Beyond secondary prevention: Identifying the high-risk patient for primary prevention: Executive summary. *Circulation, 101,* 111–116.

The Society for Surgery of the Alimentary Tract (SSAT). (2006). *Treatment of gallstone and gallbladder disease*. Retrieved May 15, 2011, from http://www.ssat.com/cgi-bin/chole7.cgi

Sontheimer, R.D., & Kovalchick, P. (1998). Cutaneous manifestations of rheumatic diseases: Lupus erythematosus, dermatomysositis, scleroderma. *Dermatology Nursing, 10,* 81–97.

Stampfer, M.J., Hu, F.B., Manson, J.E., Rimm, E.B., & Willett, W.C. (2000). Primary prevention of coronary heart disease in women through diet and lifestyle. *New England Journal of Medicine, 343,* 16–22.

Stankus, S.J., Dlugopolski, M., & Packer, D. (2000). Management of herpes zoster (shingles) and postherpetic neuralgia. *American Family Physician, 61*, 2437–2444.

Stevens, D., Bisno, A., Chambers, H., Everett, D., Patchen, D., Goldstein, E., et al. (2005). Practice guidelines for the management of skin and soft tissue infections. *Clinical Infectious Diseases, 41,* 1373–1406.

Stoller, W.A. (2002). Individualizing insulin management. *Postgraduate Medicine, 111,* 51–66.

Strauss, J.S., Krowchuk, D.P., Leyden, J.J., Lucky, A.W., Shalita, A.R., Siegfried, E.C., et al. (2007). Guideline of care for acne vulgaris management. *Journal of the American Academy of Dermatology, 56*(4), 651–663.

Stulberg, D.L., Penrod, M.A., & Blatny, R.A. (2002). Common bacterial skin infections. *American Family Physician, 66*(1), 119–125.

Talley, N.J., & Vakil, N. (2005). Guidelines for the management of dyspepsia. *American Journal of Gastroenterology, 100,* 2324–2337.

Thiboutot, D. (2000). New treatments and therapeutic strategies for acne. *Archives of Family Medicine, 9,* 179–187.

Thomas, D.J. (2011). Abdominal problems. In L.M. Dunphy, J.E. Winland-Brown, B.O. Porter, & D.J. Thomas (Eds.), *Primary care: The art and science of advanced practice nursing* (3rd ed., pp. 492–581). Philadelphia: F. A. Davis Company.

Tigges, B.B. (2000). Acute otitis media and pneumococcal resistance: Making judicious management decisions. *Nurse Practitioner, 25,* 69–85.

Toft, A.D. (2001). Subclinical hyperthyroidism. *New England Journal of Medicine, 345,* 512–516.

Toner, C., & Krivda, S. (2009). Pseudomonas folliculitis. *Medscape*. Retrieved from http://emedicine.medscape.com/article/1053170-treatment

U.S. Department of Health and Human Services (USDHS). (2010). *How tobacco smoke causes disease: The biology and behavioral basis for smoking-attributable disease: A Report of the surgeon general.* Atlanta, GA: U.S. Department of Health and Human Services, Centers for Disease Control and Prevention, National Center for Chronic Disease Prevention and Health Promotion, Office on Smoking and Health.

U.S. Department of Health and Human Services (USDHS). (2011). Public Health Service, Centers for Disease Control and Prevention, National Center for Chronic Disease Prevention and Health Promotion, Office on Smoking and Health. *Tobacco-Related Mortality.* Retrieved June 10, 2011, from http://www.cdc.gov/tobacco/data_statistics/fact_sheets/health_effects/tobacco_related_mortality/

U.S. Preventive Services Task Force. (2002). Aspirin for the primary prevention of cardiovascular events: Recommendations and rationale. *American Family Physician, 65,* 2107–2110.

U.S. Preventive Services Task Force (USPSTF). (2004a). *Screening for hepatitis B infection: A brief evidence update for the U.S. Preventive Services Task Force.* Retrieved May 24, 2011, from http://www.uspreventiveservicestaskforce.org/3rduspstf/hepbscr/hepbup.pdf

U.S. Preventive Services Task Force (USPSTF). (2004b). Screening for hepatitis C: Recommendation statement. *Annals of Internal Medicine, 140*(6), 462–464.

U.S. Preventive Services Task Force (USPSTF). (2004c). *Screening for thyroid disease: Recommendation statement.* Rockville, MD: Agency.

U.S. Preventive Services Task Force (USPSTF). (2008). *Screening for lipid disorders in adults recommendation statement.* Retrieved June 10, 2011, from http://www.uspreventiveservicestaskforce.org/uspstf08/lipid/lipidrs.htm

U.S. Preventive Services Task Force (USPSTF). (2009). *Screening for hepatitis B infection in pregnancy.* Retrieved May 24, 2011, from http://www.uspreventiveservicestaskforce.org/uspstf09/hepb/hepbpgrs.htm

Usatine, R., & Riojas, M. (2010). Diagnosis and management of contact dermatitis. *American Family Physician, 82,* 259–255.

Usatine, R., & Tinitigan, R. (2010). Nongenital herpes simplex virus. *American Family, Physician, 82,* 1075–1082.

Vaidya, B., & Pearce, S. (2008). Management of hypothyroidism in adults. *British Medical Journal, 337,* a801. doi:10.1136/bmj.a801. Retrieved from http://www.bmj.com.floyd.lib.umn.edu/content/337/bmj.a801.full?sid=44dd0555-71bd-4ca4-bb81-190a728892fd

Vakil, N., van Zanten, S.V., Kahrilas, P., Dent, J., Jones, R., Global Consensus Group. (2006). The Montreal definition and classification of gastroesophageal reflux disease: A global evidence based consensus. *American Journal Gastroenterology, 101,* 1900–1920.

Venna, S., Fleischer, A.B., Jr., & Feldman, S.R. (2001). Scabies and lice: Review of the clinical features and management principles. *Dermatology Nursing, 13,* 257–262.

Warren-Boulton, E., Greenberg, R., Lising, M., & Gallivan, J. (1999). An update of primary care management of type 2 diabetes.*Nurse Practitioner, 24,* 14–31.

Wasley, A., Grytdal, S., & Gallagher, K. (2008). Surveillance for acute viral hepatitis: United States, 2006. *Morbidity and Mortality Weekly Report, 57,* 1–24.

Wasley, A., Kruszon-Moran, D., Kuhnert, W., Simard, E.P., Finelli, L., McQuillan, G., et al. (2010). The prevalence of hepatitis B virus infection in the United States in the era of vaccination. *Journal of Infectious Diseases, 202*(2), 192–201.

Wasley, A., Miller, J.T., & Finelli, L. (2007). Surveillance for acute viral hepatitis: United States, 2005. *Morbidity and Mortality Weekly Report, 56,* 1–24.

Waterbury, L. (2007). Anemia. In N.H. Fiebach, D.E. Kern, P.A. Thomas, & R.C. Ziegelstein (Eds.), *Barker, Burton, and Zieve's principles of ambulatory medicine* (7th ed., pp. 819–836). Philadelphia: Lippincott Williams & Wilkins.

Weichert, G.E. (2004). An approach to the treatment of anogenital pruritus. *Dermatologic Therapy, 17*(1), 129–133.

Weinstein, A., & Berman, B. (2002). Topical treatment of common superficial tinea infections. *American Family Physician, 65,* 2095–2102.

Werth, V. (2001). Current treatment of cutaneous lupus erythematosus. *Dermatology Online Journal, 7,* 2.

Whitley, R.J., & Gnann, J.W. (1999). Herpes zoster: Focus on treatment in older adults. *Antiviral Research, 44,* 145–154.

Whitmore, S.E. (2007). Common disorders of the skin. In N.H. Fiebach, D.E. Kern, P.A. Thomas, & R.C. Ziegelstein (Eds.), *Barker, Burton, and Zieve's principles of ambulatory medicine* (7th ed., pp. 1879–1930). Philadelphia: Lippincott Williams & Wilkins.

Williams, M.A., Fleg, J.L., Ades, P.A., Chaitman, B.R., Miller, N.H., Mohiuddin, S.M., et al. (2002). Secondary prevention of coronary heart disease in the elderly (with emphasis on patients >75 years of age). *Circulation, 105,* 1735–1743.

Wilson, B.A., Shannon, M.A., & Shields, K. (2012). *Pearson nurses' drug guide*. Upper Saddle River, NJ: Pearson Prentice Hall.

Wilson, P.W.F., & Meigs, J.B. (2008). Risk of type 2 diabetes mellitus and coronary heart disease: A pivotal role for metabolic factors. *European Heart Journal, 10*(Suppl. B), B11–B15. doi:10.1093/eurheartj/sum043

Winland-Brown, J.E., Porter, B.O., & Allen, S. (2011). Skin problems. In L.M. Dunphy, J.E. Winland-Brown, B.O. Porter, & D.J. Thomas (Eds.), *Primary care: The art and science of advanced practice nursing* (3rd ed., pp. 145–244). Philadelphia: F. A. Davis Company.

Winterfield, L., Menter, A., Gordon, K., & Gottlieb, A. (2005). Psoriasis treatment: Current and emerging directed therapies.*Annals of Rheumatological Diseases, 64,* 1187–1190. doi:10.1136/ard.2004.032276

Yang, Y.X., Lewis, J.D., Epstein, S., & Metz, D.C. (2006). Long-term proton pump inhibitor therapy and risk of hip fracture.*Journal of the American Medical Association, 296,* 2947–2953. doi:10.1001/jama.296.24.2947

Yanovski, S.Z., & Yanovski, J.A. (2002). Obesity. *New England Journal of Medicine, 346,* 591–602.

Yen, P.M. (2007). Thyroid disorders. In N.H. Fiebach, D.E. Kern, P.A. Thomas, & R.C. Ziegelstein (Eds.), *Barker, Burton, and Zieve's principles of ambulatory medicine* (7th ed., pp. 1336–1366). Philadelphia: Lippincott Williams & Wilkins.

Yeung-Yue, K.A., Brentjens, M.H., Lee, P.C., & Tyring, S.K. (2002). The management of herpes simplex virus infections. *Current Opinion in Infectious Diseases, 15,* 115–122.

Youngquist, S., & Usatine, R. (2001). It's beginning to look a lot like Christmas. *Western Journal of Medicine, 175,* 227–228.

Yuen, E., Romney, M., Toner, R.W., Cobb, N.M., Katz, P.O., Spodik, M., et al. (2010). Prevalence, knowledge and care patterns for gastrooesophageal reflux disease in United States minority populations. *Alimentary Pharmacology and Therapeutics, 32,* 645–654.

Zieve, P.D. (2000). Disorders of hemostasis. In L.R. Barker, J.R. Burton, & P.D. Zieve (Eds.), *Principles of ambulatory medicine* (5th ed., pp. 634–642). Philadelphia: Lippincott Williams and Wilkins.

CHAPTER ❖ 24

COMMON MEDICAL PROBLEMS: MUSCULOSKELETAL INJURIES THROUGH URINARY TRACT DISORDERS

Gwendolyn Short

Eighty percent of the population will experience low back pain during their lifetime. It is the fifth most common reason for clinical office visits in the United States. It is second only to the common cold in lost days of work and is the leading cause of disability in those under 45 years of age.

Highlights

- Musculoskeletal Conditions
- Neurological Disorders
- Ophthalmologic Disorders
- Pulmonary Disorders
- Urinary Tract Disorders

❖ INTRODUCTION

This chapter continues the coverage of usual medical problems found in the general primary care practice. Chapter references provide guidance for finding more in-depth information.

MUSCULOSKELETAL CONDITIONS

Whether physically active or sedentary, clients often visit a primary care setting complaining of aches in muscles, back, arms, wrists, legs. This section discusses the following: ankle sprain and knee sprain, acute low back pain, carpal tunnel syndrome, bursitis, fibromyalgia, gout, osteoarthritis, rheumatoid arthritis, and systemic lupus erythematosus.

ANKLE SPRAIN AND KNEE SPRAIN

Ankle sprain and knee sprain are the two most common sports-related injuries. The lateral ligaments of the ankle are most often involved in a sprain. Knee sprain typically involves the medical or lateral collateral ligament or the meniscus.

Epidemiology

The majority of all sports-related injuries involve the ankle. Once an ankle injury has occurred, the ankle is four times as likely to be injured again (Liu & Nguyen, 1999). Activities that involve running and jumping, such as basketball, volleyball, and dance, place the female athlete at risk for ankle sprain. Knee injuries occur in sports where the leg is planted and the body pivots, such as basketball, skiing, tennis, ice skating, and dance (Safran, Benedetti, Bartolozzi, & Mandelbaum, 1999).

Subjective Data

Ask the client to describe in detail the circumstances of the injury. Most ankle sprains occur when the foot is plantar-flexed and inverted. Eversion injuries are usually more severe and may involve fracture of the ankle mortise joint. The client may have continued her activities and noted pain and swelling only after several hours. Any report of a popping noise or sensation of tearing at the time of injury is significant for extensive ligament tear and disruption in both knee and ankle injuries. Ask about treatment following trauma (ice, elevation, medication) and any history of previous injuries.

Objective Data: Ankle Sprain

Physical Examination. Observe for deformity, ecchymosis, and swelling. Observe gait if the client is able to bear weight.

Range of Motion. Move the joint through its range of motion if possible (the client may have to be distracted). In assessing the ankle, cradle it in your hand and palpate the medial and lateral malleoli and the fifth metatarsal. Flex and extend the ankle. Assess resistance to anterior and varus stress.

Grade I sprain:	Mild pain and tenderness; little or no swelling; caused by overstretching or slight tearing of the ligament/muscle/tendon with no instability
Grade II sprain:	Slight to moderate instability; moderate pain and tenderness; moderate swelling and ecchymosis; caused by incomplete tearing of the ligament/muscle/tendon
Grade III sprain:	Significant instability; marked pain and tenderness; marked swelling and ecchymosis; caused by a complete tear or rupture of a ligament/muscle/tendon; must be referred to an orthopedist

Diagnostic Tests. Films are indicated if the client has point tenderness of the medial or lateral malleolus and if she is unable to bear weight right after the injury. X-ray the foot if there is tenderness at the base of the fifth metatarsal.

Differential Medical Diagnoses

Ankle fracture (x-ray confirms), fracture of the fifth metatarsal (x-ray confirms), gout (not associated with trauma).

Plan

Psychosocial Interventions. If the client is a competitive athlete or dancer, injury may cause great anxiety and possibly loss of income. Reassure her that with rest and careful rehabilitation, recovery is usually complete.

Medication. Nonsteroidal anti-inflammatory drugs (NSAIDs) such as Ibuprofen 600 mg orally three times a day for 7 to 10 days are often helpful. If NSAIDs are

TABLE 24–1. General Recommendations for Use of Nonsteroidal Anti-Inflammatory Drugs (NSAIDs)

Current evidence indicates that selective COX-2 inhibitors have important adverse cardiovascular effects, including increased risk for myocardial infarction, stroke, heart failure, and hypertension. Use of COX-2 inhibitors for pain relief should be limited to patients who have no appropriate alternatives, using the lowest dose for the shortest time necessary (Antman et al., 2007).
A stepped approach to pharmacologic therapy should be considered:
Acetaminophen, aspirin, tramadol, short-term narcotic analgesics
Nonacetylated salicylates (Disalcid, Trilisate)
Non-cyclooxygenase (COX)-2 selective NSAIDs
NSAIDs with some COX-2 activity (diclofenac, ibuprofen)
COX-2 selective NSAIDs (Celebrex)
Addition of aspirin and proton pump inhibitors for patients at elevated risk of thrombotic events with NSAID use
Regular monitoring for side effects of NSAIDs
Reduction of dose or discontinuance of the offending NSAID

contraindicated, acetaminophen may be used for pain control. (See Table 24–1 for further discussion of NSAID use.) If sprain is severe, short-term use of narcotic analgesics may be indicated.

Lifestyle. Rest, ice, compression, and elevation, commonly referred to in the medical community as the acronym RICE, are ordered for the first 48 to 72 hours postinjury to reduce swelling and pain. If the sprain is grade II, non-weight bearing is advised for 72 hours. Begin gentle range-of-motion exercises after 48 hours. Start strengthening exercises as soon as pain and swelling subside. Begin with calf and peroneal muscle stretches. Pool exercises may help if pain and stiffness prevent full stretches. Cross-training by cycling and stationary cross-country ski machines increase all-over muscle tone and endurance. Encourage the client to recondition slowly and not overdo. Advise her that pain of reinjury may be masked by analgesics.

Wrapping with elastic bandage is not considered effective support when the client is returning to previous level of activity. If used in combination with high-top shoes, efficacy is increased. Taping is often used but may lose support capability during exercise. Lace-up supports and semirigid stirrup supports have been shown to prevent reinjury (Liu & Nguyen, 1999).

Official Disability Guidelines (Work Loss Data Institute, 2011), updated annually, recommends the following work restriction guidelines:

Ankle strapping/soft cast, mild sprain (grade I): 1 day

Ankle strapping/soft cast, severe sprain (grade II–III), sedentary/modified work (10 days crutches): 4 to 5 days

Ankle strapping/soft cast, severe sprain, manual/standing work: 21 days

Follow-Up

Evaluate after 72 hours. Clients with grade I injuries may be able to start rehabilitation at this point. Grade II sprains should be examined for compartment syndrome, manifested by increased swelling, pain, and restriction of movement. Reassess grade II sprains at 7 days postinjury for possible return to weight bearing and rehabilitation or, if indicated, referral to orthopedics/physical therapy.

Approximately 10 to 20 percent of all ankle sprains either will fail conservative management or will be severe enough to require orthopedic evaluation.

Objective Data: Knee Sprain

Physical Examination

- *Range of motion:* Ask the client to flex and extend the knee. Typically, she will not be able to extend fully. If the patella was dislocated at the time of trauma (common in women), it will relocate on extension.
- *Palpation:* The client will complain of intense pain when the patella is pushed laterally. Palpate the knee for tenderness and effusion. (See discussion of technique in section Bursitis.) Large effusions appear just above the patella and are obvious. Small effusions can be detected by applying pressure to the lateral patella and observing for a bulge medially. Assess for instability during varus and valgus stress, with the ankle held under the elbow of the examiner and with the client supine. Joint laxity indicates injury to the medial and/or lateral collateral ligaments (Martin-Plank, 2011).

The most reliable and accurate test for instability of the anterior cruciate ligament is Lachman's test. The client is supine and flexes the knee 15 to 20°. The examiner places one hand on the proximal tibia and one hand on the distal femur. She or he shifts the tibial plateau anteriorly while holding the femur stationary. A soft end point to the maneuver or anterior translation indicates a tear of the anterior cruciate ligament.

Diagnostic Tests. X-ray the knee only if there was direct trauma to the patella and if a fracture or avulsion injury is suspected. For soft tissue injuries with high suspicion of cruciate ligament tear, magnetic resonance imaging (MRI) is indicated.

Differential Medical Diagnoses

Knee fracture (x-ray confirms), bursitis (palpable swelling and warmth on the patella, may not have history of trauma), meniscal tear (swelling and pain along joint line, locking or popping with varus/valgus stress), cruciate ligament tear (laxity with full extension on Drawer sign test and Lachman's maneuver).

Plan

Refer the client with patellar fracture and cruciate and collateral ligament tears to an orthopedist immediately.

Psychosocial Interventions. See section Ankle Sprain.

Medication. See section Ankle Sprain.

Lifestyle. Rest, ice, compression, and elevation are ordered for first 72 hours. Knee immobilizer more effective than elastic bandage. Continue immobilizer or wrap until ligament tenderness and swelling have resolved (may take 2–6 weeks). Weight bearing as tolerated. Isometric quadriceps exercises with tensing of the quadriceps muscle 10 times every hour. Gradual rehabilitation lasting about twice as long as the period of immobilization. Advise the client to start with straight leg raising 10 repetitions three times a day; may add handweight held on the quadriceps as tolerated (avoid ankle weights). Taping 6 in. above and below the joint line or use of short padded knee brace may be indicated when client resumes previous activity to prevent reinjury (Byank & Beattie, 1999).

Follow-Up

Evaluate in 72 hours for decrease in swelling and pain. If range of motion has decreased and pain has increased, refer to orthopedics. Meniscal tears that do not respond may require arthroscopy.

ACUTE LOW BACK PAIN

Acute low back pain is a very common, usually benign and self-limited disorder. It may arise as a result of myofascial strain, degenerative change, or injury to the spine with or without nerve impingement. It may also accompany a serious underlying systemic disorder.

Epidemiology

Eighty percent of the population will experience low back pain during their lifetime, and 90 percent of these acute low back pain episodes will resolve within 6 weeks, regardless of treatment (University of Michigan Health System, 2005). Fifty percent of those of working age will report back problems every year. It is second only to the common cold in lost days of work and is the leading cause of disability in those under 45 years of age (Philadelphia Panel, 2001).

Subjective Data

An episode of acute low back pain is considered as an episode lasting less than 4 weeks (Chou et al., 2007). The health history is key to rule out more serious underlying disorders. Important information includes age, provocative event, onset, character and radiation of pain, previous history of cancer or other serious medical condition, unexplained weight loss, pain that is worse at rest, response to self-care or previous therapy, history of intravenous drug use, and history of urinary disorder. Only 2 percent of acute low back pain is due to nonmechanical causes, such as systemic disease or infection.

Typically, the client reports onset after physical activity such as heavy lifting. It is made worse by twisting or bending. The pain may be localized to the lumbarsacral spine or may extend down the posterior thigh to the knee. Disc herniation with sciatic impingement causes unilateral radiation below the knee with numbness or weakness. Cauda equina compression, a surgical emergency, causes saddle anesthesia, bilateral leg weakness, and loss of bladder and/or bowel control. The client is referred immediately to a neurosurgeon.

Other elements to elicit in the health history include occupational history, present work status, any pending litigation or compensation issues, previous rehabilitation for back problems, substance abuse, and depression.

Objective Data

Physical Examination

- *General appearance:* Observe posture, gait; ask the client to walk on toes, on heels, and/or balance on one foot.
- *Spine:* Inspect for deformity. Observe range of motion for limitation. Palpate for tenderness.
- *Lower extremities:* Observe for quadriceps wasting. If there are lower extremity symptoms or signs, test deep tendon reflexes and great toe dorsiflexion strength.
  - Palpate the spine for tenderness.
  - The straight leg raising test is positive if the nerve root is irritated. It has low specificity but high sensitivity for herniation at the L4-5 and L5-S1 level. The client is supine, and the examiner raises the leg. It is positive if radicular pain is elicited before the leg reaches 60° or fewer.
- *Abdomen:* Examine for tenderness and auscultate for abdominal bruit.

Diagnostic Tests. Radiologic studies are not routinely ordered unless pathological fracture, infection, tumor, or traumatic injury is suspected. In the latter case, imaging may be important if litigation is a possibility. Anteroposterior and lateral lumbar films are the selected views.

MRI in clients with nerve root impingement signs is usually ordered only if results would change the course of therapy or if surgery is being considered.

Radionuclide bone scan is ordered only if high suspicion for osteomyelitis or metastasis.

Complete blood count (CBC) may be indicated if infection is suspected (Department of Veterans Affairs, 1999).

Differential Medical Diagnoses

Myofascial strain, herniated disk, compression fracture, fibromyalgia, osteoarthritis, spondylolisthesis, ankylosing spondylitis (rare in women), osteomyelitis, iatrogenic (from excessive bed rest or inactivity), pyelonephritis, bleeding aortic aneurysm, cancer of the pancreas, pelvic inflammatory disease, tumor of the pelvis, multiple myeloma, various psychosocial factors such as mood disorder, drug-seeking behavior, interpersonal, or occupational stress.

Plan

Psychosocial Interventions. Reassure the client that acute low back pain is in most cases a self-limited problem. In 90 percent of the cases, it resolves within 6 weeks, no matter what interventions are used (Della-Giustina, 1998). The drug-seeking client and the client with depression should be referred appropriately.

Medication. NSAIDs and analgesics such as acetaminophen are used as first-line agents to manage pain. They can be used singularly or concurrently. If used concurrently, explain to the client that she should alternate the NSAID and other analgesic. If muscle spasms are present, muscle relaxants may be used for 2 to 3 days. These medications are not considered as first-line therapy, but may be used short term if NSAIDs and/or acetaminophen are ineffective.

Sciatic pain from nerve root impingement may not respond to these drugs, and a brief course of a benzodiazepine such as diazepam may be effective. Opioid analgesics are not considered first-line therapy, but may be used short term if the pain does not respond to an NSAID or acetaminophen. Because benzodiazepines and opioids can lead to abuse, an assessment of the patient's abuse potential must be assessed. Tramadol is an effective nonnarcotic pain reliever, but has also been shown to have abuse potential, so should be regarded similarly.

Systemic steroids are not recommended for treating low back pain. Both the oral and intravenous routes have been found to be ineffective and are associated with hyperglycemia (Chou et al., 2007).

Nonpharmacological Interventions. Current clinical practice guidelines recommend continuation of normal activities as tolerated as the most beneficial intervention for patients with acute low back pain (Chou et al., 2007; Philadelphia Panel, 2001). While the evidence is weak, local application of ice and/or heat for 15 to 30 minutes four times a day may be beneficial (French, Cameron, Walker, Reggars, & Esterman, 2006). Additional therapies, including yoga, massage, spinal manipulation, exercise, cognitive-behavioral, or relaxation, have shown to be somewhat helpful in chronic low back pain; there is no evidence to support their use during the acute episodes (Chou et al., 2007).

Bed rest with bathroom privileges for more than 3 days may lead to more disability from deconditioning (Philadelphia Panel, 2001). Exercises are not indicated during the acute phase of pain and muscle spasm, but passive flexion and extension of the spine may provide relief. It is recommended the client do these for 5 minutes every hour as tolerated.

Diet/Lifestyle. The working client should return to work within 4 to 7 days. If her job involves heavy lifting, a review of proper body mechanics is indicated. Referral to a physical therapist may be necessary for a program of exercises and work conditioning. The obese client will benefit from weight loss. Strengthening of the abdominal muscles is indicated for all clients with chronic low back pain. Swimming pool exercises such as walking with water resistance against the trunk are helpful when weightbearing exercises are not well tolerated due to lower extremity weakness.

Follow-Up

Reevaluate the client after 2 weeks for response to therapy and return to normal activities. Refer to a physician those who complain of no improvement or a worsening of symptoms.

CARPAL TUNNEL SYNDROME

Carpal tunnel syndrome (CTS) is the most common entrapment neuropathy and is caused by compression of the medial nerve at the wrist. Although some consider CTS to be a work-related repetitive use disorder, research studies have not consistently reached that conclusion (England, 1999; Olney, 2001; Stevens, Witt, Smith, & Weaver, 2001; Szabo, 1998).

Epidemiology

Prevalence estimates in the United States indicate that 1 to 4 percent of men and 3 to 5 percent of women have symptomatic, electrophysiologically confirmed CTS, creating an overall prevalence of 4 to 10 million people (Lawrence et al., 2008). Prevalence increases with age.

Diabetes, rheumatoid arthritis, collagen vascular disorders, pregnancy, menopause, obesity, and hypothyroidism are medical conditions associated with CTS (England, 1999; Olney, 2001; Stevens et al., 2001; Szabo, 1998).

Subjective Data

The client complains of numbness, tingling, and pain in the hand that may radiate to the wrist and distal arm. The diagnostic hallmark is numbness and pain that wakes her up at night. Pain also occurs with activities that involve flexion or extension of the wrist. Fine motor coordination may be affected, causing her to drop things. The numbness and tingling is relieved by shaking the wrist in the manner of shaking down a mercury thermometer. When asked to pinpoint the areas of the hand most affected, she will identify the thumb, index, and middle fingers. She may not have pain.

Objective Data

Physical Examination. Examine base of the thumb for thenar atrophy.

Tinel's and Phalen's tests are sensitive and specific in the diagnosis.

Phalen's sign is positive when flexing the wrist 90° for 30 to 60 seconds causes numbness and tingling in the thumb and first two or three fingers.

Tinel's sign is positive when tingling symptoms are reproduced by tapping with fingers or reflex hammer over the carpal tunnel area.

Assess grip and pinch strength and sensitivity to touch. Assess for associated medical conditions such as rheumatoid arthritis, hypothyroidism, and diabetes.

Diagnostic Tests. Electromyography and nerve conduction studies will confirm the diagnosis. In most primary care settings, these tests are not ordered unless other complicating factors such as cervical disc disease or possible work compensation is at issue. Diabetics may also require more extensive studies and referral to a neurologist if there is a question of peripheral neuropathy.

Differential Medical Diagnoses

Cervical radiculopathy (pain above the shoulder, numbness and tingling occur with cough, sneeze). Ulnar neuropathy (pain in ulnar nerve distribution). Thoracic outlet syndrome (weakness of hand muscles, sensory loss over ulnar region of hand and forearm). Peripheral neuropathy of diabetes (history, numbness not position dependent).

Plan

Psychosocial Interventions. The diagnosis of CTS may have serious implications for the client's occupational or recreational activities. It is important to be sensitive to these issues and provide reassurance and support. Early intervention and ergonomics are key.

Medication. NSAIDs may help in early disease and during acute flares. See Table 24–1 for additional discussion of safe NSAID use. Steroid injections of the wrist by an experienced practitioner thoroughly familiar with the carpal tunnel may relieve pain and numbness for weeks to years. Usual dose is triamcinolone 20 to 40 mg. See discussion of steroid injections under section Bursitis.

Vitamin B_6 (pyridoxine) has no therapeutic effect in documented clinical trials. In large doses, it can be neurotoxic. Those who do report decrease in symptoms may have underlying peripheral neuropathy.

Diet/Lifestyle. Ergonomic interventions such as positioning keyboards to minimize wrist flexion, wearing wrist support during provocative activities will usually help. Wrist splinted in neutral position with palmar support worn at night is useful in early disease.

Follow-Up

Reevaluate the client in 10 to 14 days. If no improvement is noted or if the client has long-standing history, refer to an orthopedic surgeon. Age of 50, duration of disease more than 10 months, and unrelenting numbness and tingling are poor prognosticators for success of conservative management. Refer the client with probable coexisting morbidity, as indicated by positive rheumatoid factor or antinuclear antibody, to a rheumatologist.

BURSITIS

Bursitis is an inflammation of the bursa, the fibrous sac that lies between some tendons and bones and acts as a cushion. The bursa is lined with a membrane that secretes synovial fluid. The most common causes of bursitis include trauma (acute and repetitive injury), infection, and arthritic conditions. The shoulder, elbow, hip, knee, and ankle are commonly affected sites.

Epidemiology

At least 150 bursal sacs exist in the body (Martin-Plank, 2011). Clients of all ages and levels of activity are affected: the daily jogger, the dance student, the golfer or softball player, the client with osteoarthritis or rheumatoid arthritis, the childcare provider who spends a lot of time on her knees. Essentially, any client who participates in activities that place continuous, repetitive stress on joints and muscles is at risk for bursitis.

Subjective Data

The client notes an abrupt onset of swelling and localized point tenderness over the affected bursa. There is usually an aching pain and pain on range of motion, but inflammation of the olecranon bursal sac (resembling a goose egg at the tip of the elbow) may cause no pain. The client typically has a history of repeated minor trauma or overuse.

Be sure to ask her about any recent unexplained fever; history of rheumatoid arthritis, systemic lupus erythematosus, or gout; past medical history; surgical history; occupational and recreational activities.

Objective Data

Physical Examination. Inspect the affected site for swelling, erythema. Observe the client's moving the adjacent joint through active range of motion for limitations.

Shoulder Pain. Shoulder pain is assessed by having the client perform a series of movements. First, ask her to raise her arms up over her head, or as high as possible. Note the height of the arm raise and the presence of pain, if any. Have the client reach across her chest to touch the opposite shoulder and reach behind her neck to touch the opposite superior scapula (adduction and external rotation). Ask the client to place her arm and hand behind her back and reach for the opposite inferior scapula (adduction and internal rotation). The examiner should also assess passive range of motion and resisted movements. In the case of olecranon bursitis, the examiner will examine the olecranon process of the ulna for swelling and painless passive extension and flexion of the elbow (student's or miner's elbow) (Martin-Plank, 2011).

Knee. To evaluate the knee, ballotte the patella. This is done by milking the fluid into the space between the patella and the femur. Start about 15 cm above the superior margin of the knee and slide the index finger and thumb along the sides of the femur. While maintaining pressure on the kneecap, tap the patella. An effusion is present if the fingers on either side of the patella feel the tap. In bursitis no effusion is present, and the fluid cannot be milked into the space beneath the patella.

Hip. The evaluation of the hip for trochanteric or ischial bursitis includes full active and passive range of motion of the hip and palpation of the greater trochanter and ischial tuberosity for point tenderness.

All Affected Joints. Observe for erythema. Palpate the site for crepitus, tenderness, and warmth. Note degree of range of motion if possible for comparison on follow-up. Test extremity for strength and pain at extremes of range of motion. If bursitis is chronic, supporting muscles may have atrophied from underuse and weakness.

Diagnostic Tests

Arthrocentesis. If infection is suspected, aspirate fluid must be sent for analysis: cell count, appearance, culture, microscopy (presence of crystals), gram stain.

Complete Blood Count. To rule out infection.

Other Tests. May include an erythrocyte sedimentation rate, antinuclear antibody, rheumatoid factor, and/or uric acid based on differential diagnosis.

Radiographs. Usually not necessary unless there was acute trauma that preceded the pain, obvious deformity, instability, or conservative treatment for 2 to 3 weeks has failed.

Magnetic Resonance Imaging. Indicated only when surgery is considered.

Bone Scan. In the case of lower extremity pain if the diagnosis is in doubt and the management would be changed, a bone scan may be indicated to rule out stress fracture, avascular necrosis, and osteomyelitis.

Differential Medical Diagnoses

Osteoarthritis, rheumatoid arthritis (see discussions of these conditions for defining features).

Upper extremity pain: Fracture, shoulder dislocation, rotator cuff tear, adhesive capsulitis, referred pain from neck injury, Pancoast tumor of the lung, pneumonia or pleural effusion.

Lower extremity pain: Sciatica, lumbar disc disease, avascular necrosis of the femoral head, pelvic stress fracture, pelvic tumor, meniscal tear, thrombophlebitis, ligamentous injury or tear, Achilles tendinitis, Reiter's syndrome.

Plan

Psychosocial Interventions. If occupational or recreational factors have contributed to development of bursitis, the client may have concerns about future disability. Advise her that with rest, medication, and following suggested rehabilitation, bursitis can be managed and controlled without permanent damage.

Medication. NSAIDs are the first-line medications for control of pain and reduction of inflammation. The usual course of treatment is for 4 to 6 weeks if the symptoms have been present for fewer than 3 weeks and there is no significant loss of motion in the joint. See Table 24–1 for a further discussion of safe NSAID use.

Infectious Bursitis

ANTIBIOTICS. In the case of infectious bursitis, consultation may be necessary. If outpatient treatment, start the patient immediately on an antibiotic that covers staphylococcus, such as dicloxacillin 500 mg qid or cephalexin 500 mg qid, pending culture result. Continue antibiotics for 14 days. Consult a pharmacology text for further information on these medications.

Chronic Bursitis

STEROID INJECTION. In chronic bursitis or when conservative management fails, injection of a corticosteroid such as betamethasone 6 mg or triamcinolone 20 to 40 mg mixed with 3 cc of lidocaine into the bursa at the point of maximal tenderness provides rapid pain relief. Only those practitioners experienced in the procedure should attempt this. A referral to a sports medicine or orthopedic specialist may be needed at this point.

- *Adverse effects:* Complications include infection, tendon rupture, fat atrophy, skin pigment change, hyperglycemia. The client must be informed of possible adverse effects before the procedure.

Injections can be repeated in 6 to 8 weeks. If there is no improvement after the second injection, the client must be referred. In many cases, referral to a rheumatologist is helpful in order to rule out any associated diseases (Martin-Plank, 2011).

Nonpharmacological Treatment. The acronym *PRICEMM* (protection, relative rest, ice, compression, elevation, medication, and modalities) is helpful to guide the treatment of bursitis (Butcher, Salzman, & Lilligard, 1996; Byank & Beattie, 1999).

- *Protection:* For heel and knee bursitis, foam padding or bracing of the site can protect from friction injury. Retrocalcaneal bursitis often results from poorly fitting shoes or worn heel counters. Ice skaters and distance runners are groups at risk.

Bursitis of the hip, especially ischiogluteal bursitis (Weaver's bottom), is aggravated by prolonged sitting and is distinguished by pain in the gluteal region. The client may benefit from sitting on a foam pad or "doughnut" cushion.

Clients with bursitis of the shoulder may use a sling to support the weight of the arm, but this must be removed three or four times a day to prevent adhesive capsulitis.

- *Relative rest:* Encourage the client to engage in alternative exercise activities such as swimming.

In the case of shoulder bursitis, the client should perform pendulum circles with the affected arm three times a day. Later, advance to more frequent light resistance range-of-motion exercises using a towel or elastic bands. Do these for 10 minutes twice a day.

For bursitis of the knee, strengthening the quadriceps and the hamstring muscles is important.

- *Ice:* Place ice on affected site for 10 minutes twice a day or more, especially before aggravating activities.
- *Compression and elevation:* Ace bandage is applied and extremity is elevated.
- *Modalities:* May include ultrasound and/or high-voltage electrical stimulation under the direction of a physical therapist. Also if muscle weakness or loss of range of motion, refer for physical therapy (Butcher et al., 1996; Martin-Plank, 2011).

Diet/Lifestyle. If the client is obese, weight loss and exercise are encouraged to prevent future exacerbations or progression to chronic bursitis. Dedicated athletes should cross-train in activities that do not stress the affected site and may benefit from referral to sports medicine clinician. Clients whose occupation aggravates the bursa, such as workers who must raise the arm over the head repetitively, should implement a program to strengthen surrounding muscle groups.

Follow-Up

Reevaluate in 7 days or in 2 weeks if steroid injection is used. Continue therapy for 14 more days if a response is noted. If no improvement noted, consult with a physician for further workup, need for steroid injections, or referral.

FIBROMYALGIA

Fibromyalgia is a common, often underdiagnosed, pain syndrome characterized by generalized musculoskeletal pain. It is defined by tender points on the axial skeleton in all four body quadrants. There are several other syndromes often associated with fibromyalgia, including migraine headaches, irritable bowel syndrome, and affective disorders. A major component of fibromyalgia appears to be an alteration in processing of pain in the central nervous system. Low cortisol levels, elevation of substance P (a neurotransmitter involved in pain perception), and altered serotonin levels are thought to contribute to the symptoms seen in fibromyalgia (Clark & Odell, 2000; Millea & Holloway, 2000).

Epidemiology

Fibromyalgia is thought to affect as many as 6 million people in the United States. At least 10 percent of clients seen in primary care may have the disorder, which affects 3.4 percent of all women but only 0.5 percent of all men (Clark & Odell, 2000; Millea & Holloway, 2000).

Subjective Data

The client's history supplies important clues to the diagnosis. The usual presenting complaints are widespread joint pain and overwhelming fatigue. The client may have visited several other providers and/or the emergency room to find an explanation for her condition. She may have been prescribed NSAIDs, which did not provide lasting pain relief. Common features include allodynia (pain from a stimulus that does not typically cause pain), hyperalgesia (exaggeration or prolonged response to a stimulus that is normally painful), and wind-up pain (pain worse with repetition of pressure) (Huynh, Yanni, & Morgan, 2007).

It is important to review all systems because a constellation of other disorders has been associated with fibromyalgia. Their presence is not required for diagnosis but strongly suggests it.

Neurological. Higher incidence of migraine and tension headaches; fleeting parasthesias; difficulty concentrating; short-term memory difficulty; sensitivity to loud noise.

Cardiopulmonary. Noncardiac chest pain, palpitations, mitral valve prolapse; higher incidence of multiple chemical and environmental sensitivities, rhinitis, nasal congestion.

Gastrointestinal. Irritable bowel syndrome, heartburn, esophageal dysmotility.

Genitourinary. Dysmenorrhea, urinary frequency, urgency, interstitial cystitis.

Psychological. Higher incidence of depression and somatization; difficulty sleeping.

Objective Data

Physical Examination

Criteria for Diagnosis. History of pain for at least 3 months in all four quadrants of the axial skeleton.

Pain in 11 of 18 paired muscle-tendon sites, elicited by 4 kg (about 9 lb) of firm digital palpation pressure:

- Occiput
- Cervical spine C5–C7
- Trapezius muscle
- Supraspinatus muscle
- Second rib at costochondral junction
- Lateral epicondyle
- Upper outer gluteal muscle
- Greater trochanter
- Knees at medial fat pad

Satisfying these criteria has a sensitivity and specificity of nearly 85 percent in differentiating fibromyalgia from other chronic musculoskeletal pain syndromes (Goldenberg, Burckhardt, & Crofford, 2004).

Examine all joints identified as painful for swelling, warmth, synovitis, instability, and deformity.

Diagnostic Tests. There is no specific laboratory or diagnostic test to establish the diagnosis. Fibromyalgia is not a diagnosis of exclusion (Huynh et al., 2007). Diagnosis is based on history, presence of tender points, and absence of inflammation. Screening tests for other conditions may be indicated, including CBC, erythrocyte sedimentation rate, blood chemistry panel, and thyroid panel. Imaging studies are usually not necessary or helpful.

Differential Medical Diagnoses

Rheumatoid arthritis, systemic lupus erythematosus (joint inflammation, elevated sedimentation rate), hypothyroidism (high thyroid-stimulating hormone), polymyalgia rheumatica (shoulder and girdle pain and weakness, anemia, high sedimentation rate, age greater than 50), polymyositis (weakness), myofascial pain syndrome (pain arises from pressure to trigger points, which also causes twitching in the taut muscle and may feel nodular to the examiner) (Millea & Holloway, 2000).

Plan

Psychosocial Interventions. The client may feel overwhelming relief that a diagnosis has been made. Reassure her that although fibromyalgia is a chronic disease for which there is no cure, it is not progressive. She can make an enormous difference in the quality of her life by adopting healthy lifestyle measures. Encourage her to take an active role in devising the plan of care. Referral to Internet resources, such as the Fibromyalgia Network (www.fmnetnews.com), will help the patient establish a knowledge base and learn self-care strategies.

Medication

Amitryptiline. 10 mg orally 1 to 2 hours before bedtime. Dosage may be increased by 10 mg qhs per week to a maximum of 50 mg qhs.

- *Mechanism of action:* Amitryptiline is a tricyclic antidepressant that affects serotonin activity and is thought to potentiate endogenous opioids (endorphins). These two mechanisms may account for amitryptiline's analgesic effect in chronic pain syndromes.
- *Adverse effects:* Include vivid dreams or nightmares for the first few nights, hungover feeling in the morning. Other adverse effects include dry mouth, constipation, and nausea.
- *Expected outcome:* The client will note improved and more restful sleep. Advise her that it may take several weeks and some titration of the medication to achieve maximal effect.
- *Client teaching:* Advise the client to keep sleep diary and note dosage at which sound sleep with minimal hangover is achieved. Advise her of additive effects of alcohol, antihistamines, sedatives, and tranquilizers.

Cyclobenzaprine (Flexeril). 10 mg taken at bedtime may be prescribed if the client is unable to tolerate amitriptyline. Titrate to maximum dose of 40 mg/day. Contraindications, adverse effects, and client teaching are similar to amitriptyline. May cause significant somnolence in some clients.

Antidepressents. Fluoxetine (Prozac), duloxetine (Effexor), and paroxetine (Paxil) may prove helpful in improving sleep quality and functional status (Clark & Odell, 2000; Huynh et al., 2007; Millea & Holloway, 2000).

Narcotic Analgesic. Should be avoided.

Non-Narcotic Analgesic. NSAIDs are not typically helpful. Tramadol alone, or when combined with acetaminophen, has been demonstrated to be effective.

Other. Pregabalin (Lyrica) and gabapentin (Neurontin) have shown to be beneficial.

Lifestyle/Diet. The cornerstone of treatment is promotion of adequate rest and appropriate exercise. Among the nonpharmacological therapeutics, physical activity and cognitive behavioral therapy have shown the strongest evidence for improvement of fibromyalgia symptoms. Encourage the client to start a daily program of aerobic exercise, initiated during a relatively pain-free time period and concurrent with medical intervention (Huynh et al., 2007). Examples include water exercises, stationary cycling, and cross-country skiing machines. Advise the client to avoid caffeine and alcohol before bedtime. Advise the client that results do not occur quickly, and it may take several weeks or months before significant difference is appreciated.

Follow-Up

Regularly scheduled visits during flares are recommended, at 1- to 2-week intervals. During each visit, focus on self-help strategies such as time management to ensure adequate sleep and daily exercise routine. Encourage the client to keep diary of activities and symptom occurrence. The Fibromyalgia Impact Questionnaire can be helpful to determine symptoms severity, as well as to identify reasonable outcomes (Huynh et al., 2007).

GOUT

Gout, a disease of abnormal uric acid metabolism, is characterized by increased production or reduced excretion of uric acid from the blood stream. The excess uric acid is converted to sodium urate crystals that precipitate and become deposited in joints or other tissue. The four stages of gout are asymptomatic hyperuricemia, acute gouty arthritis, symptom-free periods between attacks, and chronic tophaceous gouty arthritis (Thomas, 2007).

Epidemiology

Gout is more common in men than in women. However, after onset of menopause, the incidence in women equals that in men. A systematic review of the literature by Singh, Reddy, and Kundukulam (2011) finds that risk factors for an episode of acute gout include alcohol consumption, especially beer and hard liquor; dietary meat and seafood; sugar sweetened soft drinks; consumption of foods high in fructose; and use of thiazide and loop diuretics. Hypertension, renal insufficiency, hypertriglyceridemia, hypercholesterolemia, hyperuricema, diabetes, obesity, and early menopause were each associated with a higher risk of incident gout and/or gout flares. Transplant recipients may have decreased renal function, and take medication that decreases uric acid excretion (especially cyclosporine). They are at high risk of developing gout.

Subjective Data

In the first stage of gout, the client will be asymptomatic. Hyperuricemia is detected during routine blood and urine screening. In the acute attack, the client complains of sudden onset of severe monarticular pain with swelling and erythema. She may report a low-grade fever and malaise. The joints most commonly affected are the first metatarsophalangeal joint, the ankle, the elbow, and the knee. The attack may have followed an episode of excessive alcohol intake, high purine diet, initiation of diuretic therapy for hypertension, renal dysfunction, surgery, or infection. Typically, the initial attack is followed by a period of remission of months to years. If the client reports a history of gout, she may present with polyarticular symptoms that may be indistinguishable from rheumatoid arthritis. Be sure to include a thorough sexual history, illicit drug use, surgical history (especially joint replacement), and risk of immunocompromise.

Objective Data

Physical Examination

- *General appearance:* Typically, the initial attack is monoarticular and affects the great toe (podagra).
- *Inspection:* The affected joint will be quite swollen and perhaps dusky red.
- *Palpation:* Joint is warm or even hot to touch and exquisitely tender. The client may not be able to tolerate anything touching the site, such as sheets, socks, or other articles of clothing.

  Tophi, nodular deposits of monosodium urate monohydrate crystals, may be found on the helix of the ear, the ulnar aspect of the forearm, Achilles tendon, and olecranon bursa.
- *Range of motion:* It may not be possible to move the joint through its range of motion due to pain.

Diagnostic Tests

Arthrocentesis. Diagnosis is confirmed by aspiration of the joint and microscopic inspection for crystals. If a reliable history of recurrent gouty attacks is given, it may not be necessary to tap the joint.

Serum Uric Acid Level, Complete Blood Count, Erythrocyte Sedimentation Rate. May be drawn, but these tests do not confirm diagnosis. Serum uric acid is almost always elevated > 6.0 mg/dL in women.

X-rays. Generally not indicated for the acute attack but in later disease may show punched out areas in the bone due to radiolucent urate tophi.

Differential Medical Diagnoses

Cellulitis (client able to move joint through range of motion, pain is superficial), septic joint (differentiated by arthrocentesis), pseudogout (crystals in aspirate are calcium pyrophosphate, uric acid level is normal), rheumatoid arthritis (differentiated by aspirate) (Kwoh et al., 2002; Lee & Weinblatt, 2001).

Plan

Psychosocial Interventions. If the client has a high alcohol intake, advise her that alcohol may precipitate gouty attacks and should be used with caution. If she is unable to control her intake, refer for substance abuse counseling.

Medication. Pharmacological intervention is based on stage of illness.

Asymptomatic Hyperuricemia. Asymptomatic hyperuricemia requires no medication. See following for diet and lifestyle management. If the client is taking a diuretic, it may contribute to hyperuricemia.

Acute Gout. The acute attack is typically treated with an NSAID, often indomethacin 25 to 50 mg tid continued until the attack resolves (5–10 days). In patients with increased risk of peptic ulcers, bleeds or perforations, coadministration of gastro-protective agents such as proton pump inhibitors (PPIs) (omeprazoles, etc.) may reduce the risk of gastrointestinal (GI) bleeding associated with NSAID use. Single-dose intramuscular betamethasone 7 mg or triamcinolone acetonide 60 mg and IV methylprednisolone 125 mg have also been found to be effective.

Avoid NSAIDs in patients with creatinine clearance (CrCL) < 50 mL/min, peptic ulcers, hepatic dysfunction, congestive heart failure, and those on anticoagulation therapy (Management of Gout, 2010). If the client is unable to take NSAIDs (e.g., transplant recipients), intra-articular injection of triamcinolone 10 to 40 mg (depending on the size of the joint) is effective and provides relief in 6 to 12 hours. Joint aspiration is required, however, to rule out the septic joint.

Prednisone. Oral prednisone 40 to 60 mg/day for 1 week.

Colchicine. May also be used in the acute attack, but it has fallen out of favor due to the high incidence (80 percent) of significant and often serious GI symptoms, such as nausea, vomiting, diarrhea, and abdominal cramping. It is most effective if taken early in the attack (first few hours). The latest thinking is that taking more than three 0.6 mg tablets for acute gout is not more effective, and it increases adverse effects (Management of Gout, 2010).

Chronic Gout. Colchicine can be used prophylactically at 0.6 mg bid to prevent flare-ups. Contraindication to use of colchicine includes serious renal, hepatic, cardiac disease, blood dyscrasias, or inflammatory bowel disease.

Uric Acid–Lowering Agent. Uric acid lowering agent such as allopurinol may be indicated if serum uric acid levels remain high (8.5–9.0 mg/dL) after diet modification and alcohol avoidance. Several uric acid lowering agents have been approved and marketed in recent years, with similar efficacy to allopurinol, but that cost much more. Monitor CBC, serum uric acid levels, hepatic, and renal function at onset of treatment and periodically thereafter. Dosing is 100 to 300 mg orally per day, and client must be advised to drink 10 to 12 glasses of water per day to maintain urine output.

Triamcinolone. If client is unable to take NSAIDs, steroid injection of triamcinolone 10 to 40 mg, depending on the size of the joint, may provide relief. Before injection, joint aspiration for gram stain and microscopic examination for crystals should be done to rule out sepsis (see discussion under Bursitis).

Diet/Lifestyle. The obese client should be advised on weight loss. Stress the importance of avoiding liquid fad diets or fasts. Hyperuricemia is associated with obesity and hyperlipidemia. Dietary sources of purines do not cause gouty attacks, but a low cholesterol diet is important in maintaining health. Dairy intake, folate intake, and coffee consumption have been associated with a lower risk of incident gout, and in some cases a lower rate of gout flares. A high liquid intake is important to aid urate excretion and minimize formation of urate stones in the kidney. Bed rest is important in the acute attack. Cold compresses and elevation of the extremity may increase comfort.

Follow-Up

Evaluate the client in 7 to 10 days. After the initial attack, if a second attack occurs within 6 months, refer to a rheumatologist.

OSTEOARTHRITIS

Osteoarthritis, or degenerative joint disease (DJD), usually becomes symptomatic at age 40 to 50 years. The onset is insidious, the changes in joints slowly progressive. It begins with joint space narrowing followed by osteophyte formation. Virtually all individuals over the age of 70 are affected.

Epidemiology

Of all the arthritic conditions in the United States, osteoarthritis is the most common (Altman, Hochberg, Moskowitz, & Schnitzer, 2000; Felson & Nevitt, 1999). Between 10 and 15 percent of the adult population aged 30 or older have symptoms of osteoarthritis in at least one joint. The most commonly affected joints are the knees and hips. Although osteoarthritis is more prevalent among men initially, by the age of 50 the disease affects women more than men (Felson & Nevitt, 1999).

Subjective Data

Important areas to cover in the symptom history include onset, nature, and duration of the pain. Be sure to include issues of lifestyle, obesity, and/or occupational factors that may contribute to the condition.

The client complains of increased pain with use. Although she may find pain is more severe in the knee or the hip, the hands and the feet are the most common sites of early arthritic changes. She may also note morning stiffness. This usually lasts fewer than 30 minutes. Going up or down stairs, bending, or kneeling may have become increasingly difficult. A family history of arthritis or a previous injury to the affected joint may exist. Ask her about former or current activities, such as jogging, weight or fitness training, or dancing.

Objective Data

Physical Examination. The physical exam focuses on the affected joint(s).

Gait. Observe the client's gait for antalgia.

Inspect for erythema, deformity, muscle atrophy, or swelling.

Palpate the joint for warmth, swelling, and tenderness. *Inflammation* manifested by warmth, swelling, or effusion requires further evaluation to rule out infection, inflammatory processes such as rheumatoid arthritis or gout, or autoimmune disease (see following Differential Medical Diagnoses).

Range of Motion. Move the joint through its active and passive range of motion, noting limitation, crepitus, and client's expression of pain.

Diagnostic Tests. The most important question to answer before ordering a specific test or an x-ray is whether the outcome of the test will alter the plan of care or the prognosis of the client. If the pain is recent in onset (within the last few weeks) and the joint does not appear inflamed or unstable, no further diagnostic tests are indicated.

Radiographic Evaluation. Indicated if the pain has persisted despite conservative management, if trauma preceded the pain, or the joint appears unstable.

Laboratory Tests. Erythrocyte sedimentation rate, antinuclear antibody titer, serum uric acid, and/or rheumatoid factor should be drawn if a high suspicion of rheumatoid arthritis, gout, or systemic lupus erythematosus is raised. These tests should not be used to screen because of their low specificity.

Arthrocentesis. Fluid aspirate must be tested to rule out infection if the joint is warm, an effusion is present, and the client reports a history of fever, recent unprotected sex, or sexually transmitted disease.

Differential Medical Diagnoses

See Table 24–2.

Diagnosis is usually based on physical exam, lack of systemic or constitutional symptoms such as malaise or fever, and minimal joint inflammation.

Rheumatoid arthritis presents with the warm spongy joint enlargement of synovitis as opposed to the bony hard and cool enlargement in osteoarthritis.

Systemic lupus erythematosus usually features discoid skin lesions or malar rash and complaints of extreme fatigue, anorexia, and weight loss.

Gout has an acute onset usually with monarticular involvement, especially the first metatarsophalangeal joint.

Other bone diseases: Always be alert to the possibility that pain, especially back pain, may be due to other bone diseases such as osteoporosis, metastatic neoplasia, or multiple myeloma. Suspicion is raised by history and lack of response to conservative therapy.

Plan

Psychosocial Interventions. A diagnosis of arthritis for a woman in her 30s or 40s is distressing in view of the chronicity and progressive character of the disease process. Reassure her that with pharmacological management of her pain and with promotion of overall fitness and control of body weight, arthritis need not significantly alter her lifestyle.

Medication. Analgesics such as acetaminophen and topical NSAIDs should be considered before oral NSAIDs, cyclooxygenase 2 (COX-2) inhibitors, or opioids (National Collaborating Centre for Chronic

TABLE 24–2. Comparison of Osteoarthritis and Rheumatoid Arthritis

	Osteoarthritis	Rheumatoid Arthritis
Onset	Age 50–55 years (men often earlier)	Age 20–60 years
M/F ratio	Men = Women	Women two to three times greater than men
Constitutional symptoms	Absent	Present
Joints affected	Hips, knees, spine, DIP, PIP, MTP	Wrists, MCP, PIP, MTP
Pattern	Asymmetrical, often monoarticular in weightbearing joints	Symmetrical, often polyarticular
Other signs	Crepitus	Swelling, warmth, tenderness
	Heberden's nodes on dorsum of DIP	Deformities such as swan's neck and boutonniere of fingers
	Osteophyte formation and joint space narrowing on x-ray	Rheumatoid nodules on bony prominence especially elbows
Laboratory tests	None indicated	Elevated sedimentation rate + Rheumatoid factor

DIP—distal interphalangeal joint
MCP—metacarpophalangeal joint
MTP—metatarsophalangeal joint
PIP—proximal interphalangeal joint

Sources: Altman et al., 2000; Ignatavicius, 2001; Kwoh et al., 2002; Lee & Weinblatt, 2001.

Conditions, 2008). While acetaminophen does not have anti-inflammatory properties, several studies have shown that it may be as effective as an NSAID in relieving pain of osteoarthritis (Altman et al., 2000). Recommended dose of acetaminophen is 325 to 65 mg po every 4 hours, not to exceed 4 g per day for 1 month, or 2.6 g daily for long term use.

Nonsteroidal anti-inflammatory medications have fallen out of favor over the past few years because of the not uncommon and potentially dangerous adverse reaction of GI bleeding. Additional adverse reactions include headache, peripheral edema, tinnitus, prolonged bleeding time, and bronchospasm. However, if pain control is not achieved with lifestyle changes, acetaminophen, and topical NSAID use, then a standard NSAID or a COX-2 inhibitor may be useful. Co-prescription of a PPI may help decrease the incident of gastric side effects. However, routine use of the PPI with the NSAID is not recommended because of possible increased fracture risk (Vestergaard, Rejnmark, & Mosekilde, 2006).

Intra-articular injection of steroids is usually not indicated unless there is an associated synovitis caused by accumulation of intra-articular debris, evidence of tendinitis, or trochanteric bursitis. Steroid injection is difficult and should be attempted only by the skilled practitioner after consultation with physician and appropriate radiologic studies.

Glucosamine and chondroitin are two supplements that have been used by many to diminish arthritis joint pain. Current guidelines do not support their use. However, many people continue to report the benefits they receive from this supplement. A reasonable approach by the health care provider, then, is to suggest 8 to 12 weeks of use, then discontinue if there does not seem to be much benefit.

Diet/Lifestyle. Modest weight loss, even as little as 10 percent of body weight, may dramatically improve osteoarthritis symptoms in weightbearing joints. Therefore, weight loss for individuals who are overweight or obese is an essential component to arthritis management. Exercise programs consisting of aerobic and muscle-strengthening activities can reduce pain and improve function and are also considered as first-line strategies in dealing with arthritis pain. If the client is unable to tolerate traditional low-impact aerobics and weight training, refer her to an aquatic program. Many community pools and health clubs offer a full range of water aerobic and weight-training programs. The buoyancy and resistance offered by the water reduces jarring of joints but allows for full range of motion. One documented advantage of aerobic and weight-training programs is better proprioception and reduced sensory dysfunction in knee joints (Altman et al., 2000). This may lead to fewer knee injuries or falls.

Specific exercises that strengthen supporting muscles such as the quadriceps are beneficial. Clients can be shown how to do these exercises while sitting down. Non-weightbearing exercises such as swimming and stretching promote and maintain flexibility. Canes and walkers can reduce joint load and improve mobility in those with advanced disease. Client teaching on proper body mechanics in the use of assistive devices is required. Referral to a physical or an occupational therapist may be indicated, especially if limitations in activities of daily living are noted. This service is often covered by insurance.

Follow-Up

Follow-up at 1 to 2 weeks for evaluation of therapy and any adverse effects of medications. If high risk for GI bleed, obtain baseline CBC. Monitor renal function, liver function, and CBCs at 3-month intervals if on daily medication. Refer to an orthopedic surgeon if pain is intolerable with medication or if significant loss of movement and disability.

RHEUMATOID ARTHRITIS

Rheumatoid arthritis is a chronic inflammatory disease of the joints affecting the synovial membrane and tendon sheath. There is no known cause. Although rheumatoid arthritis has systemic manifestations, the hallmark of the disease is synovitis of the peripheral joints in a symmetric distribution. This usually results in cartilage destruction, erosion of the bone, and joint deformities. The course is unpredictable. Some individuals have mild disease with little joint damage, while others experience crippling disease and nerve compression syndromes.

Epidemiology

Rheumatoid arthritis affects 1 percent of the adult population and is responsible for 9 million office visits annually. Women are affected more than men, in a 2.5:1 ratio. It is a disease of middle age, commonly noted among 40- to 70-year-olds (Kwoh et al., 2002; Lee & Weinblatt, 2001).

Subjective Data

The client commonly reports a prodrome of extreme fatigue, anorexia, weight loss, weakness, and mild musculoskeletal pain. She may have a history of low-grade fever. Inflammatory changes of swelling and erythema in several joints such as the hands, wrists, and knees appear in a symmetric pattern. These changes may emerge gradually over a period of weeks or months. The defining features of rheumatoid arthritis are morning stiffness lasting more than 1 hour and symmetric peripheral joint swelling and pain.

Objective Data

Physical Examination. Inspection of the affected sites reveals swelling and often erythema. Palpation elicits tenderness, and the joint is warm to touch. Range of motion may be limited due to accumulation of synovial fluid and pain. If disease is in later stages, soft tissue contractures can result in deformities. Examples of these are radial deviation of the wrist with ulnar deviation of the fingers, swan neck, and boutonniere deformities of the digits, involving the proximal intraphalangeal (PIP) and distal interphalangeal (DIP) joints. Deformities can also develop in the feet.

Extraarticular manifestations of disease process include rheumatoid nodules on extensor surfaces, especially the elbow and lower arm, the Achilles tendon and the occiput; muscle atrophy; rheumatoid vasculitis; pleuropulmonary inflammation; scleritis; and osteoporosis.

Diagnostic Tests. Results of diagnostic tests may be misleading, and no test is specific for diagnosis. Diagnostic criteria differ, according to source. In order to make an early diagnosis, and hopefully to prevent joint damage, the National Collaborating Centre for Chronic Conditions (2009) guideline for management of rheumatoid arthritis recommends that persistent synovitis, in the absence of any other pathology, should be treated as rheumatoid arthritis. For treatment purposes, rheumatoid arthritis is categorized into two categories, with regard to symptoms: recent onset (less than 2 years) and established (2 years or longer). With recent onset of symptoms, and without a clear diagnosis, referral to a specialist needs to be made. An urgent referral needs to be made if the small joints of the hands or feet are affected; more than one joint is affected; and there has been a delay of 3 months or longer between onset of symptoms and seeking medical advice.

Seventy to 90 percent of persons with rheumatoid arthritis test positive for rheumatoid factor. If the client is tested early in her disease, she may have a negative rheumatoid factor test. Retest in 6 months. In healthy older clients, rheumatoid factor may be present in 10 to 25 percent of persons older than 70 who do not have the disease (Haque & Bathon, 2007). There is no correlation between rheumatoid factor levels and the extent of disease. Other disease entities with similar presentation may generate rheumatoid factor, such as systemic lupus erythematosus, sarcoidosis, mononucleosis, and hepatitis B. Therefore, rheumatoid factor is not useful as a screening test but can confirm diagnosis.

Complete Blood Count. May reveal a normochromic normocytic anemia. Erythrocyte sedimentation rate is increased in active disease.

Radiographic Evaluation. Radiographs of the hands and feet are recommended because these are the joints frequently affected. Radiographs of other affected joints are also recommended. These radiographs can serve as baseline indicators for future comparisons. Also, active disease may cause insidious joint damage not noted during the examination, so periodic radiographs help monitor the success of treatment in preventing or slowing joint damage (Kwoh et al., 2002).

Differential Medical Diagnoses

Osteoarthritis has minimal joint inflammation, lacks constitutional symptoms, and affects weightbearing joints (see Table 24–2).

Systemic lupus erythematosus has a similar presentation and age of onset and may be differentiated by malar rash or characteristic discoid lesions, positive antinuclear antibody, and antibody to double stranded DNA.

Gout is monarticular, more common in men.

Plan

Psychosocial Interventions. Diagnosis of a chronic disease with an unpredictable course is a major life stressor in addition to the pain and fatigue that accompany it. Reassure the client that the goals of therapy include pain management, preservation of function, and control of destructive processes. Be alert for signs of depression that may necessitate referral for counseling. Encourage the client to join a support group. Reassure her that even though you may refer her to a rheumatologist and/or physical therapist, you will continue to provide primary care and case management.

Medication. The goal of treatment is to control rheumatoid arthritis because it cannot be cured. Preservation of joint function is important. Disease-modifying antirheumatic drugs (DMARDs) are the first-line treatment for rheumatoid arthritis. DMARDs include D-penicillamine, gold, hydroxychloroquine, minocycline, etanercept, and infliximab (Ignatavicius, 2001). Methotrexate is one of the oldest DMARDs and is usually administered orally once a week (7.5 to 25 mg). Onset of medication is 4 to 8 weeks. Side effects (alopecia, stomatitis, GI intolerance, anemia) can be minimized by adding folic acid (1 mg/day) or folinic acid (5 mg/week) (Lee & Weinblatt, 2001). Acetaminophen can be useful for pain management, and if ineffective an NSAID can be initiated for appropriate patients. NSAID use should begin at the lowest therapeutic dose, with careful consideration of adding a PPI, depending on the patient's risk factors.

Nonpharmacological Interventions. Rheumatoid arthritis management should be conducted by a multidisciplinary team and needs to include referral to a licensed physical therapist for pain management, physical conditioning, and preservation of function. The therapist can provide a home therapy routine as well as adaptive devices to assist with activities of daily living (Ignatavicius, 2001; Kwoh et al., 2002; Lee & Weinblatt, 2001).

Lifestyle/Diet. Although diet claims for relief and even cure of arthritis abound, there is no scientific basis for these claims. Advise that a sensible diet that includes a wide variety of foods and a program of physical conditioning and overall health maintenance assures the best outcome. Encourage adequate rest periods to decrease joint inflammation.

Follow-Up

Once the initial diagnosis is made, follow-up is based on disease progression. All clients should be reevaluated in 4 to 8 weeks for response to therapy. If treatment is not successful within the first 3 months, refer to a physician or rheumatologist for combination therapy and more aggressive management (Kwoh et al., 2002). Most clients have a disease pattern of periodic exacerbations with periods of remission. About 15 percent have remission after an initial flare without major deformity developing. Predictors of future disability include age, female sex, radiologic pathology, and increased titers of rheumatoid factor (Lee & Weinblatt, 2001).

SYSTEMIC LUPUS ERYTHEMATOSUS

Systemic lupus erythematosus is a disorder of unknown etiology that can affect almost any organ system. It is characterized by damage to cells and tissue caused by immune complexes and pathogenic autoantibodies.

Epidemiology

Systemic lupus erythematosus is generally a disease of women in their childbearing years, specifically, ages 15 to 25; 90 percent of all cases fall into this category. It is more common in African Americans. The incidence rates are 1 to 25 per 100,000 in North America, South America, Europe, and Asia (Schur & Hahn, 2011). The increased frequency of systemic lupus erythematosus among women has been attributed to an estrogen hormonal effect that impacts women most significantly in their childbearing years. There appears to be a genetic predisposition (McAlindon, 2000).

Subjective Data

The client may present with a variety of clinical presentations, including a malar or discoid rash (50%); oral ulcers (30%); generalized joint pain, especially of the hands; fever and malaise; pleurisy (20–40); and nephropathy, varying from mild proteinuria and mild hematuria to renal failure. Multiple system involvement may also be indicated by chest pain and nonspecific GI complaints (anorexia, weight loss, nausea). Be sure to ask about medication use. Several drugs cause a syndrome resembling lupus, especially procainamide and hydralazine. Other drugs that have been implicated more rarely include isoniazid, chlorpromazine, d-penicillamine, methyldopa, and oral contraceptives. Discontinuation of the offending drug usually resolves clinical symptoms in a few weeks (Clark, Queener, & Karb, 2000).

Objective Data

Vital Signs. Temperature may be slightly elevated.

Physical Examination. If suspicion of systemic lupus erythematosus is high, a thorough head to toe physical exam is indicated, including weight.

- *Skin:* The rash of systemic lupus erythematosus is more often malar in a butterfly shape than discoid (as in discoid lupus). It is flat or slightly raised, erythematous, appearing over the cheeks and the bridge of the nose but can extend to the chin, ears, or any sun-exposed area. The client may also have aphthous ulcers in the buccal mucosa and vasculitic skin lesions such as purpura, infarcts (splinter hemorrhages) of skin, digits, or nail and leg ulcers. Twenty percent of those with systemic lupus erythematosus have discoid lupus lesions. (See discussion of cutaneous lupus erythematosus in Chapter 23.) The client may have patchy alopecia (Klippel & Arayssi, 2000).
- *Eyes:* The eye and retina should be examined for episcleritis, conjuctivitis, swelling of the optic disc, and vascular abnormalities.
- *Heart:* Cardiac involvement is indicated by the presence of a pericardial friction rub, gallop rhythm, or new onset of murmur.

- *Lungs:* Pulmonary manifestations include adventitious lung sounds, pleural rub, and increased respiratory rate.
- *Abdomen:* Palpate the abdomen for tenderness and note any guarding. Clients with systemic lupus erythematosus are at risk for peritonitis and pancreatitis.
- *Musculoskeletal exam:* Musculoskeletal manifestations include joint swelling, especially the PIP, metacarpophalangeal (MCP) joints of the hands, the wrists, and knees. The client may have only hand and feet puffiness and tenosynovitis.
- *Neurological exam:* Perform a thorough neurological examination, concentrating on cognitive function, cranial nerves for palsy, and cerebellar dysfunction.

Diagnostic Tests. *Urine pregnancy test* for all women of childbearing age.

Routine urinalysis to detect proteinurea, hematuria.

Antibody to double stranded DNA (most specific test to detect systemic lupus erythematosus).

Antinuclear antibody (most sensitive test to detect systemic lupus erythematosus). Antinuclear antibody titer may remain positive for years.

Chest x-ray if indicated to detect effusion.

ECG or echocardiogram if indicated to detect pericarditis, endocarditis, valvular abnormality.

Flat plate of the abdomen if ascites, liver enlargement.

Complete blood count to detect anemia.

Serum chemistries to assess renal and hepatic function.

Differential Medical Diagnoses

Rheumatoid arthritis; skin disorders such as urticaria, erythema multiform, rosacea; scleroderma; multiple sclerosis. Always consider drug-induced lupus, from procainamide, hydralazine, and less frequently isoniazid, chlorpromazide, d-penicillamine, methyldopa, oral contraceptives (Clark et al., 2000).

If client is diagnosed with systemic lupus erythematosus, she is referred to a specialist for further management.

She may be followed by a rheumatologist, nephrologist, cardiologist, pulmonologist, or neurologist based upon the stage and manifestation of disease.

Plan

Psychosocial Interventions. Systemic lupus erythematosus is a chronic disease with no known cure. Its course is unpredictable with emissions and flares. The overall survival rate is about 85 percent over 10 years (Trager & Ward, 2001).

The client will need a high degree of support and empathy from the provider. She may go through denial, anger, despair. If pregnant, she will need information and counseling on how the pregnancy may affect the course of her disease. She may have to consider terminating the pregnancy. Assure her that even though she is seen by various specialists, you are available for support and education.

Medication. Drug therapy based on systemic manifestations of disease.

Anti-Inflammatory Agents. Most clients with mild systemic lupus erythematosus are treated with NSAIDs and topical corticosteroids for joint pain and skin rashes.

Hydroxychloroquine. An antimalarial drug, this medication is also used to treat the skin rash of systemic lupus erythematosus.

Systemic Steroids. Those with complications of diseases such as thrombocytopenic purpura, hemolytic anemia, myocarditis, pericarditis, and nephritis are treated with glucocorticoids. During acute exacerbations, doses may be given every 8 to 12 hours. When disease is controlled, one morning dose of prednisone or other short-acting glucocorticoid is given and tapered down to the lowest dose that suppresses acute flare (Clark et al., 2000).

Immunosuppressive Agents. These medications include azathioprine, cyclophosphamide, methotrexate, and mycophenolate.

Diet/Lifestyle. The practitioner can be a very important resource for the client in promoting healthy diet and lifestyle to retard disease progression. Infection and renal disease are the major causes of death in those with systemic lupus erythematosus. Adequate rest and nutrition, a positive outlook, protection of joints, regular exercise as tolerated, use of sunscreen on skin (or remaining out of the sun) are key to maintaining optimum health in the presence of illness.

Follow-Up

The practitioner should continue to follow the client for routine health care including an annual well-woman exam, mammogram, and treatment of episodic illness.

NEUROLOGICAL DISORDERS

The term *neurological disorders* casts a broader net than one might first suppose, since within its boundaries can be found everything from the common headache to seizures and Parkinsonism. This section encompasses information on headache, fever, dizziness and vertigo, Bell's palsy, two alterations in consciousness—syncope and seizures—and Parkinsonism and essential tremor.

TABLE 24–3. Red Flag Symptoms for Dangerous Headaches

No recognizable benign pattern for headaches
Client description: "Worst headache ever"
Onset of headache with exertion (cough, strain, Valsalva maneuver)
Vomiting without nausea
Personality changes (decreased alertness or cognition)
Any abnormality on physical exam
Neck not supple, pain with flexion
Fever
Focal neurological signs
Seizure(s)
Sudden change in headache pattern especially in those over age 50
Progression of symptoms

HEADACHE

Headache is one of the most common complaints leading to office and emergency room visits. It accounts for many lost work days and disruptions in family relationships. This section focuses on the two most common types: tension and migraine. Most experts agree that tension and migraine headaches are on a continuum, with some overlap and shared characteristics and etiologies.

Prior to discussing the common and more benign headaches, it is best to understand less common headache variants and potentially more dangerous headaches requiring referral and further diagnostic testing.

Some headaches are due to organic causes such as brain tumors, bleeding, or meningitis. These headaches usually present with some of the "red flags" listed in Table 24–3. If these red flags are present, prompt imaging and consultation with a neurologist is necessary (C.J. Johnson, 2007; G.D. Johnson, 1998).

Uncommon Headache Variants

Several uncommon headache variants must be considered in diagnosis: cluster headaches, complex migraines, and headaches caused by pseudotumor cerebri, temporal (giant cell) arteritis, and subarachnoid hemorrhage.

Keep in mind that systemic illnesses can affect headaches and that anxiety about the cause of the headache may magnify or distort the clinical features. Look at the total picture including the possibility of referred pain from sinus infections or dental infections.

Cluster Headaches. Cluster headaches are an uncommon variant type of migraine. Reports show that cluster headaches occur two to seven times more often in men than women. Attacks usually begin between ages 20 and 50 and occur in "clusters," usually nightly in 6-week cycles. The pain often begins 1 to 2 hours after falling asleep and wakes the client up. Excruciating pain lasts about 1 hour and is described as "boring" around one eye. Tearing and nasal congestion often occur on the affected side. In contrast to migraine, those affected are restless, often getting out of bed and pacing. Cluster headaches are frequently triggered by alcohol or histamine. Refer the client to a neurologist (C.J. Johnson, 2007).

Complex Migraine Headaches. Complex migraines are associated with focal neurological signs, which may continue after the prodrome and into or past the headache phase. They may be confused with stroke. Always refer the client to a neurologist.

An unusual variation in young people is the basilar migraine. The client may complain of vertigo, double vision, and numbness and may have an ataxic gait, visual field changes, and changes in level of consciousness (C.J. Johnson, 2007).

Pseudotumor Cerebri. Headaches may be caused by pseudotumor cerebri (benign intracranial hypertension). The intracranial hypertension, often of unknown etiology, is most often seen among children or obese young women. It has been associated with use of tetracycline, vitamin A, corticosteroids, and oral contraceptives as well as pulmonary disease and endocrine disturbances. A client is in no apparent distress. She may report "mild headache"; papilledema is noted on the physical exam. Partial or complete visual loss may occur if not treated. Refer the client to a neurologist immediately.

Temporal Arteritis. Headaches may also result from temporal (giant cell) arteritis. The arteritis is of unknown etiology and occurs primarily after age 50. Clients may have associated fever, malaise, and muscle aches, especially in the shoulders and hips. Clients usually, although not always, have a headache. Visual symptoms such as diplopia occur among 50 percent. Temporal arteritis is also associated with proximal muscle weakness (polymyalgia rheumatica). Tenderness over the temporal artery and rarely the occipital artery may be elicited. The erythrocyte sedimentation rate is dramatically elevated, often greater than 100 mm per hour. Refer the client to a neurologist immediately. Treatment with steroids is initiated to prevent blindness.

Subarachnoid Hemorrhage. Subarachnoid hemorrhage may be reported as a sudden onset of the "worst headache of my life."

This may be followed by nausea, vomiting, and a decreasing level of consciousness. The hemorrhage is usually secondary to trauma, a ruptured aneurysm or congenital arteriovenous malformation. Subarachnoid hemorrhage is most common between ages 25 and 50. The individual may collapse and lose consciousness. Neck stiffness and neurological signs almost always occur. Refer the client to a neurologist immediately or an emergency room for an emergent computed tomography (CT) scan.

Tension Headaches

The pathophysiology of tension headaches is poorly understood. Although once referred to as muscle contraction headaches, current research indicates that muscle contraction is not always present with this type of headache. Stress or tension is almost always involved, but the exact pathophysiology is unknown. Tension headaches can be episodic or chronic daily headaches.

Epidemiology. Studies reveal that tension headaches are the most prevalent of all headache types. They are more common in women than in men and decrease in frequency with age (C.J. Johnson, 2007). Episodic tension headaches are the classic stress-related headaches. Chronic daily headaches, on the other hand, are often associated with depression that requires treatment.

Subjective Data. A headache history, taken with interest and concern, is the key to the diagnosis. Patterns should be established (see Table 24–4). Rule out a history of trauma, neurological signs, and concurrent disorders.

Have the client keep a headache diary. She should record the day and time of the headache and surrounding events, such as diet, physical activity, and menstrual cycle. Assessing sleep patterns and intake of caffeine and alcohol is especially helpful. She should note aggravating and relieving factors. Have her record the time and dose of any medication taken, both prescribed and over the counter. This not only helps the health care provider to complete a more thorough history, but educates the patient that she may have some control over her headache triggers.

When taking a history, it is important to have a client identify different types of headaches, as she may easily have more than one. Ask her to describe specific symptoms (see Table 24–4).

Objective Data. Data are based on a complete physical examination and, in some instances, diagnostic tests. Physical examination includes examination of the nervous system and eyes, nose, and throat (see Table 24–5).

Usually no diagnostic tests are indicated for tension headaches. For any patient older than 40 with a new type of headache, order a CBC and erythrocyte sedimentation rate to rule out temporal arteritis.

Differential Medical Diagnoses. Temporomandibular joint syndrome, chronic myositis, cervical osteoarthritis, migraines, perimenstrual headache, cluster headache, cranial masses (tumors, edema), sinusitis, tooth abscess, temporal arteritis, pseudotumor cerebri, depression.

Plan

Psychosocial Interventions. It is crucial to reassure the client that tension-type headaches are usually not associated with any severely negative consequences. A thorough physical exam can greatly decrease the woman's anxiety level. Once reassured, she can better focus on lifestyle changes and stress management techniques that might help to decrease the frequency of headaches.

Medication. NSAIDs are very helpful for tension headaches as well as migraine and perimenstrual headaches. Ibuprofen is the first choice; naproxen sodium is helpful for perimenopausal headaches. Refer to the

TABLE 24–4. Headache Symptom Patterns in History

Symptom	Migraine Headache	Tension Headache
Onset	10% have aura; may awake with headache	Gradual; often begin during times of stress
Duration	Usually 8–12 hours; range 3 hours to rarely 3 days	Usually 8–12 hours; may last days, weeks, months
Frequency	Usually one or two per month or fewer with pain free periods; rarely one per week	Wide range (daily to rarely)
Pain location	Approximately 60% unilateral; may switch side or become bilateral	Approximately 90% bilateral; frontal area, "hat band" area, or back of neck
Pain quality	Throbbing; moderate to severe	Constant; nagging to severe
Associated symptoms	Nausea, vomiting photophobia, phonophobia	Varied from mild intolerance to light and noise to nausea and anorexia
Triggers	Stress; menses; alcohol; food; "letdown" after stress	Stress
Relieving factors	Rest in dark room; sleep	Relaxation exercise; Tylenol/NSAID

NSAID—nonsteroidal anti-inflammatory drug

TABLE 24–5. Physical Exam for Headache

General appearance: Note affect, photophobia.
Vital signs: Blood pressure and temperature must be charted.
Blood pressure: Hypertension (HTN) can cause headaches; pain with diastolic > 120–140. HTN may aggravate migraine.
Temperature: Fever, rule out meningitis, arteritis, sinusitis, abscess.
Mental status: Usually assessed within framework of interview.

Cranial Nerves[a]	Head, Eyes, Ears, and Throat
(If normal, efficient charting states "cranial nerves II–XII intact.")	
I. Olfactory: usually not done	
II. Optic: visual acuity, visual fields by confrontation	Disc flat (rule out papilledema)
III, IV, VI. Oculomotor, trochlear, abducens	
PERRLA, EOMs, note ptosis of upper lids	
V. Trigeminal	Palpate "click" from temporomandibular joint
Motor—palpate masseter, open and close jaw	Palpate temporal area (rule out arteritis)
Sensory—touch forehead, cheek, jaw	
VII. Facial	Check tenderness over sinuses (rule out sinusitis)
Observe facial symmetry	
Raise eyebrows, frown	
Close eyes, resist opening	
Smile, puff out cheeks	
VIII. Acoustic: hearing watch tick	Look at tympanic membrane
IX, X. Glossopharyngeal, vagus	Check teeth
Symmetrical movement soft palate	
XI. Spinal accessory	Check nodes
Atrophy, shrug upward against hands	Check neck stiffness
Turn head against your hands	Bruits
	Tender neck muscles
XII. Hypoglossal	
Tongue movement, fasciculations	
Screening motor and cerebellar function	
Walk: note gait, heel/toe walk	
Hop on one foot, Romberg	
Deep knee bend, check arms pronator drift	
Finger to nose	
Screening sensory	
Pain and vibration (tuning fork), hands and feet	
Stereognosis	
Reflexes	
Check deep tendon reflexes, Babinski, and other systems if indicated by history	

EOM—extraocular movement
PERRLA—pupils equal, round, reactive to light and accommodation
[a] For efficiency, examine cranial nerves and head, eyes, ears, nose, and throat system simultaneously.

previous discussion of NSAIDs in section Musculoskeletal Conditions. Treatment guidelines for headache are available through the Institute for Clinical Systems Improvement (2011) organization at http://www.icsi.org/headache.

- *Side effects:* GI distress and bleeding may occur. A thorough patient assessment is needed prior to recommendation of NSAIDs.
- *Contraindications:* Do not administer to those clients with a history of peptic ulcer disease, bleeding disorders, pregnancy, kidney problems, or allergic reactions to NSAIDs.
- *Anticipated outcome on evaluation:* Headache is relieved.
- *Client teaching:* Advise the client that NSAIDs are most effective when taken at onset of pain. Encourage her to break the pain cycle and give adequate amounts of medication. Narcotics should not be given for this diagnosis, as clients may become physically dependent and experience withdrawal and rebound headaches.

Note: Chronic daily headaches are often drug-rebound headaches caused by overuse of analgesics, especially narcotics, acetaminophen, and ibuprofen. Anyone taking these medications more than four times a week is at risk.

Lifestyle/Dietary Changes. The client may require support in evaluating current life situation and stressors. Help her to prioritize activities and to let go of unnecessary tasks and difficulties. Teach general stress management principles and coping mechanisms. Refer the client for counseling if indicated.

Dietary changes may be applicable if over- or undereating is a source of tension or stress, or if specific foods (high in caffeine or sugar) are noted to trigger the headache.

Exercise or other physical activity is an effective stress reducer. Encourage and support lifestyle changes that incorporate 30 minutes of aerobic exercise at least 5 days a week.

Follow-Up. Plan a follow-up visit 2 weeks after the initial visit to support and reassess the client. If headaches have not significantly improved or if the client has experienced any new symptoms, such as those listed in Table 24–4, refer her to a neurologist. Headache may be an indicator of other psychological problems such as depression. One study found a significant correlation between a history of childhood sexual assault and headaches in adulthood in women (Golding, 1999).

Migraine Headaches

Migraine headaches are recurrent and episodic, accompanied by nausea and/or vomiting and photophobia. According to the International Headache Society classification at least two of the following features must also be present: unilateral location, pulsating quality, moderate to severe intensity, and aggravated by physical activity (C.J. Johnson, 2007; Silberstein, 2000).

The pathogenesis of migraine is thought to be composed of three phases. The first phase begins in the brainstem. The second phase involves vasomotor activation (constriction and dilatation) of arteries both inside and outside the brain. The third phase starts with activation of the brain's head and face pain processing center and the subsequent release of neuropeptides. Pain can be generated during any one of these phases. Most studies of the etiology of migraine pain now focus on disturbances in serotonergic mechanisms as the primary cause (G.D. Johnson, 1998).

In migraines with an aura, previously called "classic migraines," focal neurological symptoms usually precede the headache and may last up to about 20 minutes. Auras are often visual; they may include visual field deficits, a scintillating scotoma (a luminous patch with irregular outline in the visual field), or a fortification spectrum (a dark patch with zigzag outline). Other neurological auras, such as aphasia and hemiplegia, occur occasionally. When the aura fades, the headache usually begins.

Migraines without an aura, previously called "common migraines," have the features of classic migraines, such as throbbing pain, nausea, vomiting, photophobia, and phonophobia, but no aura.

Perimenstrual headaches occur either 2 to 3 days before onset of menses or during the first days of flow. They are frequently severe, usually without aura, and accompanied by nausea and vomiting. It is hypothesized that they are related to fluctuations in estrogen and serotonin levels. Many women consider them as part of premenstrual syndrome (PMS) and may fail to report them (Boyle, 1999).

Epidemiology. The overall incidence of migraine is 18 percent in women and 6 percent in men (Silberstein, 2000). There is usually a strong positive family history. It is more common in women than in men by a ratio of 3:1. Onset is often in childhood, usually at the time of puberty, generally decreasing in frequency after menopause. Pregnancy may relieve or intensify migraine (C.J. Johnson, 2007; Silberstein, 2000). The use of oral contraceptives may be a risk factor for more frequent, more intense migraines; on the other hand, oral contraceptives may make migraines better. Women with neurological symptoms accompanying the headache (other than visual aura) should not take oral contraceptives. Those on hormone replacement with estrogen who report new onset of migraine or an increase in incidence may need an adjustment in dosage or a change from conjugated to pure estrogen (Boyle, 1999).

Subjective Data. Obtaining a complete history is essential (see Table 24–4). The history is used to differentiate between migraines and tension headaches because their treatments differ. The criteria for migraine without an aura include a recurring idiopathic headache with at least two of the following: nausea (with or without vomiting), unilateral pain, throbbing, photophobia or phonophobia, association with menstrual cycle, and positive family history.

Objective Data. A physical examination is done (see Table 24–5). For recurrent migraines, no diagnostic workup is necessary. For an initial diagnosis, a CBC and chemistries may be helpful. Anemia, electrolyte imbalance, and increased calcium can aggravate migraines.

Differential Medical Diagnoses. See section Tension Headaches.

TABLE 24–6. Overview of Medications for Migraines[a]

Abortive Measures: Appropriate for clients experiencing occasional headaches, not more than one a month. These can be used according to headache severity.

Mild: Acetaminophen/ASA/NSAIDS/triptans

Moderate: DHE/ergotomine/lidocaine nasal
Severe: Antiemetics/DHE/ketorolac IM

Preventive Measures: Indicated for three or more attacks per month or one prolonged attack per month. Give adequate trial of 3 to 6 months of therapy.

Beta blockers: Numerous types (propranolol, long-acting preparation increases compliance). Effective in 50% of cases.

Caution: Contraindicated with such conditions as asthma and congestive heart failure.

Tricyclics: Numerous types (amitriptyline [Elavil] often used, starting with a 25 mg dose at bedtime, increasing as necessary).

NSAIDs: Ibuprofen, naproxen sodium, aspirin. Observe for gastrointestinal side effects.

Calcium channel blockers: Numerous types (verapamil [Calan, Isoptin] po 240–360 mg per day). Usually ordered by a neurologist.

For up-to-date headache treatment guidelines, consult the Institute for Clinical Systems Improvement at http://www.ics.org/hedache (2011).

[a]Please consult a current pharmacotherapeuties text for details.

Plan

Psychosocial Interventions. Psychosocial intervention is critical, especially for a client who has migraines with an aura, as these can be very frightening. Reassure the client that she is not having a stroke and involve her as an active participant in measures to prevent and abort attacks.

Medication. See Table 24–6.

Lifestyle/Dietary Changes. Focus primarily on what triggers the migraine. Often there is a "let-down" trigger; for example, the headache starts Saturday morning following a stressful week. Counsel the client to readjust her lifestyle, and help her with stress management.

Diet may be a factor in the occurrence of migraines. The most common triggers are chocolate, alcohol, and aged cheeses. Ask the client to keep a diary of foods eaten and to avoid foods associated with the onset of migraine. Encourage her to eat at regularly scheduled intervals; a drop in blood sugar level may trigger a headache.

Advise the client that physical activity, including aerobic exercise for 30 minutes three to five times a week, helps to reduce stress.

Follow-Up. Teach the client the warning signs of headaches with serious underlying causes (see Table 24–3). If such a warning sign occurs, refer her to a neurologist immediately. Otherwise, arrange to see the client about every 4 to 6 weeks until the migraines improve. If no improvement is seen in 8 weeks or the migraines worsen, refer her to a neurologist.

FEVER

Body temperature is regulated between 97 to 99°F (36 to 37.2° C). When heat production exceeds heat dissipation, for example, during vigorous exercise, the core body temperature may rise above this range until regulatory mechanisms such as sweating, hyperventilation, and vasodilatation promote heat loss and return the body temperature to normal. A sustained elevation of body temperature is called fever and represents a regulated rise to a new set point. Fever of unknown origin (FUO) is a temperature greater than 101.3° F (38.5° C) that occurs on at least three occasions during a three-week period in a person whose diagnosis is not apparent after one week (Porter & Winland-Brown, 2011). It should be noted that in the vast majority of occurrences the diagnosis is either readily apparent after a history and physical exam or becomes evident within a few days.

Epidemiology

The febrile response in children is greater than in adults; in older people, it may be absent even in bacterial illnesses.

The setting in which the fever occurs is also important. Acute fever in a traveler to Southeast Asia or Africa may be due to malaria or an insect-borne virus. A college student with fever is likely to have a viral infection or mononucleosis. An older person recently hospitalized may have urinary tract infection (UTI), pneumonia, phlebitis, or wound infection. Someone with an immune disorder may have an infection caused by an opportunistic agent.

Subjective Data

A symptom history may suggest the cause of fever, especially upper respiratory congestion, myalgias, GI upset, ear pain, cough, painful or frequent urination, or rash.

In the absence of these symptoms, inquire about recent use of major tranquilizers such as haloperidol and fluphenazine or antibiotic use. Neuroleptic malignant syndrome is a rare but potentially life-threatening reaction to these drugs. Serum sickness may follow antibiotic treatment and is usually accompanied by rash and arthralgias. Also inquire about illicit drug use and possible occupational exposures to infected animals or chemicals.

Older patients may report no other symptom than fever but suspect tuberculosis (TB), occult neoplasm, or UTI.

Objective Data

Physical Examination. A thorough head to toe exam of all organ systems is necessary if the etiology of the fever is not elicited by the history. If the fever is high (greater than or equal to 102°F or 39°C) with few systemic complaints, look for a bacterial infection of the chest, throat, or abdomen. If there is a low-grade fever (less than or equal to 101.5°F or 38.6°C) associated with systemic complaints and few focal findings, it is due to a virus.

Do not neglect the dental exam. Abscessed devitalized teeth may cause fever without pain.

Fever after an upper respiratory infection (URI) suggests sinusitis. Shaking chills suggest pyelonephritis or pneumonia.

Diagnostic Tests. Laboratory studies are indicated by the results of the history and physical. These may include CBC with differential, urinalysis; monospot (detects mononucleosis); erythrocyte sedimentation rate (elevated in inflammatory condition such as rheumatoid arthritis, inflammatory bowel disease); liver function tests (elevated in hepatitis); antistreptolysin; titers (elevated in recent streptococcal infection); Lyme titer; and cultures of blood, stool, urine, and throat.

Radiographic Studies. A chest x-ray or flat plate of the abdomen may also be useful.

If endocarditis is suspected, order an ECG (electrocardiogram) and possibly an echocardiogram if valvular involvement is likely.

TB skin test with controls should be placed when appropriate and especially if no obvious etiology is found.

Human immunodeficiency virus (HIV) test is indicated if high-risk behaviors are elicited by history.

Differential Medical Diagnoses. See Table 24–7.

Plan

Psychosocial Interventions. Reassure the client that you will continue to follow her closely and inform her of all test results. Answer all questions as fully and candidly as possible and provide an office telephone number.

Medication. Antipyretics such as acetaminophen or ibuprofen may be taken for comfort and are best given on a regular schedule as opposed to as needed. The etiology of the fever will guide the prescription of other medications.

Lifestyle/Diet Changes. Tepid water baths and plenty of fluids (at least 8 oz of water or juice every hour while awake) will promote comfort and prevent dehydration. Ask the client to keep a temperature diary by checking body temperature at least three times a day before taking antipyretic medications.

Follow-Up

Telephone follow-up within 2 to 3 days. Schedule appointment in 1 week to review findings and assess response to any medications prescribed. If no obvious cause is found after completion of initial diagnostic testing, consult or refer for further evaluation.

DIZZINESS/VERTIGO

Dizziness is a sensation of disequilibrium or altered orientation in relation to one's surroundings. Dizziness as lightheadedness must be distinguished from vertigo. Dizziness may be a sensation of generalized weakness (presyncopal light-headedness) or an inability to maintain balance (disequilibrium). Vertigo is a hallucination of movement. With objective vertigo, the client has the sensation of the room spinning; with subjective vertigo, she has the feeling of her own body spinning when her eyes are closed (Hasso et al., 1999; Magaziner & Walker, 2007).

Epidemiology

Dizziness as a chief complaint accounts for 1 percent of office visits per year. Up to one-third are diagnosed as vestibular in origin, one-fifth are attributed to hyperventilation, and the remainder to neurologic, psychiatric, and cardiovascular etiologies. It is a frequent complaint of older people and may be a predictor of risk for falling, morbidity, and/or functional decline. (Hasso et al., 1999).

The key to differentiating self-limiting versus more serious causes of dizziness is to obtain a thorough history and perform a careful examination.

Subjective Data

The client may have difficulty clarifying what she means by "feeling dizzy." Important questions include the following: Are you spinning? Is the room spinning? Is the dizziness most noticeable when you first stand, sit up, or turn your head? Did the dizziness start suddenly, or has it gone on for a while? How long does the feeling last? What makes the dizziness decrease? What kind of medicines are you taking and for how long have you taken them?

TABLE 24–7. Differential Diagnosis of Fever

Etiology	Symptoms and Associated Factors	Physical Findings
Upper Respiratory Infection:		
Viral	Mild fever Temp 101.5° F (38.6° C) Sore throat, rhinitis, ear fullness Systemic symptoms	Cough, oropharynx injected (no exudate)
Bacterial	High fever—Temp 102° F (39° C) More common in children Pronounced localized symptoms	Tonsillar exudate Bulging tympanic membrane
Other viral syndromes (influenza gastroenteritis)	Mild fever	Minimal physical findings
Drug reaction	Muscle aches, nausea, vomiting, diarrhea Often high fever Occasionally rash Use of over-the-counter or prescription drug	Fever abates when drug stopped
Urinary tract infection	Often high fever and chills, backache, urinary frequency and urgency Often hematuria	Costovertebral angle and suprapubic tenderness
Chronic hepatitis	Intravenous drug use Low-grade fever Fatigue, anorexia	Right upper quadrant tenderness Hepatomegaly Jaundice
Tuberculosis	Low-grade fever Weight loss Night sweats May have been incarcerated	Chest findings + skin test for purified protein derivative (PPD)
Infectious mononucleosis	Young adult Low-grade fever Fatigue	Pharyngitis Adenopathy Splenomegaly
Chronic fatigue syndrome	Debilitating fatigue lasting more than 6 months Mild recurrent or persistent low-grade fever for 6 months Sore throat, muscle weakness, myalgia, migratory arthralgia without swelling or redness Neuropsychologic complaints	Nonexudative pharyngitis Posterior or anterior cervical adenopathy 2 cm or more Low-grade fever on two separate occasions

Sources: Auwaerter, 2007; Porter & Winland-Brown, 2011; Waterbury, 2007.

Significant associated symptoms will assist in the correct diagnosis, especially nausea, tinnitus, ear fullness, one-sided weakness, double vision, facial numbness, numbness, or tingling of the extremities. It is also important to ask if the dizziness has been followed by loss of consciousness or seizure activity. If pregnancy is a possibility, a sexual history and evaluation of contraceptive measures are needed.

Objective Data

Physical Examination

- *Vital signs:* Postural blood pressure readings.
- *Head and neck:* Auscultate for carotid bruit. Examine ear canal and tympanic membrane. Test hearing acuity with 512 Hz tuning fork.
- *Full neurological exam:* Includes evaluation of the cranial nerves (sensory and motor), assessment of cerebellar function, and sensory/motor function. Observe gait for spasticity, ataxia, antalgia, and foot drop.
- *Specific provocative tests and maneuvers:* May also aid in correct diagnosis. Having the client hyperventilate for a minute or two may reproduce symptoms if no focal abnormalities are found on exam. The Dix-Hallpike maneuver is done on clients with positional vertigo (those whose vertigo disappears at rest). It involves rapid change from the sitting position to lying down with the head turned to one side and the neck extended over the end of the exam table 30 to 45°. A diagnosis of paroxysmal positional vertigo can be established with any of the following findings:
- Subjective vertigo.
- *Nystagmus* preceded by a latent period of several seconds after completion of the Dix-Hallpike maneuver. Care should be used in doing this maneuver and should not be performed on frail patients or those with atherosclerotic disease (Magaziner & Walker, 2007).

Diagnostic Tests. If a cardiovascular cause of dizziness is suspected, a 12-lead ECG is appropriate to rule out arrhythmias and conduction disorders.

If focal neurological deficits are found during the physical exam, CT of the head and/or audiogram may be ordered to rule out hemorrhage or tumor.

Pregnancy test, beta human chorionic gonadotropin (HCG), is ordered as needed for women of reproductive age.

Differential Medical Diagnoses of Dizziness/ Lightheadedness and Vertigo

Many physical and psychological maladies have symptoms that include dizziness or vertigo. Otitis media, reactive hypoglycemia, migraine headaches, and orthostatic blood pressure may cause sensations of dizziness or lightheadedness. Many medications, especially antihypertensives, are responsible for symptoms of dizziness or lightheadedness. Afflictions of the inner ear structures, such as Ménière's disease, labryinthitis, and acoustic neuroma cause vertigo. Anxiety and associated hyperventilation cause lightheadedness. Sick sinus syndrome results in recurrent episodes of dizziness. Consult or refer for further evaluation if cardiac etiology is suspected or if focal neurologic deficits are noted.

Plan

Psychosocial Interventions. If a benign or self-limiting etiology is found, client reassurance is most important. Older people may need family support with medication use. Emphasize importance of making the home environment safer to prevent falls. If referral to a cardiologist, neurologist or ear, nose, throat (ENT) surgeon is indicated, reassure the client that you will be available for her other health needs and as a resource.

Medication. Positional vertigo: Meclizine HCl 25 mg, one po every 6 hours as needed for dizziness.

- *Adverse effects:* Drowsiness, dry mouth, blurred vision, nausea, constipation, diarrhea.
- *Contraindications:* Known hypersensitivity. Use with caution in older people due to sensitivity to antihistamine effects; may increase dizziness, cause sedation or hyperexcitability. Use with caution in glaucoma, asthma.
- *Client teaching:* May potentiate effects of alcohol or other central nervous system depressants.

If otitis media is diagnosed, appropriate antibiotics are given (see discussion of otitis media in Respiratory Infections).

Ménière's disease is treated with diuretics, such as hydrochlorothiazide 50 to 100 mg daily (see previous discussion of diuretics under hypertension) and a low salt diet.

Lifestyle Changes. If vertigo is acute, bedrest and a low salt diet are helpful. Advise the client to use care in movement. Driving may have to be curtailed until the symptoms resolve. Provocative head maneuvers such as the Dix-Hallpike (five repetitions performed twice a day) may habituate the vestibular response of positional vertigo. If symptoms persist, the patient may be referred for vestibular rehabilitation therapy (VRT), which has shown to be helpful as a nonpharmacologic approach to symptom relief.

Follow-Up

Refer those with labyrinthine, cardiovascular, psychiatric, and neurologic disorders to an appropriate health care provider. Telephone follow-up to assess alleviation of acute symptoms may be warranted. Anyone who is not referred should be seen within 7 to 10 days.

BELL'S PALSY

Bell's palsy is an idiopathic facial paralysis of the seventh cranial nerve. Its pathogenesis is unknown. There is no evidence to support the theory that it is related to reactivation of the herpes simplex virus, but the benefits of acyclovir treatment lend credence to the possibility that Bell's palsy may have a viral etiology (Grogan & Gronseth, 2001).

Epidemiology

Bell's palsy has an annual incidence of 15 to 30 per 100,000 and occurs equally in men and women; peak incidence appears to be in the fifth decade (Tiemstra & Khatkhate, 2007). Eighty percent recover with full or near-normal function, but 8,000 persons per year retain permanent facial weakness (Grogan & Gronseth, 2001).

Subjective Data

The client may report a sudden onset of pain behind the ear that precedes the paralysis by a day or two. Taste sensation may be diminished or absent. She may also find that her sense of hearing is heightened. She may complain of tearing and inability to close the eye on the affected side. Eating may be difficult.

Objective Data

Physical Examination. The affected side of the face is expressionless with smoothing of forehead wrinkles and flattening of the nasolabial fold. The corner of the mouth sags on the affected side, and the mouth is drawn to the unaffected side. The ipsilateral eyebrow may be raised or lowered. The client will be unable to wink, but on attempt, the eye will rotate upward. There may be a pooling of tears in the lower eyelid. Either side of the face can be affected, and the extent of paralysis can range from mild to complete.

A complete neurological exam to determine if other neurological deficits are present is necessary. The ear and surrounding area should also be evaluated.

Differential Medical Diagnoses

Herpes zoster may also produce a facial palsy, but a vesicular eruption is present. Acoustic neuromas can produce palsy, but hearing loss accompanies this disorder. Bilateral palsy, facial weakness that progresses slowly over several weeks and/or persists more than 6 months, focal neurological signs discovered during the physical exam suggest other more serious diagnoses, such as stroke or infarct, tumor, or multiple sclerosis.

Plan

Psychosocial Interventions. Client reassurance of good recovery in several weeks to months is important. Eighty percent have full recovery in a few months (Grogan & Gronseth, 2001). Incomplete paralysis in the first week is the most favorable prognostic sign. Body image may suffer as client waits for resolution.

Medication. Research supports the early use of prednisone, 1 mg/kg (maximum: 70 mg) in two divided doses for 6 days, followed by a four-day taper. Symptoms also responded to combined treatment with acyclovir (800 mg po five times a day for 7 to 10 days) (Grogan & Gronseth, 2001). Many subjects in research studies experienced spontaneous improvement without treatment, leaving the examiner to conclude that medications may not be necessary. Aside from emotional support to the woman and possible placebo affects, the steroids may at least reduce any discomfort present with Bell's palsy.

Lifestyle/Comfort Measures. Liquid tears may protect the eye from excessive drying, and an eye patch should be worn at night.

Follow-Up

Telephone follow-up is suggested within 2 weeks. The client should return for office evaluation in 6 to 8 weeks. Consult or refer if there is residual paralysis.

ALTERATIONS IN CONSCIOUSNESS

Syncope

Syncope is sudden loss of consciousness and postural tone that resolves rapidly and spontaneously. It arises from an interruption in the flow of blood to the brain. If cerebral tissue is deprived of glucose or oxygen for more than 5 seconds, syncope can occur. If the event lasts more than 15 seconds, tonic movements can occur that may resemble seizure activity (Magaziner & Walker, 2007). The challenge to the provider is to determine if syncope is due to underlying cardiovascular disease or another serious cause.

Epidemiology. Syncope is a relatively common complaint and may account for 3 percent of emergency room visits and up to 6 percent of hospital admissions. Most studies show that in at least 40 percent of individuals with syncope, no cause will be identified (Magaziner & Walker, 2007). Up to half of all adults will experience a syncopal episode during their lives. In older people, the incidence is increased because of decreased blood flow to the brain, a result of the aging process (Magaziner & Walker, 2007).

Subjective Data. A complete history including a detailed account of the syncopal episode, premonitory symptoms, and postsyncopal recover period is crucial to identifying a potential cause. Other factors to note are associated symptoms such as angina, palpitations, nausea, visual changes, numbness in the face, or extremities.

Ask if the event was preceded by exertion, heat exhaustion, dehydration, or emotional stress. Tachyarrhythmias usually have an abrupt onset with no warning and lead to a fall, which may result in injury. Neurogenic syncope or seizure may be preceded by an aura and followed by confusion, drowsiness, and incontinence. Often the event is not witnessed and details may not be provided.

Ask the client about her medications purchased over the counter.

Past medical history may elicit key factors such as history of myocardial infarction or seizure disorder.

Objective Data

Physical Examination. Thorough cardiac and neurologic exams are key.

CARDIOVASCULAR. Blood pressure readings in both arms sitting, supine, and standing must be obtained. The client's blood pressure is measured in both arms 5 minutes after she has stood up from a supine position. A fall of 30 mmHg in the systolic blood pressure is significant for orthostatic hypotension. Important parts of the exams to differentiate cardiac from noncardiac causes include heart rate and rhythm to detect arrhythmia, presence of bruit or murmur, character of peripheral pulses, presence of edema, or adventitious lung sounds indicating congestive heart failure.

NEUROLOGICAL. Includes evaluation of gait, presence of nystagmus, assessment of cranial nerves, cerebellar function, mental, and/or emotional status.

Diagnostic Tests

12-LEAD ECG. The single most important diagnostic test to differentiate cardiac from noncardiac causes of syncope is the 12-lead ECG. If the office ECG is normal and a cardiac cause is strongly suspected, ambulatory ECG (Holter monitoring), may be necessary.

ECHOCARDIOGRAM. If a murmur is auscultated and the syncopal event occurred with exertion, an echocardiogram may detect left ventricular outflow tract abnormality.

Carotid dopplers are indicated if a carotid bruit is detected.

Routine blood tests are usually not helpful unless anemia, hypoglycemia, or electrolyte abnormality is strongly suspected.

Head CTs are not helpful in diagnosis unless focal neurological findings are present; likewise electroencephalograms (EEG) are generally not diagnostic.

Differential Medical Diagnoses. Cardiac causes of syncope can be due to obstruction, ischemia, or arrhythmia. Clients with obstructive causes often report syncope with exertion. This occurs when cardiac output is fixed by aortic stenosis or hypertrophic obstructive cardiomyopathy. Pulmonary hypertension can also cause exertional syncope.

Bradyarrhythmias from complete heart block or other high-grade atrioventricular block can present with syncope unrelated to posture. Sick sinus syndrome (characterized by sinus bradycardia and sinus pause that is preceded by supraventricular tachycardia) is suspected in the client who complains of palpitations just prior to the syncope.

Tachyarrhythmias, especially self-terminating ventricular tachycardia, are common in clients with coronary artery disease and reduced left ventricular function. It can be life threatening if the rhythm converts to ventricular fibrillation. Torsades de Pointes, an arrhythmia associated with prolongation of the QT interval, is a cause of syncope. It may result from certain medications such as antiarrhythmic agents, antidepressants; the interactions of common drugs such as terfenadine with erythromycin; from metabolic abnormalities (hypokalemia, hypomagnesemia, hypocalcemia); and drug use (cocaine, sympathometrics).

Wolf-Parkinson-White syndrome, a supraventricular tachycardia, can be diagnosed by 12-lead ECG.

Ischemic events such as acute angina and infarct can present as syncope. The client may have not have had any preceding chest pain.

Consider cardiac origin of syncope in any client with organic heart disease, especially older people and in those with no premonitory symptoms who collapse abruptly.

Cerebrovascular disease causing temporary interruption of blood flow to the vertebral or basilar arteries is detected by neurological exam. Focal findings may include vertigo, cranial nerve abnormalities, and bilateral sensory motor abnormalities.

Noncardiac causes include vasovagal syncope, which is the most common type in healthy young women. It is often preceded by pain, fear, and emotional stress. It may be accompanied by tonic clonic movements or muscle twitches and may be mistaken for seizures. Rapid recovery and lack of confusion or drowsiness differentiate it from seizure activity.

Situational syncope is also mediated by autonomic reflex mechanisms. Examples include cough, micturition, and defecation syncope.

Drug-related syncope can be caused by diuretics, antihypertensives, antiarrhythmics, cocaine, or alcohol.

With improved diagnostic methods and tools now available the number of patients whose syncopal episodes are considered to be related to psychiatric problems has decreased significantly (Magaziner & Walker, 2007).

Plan. Consult for further diagnostic workup, if indicated, and refer any client with suspected cardiac or neurological causes of syncope.

Psychosocial Interventions. Reassurance is offered to the client with noncardiac, nonneurologic syncope. If an underlying psychiatric disorder is suspected, suggest referral for counseling.

Medication. The client who is referred to cardiology or neurology may be placed on a variety of medications, depending on the underlying etiology of the syncope. The practitioner should become familiar with these agents and provide medication teaching if needed. Be especially alert for interactions with other medications the client may be prescribed or take as over-the-counter remedies.

If the cause of the syncope is a result of medications the client was taking at the time of the event, adjustment in dosage or stopping the medication may be necessary.

Lifestyle Changes. If substance abuse is present, advise the client of the consequences of continued abuse and refer to appropriate drug treatment program. Recommend stress reduction measures. In the older or frail client who is at risk for recurrence, fall precautions are needed. Some clients may have to stop driving.

Follow-Up. Telephone or office follow-up in 7 to 10 days is recommended for those not scheduled for further workup. Alert them that recurrent syncope requires further diagnostic testing.

Seizures

A seizure is a paroxysmal, transient change in neurologic function caused by a disturbance in the electrical activity of the brain. Chronic, recurrent seizures are diagnosed as epilepsy. Seizures are classified as simple, complex partial, absence, and generalized tonic-clonic seizures. The seizure may entail a brief lapse of attention or a period of several minutes of loss of consciousness with abnormal movements.

Epidemiology. Epilepsy is usually diagnosed between 5 and 20 years of age but can start later in life as a result of trauma or disease. Epilepsy affects about 2 million people in the United States and costs about $15.5 billion in direct medical costs (Centers for Disease Control and Prevention [CDC], 2011d). The incidence of seizures rises sharply in the older population, approaching 140 per 100,000 in persons aged 80 and up (Rowan, 1998). One third of people with epilepsy and recent seizures have not seen a neurologist in the past year (CDC, 2011d). And, more than one third of people with epilepsy continue to have seizures despite treatment.

Subjective Data. First ask the client whether she has ever been diagnosed with a seizure disorder and if she is still taking anticonvulsant medication. If the answer is no, then a detailed account of events or sensations that preceded and followed the seizure is key. A febrile illness, headache, or mental confusion suggests an acute infection. Headache with vomiting and a neurological deficit point to a tumor or an intracranial bleed. Recent heavy use of alcohol or barbiturates with sudden withdrawal can trigger seizures. It is also important to ask about prior history of head trauma, kidney disease, or cardiovascular disease. Assess risk factors for HIV. In the older patient, Alzheimer's disease (AD) may be a cause.

Some clients may have a prodrome or premonition of an impending seizure but memory of this may be lost in the postictal state.

Prodromal symptoms include headache, mood change, fatigue, and myoclonic jerking. These precede the seizure by several hours and are not considered part of the aura that immediately precedes the seizure.

If the seizure was witnessed, ask for a description. Partial seizures affect only part of the brain. Simple partial seizures may be characterized by focal motor symptoms such as convulsive jerking or altered sensation such as parasthesias or tingling that spread to other parts of the extremity or body. Consciousness is not impaired. Complex partial seizures are characterized by impairment of consciousness along with the symptoms and signs of simple seizures.

Generalized seizures involve the whole brain. Absence seizures have an abrupt onset of unresponsiveness to external stimuli that may be very brief. Typically, they begin in childhood. Myoclonic seizures are distinguished by single or multiple myoclonic jerks. Tonic-clonic seizures (grand mal) are characterized by sudden loss of consciousness, rigidity (tonic phase) lasting about a minute followed by clonic jerking of the muscles lasting 2 to 3 minutes. Immediately after the seizure, the client may recover consciousness, fall asleep, or have another seizure. The postictal state is characterized by stupor or confusion. Often the client is incontinent during the seizure or may have suffered injury from a fall or from tongue biting (Kaplan, 2007).

Objective Data

Physical Examination. A complete neurological and cardiovascular exam may reveal no abnormalities, especially in younger women.

Note body temperature. Assess for nuchal rigidity.

Examine the skin for signs of alcohol or drug abuse (jaundice, needle marks). Subcutaneous nodules and café-au-lait spots may indicate the presence of neurofibromatosis.

Perform a complete cardiovascular examination to distinguish seizure from syncope (see previous section).

A thorough neurological examination may reveal focal neurological deficits that point to a space occupying lesion, such as tumor or abscess, chronic subdural hematoma, or to arteriovenous malformation. Assess mental status, especially in older people, for signs of AD.

Diagnostic Tests. Diagnostic tests are selected on the basis of prior history and physical exam. Blood chemistries that measure liver and kidney function, blood glucose, and anticonvulsant medication levels may be indicated as well as a CBC. In high risk populations, an HIV test may be appropriate. If a cardiovascular cause is suspected, an ECG is needed to complete the workup.

Any woman with a new onset seizure needs an EEG and a CT scan with and without contrast or MRI.

Differential Medical Diagnoses

- *Syncope:* See previous section.
- *Transient ischemic attacks:* These last longer than seizures and are accompanied by weakness or numbness, not by abnormal motor activity.
- *Migraine headache:* Can present with aura preceding the headache that can make it difficult to distinguish from partial seizures. There are also migraine equivalents, which may be characterized by hemiparesis, numbness, and/or aphasia without headache. Usually the symptoms and signs develop more slowly (over several minutes) and the time factor helps distinguish from seizure activity.
- *Panic attacks:* These may be harder to distinguish from absence or simple seizures but psychiatric history may provide clues.
- *Orthostatic syncope:* Usually occurs after a change in posture, lasts a few seconds, and is followed by prompt recovery as opposed to postictal confusion.
- *Pseudoseizures:* May be hysterical conversion reaction or malingering. They are usually neither preceded by a tonic phase nor followed by postictal behavior. The EEG is usually normal.
- *Generalized tonic-clonic seizures:* May occur 48 hours after withdrawal from alcohol in the client with a history of chronic or high intake. Treatment with anticonvulsants is generally not required unless status epilepticus occurs. As long as the client abstains from alcohol, seizure should not recur.

Plan

Referral. Consultation and/or referral may be warranted for any client who is suspected to have had a seizure. MRI, CT scan, and/or EEG may be ordered before referral to a neurologist. If the underlying cause is infection, admission to the hospital may be indicated. If the underlying etiology is cardiovascular, refer to a cardiologist for further workup. The client with an alcohol withdrawal seizure should be referred for detoxification and rehabilitation.

Medication. Anticonvulsant medication is selected by the neurologist, based on the type of seizure. Once stabilized on a dose, she usually returns to the care of the primary care provider.

The practitioner should be familiar with the more commonly prescribed anticonvulsant medications such as phenytoin and carbamazepine. These medications are effective and affordable. However, newer anticonvulsant medications—lamotrigine, oxcarbazepine, and others—have fewer adverse reactions with improved safety profiles, and so are being used as first-line agent much more frequently. For more complete information, consult a pharmacology reference.

Diet/Lifestyle. The client with well-controlled seizure disorder is capable of leading a normal life, including work, school, and driving (depending on state laws). She should be counseled regarding the importance of healthy eating and rest patterns to maintain optimal health. Confront possible alcohol and illicit drug use openly and advise client of risks. Preconception counseling and consultation with the neurologist before pregnancy is advisable.

Follow-Up. For the person with an isolated seizure and no further workup scheduled, telephone follow-up in 7 days is suggested. Follow-up office visit in 3 months is warranted as well as immediate follow-up should the seizure recur. Telephone follow-up is advised after client is seen by a neurologist or other specialist to become familiar with treatment plan.

PARKINSONISM AND ESSENTIAL TREMOR

Tremor is a purposeless, rhythmic movement resulting from the involuntary alternating contraction and relaxation of opposing groups of skeletal muscles. Essential or familial tremor is usually inherited and has no other associated features. Parkinsonism is a movement disorder characterized by tremor, rigidity, and bradykinesia. It is slowly progressive and caused by an imbalance of the neurotransmitters dopamine and acetylcholine.

Epidemiology

Essential tremor and Parkinsonism are common disorders. Familial essential tremor is often inherited in an autosomal dominant pattern. It can appear at any age. Parkinsonism affects 1 in 100 adults over 50 years of age. It can be found in equal numbers of males and females and occurs in all ethnic groups (Olanow, Watts, & Koller, 2001).

TABLE 24–8. Folstein Mini-Mental State Examination

Maximum Score	Client Score	Questions
5		"What is the (year) (season) (date) (day) (month)?"
5		"Where are we?" Name of (state) (county) (city or town) (place, such as hospital or clinic) (specific location, such as floor or room).
3		The examiner names three unrelated objects clearly and slowly, then asks the client to name all three of them. The client's response is used for scoring. The examiner repeats them until client learns all of them if possible.
5		"Begin with 100 and count backwards by subtracting 7." Stop at 65 (five responses).
3		If the client learned the three objects mentioned earlier, ask her to recall them now.
2		The examiner shows the client two simple objects, such as a wrist watch and pencil, and asks her to name them.
1		"Repeat the phrase, 'No ifs, and, or buts.' "
3		The examiner gives the client a piece of blank paper and asks her to follow the three-step command: "Take the paper in your right hand, fold it in half, and put it on the floor."
1		On a blank piece of paper, the examiner prints the command "Close your eyes," in letters large enough for the client to see clearly, then asks her to read it and follow the command.
1		"Make up and write a sentence about anything." This sentence must contain a noun and a verb.
1		The examiner gives the client a blank piece of paper and asks her to draw a symbol (two interlocking pentagons). All 10 angles must be present and 2 must intersect.
Total Possible = 30	Client's Total =	(If total score is 23 or below, further evaluation may be indicated.)

Source: Folstein, Folstein, & McHugh, 1975.

Subjective Data

Important questions to ask the client: What parts of the body are involved? Does the tremor occur with movement (intentional tremor) or at rest? Does the tremor only affect one side of the body, or is it symmetrical? Does any other member of the family have a similar disorder? Does emotional stress make the tremor worse, and does alcohol make it less noticeable? Are there any other associated complaints such as hoarseness, dysphagia, drooling, depression, nightmares, slowed movement, problems cutting food, turning in bed, and buttoning clothing? Do you use caffeine, stimulant drugs, drink alcohol, take theophylline, and/or anticonvulsants?

Objective Data

Physical Examination. A complete neurological exam is performed, including assessment for cognitive impairment.

Begin with observation of the client's gait, posture, and facial expression. The client with Parkinson's disease takes small, shuffling steps, with little swinging of the arms. The posture is stooped. She may have difficulty stopping and turning around. The facial expression may be fixed with little blinking. Examine the skin for signs of seborrhea of the scalp and face (common in Parkinson's disease).

Examine the mouth and lips for tremor and drooling.

Assess the extremities for strength and deep tendon reflexes. There is usually no weakness and no alteration of deep tendon reflexes.

Observe the tremor. The benign essential tremor will involve one or both hands and/or the head. It persists at rest but worsens with use of the affected hand. No other abnormalities are noted during the exam.

The tremor of Parkinson's disease often becomes less apparent with activity. In early disease, it is confined to one limb or one side of the body. Emotional stress may exacerbate it.

Assess for rigidity. The client with Parkinsonism exhibits increased resistance to passive movement. She may have difficulty arising from a sitting position.

Assessment of cognitive function may be incorporated into the rest of the exam. If deficits are found, more in depth testing may be needed such as the Folstein Mini-Mental Status Examination (see Table 24–8).

Diagnostic Tests. Selected on basis of examination findings but may include rapid plasma reagent (RPR), vitamin B-12 and folate levels, CBC, blood chemistries for electrolyte levels and liver function, thyroid stimulating hormone.

Differential Medical Diagnoses

Huntington's disease involves rigidity and bradykinesia but is distinguished by choreic movements, which are irregular and jerky, as opposed to tremor, which is rhythmic. It is an inherited disease.

Depression may present with expressionless face and slowed movement. It can be difficult to distinguish from early Parkinson's disease and may coexist at the time of diagnosis.

Progressive supranuclear palsy (PSP) and multiple system atrophy (MSA) appear clinically similar to PD. PSP can be differentiated from PD by the woman's inability to move her eyes in vertical planes, especially downward. Clients with consistent orthostatic hypotension that cannot be attributed to other causes (e.g., dehydration, medications) may have MSA (Olanow et al., 2001).

Plan

Consult and/or refer to neurologist if Parkinsonism is suspected. Initial management may be at the primary care level, but expert evaluation and intervention should be obtained within 2 to 6 weeks following preliminary diagnosis.

Psychosocial Interventions. Reassure the client with essential tremor that though the tremor may become progressively worse with age, no other functional abnormalities are associated with this disorder. Provide emotional support to the client and her family affected with Parkinsonism. This is a progressive, debilitating illness. Not only does it affect motor function, 15 to 30 percent of clients develop dementia (Kaye, 1998). Anticipatory guidance is key to the plan. Refer family to support and information groups, such as the Parkinson's Disease Foundation, the National Parkinson's Foundation, and the American Parkinson's Disease Association, Inc.

Medication. Essential tremor has been shown to respond to first-line treatment with propranolol (short or long acting form), and primidone, although 30 percent of all patients are likely to be nonresponders (Treatment of essential tremor, 2006).

Pharmacologic intervention for Parkinsonism is based on restoring dopaminergic function through the use of levodopa (which is metabolized to dopamine) combined with carbodopa (a dopa-decarboxylase inhibitor), which inhibits levodopa metabolism outside the brain (Olanow et al., 2001).

Current clinical management guidelines suggest that either levodopa or a dopamine agonist can be used as first-line therapy for clients with early symptoms of Parkinson's Disease (National Collaborating Centre for Chronic Conditions, 2006). Refer to a pharmacology text for further discussion and current research on these medications.

Parkinsonism Medication

CARBODOPA-LEVODOPA (SINEMET OR SINEMET CR)

- *Administration:* Available in several dosage combinations and as an immediate release and a controlled release form. Dosage will depend on stage of disease and diurnal progression of symptoms. See pharmacology text for further discussion on adjusting dosage.
- *Adverse effects:* Worsening of Parkinsonism symptoms, dyskinesias, cardiac rhythm irregularities, orthostatic hypotension, spasm or closing of eyelids, severe nausea, and vomiting. In clients with dementia, may cause hallucinations and psychosis.
- *Contraindications:* Known hypersensitivity, asthma, emphysema, severe cardiovascular disease, narrow-angle glaucoma, malignant melanoma, history of myocardial infarction.
- *Expected outcome:* Improvement in ability to perform activities of daily living.
- *Client teaching:* Adverse effects, signs of toxicity (muscle twitching and blepharospasm are early signs).

Selegiline, a monamine oxidase-B inhibitor, has been tested for potential neuroprotective properties. Some neurologists advocate the use of selegiline prior to treatment with levodopa (Olanow et al., 2001). Researchers have found that selegiline improves the symptoms of PD initially and may initially delay the need for levodopa therapy. This drug, however, does not slow or prevent the development of levodopa complications once levodopa is begun (Jankovic, 2000). Refer to a pharmacology text for further information.

Other medications may be added based on associated symptoms and progression of disease. These are best initiated in consultation with a neurologist.

Lifestyle/Diet. Clients with essential tremor should be advised to avoid self-medication with alcohol. If tremor is not well controlled with medication, client may have problems with handwriting and other manual skills. Be sensitive to impact on social and professional life.

Help with activities of daily living in the form of assistive devices may help client with Parkinsonism maintain independence. These measures may include rails and banisters in the home, eating utensils with large handles, nonskid mats for table and bath, and communication devices to enhance speech. Client may need special texturized diet if swallowing difficulties are present.

Occupational and physical therapy referrals may be appropriate.

Follow-Up

The client diagnosed with essential tremor should be seen in 2 weeks for response to medication and possible adjustment of dosage.

Client with Parkinson's Disease should be seen within 2 to 3 days of initiation of carbodopalevodopa to assess response and to observe for toxicity. Evaluation and follow-up by a neurologist is considered essential. Continue to provide primary care services.

DEMENTIA/ALZHEIMER'S DISEASE

Dementia is a progressive organic mental disorder with characteristic behaviors and cognitive decline. The hallmark is short-term memory loss, but associated features may include impaired judgment, impaired abstract thinking, language or motor function disturbance, and/or personality change. It must be distinguished from delirium or acute confusional state, which is usually reversible when the underlying cause is corrected. A major irreversible cause of primary dementia in older people is AD. Other causes of dementia are listed in Table 24–9.

Epidemiology

Dementia affects 1 in 10 U.S. adults over the age of 65. It is probably the most feared problem of aging. Alzheimer's accounts for 60 to 70 percent of irreversible dementia. It is age related, has an insidious onset, and may follow a familial pattern. While earlier studies indicated that women who took estrogen during the peri- or postmenopausal stage may be less likely to develop AD (Friedland & Wilcock, 2000; Hebert, Beckett, Scherr, & Evans, 2001), current research does not show this to be the case (Hogervorst, Yaffe, Richards, & Huppert, 2009).

Multi-infarct dementia accounts for 15 to 20 percent of dementias, is more common in men, and is associated with hypertension and transient ischemic attacks (TIAs). About 11 percent of dementias are reversible or partially reversible. The clients more likely to have a reversible dementia are those with recent acute onset, rapid deterioration, atypical presentation, multiple drug use or polypharmacy, history of depression, and onset younger than 60 to 70 years old (Friedland & Wilcock, 2000; Rockwood, 2000).

TABLE 24–9. Causes of Dementia

Probably Irreversible Causes
Alzheimer's disease
Multi-infarct dementia
Alcohol
Parkinson's disease
Huntington's disease
Mixed (Alzheimer's and multi-infarct)
Trauma
Anoxia
Potentially Reversible Causes
Depression
Normal-pressure hydrocephalus
Drugs
Neoplasm
Metabolic
Infections
Subdural hematoma

Sources: Friedland & Wilcock, 2000; Rockwood, 2000.

Subjective Data

A complete health history is needed in the assessment of dementia and preferably taken in the presence of an independent informant who can supplement the history.

The first symptom noted is forgetfulness or loss of short-term memory. This must be distinguished from the benign senescent forgetfulness that sometimes accompanies aging and from depression. Progression of symptoms differentiates benign senescent forgetfulness from the short-term memory loss of Alzheimer's. The family may begin to note increasing difficulty with daily activities such as balancing the checkbook, dressing appropriately, cooking. The client may have some loss of expressive and comprehensive language including word finding difficulty. She may have undergone a personality change, becoming more irritable and impatient; she may be paranoid in her thinking at times. At this point, the family may bring the client in for evaluation. The client herself may have no specific complaint but may become agitated when asked simple questions that she is unable to answer. It is important to review prescription and nonprescription medications taken and alcohol intake.

Objective Data

Physical Examination

- *General appearance:* Begin with careful observation of the client, paying special attention to gait, affect and facial expression, initiation or fluency of speech. Physical appearance may resemble Parkinsonism with stooped gait, masklike face, and slowed movement.
- A *complete cardiovascular exam* focuses on blood pressure and the presence of carotid bruits.
- The *neurological exam* focuses on motor, sensory, hearing, vision, cranial nerves, tremor, reflexes, and cerebellar function.

The client in the early stages of Alzheimer's may have an essentially normal exam up to this point.

Diagnostic Tests. A Folstein or other Standard Mini-Mental Test (see Table 24–8) to assess cognitive function will aid in the diagnosis, but be aware that educational and cultural differences may make scoring difficult.

Standard lab tests to order include CBC, B_{12} and folate, thyroid function, biochemical profile. Consider an RPR or HIV test if high risk for syphilis or acquired immunodeficiency syndrome (AIDS) dementia.

Order CT or MRI if tumor, subdural hematoma, stroke, hydrocephalus, or multi-infarct dementia is suspected. There is no imaging modality available to definitively diagnose AD.

Differential Medical Diagnoses

The cognitive changes that can occur with depression can often be mistaken for signs of dementia, so a depression screening is often indicated. A referral for neuropsychiatric testing can be a valuable step at arriving at an appropriate diagnosis.

The client with normal pressure hydrocephalus may have gait disturbance (broad-based stance) and incontinence.

Creutzfeldt-Jacob disease is a rare, rapidly progressive fatal neurological disease characterized by behavior change, myoclonus, and rigidity.

Parkinson's disease may manifest with early symptoms of dementia when neuromuscular features are not prominent.

Huntington's disease is diagnosed on the basis of family history and the accompanying movement disorder. Onset is 20 to 50 years of age.

Korsakoff's syndrome due to chronic alcohol use involves memory loss and some impairment of cognitive function. It is associated with thiamine deficiency and has a sudden onset.

Tumor, multi-infarct, and subdural hematoma are differentiated on the basis of the imaging modality used.

Plan

Psychosocial Interventions. The practitioner must approach the client and her family with tact and understanding. First, the diagnosis must be made clear. The practitioner should emphasize that maintaining optimal health status for the client will improve the quality of life for both family and client. The practitioner should provide the client and family with resources to help educate them about AD; the Alzheimer's Association [www.alz.org, (800) 272-3900] is a good place to start. The practitioner will need to convey to the family/caregivers the importance of establishing proxy decision makers for future financial and health concerns. It is usually easier to enlist the client's cooperation during the early stages of AD than in later stages, when paranoia may prove to be an obstacle. Attorneys, financial planners, and other professionals are good resources for help in managing her affairs.

Family members may be overwhelmed with the task of caring for a person with dementia. At every visit, take time to talk to caregivers and be alert for caregiver stress or possible elder abuse. Reiterate the importance of maintaining a safe environment. A bracelet with the client's name, address, and phone number is a must, especially if she wanders off. Refer family members to respite services; respite services range from a few hours during an afternoon to entire weekends. Some nursing homes and assisted living facilities offer varying degrees of respite and adult day programs for cognitively impaired older people.

Medication

Cholinesterase inhibitors—donepezil, rivastigmine, and galantamin—are the primary medications used in the management of the dementia of AD. This class of medication has shown some benefit in enhancing cognitive function in those with mild to moderate AD. However, recent studies (Gill et al., 2009) have shown a tendency for these medications to have an adverse reaction of bradycardia and subsequent episodes of fainting and falls, thus requiring close monitoring of clients taking these medications.

Antidepressants, such as secondary amine *tricyclic antidepressants* (nortriptyline and desipramine) or one of the selective serotonin reuptake inhibitors, may improve quality of life significantly in early disease. See Chapter 25 for further information on these medications.

Diet/Lifestyle. A healthy and varied diet, adequate rest, maintenance of regular elimination, and skin hygiene are vitally important areas for the client, especially when she is unable to provide these for herself. Advise family to avoid using antihistamines for sleep problems. These medications have a high potential to cause confusion. Instead suggest limiting chocolate, colas, tea, and coffee that contain caffeine. Providing a safe environment is key as well as including client in family or community activities as much as possible. Activities that target cognitive function, physical activity, and overall well-being should be encouraged.

Follow-Up

Once the diagnosis is made, a follow-up visit in 2 weeks is suggested to ascertain how the client and her family are adjusting to the diagnosis. Consult with a neurologist if signs of psychosis appear or if the client shows increasing agitation and behavioral disturbances. Schedule regular visits every 3 months or more often based on the client's status (Friedland & Wilcock, 2000).

OPHTHALMOLOGICAL DISORDERS

CONJUNCTIVITIS

The most common eye problem encountered in primary care is a red eye. The redness is caused by injection of the conjunctival, episcleral, or ciliary blood vessels. In evaluating the client, it is important to remember that common problems are common; that is, that conjunctivitis caused by a virus, bacteria, or allergen is usually the diagnosis. It is imperative, however, to rule out other more serious disorders. As always, a good history and physical exam are keys to diagnosis.

Epidemiology

Several species of bacteria normally colonize the conjunctival sac, most commonly *Staphylococcus albus* and *aureus, Corynebacterium,* and *Streptococcus.* Acute bacterial conjunctivitis may be caused by an overgrowth of *Staphylococcus aureus.* It may also be caused by pneumococcal infection, especially in colder weather, and by *Haemophilus* in warmer regions of the United States. In younger individuals, *Haemophilus* is more often the causative organism than *Staphylococcus aureus.* Other bacteria implicated in acute conjunctivitis include *Neisseria gonorrhoeae, Neisseria meningitidis, Escherichia coli,* and *Proteus* species. Chronic bacterial conjunctivitis is usually caused by *Staphylococcus aureus* or by *epidermidis* or by *Streptococcus pyogenes.* It is often associated with blepharitis.

Sexually active young adults are at risk for inclusion conjunctivitis caused by *Chlamydia* contamination of the eye after sexual contact and at risk for the hyperacute conjunctivitis caused by *Neisseria gonorrhoeae.* Alcoholics and other individuals with nutritional deficiencies are at risk for all types of infectious conjunctivitis.

Viruses are the causative organism in most cases of infectious conjunctivitis. Most commonly implicated are the adenoviruses. A more serious form of viral keratoconjunctivitis is caused by the herpes simplex virus that may spread to the eye after contact with genital lesions. Herpes zoster may also spread to the eye (Schachat, 1999c).

Seasonal conjunctivitis is a recurrent, transient, and self-limiting allergic conjunctivitis associated with a particular time of year and allergen (Quinn et al., 1999). Vernal conjunctivitis, on the other hand, is a much more severe inflammation associated with dry, warm climates. It is more in young males (< 20 years of age) of African descent and usually lasts 4 years. It may exhibit a seasonal pattern in more temperate climates (Quinn et al., 1999).

Subjective Data

Important questions to ask:

Do you wear contact lenses? Contact lens wearers are at higher risk for infectious conjunctivitis, especially bacterial. Often they continue to wear the lens and are at risk for infection by anaerobes and for corneal ulceration.

When did the redness first appear? Which eye? The onset of viral and acute bacterial conjunctivitis as well as inclusion conjunctivitis is abrupt, often affecting one eye and after several days spreading to the other eye by autoinoculation. Irritant conjunctivitis follows contact with a trigger such as a chemical.

Is there any change or loss of vision? Blurred vision may occur with inclusion conjunctivitis. Epidemic keratoconjunctivitis caused by several *adenovirus* types may be associated with formation of a pseudomembrane that reduces vision. *Herpes* infection of the eye may also cause decreased visual acuity especially if not treated promptly.

Any discharge? Copious, thick exudate is the hallmark of gonococcal conjunctivitis. Mucopurulent to mucoid discharge accompanies other forms of infectious conjunctivitis. Allergic conjunctivitis causes tearing.

Any pain? Foreign body sensation? Pruritis? Gonococcal conjunctivitis is accompanied by discomfort, swelling of the eyelid, and tenderness. Chronic bacterial conjunctivitis and *herpes* virus keratoconjunctivitis may cause a foreign body sensation. If treatment of *Chlamydial* conjunctivitis is delayed, iritis may develop resulting in photophobia. Allergic conjunctivitis is characterized by often intense pruritis.

Previous eye injury, head trauma, infection, or surgery? Viral conjunctivitis often follows an URI. Previous eye surgery may put client at risk for bacterial conjunctivitis. Eye injury puts client at risk for subsequent iritis and corneal abrasion (which must be differentiated from the red eye of conjunctivitis).

Any contact with infected genital secretions? Always retain high suspicion of sexually transmitted etiology of conjunctivitis in sexually active client. *Gonococcal, Chlamydial,* and *herpes* virus conjunctivitis require prompt diagnosis and referral to an ophthalmologist to prevent serious consequences including loss of vision.

Any chronic disease? Medications taken routinely? Immunocompromised individuals are at higher risk for infectious conjunctivitis. Clients with psoriasis or seborrhea are more prone to chronic conjunctivitis. Conditions associated with increased risk of iritis include herpes zoster, herpes simplex infections, Lyme disease, TB, syphilis, and autoimmune disease such as inflammatory bowel disease and sarcoidosis.

Any association with occupation or hobby? Welders who do not wear protective eyeglasses are at risk for a punctate keratitis (arc welder's eye), which presents with redness and photophobia. Irritant or allergic conjunctivitis may follow accidental exposure to chemical used in a hobby or craft.

Any family member with similar problem? Viral conjunctivitis is highly contagious.

Objective Data

Physical Examination. Appearance of the eye and lids. Conjunctival (bulbar and palpebral) injection is the hallmark of conjunctivitis. Lids may be very swollen in gonococcal conjunctivitis, erythematous in chronic bacterial conjunctivitis with crusting at the base of the eyelash (see Table 24–10).

Chlamydial inclusion conjunctivitis produces follicles on the palpebral conjunctiva, especially on the lower lid. Marked swelling of the conjunctiva occurs in allergic conjunctivitis. Examine for exudate. The exudate of gonococcal conjunctivitis is thick, copious, and accumulates in the lashes. Acute bacterial conjunctivitis is characterized by thinner mucopurulent discharge. The exudate of viral and allergic conjunctivitis is watery.

Compare pupils for equality of size, important in differentiating conjunctivitis from iritis and glaucoma. Conjunctivitis causes no inequality. In iritis, pupil is small and unequal.

Examine for swelling of preauricular nodes present in viral conjunctivitis, including herpes keratoconjunctivitis.

Evert eyelid to examine for foreign body that may have triggered injection of the conjunctiva.

Evaluate extraocular movements, test pupillary reaction, visual fields.

Direct ophthalmoscopy of fundus and disc. Flashlight examination of anterior chamber.

Diagnostic Tests

Visual Acuity. It is imperative to assess visual acuity. If this is not done, a serious mistake in diagnosis may occur, placing the practitioner at risk for negligence. If the client has forgotten or lost her corrective lenses, a pinhole disk may be used to optimize acuity.

Client with chemical conjunctivitis caused by acid or alkali needs pH measurement of conjunctival secretion after initial irrigation with large amounts (1 to 2 L) of normal saline or water. If pH is less than or greater than 6.8 to 7.0, continue to irrigate to prevent permanent damage and refer immediately to an ophthalmologist.

Fluorescein Staining. Fluorescein staining of conjunctiva and examination by slit lamp or Wood's Lamp for epithelial staining defect if corneal injury suspected. Fluorescein staining assists in the diagnosis of herpes keratoconjunctivitis, which has a characteristic dendritic appearance.

If gonococcal or Chlamydial infection is suspected, confirmation by stained smear and culture is needed. Prompt diagnosis and treatment prevent blindness.

Acute bacterial conjunctivitis and chronic conjunctivitis are usually diagnosed by examination and history; however, if there is doubt about the causative organism a culture and sensitivity should be obtained.

TABLE 24–10. Objective Findings in Conjunctivitis

	Viral	Bacterial	Chlamydia	Allergic
Exudate	Serous	Copious mucopurulent or mucoid NOTE: Gonococcal conjunctivitis drainage is copious and purulent	Thin, serous	Watery profuse
Unilateral vs. bilateral	Bilateral NOTE: HSV unilateral	Unilateral	Often unilateral	Bilateral
Associated features	Enlarged preauricular nodes	Blepharitis	Urethritis	Asthma
	Pharyngitis	Hordeolum	Prominent follicles upper and lower lids	Atopy
	Abrupt onset	Eyelids stuck together		Itchy eyes
	Palpebral conjunctiva injected		Nontender preauricular node	Swollen eyelids
	HSV: Dendritic pattern if fluorescein stained		May have mild keratitis	Chemosis (edema) of cornea and conjunctiva

HSV—herpes simplex virus

Sources: Quinn et al., 1999; Schachat, 1999a, 1999c.

TABLE 24–11. Differential Diagnoses of Red Eye

	Conjunctivitis	Corneal Abrasion	Iritis	Acute Glaucoma
Signs and Symptoms				
Pain	Mild	Moderate to severe	Moderate to severe	Severe (often with nausea and vomiting)
Foreign body sensation	Mild	Moderate to severe	None	None
Vision	Normal	Blurred	Blurred with photophobia	Greatly reduced
Pupil size	Normal	Normal	Small and fixed in affected eye	Dilated
Other information	May follow upper respiratory infection	Hx important for foreign body, abrasion, contact lens wear, use of arc welding equipment	"Ciliary flush" redness from iritis extends into cornea. Urgent referral to an opthalmologist needed.	Anterior chamber shallow

Sources: Quinn et al., 1999; Schachat, 1999b, 1999c.

Differential Medical Diagnoses

Iritis presents with intense photophobia, redness localized around the cornea, and smaller unequal pupil of the affected eye (see Table 24–11).

Acute angle closure glaucoma causes diminished vision, hazy or steamy cornea, dilated unequal pupil in the affected eye, with redness around the cornea.

Scleritis, an inflammatory condition of the deeper vessels of the sclera, is characterized by pain, no exudate, and a localized redness, often most intense in the superior globe of the eye.

Corneal abrasion and foreign body are diagnosed by history, foreign body sensation, and epithelial staining defect on staining and slit lamp or Wood's Lamp examination.

Plan

The client with acute angle closure glaucoma, foreign body that has penetrated the cornea or is not removed by irrigation, iritis, scleritis, or keratoconjunctivitis caused by herpes virus or arc welding is referred immediately to an ophthalmologist.

Psychosocial Interventions. Reassure client eye tissue heals very quickly; with adherence to treatment regimen, good outcome is expected. Client may be sensitive about appearance, especially if exudate is present. She should avoid mascara and eyeliner until conjunctivitis resolved. She may need a work excuse if she works in health care setting, food service, or childcare. If conjunctivitis is due to sexually transmitted disease, advise client that partner(s) need treatment.

Medication. *Viral Conjunctivitis*

NORMAL SALINE EYE DROPS

- *Administration:* Two drops each eye every 2 to 3 hours for as long as needed.
- *Side effects:* May experience transient stinging of eyes.
- *Contraindication:* None.
- *Expected outcome:* Advise the client it may take 7 to 10 days before conjunctiva clear.

Note: Ophthalmologists recommend that antibiotic eye drops not be used for the treatment of viral conjunctivitis due to the potential for allergic response. Agents such as sodium sulfacetamide and erythromycin have low potential; gentamicin, neomycin, and tobramycin have high potential. If it is difficult to distinguish whether conjunctivitis is due to virus or bacteria treat with an agent with a low potential for allergic response.. If client is at risk for bacterial superinfection, treat with low potential agent and evaluate after 3 to 5 days for response.

Allergic Conjunctivitis. There are numerous products now available for treatment of "itchy eyes," some of which are available over the counter, others only by prescription. Naphazoline is just one of these products, and its use is described here.

NAPHAZOLINE HYDROCHLORIDE.
Ophthalmic solution 0.1 percent.

- *Administration:* Instill one to two drops each eye every 3 to 4 hours for relief of itching and redness.
- *Adverse effects:* Transient stinging, pupillary dilation, hyperemia, increased or decreased intraocular pressure.
- *Contraindications:* Sensitivity to ingredients, history of glaucoma.
- *Expected outcome:* May be a recurrent problem, but medication should relieve symptoms.
- *Client teaching:* Advise the client to report blurred vision, eye pain, lid swelling, and discontinue use if occurs. Use of cool compresses as needed for added comfort. May add oral antihistamine such as Benadryl if severe itching.

Chemical Conjunctivitis. Cool compresses for 15 to 20 minutes several times a day and use of topical vasoconstrictor solution such as naphazoline hydrochloride solution (see prior information).

Note: If chemical trigger is acid or alkali, immediately irrigate eye with normal saline or water, measure pH. When neutral pH achieved, examine fluorescein-stained eye with slit lamp and/or refer to an ophthalmologist.

Acute Bacterial Conjunctivitis. As with formulations for treatment of allergic conjunctivitis, there are currently many available antibiotic preparations for treatment of bacterial conjunctivitis. These are typically prescribed based on factors such as the client's known allergy history to medications, and what formulation will be most accessible through the client's health insurance plan. Sodium sulfacetamide is available in a generic form, so therefore more affordable, and is described here.

SODIUM SULFACETAMIDE.
(Sulamyd—10 percent) solution.

- *Administration:* Two drops in the eye every 3 hours while awake for 5 to 7 days.
- *Adverse effects:* Blurred vision, transient burning, and stinging. Hypersensitivity, intense itching, and/or burning.
- *Contraindication:* Known sensitivity to sulfonamides.
- *Expected outcome:* Symptoms usually resolve in a couple of days.
- *Client teaching:* Advise the client not to let dropper touch eye, remove exudate with warm, clean cloth before instilling drops. Teach signs/symptoms of sensitivity and advise client to discontinue use immediately and call practitioner if sensitivity develops. Wait 10 minutes before using another eye preparation.

Hyperacute Bacterial Conjunctivitis. Hyperacute bacterial conjunctivitis due to *Neisseria gonorrhoeae* must be referred to an ophthalmologist for topical and systemic antibiotic therapy to prevent corneal damage and systemic spread.

Note: If the client is allergic to sulfonamides, erythromycin ophthalmic ointment may be used four times a day for the same duration of time. See the following for adverse effects and client teaching.

Chronic Bacterial Conjunctivitis

ERYTHROMYCIN OPHTHALMIC OINTMENT

- *Administration:* Apply to lower lid inner canthus to outer canthus four times a day for at least 2 weeks.
- *Adverse effects:* Blurred vision, transient burning, and stinging.
- *Contraindication:* Known sensitivity to erythromycin.
- *Expected outcome:* Reduces bacterial count but may recur.
- *Client teaching:* Advise the client to clean eyelashes with neutral soap such as baby shampoo (see Blepharitis for details) before applying ointment. Advise client scrupulous hygiene may help prevent recurrence.

Inclusion Conjunctivitis (Chlamydial Conjunctivitis). Requires referral to an ophthalmologist for systemic therapy and confirmation of diagnosis. If there is any doubt about the diagnosis, refer. Sexually active women may have no associated symptoms, such as vaginal discharge. Diagnosis is based on suspicion, prominent follicles on lower palpebral conjunctival sac, and confirmation by Giemsa-stained conjunctival scraping. Treatment is with Doxycycline 100 mg twice a day for 3 to 5 weeks.

Lifestyle. Clients with infectious conjunctivitis should avoid spread by not sharing towels, washcloths, and makeup. Advise client to discard any eye makeup used at time of onset of symptoms.

Frequent handwashing is emphasized, and always after touching eyes. May not return to work until exudate resolved if employed in health care, childcare, or food service.

Clients with allergic conjunctivitis should try to determine trigger(s) and avoid as much as possible.

If conjunctivitis is associated with sexually transmitted disease, advise client on other risks of unprotected sex such as pelvic inflammatory disease, sterility, and HIV infection.

CORNEAL ABRASION

Corneal abrasion is caused by disruption of the epithelial covering of the cornea. It may follow trauma, any superficial contact such as with dust, debris, or prolonged exposure to ultraviolet light such as sunlight, sunlamp, or welder's arc.

Epidemiology

Contact lens wearers are at higher risk for abrasion (and ulceration) not only because insertion of the lens may result in abrasion but also because the cornea over time may become less sensitive to insult and treatment may be delayed. Clients in occupations involving prolonged exposure to dirt, dust, debris, sunlight, and wind are also at higher risk for corneal abrasion.

Subjective Data

Client reports history of trauma, severe pain, foreign body sensation, and photophobia.

Objective Data

Physical Examination. Diffuse or localized redness. May have profuse tearing. Client may be unable to open eye for examination if pain is severe. Oblique illumination of the cornea by penlight may reveal irregular area on corneal surface. Always evert eyelid to examine for foreign body.

Diagnostic Tests

Visual Acuity. Is recorded. (Practitioner may have to instill one to two drops topical ophthalmic anesthetic such as procainamide before starting examination.)

Fluorescein Staining. Fluorescein strip is dampened with sterile normal saline and lightly touched to the conjunctival surface of lower lid. After stain is blinked into surface of the eye, cornea is examined with slit lamp or Wood's lamp. Epithelial staining defect appears as deep green with cobalt blue filter.

Differential Medical Diagnoses

Herpes simplex keratitis. Suspect if previous history of herpes keratitis, coexisting fever blister or herpes genitalis, vague or absent history of trauma, dendritic corneal stain pattern.

Ultraviolet keratitis. History of exposure to sunlight, snow, sunlamp, or welder's arc without adequate eye protection. Symptoms occur 6 to 12 hours after exposure. Client complains of intense pain and photophobia and may be unable to open eyes. Staining reveals diffuse punctate pattern of both corneas.

Plan

Refer immediately any client with herpes keratoconjunctivitis or ultraviolet keratitis to an ophthalmologist. Consult and/or refer to an ophthalmologist if corneal abrasion. Deep or extensive abrasions, corneal ulceration, contact lens wearers should always be referred for follow-up with an ophthalmologist.

Psychosocial Interventions. Reassure client that cornea heals very rapidly but emphasize strict adherence to treatment plan to prevent complications such as ulceration and infection.

Medication

Erythromycin Ophthalmic Ointment. Is used to prevent infection.

- *Administration:* Apply to lower lid.
- *Contraindication:* Sensitivity to erythromycin (rare).
- *Expected outcome:* Superficial abrasion usually heals within 24 to 48 hours without complication.
- *Client teaching:* Advise the patient not to drive. She should rest at home, and keep unaffected eye closed as much as possible. She should be seen the next day by the practitioner (if skilled in using slit lamp) or referred to an ophthalmologist (always if contact lens wearer).

Lifestyle Changes. If the client is a contact lens wearer and has recurrent episodes of conjunctivitis, irritation, or abrasion, advise her to return to ophthalmologist or optometrist who originally prescribed lenses for further evaluation.

Follow-Up

Client is always examined the next day using slit lamp or Wood's lamp after fluorescein staining. If staining defect remains or if client continues to complain of foreign body sensation or pain, consult with an ophthalmologist immediately. Request copy of visit note and treatment plan if referred to an ophthalmologist in order to ensure continuity of care.

DISORDERS OF THE EYELID

Hordeolum and Chalazion

A hordeolum is an abscess of the meibomian gland (internal hordeolum) or the gland at the base of the lash (external hordeolum or sty). It can occur on the upper or the lower lid. It is caused by *Staphylococcus.* If the abscess is internal, it can press on the conjunctiva and cause a cellulitis of the lid.

A chalazion is a granulomatous inflammation of the meibomian gland that is caused by an internal hordeolum.

Epidemiology. Both conditions are common in children and adults. Clients with compromised immunity such as diabetics may be more prone to develop hordeolum.

Subjective Data. The client with hordeolum may complain of pain in proportion to the degree of swelling. If a chalazion is large, it may press on the eyeball and cause pain, conjunctival injection, or even blurring of vision.

Objective Data. Hordeolum causes a red, tender swelling of the lid, usually arising from the skin surface. If the hordeolum is internal (less common), it is larger and can press on the conjunctiva. If the entire lid becomes swollen, it can progress to a cellulitis. Chalazion is a small nontender nodule that can be palpated within the upper or lower eyelid. If the lid is everted, a corresponding area of redness is seen. A chalazion may become infected, and the presentation would be similar to a hordeolum with painful swelling.

Physical Examination. Inspection of the eyelid and everting the lid usually confirm the diagnosis. If the hordeolum is internal, the cornea should be examined for abrasion (see previous section).

Diagnostic Test. None is indicated.

Differential Medical Diagnoses. Chalazion and hordeolum are often confused. Chalazion tend to be smaller and chronic; they are usually not painful unless they are quite large. Hordeolum presents with pain and localized redness.

Blepharitis (see following) involves the whole eyelid and is usually accompanied by scaling, itching, and burning.

Plan

Psychosocial Interventions. Both hordeolum and chalazion can be disfiguring and cause body image concerns. Reassure the client that if conservative measures do not resolve the conditions, prompt referral to the ophthalmologist will follow.

Medication and Treatment

HORDEOLUM

- Bacitracin or erythromycin ophthalmic ointment instilled into the conjunctival sac every 3 hours (see section Conjunctivitis).
- Sodium Sulfacetimide Solution (Sulamyd-10) If drops preferred and the client not allergic to sulfa, may be prescribed, two drops in affected eye every 3 hours while awake (see section Conjunctivitis).
- Warm compresses applied for 15 minutes to the affected eye three or four times a day are also helpful to reduce swelling. If the acute stage is not resolved within 48 hours, refer to an ophthalmologist for incision and drainage.

CHALAZION

- Erythromycin ophthalmic ointment. If the chalazion is large or if it appears to be infected, inflamed, or affects vision, treat with erythromycin ophthalmic ointment and refer to an ophthalmologist.
- Small chalazion may be treated with warm compresses, as described earlier.

Lifestyle. Ophthalmic ointment may cause blurred vision and impair driving and close work. Advise client not to rub, scratch or touch eye, wash hands before and after applying medication or compresses.

Follow-Up. If hordeola recur, client may have a chronic Staphylococcal infection of the eyelid. In addition, recurrent eyelid lesions may be basal cell carcinoma. Refer to an ophthalmologist.

Blepharitis

Blepharitis is an inflammation of the lid margins that is usually chronic. There may be acute exacerbations and infectious flare-ups.

There are two types of blepharitis, anterior and posterior. Anterior blepharitis involves the eyelid skin, lashes, and glands. It may be chronic with swelling of the lids along the lash line and scaling of the skin. It is often associated with seborrhea and dandruff. There can be acute flare-ups of anterior blepharitis caused by *Staphylococci.*

Posterior blepharitis is an inflammatory condition of the eyelids caused by dysfunction of the meibomian glands.

Epidemiology. Blepharitis is the most common disorder of the eyelids. The client often has associated seborrhea, dandruff, and/or acne rosacea.

Subjective Data. The client usually complains of burning, itching, and irritation. She may also have noted mucous discharge if the meibomian glands are inflamed.

Objective Data

Physical Examination. In anterior blepharitis, the client's eyes are red-rimmed and the conjunctiva may be injected. Scales may be seen clinging to the eyebrows and eyelids. If there is an acute flare, there may be a loss of lashes. The redness and crusting will be more pronounced.

In posterior blepharitis, telangiectasias can be seen on the lid margins. The openings of the meibomian glands may be plugged, inflamed, and exudative. Associated tears may be greasy. There may be mild entropion of the lid margin.

Diagnostic Test. Usually not indicated. Physical exam confirms the diagnosis.

Differential Medical Diagnoses. See section Hordeolum and Chalazion.

Plan

Psychosocial Interventions. Reassure the client that even though this is a chronic condition, flare-ups can be minimized with meticulous hygiene and self-care. Body image concerns should be explored because of the scaling and redness of the lids.

Medication and Treatment

ANTERIOR BLEPHARITIS

- If the client has frequent exacerbations, nightly application of erythromycin or bacitracin ophthalmic ointment applied with a cotton swab to the lid margin may be indicated (see section Conjunctivitis).
- Tar or selenium shampoo daily controls scaling of the scalp.
- Acute flare of anterior blepharitis is treated with sodium sulfacetamide (Sulamyd-10) drops every 2 to 3 hours while awake or erythromycin ointment applied four times a day (see section Conjunctivitis).
- The cornerstone of treatment is scrupulous hygiene of the scalp, eyebrows, and lid margins. Scales should be removed from the lashes and eyebrows with a damp cotton applicator dipped in baby shampoo twice a day. Advise the client to pull the lower lid down so that lash margins are thoroughly scrubbed. Follow with warm water cloth to rinse. If scales adhere to lashes, advise client to apply warm compresses for several minutes before swabbing with baby shampoo to loosen scales.

POSTERIOR BLEPHARITIS

- Inflammatory flares may require systemic therapy with erythromycin 250 mg four times a day or tetracycline 250 mg twice a day.
- Consult with an ophthalmologist regarding use of topical steroid drops.
- Mild posterior blepharitis may only require daily expression of meibomian glands by gentle pressure to lids followed by cleansing regimen as described previously.
- Client with associated entropion may require referral to an ophthalmologist for surgery if lashes rub on cornea.

Lifestyle Modifications. Advise the client to use hypoallergenic cosmetics and not to share eye makeup. She should avoid rubbing the eyes and wash hands often especially after touching eye area.

Follow-Up. During acute flares evaluate for response to therapy in one week. Encourage client to call if inflammation starts in order to initiate therapy promptly.

UVEITIS

Uveitis is an inflammation of the uveal tract of the eye, which includes the iris, ciliary body, and choroid. Uveitis is most often confined to the anterior structures of the iris and ciliary body. Posterior uveitis is rare and usually does not present with a painful red eye but with complaint of decreased vision and spots in the visual field (Schachat, 1999c).

Epidemiology

In the client without accompanying systemic illness, the most common cause of acute anterior uveitis is trauma. Systemic disorders associated with anterior uveitis include the HLA-B27 complexes (sarcoidosis, psoriasis, inflammatory bowel disease, ankylosing spondylitis, Reiter's syndrome). Herpes simplex and herpes zoster may also cause anterior uveitis. Posterior uveitis may be caused by sarcoidosis (usually bilateral involvement), TB, syphilis, toxoplasmosis, and leprosy. In many cases of anterior uveitis, no underlying cause is determined (Perez & Foster, 2001).

Subjective Data

In anterior uveitis, the client complains of eye pain, redness, photophobia, and blurred vision. She may deny history of trauma or coexisting illness. In posterior uveitis, the client presents with complaint of gradual diminution of vision, spots appearing in the visual field, and no inflammation or pain.

Objective Data

Physical Examination. In acute anterior uveitis, the affected pupil is small and may be irregular. The conjunctiva is injected around the limbus. Profuse tearing may be present. In posterior uveitis, the eye appears normal or quiet.

Diagnostic Tests

Visual Acuity. Always record visual acuity. If client has forgotten or lost corrective lenses, a pinhole disk may be used to optimize acuity. Acuity in the affected eye is diminished from baseline.

Slit Lamp Examination. Slit lamp examination of the anterior chamber reveals inflammatory cells and flare.

Note: The practitioner who is not skilled in the use of a slit lamp should not attempt to examine the client and referral needs to be made to an ophthalmologist.

Plan

Refer immediately to an ophthalmologist. Treatment involves use of topical mydriatic and cycloplegic agents that dilate the pupil and paralyze the ocular muscles of accommodation and use of topical corticosteroids to suppress inflammation.

GLAUCOMA

Glaucoma is a condition of abnormally elevated pressure within the eye caused by an obstruction of outflow of the aqueous humor. Acute (angle-closure) glaucoma occurs when the obstruction arises from the iris and blocks the exit of aqueous humor from the anterior chamber. It is acute in onset, occurring with pupillary dilatation, and is an ophthalmology emergency. The client must be referred immediately to prevent vision loss and damage to the optic nerve. Open angle glaucoma develops slowly from an obstruction within the canal of Schlemm. Over time it too can cause optical nerve damage and blindness if not detected and treated appropriately.

Epidemiology

Glaucoma is the second most common cause of irreversible blindness in the United States, and currently affects more than 2 million individuals in the United States (Eye Diseases Prevalence Research Group, 2004). There are two major types of glaucoma, primary and secondary. Primary open angle and primary acute angle closure (angle-closure glaucoma) are seen most commonly in primary care. Primary open angle glaucoma is the most common cause of glaucoma in the United States and is responsible for 20 percent of blindness (Friedman, 2007; Schachat, 1999b).

Open angle glaucoma is more common among African Americans with earlier onset and more severe damage at time of diagnosis. The risk of glaucoma increases with age and has a hereditary pattern. Risk factors for damage to the optic nerve due to open angle glaucoma include the following: elevated intraocular pressure; enlargement of the optic cup; vascular abnormalities, for example, hypertension, diabetes, and migraine; myopia; and use of steroids (Schachat, 1999b).

Subjective Data

Acute angle closure glaucoma presents with sudden onset of extreme pain and blurred vision. Client may associate onset with sitting in darkened theater, time of stress, or having pupil dilated during ophthalmoscopic examination. She may experience nausea and abdominal pain.

Open angle glaucoma has an insidious onset and there are no symptoms in the early stages. Later the client may note constriction of the visual field with central vision preserved. She may note haloes around lights if the intraocular pressure is markedly elevated.

Objective Data

Physical Examination. Acute angle closure glaucoma causes a red eye, steamy-appearing cornea, and a moderately dilated pupil that is nonreactive to light. The globe feels hard when lightly touched. The client with open angle glaucoma has a normal-appearing eye. The nurse practitioner in primary practice may not be skilled in tonometric measurement to assess intraocular pressure but she or he can perform the most useful method of screening, ophthalmoscopic examination of the optic disk. The average cup to disk ratio is 0.3 and is equal bilaterally. Examine disk for narrow rim and hemorrhage. An enlarged cup or an asymmetric cup-to-disk ratio is grounds for referral to an ophthalmologist for visual field and tonometric analysis (Schachat, 1999b).

Assessment of visual fields by confrontation may be done but may not be reliable. Constriction of vision is gradual and subtle. Thorough examination is done with specialized equipment usually not found in primary practice and requires 10 to 20 minutes per eye.

Diagnostic Tests

Visual Acuity. Central vision is usually preserved, but every good eye exam begins with acuity.

Visual Fields by Confrontation. Detects tunnel vision through use of special instrument used by trained personnel in optometrist or ophthalmologist's office.

Tonometry. Examination of intraocular pressure using tonometry is not recommended for the primary care provider, because common handheld devices alone are not sensitive or specific enough to accurately assess intraocular pressure. Instead, visualization of the optic disc through a dilated lens, measurement of intraocular pressure, and visual field assessment by an optometrist or ophthalmologist result in better screening outcomes for glaucoma. Clients who are at high risk (African American age 40 or older, all adults age 65 or older) should receive glaucoma screening every year or two (Schachat, 1999b).

Differential Medical Diagnoses

See Table 24–11.

- *Acute angle closure glaucoma:* Client complains of intense pain and photophobia, pupils are unequal, cornea has steamy appearance.
- *Optic neuritis:* Sudden loss of vision, pain especially with eye movement, usually central vision lost. Associated with underlying disorder as multiple sclerosis, sarcoidosis, and systemic lupus erythematosus.

Plan

The client with acute angle closure glaucoma is referred immediately to an ophthalmologist. It is an ocular emergency and is usually treated by laser iridotomy to reduce pressure. Subsequent treatment is the same as open angle glaucoma.

If open angle glaucoma is suspected, the client is referred for outpatient ophthalmologic evaluation as soon as possible.

Psychosocial Interventions. A diagnosis that carries with it the risk of blindness is very frightening. Reassure the client that with early diagnosis, treatment, and careful follow-up, glaucoma can be managed. A high level of compliance is necessary and the medications can be very expensive. Assessment of the client's support system and social situation is important to promote a favorable outcome.

Medication. Prostaglandin analogs and beta blockers are the most frequently used initial eye drops for lowering intraocular pressure in patients with glaucoma. Prostaglandin analogs are the most effective and can be considered as initial medical therapy unless other considerations such as cost, side effects intolerance, or patient refusal preclude this.

Prostaglandin Analogs or Topical Beta Adrenergic Blocker

- *Expected Outcome.* Ophthalmologists will monitor response to therapy and adjust dosage until maintenance drug regimen is determined. The practitioner should assess adherence and barriers to the treatment plan. He or she should examine the optic disc during periodic screenings between eye doctor visits for any changes.
- *Client Teaching.* Inform the client that glaucoma can be managed but not cured. Therefore, adherence to dosage and administration of eye drops is crucial. Inform client to report any adverse effects promptly.

Miotics Pilocarpine. This is the most widely used agent. It lowers intraocular pressure through contraction of the sphincter muscle of the iris, resulting in pupil constriction.

- *Administration:* One or two drops in the eye four times per day.
- *Side effects:* Blurred vision, increased bronchial secretions, nausea, vomiting, and diarrhea.
- *Contraindications:* Known hypersensitivity, overt congestive heart failure.
- *Expected outcome:* See aforementioned.
- *Client teaching:* See prior information. Warn patient about blurred vision and driving or operating equipment.
- *Surgical interventions:* Argon laser trabeculectomy may be performed on those for whom optimal pressure has not been achieved with topical medications or who are unable to tolerate these agents. It is done on an outpatient basis under topical anesthesia. Glaucoma filtration surgery is reserved for those clients who have failed all other methods. It involves establishing an alternative exit for aqueous humor. It can be done on an outpatient basis (Schachat, 1999b).

Follow-Up

Request notification from ophthalmologist of any change in treatment regimen and timing of follow-up visits. Assess client adherence to plan of care.

CATARACTS

A cataract is an opacity of the lens of the eye. Because lens fibers are produced throughout a lifetime and none is lost, the density of the lens increases with age. A cataract may or may not be associated with visual impairment. The specific changes in vision that result are loss of contrast sensitivity and glare.

Epidemiology

Incidence of cataract increases with age after the age of 50. It is estimated from several studies that the prevalence is close to 50 percent in individuals over 75 years old. Risk factors associated with development include exposure to ultraviolet-B radiation; diabetes; smoking; heavy alcohol use; history of trauma; retinal detachment; prolonged systemic steroid therapy; and certain systemic illnesses such as diabetes, myotonic dystrophy, and atopic dermatitis (Schachat, 1999a).

Subjective Data

The client may complain of impaired vision, "like a fog over my eyes." The location of the opacity often determines whether near vision or far vision is affected. The client with a central opacity complains of glare because pupillary constriction causes light to enter the area most opacified. She may report that she sees better in low light than in well-lighted rooms. She may have stopped driving at night due to the glare from oncoming head-lights. Color vision may be impaired. There is no complaint of pain or redness.

Objective Data

Physical Examination. Conjunctiva are clear.

- *Funduscopic examination:* As the cataract becomes denser, the retina becomes harder to visualize.

Diagnostic Tests

- *Visual acuity:* May or may not be affected depending on location of opacity.

Differential Medical Diagnoses

Glaucoma, retinal vascular occlusive disorders, macular degeneration.

Plan

Refer client to an ophthalmologist for further evaluation. Other retinal disorders may be present.

Psychosocial Interventions. Reassure the client that early detection and regular follow-up with an ophthalmologist improves outcome. Advise client surgery may not be indicated immediately.

Medication. None.

Nonsurgical Measures. Changing eyeglass prescription as needed, especially when myopia is induced by the cataract. Bifocals, magnifying lenses, and appropriate lighting may be helpful until surgery is performed.

Surgery. The decision to perform surgery is based on clinical judgment and visual acuity, usually when acuity is reduced to 20/50 or less (based on state driving laws requiring better vision to drive). Current standard of care technique involves ultrasonic fragmentation of the lens nucleus with implantation of an intraocular lens. Postoperative complications include risk of infection, glaucoma, retinal detachment, hemorrhage, and posterior capsular opacification. In 95 percent of cases acuity is improved (Schachat, 1999a).

Lifestyle. Before surgery the client may have curtailed some activities such as night driving, hobbies, and reading. She may experience the loss of independence or income.

Follow-Up

Usually followed by an ophthalmologist for 6 to 8 weeks after surgery. The practitioner should continue to monitor vision and perform functional assessments at each visit after release from the surgeon. Be alert for posterior capsular pacification, which can develop several months to several years after removal of the lens. Signs and symptoms same as for cataracts.

PULMONARY DISORDERS

This section on disorders associated with the lung covers asthma and influenza as well as the lower respiratory tract infections, pneumonia, and acute bronchitis.

ASTHMA

Asthma is a chronic inflammatory disorder of the airways. Chronic inflammation is responsible for increased airway hyperresponsiveness to a variety of stimuli, for recurrent symptoms, airway narrowing, and respiratory symptoms. Inflammation is responsible for acute bronchoconstriction, swelling of the airway wall, chronic mucus plug formation, and airway wall remodeling. Asthma can begin in response to sensitizing agents and the development of atopy later in life. Atopy is considered to be the strongest risk factor for the development of asthma (Jablonski, 2000).

It is important to understand that any client with asthma, regardless of severity, may develop an acute severe asthma exacerbation. The clients most at risk are those with a history of multiple hospital admissions, past intubation, multiple psychosocial problems, a recent decrease in corticosteroids, and noncompliance with lifestyle modifications and medications.

Effective management of asthma relies on four integral components: measurement of lung function to assess and monitor the client's asthma, pharmacologic therapy, environmental measures to control allergens and irritants, and client education (U.S. Department of Human Services [USDHS], 2011).

An acute asthma exacerbation has an early and a late phase response. The early/bronchoconstrictive phase is characterized by the rapid development of reversible airway obstruction in response to a stimulus, usually within minutes but may occur up to 2 hours later.

The late phase response can occur 6 to 12 hours later. It is an inflammatory response less likely to respond to bronchodilators.

Epidemiology

Asthma affects more than 17 million adults, and 7 million children under the age of 18 in the United States (USDHS, 2011). A disproportionate number of women, children, racial minorities, and individuals with low incomes are affected by asthma. Asthma was the most common chronic health condition of individuals hospitalized in the United States during 2009 with the H1N1 influenza virus (USDHS, 2011). Asthma is associated with predisposing and causal factors and can vary in severity.

Subjective Data

The client may report a history of any of the following: chest tightness, shortness of breath, dyspnea on exertion, or a nonproductive cough. The symptoms may occur with exercise, exposure to animals with fur, smoke, pollen, changes in temperature, strong emotional expression, aerosol chemicals, and dust mites. Many clients will have a history of childhood asthma, a history of seasonal allergies, and/or a family history of asthma.

Objective Data

Physical Examination. The physical examination between exacerbations may be normal.

Evaluate the client for signs of atopy: eczema, allergic conjunctivitis, rhinitis, coughing, and sneezing.

During an exacerbation, the client may exhibit signs of acute respiratory distress such as wheezing, coughing, tachycardia, and anxiety.

Diagnostic Tests. In clients with mild to moderate asthma, all laboratory tests may be normal. Well-controlled asthma blood gases will be normal. During an exacerbation, mild to moderate hypoxia and hypocapnia with a respiratory alkalosis may be present. During a severe exacerbation, respiratory acidosis may be present.

Measurement of lung function for diagnosing asthma is analogous to measurement in other chronic disease. For most, peak expiratory flow (PEF) correlates well with FEV1 (NHLBI, 1999). Regular home monitoring can help clients detect early signs of deterioration.

Differential Medical Diagnoses

Cardiac disorders, allergic rhinitis/sinusitis, sarcoidosis, chronic obstructive pulmonary disease (COPD), airway obstruction, cystic fibrosis pulmonary embolism, gastroesophageal disorders, cough associated with angiotensin converting enzyme inhibitors, obesity.

Plan

Treatment must be individualized with consideration to medication, risk reduction, and severity of disease. The National Heart Lung and Blood Institute (NHLBI) has established guidelines for the diagnosis, treatment, and ongoing management of asthma. Refer to its website at http://www.nhlbi.nih.gov/guidelines/asthma/.

Psychosocial Intervention. Clients with asthma frequently have poor recognition of their symptoms and poor perception of severity, especially if their asthma is severe and long standing. Clients frequently are concerned with lost time from work and decreased productivity. The client may also need to consider a job change away from triggering agents.

Medication. Medication choice focuses on airway inflammation associated with both acute and chronic asthma. The goal is to focus on preventive use of avoidance strategies and anti-inflammatory drugs to treat the underlying disease process rather than only the acute consequences. Clients with asthma are at risk for influenza and pneumonia; influenza and pneumovax vaccines are recommended.

Client Education. Stress avoidance of known triggers, proper use of metered dose inhalers, use of peak flow monitors, and smoking cessation.

Follow-Up

Follow-up of acute exacerbations should be individualized based on severity and client comfort and reliability.

Asymptomatic clients should be followed on an as-needed basis with emphasis placed on continued client education.

INFLUENZA

Influenza, an acute, usually self-limiting, URI, may be caused by influenza A, B, or C virus. Strains of the A virus are the most common and most virulent. B virus infection has some increased association with Reye's syndrome. C virus infection is a mild illness, usually not significant or identified clinically. Influenza caused by the H1N1 virus ("swine flu") is a more recently identified strain of influenza that was first identified in April of 2009 (CDC, 2011b). The World Health Organization declared the H1N1 outbreak a pandemic (global outbreak) in June of 2009.

Epidemiology

Etiology of the influenza virus reveals the unique ability to vary antigenically from year to year, hence the terms antigenic drift (minor variations) and antigenic shift (major variations). Prior exposure provides limited immunity. Epidemics occur every 2 to 3 years; about every 10 years, the strains vary dramatically and produce a "pandemic" (Prisco, 2002).

Transmission is primarily through aerosolized particles from a cough or sneeze, although the virus can be spread by clothing or hand contact. The incubation period is about 18 to 72 hours. Infectious viral shedding occurs for 10 days but is most prominent in the first 48 hours of illness.

In an epidemic year, 20 to 30 percent of the population may contract influenza. Deaths are usually due to pneumonia (influenza pneumonia is the sixth leading cause of death in the United States) or to cardiovascular decompensation related to the influenza (Couch, 2000).

Groups at risk for influenza complications include persons over 65, persons with chronic cardiac or pulmonary disorders (e.g., asthma), persons with chronic metabolic disorders (e.g., diabetes mellitus), renal dysfunction, immunosuppression, and nursing home residents (Couch, 2000).

Subjective Data

History reveals the four hallmarks of influenza: headache; myalgias, especially in the legs and back; fever, often to 102 to 104° F for 3 to 4 days or longer; and nonproductive cough, which usually is not prominent at the beginning of illness but increases over time. Watery eyes and dry throat may be present, but nasal symptoms are usually absent.

Objective Data

Physical Examination. The client may be flushed and sweating. She appears ill. High fever is common, usually greater than 102° F, but rarely 106° F or higher. Heart and respiratory rates are increased.

The eyes, ears, nose, and throat usually appear normal. The lungs are clear. If crackles or rhonchi are heard, obtain a chest x-ray to rule out influenza pneumonia.

Monitor the heart to assess cardiovascular status. Influenza may precipitate cardiovascular failure in cardiac clients.

Diagnostic Tests. A variety of influenza tests are currently available, including those that can be run within a clinic setting at the point of care. Recommendations for testing are fairly broad, and include individuals with respiratory symptoms and fever, with special focus on those who have underlying immunosupression, children, and older people (AHRQ, 2011).

Differential Medical Diagnoses

Parainfluenza virus, respiratory syncytial virus, adenovirus, and other viral syndromes. In the absence of an epidemic, it is difficult to identify influenza from many other viral syndromes. Note that influenza is always associated with cough.

Plan

Psychosocial Interventions. Inform the client about the expected course of disease, and teach the warning signs of influenza, pneumonia, and cardiac complications. Reassure her that taking acetaminophen is permitted. Aspirin, however, should be avoided because of its association with Reye's syndrome. Comfort will be increased and myalgia decreased if fever is controlled.

Medication. Medication is administered for prophylaxis and treatment.

Antiviral Drugs. Influenza viruses and their susceptibilities to available antiviral medications evolve rapidly and vary between communities (AHRQ, 2011). Current and updated information on antiviral resistance and recommendations on antiviral use can be found at http://www.cdc.gov/flu (CDC, 2011c). The most common antiviral medications include zanamivir, rimantadine, and oseltamivir, and use of these medications is dependent on the subtype of influenza infection, and the community resistant pattern. If subtype information is unknown, influenza A should be treated either with zanamivir, or with a combination of oseltamivir and rimantadine; influenza B should be treated only with oseltamivir or zanamivir (AHRQ, 2011).

Influenza Trivalent Vaccine. Current CDC recommendations include universal influenza vaccine for all those over 6 months of age. Special attention should be made to vaccinate pregnant women; children under age 5, but especially under age 2; people older than age 50; people with underlying chronic illnesses; those living in nursing homes or other institutional facilities; and people who live with or who take care of those whom are at risk for significant complications from the flu, including health care workers, caregivers of infants 6 months of age or younger, and household contacts of individuals who might suffer significant complications. A nasal spray vaccine is available for individuals aged 2 to 49. The vaccine provided during the 2010 to 2011 flu season also included protection against the H1N1 virus and may continue to do so in subsequent years.

Lifestyle Changes. Encourage the client to increase intake of fluids to prevent dehydration, to get adequate bed rest, and to avoid contact with others; discourage smoking.

Follow-Up

Influenza pneumonia occurs approximately 1 week after the onset of influenza symptoms. It is characterized by severe dyspnea, cyanosis, and often scanty blood-tinged sputum. The lungs may sound clear, evaluation by chest x-ray and pulse oximetry will assist in determining severity of illness. Pneumonia, which can occur at any age, accounts for one-half of the deaths associated with influenza. If you suspect pneumonia, refer the client for possible hospital admission.

Preventing influenza is crucial, and the majority of patients need to be encouraged to receive the influenza vaccine on a yearly basis. Those who should not receive the vaccine include those with a severe allergy to chicken eggs; those who have experienced a severe reaction to a previous influenza vaccine; those who have developed Guillain-Barre syndrome within 6 weeks of a previous influenza vaccine; those under 6 months of age; and those who have a moderate to severe fever (who should wait until the fever resolves).

LOWER RESPIRATORY TRACT INFECTIONS: PNEUMONIA AND ACUTE BRONCHITIS

Pneumonia is defined as an acute infection of the alveolar spaces or interstitial tissues (or both) of the lung. There are four classifications of pneumonia: typical, or classic bacterial, pneumonia; atypical pneumonia; aspiration pneumonia; and hematogenous pneumonia. This section focuses on the two types seen most often in primary care, typical and atypical.

TABLE 24–12. Pneumonia Pathogens Observed in Primary Care

Classic	Atypical
Common	
Streptococcus pneumoniae (also called pneumococcal)	Mycoplasma pneumonia Viral
Uncommon	
Haemophilus influenzae	Legionella pneumophila
Staphylococcus aureus	Chlamydia psittaci
Klebsiella pneumoniae	Francisella tularensis

Sources: Bartlett, Davell, & Mandell, 2000; Boldt & Kiresuk, 2001.

Acute bronchitis has been defined as an acute, usually transient, inflammation of the tracheobronchial tree. It most often occurs in response to a viral infection, to a noxious stimulus, or to the use of certain medications. Secondary bacterial bronchitis can be a complication of a viral respiratory infection. Invaders include the usual respiratory pathogens, such as Streptococcus pneumonia, Hemophilus influenza, Chlamydia pneumonia, and Mycoplasma pneumonia (see Table 24–12).

Epidemiology

The prevalence of pneumonia varies from 8 to 15 cases per 1,000 annually and has a disproportionate impact on the very young and the very old. The incidence of pneumonia also varies with the season, with increased illness during the winter months. While variable between communities, the causative agent that causes the most cases of pneumonia worldwide is streptococcus pneumoniae (Marrie, 2010). Acute bronchitis is more common; a large percentage of cases are caused by viral pathogens or atypical pathogens.

Subjective Data

The symptoms reported by clients with pneumonia and acute bronchitis are compared in Table 24–13.

Pneumococcal pneumonia has a classic history of a sudden onset of rigor and fever of 101 to 106° F. Clients report a rusty-colored or purulent sputum, chest pain, and shortness of breath.

Mycoplasma pneumonia, on the other hand, has a less dramatic clinical picture and history. The cough is paroxysmal and may be nonproductive. Fatigue and shortness of breath are common.

Questions to ask include the following: How long has the cough lasted? Was the cough preceded by a URI? Have you missed work or school? Do you have

TABLE 24–13. History and Examination to Differentiate Pneumonia and Acute Bronchitis

Symptoms/Signs	Bronchitis	Pneumonia
History		
Onset	Gradual, over 5–10 days, usually preceded by URI	Acute onset, ± preceding URI
Fever	Mild or absent	Usually 101–106° F
Chills	Mild, recurring, or intermittent	True "rigor," teethratting chill
Chest pain	Vague "tightness" or chest congestion	Intense, pleuritic, localized
Sputum	Scant to copious	"Rusty" colored in pneumococcal or mucopurulent
Dyspnea	Rare	Common
Examination		
General appearance	Not toxic, no apparent distress	Often toxic, weak, may use accessory muscles
Vital signs	Often normal	Often tachycardia, tachypnea, fever
HEENT*	Heart	Normal or findings consistent with URI
Lungs		Crackles, won't clear with cough; signs of consolidation (E to A changes, dull to percussion) ± rub
Heart	At normal baseline	Tachycardia

HEENT—head, eyes, ears, nose, and throat
URI—upper respiratory infection
Sources: American Thoracic Society, 2001; Bark, Curhan, & Rimm, 2000; Bartlett et al., 2000.

an underlying respiratory disorder? Did the cough begin abruptly? Did the cough begin after the initiation of a new medication?

Objective Data

Physical Examination. Positive findings on exam can be found in Table 24–13.

Diagnostic Tests

Labwork. Is ordered only if pneumonia is suspected. The serum white blood count is often higher than 12,000 in pneumonia and normal in bronchitis. Cold agglutinins are found in 75 percent of cases of Mycoplasma pneumonia (titer of 1:64 or greater). Arterial blood gases can be useful in determining severity of illness.

Chest X-ray. Is indicated if pneumonia is suspected and will guide treatment and follow-up. Lobar or segmental consolidation is strongly suggestive of Pneumococcal pneumonia. The chest x-ray may be falsely negative if the client is dehydrated.

Gram Stain. A gram stain of sputum may be helpful if an adequate sample is obtained. Good smears have fewer than 10 squamous epithelial cells and more than 25 neutrophils per high power field. These results can guide empirical therapy if one organism predominates. Gram-positive diplococci suggests Streptococcus pneumonia; gram-negative coccobacilli suggests Haemophilus influenzae; and absence of a predominant bacterium with neutrophils suggests Mycoplasma pneumoniae.

A sputum culture, if carefully obtained, will confirm the diagnosis and is critical for immunocompromised clients.

Differential Medical Diagnoses

Asthma, exposure to noxious substances, allergic rhinitis, gastroesophageal reflux disorder, medication induced, aspiration, other infectious causes, pulmonary edema, and foreign body.

Plan

Psychosocial Interventions. Reassure the client and teach her the warning signs of potential complications. In addition, advise her to notify the health care provider immediately if symptoms of complications develop (see Table 24–14).

Medication. Antibiotics are used in treatment. Pneumonococcal vaccine is used in prevention.

Antibiotics. The use of antibiotics is not recommended in treatment of bronchitis. Patient education is often necessary to remind her that bronchitis is typically caused by a virus. The cough associated with acute bronchitis can sometimes last for several weeks, so an antitussive medication is helpful. A short-term beta agonist MDI can be used effectively for those patients with wheezing as a

TABLE 24–14. Criteria for Outpatient Management of Pneumonia[a]

1. Able to take fluids and oral medications.
2. Not toxic, no respiratory distress, only single lobe involvement.
3. No underlying chronic disease, such as chronic obstructive pulmonary disease or diabetes.
4. Pneumonia not related to aspiration (alcoholism or sedation, for example).
5. Adequate support system at home to provide care, observation, and immediate transportation to hospital if condition worsens.

[a] Client must meet the following criteria.
Sources: American Thoracic Society, 2001; Bark et al., 2000; Bartlett et al., 2000.

primary symptom. Mucolytic agents have not been shown to be effective.

- *Pneumococcal polysaccharide vaccine:* This is recommended for healthy adults over 65; anyone with heart, lung, liver, or renal disease; diabetics; alcoholics; immunocompromised adults (including clients with HIV and splenectomized clients); and children older than 2 years who have risk factors such as sickle cell disease, HIV, and nephrotic syndrome.

Lifestyle Changes. Advise the client to humidify the environment if possible, to increase the intake of fluids, to get proper nutrition, and to rest. Encourage smoking cessation and exposure to secondhand smoke.

Follow-Up

Any client with pneumonia should be reevaluated every 24 hours. Most clients with pneumonia should be afebrile in 72 hours. Refer for hospitalization any client who does not rapidly improve. Possible complications of pneumonia include pleural effusion, emphysema (suspect a lung abscess if fever persists), disseminated intravascular coagulation, and nephritis.

Clients with bronchitis should gradually improve and the cough resolve over the course of several weeks. Any client with a cough lasting more than 6 weeks requires a chest x-ray to rule out other conditions such as lung cancer, lymphoma, TB, and pulmonary edema. If the x-ray is negative, consider asthma.

CHRONIC OBSTRUCTIVE PULMONARY DISEASE

COPD refers to several pulmonary disorders with airway obstruction as the common denominator. The two most common disorders, emphysema and chronic bronchitis, will be addressed here. Chronic bronchitis is characterized by cough and hypersecretion (phlegm production) for at least 3 months of the year for 2 consecutive years with airway obstruction documented by spirometry. Emphysema is characterized by abnormal permanent enlargement of the airspaces distal to the terminal bronchiole, destruction of their walls, without obvious fibrosis. Most clients with COPD demonstrate features of coexistent chronic bronchitis (pink puffer) and emphysema (blue bloater). Pure forms of chronic bronchitis and emphysema are rare (Barnes, 2001).

Cigarette smoking is the single most important risk factor for the development of COPD. Clients with COPD may exhibit signs of bronchial hyperresponsiveness with episodes of wheezing in addition to their baseline airway obstruction (Doherty, 2002).

Epidemiology

COPD is the fourth leading cause of death in the United States, and mortality from COPD has doubled for women over the past 20 years to that now equivalent to men; more than half of patients with COPD die within 10 years of diagnosis. While death rates for COPD have declined among men in the United States between 1999 and 2006, there has been no significant change among death rates in women (CDC, 2011a). Cigarette smoking is the most common cause of COPD. Cigar and pipe smoking also increase risk but to a lesser extent. Host susceptibility is a key factor since approximately 15 percent of smokers develop COPD. Males are affected more often than females, but this is changing as more females continue to smoke. Chronic exposure to coal, cement, grain dusts, or acid fumes could result in chronic bronchitis (Barnes, 2001; Blanchard, 2002; CDC, 2011a; Rennard, 2002).

Subjective Data

The client will give a history of smoking or chronic occupational exposure. She will usually be over 50 but may be significantly younger relative to the age of onset and number of cigarettes per day.

Chronic bronchitis is characterized by cough, phlegm production (white/gray, worse in the morning), and dyspnea. Clients with emphysema will complain of dyspnea and little productive cough.

Objective Data

Physical Examination Typically, a diagnosis of COPD is not made from the physical exam. Physical signs of airflow obstruction are not usually seen until significant lung damage has occurred, and detection of these physical signs has relatively low sensitivity and specificity

(National Guideline Clearinghouse [NGC], 2010). However, with advanced or prolonged disease, the following may be observed on physical exam.

- *General:* Normal body weight with chronic bronchitis. Weight loss with emphysema.
- *Skin:* Cyanosis with advanced disease.
- *Neck:* Jugular venous distention.
- *Lungs:* Tachypnea, accessory muscle use, pursed lip breathing, wheezing, rhonchi that shift with cough, decreased breath sounds.
- *Heart:* Positive S-3 or S-4 with advanced disease.
- *Abdomen:* Accessory muscle use. Enlarged liver with advanced disease.
- *Extremities:* Lower extremity edema with advanced disease.

Diagnostic Tests. Pulmonary function tests (PFTs) to assess for obstruction. Arterial blood gases to assess oxygenation. An oxygenation saturation of less than 88 percent and a PaO_2 of less than 55 are indicative of severe hypoxemia requiring supplemental oxygen (Blanchard, 2002). A CBC may demonstrate polycythemia. A chest x-ray may demonstrate overdistended lungs.

Differential Medical Diagnoses

Asthma, congestive heart failure, sarcoidosis, interstitial lung disease, cystic fibrosis, sleep apnea, and cardiac disease.

Plan

Encourage smoking cessation. Studies show a significant improvement in lung function and slowing of the rate of decline in FEV1.

Psychosocial Interventions. Involve the client in decisions concerning treatment. Acknowledge COPD is a chronic debilitating disease that can be treated and quality of life can be improved. Discuss the possibility of progression of the disease. Discuss with the client and her significant others advanced directive wishes.

Depression, fear, and chronic fatigue are common occurrences in clients with COPD and are frequently related to the client's emotional state, not pulmonary dysfunction. Inability to carry out activities of daily living can lead to low self-esteem. Assess the client's emotional state at frequent intervals.

Medication. Short acting beta-agonists (e.g., albuterol), long acting beta-agonists (e.g., ipratropium), and inhaled corticosteroids (ICS) are all effective in treating COPD (NGC, 2010). Recommendations for treating COPD are similar as for those for treating asthma, as agents are added with progression of symptoms.

Other Medications. Encourage the client to receive the influenza vaccination annually. The client should receive a Pneumovax injection at the time of diagnosis and every 5 years after, until age 65. These injections will decrease the risk of further lung damage and possible progression of COPD.

Oxygen. Home oxygen therapy has been documented to increase the life span and improve quality of life in hypoxemic clients, when used for 15 hours per day or longer. Oxygen is indicated when the PaO_2 reaches 55 or below and/or the O_2 saturation reaches 88 percent or below. The dosage of oxygen should be the liters per minute needed to attain a PaO_2 between 65 and 80 mmHg. The usual dose is 2 l per minute.

Lifestyle/Dietary Changes. Encourage the client to increase her hydration to 2 to 4 L in 24 hours to thin secretions and facilitate expectoration. The client with COPD has increased nutritional needs at a time when her disease may make her feel anorexic secondary to increased work of breathing, diaphragm pressure. Encourage the client to eat small, frequent, high-calorie meals. A nutrition consult may be helpful. Encourage frequent regular exercise. The American Lung Association and local hospitals frequently offer support groups.

Follow-Up

Regular follow-up is recommended to assess for progression of disease, nutritional status, psychosocial status, medication usage, and polycythemia. Annual PFTs and arterial blood gases may be needed to assess the client's current status, or to document the continued need for oxygen therapy.

URINARY TRACT DISORDERS

This section discusses three common disturbances: UTI, interstitial cystitis, and urinary incontinence (UI).

URINARY TRACT INFECTION

UTI denotes the presence of microorganisms anywhere from the kidney (acute pyelonephritis), to the bladder (cystitis), to the distal urethra (urethritis). Urine is sterile, with the possible exception that the normal urethra may be colonized by diphtheroids, lactobacillus, and alpha hemolytic streptococci. Ascent of pathogenic bacteria typically begins with the rectal flora moving upward to the vaginal introitus, distal urethra, bladder, and finally, occasionally, the kidney.

With repeated infections, it is important to differentiate between reinfection and relapse. In relapse, subsequent infections are caused by the same organism and serotype responsible for the initial infection. Relapse usually occurs within 6 weeks of treatment. Reinfection, on the other hand, results from infection from a different organism, and serotype and is more common than relapse (Murphy, 2007).

Epidemiology

Etiology. In a bladder infection, a combination of specific host and pathogen factors are involved. In healthy women, a few serotypes of *E. coli* are responsible for more than 85 percent of bladder infections, yet these serotypes constitute only 1 percent of rectal flora. A specific interrelationship between bacterial adhesion and epithelial cell receptors in women may predispose them to infection (Eriksen, 1999; Madersbacher, Thalhammer, & Marberger, 2000).

Periurethral cells in infection-prone women more readily bind *E. coli* cells than do periurethral cells in women who are not prone to infection. In women with recurrent UTIs, periurethral tissue is laden with pathogenic bacteria. Any additional factor, such as the motion of sexual intercourse, may cause these women to develop infection. Surface mucin that coats the bladder helps prevent bacterial attachment. That lining, however, may decrease with age and falling estrogen levels (Eriksen, 1999; Madersbacher et al., 2000).

Sexual activity places women at risk for all types of UTIs. The risk for cystitis is highest with vaginal intercourse. Any manipulation of the urethra, however, such as oral sex and masturbation, has some associated risk. Voiding prior to intercourse has not been shown to decrease risk of infection; however, voiding after intercourse decreases infection rates (Madersbacher et al., 2000; Murphy, 2007). Diaphragm and spermicide use greatly increases risk. Studies have suggested that diaphragms and spermicides may predispose women to UTIs by altering vaginal flora (Eriksen, 1999; Madersbacher et al., 2000; Murphy, 2007).

Transmission. Most often women serve as their own reservoir for pathogenic bacteria. Bacterial growth in the urinary tract of women is primarily related to urethral manipulation, most often as a result of intercourse. Residual urine, blockage of urine flow, or decreased voiding due to dehydration can also promote bacterial growth. Common pathogenic organisms in the urinary tract of women are listed in Table 24–15.

TABLE 24–15. Common Pathogenic Organisms in Women

Gram-Negative Pathogens	Gram-Positive Pathogens
Escherichia coli (responsible for > 85% of UTIs)	*Staphylococcus saprophyticus* (previously thought not to be a pathogen; now second most common cause of UTI in women)
Proteus mirabilis (a urea-splitting organism, associated with stone formation)	*Staphylococcus aureus*
Klebsiella species	Group A beta hemolytic streptococci Enterococci

UTI—urinary tract infections
Sources: Madersbacher et al., 2000; Murphy, 2007.

Urethritis may be caused by sexually transmitted diseases, primarily gonorrhea, chlamydia, and herpes. Urethritis and dysuria in males are usually secondary to sexually transmitted diseases; therefore, male partners with suspected UTIs should be carefully assessed and treated for sexually transmitted diseases as appropriate. Some men develop dysuria in the presence of *Ureaplasma urealyticum,* which is not currently considered a cause of sexually transmitted disease.

Incidence. Approximately 20 percent of women will experience a lower UTI. Among women with a UTI, 25 percent with an acute uncomplicated infection will have a recurrence (Madersbacher et al., 2000; Schwartz, Wang, Eckert, & Critchlow, 1999). UTIs may occur at any time in the life span, but are more common with increasing age. The high prevalence rate with increased age is associated with falling estrogen levels, bladder emptying problems, an increase in chronic systemic problems, concurrent diseases, bowel incontinence, overuse of catheters, and poor nutrition (Eriksen, 1999; Nicolle, 2000).

Subjective Data

After data are collected, the primary care provider must discern whether symptoms are vaginal or urinary (see Table 24–16) and whether the upper urinary tract is involved (see Table 24–17). It is important to review a woman's history of UTIs or urinary problems and any recent medications. Current use of antibiotics will yield negative urine findings, and medications such as pyridium can make urine orange or green, be over-the-counter

TABLE 24–16. Historical Clues to Dysuria

Cystitis	Vaginitis	Urethritis
Abrupt onset	Gradual onset	Gradual onset
Internal dysuria	External dysuria	Internal dysuria
Change in voiding: frequency, urgency, small volumes, possibly nocturia, and/or incontinence	No change in voiding pattern	May have some change in voiding pattern, no nocturia
Symptoms aggravated by voiding	Symptoms more continuous	Symptoms primarily associated with voiding
May have grossly bloody or odorous urine	No change in urine appearance	No change in urine appearance
No vaginal discharge	Vaginal discharge odor, itch, or irritation	May or may not have vaginal discharge or bleeding
10% complain of suprapubic tenderness	No abdominal symptoms	Abdominal pain if associated with pelvic inflammatory disease

TABLE 24–17. Differentiation of Upper and Lower Urinary Tract Infections by means of History and Physical Examination

Lower UTI (Cystitis)	Upper UTI (Acute Pyelonephritis)
Usually sudden onset	Often gradual onset over > 5 days
Dysuria and voiding symptoms	± Voiding symptoms
No systemic symptoms	Fever, chills, nausea, vomiting
No costovertebral angle tenderness	Often costovertebral angle tenderness
Serum WBC count normal	Serum WBC count often elevated
No WBC casts	May have WBC casts

UTI—urinary tract infection
WBC—white blood cell

medications such as those containing phenylpropanolamine or pseudoephedrine, which may impair bladder emptying (Clark et al., 2000).

An accurate sexual history is crucial. Women do not always volunteer important information such as having vaginal discharge or a new sex partner and, consequently, need to be questioned carefully. Women can usually discern whether dysuria is internal or an external burning as the urine passes over the labia. Vaginal infections, such as *Trichomonas, Candida,* bacterial vaginosis, and herpes simplex, may cause external dysuria.

Most often, urethritis in women is caused by *Chlamydia trachomatis,* the most prevalent bacterial sexually transmitted disease in the United States. Infrequent infections of the urethra may include *Neiserria gonorrhoeae, Trichomonas,* herpes simplex, and *Candida.*

Dysuria occurring gradually over 5 to 7 days is more characteristic of urethritis and acute pyelonephritis than cystitis, which usually has an abrupt onset. Urethritis symptoms, such as dysuria, with no recognized pathogens and no pyuria may be secondary to trauma or postmenopausal estrogen deficiency (Murphy, 2007).

Accurate discrimination between upper and lower UTIs by means of a history or physical exam is difficult. Because pyelonephritis can cause permanent renal damage or death, if untreated, it is crucial to try to make the correct diagnosis using a history (see Table 24–17). Differences may distinguish lower UTI (cystitis) from upper UTI (acute pyelonephritis). The typical presentation of acute pyelonephritis is abrupt onset of fever and flank pain; it may also be associated with generalized symptoms, such as nausea, vomiting, and chills. Pain may be perceived as low back or abdominal. Women with acute pyelonephritis may have no symptoms of dysuria or other common bladder symptoms.

History must confirm the presence or absence of any systemic symptoms: fever, chills, nausea, vomiting, diarrhea, headache, or malaise. Be sure to ask about any previous history of pyelonephritis or kidney stones. Cystitis is rarely associated with fever or systemic symptoms; therefore, the presence of fever or systemic symptoms is strongly suspicious of pyelonephritis. Risk factors for upper UTIs also need to be assessed.

Objective Data

Physical Examination. The client is generally assessed; occasionally a pelvic exam is necessary.

- *General appearance:* A client with acute pyelonephritis may appear toxic.
- *Vital signs:* Blood pressure and temperature are elevated.
- *Costovertebral angle tenderness:* Determine whether it is present.
- *Abdomen:* Check for suprapubic tenderness; a more extensive exam is done if the abdomen is very tender or if the bladder is palpable from distention.
- *Pelvic exam:* A pelvic exam may or may not be indicated based on the history and results of lab tests. When it is done, examine Skene's and periurethral glands. A pelvic exam may be necessary if the client has a history of external dysuria or gradual-onset dysuria especially with vaginal discharge or other vaginal symptoms; new or multiple sex partners; or internal dysuria (but the urinalysis appears benign with no pyuria).

Diagnostic Tests. Methods of testing include urine dipstick urinalysis, urine culture and sensitivity, vaginal wet mounts, and various cultures. The leukocyte esterase dipstick detects pyuria associated with infection. A positive reading on the leukocyte esterase dipstick correlates with 10 or more WBCs per cubic millimeter (Sacher & McPherson, 2000).

Urinalysis is the cornerstone of diagnosis. It is important to teach women how to collect a urine specimen* and to examine urine within one hour of collection, because bacteria multiply (see Table 24–18).

Although a urine culture and sensitivity test is beneficial in determining the type of bacteria and its sensitivity to antibiotics, a urine culture and sensitivity test is not routinely done unless the client does not improve with treatment or the clinical picture is unclear. In cases of treatment failures, a culture and sensitivity test may be warranted to identify the causative organism and prescribe the best antibiotic.

With uncomplicated cystitis, urine pretreatment cultures are not recommended unless the diagnosis is in question. The purpose of posttreatment cultures is to rule out relapses or untreated foci of infection.

*Studies reported in the *Journal of Pediatrics, American Journal of Medicine,* and *New England Journal of Medicine* have shown that the procedure to obtain a clean catch urine specimen does not reduce bacterial contamination of urine cultures. A study of 100 women was reported in 1993 by the University of Virginia Health Sciences Center. It confirmed that to obtain a good urine sample for culture, it is not necessary to first clean the urinary meatus or to hold the labia apart while voiding.

Pretreatment urine cultures are recommended in specific circumstances.

- All complicated UTIs, including suspected pyelonephritis, history of structural abnormalities, and history of frequent urinary problems/infections
- Uncertain diagnosis
- Symptoms present longer than 7 days
- History of UTI within preceding 3 weeks (possible relapse)
- History of recent catheterization or urologic surgery
- Pregnancy or suspected pregnancy
- Diabetes or other immunocompromising disorders

Posttreatment cultures are recommended in the following circumstances.

- Failure to improve with treatment
- Diagnosis of acute pyelonephritis
- Presence of complications

Vaginal wet (KOH and saline) mounts are used to rule out *Trichomonas, Candida,* and *bacterial vaginosis* (see Chapters 3 and 14).

STD cultures are done to rule out gonorrhea and chlamydia.

Differential Medical Diagnoses

Primary differential diagnoses are urethritis cystitis and pyelonephritis (see Tables 24–16 and 24–17). Differential

TABLE 24–18. Urinalysis Findings Altered by Urinary Tract Infections

Color/appearance	Often dark, turbid with foul smell; may be grossly bloody (hemorrhagic cystitis)
Dipstick	
Specific gravity	If too dilute, may be false-negative reading (i.e., low count of WBCs, RBCs, and bacteria).
pH	If very high pH, may be associated with urea stone-forming *Klebsiella;* low pH retards bacterial growth
Nitrites	Confirms presence of bacteria that convert nitrates to nitrites (does not always mean infection if asymptomatic; see asymptomatic bacteriuria section)
Protein	May have 1+ or 2+ protein with lower UTI; however, 3+ or 4+ urine deserves special attention and follow-up to rule out kidney damage. Vaginal secretions may contaminate urine and give false positive for some protein; deserves follow-up
Leukocyte esterases	Quick way to determine pyuria, not as accurate as microscopic.
Microscopic Exam	Usually performed on spun urine; in women, normal urinary sediment may contain one or two RBCs and up to four WBCs per high-power field
RBCs	40–60% of women with cystitis have some microscopic hematuria; most common cause of hematuria is infection; also seen with stones, glomerulonephritis, neoplasm, tuberculosis
WBCs	May come from any part of urinary tract; "clumping" may be seen in infection; presence of 5–10 WBCs per high-power field is suspicious for UTI, although false positives are common in women
Bacteria	Usually visible in true infection
Casts	RBC and/or WBC casts indicate kidney involvement
Epithelial cells and mucous	Large amounts of either suspicious for vaginal contamination

RBC—red blood cell
UTI—urinary tract infection
WBC—white blood cell

diagnoses also include asymptomatic bacteriuria, interstitial cystitis, and renal calculi.

Asymptomatic Bacteriuria. Asymptomatic bacteriuria is defined as bacteria in the urine with no symptoms of UTI. Whether to treat is debatable. Current recommendations are to treat pregnant women as if the condition were a UTI. Older women who have a high incidence of bacteriuria have not been harmed by asymptomatic bacteriuria nor do they benefit from treatment. In fact, treatment is expensive and may cause drug toxicity (Murphy, 2007).

Interstitial Cystitis. Interstitial cystitis is a syndrome of painful bladder without infection, characterized by urinary frequency, urgency, nocturia, and bladder pressure sensations that are often relieved by voiding. The urologist diagnoses interstitial cystitis by excluding other causes of painful bladder (cancer, TB, cystitis, herpes). Diagnosis is supported when cystoscopy reveals mucosal bleeding after distention of the bladder. Etiology is uncertain. (See Interstitial Cystitis in this chapter.)

Renal Calculi. Renal calculi, called kidney stones, may cause intermittent flank pain or pain that radiates around the abdomen. They are associated with hematuria. Clients may develop superimposed UTIs. Most calculi are composed of calcium oxalate and phosphate and can be visualized on x-ray of the kidney, ureter, and bladder. Uric acid stones, on the other hand, do not show up on x-rays and are associated with urea-splitting bacteria, such as *Proteus mirabilis.* UTIs with *Proteus* must be evaluated to rule out calculi (Spector, 2007).

Plan

Psychosocial Interventions. Discuss pain/discomfort management with the client and explain the mechanisms of UTIs. Reassure her that a UTI is not a sexually transmitted disease, although intercourse may be mechanically related to the condition. Inform the woman so that she can identify her own precipitating factors and use appropriate preventive measures.

Medication. Table 24–19 lists the management options for cystitis and Table 24–20 describes outpatient management of acute pyelonephritis.

Surgical Interventions. Women with recurrent cystitis rarely have anatomic abnormalities that require surgical intervention. Referral to a urologist, however, is suggested for women with recurrent problems who have a history of childhood infections, more than one episode of acute pyelonephritis, possible nephrolithiasis, relapsing infections, infections caused by *Proteus mirabilis,* or painless hematuria. Prolapse of the bladder, uterus, or rectum in older women may cause bladder outlet obstruction and impaired emptying resulting in urine stasis and increasing the risk of infection. These women may benefit from referral for urodynamic studies (Murphy, 2007).

Lifestyle Changes. Teach the client healthy voiding practices: void at first urge, void after intercourse. Encourage the client to make these practices routine. Advise her to maintain adequate hydration and to avoid use of contraceptive methods associated with increased UTI risk, such as a diaphragm.

Older women may benefit from use of estrogen cream therapy, 2 g intravaginally twice a week, or use of an estrogen releasing, silicone vaginal ring. A recent trial demonstrated the efficacy of an estradiol-releasing ring on reducing UTIs in postmenopausal women. The silicone ring, containing 2 mg of estradiol, remains in the vagina for 12 weeks, during which time a steady amount of hormone is released. The subjects used the ring for 36 weeks. The investigator discovered that 80 percent of the control group and 51 percent of the experimental group developed UTIs during the study. Vaginal atrophy and irritation, and UTIs have been shown to be significantly reduced with use of an estrogen releasing ring (Eriksen, 1999).

Follow-Up

Women should feel much improved within 24 to 48 hours of starting medication; if not, they should be instructed to telephone or return to the clinic. Teach clients the warning signs and symptoms of pyelonephritis and instruct them to telephone immediately if any of the symptoms develop.

For management of urethritis and vaginitis, see Chapter 11. For pregnant women, aggressive screening for UTI and treatment are recommended. UTIs and asymptomatic bacteriuria in pregnancy are associated with increased fetal and maternal morbidity.

INTERSTITIAL CYSTITIS

Interstitial cystitis is a chronic, painful bladder disorder whose course is unpredictable. It is characterized by urinary frequency, urgency, nocturia, and suprapubic pain in the absence of urinary pathogens. The etiology is unknown, but most accepted theories involve an initial insult to the bladder wall by toxin, allergen, or immunologic agent that causes an inflammatory response.

TABLE 24–19. Treatment Options for Uncomplicated and Recurrent Cystitis[a]

	Uncomplicated Cystititis: Rare or Infrequent Episodes of Cystitis
First-Line Medications	
1. Single-dose therapy	No longer recommended due to low rates of cure.
2. Three-day treatment	
Advantages	New area of study that combines decreased cost and decreased side effects.
Disadvantages	Twice the side effect rates as single dose; more research on effectiveness needed.
Medications of choice	TMP/SMX double-strength tablets bid × 3 days or nitrofurantoin (Macrodantin) 50–100 mg qid × 3 days.
Client teaching	Call to return to clinic quickly if not improved or symptoms reappear.
3. Traditional 7- to 10-day treatment	
Advantages	Only a 5% failure rate; most research done with this approach.
Disadvantage	Twice the side effect rate of single dose, increased cost, decreased compliance.
Medication of choice	TMP/SMX DS bid × 7 days or nitrofurantoin 50 mg qid × 7 days.
Client teaching	Encourage finishing medication as ordered; if side effects occur, stop medications and telephone primary health care provider.
Second-Line Medications	
Several new, expensive medications are now available for urinary tract infections. They should be reserved for clients with allergies or with resistant organisms, for example, ciprofloxacin (Cipro) 250 or 500 mg bid × 7 days or norfloxacin (Noroxin) 400 mg bid × 7 days.	
	Recurrent Cystitis: Arbitrarily Defined as Three or More Episodes of Cystitis Per Year
1. Postcoital prophylaxis	
Indications	Highly effective for the 85% of women who have onset of symptoms 24 to 48 hours after intercourse; intercourse does not occur as frequently as daily.
Medications	Oral antibiotic is taken just prior to or just after intercourse.
Options	50 mg nitrofuraniton, 250 mg cephalosporin, half single-strength TMX/SMX.
2. Intermittent self-start therapy	Client must be motivated and reliable about following directions.
Indications	Home dipslide cultures are prepared by client at onset of symptoms and the client self-starts traditional first-line antibiotics as prescribed; dipslides are inexpensive and save cost of two office visits; client must demonstrate a clear knowledge of the procedures and the signs of relapse and pyelonephritis. 3-day course of traditional antibiotics
Medications	TMP/SMX double strength bid × 3 days or nitrofurantoin 50–100 mg qid × 3 days po
3. Low-dose continuous prophylaxis	
Indications	Method of choice with high or daily sexual frequency; absence of any infection must be documented by urine culture prior to start.
Medications	Cephalexin (Keflex) 250 mg, trimethoprim 100 mg, TMP/SMX ½ tablet single strength. Given daily at bedtime or three times weekly; nitrofurantoin avoided, as long-term exposure may cause hypersensitivity reactions in the lung and kidney maybe an option during pregnancy; breakthrough infections treated with the full traditional 7-day therapy as indicated.

TMP/SMX—trimethoprim—sulfamethoxazole (Bactrim)

[a] See a current pharmacotherapeutics text for details.

Sources: Madersbacher et al., 2000; Murphy, 2007; Schaeffer & Stuppy, 1999.

Interstitial cystitis is frequently misdiagnosed as psychogenic in origin or goes undiagnosed for years. It can profoundly affect the client's ability to work and to maintain a home, family, and satisfying sexual relationship. There is no uniformly effective treatment; however, an individualized management plan that actively involves the client helps prevent permanent disability (Moldwin & Sant, 2002).

Epidemiology

Interstitial cystitis is estimated to affect between 3 to 8 million women in the United States ages 18 and older (Berry et al., 2011). Ninety percent of overall interstitial cystitis sufferers are female, and the majority of them are between the ages of 40 and 60 (Henderson, 2000). Persons with interstitial cystitis may spend 4 to 7 years and visit five physicians before receiving the appropriate diagnosis (Henderson, 2000; Parsons, 2002).

Theories of Etiology. Currently accepted theories of the origin of interstitial cystitis include epithelial cell dysfunction, mast cells, neurogenic causes, infection, and genetics.

Glycosaminoglycans provide a protective coating to the bladder urothelium, preventing the urine from leaking through and damaging nerves and muscles. It is hypothesized that the glycosaminoglycan layer is more permeable in persons with interstitial cystitis and that the leaking urine irritates nerves and creates the symptoms associated with the condition (Henderson, 2000; Parsons, 2002; Warren & Keay, 2002). Several studies have shown that the instillation of solutions into the bladders of persons with interstitial cystitis resulted in either absorption of solutes into the bloodstream from the bladder (which did not occur in healthy controls without the condition) or irritation of the bladder (which did not occur in healthy

TABLE 24–20. Acute Pyelonephritis: Outpatient Management[a]

Criteria for Outpatient Management[b]

1. Diagnosis is secure (consult with physician)
2. No underlying, complicating disease, such as diabetes
3. Not pregnant
4. No history of recent urinary tract instrumentation
5. Not toxic, must be able to tolerate oral therapy and fluids
6. Follow-up must be easily accessible in 24 hours
7. Culture and sensitivity must be sent the day treatment is initiated

Medications

1. Must be broad spectrum (ampicillin and first-generation cephalosporins should not be used) trimethoprim—sulfamethoxazole (Bactrim) double strength bid or ciprofloxacin hydrochloride (Cipro) 500 mg bid for 14 days
2. Addition of a stat dose of intramuscular gentamicin (dose based on weight) or ceftriaxone 1 GM, IM used by some clinicians
3. Client should improve substantially in the first 24 hours; consult/refer if not improved.

[a] Consult a pharmacotherapeutics text for details.
[b] Woman must meet these criteria to attempt outpatient management.

controls without the condition) (Chai, 2002; Parsons, 2002; Warren & Keay, 2002).

Mast cells are thought to be involved in the etiology of interstitial cystitis, but their role remains elusive. These cells may interact with existing nerve cells in the bladder lining, resulting in an up-regulation of nerve cells and thus increased pain pathways. Substance P, a small chain peptide, is also thought to play a part in interstitial cystitis (Parsons, 2002; Warren & Keay, 2002). Because some individuals with interstitial cystitis have responded to treatment with antibiotics, investigators believe that an organism or organisms may be responsible for the condition (Warren & Keay, 2002). On the other hand, the occurrence of interstitial cystitis in identical twins and the relative lack of the condition in fraternal twins points to a possible genetic predisposition (Warren & Keay, 2002). Finally, like many diseases, interstitial cystitis may be the result of multiple pathologies (Moldwin & Sant, 2002).

Subjective Data

The client may have consulted several health care providers in the past several months or years without getting relief from her symptoms. She will report urgency, frequency, and acute suprapubic pain. She may have to void every hour while awake and several times at night. She may complain of painful intercourse. Because of these disruptions in her life, she may be sleep deprived, anxious, depressed, and suffer from social isolation. She may describe periods of flare in symptoms right before her menses, at menopause, with certain foods, and/or at times of stress.

Be sure to ask about coexisting conditions such as migraine headaches, irritable bowel syndrome, fibromyalgia, chronic fatigue syndrome, allergies, and hypersensitivities to foods and medications. Review gynecologic history for previous UTIs, pelvic inflammatory disease, vaginal infections, bladder instrumentation, hysterectomy, laporoscopic procedures. Ask her about both traditional and nontraditional treatments she has tried and the outcomes.

Objective Data

Physical Examination. The physical exam focuses on the abdomen and pelvis.

- *General appearance:* The client may seem anxious. Her gait may be slow and measured to avoid jarring pain.
- *Vital signs:* Afebrile.
    - Palpate the back for costovertebral angle and lower back tenderness.
    - Percuss the abdomen for bladder distension and palpate for suprapubic tenderness and masses.
    - Pelvic Exam. Because interstitial cystitis is a diagnosis of exclusion, a complete pelvic exam is indicated to rule out infection, pelvic inflammatory disease, uterine and adnexal masses. Be sure to examine the urethra, Bartholin's, and Skene's glands.

Diagnostic Tests. Urinalysis to detect infection, hematuria. Urinanalysis will be normal with interstitial cystitis.

Pregnancy test, wet prep, gonorrhea, and/or chlamydia cultures as indicated by exam.

Differential Medical Diagnoses

- *Cystitis:* Presence of white blood cells and bacteria in urine sediment.
- *Renal calculi:* Presence of hematuria, colicky flank pain.
- *Pelvic or vaginal infection* indicated by exam, wet prep, cultures.
- *Pelvic masses* such as fibroid tumor, ovarian cyst detected by examination, history.
- *Genital herpes* indicated by history and presence of lesions.
- *Tubercular cystitis* and bladder detected on cystoscopy (see following).

Plan

Diagnosis/Management. The client is referred to the urologist for cystoscopy under general anesthesia. Diagnosis is made on the basis of presence of fissures, hemorrhage, and/or ulcers in the bladder wall and biopsy showing inflammatory process (presence of mast cells).

Psychosocial Interventions. Reassurance and support of the client are the first steps in alleviating some of her discomfort. She may feel overwhelming relief that her pain is considered real and not "all in her head." Actively involve her in the plan of care. Ask her to keep a diary of voiding patterns, symptoms, and flares with pain scales and associated conditions such as onset of menses, periods of high stress. When the diagnosis is confirmed by a urologist, refer her to the Interstitial Cystitis Association, a nonprofit organization that provides information and support and funds research.

The Interstitial Cystitis Association
100 Park Avenue, Suite 108-A
Rockville, Maryland 20850
www.ichelp.org

Medication. There is no definitive medical treatment for interstitial cystitis. Occasionally, the dilatation of the bladder during diagnostic cystoscopy results in relief of symptoms.

Pentosan Polysulfate Sodium (Elmiron). This polysaccharide is structurally similar to heparin but with one-fifteenth of its anticoagulant properties. The drug is taken orally, 100 mg three times a day (Moldwin & Sant, 2002). Studies have shown that up to 900 mg in three divided doses may be needed for control of symptoms (Parsons, 2002). Common side effects include dyspepsia, reversible alopecia, and increased bruising. Please consult a pharmacology text for additional information.

Amitriptyline. 10 to 75 mg po at night is used for its analgesic and anticholinergic properties (Moldwin & Sant, 2002). See previous discussion of amitriptyline in section Fibromyalgia.

Hydroxyzine (Atarax). 25 to 50 mg po at night may be prescribed for its anticholinergic property of inhibiting mast cell production (Moldwin & Sant, 2002).

Steroids. This class of drugs is used for its anti-inflammatory effect.

Oxybutinin. The anti-spasmodic effects of this medication helps to reduce bladder spasm.

TABLE 24–21. Dietary Modifications for Interstitial Cystitis

Foods to Avoid	
Chocolate	Alcoholic beverages
Soy sauce	Hot, spicy foods
Fruits, especially citrus or foods with citric acid	Coffee, tea, all caffeine
	Carbonated soft drinks
Artificial sweeteners	Avocado
Brewer's yeast	Cheese (especially aged)
Chicken liver	Corned beef
Fava and lima beans	Mayonnaise
Pickled herring	Onions (small amount for flavoring acceptable)
Rye bread and rye products	
Yogurt	Vitamins with aspartate, yeast, synthetic vitamin D
Sour cream	
High animal protein meals	Fermented foods
Vinegar and vinegar products	Tap water
Sprouts of any kind	Foods with molds
Foods with chemical additives	Fried foods
Hydrogenated fats including margarine or shortening	Smoked foods

There are no controlled studies suggesting that dietary changes can relieve symptoms; however, many clients identify acid foods or fluids with exacerbation of symptoms.
Source: Moldwin & Sant, 2002.

Instillation Therapy. Intravesical or bladder instillation therapy is a procedure performed by a urologist that involves instilling into the bladder a liquid medication, such as an anti-inflammatory or an anesthetic. Ongoing studies are looking at comparing the effects of different types of medications.

Lifestyle Changes. Because no medication appears to show consistent relief of symptoms, an individualized approach to the client involving a self-care regimen is recommended.

The most effective plans include the following:

- *Dietary modifications:* Avoid high acid foods and fluids that contain high fat and low carbohydrates (see Table 24–21). Obviously, eliminating all of the food in Table 24–21 would be impossible. Some persons with interstitial cystitis have no food sensitivities. Advise the client to begin with a bland diet and slowly add foods, paying attention to any symptoms that begin within 30 minutes to 6 hours after ingestion (Moldwin & Sant, 2002). If symptoms occur, have her eliminate that food until symptoms lessen, then proceed with more additions. Including high fiber foods may also be helpful. Encourage the client to drink 64 oz of water daily. Many interstitial cystitis sufferers restrict their fluid intake, thinking that this will minimize their symptoms. Instead, water restriction results in concentrated urine, which may aggravate their symptoms (Moldwin &

Sant, 2002). Encourage eating several small meals per day instead of large meals.

- *Nutritional supplements:* Vitamins A, B_6, and C may have protective effects on the bladder. Vitamin E is a natural vasodilator. Magnesium may have antianxiety properties.
- *Stress reduction:* Stress is the most significant factor for flare of symptoms. Adequate rest, exercise, participation in support group, and relaxation techniques such as yoga and deep-breathing are recommended.
- *Bladder retraining:* Used when pain is absent or at lower level. Method is to increase time between voids in intervals, for instance, 10 to 15 minutes longer each time.

Set goal with client for target time between voids based on voiding pattern before treatment began. Teach her how to do Kegel's exercises (Moldwin & Sant, 2002) (see section Urinary Incontinence).

Follow-Up

Continue to follow for primary health care. As with other pain syndromes, it is better to schedule client for regular visits to assess response to therapy. A suggested interval may be every 2 weeks at the beginning of the treatment plan and then monthly. Maintain close communication with urologist.

URINARY INCONTINENCE

Urinary incontinence is the involuntary loss of urine that is demonstrable and that is sufficient to be a social or hygienic problem (Luft & Vriheas-Nichols, 1998). It is a common and costly problem in younger and older women. It has significant psychosocial and economic impact on the individual, her caregivers, and society. It is estimated that less than half the individuals with UI consult health care providers about the problem. This may be due to its acceptance as a natural condition of aging, the availability of absorbent products (minipads and Depends), and lack of information on treatment options and benefits (DuBeau, 2000; Luft & Vriheas-Nichols, 1998).

Appropriate management can result in significant improvement. Development of an effective treatment plan depends on accurate identification of the subtype of UI.

Subtypes

Control of bladder function is maintained by voluntary and involuntary mechanisms. The detrusor muscles of bladder and internal urethral sphincter are under autonomic nervous system control, which may be modulated by cerebral cortex connections. The external urethral sphincter and pelvic floor muscles are under voluntary control.

Other factors that contribute to urinary continence include adequate estrogen, which may help maintain bladder sphincter tone; adequate bladder capacity, elasticity, and smooth muscle tone; maintenance of an acute posterior urethravesicular angle to support the bladder neck and urethra.

Subtypes of UI are based on compromise of aforementioned mechanisms.

Urge incontinence is the involuntary loss of urine associated with a strong desire to void. It is caused by *detrusor instability* due to involuntary detrusor contractions. These involuntary contractions may be caused by a neurological disorder such as stroke or multiple sclerosis, or occur as part of the aging process.

Stress urinary incontinence (SUI) is involuntary loss of urine during coughing, sneezing, laughing, or other physical activities that increase intra-abdominal pressure. The most common cause of SUI in women is urethral hypermobility or significant displacement of the urethra and bladder when intra-abdominal pressure is increased. Other causes include intrinsic urethral sphincter weakness, which may be congenital or acquired after trauma or radiation therapy, multiple incontinence surgical procedures, spinal cord lesion, or hypoestrogenism.

In older women UI is most often a combination of urge and stress incontinence. It is important to identify which component is most bothersome in order to target treatment.

Overflow incontinence is the result of overdistention of the bladder. It usually presents with frequent or constant dribbling or urge/stress incontinence symptoms. It is caused by underactive or a contractile detrusor or by bladder outlet obstruction. Medications (diuretics, anticholinergics, psychotropics, alpha-adrenergic blockers), neurologic conditions such as diabetic neuropathy, spinal cord injury, or radical pelvic surgery causing prolapse of pelvic organs may impair or alter the innervation of the detrusor muscle. Overflow incontinence secondary to outlet obstruction is rare in women.

Other types of incontinence include functional incontinence caused by factors outside the urinary tract such as chronic physical or cognitive impairment and unconscious or reflex incontinence common in paraplegics (Finucane, 1999).

Epidemiology

UI affects women to a much greater extent than men in the United States and worldwide, and its prevalence among both women and men is increasing (Markland,

Richter, Fwu, Eggers, & Kusek, 2011). From 2001 to 2008, the prevalence of UI in women increased from 49.5 to 53.4 percent, and in men from 11.5 to 15 percent.

Risk factors for development of UI in women include increasing age, increased parity, immobility, impaired cognition, obesity, medications (diuretics, anticholinergic agents, psychotropics, narcotic analgesics, alpha-adrenergic blockers), hysterectomy, smoking, alcohol use, fecal impaction, estrogen depletion, pelvic muscle weakness, and childhood nocturnal enuresis. Of these factors that are modifiable, obesity and hysterectomy may have the most impact on prevention of daily incontinence (DuBeau, 2000; Finucane & Wright, 2007; Luft & Vriheas-Nichols, 1998).

Subjective Data

Information should include a focused medical, neurologic, and genitourinary history that includes the risk factors cited previously and a review of medication use, both prescribed and over the counter.

Ask detailed questions about the associated symptoms and factors of her incontinent episodes including the following:

- Duration and characteristics (stress, urge, dribbling)
    - What symptoms are most bothersome to the client
    - Frequency, timing, and amount of continent and incontinent voids, for example, dribbles in underpants versus soaking through clothing
    - Triggers of incontinence (cough, exercise, surgery, trauma, new medication)
    - Other lower urinary tract symptoms such as nocturia, dysuria, hesitancy, weak and/or thin stream, hematuria, suprapubic pain
    - Fluid intake, especially coffee or other caffeine containing foods and fluids
    - Alterations in bowel, sexual function
    - Previous treatment and outcome
    - Amount of absorbent pads, briefs (Depends) used
    - Expectations of treatment
    - Psychosocial evaluation of mental status, mobility, living environment

Objective Data

Physical Examination

- Vital signs for hypertension, elevated temperature.
- Gait for mobility.
- Neuromuscular assessment to detect abnormalities that suggest multiple sclerosis, stroke, spinal cord lesion, and to assess cognition, strength, and manual dexterity.
- Cardiovascular status for presence of edema that may contribute to nocturia.
- Lungs for crackles or wheezes that may indicate congestive heart failure, COPD, asthma that may contribute to cough.
- Abdominal examination to assess for organomegaly, masses, diastesis recti, bladder distension, or other factors that may affect intra-abdominal pressure.
- Rectal examination to assess sphincter tone, presence of fecal impaction, rectal mass.
- Pelvic examination to assess perineal skin, genital atrophy, pelvic organ prolapse (cystocele, rectocele, uterine prolapse), pelvic mass. Palpate anterior vaginal wall for discharge from urethra or tenderness, which suggests diverticulum, carcinoma, or inflammation of the urethra.

Diagnostic Tests. Urinalysis to detect hematuria (infection, cancer, stone), glucosuria (polyuria), pyuria, and bacteria.

Cough Stress Test. Test is done when bladder is full but before urge to void is strong. Done in lithotomy position. Examiner observes for urine loss from urethra while client coughs vigorously. If instant loss, SUI likely. If leakage delayed or persists after cough, detrusor instability may be cause of UI. If no leakage and symptoms suggest SUI, perform test in upright posture.

Postvoid Residual (PVR). Can be done by catheterization or pelvic ultrasound. Observation of urine stream can be noted for hesitancy, straining, and slow or interrupted stream. Measure postvoid residual within a few minutes after voiding. It is generally accepted that PVRs fewer than 50 cc are normal. If repetitive PVRs range from 100 to 200cc, then inadequate emptying is diagnosed. One measure of PVR may not be sufficient.

If transient, reversible, or modifiable causes of UI have been detected, client may need no further evaluation and may be treated with trial of medications and behavioral modalities described subsequently.

Plan

Those who should be referred to a urogynecologic specialist include the following:

- Those whose UI persists after initial therapeutic trial
- Uncertain diagnosis (lack of correlation between symptoms and findings)

- Consideration of surgical referral especially if failure of previous surgery
- Hematuria without infection
- Comorbid conditions such as incontinence with recurrent symptoms of UTI, persistent difficulty emptying bladder, history of radical pelvic surgery, symptomatic pelvic prolapse, abnormal PVR, neurological condition (Finucane, 1999).

Psychosocial Interventions. Because UI is so common and underreported, it is suggested that questions about bladder function be a routine part of the annual gynecologic exam for women of all ages. Not only can this lead to prompt treatment of reversible causes of UI but also can relieve client hesitancy in bringing the subject up.

Client education about causes and initial therapy are important in order to reassure her that certain modalities may relieve or resolve her incontinence. Be realistic. In some clients, incontinence may never be cured but may only be manageable. Advise client that corrective surgery or bladder tuck may not cure incontinence. Be sure to refer her to support groups such as

National Association for Continence
Charleston, South Carolina
www.nafc.org

Medication

Stress Urinary Incontinence

ESTROGEN. Postmenopausal women in whom stress incontinence is related to intrinsic sphincter atrophy may benefit from estrogen replacement as the initial therapy. (See hormone replacement therapy in Chapter 18.) The estrogen may be administered orally, transdermally, or intravaginally. Some reports suggest topical estrogen may bring faster relief by local effect. Remember women with intact uteri should be given a progestin.

- *Expected outcome:* Advise her that beneficial effects may not occur earlier than 6 to 12 weeks after initiation of treatment.

IMIPRAMINE. Alternative is imipramine (Tofranil). An anticholinergic and alpha-adrenergic agonist. May be of benefit. No large scale studies to support its use.

- *Administration:* 75 mg po daily if first-line medications fail or are contraindicated. Nighttime dose may be used to avoid daytime drowsiness.
- *Adverse effects:* Nausea, drowsiness or insomnia, weakness, fatigue, postural hypotension.
- *Contraindications:* Known hypersensitivity to tricyclic antidepressants, recovery phase of myocardial infarction. Caution with cardiovascular disease.

Urge Incontinence With Detrusor Instability

ANTICHOLINERGIC AGENTS. First-line medications are anticholinergic agents that work by blocking bladder contractions and relaxing sphincter muscle. Examples of these include oxybutynin (Ditroopan & Ditropan XL) and tolterodine tartrate (Detrol).

Overflow Incontinence Due to Detrusor Hypomobility (When Obstruction Is Ruled Out). Is usually the result of neurological disorders such as diabetic neuropathy. Anticholinergics and tricyclic antidepressants should be avoided. Pharmacologic intervention is usually ineffective except for Bethanecol.

BETHANECOL. (Urecholine) 10 to 25 mg three to four times a day (Clark et al., 2000).

- *Mode of action:* Cholinergic agonist that stimulates muscarinic receptors of parasympathetic nervous system. Increases tone of detrusor muscle resulting in contraction, decreased bladder capacity, and subsequent urination.
- *Adverse effects:* Abdominal pain, diarrhea, bradycardia, hypotension, bronchoconstriction.
- *Contraindications:* Known hypersensitivity, coronary artery disease, peptic ulcer, Parkinsonism, asthma.
- *Expected outcome:* Advise client may be ineffective. Check postvoid residual urine volumes before and after treatment to assess efficacy.

Behavioral Interventions

- *Habit training* is targeting scheduled voids to match client's voiding habits as observed by caregiver. It can achieve good results with those who are homebound and have a caregiver.
- *Bladder training* is recommended for management of urge incontinence and mixed stress and urge incontinence. Client is advised to resist urge to void or postpone voiding and urinate on a fixed schedule. Initial goal is usually set for 2 to 3 hours between voids while awake. Adjustment of fluid intake may be needed. Goal is to increase intervals over a period of several months.

- *Pelvic muscle exercises* are especially useful for SUI and urge incontinence. The first step is to make the client more aware of muscle function. The examiner teaches the woman how to do the exercises by inserting the gloved finger into vagina and instructs client to tighten muscles around finger. Client is advised to sustain contraction for at least 2 to 4 seconds followed by an equal period of relaxation. She is instructed to perform these exercises with five repetitions every half-hour during the day, or alternatively, for 10 minutes twice a day. The key is consistency. Advise her to contract these muscles before and during situations when leaking occurs (e.g., cough, sneeze, laughter, exercise). Other behavioral modalities that may be of benefit include biofeedback, vaginal weight training, and pelvic floor electrical stimulation. These may be used in conjunction with pelvic muscle exercises. Consult urogynecologist for referral.

Diet/Lifestyle. Client education regarding factors that may impact incontinence include the following:

- Avoiding excessive alcohol and caffeine.
- Use of fiber and stool softeners to avoid constipation.
- Medications that may have adverse effects on incontinence, including diuretics, psychotropic agents, narcotic analgesics, over-the-counter products for appetite control and colds, and calcium channel blockers.
- Control of blood sugar to prevent polyuria.
- If prescribed diuretics are part of treatment for coexisting medical conditions, edema dosages may be minimized by use of nonpharmacologic interventions such as use of support stockings, leg elevation, and sodium restriction.
- Barriers to reaching toilet and environmental alterations such as bedside commode.

Follow-Up

Telephone follow-up in 1 week to assess adherence and barriers to treatment plan. Office visit in 2 weeks. Try initial treatment for 4 to 6 weeks. If no improvement, refer to urogynecologist for further urodynamic studies.

REFERENCES

Agency for Healthcare, Research, and Quality (AHRQ). (2011). *Seasonal influenza in adults and children. Diagnosis, treatment, chemoprophylaxis, and institutional outbreak management: Clinical practice guidelines by the Infectious Diseases Society of America.* Retrieved July 6, 2011, from http://www.guideline.gov/content.aspx?id=14173&search=influenza

Altman, R.D., Hochberg, M.C., Moskowitz, R., & Schnitzer, T.J. (2000). Recommendations for the medical management of osteoarthritis of the hip and knee: American College of Rheumatology Subcommittee on Osteoarthritis Guidelines. *Arthritis and Rheumatism, 43,* 1905–1915.

American Thoracic Society. (2001). Guidelines for the management of adults with community-acquired pneumonia. *American Journal of Respiratory and Critical Care Medicine, 163,* 1730–1754.

Antman, E.M., Bennett, J.S., Daughterty, A., Furberg, C., Roberts, H., & Taubert, K.A. (2007). Use of nonsteroidal anti-inflammatory drugs: An update for clinicians: A scientific statement from the American Heart Association. *Circulation, 115*(12), 1634–1642.

Auwaerter, P.G. (2007). Approach to the patient with fever. In N.H. Fiebach, D.E. Kern, P.A. Thomas, & R.C. Ziegelstein (Eds.), *Barker, Burton, and Zieve's principles of ambulatory medicine* (7th ed., pp. 457–464). Philadelphia: Lippincott Williams & Wilkins.

Bark, J., Curhan, G.C., & Rimm, E.B. (2000). A prospective study of age and lifestyle factors in relation to community-acquired pneumonia in U.S. men and women. *Archives of Internal Medicine, 160,* 3082–3088.

Barnes, P.J. (2001). Chronic obstructive pulmonary disease. *New England Journal of Medicine, 343,* 269–280.

Bartlett, J.G., Davell, S.F., & Mandell, L.A. (2000). Guidelines for the management of community acquired pneumonia in adults. *Clinical Infectious Disease, 31,* 347–382.

Berry, S.H., Elliott, M.N., Suttorp, M.S., Bogart, L.M., Stoto, M.A., Eggers, P., et al. (2011). Prevalence of symptoms of bladder pain syndrome/interstitial cystitis among adult females in the United States. *Journal of Urology, 186,* 540–544.

Blanchard, A.R. (2002). Treatment of COPD exacerbations. *Postgraduate Medicine, 111,* 65–75.

Boldt, M.D., & Kiresuk, T. (2001). Community-acquired pneumonia in adults. *Nurse Practitioner, 26,* 14–23.

Boyle, C.A. (1999). Management of menstrual migraine. *Neurology, 53,* S14–S18.

Butcher, J., Salzman, K., & Lilligard, W. (1996). Lower extremity bursitis. *American Family Physician, 53,* 2317–2324.

Byank, R.P., & Beattie, W.E. (1999). Exercise-related musculoskeletal problems. In L. R. Barker, J.R. Burton, & P.D. Zieve (Eds.), *Principles of ambulatory medicine* (5th ed., pp. 939–959). Philadelphia: Lippincott Williams & Wilkins.

Centers for Disease Control and Prevention (CDC). (2011a). *Data and statistics: Chronic obstructive pulmonary disease (COPD).* Retrieved August 1, 2011, from http://www.cdc.gov/copd/data.htm

Centers for Disease Control and Prevention (CDC). (2011b). *H1N1 flu.* Retrieved August 3, 2011, from http://www.cdc.gov/H1N1flu/

Centers for Disease Control and Prevention (CDC). (2011c). *Seasonal influenza: Key facts about seasonal flu vaccine*. Retrieved July 6, 2011, from http://www.cdc.gov/flu/protect/keyfacts.htm

Centers for Disease Control and Prevention (CDC). (2011d). *Targeting epilepsy: Improving the lives of people with one of the nation's most common neurological conditions*. Retrieved August 1, 2011, from http://www.cdc.gov/chronicdisease/resources/publications/AAG/epilepsy.htm

Chai, T.C. (2002). Diagnosis of the painful bladder syndrome: Current approaches to diagnosis. *Clinical Obstetrics and Gynecology, 45,* 250–258.

Chou, R., Qaseem, A., Snow, V., Casey, D., Cross, T., Shekelle, P., et al. (2007). Diagnosis and treatment of low back pain: A joint clinical practice guideline from the American College of Physicians and the American Pain Society. *Annals of Internal Medicine, 147*(7), 478–491.

Clark, J.B.F., Queener, S.F., & Karb, V.B. (2000). *Pharmacological basis of nursing practice* (6th ed.). St. Louis: Mosby.

Clark, S., & Odell, L. (2000). Fibromyalgia syndrome: Common, real and treatable. *Clinician Reviews, 10,* 57–64.

Couch, R.B. (2000). Prevention and treatment of influenza. *New England Journal of Medicine, 343,* 1778–1787.

Della-Giustina, D. (1998). Guidelines for treating common—and uncommon—back pain syndromes. *Consultant, 38,* 1528–1537.

Department of Veterans Affairs. (1999). *Low back pain or sciatica in the primary care setting*. Bethesda, MD: Department of Veterans Affairs.

Doherty, D.E. (2002). Early detection and management of COPD. *Postgraduate Medicine, 111,* 41–60.

DuBeau, C.E. (2000). Urinary incontinence. In J.G. Evans, T.F. Williams, B.L. Beattie, J.P. Michel, & G.K. Wilcock (Eds.), *Oxford textbook of geriatric medicine* (2nd ed., pp. 677–689). Oxford: Oxford University Press.

England, J.D. (1999). Entrapment neuropathies. *Current Opinion in Neurology, 12,* 597–602.

Eriksen, B. (1999). A randomized, open, parallel-group study on the preventive effect of an estradiol-releasing vaginal ring (Estring) on recurrent urinary tract infections in postmenopausal women. *American Journal of Obstetrics and Gynecology, 180,* 1072–1079.

Eye Diseases Prevalence Research Group. (2004). Prevalence of open-angle glaucoma among adults in the United States. *Archives of Ophthalmology, 122,* 532–538.

Felson, D.T., & Nevitt, M.C. (1999). Estrogen and osteoarthritis: How do we explain conflicting study results? *Preventive Medicine, 28,* 445–448.

Finucane, T.E. (1999). Geriatric medicine: Special considerations. In L.R. Barker, J.R. Burton, & P.D. Zieve (Eds.), *Principles of ambulatory medicine* (5th ed., pp. 82–98). Philadelphia: Lippincott, Williams, & Wilkins.

Finucane, T.E., & Wright, E.J. (2007). Urinary incontinence. In N.H. Fiebach, D.E. Kern, P.A. Thomas, & R.C. Ziegelstein (Eds.), *Barker, Burton, and Zieve's principles of ambulatory medicine* (7th ed., pp. 807–815). Philadelphia: Lippincott Williams & Wilkins.

Folstein, M.J., Folstein, S., & McHugh, P.R. (1975). Mini-mental state: A practical method for grading the cognitive status of patients for the clinician. *Journal of Psychiatric Research, 12,* 189–198.

French, S., Cameron, M., Walker, B., Reggars, J., & Esterman, A. (2006). Superficial heat or cold for low back pain. *Cochrane Database Systematic Review*, 1, CD004750.

Friedland, R.P., & Wilcock, G.K. (2000). Dementia. In J.G. Evans, T.F. Williams, B.L. Beattie, J.P. Michel, & G.K. Wilcock (Eds.), *Oxford textbook of geriatric medicine* (2nd ed., pp. 922–932). Oxford: Oxford University Press.

Friedman, D.S. (2007). Glaucoma. In N.H. Fiebach, D.E. Kern, P.A. Thomas, & R.C. Ziegelstein (Eds.), *Barker, Burton, and Zieve's principles of ambulatory medicine* (7th ed., pp. 1808–1815). Philadelphia: Lippincott Williams & Wilkins.

Gill, S., Anderson, G., Fischer, H., Bell, C., Li, P., Normand, S., et al. (2009). Syncope and its consequences in patients with dementia receiving cholinesterase inhibitors: A population-based cohort study. *Archives of Internal Medicine, 169,* 867–873.

Goldenberg, D.L., Burckhardt, C., & Crofford, L. (2004). Management of fibromyalgia syndrome. *Journal of the American Medical Association, 292,* 2388–2395.

Golding, J.M. (1999). Sexual assault history and headache: Five general population studies. *Journal of Nervous and Mental Disease, 187,* 624–629.

Grogan, P.M., & Gronseth, G.S. (2001). Practice parameter: Steroids, acyclovir, and surgery for Bell's palsy (an evidence-based review): Report of the Quality Standards Subcommittee of the American Academy of Neurology. *Neurology, 56,* 830–836.

Haque, U.J., & Bathon, J.M. (2007). Rheumatoid arthritis. In N.H. Fiebach, D.E. Kern, P.A. Thomas, & R.C. Ziegelstein (Eds.), *Barker, Burton, and Zieve's principles of ambulatory medicine* (7th ed., pp. 1234–1279). Philadelphia: Lippincott Williams & Wilkins.

Hasso, A.N., Drayer, B.P., Anderson, R.E., Braffman, B., Davis, P.C., Deck, M.D.F., et al. (1999). *American College of Radiology appropriateness criteria: Vertigo and hearing loss*. American College of Radiology [Online]. Retrieved June 6, 2002, from http://www.acr.org

Hebert, L.E., Beckett, L.A., Scherr, P.A., & Evans, D.A. (2001). Annual incidence of Alzheimer disease in the United States projected to the years 2000 through 2050. *Alzheimer Disease and Associated Disorders, 15,* 169–173.

Henderson, L.J. (2000). Diagnosis, treatment, and lifestyle changes of interstitial cystitis. *AORN Journal, 71,* 525–530.

Hogervorst, E., Yaffe, K., Richards, M., & Huppert, F.A.H. (2009). Hormone replacement therapy to maintain cognitive function in women with dementia. *Cochrane Database of Systematic Reviews*, 1, CD003799.

Huynh, C.N., Yanni, L.M., & Morgan, L.A. (2007). Fibromyalgia: Diagnosis and management for the primary healthcare provider. *Journal of Women's Health, 17*(8), 1379–1387.

Ignatavicius, D.D. (2001). Rheumatoid arthritis and the older adult. *Geriatric Nursing, 22,* 139–142.

Institute for Clinical Systems Improvement. (2011). *Health care guideline: Diagnosis and treatment of headache.* Retrieved August 3, 2011, from http://www.icsi.org/headache

Jablonski, R.A.S. (2000). Discovering asthma in the older adult. *Nurse Practitioner, 25,* 14–39.

Jankovic, J. (2000). Parkinson's disease therapy: Tailoring choices for early and late disease, young and old patients. *Clinical Neuropharmacology, 23,* 252–261.

Johnson, C.J. (2007). Headaches and facial pain. In N.H. Fiebach, D.E. Kern, P.A. Thomas, & R.C. Ziegelstein (Eds.), *Barker, Burton, and Zieve's principles of ambulatory medicine* (7th ed., pp. 1484–1503). Philadelphia: Lippincott Williams & Wilkins.

Johnson, G.D. (1998). Medical management of migraine-related dizziness and vertigo. *Laryngoscope, 108,* 1–28.

Kaplan, P.W. (2007). Seizure disorders. In N.H. Fiebach, D.E. Kern, P.A. Thomas, & R.C. Ziegelstein (Eds.), *Barker, Burton, and Zieve's principles of ambulatory medicine* (7th ed., pp. 1504–1530). Philadelphia: Lippincott Williams & Wilkins.

Kaye, J.A. (1998). Diagnostic challenges in dementia. *Neurology, 51,* S45–S52.

Klippel, J.H., & Arayssi, T. (2000). Connective tissue disorders. In J.G. Evans, T.F. Williams, B.L. Beattie, J.P. Michel, & G.K. Wilcock (Eds.), *Oxford textbook of geriatric medicine* (2nd ed., pp. 585–593). Oxford: Oxford University Press.

Kwoh, C.K., Anderson, L.G., Greene, J.M., Johnson, D.A., O'Dell, J.R., Robbins, M.L., et al. (2002). Guidelines for the management of rheumatoid arthritis: American College of Rheumatology Subcommittee on Rheumatoid Arthritis Guidelines. *Arthritis and Rheumatism, 45,* 328–346.

Lawrence, R.C., Felson, D.T., Helmick, C.G., Arnold, L.M., Choi, H., Deyo, R.A., et al. (2008). Estimates of the prevalence of arthritis and other rheumatic conditions in the United States: Part II. *Arthritis and Rheumatism, 58*(1), 26–35.

Lee, D.M., & Weinblatt, M.E. (2001). Rheumatoid arthritis. *Lancet, 358,* 903–911.

Liu, S.H., & Nguyen, T.M. (1999). Ankle sprains and other soft tissue injuries. *Current Opinion in Rheumatology, 11,* 132–135.

Luft, J., & Vriheas-Nichols, A.A. (1998). Identifying the risk factors for developing incontinence: Can we modify individual risk? *Geriatric Nursing, 19,* 66–70.

Madersbacher, S., Thalhammer, F., & Marberger, M. (2000). Pathogenesis and management of recurrent urinary tract infection in women. *Current Opinion in Urology, 10,* 29–33.

Magaziner, J.L., & Walker, M.R. (2007). Dizziness, vertigo, motion sickness, syncope and near syncope, and disequilibrium. In N.H. Fiebach, D.E. Kern, P.A. Thomas, & R.C. Ziegelstein (Eds.), *Barker, Burton, and Zieve's principles of ambulatory medicine* (7th ed., pp. 1531–1553). Philadelphia: Lippincott Williams & Wilkins.

Management of gout. (2010). *Pharmacist's Letter/Prescriber's Letter, 26*(11), 261102.

Markland, A.D., Richter, H.E., Fwu, C.W., Eggers, P., & Kusek, J. (2011). Prevalence and trends of urinary incontinence in adults in the United States, 2001–2008. *Journal of Urology, 186*(2), 589–593.

Marrie, T.J. (2010). Epidemiology, pathogenesis, and microbiology of community acquired pneumonia in adults. *UpToDate*. Retrieved July 6, 2011, from http://www.uptodate.com/contents/epidemiology-pathogenesis-and-microbiology-of-community-acquired-pneumonia-in-adults

Martin-Plank, L. (2011). Musculoskeletal problems. In L.M. Dunphy, J.E. Winland-Brown, B.O. Porter, & D.J. Thomas (Eds.), *Primary care: The art and science of advanced practice nursing* (3rd ed., pp. 735–829). Philadelphia: F. A. Davis Company.

McAlindon, T. (2000). Update on the epidemiology of systemic lupus erythematosus: New spins on old ideas. *Current Opinion in Rheumatology, 12,* 104–112.

Millea, P.J., & Holloway, R.L. (2000). Treating fibromyalgia. *American Family Physician, 62,* 1575–1587.

Moldwin, R.M., & Sant, G.R. (2002). Interstitial cystitis: A pathophysiology and treatment update. *Clinical Obstetrics and Gynecology, 45,* 259–272.

Murphy, P.A. (2007). Genitourinary infections. In N.H. Fiebach, D.E. Kern, P.A. Thomas, & R.C. Ziegelstein (Eds.), *Barker, Burton, and Zieve's principles of ambulatory medicine* (7th ed., pp. 528–537). Philadelphia: Lippincott Williams & Wilkins.

National Collaborating Centre for Chronic Conditions. (2006). *Parkinson's disease. National clinical guideline for diagnosis and management in primary and secondary care.* London: Royal College of Physicians.

National Collaborating Centre for Chronic Conditions. (2008). *Osteoarthritis: The care and management of osteoarthritis in adults* (Clinical Guideline No. 59). London: National Institute for Health and Clinical Excellence.

National Collaborating Centre for Chronic Conditions. (2009). *Rheumatoid arthritis: The management of rheumatoid arthritis in adults* (Clinical Guideline No. 79). London: National Institute for Health and Clinical Excellence.

National Guideline Clearinghouse (NGC). (2010). Diagnosis and management of stable, chronic pulmonary obstructive disease. *National Guideline Clearinghouse*. Retrieved July 6, 2011, from http://www.guideline.gov

National Heart, Lung and Blood Institute (NHLBI). (1999). *Data fact sheet: Asthma statistics*. Bethesda, MD: U.S. Department of Health and Human Services.

Nicolle, L.E. (2000). Urinary tract infection. In J.G. Evans, T.F. Williams, B.L. Beattie, J.P. Michel, & G.K. Wilcock (Eds.), *Oxford textbook of geriatric medicine* (2nd ed., pp. 700–712). Oxford: Oxford University Press.

Olanow, C.W., Watts, R.L., & Koller, W.C. (2001). An algorithm (decision tree) for the management of Parkinson's disease: Treatment guidelines. *Neurology, 56,* S1–S88.

Olney, R.K. (2001). Carpal tunnel syndrome: Complex issues with a "simple" condition. *Neurology, 56,* 1431–1432.

Parsons, C.L. (2002). Interstitial cystitis: Epidemiology and clinical presentation. *Clinical Obstetrics and Gynecology, 45,* 242–249.

Perez, V.L., & Foster, C.S. (2001). Uveitis with neurological manifestations. *International Ophthalmology Clinics, 41,* 41–59.

Philadelphia Panel. (2001). Philadelphia Panel evidence-based clinical practice guidelines on selected rehabilitation interventions for low back pain. *Physical Therapy, 8,* 1641–1675.

Porter, B.O., & Winland-Brown, J.E. (2011). Hematologic and immune problems. In L.M. Dunphy, J.E. Winland-Brown, B.O. Porter, & D.J. Thomas (Eds.), *Primary care: The art and science of advanced practice nursing* (3rd ed., pp. 907–1002). Philadelphia: F. A. Davis Company.

Prisco, M.K. (2002). Update your understanding of influenza. *Nurse Practitioner, 27,* 32–38.

Quinn, C.J., Mathews, D.E., Noyes, R.F., Oliver, G.E., Thimons, J.J., & Thomas, R.K. (1999). *Optometric clinical practice guideline: Care of the patient with conjunctivitis*. St. Louis, MO: American Optometric Association.

Rennard, S.I. (2002). Overview of causes of COPD. *Postgraduate Medicine, 111,* 28–38.

Rockwood, K. (2000). Disordered levels of consciousness and acute confusional states. In J.G. Evans, T.F. Williams, B.L. Beattie, J.P. Michel, & G.K. Wilcock (Eds.), *Oxford textbook of geriatric medicine* (2nd ed., pp. 932–937). Oxford: Oxford University Press.

Rowan, A.J. (1998). Reflections on the treatment of seizures in the elderly population. *Neurology, 51,* S28–S33.

Sacher, R.A., & McPherson, R.A. (2000). *Widmann's clinical interpretation of laboratory tests* (11th ed.). Philadelphia: F. A. Davis Company.

Safran, M.R., Benedetti, R.S., Bartolozzi, A.R., & Mandelbaum, B.R. (1999). Lateral ankle sprains: A comprehensive review. Part 1: Etiology, pathoanatomy, histopathogenesis, and diagnosis. *Medicine and Science in Sports and Exercise, 31,* S429–S437.

Schachat, A.P. (1999a). Common problems associated with impaired vision: Cataracts and age-related macular degeneration. In L.R. Barker, J.R. Burton, & P.D. Zieve (Eds.), *Principles of ambulatory medicine* (5th ed., pp. 1473–1480). Philadelphia: Lippincott Williams & Wilkins.

Schachat, A.P. (1999b). Glaucoma. In L.R. Barker, J.R. Burton, & P.D. Zieve (Eds.), *Principles of ambulatory medicine* (5th ed., pp. 1481–1487). Philadelphia: Lippincott Williams & Wilkins.

Schachat, A.P. (1999c). The red eye. In L.R. Barker, J.R. Burton, & P.D. Zieve (Eds.), *Principles of ambulatory medicine* (5th ed., pp. 1488–1498). Philadelphia: Lippincott Williams & Wilkins.

Schaeffer, A.J., & Stuppy, B.A. (1999). Efficacy and safety of self-start therapy in women with recurrent urinary tract infections. *Journal of Urology, 161,* 207–211.

Schur, P.H., & Hahn, B.H. (2011). *Epidemiology and pathogenesis of systemic lupus erythematosus*. Retrieved August 2, 2011, from http://www.Uptodate.com/contents/epidemiology-and-pathologensis-of-systemic-lupus-erythematosus

Schwartz, M.A., Wang, C.C., Eckert, L.O., & Critchlow, C.W. (1999). Risk factors for urinary tract infection in the postpartum period. *American Journal of Obstetrics and Gynecology, 181,* 547–553.

Silberstein, S.D. (2000). Practice parameter: Evidence-based guidelines for migraine headache (an evidence-based review): Report of the Quality Standards Subcommittee of the American Academy of Neurology. *Neurology, 55,* 754–762.

Singh, J.A., Reddy, S.G., & Kundukulam, J. (2011). Risk factors of gout and prevention: A systematic review of the literature. *Current Opinion in Rheumatology, 23*(2), 192–202.

Spector, D.A. (2007). Urinary stones. In N.H. Fiebach, D.E. Kern, P.A. Thomas, & R.C. Ziegelstein (Eds.), *Barker, Burton, and Zieve's principles of ambulatory medicine* (7th ed., pp. 754–765). Philadelphia: Lippincott Williams & Wilkins.

Stevens, J.C., Witt, J.C., Smith, B.E., & Weaver, A.L. (2001). The frequency of carpal tunnel syndrome in computer users at a medical facility. *Neurology, 56,* 1568–1570.

Szabo, R. (1998). Carpal tunnel syndrome as a repetitive motion disorder. *Clinical Orthopaedics and Related Research, 351,* 78–79.

Thomas, P.I. (2007). Crystal-induced arthritis. In N.H. Fiebach, D.E. Kern, P.A. Thomas, & R.C. Ziegelstein (Eds.), *Barker, Burton, and Zieve's principles of ambulatory medicine* (7th ed., pp. 1228–1233). Philadelphia: Lippincott Williams & Wilkins.

Tiemstra, J.D., & Khatkhate, N. (2007). Bell's palsy: Diagnosis and management. *American Family Physician, 76*(7), 997–1002.

Trager, J., & Ward, M.M. (2001). Mortality and causes of death in systemic lupus erythematosus. *Current Opinion in Rheumatology, 13,* 345–351.

Treatment of essential tremor. (2006). *Pharmacist's Letter/Prescriber's Letter, 22*(3).

University of Michigan Health System. (2005). *Guidelines for clinical care: Acute low back pain.* Retrieved March 7, 2011, from http://cme.med.umich.edu/pdf/guideline/backpain03.pdf

U.S. Department of Human Services (USDHS). (2011, May 3). World asthma day: NIH research advances help people with asthma. *NIH News: National Institute of Health*. Retrieved from http://www.nih.gov/news/health/may2011/niehs-03.htm

Vestergaard, P., Rejnmark, L., & Mosekilde, L. (2006). Proton pump inhibitors, histamine H_2 receptor antagonists, and other antacid medications and the risk of fracture. *Calcified Tissue International, 79*, 76–83.

Warren, J.W., & Keay, S.K. (2002). Interstitial cystitis. *Current Opinion in Urology, 12,* 69–74.

Waterbury, L. (2007). Selected disorder of lymph nodes and lymphocytes. In N.H. Fiebach, D.E. Kern, P.A. Thomas, & R.C. Ziegelstein (Eds.), *Barker, Burton, and Zieve's principles of ambulatory medicine* (7th ed., pp. 861–866). Philadelphia: Lippincott Williams & Wilkins.

Work Loss Data Institute. (2011). Ankle & foot (acute & chronic). In *Official disability guidelines* (16th ed., p. 146). Corpus Christi, TX: Author.

CHAPTER ❖ **25**

PSYCHOSOCIAL HEALTH CONCERNS FOR WOMEN

Anne L. Bateman ◆ *Eugenia "Jeanie" Zelanko*

You must be the change you wish to see in the world.—Mahatma Gandhi. Promoting the integration of primary care and mental health services for women increases the understanding of the essential part of mental health in women's overall health.

Highlights

- Cultural Considerations
- The Stress Response
- Grieving and Loss
- Mood Disorders
- Anxiety Disorders
- Schizophrenia and Other Psychotic Disorders
- Personality Disorders
- Chemical Abuse, Dependency, and Addiction
- Women in the Military
- Eating Disorders
- Sleep Dysregulation
- Violence and Abuse
- Homelessness

❖ INTRODUCTION

To understand overall women's health, the primary care provider must consider the burden of mental illnesses on their lives. The body of evidence from research, public policy analysis, and clinical practice has underscored the critical importance of mental health to the overall health of women. Advances have been made in our understanding of mental illness. Effective treatment options and promising approaches for promoting mental health have improved the quality of life for those living with a mental illness (Rapport, Clary, Fayyad, & Endicott, 2005). These advances have emphasized the critical role of gender in determining the risks and course of treatment of mental illness. Newer models of treatment are recovery oriented and strengths based, and include the active participation of women in their treatment (U.S. Department of Health and Human Services [USDHHS], 2009).

Community education and better support systems offer women the opportunity to learn new skills and behaviors that can reduce the incidence of psychosocial problems and their associated morbidity and mortality. With knowledge and understanding of the issues affecting women today, the primary care provider can facilitate women's access to necessary services (Substance Abuse and Mental Health Services Administration [SAMHSA], 2011). Although more resources are available to improve the mental health of women, additional resources are necessary to meet the needs of at-risk women who are poor, have limited access to health care, and live in underserved areas. The HHS Office on Women's Mental Health is a collaborative effort of a variety of HHS organizations with the purpose of using an evidence-based approach to increase the current understanding of issues affecting the mental health of women and girls. A study, *The Women's Mental Health Initiative*, has been started to examine sex and gender differences in mental health (USDHHS, 2009).

The *Diagnostic and Statistical Manual of Mental Disorders*, fourth edition, text revision (*DSM-IV-TR*) is the index used for the classification of psychiatric disorders based on specific diagnostic criteria. It also provides a standardized nomenclature to classify and identify patients with various mental health symptomatology. This chapter references the *DSM-IV-TR* and provides an overview of some of the biopsychosocial issues common to women's lived experience. Identifying women at risk for mental health problems and managing their care are important roles for primary care providers.

CULTURAL CONSIDERATIONS

Health and illness are influenced by an individual's ethnic and cultural heritage as well as religious beliefs and spirituality. These beliefs influence one's explanation of the cause of mental illness, its severity, and acceptable choices for treatment. In addition, the family system has a significant effect on the course of the disorder (Rapport et al., 2005).

Different cultures perceive mental illness and psychosocial issues in different ways. For example, most Hispanic and Southeast Asian cultures attribute psychosis to be an act of a spiritual influence, usually negative.

There are many complex social and ethnic minority groups in the United States and Canada and it is important for the primary care provider to understand the cultural patterning of the population served. Some of the social-environmental factors that have an impact on an individual's lived experience include poverty, racism, generational differences in sexual mores and behavior, and stress of resettlement and acculturation. In the delivery of quality health care, this understanding is referred to as cultural competence; this sensitivity to the cultural beliefs helps the primary care provider more effectively identify the psychosocial needs of the client and her family. In addition, it is important to consider the unique metabolic considerations for certain ethnic groups that impact psychopharmacology (Campinha-Bacote, 2002). The primary care provider is encouraged to maintain cultural competence to better understand the issues related to the individual lived experience for all clients (Bateman, 2006).

THE STRESS RESPONSE

All women and men are at risk for stress related to the biopsychosocial challenges that are part of their day-to-day lives. It is an individual expression in response to any number of events. Stress occurs when the adaptive or coping mechanism of the individual is overwhelmed by life events. The event is not always negative; it may be positive, such as marriage, a promotion, or the birth of a child. How the event affects the individual is dependent upon an intertwining of forces involved such as number of stressors, perceptions of those stressors, emotional and physiological responses to those perceptions, and success with efforts to cope. The degree to which a certain stressor causes stress is also determined by the perception of that stressor. Stressors may include interpersonal problems, time demands, and internal conflicts.

Stress had been implicated in the pathophysiology of atherosclerotic processes, heart disease, hypertension, and stroke (Kopp, 1999). While direct evidence that stress causes cardiovascular dysfunction or disease is not always conclusive, there is enough evidence to be concerned about stress levels in patients and to make recommendations for stress reduction (Institute of Medicine, 2001). In women, extreme emotional stress has been related to the development of a reversible cardiomyopathy called takotsubo cardiomyopathy or more commonly stress-induced cardiomyopathy. It mimics an acute myocardial infarction in presentation, is more common in women over age 50, and may be misdiagnosed initially (Beale, 2009).

Risk factors for adverse reaction to stress can include an inadequate support system, ineffective coping skills, and psychopathology. Health is not just a biological phenomenon; it also reflects a woman's adaptation to biopsychosociocultural factors in her life. Health care providers who strive to promote women's wellness, vitality, and overall well-being will help clients improve their quality of life. Stress assessment and reduction are important interventions.

SUBJECTIVE DATA

Women who experience chronic stress and trauma have a variety of reactions. Neurobiological factors *that impact the individual stress response* include developmental stage, genetic predisposition, gender, and processes that affect temperament, immune responses, and neuroendocrine activation. These factors impact the person's ability to cope and adapt to traumatic events and increase the risk of various stress-related medical and psychiatric disorders, such as gastrointestinal (GI) disturbances, depression, and substance abuse. Responses to traumatic events vary and are mediated by diverse influences, such as neurobiological, psychological, and cognitive factors. Complex responses are essential for survival and aim to establish homeostasis by reducing exposure to the stressor or its deleterious effects (Antai-Otong, 2002).

DIFFERENTIAL MEDICAL DIAGNOSES

The differential assessment takes into consideration that a woman living with chronic stress is at risk for numerous medical issues that are directly attributable to the stress response (see Table 25–1). Treatment of any of these disorders will have limited success as long as the source of the stress persists (USDHHS, 2009).

PLAN

During an acutely stressful event, frequent clinic visits may be necessary and the decision to refer the client to a mental health specialist is contingent upon many factors. The provider's expertise in managing the severity of the client's symptoms is important to achieving a positive outcome. Immediate referral is indicated for any client who displays behaviors that are dangerous to self or others. In addition, primary care providers are mandated reporters in situations where there is reason to believe that the client is at risk of hurting a child, an older person, or a disabled adult. The clinician needs to be familiar with the statute governing reporting in his or her state.

The client will benefit from receiving counsel about ways to avoid or manage stressful situations. If a stressful situation is unavoidable, discuss ways to minimize the degree of stress by altering the stressor. The client may need to develop coping skills to help her deal with the specifics of the situation. Improved coping is achieved through taking steps toward a healthier lifestyle: including sleep, balanced nutrition, exercise, and relaxation (Martin, 2002).

GRIEVING AND LOSS

The process of grieving follows a predictable course in most situations; however, there is no typical time or way to grieve, just as there is no typical

TABLE 25–1. Stress-Related Disorders

Coronary artery disease	Chronic pain headaches	IBS	Anxiety
			Depression
Hypertension	Rheumatoid arthritis	Ulcers	Insomnia
Asthma		Eczema	Fatigue
Muscle tension	Back pain	Obesity	Substance abuse

Source: Sadock & Sadock, 2007.

loss. Kubler-Ross (1969) developed a framework for understanding the grieving process. She described five stages of grieving—denial, anger, bargaining, depression, and acceptance. In normal grieving, the individual progresses through these stages without treatment or intervention. Although some individuals may not experiences all five stages, most clients eventually move to the final stage of acceptance without complications.

Unfortunately, Western society often considers an appropriate level of sadness to be a problem that requires fixing. Normal depression is the sadness we feel at certain times in our lives as a response to a real or perceived loss. Similarly, anger is a natural reaction to the unfairness of loss and is an indication that the individual is progressing through the grieving process. Again the reaction is individual and it is important to provide support and guidance that best meets the needs of the individual (Kubler-Ross & Kessler, 2005).

EPIDEMIOLOGY

All individuals experience loss as part of daily living and with any loss comes some degree of grieving. The loss may be real, perceived, or anticipated. Loss of a relationship through separation, divorce, or death can precipitate a response similar to the threat of loss of health, loss of income, and homelessness. Individual response is a result of the impact of the loss.

Etiology

How one grieves is dependent upon one's coping ability and available supports. Individuals with a history of ineffective coping with change and who perceive a lack of supports have a greater incidence of dysfunctional grieving. Understanding the process of grieving and loss from the perspective of the individual's lived experience will enhance the health care provider's ability to better meet individual need. It is also important to be aware of how culture may influence the grieving process (Bateman, 1999) (see Table 25–2).

TABLE 25–2. Grieving and Loss

Spanish-Speaking Groups	African Americans	Ethnic Chinese-Related Groups	Southeast Asian Refugees
◆ Need to complete the relationship to free the person's spirit after death; important to say goodbye ◆ Wakes lasting several days offer a mechanism for support and the expression of grief ◆ Predominant religion Roman Catholic with rituals such as masses, rosaries, and novenas ◆ Sometimes grief is expressed as *elstaque*—seizure-like behavior, hyperkinetic episodes, a display of aggression, and stupor ◆ Machismo—the keeping of feelings of suffering may prevent bereaved Hispanic men from being receptive to griefcounseling, and they may resent being told "it's okay to cry" ◆ Economic stress may prevent the family from fulfilling the desire to accompany the body of the deceased to their homeland ◆ Desire to protect the dying and the bereaved from the details ◆ Often rally together and take turns in shifts of vigil around hospitalized loved one	◆ Patterns of coping with death vary widely ◆ Likely to rely on friends, church members, neighbors, and nonrelatives when faced with death of a loved one ◆ Extended family does not predominate among either rural or urban African Americans ◆ Preponderance of female-headed single-parent family units ◆ Less likely to express grief overtly and publicly ◆ Fewer die in bed of old age or illness; more likely to die violently than Whites	◆ Tend to be stoic and fatalistic when faced with terminal illness and death ◆ Recognize the family as the basic social unit ◆ *Wu-fu* (five kinds of clothing) defines degrees of relationships and determines the severity of mourning in terms of closeness and importance of the deceased to the mourner ◆ Traditionally follow a system of double burial; the initial burial in a coffin lasts 7 years, after which the remains are exhumed and stored in an urn for years; reburial in an elaborate tomb marks the second burial after which the deceased is able to have beneficial effect on descendants ◆ Many Chinese Americans have adopted an American Christian religion while maintaining non-Christian cultural beliefs related to death, dying, and burial ◆ Many are Mahayana or Therevada Buddhist	◆ Many refugees have lost close family members as a result of war ◆ Traditional mourning practices must be modified in the United States ◆ Many variations in mourning among subgroups exist including color of mourning clothes and the duration for which they are worn, commemorative celebration on the anniversary of death, and marriage of the deceased person's spouse and children ◆ Special preparation of the body, including placement of a coin in the deceased's mouth to help the spirit at various stages of its journey and the use of divination when choosing the grave site ◆ Many Vietnamese are Mahayana or Therevada Buddhist and Hmong and other hill tribes are animist in their beliefs

Source: Bateman, 1999.

Grieving becomes dysfunctional with the presence of some of the following predisposing factors as described by Worden (1991):

- A relationship with the loss that was ambivalent, narcissistic, or dependent, such as the loss of a relationship that was troubled or a job that was unfulfilling
- Circumstances surrounding the loss that were uncertain, sudden, or overcomplicated, such as the loss of an unwanted pregnancy or a partner who was abusive
- A history of depressive disorder or previous complicated grief response
- A conflict between the view of oneself as being strong and the arousal of feelings of dependency and neediness such as the loss of a professional career
- A loss that is socially unspeakable or socially negated such as the diagnosis of HIV

SUBJECTIVE DATA

Few women who seek medical care will be able to specifically identify grieving as the source of their presenting symptoms. A woman may describe decreased sleep and appetite, loss of energy, fatigue, aches, and pains. She will often ruminate about the specifics surrounding the loss. In the initial stages of grieving a loss, this behavior can be expected; however, if the individual is unable to return to her previous level of functioning within 6 months, the health care provider should consider prolonged grief. Occasionally, the grief response becomes dysfunctional and there is an exacerbated or delayed emotional reaction in one stage or the other resulting in severe depression or anger.

OBJECTIVE DATA

A woman dealing with grieving and loss may present emotionally distraught, fatigued with difficulty concentrating. She may have lost weight and report feeling overwhelmed by even the thought of doing day-to-day activities. She may be in denial and not want to talk about the situation or she may be angry and irritable while another may appear unemotional and disconnected from the loss.

DIFFERENTIAL DIAGNOSIS

It is important that any medical issues be ruled out. A complete physical exam with laboratory studies (e.g., complete blood count, comprehensive metabolic panel, and thyroid-stimulating hormone) is indicated.

PLAN

The goal of treatment and intervention for grieving and loss is to reduce the acute symptoms and to minimize the long-term residual effects. In mild to moderate grief, medication is usually unnecessary because it is important that the grieving individual feel the emotions associated with the loss; however, referral to grief support can be helpful in the early stages (Bateman, 1999). Occasionally in the acute stages, medication for anxiety and sleep may be needed. For prolonged or dysfunctional grieving, medication and referral to a mental health professional are indicated.

MOOD DISORDERS

In 2008, the National Institute of Mental Health (NIMH) estimated that in a 12-month period, 9.5 percent of the general population could be diagnosed as having a mood disorder. Severe mood disorders include major depressive disorder and bipolar disorders I and II. It is estimated that 50 percent of the women in the United States experience symptoms of a mood disorder at some time during their life. Almost 50 percent of individuals with mood disorders can be classified as severe. Mood disorders have a high comorbidity with acute and chronic medical conditions. They can also be induced by certain medications (i.e., interferon, isotretinoin, chronic opiate analgesic therapy, beta blockers, or recreational drugs such as cannabis and alcohol) (NIMH, 2008b).

MAJOR DEPRESSIVE DISORDER

Major depression occurs as a single or recurrent episode that is independent of life events. It is characterized by a depressed mood or loss of interest or pleasure in usual activities. The individual will show impaired social and occupational functioning that has existed for at least 2 weeks, no history of manic behavior, and symptoms that cannot be attributed to use of substances or general medical condition (American Psychiatric Association [APA], 2000).

Epidemiology

The NIMH (2008a) has reported that at any time during the year, 8.1 percent of women in the United States experience symptoms of major depression. Hispanic women appear to experience symptoms of depression almost twice as often as white non-Hispanic women. Native American women experience depression at almost the same rate as Hispanic women. African American women are 50 percent more likely to experience depression when compared to their white non-Hispanic counterparts. Approximately 10 percent of women between the ages of 45 and 64 have experienced at least one episode of major depression. Symptoms of depression are often the side effect of chronic medical disorders and the treatment including medications such as corticosteroids, antivirals, and medications for cancer treatment.

Etiology. The likelihood of inheriting genetic factors associated with depression is 42 percent for women and 29 percent for men (Kendler, Gatz, Gardner, & Pedersen, 2006). Neurobiological research has described the neurochemistry of the brain as important to the cause of major depression. Additional theories involve the monoamine, deficiency that impacts levels of serotonin and norepinephrine, and the hypothalamic-pituitary, cortisol systems that influence levels of cortisol and the brain's perception of stress and feeling overwhelmed by one's environment. Any alteration in the neurochemicals in the brain, serotonin, norepinephrine, dopamine, monoamine, gamma-aminobutyric acid, acetylcholine, glutamate, and monoamine will directly effect mood regulation (NIMH, 2002).

Subjective Data

A woman may experience depressed mood or loss of interest or pleasure in most of her usual activities. Behavioral issues may include decreased productivity, weight gain or loss, increased tearfulness, vague physical complaints, or decreased libido. In some cases, there may be complaints about increased difficulty getting along with people at home or at work that has resulted in problems with important relationships. There may have been recent episodes of road rage, physical aggression, and illicit activity.

Objective Data

The depressed client may be over- or underweight, be unkempt, have restricted affect, or move sluggishly. Dirty, unkempt hair and fingernails that appear brittle or dry are common in the severely depressed individual. Scars may be visible on the wrists or other parts of the body. The eyes may appear dull with a fixed gaze, poor eye contact, circles present under eyes from lack of sleep, and pale conjunctiva and mucosa. Oral hygiene may be poor. The thyroid may be palpable. Mood disorders such as depression may be associated with menstrual irregularities. de Niet et al. (2010) found that women with polycystic ovary syndrome often suffered from low self-esteem because of the body image issues associated with the syndrome.

Differential Medical Diagnoses

Differentials include chronic medical illness (such as hypothyroidism), early onset dementia, head injury, premenstrual syndrome, depressive side effects from medication, and substance abuse.

Physical Examination. A complete physical examination is done with a focus on ruling out any chronic medical illness. Several diagnostic tests may be performed, including those ruling out substance abuse. Begin with evaluation of the client's general appearance. She may be over- or underweight, be unkempt, have poor affect, or move sluggishly.

- *Skin, nails, and hair:* Hair may be dirty and uncombed, and nails brittle and dry. Scars may be visible on the wrist or other parts of the body.
- *Eyes:* The eyes may appear dull with a fixed gaze, poor eye contact, circles present under eyes from lack of sleep, and pale conjunctiva and mucosa.
- *Mouth:* Oral hygiene may be poor.
- *Neck:* Thyroid may be palpable or with nodules.
- *Nervous system:* See Violence and Abuse section. Mental status may require qualitative scales to determine degree of depression.

Diagnostic Tests. Test to consider will vary according to presentation. Hematocrit and hemoglobin tests rule out anemia. The thyroid panel rules out thyroid disease. See Violence and Abuse section for specific tests.

In order to meet the *DSM-IV-TR* criteria for major depressive disorder, four of the following symptoms must be present during the same 2-week period and represent a change from the individual's previous level of functioning:

- significant weight loss or gain
- changes in appetite
- sleep disturbances
- psychomotor agitation or retardation

- fatigue or loss of energy
- feelings of worthlessness or inappropriate guilt
- diminished ability to concentrate
- recurrent thoughts of death

Plan

The individual who is depressed is assessed for any degree of safety risk at each visit. If there is evidence or endorsement by the client of imminent risk of serious harm to self or others, then a referral to additional services is indicated. Mild to moderate depression can be managed in the primary care setting with antidepressant such as the selective serotonin reuptake inhibitor (SSRI) and serotonin–norepinephrine reuptake inhibitor medications that include sertraline, fluoxetine, citalopram, bupropion, Effexor, or Cymbalta. If the individual fails to respond in 4 to 6 weeks, a referral to a mental health provider for further evaluation is indicated.

Nursing Implications. The health care provider must give full attention to the client in the privacy of an office. If the client does not feel comfortable, she will probably not be honest about her problem. A nurse practitioner may provide care for a mildly depressed woman usually in collaboration with a physician, but referral should be made to a qualified mental health professional for a seriously depressed woman. It is critical to know when to refer. *Always refer a client if suicidal ideation is expressed.*

BIPOLAR DISORDER

Bipolar mania, hypomania, and depression are symptoms of bipolar disorder. The dramatic mood swings of bipolar disorder do not follow a set pattern. Depression does not always follow mania. A person may experience the same mood state several times—for weeks, months, even years at a time—before suddenly having the opposite mood. Also, the severity of mood phases can differ from person to person.

Hypomania is a less severe form of mania. Hypomania is a mood that many don't perceive as a problem. It actually may feel pretty good. You have a greater sense of well-being and productivity. However, for someone with bipolar disorder, hypomania can evolve into mania—or can switch into serious depression.

Epidemiology

The term *bipolar disorder* is used to define a category of mood disorders that includes bipolar I and bipolar II, and several subcategories. In the general population, the prevalence of bipolar disorder is estimated to be 4.5 percent for both men and women with the first episode usually occurring between 18 and 29 years of age (Kessler et al., 2005).

Etiology. As with other psychiatric disorders, the origins of bipolar disorder are multifactorial. In addition to the neurochemical influence, life events and the absence of psychosocial supports play a significant role in the development of disorders on the bipolar spectrum.

Subjective Data

A woman experiencing a disorder on the bipolar spectrum may report feeling like she is on a roller coaster swinging from feeling high, upbeat, or irritable with anxiety or unexplained anger to extreme sadness and being so depressed that she is unable to function or get out of bed. She may express feelings of not wanting to be around or wishing she would not wake up, which puts the client at risk of hurting herself.

Objective Data

When assessing the client for symptoms of any mood disorder, data is collected from a variety of sources. Information is gathered from direct observation, client and family input, physical assessment and lab values, mental status exam, current medications, medical and psychiatric history, and use of alcohol or any recreational drugs. Explore current stressors and any recent losses or changes in her living situation. Ask specifically about any thoughts about hurting herself or others. If you have any concerns about safety, refer for further psychiatric assessment as indicated.

Diagnostic Criteria

In order to meet the *DSM-IV-TR* criteria for bipolar disorder I, four of the following symptoms must be present and represent a change from the individual's previous level of functioning:

- a discrete period of elevated or irritable mood that lasts at least 1 week
- includes at least three symptoms of mania
- may include diminished sleep, grandiosity, pressured sleep, tangentiality, irritability, being overly focused on goal-directed activities, agitation, or over seeking pleasurable activities likely to result in negative outcomes
- followed by a return to a normal (euthymic) state

Bipolar II disorder is a bipolar spectrum disorder characterized by at least one hypomanic episode and at least one major depressive episode; with this disorder, depressive episodes are more frequent and more intense than manic episodes. It is believed to be underdiagnosed because hypomanic behavior often presents as high-functioning behavior. Those with bipolar II are at highest risk of suicide among the bipolar spectrum. Hypomania in bipolar II may manifest itself in disorganized racing thoughts, irritability, anxiety, insomnia, or all of these combined. Because these agitated symptoms are negative, it may be difficult to distinguish a bipolar II hypomanic state from depression. Hypomania is often regarded as an elation of mood; however, mood may be negative in bipolar II hypomania. Moods that oscillate in the depressive spectrum are common, and very rarely does a person with bipolar II experience hypomanic euphoria. To a clinician psychologist specializing in mood disorders, highly confident ambition might appear to be symptomatic of hypomania only if the individual's goals are viewed as unrealistic.

The term *cyclothymia* is sometimes used when describing individuals with mood variability. However, cyclothymia differs from bipolar I or II in that the individual experiences numerous periods of hypomania and depression without a full mania or major depressive episode (APA, 2000).

Plan

Assess the client for any safety risk at each visit and refer to additional services as indicated. The symptoms of bipolar disorder are often difficult to manage and the medication regime is complex. The treatment involves the concomitant use of a variety of agents such as a mood stabilizer such as lithium, antipsychotics such as Seroquel and Abilify, and antiepileptic medications such as Lamictal and Depakote. The antidepressants may be included but must be used with caution for the individual with a bipolar manic disorder. The client who fails to demonstrate significant improvement after 6 to 8 weeks of monotherapy should be referred to a mental health prescriber for further evaluation and augmentation strategies (Sadock & Sadock, 2007).

Nursing Implications. Managing the depression, mania, and hypomanic symptoms associated with the bipolar disorders can be a challenge. The primary care provider provides the client a safe and emotionally supportive environment to talk about her situation. Help the client understand the importance of continuing treatment for a minimum of 4 months to 1 year or longer. In addition, it is important for the provider to have a clear understanding of the symptoms, treatment, and available resources to meet the client's need.

ANXIETY DISORDERS

Anxiety disorders are the most frequently occurring psychiatric disorder in the general population of the United States (Kessler et al., 2005). Anxiety is associated with substantial social and vocational impairment as well as physical disorders. Many individuals with anxiety are high users of primary care services due to chest pain, difficulty breathing, and pain-related concerns. They also may have psychiatric comorbidity, particularly major depression. Anxiety disorders are also associated with adverse health behaviors, such as smoking, sedentary lifestyle, and substance abuse that may contribute to the high levels of medical comorbidity found in clients with anxiety disorders.

EPIDEMIOLOGY/ETIOLOGY

There are numerous risk factors for the development of an anxiety disorder including life situations and family history. Anxiety disorders affect about 40 million American adults age 18 years and older (about 18%) in a given year (Kessler et al., 2005).

Unlike the relatively mild, transient anxiety experienced during a stressful event, anxiety disorders last at least 6 months and can get worse if they are not treated. Anxiety disorders commonly occur concurrently with other psychiatric or physical disorders, chronic illness, or substance abuse. These disorders may mask or exacerbate the symptoms of anxiety and need to be resolved before there can be adequate treatment of the anxiety disorder (Kroenke, Spitzer, Williams, Monahan, & Lowe, 2007). In addition, some recreational drugs and prescribed medications may precipitate or exacerbate the client's symptoms.

The *DSM-IV-TR* classifies ten subtypes of anxiety disorders, including generalized anxiety disorder, obsessive-compulsive disorder (OCD), panic disorder, agoraphobia, social phobia, post-traumatic stress disorder, anxiety secondary to medical condition, acute stress disorder, substance-induced anxiety disorder, and simple phobia. Only a selected few of these subtypes will be discussed in this chapter. Very often one type of anxiety disorder may precipitate or exacerbate the symptomatology of another.

- *Panic disorders:* Panic disorders are short-lived, recurrent, unpredictable episodes of intense anxiety accompanied by physiological symptomatology. Episodes of apprehension, fear, and a sense of doom may be precipitated by a stimulus or may arise spontaneously (APA, 2000). The ratio is 2:1 for prevalence of anxiety among women compared to men; the onset is between late adolescence and mid-30s (late adulthood) and it affects between 1 and 2 percent of the general population with some studies reporting as high as 3.5 percent (Kroenke et al., 2007).
- *Generalized anxiety disorder:* Generalized anxiety is defined as unrealistic or excessive anxiety and worry about two or more life circumstances occurring for 6 months or longer. This disorder does not develop into panic attacks or phobias and is not due to physiological effects of a substance or a general medical condition (APA, 2000). Approximately 4.0 million U.S. adults ages 18 to 54, or about 2.8 percent of this age group in a given year, have generalized anxiety disorder and the risk is highest between childhood and middle age (Kroenke et al., 2007).
- *Agoraphobia:* Agoraphobia involves intense fear and avoidance of any place or situation where escape might be difficult or help unavailable in the event of developing sudden panic-like symptoms (APA, 2000). Approximately 3.2 million U.S. adults ages 18 to 54, or about 2.2 percent of this age group in a given year, have agoraphobia (Kroenke et al., 2007).
- *Phobic disorders:* Phobic disorders are based on the defense mechanism of displacement. Clients transfer their feelings of anxiety from the true object to one that can be avoided. A specific phobia can develop as a specific disorder or in combination with other disorders in this category and involves marked and persistent fear and avoidance of a specific object or situation (APA, 2000). Approximately 6.3 million U.S. adults ages 18 to 54, or about 4.4 percent of people in this age group in a given year, have some type of specific phobia. Severity depends upon the impact of the phobia on activities of daily living (Kroenke et al., 2007).
- *Obsessive-compulsive disorder*: OCD involves an irrational idea or impulse that persistently intrudes into awareness. The client recognizes its absurdity, but anxiety is relieved only with ritualistic performance, impulse, or entertainment of an idea (APA, 2000). In the general population in the United States, there is a 2.5 percent lifetime prevalence of OCD and the disorder occurs equally in women and men (Kroenke et al., 2007).

SUBJECTIVE DATA

With mild anxiety, the client may complain about restlessness, fatigue, sleep disturbances, irritability or edginess, exaggerated startle response, difficulty concentrating, fear of being in places or situations from which escape might be difficult. More severe anxiety or panic disorder may produce symptoms that involve multiple organ systems and cause diagnostic confusion and frequent medical consultation and testing (APA, 2000). In taking a history, explore the client's chief complaint, including precipitating factors, duration of symptoms, and any techniques used to manage symptoms. The client may have a positive history and treatment for acute or chronic illness such headaches, thyroid disorder, pulmonary disease, GI disorders, insomnia, and the use of caffeine or nicotine and over-the-counter weight control drugs.

OBJECTIVE DATA

An extensive physical examination is done and a variety of diagnostic tests are performed.

Physical Examination

- *General appearance:* The client may appear restless, trembling, or emotional.
- *Eyes:* Circles under the eyes indicate a lack of sleep. Nystagmus may be elicited with different maneuvers.
- *Ears:* Rule out otitis externa or media.
- *Mouth:* Rule out large tonsils, lesions, and polyps in throat causing difficulty swallowing.
- *Neck:* Enlarged, tender, or nodular thyroid indicates thyroid disorder.
- *Skin:* Skin may be cold, clammy, sweaty, flushed, or pale.
- *Chest:* Respiratory rate may be increased. The client may hyperventilate. Wheezing may indicate asthma.
- *Vascular system:* Blood pressure and heart rate may be increased. A murmur, gallop, or click may indicate mitral valve prolapse or arrhythmias. Rule out heart disease with chest pain.
- *Abdomen:* The client may experience pain with palpation. Bowel sounds may be absent or hyperactive.

- *Musculoskeletal system:* Gait may be unsteady. Joints may be red and edematous and a source of pain. Muscle strength may be abnormal. Signs of trauma may be evident.
- *Nervous system:* Examination may reveal hyperreflexia, positional vertigo, and abnormal cranial nerve findings.

Diagnostic Tests

- Electrocardiogram
- Electroencephalogram
- Urinalysis to rule out urinary tract infection and diabetes
- Thyroid panel as indicated
- Complete blood count to rule out anemia and infection
- Electrolytes as indicated
- Glucose tolerance test to rule out diabetes and hypoglycemia
- Upper and lower GI series if indicated

DIFFERENTIAL MEDICAL DIAGNOSES

Hyperthyroidism, hypoglycemia, cancer, organic brain syndrome, depression, substance abuse, hypertension, side effects of prescription or over-the-counter medication, physical or sexual abuse (see Table 25–3).

PLAN

Generally, it is important to emphasize healthy lifestyle behaviors such as reducing stress whenever possible, decreasing caffeine intake, avoiding alcohol or illicit drugs, increasing exercise, and assuring quality sleep. During an acute anxiety episode, stay with the client, decrease environmental stimuli, and, above all, remain calm. Acknowledge and express acceptance of anxiety and encourage relaxation techniques and guided imagery to help decrease the acute symptoms.

TABLE 25–3. Medical Disorders That Resemble Anxiety Disorders

Hyperthyroidism	Hypoglycemia
Cancer	Organic brain syndrome
Depression	Substance abuse
Hypertension	Physical or sexual abuse
Prescription or over-the-counter medication side effects	

Source: Sadock & Sadock, 2007.

Nursing Implications

Showing genuine concern and empathy increases the chance that the client will perceive the health care provider as sympathetic to her problem. Using open-ended questions when interviewing allows the client to disclose information she may not otherwise have revealed and allows her to prioritize her concerns.

Medication

The psychopharmacological treatment for anxiety disorders includes the SSRIs, benzodiazepines, tricyclic antidepressants, and beta-adrenergic blocking agents. Cognitive-behavioral therapy in conjunction with medication is the treatment of choice for anxiety disorders. Clients with comorbid psychiatric disorders or substance abuse should be referred to a mental health specialist for consultation. See Table 25–4 for psychopharmacological treatment for anxiety.

Psychosocial Intervention

During an acute anxiety episode, stay with the client, decrease environmental stimuli, and, above all, remain calm. Counseling that focuses on the present, using reflection and clarification, is most effective. Deal with issues of fears, self-concept, self-esteem, problem solving, and coping mechanisms. Acknowledge and express acceptance of anxiety. Relaxation techniques and imagery may help decrease anxiety. Assist the client to identify sources of anxiety, to develop plans to deal with them, and to modify her lifestyle. Generally, it is important to emphasize healthy lifestyle behaviors, avoiding stress when possible, decreased caffeine, no alcohol or illicit drugs, proper exercise, and sleep. Social support is known to be helpful in reducing anxiety symptoms. Knowing that she has a condition that is treatable provides immense relief, as many people think they are going crazy.

FOLLOW-UP

Close monitoring is recommended when initiating psychopharmacological treatment for any of the anxiety disorders. Refer for mental health services depending upon severity of symptomatology, increased risk to self or others, and less than desirable response to initial treatment in 4 to 6 weeks.

TABLE 25–4. Medications Used for Anxiety

Classification	Indication	Side Effects	Caution	Examples	Contraindicated
Benzodiazepine	Rapid onset Short-term use	Drowsiness Dizziness Fatigue confusion Disorientation Addiction Sedation Increased anxiety	Rebound anxiety Short-term use Dependency Withdrawal Ethanol use	Lorazepam Clonazepam	Pregnancy
Selective serotonin reuptake inhibitor	2–3 week onset	Drowsiness fatigue Gastrointestinal distress		Sertraline Citalopram Fluoxetine Paroxetine	Pregnancy
Tricyclics	2–3 week onset	Sedation Orthostatic hypotension Anticholinergic effects	Suicidal ideation Urinary retention		Pregnancy
Beta adrenergic blocker	Reduce peripheral symptoms	Bradycardia Hypotension		Propranolol	Congestive heart failure First-degree block
Buspirone	2–3 week onset	Dizziness Headache Gastrointestinal upset Nervousness		Buspar	Pregnancy Ethanol use

Source: Stahl, 2008.

POST-TRAUMATIC STRESS DISORDER

Post-traumatic stress disorder (PTSD) is estimated that the majority of the general population in the United States has experienced some type of traumatic event. Less than 10 percent of the trauma victims develop PTSD and the sequelae of related mood and affect disorders. Females are at higher risk for developing PTSD than males (Breslau, 2009; Kroenke et al., 2007). Symptoms of PTSD may develop following a traumatic experience. The affected individuals often reexperience the traumatic event with persistent distressing memories or dreams, insomnia, exaggerated startle response, and hypervigilance. They may relive the experience as if it were happening now following cues that remind them of the event such as sights or sounds. They will avoid stimuli associated with the event or exhibit a numbed general responsiveness.

Subjective Data

According to the *DSM-IV-TR* (APA, 2000), a client must meet the following diagnostic criteria for PTSD: A person must have experienced a traumatic event in which both of the following were true—(1) the person experienced, observed, or was involved with an event where harm or death was threatened and (2) intense fear, helplessness, or horror were the primary affects. Symptoms may include any of the following: (1) persistent distressing memories of the event, (2) recurrent upsetting dreams, (3) reliving the experience as if it were happening now, (4) psychological distress following cues that remind the client of the event, (5) persistent avoidance of specific things that remind the client of the event, and (6) symptoms of increased arousal (e.g., insomnia, exaggerated startle response).

Objective Data and Differential Medical Diagnoses

See Anxiety Disorders, Major Depressive Disorders, and Violence and Abuse sections.

Plan

The initial challenges of psychiatric treatment are to assess the meaning of the traumatic event and acknowledge its emotional impact on the individual. Immediate interventions must include education about normal stress responses (see Table 25–1) and healthy ways of managing the stress response. Anticipating stress-related responses for the individual will help alleviate further negative response. Symptoms of serious psychiatric symptoms, such as suicidal risk, major depression, and exacerbation of PTSD, warrant referral to a mental health professional. An ongoing assessment of the client's perception of the traumatic event and the interventions is important to evaluate efficacy of treatment plan.

Psychosocial Intervention. Focus on counseling that emphasizes the here and now and strengthens existing defenses. Helping clients to clarify the problem allows them to begin viewing it within its proper context and facilitates decision making. Instructing clients about stress-reduction techniques and encouraging them to develop relaxation and exercise programs may help them to reduce stress by providing other outlets for their feelings.

Medication. SSRIs are efficacious in the treatment of PTSD (see Table 25–4).

Follow-Up

As with anxiety, referral depends on the severity of symptoms and functional impairment and the client's response to interventions in a 4- to 6-week period. Group and individual psychotherapy are often needed for PTSD. Refer the client to a mental health provider for medication and therapy as indicated.

SCHIZOPHRENIA AND OTHER PSYCHOTIC DISORDERS

The *DSM-IV-TR* (APA, 2000) identifies various types of schizophrenia and psychotic disorders. Differential diagnosis is made according to the total clinical picture. The spectrum of psychotic disorders includes a cluster of symptoms that are associated with varying degrees of loss of contact with reality and include:

- disintegration of thought processes and emotional responsiveness
- auditory hallucinations and bizarre delusions
- disorganized speech and thinking with often incoherent communication
- tumultuous interpersonal relationships and social impairment
- marked difficulties in educational, occupational, social situations, and anhedonia
- regressive and primitive behaviors with bizarre mannerisms
- flattened or inappropriate affect

The *DSM-IV-TR* (APA, 2000) classifies schizophrenia and psychotic disorders into subgroups including:

- *Paranoid type:* Where delusions and hallucinations are present but thought disorder, disorganized behavior, and flat affect are absent.
- *Disorganized type:* Where thought disorder and flat affect are present together.
- *Catatonic type:* The client may be almost immobile or exhibit purposeless movement. Symptoms can include catatonic stupor and waxy flexibility.
- *Undifferentiated type:* Psychotic symptoms are present but the criteria for paranoid, disorganized, or catatonic types have not been met.
- *Residual type:* Positive symptoms at a low intensity only.
- *Brief psychotic disorder:* Sudden onset of psychotic symptoms that may or may not be preceded by a severe stressor, lasting from 1 day but less than 1 month with full return to the premorbid level of functioning.
- *Schizophreniform disorder:* The essential features are identical to those of schizophrenia, with the exception that the duration is less severe and lasts less than 6 months.
- *Schizoaffective disorder:* Manifested by schizophrenic behaviors, with a strong element of symptomatology associated with mood disorders (depression and mania).
- *Delusional disorder:* The presence of one or more nonbizarre delusions that persist for at least 1 month. Delusional disorders include erotomanic type (someone of higher power is in love with them), grandiose type (irrational ideas regarding their own worth, talent, knowledge, or power), jealous type (centers on the idea that the person's sexual partner is unfaithful, which is irrational and without cause), persecutory type (most common delusion, belief that of being malevolently treated in some way, conspired against, cheated, spied on, followed, poisoned, or maliciously maligned), somatic type (belief of some physical defect, disorder, or disease such as a foul odor, insect infestation, parasite, misshapen body part, or dysfunctional body part).
- *Shared psychotic disorder: Folie à deux*, a delusional system that develops in a second person as a result of a close relationship with a person who has a psychotic disorder.
- *Psychotic disorder due to a general medical condition:* Specify disorder, with delusions or hallucinations,

substance-induced psychosis, not directly attributed to delirium or chronic, progressing dementia.

- *Psychotic disorder NOS:* Psychosis not otherwise specified.

EPIDEMIOLOGY

The NIMH (2008c) reports that 1.1 percent of the U.S. population is affected by schizophrenia. The prevalence of schizophrenia is higher for men than for women (Longnecker et al., 2010). The onset of symptoms typically occurs in young adulthood.

Etiology

Genetics, early environmental influences, neurobiology, and psychological and social processes appear to be important contributory factors to the development of a psychotic disorder; some recreational and prescription drugs appear to cause or worsen symptoms, or in some cases hasten the onset of schizophrenia (March & Susser, 2006).

In studies of monozygotic and dizygotic twins, the rate of schizophrenia in monozygotic twins was 40 to 50 percent. Genetic mapping studies have demonstrated that three anomalies in the X chromosome appear to be the most common genetic defect. However, although these three anomalies appear most common, others have been implicated (Tandon, Keshavan, & Nasrallah, 2008).

Environmental factors have also been found to have a significant role in the development of schizophrenia including injury, viral infection, pollution, and stress. Events in early development including obstetrical complications and prenatal infections have been documented as possible causes. In later development, a stressful lifestyle and urban living may contribute to the development of the disorder.

The neurochemical pathways in the brain have been extensively researched. The neurotransmitter most implicated in schizophrenia is dopamine. Increases or decreases affect the individual's ability to function day to day (Stahl, 2008). These increases or decreases in dopamine production along the mesolimbic dopamine pathway have been associated with both positive and negative symptoms.

The positive symptoms of schizophrenia are those that affect content and form of thought, perception, and sense of self. Positive symptoms include hallucinations and delusions, distortions, and disorganization in thought, speech, and behavior including agitation. The negative symptoms are those that impact affect, volition, and psychomotor behavior. Negative symptoms include passivity, social isolation, inability to experience pleasure, lack of goal-directed behavior, inability to communicate, flattened affect, and inability to physically express emotion such as laughing and smiling (APA, 2000).

Decreases in dopamine along the mesocortical dopamine pathway are thought to be responsible for impaired attention and difficulty with abstract thinking. Decreased dopamine activity along the third dopamine pathway, the nigrostriatal pathway, is associated with the atypical posturing (i.e., waxy flexibility). The fourth dopamine pathway, the tuberoinfundibular dopamine pathway, is important because it is responsible for the production of prolactin. Although prolactin itself is not implicated in schizophrenia, many of the medications used to treat schizophrenia block the dopamine receptors along the tuberoinfundibular dopamine pathway and lead to galactorrhea or sexual dysfunction in men and women, as well as amenorrhea (Stahl, 2008).

Psychosis may be seen as part of schizophrenia or other disorder that manifests psychotic symptoms. The causes of psychosis may be psychiatric or medical in nature.

SUBJECTIVE DATA

The client who presents with symptoms of psychosis will often present with a variety of physical complaints. The client may report being acutely aware of things in her environment such as increased sensitivity to noise, lights, or being touched. Often, she may misinterpret stimuli in her environment. Hearing voices or less commonly seeing things that aren't there are frequent descriptions of the hallucinations experienced by individuals with any of the psychotic disorders. Rarely, psychotic individuals will report olfactory hallucinations such as unusual smells that others don't smell or a crawling sensation or that others are touching them which are more suggestive of a neurological disorder.

OBJECTIVE DATA

A comprehensive assessment of the individual who presents with psychotic symptoms is crucial to identifying whether the client is truly schizophrenic. The client often presents with poor hygiene and/or odd or inappropriate dress. She may be irritable or slow to provide answers to questions asked of her. Speech may be overproductive or underproductive and the client may stop her conversation for a brief moment and then resume it. She may change the topic of conversation without warning and go off on a tangent or describe life events that sound unreasonable. She is usually circumstantial and provides a large amount of information that may be irrelevant. The psychotic client may be concrete in her thinking and provide overly simplistic responses to direct questions. She may report recent job loss or failure to fulfill personal obligations. Ambivalence, apathy, disorganization, poor insight, and poor judgment with difficulty making decisions are common.

DIFFERENTIAL MEDICAL DIAGNOSIS

With an acute onset of psychotic symptoms, a medical precipitant should be ruled out. Initially, psychosis and delirium may manifest with similar symptomatology. Delirium is a medical emergency, and once the medical cause is resolved, further assessment of the psychotic symptoms is indicated. Unlike the hallucinations associated with a psychiatric-induced psychosis, the individual with delirium usually experiences tactile or olfactory hallucinations. A complete physical assessment with toxicology screening is indicated.

Substance-induced psychosis may be the result of using alcohol, recreational drugs, or some prescribed medications, such as steroids. It is recommended that the client be monitored for a return of these symptoms despite the fact symptoms have resolved following withdrawal of the offending agent (Drake et al., 2011).

PLAN

The plan for treating the symptoms of psychosis is based on the origin. Treatment for psychotic disorders involves the use of antipsychotic medications and supportive psychosocial interventions as indicated to preserve independence and quality of life. Antipsychotic medications are also referred to as neuroleptics and are major tranquilizers. Without drug treatment, 80 percent of the individuals who have experienced a psychotic episode relapse within 1 year. This relapse rate can be reduced to about 30 percent with continuous medication (Kessler et al., 2005).

The typical antipsychotics work by blocking the postsynaptic dopamine receptors in the basal ganglia, hypothalamus, limbic system, brainstem, and medulla. This blocking of numerous receptors is responsible for the wide spectrum of side effects.

The atypical antipsychotics have a more favorable side effect profile. They are weaker dopamine receptor agonists than the conventional antipsychotics, but are more potent antagonists of the serotonin type 2A (5-HT$_{2A}$) receptors. Dopamine blockade occurs more readily in the mesolimbic pathway than in the nigrostriatal pathway and exerting antipsychotic action. Some of the medications used for the treatment of the psychotic disorders are listed in Table 25–5.

The alterations in mental status are difficult for the individual. Frequently, the client is aware that the thoughts and behaviors are not supported by those around them, which contributes to further distress. Delusions and auditory hallucinations can be troubling and often overwhelming. These factors put the individual at risk for self-injurious behaviors and suicide.

Nursing Implications

The client with a psychotic disorder who is adequately medicated and stabilized often develops the notion that she is better and may want to stop her medication. Noncompliance with medication protocols is a significant cause of negative treatment outcomes. Teaching and regular evaluation of the client and her medications is crucial to positive outcomes.

The psychotic individual often develops odd ideas about her own health status and the side effects of the medications. For example, she may be unable to differentiate between appropriate and inappropriate fluid intake and may experience volume overload. The result may be hypernatremia, which leads to confusion and disorientation.

Metabolic syndrome and weight gain are significant risks associated with the atypical antipsychotic medications. Regular assessment of diet and physical activity as well as assessment for weight gain is important. Regular monitoring with serum studies including metabolic profile, prolactin levels, kidney, and liver function is also needed.

All women of childbearing age with schizophrenia or other psychotic disorders should be counseled about the use of these medications during pregnancy and lactation and the risk to the developing fetus. However, pregnancy is often unplanned or unexpected, and a risk-benefit analysis of continuing medication should be done on a case-by-case basis. Consultation with a psychiatric provider with a subspecialty in obstetrics and lactation is recommended.

Thus, assistance with managing stress, family issues, vocational counseling, and identifying and utilizing

TABLE 25–5. Antipsychotic Medications

Classification	Indication	Side Effects	Examples	Contraindicated
Typical antipsychotics				
Phenothiazines		Anticholinergic side effects, nausea, skin rash, sedation, orthostatic hypotension, tachycardia, photosensitivity, decreased libido, amenorrhea, retrograde ejaculation, gynecomastia, weight gain, agranulocytosis, extrapyramidal symptoms, tardive dyskinesia, neuroleptic malignant syndrome	Thorazine Prolixin Trilafon Compazine Mellaril Stelazine	Pregnancy
Thioxanthenes		Blurred vision, dry eyes, constipation, dry mouth, photosensitivity, tardive dyskinesia, severe muscle stiffness, fever, unusual tiredness or weakness, tachycardia, breathing difficulty, increased sweating, urinary incontinence, seizures, neuroleptic malignant syndrome	Navane	Central nervous system depression, circulatory collapse, blood dyscrasias, hypersensitivity to phenothiazines
Benzisoxazole		Anxiety, agitation, insomnia, sedation, extrapyramidal symptoms, dizziness, headache, constipation, nausea, rhinitis, rash, tachycardia, hyperglycemia	Risperdal Invega	Older people
Butyrophenone Dibenzoxazepine Dihydroindole	Fast-acting behavior management	Refer to side effects of phenothiazines	Haldol Loxitane Moban	
Atypical antipsychotics				
Dibenzodiazepine		Drowsiness, dizziness, agranulocytosis, seizures, sedation, hypersalivation, tachycardia, constipation, fever, weight gain, orthostatic hypotension, neuroleptic malignant syndrome, hyperglycemia	Clozapine (Clozaril)	
Thienobenzodiazepine		Asthenia, somnolence, headache, fever, dizziness, dry mouth, constipation, weight gain, orthostatic hypotension, tachycardia, extrapyramidal symptoms, hyperglycemia	Olanzapine (Zyprexia)	
Dibenzothiazepine		Somnolence, dizziness, headache, constipation, dry mouth, dyspepsia, weight gain, orthostatic hypotension, neuroleptic malignant syndrome, extrapyramidal symptoms, tardive dyskinesia, cataracts, lowered seizure threshold, hyperglycemia	Quetiapine (Seroquel)	
Benzothiazoly piperazine		Somnolence, headache, nausea, dyspepsia, constipation, dizziness, diarrhea, restlessness, extrapyramidal symptoms, prolonged QT interval, orthostatic hypotension, rash, hyperglycemia	Ziprasidone (Geodon)	
Dihydrocarbostyril		Headache, nausea and vomiting, constipation, anxiety, restlessness, insomnia, lightheadedness, somnolence, weight gain, blurred vision, increased salivation, extrapyramidal symptoms, hyperglycemia	Aripiprazole (Abilify)	

Source: Stahl, 2008.

community resources are important aspects of relapse prevention with the psychotic disorders. In the case of delirium, drug-induced psychosis, and psychosis due to a general medication, the focus is on eliminating the causative agent and monitoring the client for a reoccurrence of symptoms.

FOLLOW-UP

Follow-up involves regular evaluation for new onset of symptoms of psychosis. The client should be assessed for suicidal and homicidal ideation at each visit and complaints such as disturbances in sleep should be explored further to rule out decompensation. Laboratory studies including liver and kidney function, metabolic profiles, and complete blood counts should be done routinely every 3 to 6 months. Weights and blood pressures and medication compliance should be evaluated each visit. Any issues with living arrangements, finances, and relationship should be explored. As with any psychiatric disorder, the priority at follow-up is always safety.

PERSONALITY DISORDERS

The *DSM-IV-TR* (APA, 2002) defines personality disorders as mental illnesses that share several unique qualities and patterns of response to all aspects of the individual's lived experience. They contain symptoms that are enduring and play a major role in most, if not all, aspects of the person's life. While many disorders vacillate in terms of symptom presence and intensity, personality disorders typically remain relatively constant. To be diagnosed with a disorder in this category, the individual meets the following criteria:

- Symptoms have been present for an extended period of time, are inflexible and pervasive, and are not a result of alcohol or drugs or another psychiatric disorder.
- The history of symptoms can be traced back to adolescence or at least early adulthood.
- Symptoms have caused and continue to cause significant distress or negative consequences in different aspects of the person's life.
- Symptoms are seen in at least two of the following areas:
  - Thoughts (ways of looking at the world, thinking about self or others, and interacting)
  - Emotions (appropriateness, intensity, and range of emotional functioning)
  - Interpersonal functioning (relationships and interpersonal skills)
  - Impulse control

Personality disorders lead to rigidity in the client's pattern of thinking and worldview. The degree of severity of the disorder remains fairly constant throughout one's lifetime and these disorders are also frequently associated with mood and anxiety disorders, as well as substance abuse (Silk, 2010).

EPIDEMIOLOGY

Personality disorder can be a major medical and social problem. It has a reported prevalence of about 10 to 15 percent in the community, and about 50 percent of the patients were admitted psychiatrically. It is a chronic and debilitating disorder, as the symptoms usually first occur in adolescence, sometimes even earlier, peak in the early 20s, and persist for decades causing personal suffering, family dysfunction, and social difficulties including criminality and addictions. Clinically, personality disorder not only is difficult to treat, but also interferes with treatment of other comorbid psychiatric and medical conditions, increasing incapacitation, morbidity, and mortality of these patients (Lenzenweger, 2008).

Etiology

In general, in clinical populations, patients with dependent, borderline, obsessive-compulsive, avoidant, and schizotypal personality disorders are overrepresented, and patients with antisocial, schizoid, and paranoid personality disorders are underrepresented. Higher prevalences are generally seen in less-educated populations living in congested urban areas. Men more commonly have schizoid, antisocial, or obsessive-compulsive personality disorders, and women more commonly have dependent or histrionic personality disorders (Cleveland Clinic, 2011; Oldham, 2005).

Little is known about the causes of a personality disorder. Currently, there is some research into the role of genetics and the neurotransmitters, such as the dopamine reward system, but the results are inconclusive. While the information on the biological origins of personality disorder is limited, the role of environmental factors has been more extensively reviewed. The available research describes emotional neglect, traumatic experiences, and early childhood abandonment or separation from parent as contributing to these disorders (Skodol & Gunderson., 2008).

SUBJECTIVE DATA

The consistent presentation for the individual with a personality disorder is dramatic emotional reactions and tumultuous interpersonal relationships. She may be estranged from family members, have chronic work and legal issues, and have difficulty making decisions.

OBJECTIVE DATA

Although the characteristics of these personality disorders manifest in a variety of ways, the problems for the health care provider are quite similar. The individual often perceives many aspects of her lived experience as all black or all white and may become passive aggressive or angry when challenged. At times she may be emotionally overwhelmed and become self-abusive or suicidal.

PLAN

There are no pharmacologic interventions that address specific character traits of the individual with a personality disorder. Thus interventions involve medications for the symptoms of anxiety, depression, mood disorders, and sleep dysregulation. In addition, cognitive-behavioral therapy or, in some cases, dialectical behavioral therapy has been demonstrated to assist the client in identifying the relationship between personal thoughts, behaviors, and beliefs (Beck, Freeman, & Davis, 2007; Devens, 2007).

Nursing Implications

Managing the individual with a personality disorder involves a multidisciplinary approach. Often due to the challenging nature of the client's presentation and the issues surrounding her concerns, the clinician will need to be in communication with other providers involved in the care to minimize confusion. There might be an occasion where the client provides conflicting information at different times as a result of conscious or unconscious influences on how she perceives the situation. In the process, different providers of care to the client are often negatively affected by these reactive behaviors (known as *splitting*) and treatment planning becomes a challenge. Frequently, the client will give pieces of information to one provider and exclude others from the information. A comprehensive approach to treatments helps minimize negative outcomes.

Outcomes

It is difficult to measure positive outcomes when treating the client with a personality disorder. The focus is on treating the comorbid issues such as anxiety, depression, unstable mood, and substance use and abuse.

CHEMICAL ABUSE, DEPENDENCY, AND ADDICTION

The *DSM-IV-TR* (APA, 2000) makes a distinction between substance abuse and dependence; however, the treatments are similar. The diagnosis is made following a 12-month or longer pattern of continued use of a psychoactive or potentially addicting substance despite persistent or recurrent social, occupational, psychological, or physical problems that are the result, or made worse because of its use.

EPIDEMIOLOGY

The National Center for Health Statistics (2010) reported that 6.8 percent of American women over the age of 12 reported that they had used an illegal substance within the past month. Almost 19 percent of women over the age of 18 reported that they had smoked. Regular alcohol consumption was admitted to by almost 59 percent of women (Bernstein, Franco, & Freid, 2010; National Institute on Alcohol and Alcoholism, 2011).

In 2008, SAMHSA described the profile of a woman in the United States who abused alcohol as Caucasian, between the ages of 18 and 25, a high school graduate, and employed. The ethnic minority woman had 11 years of education and was unemployed. Low-income women living below the poverty level were less likely to have problems with alcohol than those above the poverty level (National Survey on Drug Use and Health [NSDUH], 2009).

It is estimated that women account for approximately 30 percent of substance abusers in the United States (Lowinson, Ruiz, Millman, & Langrod, 2005). This statistic, combined with the fact that the profile of a woman who abuses drugs is between the ages of 18 and 25, points to the issue of reproductive health in the woman who is addicted to drugs and/or alcohol. The American College of Obstetricians and Gynecologists (ACOG, 2008) reported that 12 percent of pregnant women between the ages of 15 and 44 reported consuming *some* alcohol during the previous month. The seriousness of this issue is highlighted in a CDC's *Morbidity and Mortality Weekly* report (2010b), which reported that 11 percent of pregnant women surveyed in Oklahoma and South Carolina felt they needed assistance with smoking cessation and 1 percent of those surveyed reported needing help with an alcohol or drug program. This suggests that it is imperative that the pregnant woman not only be questioned regarding her patterns of drug and alcohol intake but possibly also undergo a drug screen that includes both drugs and alcohol as part of the routine prenatal labs. The risk of relapse associated with drugs and alcohol suggests that any pregnant client who is considered at risk would benefit from periodic quantitative urine drug screens during pregnancy.

Tobacco is the drug most commonly used by women (Ruiz, Strain, & Langrod, 2007). Successful smoking cessation involves a combination of behavioral therapy and pharmacologic agents. The woman's readiness to quit is crucial to successful smoking cessation. Education regarding withdrawal symptoms that may sabotage her success is crucial to permanent smoking cessation. Common nicotine withdrawal symptoms include irritability, restlessness, hunger, drowsiness, difficulty concentrating, sleep disturbances, and strong cravings for nicotine (West, Ussher, Evans, & Rashid, 2005). Successful management of withdrawal symptoms often involves direct nicotine absorption through the use of nicotine gum, spray, or transdermal patches. The Food and Drug Administration (FDA) has not approved nicotine replacement therapy for pregnant women; however, heavy smoking during pregnancy may have greater risks than the short-term use of nicotine replacement, if replacement therapy is followed by complete nicotine abstinence. Lumley et al. (2009) found that although nicotine replacement medications were helpful in smoking cessation during pregnancy, nonpharmacological incentives for smoking cessation proved to be the most successful in helping individuals stop smoking.

A number of nonnicotine pharmacologic agents have been studied in smoking cessation. Bupropion hydrochloride (Zyban/Wellbutrin) has been shown to be effective for smoking cessation. However, bupropion is contraindicated in the presence of a history of seizures or an eating disorder. Other agents that are used include clonidine, a centrally acting adrenergic blocking agent, and lobeline, a nicotine imposter (Schaffer, 2002). The most recent addition to the field of treatment options for nicotine dependence is Chantix (varenicline). Although the medication is highly effective, clients on varenicline must be closely monitored because of reports of behavior changes, sleep disturbance, agitation, and mood disturbance.

Etiology

Women respond differently to alcohol than men due to physiological differences that decrease tolerance. Women develop adverse health consequences from the use and abuse of alcohol and other drugs over a shorter period of time and with lower consumption than men (Ruiz et al., 2007).

The available research has identified a genetic link to substance abuse disorders as well as a strong environmental influence. Women with substance abuse disorders have higher levels of depression and anxiety (Ruiz et al., 2007).

Associated Factors. Specific risk factors exist.

- An addictive parent
- Divorce or separation
- Living alone with children
- Lesbian lifestyle
- Reliance on pharmacological agents or alcohol to relax, sleep, feel more comfortable in social settings, or control unpleasant feelings
- Adolescent smoking

Incidence. Heavy drinking was reported by 5.6 percent of the population aged 12 and older, or 12.6 million people (SAMHSA, 2001). Although men have higher rates of alcoholism and other substance abuse, alcohol abuse is a significant problem for women. Among younger women in the general population, the proportion of drinkers is beginning to approximate that of men. In addition, rates of substance abuse in women may be underreported. Though older women drink less and have fewer drinking problems than older men, their use of prescribed psychoactive drugs is thought to cause more problems.

In 2000, approximately 14 million Americans reported that they currently used illegal drugs. Women used virtually the same types of illegal drugs as did men, but they used them less frequently than men did (5% versus 7.7% in 1993). Among youth aged 12 to 17 in 2000, the rate of current illicit drug use was similar for boys (9.8%) and girls (9.5%). Illicit drug use included marijuana, cocaine, heroin, hallucinogens, and inhalants, and nonmedical use of prescription-type pain relievers, tranquilizers, stimulants, and sedatives. The drug ecstasy (3,4-methylenedioxymethamphetamine) was included under hallucinogens. This drug is a growing problem, especially in adolescent women with serious health consequences. In 2000, an estimated 6.4 million persons had tried ecstasy at least once in their lifetime (SAMHSA, 2001).

Marijuana is the most commonly used illicit drug. Of the 5.7 million users of illicit drugs other than marijuana, 4.9 million were using psychotherapeutics nonmedically. Psychotherapeutics include pain relievers (3.9 million users), tranquilizers (1.0 million users), stimulants (1.8 million users), and sedatives (1.2 million users) (SAMHSA, 2008).

Among pregnant women aged 15 to 44 years, 4.4 percent reported using illicit drugs in the month prior to the survey (NSDUH, 2010). Although this rate is significantly lower than the rate among nonpregnant women aged 15 to 44 years (10.9%), the rate of use among pregnant women aged 15 to 17 years was 12.9 percent, nearly equal to the rate for nonpregnant women of the same age (13.5%) (SAMHSA, 2008). While all pregnant women should be screened for illicit drug use, adolescent and pregnant women may need specific interventions geared to reducing drug use.

In addition, cigarette smokers are more likely to use other tobacco products, illicit drugs, and alcohol than are nonsmokers. Among past month smokers in 2000, 39.4 percent were heavy alcohol users. Among nonsmokers, 14.4 percent were binge alcohol users and 3.0 percent were heavy alcohol users. Only 3.2 percent of nonsmokers were current illicit drug users, compared with 15.6 percent of smokers (SAMHSA, 2008). Tobacco addiction causes a number of preventable deaths in the United States. While the prevalence of smoking has declined to nearly 29.3 percent of the U.S. population and the health risks associated with smoking are widely known, millions of Americans continue to smoke (SAMHSA, 2001). Rates for women who smoked in 2000 remain at approximately 14.1 percent (SAMHSA, 2008) (see Table 25–6).

SUBJECTIVE DATA

Careful observation and listening may reveal symptoms of abuse of a specific substance. Histories are also essential. Symptoms of abuse are often specific to a particular substance.

Alcohol abusers often report gastritis, vomiting, and diarrhea. They may lose or gain weight. In addition, a client may report nervousness, anxiety, depression, sleep disturbances, pelvic pain, abnormal vaginal discharge, infertility, or sexual dysfunction.

Cocaine abuse may lead to sinusitis and upper respiratory infection, allergic rhinitis, nasal congestion, and epistaxis. Weight loss may be experienced. Abstinence from cocaine may produce anxiety, fatigue, depression, irritability, and sleep disturbances.

Abuse of sedative-hypnotics (benzodiazepines) may cause headaches, nausea, paranoia, and sleep disturbances. Withdrawal may cause insomnia and irritability. When used with alcohol, sedative-hypnotics increase central nervous system depressant effects.

Cannabis (marijuana) abuse may provoke fatigue, decreased motivation, panic attacks, anxiety, and paranoia. Hallucinogens can cause mood swings, memory loss, hyperactivity, and even death. Ecstasy can increase heart rate and blood and heart oxygen consumption without

TABLE 25–6. Drugs of Abuse

Drug (route)	Peak Time for Onset After Last Use	Hours Detectable in Body	Effects	Symptoms of Overdose	Withdrawal Syndrome Symptoms
Alcohol (oral)	12–24 hours	6–24 hours	Sedation, decreased inhibition, relaxation, impaired coordination and judgment, slurred speech, nausea, euphoria, depression	Respiratory depression, stupor, circulatory collapse, cardiac arrest, coma, death	Tremors; increased temperature, pulse, and respiration; psychomotor agitation; impaired attention and memory; illusions; auditory, visual, or tactile hallucinations; delusions; seizures; delirium tremens; circulatory collapse; death
Opiates (oral, inhalation, intramuscular, intravenous, smoking)			Analgesia, sedation, decreased short-term memory and concentration, slowed reaction time, constricted pupils, constipation	Respiration, depression, stupor, circulatory collapse, coma, death	Yawning, rhinorrhea, lacrimation, abdominal cramps, diaphoresis, irritability, restlessness, anxiety, disturbed sleep, body/muscle aches, nausea, diarrhea, fever, dilated pupils, increased blood pressure, pulse, respiration, dysphoria, cravings
Morphine, opiates, hydromorphone, methadone, meperidine, hydrocodone, propoxyphene	2–4 hours	1–4 days			
Heroin	10–12 hours				

(*continued*)

TABLE 25–6. Drugs of Abuse (continued)

Drug (route)	Peak Time for Onset After Last Use	Hours Detectable in Body	Effects	Symptoms of Overdose	Withdrawal Syndrome Symptoms
Central nervous system depressant			Relief of anxiety, euphoria, sedation, impaired judgment, dizziness, impaired coordination and memory	Somnolence, hypotension, hypotonia, respiratory depression, coma, cardiac arrest, death	Tremor; nightmares; diaphoresis; blepharospasm; dilated pupils; agitation, ataxia, increased respiration, and blood pressure; vomiting; delusions; anxiety/panic; decreased sensorium; confusion; delirium; seizures
Benzodiazepines Long acting Clonazepam	5–8 days	1–6 weeks			
Short acting Diazepam, lorazepam, alprazolam, oxazepam, chloraze	12–24 hours				
Barbiturates Amobarbital, butabarbital, butalbital, pentobarbital, phenobarbital, secobarbital	72 hours	2–10 days	See benzodiazepines	See benzodiazepines	See benzodiazepines
Stimulants (oral, inhalation, intravenous, smoking)	12–24 hours	1–2 days	Alertness, reduced fatigue, euphoria, central nervous system stimulation followed by depression, sleep disturbance, irritability, decreased appetite, paranoia	Cardiac arrhythmias, cardiac arrest, elevated/lowered blood pressure, chest pain; vomiting; seizures, hallucinations, confusion, impaired judgment, hypertension fever, agitation, tremor	Fatigue, insomnia, increased appetite, psychomotor retardation, agitation, severe, dysphoria, anxiety, cravings, disturbed sleep, suicide
Cocaine	4–6 hours	2–4 days			
Crack cocaine	30–60 minutes	2–4 days			
Dexedrine, amphetamines, methylphenidate	12–24 hours	1–4 days			
Caffeine	3–7 hours		Stimulation, increased mental acuity, inexhaustibility	Restlessness, nervousness, excitement, insomnia, flushing, gastrointestinal distress, muscle twitches, tachycardia, agitation	Headache, drowsiness, fatigue, craving, impaired psychomotor performance, difficulty concentrating, yawning, nausea
Cannabis, hashish (inhalation, orally i.e., "brownies")	20 hours	5–60 days	Euphoria, dysphoria, drowsiness, anxiety, panic, sensitivity to sound, heightened perception of colors, unusual body sounds	Rare	None recognized
Inhalants	Not available	Not available	Euphoria, giddiness, excitation, disinhibition, loss of consciousness, ataxia, nystagmus, dysarthria	Central nervous system depression, heart failure, coma, seizures, death	Similar to alcohol, but milder with anxiety, tremors, hallucinations, sleep disturbance

(*continued*)

TABLE 25–6. Drugs of Abuse (continued)

Drug (route)	Peak Time for Onset After Last Use	Hours Detectable in Body	Effects	Symptoms of Overdose	Withdrawal Syndrome Symptoms
Butane, propane, refrigerant gasses, spray paint, deodorants, air fresheners, fabric sprays, cooking oil sprays, nitrous oxide, chloroform, ether, cleaning agents, airplane glue, rubber cement, amyl nitrate					
Hallucinogens	7–46 hours	5–7 days	Feeling powerful, invulnerable, decrease awareness of environment, elevated pulse, respiration, blood pressure, flushing, diaphoresis, ataxia, dysarthria, decreased pain perception, paranoia, confusion, unintelligible speech	Decreased pulse, respirations, blood pressure; extreme aggression, suicidality, nausea; vomiting; rapid eye movement, blurred vision; drooling; hallucinations; seizures; coma; death	None
Phencyclidine					
Lysergic acid diethylamide					

Source: Lowinson et al., 2005.

increasing the heart's ejection fraction, putting users at risk for a heart event such as a myocardial infarction.

Abuse of opiates produces an initial sense of euphoria, followed by a sense of tranquility and then sleepiness. Tolerance and dependence develop requiring higher doses to maintain the desired level of euphoria. Opiates do not directly cause serious organ damage.

Use of tobacco causes many effects on the body. Chronic cough, wheezing, dyspnea, sore throat, and bad breath are rarely mentioned as complaints by clients. Clients do become concerned, however, about chronic obstructive pulmonary disease, asthma, cardiovascular disease, lung cancer, and other potentially fatal illnesses, all of which have been associated with tobacco use. Tobacco products also contain nicotine, which is known to cause addiction and withdrawal.

Histories are the best indicators of early substance abuse. Screening for substance abuse focuses on adverse consequences (e.g., family or marital problems, seizures, or withdrawal symptoms) rather than on physical or laboratory findings. An alcohol history may use a screening questionnaire such as the CAGE questionnaire, which looks at patterns and consequences, or the Short Michigan Alcoholism Screening Test (SMAST), which deals with consequences. Diagnosis should not rest solely on the questionnaire; rather, the questionnaire is used to determine the index of suspicion for abuse. Clients will often describe starting out experimenting with a substance, like tobacco, to go on to using more and more to achieve the same effects.

The health care provider should always approach the client in a nonbiased manner.

When questioning about abuse, *always* begin with questions about less sensitive substances:

How many cups of coffee do you drink per day?
How much tobacco do you use per day?
How many drinks per day?

Then ask about tolerance: How many drinks does it take for you to feel high? and the occurrence of blackouts. Inability to remember what happened when drinking is a probable sign of alcoholism.

The drug history includes information about prescription medication, over-the-counter medication, and illicit drugs (substance abuse may progress from alcohol, to cannabis, to cocaine, etc.). Inquire if one drug is taken in conjunction with another or with alcohol. Previous treatment for substance abuse should be noted. Has the client tried to quit smoking in the past? If so, how did she quit and how long did she maintain nonuse of the substance.

The social history includes information about marital or family problems job or promotion loss due to poor performance or absenteeism, financial difficulties, and multiple arrests for disorderly conduct or driving under influence of a drug. Inquire about behavior changes, such as termination of old friendships and loss of interest in favorite pastimes.

Past medical histories include questions about accidental injuries and illnesses related to abuse. For example, individuals who abuse cocaine have frequent urinary tract infections, sinusitis, nosebleeds, and burns if the drug is smoked; alcohol abuse may cause gastroenteritis, ulcers, hepatitis, and pneumonia; and cannabis frequently causes urinary tract infections. Smoking causes increased rates of upper respiratory and lung infections. A history of pneumonia or chronic bronchitis may be elicited.

The reproductive system and sexual history includes questions about pregnancies, abortions, sexually transmitted infections, pelvic inflammatory disease, abnormal Pap smears, menstrual irregularities, sexual dysfunction, and sexually transmitted disease (STD) and HIV risk factors. Substance use and abuse decrease inhibitions. Consequently, a woman is more likely to engage in sexual intercourse, which may increase the risk of sexual abuse. Substance abuse may lead to frequent partners if sex is exchanged for substance; intravenous drug use increases the risk of hepatitis B and HIV infection.

Family medical history includes information about mental illness, dysfunctional family, and substance abuse. Exposure to secondhand smoke should be noted.

OBJECTIVE DATA

Client history is important for diagnosis as are laboratory tests and physical examination. The individual who is abusing drugs or alcohol should have a standard laboratory studies including complete metabolic panel, thyroid-stimulating hormone, liver function, complete blood count, lipid panel, and electrocardiogram. Abnormal findings are further investigated to determine the extent of multisystem involvement and the effects of the substance use.

Abnormalities in liver function tests often include elevated serum γ-glutamyltransferase (most sensitive), alanine aminotransferase, aspartate aminotransferase, lactate dehydrogenase, amylase, alkaline phosphatase, total bilirubin, cholesterol, and triglycerides (indicative of alcoholic liver disease). Uric acid is also frequently elevated and the serum magnesium, calcium, phosphorus, and potassium usually decreased (SAMHSA, 2008).

Toxicology studies should be compared to the client's subjective reports regarding drug use patterns. Furthermore, levels of drugs present should be compared to the client's reports of the last episode of use. Although blood alcohol levels give an indication of acute alcohol intoxication, urine for alcohol glucuronide provides an indication of alcohol use for several days after the serum ethanol level has returned to zero. Some drugs of abuse (i.e., cannabis and benzodiazepines) may remain positive for days after the last use (SAMHSA, 2008).

PLAN

Psychosocial interventions

Psychosocial intervention involves encouraging the client to involve her significant others in the treatment plan to maximize success (Ivbijaro, 2010). Refer the client for a psychiatric assessment if she has concurrent mental health issues and a dual-diagnosis disorder.

Smoking cessation success may be enhanced by using behavioral therapy alone or in conjunction with nicotine replacement products or an antidepressant. First, assess the woman's readiness to quit kind and then help her plan a specific quit program. The provider must prepare her for withdrawal symptoms that may sabotage her earnest attempts. Assure her it takes most people several attempts. A partial list of withdrawal symptoms includes irritability, restlessness, hunger, drowsiness, difficulty concentrating, sleep disturbances, and strong cravings for nicotine (West et al., 2005). Nicotine replacement products are not recommended during pregnancy.

Nursing Implications

Healthy People 2020 (2011) includes identification and treatment of individuals with issues related to drug or alcohol abuse as a goal for the health of Americans. The primary health care provider is in a position to help the client recognize that she has a problem and to acknowledge the negative relationship between her substance use and the consequences. If substance use causes problems (physical, mental, legal, or financial), then the individual has a problem. Treatment should be individualized, and continue indefinitely for maximum success.

FOLLOW-UP

Once the individual has been medically stabilized and detoxed from the addicting substance, encourage the client to become involved in Alcoholics Anonymous or a similar 12-step programs. Biofeedback and relaxation training may also be helpful. Refer the client for psychiatric consultation or other social support services as indicated. For women, relapse occurs in situations involving excessive stress, inner conflicts, conflicts with others, and loss. Relapse is more likely to occur in situations where there is a conflict with others than with inner conflicts.

WOMEN IN THE MILITARY

For women in the military trauma comes from a variety of sources that include not only combat and other military experiences, but also sexual abuse and assault. In 2009, the Veterans Administration reported that 14 percent of active duty military and 17 percent of Guard and Reserve personnel were women. Like her male counterpart, a woman can experience difficulties associated with combat and military life that can contribute to the development of anxiety and depression, sleep dysregulation, and PTSD. See section on PTSD for additional information.

EPIDEMIOLOGY

Women who serve in the military experience psychological distress at a rate that is about twice that of women who are not in the military. The Department of Veterans Affairs (2011) estimated that as much as 78 percent of female military personnel experienced some form of sexual harassment and 35 percent reported having been the victim of physical assault. Women returning from combat were slightly more likely to experience psychological distress when compared to their male counterparts.

Etiology

The neurochemistry of depression and psychological trauma is no different for female veterans than women in the general population. Therefore, the primary care provider considers the impact of these life experiences when planning treatment in the same manner as the nonmilitary female client.

PLAN AND FOLLOW-UP

Although progress has been made by the military in identifying and treating the mental health needs of the active and returning military personal, the individual is not always willing or able to take advantage of mental health services. For many there continues to be a stigma associated with admitting to psychological issues or asking for help, while specialized mental health services may not be readily available. For female returning veterans, the traumatic experience may involve rape or sexual violence and their issues are no different from individuals in the civilian population who experience this type of trauma.

In the primary care setting, it is important to ask the female veteran about her experiences both in the field and upon returning home. Providing an environment that encourages her discuss her individual lived experience can be helpful in identifying need for referral for additional resources. For updated information about available resources for veterans, active military personnel and their families go to http://www.mentalhealth.va.gov or http://www.samsa.gov/militaryfamilies.

EATING DISORDERS

The three types of eating disorders are anorexia nervosa, bulimia, and obesity. The eating disorders are primarily associated with distortions in body image. Anorexic individuals refuse to maintain a body weight that is considered appropriate for their age and height (less than 85% of their expected body weight). There are two types of anorexia: restricting type and binge eating/purging type. Bulimia involves the consumption of large amounts of food within a short time period (usually 2 hours). During these episodes, individuals will often report feeling that they are out of control about what they eat or how much they eat. These individuals then use diuretics, laxatives, enemas, or engage in vigorous exercise or fasting as a means of losing weight after the episode of binging. To meet *DSM-IV-TR* criteria, these episodes must occur at least twice a week for a 3-month period. Based on clients' means of relieving themselves of what they have consumed, bulimia is categorized as either purging type or nonpurging type. Obesity is defined as a body mass index (BMI) of 30 or greater. Despite the fact that there are three types of eating disorders, treatment for all three is essentially the same.

Biologic changes in individuals with anorexia include elevated levels of endogenous opiates in the spinal fluid of individuals who have eating disorders. In addition, the dopamine level aberrations were found in women who had recovered from anorexia nervosa.

Sadock and Sadock (2007) reported that there are also increases in levels of serotonin in the brains of women with anorexia. Furthermore, individuals with anorexia may have changes in the limbic system. Abnormalities within the limbic system may be responsible for the emotional rigidity, and perfectionistic style often seen with anorexia. Other risk factors such as early feeding difficulties, symptoms of anxiety, perfectionistic traits, and parenting styles may all play a role in the development of anorexia.

Families of clients with eating disorders tend to be enmeshed, intrusive, and are often hostile toward the identified client while maintaining conflict avoidance. The issues of power and control are overriding factors in the family of the client with an eating disorder (Sadock & Sadock, 2007).

EPIDEMIOLOGY

The data from the National Comorbidity Replication Study described the lifetime prevalence of anorexia as 0.9 percent for women and 0.3 percent for men and the prevalence of bulimia was 1.5 percent for women and 0.5 percent for men. In the United States, it is estimated that of the adults 20 years of age and older, 68.3 percent are overweight with 33.9 percent of those in the obese range (CDC, 2010c). Obesity is more common in black women and white men and the prevalence in the lower socioeconomic classes is six times that in upper socioeconomic classes. The latest figures from the CDC (2010c) indicate that 5.7 percent of the U.S. adult population may be categorized as *morbidly* obese (BMI greater than 40). Mood, anxiety, impulse control, and substance abuse disorders were common comorbidities in those reporting anorexia and bulimia. Survey participants reported that the average duration for anorexia was about 1.7 years while individuals with bulimia and binge eating symptoms lasted approximately 8 years. The median age of onset was 18 to 21 years of age. Anorexia nervosa usually occurs among white females of middle-upper socioeconomic status. They may have career choice that stresses thinness, competition, perfection, or self-discipline (modeling, theater, ballet, competitive athletics); parent or sibling with eating disorder, affective disorder, or substance abuse problem; psychiatric illness or depression; or being achievement oriented, compliant, "model" child, or perfectionist. A tremendous toll is taken on the families and clients affected by this illness. Mortality from anorexia nervosa is estimated to be between 6 and 10 percent; in a hospitalized population, it is estimated to be over 10 percent. Death usually results from starvation, suicide, or electrolyte imbalance (APA, 2000).

Etiology

As with other psychiatric syndromes, the origins of the eating disorders are multifactorial (Fichter et al., 2005). Genetic factors have a predisposition to the development of an eating disorder, with a high incidence among sisters and mothers. Neuroendocrine abnormalities include hypothalamic dysfunction, elevated cerebrospinal fluid cortisol levels, and possible impairment of the dopaminergic regulation.

SUBJECTIVE DATA

The client may report feeling bloated, fatigue, constipation, diarrhea, decreased libido, cold intolerance, insomnia, sore tongue, frequent upper respiratory infections, muscle weakness and cramps, dizziness, social isolation, nausea, fainting spells. She may complain about things such as hair loss, cold intolerance, or irritability. She may deny hunger or exhaustion. There may be compulsive and excessive exercise intended to burn calories. Amenorrhea or infertility is associated with anorexia and bulimia (APA, 2000). Women often hide their symptoms so the provider should maintain a high index of suspicion especially if menstrual irregularities exist (Loomis, Griswold, Pastore, & Dunphy, 2011). An evaluation should begin when clients report missing three to six menstrual cycles.

Subtle clues may be detected by a health care provider who is attuned to the client. For example, the client may be oversensitive when weighed or have excessive concerns about being overweight, even if she appears normal or under normal weight. She may request advice about fad diets and weight loss programs, may claim she "does not have enough time to eat," may dress in oversized clothes or layers of clothing to hide weight or health (yet she denies a problem), and may be compulsive about exercise. A wide discrepancy may exist in caloric intake and expenditure, leading to caloric deficit and subsequent weight loss.

Clients who present with anorexia nervosa will most likely begin by expressing the belief that they are overweight. These women will quickly share that they have an intense fear of gaining weight. The individual with bulimia will frequently be secretive about their binge eating behavior. They recognize that their pattern of binging is abnormal, but lack the ability to control it. As a result, they will tell you that they are embarrassed or feel guilty about their behavior.

Individuals who are obese may try to avoid any discussion of their weight. They often feel guilty and embarrassed that they have not lost weight and may have in fact gained but will not volunteer any information related to their weight. When asked they may respond that they only eat a little and don't know how they could gain weight. A sedentary lifestyle and binge eating may be a factor in obesity.

Attia and Walsh (2007) note that women with anorexia may be more resistant to treatment than women with bulimia. This is in part because the anorexic is frequently in denial of her illness and does not seek treatment willingly. They will describe homes in which they were faced with pressure to succeed or perform well in all of their activities. They may describe their developmental years as being laden with intense criticism regarding less than optimal performance. They may also describe episodes of illicit activity such as shoplifting.

Thorough medical and psychosocial histories are of utmost importance. Various screening tools are available and most often used in psychotherapy: Eating Attitudes Test, Diagnostic Survey for Eating Disorders, Eating Disorder Inventory, and Bulimia Test. A pertinent history that is applicable to any eating disorder addresses at minimum the following seven topics: attitude, diet history, exercise habits, menstrual history, social history, psychological history, and binging/purging history.

OBJECTIVE DATA

The client with bulimia does not have the malnourished appearance that is a hallmark feature of the client with anorexia. Individuals with bulimia should be carefully evaluated for signs and symptoms of self-induced vomiting. They may be hoarse or have complaints of a chronically sore throat. They may have an erythematous throat because of self-induced vomiting. In addition, self-induced vomiting is often associated with enlargement of the parotid glands. Often the dental enamel shows signs of erosion. Calluses or abrasions are often present on the knuckles as a result of their efforts to induce vomiting. As with anorexia, the client with bulimia may have symptoms of dehydration.

Physical Examination

- *General appearance:* The client appears pale and emaciated and manifests delayed sexual maturation.
- *Skin:* The client may have lanugo (fine, downy hair that covers extremities and face), brittle nails, dry skin, hair loss or thinning, and carotenemia evidenced by yellowing palms and soles.
- *Throat:* Buccal mucosa may be erythematous.
- *Breasts:* Breasts may be atrophied or poorly developed.
- *Vascular system:* Arrhythmias (secondary to electrolyte abnormalities) and peripheral edema may be detected.
- *Abdomen:* The abdomen may appear scaphoid. Bowel sounds may be hypoactive.
- *Genitalia and reproductive tract:* The client may have primary or secondary amenorrhea, irregular menses (may not be identified if she takes oral contraceptives), and decreased fertility. Preterm birth and stillbirth are associated with anorexia and pregnancy.
- *Rectal area:* Hemorrhoids (secondary to constipation) may be present.
- *Musculoskeletal system:* The client may exhibit overuse injuries (stress fractures, joint or tendon problems). A client with severe anorexia is at risk for osteoporosis.
- *Nervous system:* Determine if the client is suicidal.
- *Endocrine system:* Thyroid abnormalities may be detected.

Diagnostic Tests

- *Urinalysis:* A urinalysis is done to evaluate carbohydrate metabolism and specific gravity. Elevated ketones and protein indicate low carbohydrate metabolism (due to poor intake). Specific gravity is increased if the client is dehydrated and decreased if she is drinking excessive water (common before being weighed). A urine pregnancy test is done if amenorrhea is a symptom and the client is sexually active.
- *Blood chemistry:* A complete blood count is done to determine anemia and neutropenia. A full set of electrolytes are evaluated. Individuals who vomit and use laxatives and/or diuretics usually will have significant and sometimes life-threatening electrolyte imbalances. Decreased potassium may cause arrhythmia, then death. In addition, decreased calcium, magnesium, chloride, sodium, albumin, and globulin and increased blood urea nitrogen are typical with anorexia nervosa.
- *Liver function tests:* To help rule out other causes of weight loss, some values may be affected by malnutrition.
- *Endocrine tests:* Levels of follicle-stimulating hormone and luteinizing hormone may be decreased. Prolactin, thyroid-stimulating hormone, and thyroxine levels may be normal. Thyroid function tests may be borderline low.
- *Electrocardiogram:* An electrocardiogram is indicated to determine the presence of arrhythmias, especially if the health care provider suspects poor follow-up or severe disease.

- If amenorrhea is persistent and weight loss marked, obtain a bone mineral density measure to rule out osteoporosis.

DIFFERENTIAL MEDICAL DIAGNOSES

Weight loss: rule out hyperthyroidism, malabsorption syndrome, mesenteric artery syndrome, Addison's disease, Alzheimer's disease, Crohn's disease, depression, ischemic heart disease, carcinoma, other chronic diseases. Amenorrhea, primary: rule out pituitary adenoma, ovarian failure, genital tract obstruction; secondary: rule out pregnancy, pituitary failure, weight loss, or decreased body fat due to body building or sports.

PLAN

The first priority is establishing the client's safety and restoring the client's physiologic balance. Women with an eating disorder often have difficulties with anxiety and need to learn new coping skills for managing anxiety.

The goal of therapy for eating disorders focuses on behavioral interventions that lead to in a healthy perception of food and body image as well as the demonstration of sound eating behaviors. The care of patients with an eating disorder needs to be highly structured and regimented. Short-term positive goals with anorexia are measured in terms of slow, but steady weight gain (1–4 lb/week) and stable electrolytes. With bulimia, the goals include reduction in the binge-purge cycle. A comprehensive interdisciplinary team approach is necessary for the best possible outcome and treatment that is focused on the biopsychosocial model is helpful. Primary support system participation is crucial to recovery. In addition, concurrent psychiatric issues such as mood disorders, anxiety, and impulse control issues should be addressed.

In the available literature, there is limited research into the pharmacotherapy for eating disorders and most of the studies were of limited clinical significance. To date there have been few studies into the effects of antidepressants, antipsychotics, mood stabilizers, antiseizure medications, appetite stimulants, hormone therapy, and nutritional supplements with inconclusive evidence. Currently, pharmacotherapy is aimed at addressing the presenting symptomatology, such as the mood instability, anxiety, and impulsivity that are often associated with the eating disorders. The treatment includes individual and group psychotherapy and is a long-term process for the individual with anorexia or bulimia.

FOLLOW-UP AND REFERRAL

Positive outcomes for the patient with an eating disorder are somewhat limited. Attia and Walsh (2007) reported that 50 percent of patients treated for anorexia relapse within a year of reaching a clinically acceptable weight. Over time, the cycle of relapse has a negative impact on the clients mood and affect and her primary support system. Referral to an eating disorder specialist for ongoing treatment can be effective and improve outcomes.

SLEEP DYSREGULATION

The National Institutes of Health identified sleep-related issues a priority for health care professionals. A 2004–2005 National Sleep Foundation (NSF) survey of adults aged at least 18 years found that about 21 percent thought they had a sleep problem, and about the same number (24%) stated that sleep problems negatively affected their daily lives. Among individuals who experience insomnia, 42 percent reported sleep problems nearly every night and 88 percent had difficulty sleeping for more than a year. Despite affecting millions of people in the United States, insomnia is underrecognized and many patients do not receive adequate treatment. This lack of effective sleep management can result in serious consequences for affected individuals.

The loss of even small amounts of sleep on a daily basis leads to progressive impairment of cognitive performance. Chronic restriction of sleep to 6 hours or less per night for 14 days (short-term partial sleep deprivation) was found to produce cognitive performance deficits equivalent to as much as two nights of total sleep deprivation. Even relatively moderate sleep restriction can seriously impair waking neurobehavioral functions in healthy adults, resulting in fatigue, mood changes such as depression and irritability, difficulty with concentration, and impaired daytime functioning. These symptoms diminish the quality of daily activities, resulting in a reduced ability to accomplish tasks, nodding off and poor concentration, decreased quality of work and increased work absences, relationship problems, and less enjoyment of family and social life. Daily skills such as driving are often impaired; 37 percent of licensed drivers in the NSF survey reported that they have nodded off or fallen asleep while driving a vehicle, with 13 percent having done so at least once a month. About 4 percent have reported an accident or near-accident in the previous year because of dozing off or feeling too drowsy (Kyle, Morgan, & Espie, 2010).

Physiologic control of the sleep-wake cycle is generally believed to involve two components: a homeostatic system that seeks to recover a set point when disturbed (e.g., sleep deprivation is followed by extra recovery sleep to make up for the sleep deficit) and a circadian pacemaker that is essentially independent of sleep and waking. Homeostatic regulation, a sleep-inducing substance that accumulates during waking, could enhance the activity of sleep-promoting neurons while reducing the activity of wake-producing neurons (Schultz & Steimer, 2009). During sleep, concentrations of the sleep-inducing substance would decrease (Lieberman & Neubauer, 2007).

In the primary care setting, many of the negative effects of sleep deprivation are often the chief complaint. A thorough assessment of sleep and sleep hygiene is important to rule out sleep dysregulation as a cause of the present symptoms (Doghramji, 2010) (see Table 25–7).

VIOLENCE AND ABUSE

There are several major forms of violence against women, including intimate partner violence, stalking, and sexual assault. In addition, women are exposed to war and random acts of violence such as street violence. Known psychological effects of such victimization are pervasive and involve all aspects of the women's lived experience. Variables that combine to determine the effects of victimization include type and characteristics of the assault. To understand these effects, it is important to consider the victim variables such as demographics, psychological reactions at the time of the trauma, history of previous victimization, current or previous mental health issues, and general coping style. Important also are the sociocultural factors such as poverty, social inequality, and inadequate social support (Briere & Jordan, 2011; Straus, 2004).

Violence against women is now well recognized as a public health problem and human rights violation of worldwide significance. It is an important risk factor for women's ill health, with far-reaching consequences for both their physical and mental health (Krantz & Garcia-Moreno, 2005).

INTIMATE PARTNER VIOLENCE

Four types of individual partner violence are identified based on the dyadic control context of the violence. In intimate terrorism, the individual is violent and controlling, the partner is not. In violent resistance, the individual is violent but not controlling, the partner is the violent and controlling one. In situational couple violence, although the individual is violent, neither the individual nor the partner is violent and controlling. In mutual violent control, the individual and the partner are violent and controlling. Evidence is presented that situational couple violence dominates in general surveys, intimate terrorism and violent resistance dominate in agency samples, and this is the source of differences across studies with respect

TABLE 25–7. Medications Used for Sleep Dysregulation

Classification	Indication	Side Effects	Caution	Examples	Contraindicated
Barbiturates	Anxiety, insomnia short-term use, preoperatively Seizures	Tolerance Dependence CNS depression	Older people With ethanol With other CNS depressants	Amobarbital Butabarbital Pentobarbital Phenobarbital Secobarbital	Pregnancy and lactation Cardiac, hepatic, renal, or respiratory insufficiency, suicidality, addiction
Benzodiazepines	Anxiety, insomnia	Dependence, drowsiness, lethargy, residual sedation	Decreased mental alertness, confusion, with ethanol, hepatic, respiratory, renal, cardiac disease	Temazepam, lorazepam, clonazepam	Pregnancy and lactation, addiction
Miscellaneous	Sedation, insomnia	Dependence, residual sedation	With ethanol Cardiac, hepatic, respiratory, renal disease Decreased effects with food	Zaleplon, zolpidem, eszopiclone	Pregnancy and lactation, addiction
Exception	Insomnia	Drowsiness	No physical dependence	Ramelteon	Pregnancy and lactation

Source: Hall-Porter, 2010.

to the gender symmetry of partner violence. An argument is made that if we want to understand partner violence, intervene effectively in individual cases, or make useful policy recommendations, we must make these distinctions in our research (Johnson, 2006).

Walker (2009) conducted classic studies of battered women and their relationships. She described the cycle of predictable behaviors that repeat over time. Walker's theory developed in the 1970 is based on the idea that once abusive relationships are created, repetitive patterns characterize them. She describes these predictable behaviors as the tension-building stage, the incident of abuse stage, the reconciliation stage, and the calm stage. This cycle of abuse concept is widely used in the treatment options of American domestic violence programs.

Epidemiology

One in four women (25%) has experienced domestic violence in her lifetime. Estimates range from 960,000 incidents of violence against a current or former spouse, boyfriend, or girlfriend to 3 million women who are physically abused by their domestic partner husband or boyfriend per year. Women accounted for 85 percent of the victims of intimate partner violence, men for approximately 15 percent (Bureau of Justice Statistics, 2007; CDC, 2010a).

Etiology. Domestic violence may start when one partner feels the need to control and dominate the other. Abusers may feel this need to control their partner because of low self-esteem, extreme jealousy, difficulties in regulating anger and other strong emotions, or when they feel inferior to the other partner in education and socioeconomic background. Some men with very traditional beliefs may think they have the right to control women, and that women aren't equal to men. This domination then takes the form of emotional, physical, or sexual abuse. Studies suggest that violent behavior often is caused by an interaction of situational and individual factors. That means that abusers learn violent behavior from their family, people in their community, and other cultural influences as they grow up. They may have seen violence often or they may have been victims themselves (Goldsmith, 2006; Humphries, 2009).

Subjective Data

Physical abuse can often be seen in the form of bruises and broken bones. Abuse that is emotional tends to be less noticeable. The person who is emotionally abused may be belittled, patronized, threatened, ignored, or rejected. Sexual abuse occurs when someone is forced to engage in any sexual act to which she did not consent. Neglect is a form of abuse that generally victimizes children, older people, and those who are dependent on others. It involves depriving someone of her basic physical and emotional needs.

Women present to the primary care setting with issues resulting from some aspect of violence second only to the emergency department. However, the present complaint is most often related to some other complaint such as anxiety, headaches, GI distress, or difficulty sleeping. The provider needs to be aware of the subtle indicators of abuse and violence.

Objective Data

A complete physical assessment with lab studies is important to fully evaluate physical and psychological status. Obvious signs such as new and old bruises, fractures, evidence of head injuries, and broken or missing teeth are easy to suspect violence and evaluate further. However, more subtle signs such as increased anxiety, lack of eye contact, jumpiness, and denial about the situation may be indicators of abuse.

Victims of intimate family violence represent all age, racial, religious, cultural, educational, and socioeconomic groups. They are often isolated from family members and support systems. They frequently have low self-esteem and take responsibility for the behavior of the batterer, stating "I shouldn't have said that" or "I know that makes him mad and I shouldn't have done it." The phenomenon of learned helplessness frequently sets in and the victim is unable to act in her own behalf. She comes to understand that regardless of her behavior, the outcome is unpredictable and usually undesirable.

Plan and Follow-Up

The first priority in planning for victims of intimate partner and family violence is to help them create a comprehensive safety plan. With assistance from a victim service professional, victims should create an individualized plan for safety in all situations, including a checklist of necessary items to take when leaving an abusive situation. Make available telephone numbers of available resources even if the woman is not ready to seek victim services at the time (Tozzi et al., 2003).

SEXUAL ABUSE OR RAPE

Sexual abuse or rape is forced sexual intercourse perpetrated against the will of a victim; it can occur with an intimate partner but the perpetrator can also be a stranger.

Force may be employed by physical violence, coercion, or threat of harm. Acquaintance rape usually occurs in a dating situation and is perpetrated by someone the woman knows and trusts. Sexual assault involves actions other than rape: sodomy, forced anal intercourse; oral copulation, forced copulation of mouth of one person with sexual organ or anus of another; rape with a foreign object, forced penetration of genital or anal openings with a foreign object; and sexual battery, unwanted touching of an intimate part for sexual arousal. Health care providers may be required to report assault-related injuries to law enforcement agencies (CDC, 2007).

Rape challenges a woman's ability to maintain her defenses and arouses feelings of guilt, anxiety, and inadequacy. The overwhelming experience heightens her sense of helplessness and intensifies her conflict about dependence and independence. The survivor's response is determined by her stage in life, her defensive structures, and her coping ability. Rape trauma syndrome comprises the sequential reactions of the survivor in dealing with her experience. The syndrome, described as a two- or three-stage process, helps explain how rape victims respond to their traumatic experience (Basile, Chen, Black, & Saltzman, 2007).

The immediate response, or acute phase, occurs immediately after the assault or the disclosure of assault. The survivor's lifestyle is completely disrupted and reactions are tearfulness and agitation or a relaxed calm. This stage can last as long as 3 to 6 months, with typical symptoms being anxiety, fears and phobias, suspiciousness, major depressive symptoms, feelings of inferiority, inability to think clearly, and difficulty functioning at home, work, or school. In addition to these typical symptoms, feelings of guilt, shame, embarrassment, and self-blame are common. Psychophysiological disturbances affect eating, sleeping, GI function, and sexual intimacy. Ensuring safety and regaining control over her life are the survivor's main emotional needs during this time. Medical attention is important. In a study of 1,076 victims, general body trauma was reported in 67 percent of the sample (Riggs, Houry, Long, Markovchick, & Feldhaus, 2004).

The middle phase, or readjustment stage, is a period of transition when the survivor rationalizes that she could have prevented the assault and develops unrealistic plans to avoid another.

The final stage, or reorganization phase, may last 2 years or longer and is difficult and painful. During this stage, the survivor begins to deal with the reality of her victimization and may make changes in lifestyle, relationship, and work.

Along with a two- or three-stage model of recovery, other authors discuss recovery within the broader content of PTSD as described in the *DSM-IV-TR*. (See section on PTSD for a complete discussion.) Another mental health disorder that may occur as an outcome of rape is acute stress disorder; differentiated from PTSD by the time, symptoms are exhibited. The symptoms last for at least 2 days but do not persist longer than 4 weeks after the traumatic event (APA, 2000).

Epidemiology

Risk Factors. Any woman is at risk; however, dating situations, unfamiliar partners, alcohol and drug use, and miscommunication create additional risk.

Incidence. Rape is one of the most frequently committed and underreported violent crimes in the United States. In one recent study of an emergency department population, the lifetime prevalence rate of sexual assault was 39 percent, with only 46 percent of the women reporting the crime to police. They were also more likely to report the attack to the police if the assailant was a stranger than if a partner. Certain female populations may be at an increased risk for sexual assault (CDC, 2011).

Subjective Data

Before effective treatment can be implemented with rape victims, a thorough assessment must be conducted. A client may report various physical and psychological problems. Explore a history of sexual abuse in any woman who presents with multiple physical complaints, even if associated with functional limitations.

Symptoms may include headaches, sleep disturbance, loss of appetite with weight loss or gain, eating disorders, nausea, vomiting, constipation, diarrhea, sexual dysfunction, menstrual irregularities, abnormal vaginal discharge, and urinary dysfunction. The client may report difficulty in relationships with others and in functioning at home, work, or school.

Careful recording of the details of the assault, along with the client's gynecological, sexual, and social histories, is essential. Determination of rape occurs in a court of law; therefore, the wording in the history should reflect only the client's report of the incident. It is important to record, sign, and date all information. Ask the client to sign a consent form and release of information form. Reassure the woman that answers to questions, especially those covering her sexual history, will ensure proper medical treatment. If the assault occurred within the last 72 hours, refer the client to a designated sexual assault center with trained sexual assault examiners for the completion of the assessment. The following information is for educational purposes of nonexpert examiners and for the assessment of victims who report the assault later. Detailed forms are available for the documentation of such an assessment sample (Riggs et al., 2004).

The history of assault will include date, time, location, description, use of a weapon, and type of weapon; the part of the body penetrated; the object used to penetrate (body part or foreign object); occurrence of ejaculation; and involvement of alcohol or other drugs. Record any information about the assailant. Question the client about her activities after the assault: Did she shower, change clothes, urinate, or defecate?

The past medical history includes dates of immunizations, especially tetanus and hepatitis, and prior HIV titer or status if known.

The obstetric and gynecologic history includes the date of the client's previous menstrual period, pregnancies, abortions, and miscarriages; contraceptive methods used; and history of sexually transmitted infections.

The sexual history includes information about the client's sexual activity: Was she sexually active within 1 week before or after assault? Has she been the victim of past sexual assaults (give dates)? Does she have any HIV high-risk sexual contact? Providers should use neutral language that includes the possibility of homosexual, bisexual, or heterosexual activity when asking about sexual partners.

The social history includes information about whether the survivor lives alone, has a support system, wants someone notified, needs social service assistance, or wants police notified if they are not aware of the assault.

Objective Data

Forensic evaluation refers to documentation of injuries, collection and preservation of evidence, and, with additional training, interpretation of injuries observed. Health care providers, especially in rural areas, are often the first point of contact for the women who have been raped, and therefore, should be prepared to conduct evaluation. Document findings from the physical examination and any forensic tests conducted (CDC, 2011).

Complete a thorough physical examination and STD testing after treating major injuries, no matter how much time has elapsed since the assault. If the woman has not showered or changed clothes since the assault, have her disrobe while standing on a sheet to collect any evidence. Then, give her a gown. Place any clothes that may contain evidence in a labeled paper bag.

Physical Examination

- *General appearance:* The survivor may be calm and relaxed or tearful and emotional. Notice torn and stained clothes; injuries may be visible.
- *Head, face, and throat:* There may be lacerations, abrasions, and bruising. Dried secretions may be present on the face, mouth, or ears. The client may complain of headaches.
- *Chest:* There may be bruising, lacerations, abrasions, and tenderness on palpation. Note any increased respiration, difficulty breathing, or hyperventilation.
- *Abdomen:* Bruising, lacerations, abrasions, and tenderness may be evident, indicating potential internal injuries.
- *Musculoskeletal system:* Look for potential fractures by examining the skin for lacerations, abrasions, bruising, and the back and extremities for tenderness.
- *Gastrointestinal:* Symptoms may include anorexia, nausea, vomiting, and abdominal or rectal pain.
- *Genitalia and reproductive tract:* The perineum, rectal area, and vagina may have bruises, lacerations, and abrasions. Bartholin's and Skene's glands and the urethral meatus may be tender. Uterine size, shape, and consistency may be abnormal. Note any tenderness with cervical motion and uterine and adnexal palpation. Watch for tears or pain on rectovaginal examination as suggestive of internal pelvic trauma.
- *Psychiatric:* The client may report symptoms of anxiety, depression, suicidal ideation, mood swings, phobias, sexual difficulties, uncontrollable memories or flashbacks, substance abuse, detachment from others, or dissociative symptoms.

  Use a body map to document all injuries, including their size, location, and coloration. Photographs of abrasions, with some form of identification appearing on the photographs, may be helpful if the victim plans legal action. Obtain written consent.

Diagnostic Tests. Complete within 24 to 72 hours of the assault. Forensic specimen collection is best when done by an experienced practitioner (Riggs et al., 2004). All laboratory findings are documented in the medical record. Use a Wood's light to check the perineum and thighs for blood or semen.

- Obtain gonorrhea and chlamydia cultures from the endocervix, vaginal vault, rectum, and oropharynx, as indicated by history or evidence of penetration.
- Collect urine for microscopic examination. A serum pregnancy test is preferred, if available. A urine pregnancy test is an alternative, if an enzyme-linked

immunosorbent assay and immunometric test are used. Sensitivity for urine beta-subunit human chorionic gonadotropin is 25 mIU/mL as compared to a quantitative serum test where results can be obtained with a beta-subunit radio immunoassay human chorionic gonadotropin level as little as 5 mIU/mL. Obtain cervical and rectal swabs for evidence of herpes simplex virus. Determine HIV status at this time.

- Wet mount specimens can show trichomonas, clue cells, and motile sperm for up to 72 hours. Include the pH of vaginal discharge and presence of positive whiff test.
- Collect a vaginal smear to detect sperm and p30 (prostate-specific antigen); considered more reliable than phosphatase determination.
- Bloodwork includes blood type/Rh, hepatitis antigen, rapid plasma reagin, and HIV antibody titer serum.
- Collect fingernail scrapings from each hand and save in separately labeled bag.
- Collect hair samples by combing both head and pubic hair; specimens placed in labeled bags.
- Blood and dried fluids found on the survivor's body and clothing collected and labeled for DNA fingerprinting. Saliva is collected for blood group antigen testing.

Differential Medical Diagnoses

Trauma not related to sexual assault.

Plan

Psychosocial Intervention. Refer the client for counseling. Women who do not deal realistically with rape and resolutions of issues may develop severe, long-term sequelae, such as depression, substance abuse, anxiety disorder, and suicide. If the woman desires legal action, assist the woman in contacting the proper authorities.

Medication. Offer medication for STDs or possible pregnancy.

Treatment for STDs (antibiotic prophylaxis) should be offered because of increased risk of STDs caused by *Chlamydia trachomatis*, *Neisseria gonorrhoeae*, *Treponema pallidum*, and *Trichomonas vaginalis* (Stenchever et al., 2001). See Chapter 14 for treatment guidelines. Review the risks and benefits of both treatment and observation. If the client refuses prophylactic antibiotics, then do follow-up cultures at the 6-week visit. If the client consents to prophylactic antibiotics, then treat her according to current CDC guidelines for chlamydia, gonorrhea, syphilis, and trichomoniasis. Also offer post-exposure prophylaxis for HIV.

Offer postcoital contraceptive medication to the client unless pregnancy exists or is suspected. CDC (2011) estimates the national rape-related pregnancy rate at 5 percent and states that among adult women, 32,101 pregnancies result from rape annually in the United States. Many of these pregnancies could be prevented. Emergency contraception reduces the risk of pregnancy by 75 percent. Postcoital contraceptive is a safe, effective tool in avoiding unintended pregnancy. It is offered at the time of assault, regardless of the cycle phase.

A number of options are now available for emergency contraception. The FDA has approved several specific methods (ACOG, 2001). (See Chapter 12, Managing Contraception and Family Planning, for a review of this treatment.) Perform a pregnancy test before any administration of medication. A history of thrombosis or perhaps of hypertension would be potential contraindications for some methods, especially if combination estrogen-progestin oral contraceptive options are used. Significantly fewer side effects and risks are seen with Plan B than with estrogen-progestin contraceptives. Review side effects of whichever method is provided with the client. Offer hepatitis B and tetanus vaccination if indicated.

Nursing Implications. In caring for a victim of sexual abuse or rape, it is important to understand that evaluation and treatment of the survivor require a multidisciplinary approach. If possible, a rape counselor who is present during the entire evaluation process can be helpful to provide client support.

If a woman calls and reports rape, instruct her to avoid showering or changing her clothes. Encourage her to go to the emergency room nearest her or to the health care provider's office.

Throughout her visit, explain each procedure and why it is being done and restore her sense of control. Give her options and seek consent with each procedure. Reinforce that rape was not her fault. Provide information about available social services, including a crisis hotline. Assist her to decide whether to report the crime and encourage her to seek follow-up care.

Follow-Up

A telephone call or return office visit within 24 to 48 hours of initial treatment allows for ongoing evaluation of problems and concerns. Schedule an appointment for 1 week after initial treatment to evaluate physical and emotional status. If the client has no complaints, defer the physical exam. Review all laboratory findings with the client. Inquire about counseling. If the client does not participate in counseling, encourage her to begin and provide a referral. Schedule the last visit at 4 to 6 weeks. At that time, complete a repeat physical exam, collect specimens for repeat cultures for STDs, rapid plasma reagin, and HIV antibody. Repeat HIV testing in 3-month intervals up to 1 year following exposure. Perform a pregnancy test as needed.

A sexual assault history with physical symptoms often correlate with impaired functioning and personal and social costs to the woman. In following women with a history of assault, research points to the importance of primary care provider's role in helping affected women recover from the assault. If the trauma remains unresolved and/or the abuse is chronic, referral to community services and mental health care is necessary.

HOMELESSNESS

Approximately 3 million men, women, and children are homeless at some time each year. The number of women and children living without a permanent place of dwelling is the fastest growing population among the homeless. Exactly how many women are homeless is not known. Women often remain out of sight to protect themselves against the possibility of violence (Eun-Gu Ji, 2006).

Reasons for homelessness are complex; poverty, violence, substance abuse, and mental illness are often cited as major causes. The Stewart B. McKinley Homeless Act (Pub. L. No. 100-77) defined the homeless person as one who does not have a fixed, regular, and adequate nighttime dwelling. This dwelling may be (1) a supervised or publicly operated shelter designed for temporary living quarters, (2) an institution serving as temporary residence for those requiring institutionalization, or (3) any public or private place not intended for regular sleeping quarters (National Coalition for the Homeless, July 2009).

Rarely does the literature on homeless persons distinguish health problems of women from those of men. Women cite eviction, interpersonal conflict, and loss of social support as the most common reasons for their homelessness. In contrast, men cite loss of a job, discharge from an institution, mental health problems, and substance abuse as the most common reasons. Women who are homeless are at risk for the same health problems as women who are not homeless. Due to their poverty, sense of powerlessness, and inability to access health care, however, women are particularly at risk for conditions and diseases that might be preventable if detected earlier. Pregnant women are particularly vulnerable to complications during pregnancy, labor, and postpartum periods. It is important for primary care providers to note that the use of screening tests is correlated more with access to preventive health care than to income or minority status. Homeless women are likely to experience malnutrition and related problems such as anemia. Other common health problems are infections, communicable diseases, skin complaints, poorly managed diabetes, and hypertension. Exposure to the elements, especially hypothermia, is also common (Morris & Strong, 2004).

Along with physical problems, women who are homeless experience stress, anxiety, and depression. They are also at risk for violence abuse and trauma, both physical and psychological, and use of drugs and alcohol is common. These psychological problems are complicated by limited access to health care resources. Homeless women are often underinsured and are unable to pay for many of the traditional treatments for mental health problems.

Primary care providers must work with community agencies to devise practice models that improve accessibility to care and follow-up. Systems of care that improve access to care are located in many urban areas throughout the United States. Funding, especially for health care services, continues to be a problem. Any system of care should focus on early identification of the at-risk population, provision of services that are required to reduce morbidity and mortality from acute and chronic diseases, and follow-up. Practices located near homeless shelters and streets where homeless women and their families are likely to be found will increase access to preventive health care services. Primary providers must also examine their attitudes and beliefs regarding homeless women and look for ways to create therapeutic client-provider relationships and implement health care services.

REFERENCES

American College of Obstetricians and Gynecologists (ACOG). (2001). *Clinical management guidelines for obstetricians-gynecologists*. Emergency Oral Contraception No. 25. Washington, DC: Author.

American College of Obstetricians and Gynecologists (ACOG). (2008). *All patients should be asked about alcohol and drug abuse*. Retrieved August 21, 2011, from http://www.acog.org/from_home/publications/press_releases12-12-08

American Psychiatric Association (APA). (2000). *Diagnostic and statistical manual of mental disorders* (4th ed., text rev.). Washington, DC: Author.

Antai-Otong, D. (2002). Culture and traumatic events. *Journal of the American Psychiatric Nurses Association, 8*, 203.

Attia, T., & Walsh, B.T. (2007). Anorexia nervosa. *American Journal of Psychiatry, 164*(12), 1805–1810.

Basile, K.C., Chen, J., Black, M.C., & Saltzman, L.E. (2007). Prevalence and characteristics of sexual violence victimization among U.S. adults, 2001–2003. *Violence and Victims, 22*(4), 437–448.

Bateman, A.L. (1999, October). Understand the process of grieving and loss: A critical social thinking perspective. *Journal of the American Psychiatric Nurses Association, 5*(5), 139–147.

Bateman, A.L. (2006). *Barriers to access to Mental Health Services* (STTI, Virginia Henderson International Nursing Library). Retrieved from http://www.nursinglibrary.org

Beale, A.L. (2009). Stress-induced cardiomyopathy in women. *Advance for Nurse Practitioners, 17*(11), 33–34, 36.

Beck, A.T., Freeman, A., & Davis, D.D. (2007). *Cognitive therapy of personality disorders* (2nd ed.). New York: Guilford.

Bernstein, A.B., Franco, S., & Freid, A.M. (2010). *Health, United States, 2010*. Retrieved May 11, 2011, from http://www.cdc.gov/nchs/data/hus/hus10.pdf

Breslau, N. (2009). The epidemiology of trauma, PTSD, and other posttrauma disorders. *Trauma Violence Abuse, 10,* 198–210.

Briere, J., & Jordan, C.E. (2011). Cumulative abuse: Do things add up? An evaluation of the conceptualization, operationalization, and methodological approaches in the study of the phenomenon of cumulative abuse. *Trauma Violence Abuse, 12,* 135–150.

Bureau of Justice Statistics. (2007). *Intimate partner violence, 1993–2007*. Retrieved from http://bjs.ojp.usdoj.gov/index.cfm?ty=tp&tid=971

Campinha-Bacote, J. (2002). Cultural competence in psychiatric nursing: Have you "asked" the right questions? *Journal of the American Psychiatric Nurses Association,* 8(6), 183–187.

Centers for Disease Control and Prevention (CDC). (2007). *Web-based injury statistics query and reporting system* [Online]. National Center for Injury Prevention and Control. Retrieved from http://www.cdc.gov/ncipc/wisqars/default.htm

Centers for Disease Control and Prevention (CDC). (2010a). *Intimate partner violence*. Retrieved June 5, 2011, from http://www.cdc.gov/IntimatePartner Violence/index.html

Centers for Disease Control and Prevention (CDC). (2010b). *Perceived health needs and receipt of services during pregnancy—Oklahoma and South Carolina 2004–2007*. Retrieved August 21, 2011, from http://www.cdc.gov/mmwr/pdf

Centers for Disease Control and Prevention (CDC). (2010c). *NCHS health e-stat: Prevalence of overweight, obesity, and extreme obesity among adults: United States, Trends 1960–1962 through 2007–2008.* Retrieved on May 5, 2012, from http://www.cdc.gov/nchs/data/hestat/obesity-adult-07-08/obesity-adult-07-08.htm

Centers for Disease Control and Prevention (CDC). (2011). *Sexual violence*. Retrieved September 5, 2011, from http://www.cdc.gov.SexualViolence/index.html

Cleveland Clinic. (2011). *Dependent personality disorder*. Retrieved from http://clevelandclinic.org/disorders/personality_disorders/hic_dependent_personality_disorder.aspx

de Niet, J.E., de Koning, C.M., Pastoor, H., Duivenvoorden, H.J., Valkenburg, O., Ramakers, M.J., et al. (2010). Psychological well-being and sexarche in women with polycystic ovary syndrome. *Human Reproduction, 25*(6), 497–503.

Department of Veterans Affairs. (2011). *Research on women, trauma, and PTSD*. Retrieved May 26, 2011, from http://www.ptsd.va.gov/professional/pages/women-trauma-ptsd.asp

Devens, M. (2007). Personality disorders. *Primary Care: Clinics in Office Practice, 34,* 445.

Doghramji, K. (2010). The evaluation and management of insomnia. *Clinics in Chest Medicine, 31*(2), 327–339.

Drake, R.E., Caton, C.L.M., Xie, H., Hsu, E., Gorroochurn, P., Samet, S., et al. (2011). A prospective 2-year study of emergency department patients with early-phase primary psychosis or substance-induced psychosis. *American Journal of Psychiatry, 168,* 742–748.

Eun-Gu Ji. (2006, January). A study of the structural risk factors of homelessness in 52 metropolitan areas in the United States. *International Social Work, 49*(1), 107–117.

Fichter, M.M., Katherine, A., Halmi, K., Kaplan, A.S., Strober, M., & Kaye, W.S. (2005). Symptoms fluctuation in eating disorders correlates of diagnostic crossover. *American Journal of Psychiatry, 162,* 732–740.

Goldsmith, T. (2006). The common pattern of domestic violence. *Psych Central.* Retrieved July 17, 2011, from http://psychcentral.com/lib/2006/the-common-pattern-of-domestic-violence/

Hall-Porter, J.M., Curry, D.T., & Walsh, J.K. (2010). Pharmacologic treatment of primary insomnia. *Sleep Medicine Clinics, 5*(4), 609–625.

Healthy people 2020: Understanding and improving health. (2011). Retrieved June 12, 2011, from http://www.healthypeople.gov

Humphries, D. (Ed.). (2009). *Women, violence, and the media: Readings in feminist criminology* (Vol. 6, p. 296). Boston: Northeastern University Press.

Institute of Medicine. (2001). *Health and behavior: The interplay of biological, behavioral and societal influences.* Washington, DC: National Academy Press.

Ivbijaro, G.O. (2010). Substance misuse and primary care mental house. *Mental Health in Family Medicine, 7,* 63–64. Retrieved May 11, 2011, from http://www.cdc.gov/nchs/healthy_people.htm

Johnson, M.P. (2006, November). Gender symmetry and asymmetry in domestic violence. *Violence Against Women, 12*(11), 1003–1018.

Kendler, J.S., Gatz, M., Gardner, C.O., & Pedersen, N.L. (2006). A Swedish national twin study of life time major depression and personality: Modeling the externalizing spectrum. *American Journal of Psychiatry, 163,* 109–114.

Kessler, R.C., Berglund, P., Demler, O., Jin, R., Merikangas, K., & Walters, E.E. (2005). Lifetime prevalence and age-of-onset distributions of DSM-IV disorders in the National Comorbidity Survey Replication. *Archives of General Psychiatry, 62,* 593–602.

Kopp, W.J. (1999). Chronic and acute psychological risk factors for clinical manifestations of coronary artery disease. *Psychosomatic Medicine, 61,* 476–487.

Krantz, G., & Garcia-Moreno, C. (2005). Violence against women. *Journal of Epidemiology and Community Health, 59,* 818–821.

Kroenke, K., Spitzer, R.L., Williams, J.B.W., Monahan, P.O., & Lowe, B. (2007). Anxiety disorders in primary care: Prevalence, impairment, comorbidity, and detection. *Annals of Internal Medicine, 146,* 317–325.

Kubler-Ross, E. (1969). *On death and dying.* London: Routledge.

Kubler-Ross, E., & Kessler, D. (2005). *On grief and grieving: Finding the meaning of grief through the five stages of loss* (pp. 1–4 and 7–25). New York: Scribner.

Kyle, S.D., Morgan, K., & Espie, C.A. (2010). Insomnia and health related quality of life. *Sleep Medicine Reviews, 14*(1), 69–82.

Lenzenweger, M.F. (2008). Epidemiology of personality disorders. *Psychiatric Clinics of North America, 31,* 395–403.

Lieberman, J.A., & Neubauer, D.N. (2007). Understanding insomnia: Diagnosis and management of a common sleep disorder [Special edition: October 2007]. *Journal of Family Practice, 56,* 10A.

Longnecker, J., Genderson, J., Dickinson, D., Malley, J., Elvevg, B., Weinberger, D.R., et al. (2010). Where have all the women gone? Participant gender in epidemiological and non-epidemiological research of schizophrenia. *Schizophrenia Research, 119*(1–3), 240–245.

Loomis, D.M., Griswold, K.S., Pastore, P.A., & Dunphy, L.M. (2011). Psychosocial problems. In L.M. Dunphy, B.O. Porter, J.E. Winland-Brown, & D.J. Thomas (Eds.), *Primary care: The art and science of advanced practice nursing* (3rd ed., pp. 1003–1112). Philadelphia: F. A. Davis Company.

Lowinson, J.H., Ruiz, P., Millman, R.B. & Langrod, J.G. (2005). *Substance abuse: A comprehensive textbook* (4th ed.). Philadelphia: Lippincott Williams & Wilkins.

Lumley, J., Chamberlain, C., Dowswell, T., Oliver, S., Oakley, L., & Watson, L. (2009). Interventions for promoting smoking cessation during pregnancy. *Cochrane Database of Systematic Reviews, 8*(3), CD001055. doi:10.1002/14651858.CD001055.pub3

March, D., & Susser, E. (2006). Invited commentary: Taking the search for causes of schizophrenia to a different level. *American Journal of Epidemiology, 163*(11), 979–981.

Martin, A. (2002). It's never too late to start: Seven steps toward good health. *Topics in Advanced Practice Nursing eJournal, 2*(1). Retrieved March 20, 2002, from http://www.medscape.com/viewarticle/421471

Morris, R.I., & Strong, L. (2004, August). The impact of homelessness on the health of families. *Journal of School Nursing, 20*(4), 221–227.

National Center for Health Statistics. (2010). *Health, United States, 2010: With special feature on death and dying.* Hyattsville, MD: Author.

National Coalition for the Homeless. (2009, July). *Who Is Homeless?* Retrieved September 5, 2011, from http://www.nationalhomeless.org/factsheets/who.html

National Institute on Alcohol and Alcoholism. (2011). *Women and alcohol.* Retrieved June 12, 2011, from http://pubs.niaaa.nih.gov/publications/womensfact/womensfact.htm

National Institute of Mental Health (NIMH). (2002). *Breaking ground, breaking through: The strategic plan for mood disorders research.* Retrieved June 16, 2011, from http://www.nimh.nih.gov/strategic/mooddisorders.pdf

National Institute of Mental Health (NIMH). (2008a). *Major depressive disorder in adults.* Retrieved June 16, 2011, from http://www.nimh.nih.gov/statistics/1MDD_ADULT

National Institute of Mental Health (NIMH). (2008b). *Prevalence of serious mental illness among U.S. adults by age, sex, and race.* Retrieved May 26, 2011, from http://www.nimh.nih.gov/statistics/SMI_AASR.shtml

National Institute of Mental Health (NIMH). (2008c). *Schizophrenia.* Retrieved June 16, 2011, from http://www.nimh.nih.gov/statistics/1SCHIZ.shtml

National Survey on Drug Use and Health (NSDUH). (2009). Treatment for substance abuse and mental health by race and ethnicity. *SAMSA Report.* Retrieved May 11, 2011 and June 16, 2011, from http://www.oas.samhsa.gov/2k9/163/SusUseRaceEthinicityHTML.pdf

National Survey on Drug Use and Health (NSDUH). (2010). *Results from the 2010 national survey on drug use and health: Summary of national findings.* Retrieved May 5, 2012, from http://www.samsha.gov/data/NSDUH/2k10NSDUH/2k10Results.htm#2.6

Oldham, J.M. (2005). Personality disorders. *Focus, 3,* 372–382.

Rapport, M.H., Clary, C., Fayyad, R., & Endicott, J. (2005). Quality-of-life impairment in depressive and anxiety disorders. *American Journal of Psychiatry, 162*(6), 117–118.

Riggs, W., Houry, D., Long, G., Markovchick, V., & Feldhaus, K.M. (2004). Analysis of 1076 cases of sexual assault. *Annals of Emergency Medicine, 35*(4), 358–362.

Ruiz, P., Strain, E., & Langrod, J.G. (2007). *The substance abuse handbook.* Retrieved from http://ovidsp.tx.ovid.com/sp-3.4.1b/ovidweb.cgi

Sadock, B.J., & Sadock, V.A. (2007). *Synopsis of psychiatry: Behavioral sciences/clinical psychiatry* (10th ed.). Philadelphia: Lippincott Williams and Wilkins.

Schaffer, S. (2002). Cleaning the air: Brief strategies for smoking cessation. *Topics in Advanced, Practice in Nursing and Journal, 2*(1). Retrieved March 20, 2002, from http://www.medscape.com/viewarfede/421476

Schultz, P., & Steimer, T. (2009). Neurobiology of circadian systems. *CNS Drugs, 23*(Suppl. 2), 3–13.

Silk, K.R. (2010). *Personality disorders*. Retrieved May 11, 2011, from http://www.uptodate.com/home/index.html

Skodol, A.E., & Gunderson, J.C. (2008). Personality disorders. In R.E. Hales, S.C. Yudofsky, & G.O. Gabbard (Eds.), *American psychiatric publishing textbook of psychiatry: Textbook of psychiatry* (5th ed.). Arlington: American Psychiatric Publishing.

Stahl, S. (2008). *Stahl's essential psychopharmacology: Neuroscientific basis and practical applications* (3rd ed.). Cambridge, MA: Cambridge University Press.

Straus, M.A. (2004). Prevalence of violence against dating partners by male and female university students worldwide. *Violence Against Women, 10*(7), 790–811.

Stenchever, M., Mishell, D., Herbst, A., & Droegemueller, M. (2001). *Comprehensive gynecology* (4th ed.). St. Louis, MO: Mosby.

Substance Abuse and Mental Health Services Administration (SAMHSA). (2001). *Summary of findings from the 2000 National Household Survey on drug abuse*. Office of Applied Studies, NHSDA Series H-13, DHHS Publication No. (SMA) 01-3549. Rockville, MD: Author.

Substance Abuse and Mental Health Services Administration (SAMHSA). (2008). *Treatment episode data sets: Admission by primary substance abuse by according to race/ethnicity/gender/age group TEDS 2006*. Retrieved May 16, 2011 and June 16, 2011, from http://wwwdasis.samhsa.gov/teds06/teds2k6aweb508.pdf

Substance Abuse and Mental Health Services Administration (SAMHSA). (2011, April 7). Nearly all American adults with untreated alcohol use disorders don't think they need treatment. *SAMHSA News Release*. Retrieved from http://www.samhsa.gov/newsroom/advisories/1104062257.aspx

Tandon, R., Keshavan, M.S., & Nasrallah, H.A. (2008). Schizophrenia, "just the facts" what we know in 2008. 2. Epidemiology and etiology. *Schizophrenia Research, 102*(1–3), 1–18.

Tozzi, F., Thornton, L.M., Klump, K.K., Fichter, M.M., Halmi, K.A., Kaplan, et al. (2003). Interventions for violence against women. *Journal of the American Medical Association, 289*(5), 589–600.

U.S. Department of Health and Human Services (USDHHS). (2009). *Action steps for improving women's mental health: Executive summary*. Washington, DC: Author. Retrieved July 5, 2011, from http://www.womenshealth.gov

Walker, L. (2009). *The battered woman* (3rd ed.). New York: Springer.

West, R., Ussher, M., Evans, M., & Rashid, M. (2005). Assessing DSM-IV nicotine withdrawal symptoms: A comparison and evaluation of five different scales. *Psychopharmacology, 184*, 619–627.Worden, W. (1991). *Grief counseling and grief therapy* (2nd ed.). New York: Springer.

APPENDIX ❖ **A**

EMERGENCY CHILDBIRTH AND IMMEDIATE CARE OF THE NEWBORN

Diane Marie Schadewald

INTRODUCTION

When a woman presents complaining of labor, the clinician must quickly perform an assessment to determine whether delivery of the infant is imminent or if there is time for transport. Arrangements should be made for car or ambulance transportation to the nearest facility equipped for maternal and newborn care as appropriate and possible (Cunningham et al., 2010; Varney, Kriebs, & Gegor, 2004; World Health Organization [WHO], 2011). If delivery appears imminent, the emergency response system should be activated. Those who live in remote regions who may not have rapid access to emergency care services may find these guidelines for childbirth and immediate care of the newborn especially helpful. They may also want to access the WHO guidelines for pregnancy and childbirth at www.afro.who.int/index.php?option=com_docman&task=doc_download&gid=2011.

ASSESSMENT OF LABOR STATUS

CLIENT'S HISTORY AND SUBJECTIVE ASSESSMENT OF CURRENT STATUS

Ask the client her due date, gravida, and para. If she has had previous pregnancies, were they vaginal or cesarean births? Has she had any complications during pregnancy? Ask if she has medical problems or if special tests were done for her or the fetus during pregnancy. Ask the client the time of the onset of contractions and if membranes have ruptured. If her membranes have ruptured, did she note the color? Was the amniotic fluid clear or meconium stained? Brownish-green amniotic fluid indicates the fetus has been stressed and passed meconium; the infant may need airway clearance and resuscitation immediately after birth. How long have her membranes been ruptured? Membranes ruptured longer than 24 hours place the mother and infant at risk for infection and sepsis. Ascertain the presence or absence of vaginal bleeding, fetal activity, history of allergies, and use of any medications or drugs. Has she had an ultrasound during her pregnancy; if so, was she told she had a placenta previa? If she has a placental previa, vaginal examination is contraindicated. Ask the client if she feels the urge to bear down or have a bowel movement during contractions; this could indicate that the fetal presenting part is in the vaginal vault (putting pressure on the wall of the rectum) and that birth is imminent. Never leave the laboring woman alone.

PHYSICAL ASSESSMENT

Examination of the client should include her vital signs, notation of fetal position and presentation, fetal heart rate and the duration, and quality of uterine contractions. If there are no contraindications to pelvic examination, the degree of cervical dilatation, effacement, status of the membranes, and type and station of the presenting part should be determined.

- *Is the infant's head visible?* Inspect the vulva: Bulging of the perineum, anal sphincter, or both, with separation of labia, revealing protruding membranes or crowning of the fetal head, indicates that birth is imminent.
- *Is amniotic fluid or blood present?* Leaking amniotic fluid, bloody show (blood-tinged mucus), or both indicate only that labor is in progress, not necessarily that birth is imminent. As discussed earlier, note the color of the amniotic fluid if the sac appears to have ruptured. Frank vaginal bleeding (blood flowing like a menstrual period) or dried blood on the legs indicates a possible abnormality of the placenta. In these cases, *do not* insert the fingers, a speculum, or any other object into the vagina (see Abnormal Bleeding later in this appendix).
- *Are uterine contractions effectively dilating the cervix?* Palpate the abdomen. Uterine contractions that begin every 2 minutes, last 60 to 90 seconds, and are hard (indentation is not elicited by fingertips pressing on abdomen during peak of contraction) indicate that active labor is in progress. If the client is bearing down and pushing with contractions, the fetal head is probably already out of the uterus (i.e., the cervix is fully dilated) and into the vaginal vault. Delivery is probably imminent. If sterile gloves are available and there is no frank vaginal bleeding, perform a vaginal exam, after receiving the client's permission, gently insert the index and middle fingers of one hand into the vagina until the fetal presenting part or cervix is palpable. If only the fetal head is palpable deep in the vagina close to the perineum, the cervix is completely dilated, and delivery is imminent.
- *Is the fetus tolerating the intrauterine environment?* Listen with the bell side of the stethoscope in the lower abdomen on the side where the fetal back is located. If the fetal heart rate is less than 100 beats per minute or if amniotic fluid is meconium stained (green or brown), the fetus is or has been stressed; be prepared to resuscitate the infant immediately after birth. If birth does not seem imminent, turn the client onto her side (preferably left) to allow better blood flow to her uterus and the fetus while awaiting transport. Continue to auscultate the fetal heartbeat every 5 to 10 minutes.

PROVISION OF EMOTIONAL SUPPORT AND RELAXATION COACHING

Encourage the mother to pant or blow slowly during contractions and to breathe normally between contractions. She is probably frightened and uncomfortable. Acknowledge that everything possible will be done to help her. Ask her to keep her eyes open and to watch for directions. Maintain eye contact, speak calmly, and give simple directions. Have any available support person stay by her upper body to hold her hands and assist with instructions. Give frequent feedback and reassurance.

PREPARATION FOR DELIVERY

ASSEMBLY OF AVAILABLE SUPPLIES

If a readymade delivery kit is available, open it and place it to one side within easy reach. If no kit is readily available, have someone get the following items for you: clean towels, sheets, or blankets (warm two of them if possible); bulb syringe; sterile scissors; three cord clamps, kelly clamps, or shoestrings; two pairs of sterile gloves; a bowl or sealable plastic bag; sanitary pads; 3 cc syringes with needles; alcohol wipes; vials of oxytocin (Pitocin, 10 units each) or 0.2 mg (1 cc) of methylergonovine maleate (Methergine) if available; hot water bottle (filled) or heat pack. Note: If no supplies are available, use a cloth to protect your hands from contact with body fluids. An unread newspaper can also be used to provide a clean field, as newsprint has some bacteriostatic properties.

POSITIONING OF MOTHER AND DRAPING

Wash your hands. Help the woman into a comfortable position of her choosing, with the caveat that she should be as upright as possible. Allow the woman to push with contractions as desired but do not encourage bearing down efforts. Observe the perineum while maintaining intermittent eye contact with the client and her support person.

DELIVERY OF PRESENTING PART AND CLEARANCE OF AIRWAY

When the perineum begins to be distended and the head is visible, wash your hands and put on gloves. Place the hand most comfortable for you on the presenting part, usually the crown of the head, as it protrudes from the vagina during each contraction. Provide support to the perineum with your other hand and cover the anus during delivery with a pad held by the side of your hand. Encourage the mother to breathe steadily and not push during delivery of the head. With your fingers, keep the fetal head flexed by maintaining gentle, even pressure on the head as it advances. Allowing the head to slide out of the vagina slowly minimizes perineal tearing. (It may take several contractions to complete delivery of the head.) If the amniotic sac is intact over the infant's face, remove it with your fingers. As soon as the head is born, place the fingertips of one of your hands on the back of the baby's head and then slide them down the neck, sweeping them in both directions feeling around the neck for the umbilical cord. If found and loose, pull the cord gently over the head. If the loop is too tight, have the mother pant or blow while you clamp the cord in two places; cut between the two clamps. Wipe the baby's face and head and wipe off fluid from the nose and mouth with a soft absorbent cloth. Gently suction the baby's mouth and nose with a soft rubber bulb syringe if one is available. With the next contraction, the head will align with the infant's body and externally rotate.

DELIVERY OF BODY AND IMMEDIATE CARE OF THE NEWBORN

Shift hands slightly toward the back of the infant's head. Place your hands on each side of the head so that your fingers point toward the face, with the little fingers closest to the perineum. Wait for the shoulders to rotate and then apply gentle downward pressure to deliver the top shoulder; lift the infant and deliver the lower shoulder and place the infant on mother's abdomen. (Hint: As the infant is being born, slide your bottom hand down close to the perineum so that the shoulder, arm, elbow, and hand are held close to the infant's body. The thumb on your bottom hand will be on the infant's back, your fingers will be across the infant's chest, and the infant's head will be resting on your wrist. Slide your top hand down the infant's back, slip your index finger between the infant's legs as the buttocks clear the perineum, and grasp the infant by the ankles. Of primary importance is support of each part of the infant as it delivers.) *Note the time of delivery.* Thoroughly dry the baby. Drying promotes normal respiration and provides tactile stimulation. Discard the wet cloth. If infant is not crying, observe for breathing while drying. If not breathing, immediately clamp and cut the cord as described later and move the infant to a firm warm surface and start newborn resuscitation. If breathing well, place the infant skin to skin on mother's abdomen or chest and cover with a warm, dry cloth; this will help maintain body temperature for the infant. If the mother cannot hold the infant, then place the infant in clean, warm, safe place close to the mother.

Palpate the mother's abdomen to exclude the possibility of a second infant. If second infant is suspected, renew call for emergency help and do not give oxytocin. If no suspicion of second infant and oxytocin is available, 10 units IM may be given at this point (WHO, 2011). Watch for vaginal bleeding and be prepared for delivery of the placenta.

While observing for signs of placental delivery, wash gloves or change gloves if possible. During emergency delivery, it is usually not necessary to clamp and cut the cord. However, if clamping and cutting of the cord is determined to be necessary (e.g., emergency transport will not be available for a prolonged period of time) and clamps are not available, you may use shoestrings to tie the cord. (Do not tie with thread.) The clamps or ties should be placed at a distance of around 2 cm and 5 cm from the infant's abdomen. Cut between the clamps/ties with a sterile instrument. Observe for oozing of blood from the cord. Place a second tie or clamp between the infant's abdomen and first tie or clamp as needed if oozing is present.

If necessary, a hot water bottle or heat pack covered with a towel may be used to keep the infant warm. Observe the infant for cyanosis or lethargy; stimulate as mentioned earlier if needed. Assign APGAR scores at 1 and 5 minutes. The acronym *APGAR* facilitates assessment of five components of neonates' responses: appearance, pulse, grimace, activity, and respiration.

- The APGAR is scored at 1 and 5 minutes of life.
- Five signs are evaluated and scored 0, 1, or 2.
- *10–10, indicates best possible newborn condition:* As most healthy newborns are acrocyanotic, expect a score of 8-10 or 9-10 in most cases.
- When the 5-minute score is 6 or less, some states require a 10-minute score. It is useful to obtain additional scores every 5 minutes until 20 minutes has passed or until two successive scores of 7 or higher are obtained.

- *0–2, severe asphyxia:* Infant is at high risk; requires resuscitation and further evaluation.
- *3–4, moderate asphyxia:* Infant is at moderate risk; probable resuscitation and further evaluation.
- *5–7, mild asphyxia:* Infant is at risk; possible intermittent resuscitation, and with or without further evaluation.
- *8–10, no asphyxia:* Infant is at minimal risk; routine elective procedures.

In addition to APGAR evaluation, the infant's general condition should be observed for the following characteristics. Items in parentheses indicate abnormal findings:

- *General:* Appearance, symmetry.
- *State:* Deep or light sleep, drowsy, quiet or active alert, crying.
- *Reactivity:* State changes, interactive capacity, self-consolability.
- *Color:* Pink, acrocyanosis, mottling (plethora, pallor, jaundice, cyanosis).
- *Posture:* Flexed (asymmetry, restricted movement).
- *Character of cry:* Strong, lusty (weak, high-pitched, constant, or none).
- *Skin:* Smooth, intact, elastic, warm, moist; vernix; lanugo; desquamation; Mongolian spots; milia; nevi; edema or petechiae over presenting part (pustules, lacerations, ecchymosis, rashes, café-au-lait spots, hemangiomas, meconium staining, pitting edema, poor turgor, scaling, sweating). Place gauze or cloth moistened with sterile saline over any nonintact area of skin.
- *Umbilical cord and umbilicus:* Assess cord for two arteries; one vein; gelatinous, bluish-white; umbilical hernia (two vessels, thin cord, foul odor, discharge, meconium stained).
- *Fingers and toes:* All present.
- *Respirations at rest:* Rate = 30–60; symmetric; diaphragmatic or abdominal (flaring; grunting; intercostal, supraclavicular, or substernal retractions).

DELIVERY OF PLACENTA

Observe the vaginal opening for lengthening of the cord or increased bleeding, which indicate placental separation. Do *not* pull on the cord; instead, wait for uterine contractions to push out the placenta with attached membranes, and place it in a bowl or plastic bag. Continue to monitor the mother every 5 minutes.

If emergency response is not available in a reasonable period of time, mild, controlled traction may be used for delivery of the placenta. Await signs of uterine contractions of every 2 to 3 minutes and deliver the placenta with mild, controlled traction on the cord. Place one hand above the symphysis with palm facing toward the mother's head to provide some counter traction to the uterus. Use counter traction efforts only during episodes of uterine contraction. Catch the placenta in both hands. In order to obtain all of the membranes, a gentle twisting motion may assist with separation. After expelled, check to see if it looks like the placenta and membranes are complete. If bleeding persists and the uterus is soft, massage the uterus to expel any clots. Note any lacerations of the perineum.

IMMEDIATE POSTDELIVERY CARE OF MOTHER

CONTROL OF BLEEDING

The uterine fundus should be palpable under the umbilicus. Assess for firmness. If not firm, massage the fundus with one hand while supporting the uterus with the other hand just above the symphysis pubis as described earlier for counter traction. Even if medications are not available, vaginal bleeding should be minimal if the infant is put to breast, and the uterus is kept well contracted with massage every 10 to 15 minutes. Place a sanitary pad or folded cloth firmly against the perineum. Record blood pressure, pulse, and respirations every 15 minutes; the urinary bladder should be checked for distention and emptied if needed. If the uterus is soft or is above the umbilicus, it has lost its muscle tone and is full of

APGAR Signs

Signs	0	1	2
Appearance (color)	Blue/pale	Body pink Extremities blue	Completely pink
Pulse (heart rate)	Absent	< 100	> 100
Grimace (reflex irritability)	No response	Grimace	Cough, sneeze, cry
Activity (muscle tone)	Limp	Some flexion	Flexed, active motion
Respiration (breathing efforts)	Absent	Weak, irregular gasping	Strong cry

clots. The fundus needs to be massaged (with support from the opposite hand just above the pubic bone to prevent eversion of the uterus into the vagina) until clots are expelled and the fundus is firm. If the uterus is displaced to one side of the midline, the urinary bladder may be distended and needs to be emptied. If laceration of the perineum has occurred, apply pressure over the laceration with a sterile pad or gauze and place the legs together to assist with approximation of the edges and control of bleeding. If bleeding persists beyond 5 minutes despite these efforts and transport is not yet available, suturing of the laceration may be necessary (WHO, 2011).

PHYSICAL AND EMOTIONAL RECOVERY

If the mother experiences severe shaking chills, reassure her that this reaction is normal after the hard work and anxiety of delivery. Slow, deep breathing may help alleviate the "shakes" and increase relaxation. Cover her with available blankets. Reinforce what a wonderful job she did during her labor and delivery. Encourage her to interact with her infant and support person. Assist the mother to breast-feed. Notify the receiving health care facility of the impending arrival and condition of the mother and infant.

ABNORMAL CONDITIONS

BREECH PRESENTATION

When initially assessing the vaginal opening, the buttocks may present first (breech presentation), often accompanied by meconium. This delivery should occur only in a hospital. Attempt a breech delivery only if there are no other alternatives. Prepare as usual; allow the infant's legs, buttocks, and trunk to deliver spontaneously. When the baby is born up to the umbilicus, the remainder of the baby needs to be delivered in 3 to 5 minutes to prevent anoxia. Gently pull down a loop of cord to prevent tension on the cord. If the arms do not deliver spontaneously, reach up for the hands, one at a time, and sweep them down over the face. The body will then turn to one side and the shoulders will deliver, the top shoulder followed by the bottom shoulder. The head is ready to deliver when the back is toward the ceiling. Put two fingers in the vagina below the head and press downward to make room for the baby to breathe. Have the mother push until the face starts to deliver. Then she should pant and the back of the head can be delivered slowly. Support the body in the palm of your gloved hand and on your lower arm, if unable to deliver the head transport to the nearest hospital with the mother's buttocks elevated; be prepared to resuscitate the infant if the head does deliver en route.

OTHER ABNORMAL PRESENTATION SITUATIONS

If one of the infant's arms protrudes from the vagina, provide emotional support to the mother while awaiting emergency transport to the nearest hospital's obstetric unit. This woman will not deliver spontaneously.

If a loop of umbilical cord protrudes from the vagina, cover it with moistened cloth (preferably moistened with normal saline). Have the client assume the knee-chest position on a stretcher or a car seat. (The mother and her support person will need much reassurance.) Insert a gloved hand into the vagina, and attempt to hold the presenting part off the prolapsed cord during emergency transport and until you reach the delivery operating room.

ABNORMAL BLEEDING PRIOR TO DELIVERY

If, before or during delivery, you observe blood flow rather than blood-tinged mucus, suspect a placental abnormality. While awaiting transport, keep the mother in shock position (head down, hips elevated, covered with blankets). Record blood pressure, pulse, respirations, and fetal heart rate every 10 minutes. Monitor contractions and deliver the infant as indicated, being prepared to resuscitate the infant as needed and to treat the mother for shock if pulse rises and blood pressure drops.

REFERENCES

Cunningham, F.G., Leveno, K.J., Bloom, S.L., Hauth, J.C., Rouse, D.J., & Spong, C.Y. (2010). Normal labor and delivery. In F.G. Cunningham, K.J. Leveno, S.L. Bloom, J.C. Hauth, D.J. Rouse, & C.Y. Spong (Eds.), *Williams obstetrics* (23rd ed., pp. 374–410). New York: McGraw-Hill.

Varney, H., Kriebs, J.M., & Gegor, C.L. (2004). *Varney's midwifery* (4th ed.). Sudbury, MA: Jones and Bartlett Publishers.

World Health Organization (WHO). (2011). *WHO guidelines for pregnancy, childbirth, postpartum and newborn care.* Retrieved from www.afro.who.int/index.php?option=com_docman&task=doc_download&gid=2011

The author wishes to acknowledge the contribution of Brenda T. Brickhouse and Marcia Szmania Davis, who prepared Appendixes A and B, respectively, for the third edition, as well as Mary Beth Bryant McGurin, who prepared Appendix A for the first edition

APPENDIX ❖ B

SELECTED SCREENING TOOLS FOR WOMEN'S HEALTH

Catherine Juve ◆ Diane Marie Schadewald

This appendix contains a collection of screening tools that are appropriate to use in a women's health setting. Most of these tools have been referenced in various chapters of the text. An attempt has been made to arrange the tools in order of their reference. Some of these tools are only available as online calculators and have been labeled as such. We hope you find these tools helpful for providing holistic and comprehensive care to women.

ADVERSE CHILDHOOD EXPERIENCES (ACES)

Experienced Before the Age of 18	Check if Experienced
Recurrent physical abuse	
Recurrent emotional abuse	
Contact sexual abuse	
An alcohol or drug abuser in the household	
An incarcerated household member	
Someone in the household who was chronically depressed, mentally ill, institutionalized, or suicidal	
Mother was treated violently	
One or no parents	
Emotional and physical neglect	
Calculate ACE score by adding number of categories.	

The co-principal investigators of the ACE Study are Vincent J. Felitti and Robert F. Anda.
Source: Bloom, S.L. (2010). Mental health aspects of intimate partner violence: Survivors, professionals, and systems. In A.P. Giardino & E.R. Giardino (Eds.), Intimate partner violence (pp. 207–251). STM Learning.

SUGGESTED SCREENING QUESTIONS FOR PRIMARY CARE

Routine Trauma Questions Asked in a Primary Care Setting[a]	Yes/No
• As a child or adolescent, did you live in a household in which anyone abused drugs or alcohol?	
• As a child or adolescent, did you live in a household in which anyone was mentally ill or tried to commit suicide?	
• As a child or adolescent, did you live in a household in which anyone was imprisoned?	
• As a child or adolescent, did you live in a household in which anyone assaulted anyone else in the household?	
• As a child or adolescent, did you live with a foster family?	
• Have you ever been the victim of a crime?	
• Did you suffer any form of severe physical or emotional neglect as a child?	
• Have you experienced psychological and/or verbal abuse as a child or as an adult?	
• Have you ever been physically assaulted as a child or as an adult?	
• Have you ever been sexually molested or assaulted as a child or as an adult?	
• Have you ever witnessed someone else being seriously injured or killed?	
• At any point during this (these) experience(s), did you think you were in danger of serious personal harm or of losing your life?	
• Have you ever sexually or physically assaulted someone else?	
• Have you been a civilian victim of war or witnessed any kind of atrocity?	
• What is the worst thing that has ever happened to you? Explain:	
• What is the worst thing that has ever happened to someone in your family? Explain:	
Source: Bills, L. (1995). Trauma-based psychiatry for primary care. In B.H. Stamm (Ed.), Secondary trauma stress: Self-care issues for clinicians, researchers, and educators (pp. 121–148). Lutherville, MD: Sidran Press.	

PERCEIVED STRESS SCALE

The questions in this scale ask you about your feelings and thoughts **during the last month**. In each case, you will be asked to indicate by circling *how often* you felt or thought a certain way.

Name ______________________________ Date ________

Age ________ Gender (*Circle*): **M F** Other ______________________

0 = Never 1 = Almost Never 2 = Sometimes 3 = Fairly Often 4 = Very Often

1. In the last month, how often have you been upset because of something that happened unexpectedly?.................................... **0 1 2 3 4**
2. In the last month, how often have you felt that you were unable to control the important things in your life?.. **0 1 2 3 4**
3. In the last month, how often have you felt nervous and "stressed"? **0 1 2 3 4**
4. In the last month, how often have you felt confident about your ability to handle your personal problems?.. **0 1 2 3 4**
5. In the last month, how often have you felt that things were going your way?... **0 1 2 3 4**

6. In the last month, how often have you found that you could not cope with all the things that you had to do? **0 1 2 3 4**

7. In the last month, how often have you been able to control irritations in your life? **0 1 2 3 4**

8. In the last month, how often have you felt that you were on top of things?..... **0 1 2 3 4**

9. In the last month, how often have you been angered because of things that were outside of your control? **0 1 2 3 4**

10. In the last month, how often have you felt difficulties were piling up so high that you could not overcome them?........ **0 1 2 3 4**

Scoring: Perceived Stress Scale (PSS) scores are obtained by reversing responses (e.g., 0 = 4, 1 = 3, 2 = 2, 3 = 1, & 4 = 0) to the four positively stated items (items 4, 5, 7, & 8) and then summing across all scale items. A short 4 item scale can be made from questions 2, 4, 5, and 10 of the PSS 10 item scale.

Norm Table for the PSS 10 item inventory

Category	N	Mean	S.D.
Gender			
Male	926	12.1	5.9
Female	1406	13.7	6.6
Age			
18-29	645	14.2	6.2
30-44	750	13.0	6.2
45-54	285	12.6	6.1
55-64	282	11.9	6.9
65 & older	296	12.0	6.3
Race			
white	1924	12.8	6.2
Hispanic	98	14.0	6.9
black	176	14.7	7.2
other minority	50	14.1	5.0

References

The PSS Scale is reprinted with permission of the American Sociological Association, from Cohen, S., Kamarck, T., and Mermelstein, R. (1983). A global measure of perceived stress. *Journal of Health and Social Behavior, 24*, 386–396.

Cohen, S., and Williamson, G. Perceived Stress in a Probability Sample of the United States. Spacapan, S., and Oskamp, S. (Eds.), *The Social Psychology of Health.* Newbury Park, CA: Sage, 1988.

Source: http://www.psy.cmu.edu/~scohen/

PATIENT HEALTH QUESTIONNAIRE (PHQ-2) FOR MAJOR DEPRESSIVE DISORDER

During the past month:	
Have you often been bothered by feeling down, depressed, or hopeless?	Yes or No
Have you often been bothered by little interest or pleasure in doing things?	Yes or No
Note: An affirmative answer to either question is a positive test result; a negative answer to both questions is a negative test result. If the result of PHQ-2 is positive proceed to the PHQ-9. PHQ = Patient Health Questionnaire. Copyright © Pfizer Inc. All rights reserved *Source:* http://www.innovations.ahrq.gov/content.aspx?id=2280.	

PATIENT HEALTH QUESTIONNAIRE (PHQ-9)

NAME:____________________ **DATE:**__________

Over the last *2 weeks,* how often have you been bothered by any of the following problems? *(use "✓" to indicate your answer)*	Not at all	Several days	More than half the days	Nearly every day
1. Little interest or pleasure in doing things	0	1	2	3
2. Feeling down, depressed, or hopeless	0	1	2	3
3. Trouble falling or staying asleep, or sleeping too much	0	1	2	3
4. Feeling tired or having little energy	0	1	2	3
5. Poor appetite or overeating	0	1	2	3
6. Feeling bad about yourself—or that you are a failure or have let yourself or your family down	0	1	2	3
7. Trouble concentrating on things, such as reading the newspaper or watching television	0	1	2	3
8. Moving or speaking so slowly that other people could have noticed. Or the opposite – being so figety or restless that you have been moving around a lot more than usual	0	1	2	3
9. Thoughts that you would be better off dead, or of hurting yourself	0	1	2	3
	add columns		+	+

(Healthcare professional: For interpretation of TOTAL, please refer to accompanying scoring card). TOTAL:

10. If you checked off *any problems,* how *difficult* have these problems made it for you to do your work, take care of things at home, or get along with other people?	
	Not difficult at all ____
	Somewhat difficult ____
	Very difficult ____
	Extremely difficult ____

A2663B 10-04-2005

PHQ-9 Patient Depression Questionnaire

For initial diagnosis:

1. Patient completes PHQ-9 Quick Depression Assessment.
2. If there are at least 4 ✓s in the shaded section (including Questions #1 and #2), consider a depressive disorder. Add score to determine severity.

Consider Major Depressive Disorder
- if there are at least 5 ✓s in the shaded section (one of which corresponds to Question #1 or #2)

Consider Other Depressive Disorder
- if there are 2-4 ✓s in the shaded section (one of which corresponds to Question #1 or #2)

Note: Since the questionnaire relies on patient self-report, all responses should be verified by the clinician, and a definitive diagnosis is made on clinical grounds taking into account how well the patient understood the questionnaire, as well as other relevant information from the patient.
Diagnoses of Major Depressive Disorder or Other Depressive Disorder also require impairment of social, occupational, or other important areas of functioning (Question #10) and ruling out normal bereavement, a history of a Manic Episode (Bipolar Disorder), and a physical disorder, medication, or other drug as the biological cause of the depressive symptoms.

To monitor severity over time for newly diagnosed patients or patients in current treatment for depression:

1. Patients may complete questionnaires at baseline and at regular intervals (eg, every 2 weeks) at home and bring them in at their next appointment for scoring or they may complete the questionnaire during each scheduled appointment.
2. Add up ✓s by column. For every ✓: Several days = 1 More than half the days = 2 Nearly every day = 3
3. Add together column scores to get a TOTAL score.
4. Refer to the accompanying **PHQ-9 Scoring Box** to interpret the TOTAL score.
5. Results may be included in patient files to assist you in setting up a treatment goal, determining degree of response, as well as guiding treatment intervention.

Scoring: add up all checked boxes on PHQ-9

For every ✓ Not at all = 0; Several days = 1;
More than half the days = 2; Nearly every day = 3

Interpretation of Total Score

Total Score	Depression Severity
1-4	Minimal depression
5-9	Mild depression
10-14	Moderate depression
15-19	Moderately severe depression
20-27	Severe depression

SCOFF Eating Disorders Questionnaire

The SCOFF questions[*]

1. Do you make yourself Sick because you feel uncomfortably full?
2. Do you worry you have lost Control over how much you eat?
3. Have you recently lost more than One stone (14 pounds) in a 3-month period?
4. Do you believe yourself to be Fat when others say you are too thin?
5. Would you say that Food dominates your life?

[*]One point for every "yes"; a score of ≥ 2 indicates a likely case of anorexia nervosa or bulimia.

Source: Morgan, J.F., Reid, F. & Lacey, J.H. (1999). The SCOFF questionnaire: Assessment of a new screening tool for eating disorders. *BMJ, 319,* 1467–1468. Retrieved from http://www.bmj.com/content/319/7223/1467.full.pdf?maxtoshow=&HITS=10&hits=10&RESULTFORMAT=&fulltext=scoff+questionnaire&searchid=1&FIRSTINDEX=0&resourcetype=HWCIT

PMS Symptom Tracker

Cycle Dates: ______________________________

Use this chart to track your PMS symptoms.

Day

Symptoms	1	2	3	4	5	6	7	8	9	10	11	12	13	14	15	16	17	18	19	20	21	22	23	24	25	26	27	28	29	30	31	32	33	34	35	36	37	38	39	40	41	42	43	44	45
Period																																													
Acne																																													
Breast swelling and tenderness																																													
Feeling tired																																													
Having trouble sleeping																																													
Upset stomach																																													
Cramps																																													
Bloating																																													
Constipation																																													
Diarrhea																																													
Headache																																													
Backache																																													
Appetite changes or food cravings																																													
Joint or muscle pain																																													
Trouble concentrating or remembering																																													
Tension, irritability, mood swings, or crying spells																																													
Anxiety																																													
Depression																																													
Other symptoms:																																													
Other symptoms:																																													
Other symptoms:																																													

Source: http://www.womenshealth.gov/publications/our-publications/PMS-symptom-tracker.pdf

DANGER ASSESSMENT

Jacquelyn C. Campbell, Ph.D., R.N.

Several risk factors have been associated with increased risk of homicides (murders) of women and men in violent relationships. We cannot predict what will happen in your case, but we would like you to be aware of the danger of homicide in situations of abuse and for you to see how many of the risk factors apply to your situation.

Using the calendar, please mark the approximate dates during the past year when you were abused by your partner or ex partner. Write on that date how bad the incident was according to the following scale:

1. Slapping, pushing; no injuries and/or lasting pain
2. Punching, kicking; bruises, cuts, and/or continuing pain
3. "Beating up"; severe contusions, burns, broken bones
4. Threat to use weapon; head injury, internal injury, permanent injury
5. Use of weapon; wounds from weapon

(If **any** of the descriptions for the higher number apply, use the higher number.)

Mark **Yes** or **No** for each of the following. ("He" refers to your husband, partner, ex-husband, ex-partner, or whoever is currently physically hurting you.)

___ 1. Has the physical violence increased in severity or frequency over the past year?
___ 2. Does he own a gun?
___ 3. Have you left him after living together during the past year?
3a. (If have *never* lived with him, check here___)
___ 4. Is he unemployed?
___ 5. Has he ever used a weapon against you or threatened you with a lethal weapon?
(If yes, was the weapon a gun?___)
___ 6. Does he threaten to kill you?
___ 7. Has he avoided being arrested for domestic violence?
___ 8. Do you have a child that is not his?
___ 9. Has he ever forced you to have sex when you did not wish to do so?
___ 10. Does he ever try to choke you?
___ 11. Does he use illegal drugs? By drugs, I mean "uppers" or amphetamines, "meth", speed, angel dust, cocaine, "crack", street drugs or mixtures.
___ 12. Is he an alcoholic or problem drinker?
___ 13. Does he control most or all of your daily activities? For instance: does he tell you who you can be friends with, when you can see your family, how much money you can use, or when you can take the car? (If he tries, but you do not let him, check here: ____)
___ 14. Is he violently and constantly jealous of you? (For instance, does he say "If I can't have you, no one can.")
___ 15. Have you ever been beaten by him while you were pregnant? (If you have never been pregnant by him, check here: ____)
___ 16. Has he ever threatened or tried to commit suicide?
___ 17. Does he threaten to harm your children?
___ 18. Do you believe he is capable of killing you?
___ 19. Does he follow or spy on you, leave threatening notes or messages, destroy your property, or call you when you don't want him to?
____ 20. Have you ever threatened or tried to commit suicide?
____ Total "Yes" Answers

Thank you. Please talk to your nurse, advocate or counselor about what the Danger Assessment means in terms of your situation.

Source: http://www.dangerassessment.com

Abuse Assessment Screen for Pregnancy

1. WITHIN THE LAST YEAR, have you been hit, slapped, kicked, or otherwise physically hurt by someone?	YES	NO

If YES, by whom? ____________________
Total number of times ____________________

2. SINCE YOU'VE BEEN PREGNANT, have you been hit, slapped, kicked, or otherwise physically hurt by someone?	YES	NO

If YES, by whom? ____________________
Total number of times ____________________

MARK THE AREA OF INJURY ON THE BODY MAP. SCORE EACH INCIDENT ACCORDING TO THE FOLLOWING SCALE:	SCORE
1 = Threats of abuse including use of a weapon	______
2 = Slapping, pushing; no injuries and/or continuing pain	______
3 = Punching, kicking; bruises, cuts, and/or continuing pain	______
4 = Beating up, severe contusions, burns, broken bones	______
5 = Head injury, internal injury, permanent injury	______
6 = Use of weapon; wound from weapon	______

If any of the descriptions for the higher numbers apply, use the higher number.

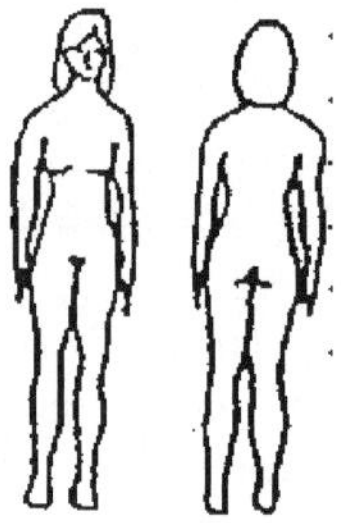

3. WITHIN THE LAST YEAR, has any forced you to have sexual activities?	YES	NO

If YES, by whom? ____________________
Total number of times ____________________

4. Have you ever been emotionally or physically abused by your partner or someone important to you?	YES	NO

If YES, by whom? ____________________
Number of times ____________________

5. Are you afraid of your partner or anyone listed above	YES	NO

Source: Nursing Research Consortium on Violence and Abuse

Edinburgh Postnatal Depression Scale[1] (EPDS)

Name: ______________________ Address: ______________________

Your Date of Birth: ______________________ ______________________

Baby's Date of Birth: ______________________ Phone: ______________________

As you are pregnant or have recently had a baby, we would like to know how you are feeling. Please check the answer that comes closest to how you have felt **IN THE PAST 7 DAYS**, not just how you feel today.

Here is an example, already completed.

I have felt happy:

- ☐ Yes, all the time
- ☒ Yes, most of the time
- ☐ No, not very often
- ☐ No, not at all

This would mean: "I have felt happy most of the time" during the past week. Please complete the other questions in the same way.

In the past 7 days:

1. I have been able to laugh and see the funny side of things
   - ☐ As much as I always could
   - ☐ Not quite so much now
   - ☐ Definitely not so much now
   - ☐ Not at all

2. I have looked forward with enjoyment to things
   - ☐ As much as I ever did
   - ☐ Rather less than I used to
   - ☐ Definitely less than I used to
   - ☐ Hardly at all

*3. I have blamed myself unnecessarily when things went wrong
   - ☐ Yes, most of the time
   - ☐ Yes, some of the time
   - ☐ Not very often
   - ☐ No, never

4. I have been anxious or worried for no good reason
   - ☐ No, not at all
   - ☐ Hardly ever
   - ☐ Yes, sometimes
   - ☐ Yes, very often

*5 I have felt scared or panicky for no very good reason
   - ☐ Yes, quite a lot
   - ☐ Yes, sometimes
   - ☐ No, not much
   - ☐ No, not at all

*6. Things have been getting on top of me
   - ☐ Yes, most of the time I haven't been able to cope at all
   - ☐ Yes, sometimes I haven't been coping as well as usual
   - ☐ No, most of the time I have coped quite well
   - ☐ No, I have been coping as well as ever

*7 I have been so unhappy that I have had difficulty sleeping
   - ☐ Yes, most of the time
   - ☐ Yes, sometimes
   - ☐ Not very often
   - ☐ No, not at all

*8 I have felt sad or miserable
   - ☐ Yes, most of the time
   - ☐ Yes, quite often
   - ☐ Not very often
   - ☐ No, not at all

*9 I have been so unhappy that I have been crying
   - ☐ Yes, most of the time
   - ☐ Yes, quite often
   - ☐ Only occasionally
   - ☐ No, never

*10 The thought of harming myself has occurred to me
   - ☐ Yes, quite often
   - ☐ Sometimes
   - ☐ Hardly ever
   - ☐ Never

Administered/Reviewed by ______________________ Date ______________________

[1]Source: Cox, J.L., Holden, J.M., and Sagovsky, R. 1987. Detection of postnatal depression: Development of the 10-item Edinburgh Postnatal Depression Scale. *British Journal of Psychiatry* 150:782-786 .

[2]Source: K. L. Wisner, B. L. Parry, C. M. Piontek, Postpartum Depression N Engl J Med vol. 347, No 3, July 18, 2002, 194-199

Edinburgh Postnatal Depression Scale[1] (EPDS)

Postpartum depression is the most common complication of childbearing.[2] The 10-question Edinburgh Postnatal Depression Scale (EPDS) is a valuable and efficient way of identifying patients at risk for "perinatal" depression. The EPDS is easy to administer and has proven to be an effective screening tool.

Mothers who score above 13 are likely to be suffering from a depressive illness of varying severity. The EPDS score should not override clinical judgment. A careful clinical assessment should be carried out to confirm the diagnosis. The scale indicates how the mother has felt ***during the previous week***. In doubtful cases it may be useful to repeat the tool after 2 weeks. The scale will not detect mothers with anxiety neuroses, phobias or personality disorders.

Women with postpartum depression need not feel alone. They may find useful information on the web sites of the National Women's Health Information Center <www.4women.gov> and from groups such as Postpartum Support International <www.chss.iup.edu/postpartum> and Depression after Delivery <www.depressionafterdelivery.com>.

SCORING

QUESTIONS 1, 2, & 4 (without an *)
Are scored 0, 1, 2 or 3 with top box scored as 0 and the bottom box scored as 3.

QUESTIONS 3, 5-10 (marked with an *)
Are reverse scored, with the top box scored as a 3 and the bottom box scored as 0.

Maximum score: 30
Possible Depression: 10 or greater
Always look at item 10 (suicidal thoughts)

Instructions for using the Edinburgh Postnatal Depression Scale:

1. The mother is asked to check the response that comes closest to how she has been feeling in the previous 7 days.
2. All the items must be completed.
3. Care should be taken to avoid the possibility of the mother discussing her answers with others. (Answers come from the mother or pregnant woman.)
4. The mother should complete the scale herself, unless she has limited English or has difficulty with reading.

[1]Source: Cox, J.L., Holden, J.M., and Sagovsky, R. 1987. Detection of postnatal depression: Development of the 10-item Edinburgh Postnatal Depression Scale. *British Journal of Psychiatry* 150:782-786.

[2]Source: K. L. Wisner, B. L. Parry, C. M. Piontek, Postpartum Depression N Engl J Med vol. 347, No 3, July 18, 2002, 194-199

Menopause Health Questionnaire (The North American Menopause Society)

Menopause is a normal event in a woman's life and is marked by the end of menstrual periods. Usually during the 40s, a gradual process leading to menopause begins. This is called the menopause transition or perimenopause. Changes in the pattern of menstrual periods are very common during this stage. Sometimes a woman can have other symptoms too, and these symptoms may extend beyond menopause. Even if a woman has no symptoms, it's important for her to understand the effects of menopause on her health.

This questionnaire is intended to help you inform your healthcare provider about your menopause experience and your general health. Working together, you can develop a plan to support your health, not only now but also in years to come. If you feel uncomfortable answering any of the questions on this form, you may wait and discuss them with your healthcare provider.

Section 1. PERSONAL INFORMATION

Date:	
Name:	
Address:	
Telephone number (home):	Telephone number (work):
Telephone number (cell):	Birth date: Age:
Ethnic/cultural background (please check what applies to you): □ Caucasian □ Black □ Asian □ Native American □ Biracial □ Hispanic/Latina □ Other (please specify)	
Marital status (circle): Single Married Divorced Widowed Committed	
Name of primary support person:	
Relationship:	
Primary support person telephone number:	
Employment status (circle): Unemployed Employed Retired Disabled If employed, occupation:	
Are you on medical leave: □ Yes □ No If yes, why? For how long?	
Who is your primary healthcare provider?	
Address:	Telephone number:

Section 2. TODAY'S OFFICE VISIT

Why are you here today?
What are your main concerns or questions you would like to have answered during your visit?
Who referred you?

Section 3. HEIGHT AND WEIGHT INFORMATION

What is your height?	
What is your maximum remembered height?	How old were you then?
What is your weight?	
What is your maximum remembered weight?	How old were you then?
What is your lowest remembered weight as an adult?	How old were you then?

Section 4. MEDICAL HISTORY

Please check if you have had problems with:

❑Migraines ❑Blood Pressure ❑Stroke ❑Cholesterol ❑Heart Attack ❑Chest pain ❑Blood clots ❑Varicose veins ❑Easy bruising ❑Anemia ❑Indigestion ❑Frequent nausea or vomiting	❑Colitis ❑Diarrhea ❑Constipation ❑Bloody or black bowel movements ❑Hepatitis ❑Liver ❑Gallbladder ❑Incontinence (urine or feces) ❑Breasts ❑Endometriosis ❑Fibroids ❑Infertility ❑Cancer	❑Diabetes ❑Thyroid ❑Asthma ❑Arthritis ❑Muscle or joint pain ❑Back pain ❑Seizures ❑Eyesight ❑Macular degeneration ❑Cataracts ❑Depression ❑Anxiety ❑Stress	❑Fatigue ❑Sleeping ❑Dizziness ❑Mood swings ❑Suicidal thoughts ❑Teeth or gums ❑Hair loss or growth ❑Skin ❑Frequent falling ❑ Losing height ❑ Broken bones ❑ Weight loss or gain

Other health problems (describe):

Section 5. MAJOR ILLNESS AND INJURY HISTORY

Date	List dates of all operations, hospitalizations, psychological therapy, major injuries, and illnesses (excluding pregnancy).
	(Please continue on back, if needed.)

Section 6. GYNECOLOGIC HISTORY

How would you describe your current menstrual status?

❑Premenopause (before menopause; having regular periods)

❑Perimenopause/menopause transition (changes in periods, but have not gone 12 months in a row without a period)

❑Postmenopause (after menopause)

Was your menopause:

❑Spontaneous ("natural")

❑Surgical (removal of both ovaries)

❑Due to chemotherapy or radiation therapy; reason for therapy: ______

❑Other (explain): ______

Age at first menstrual period: ______

Are your periods (or were your periods) usually regular? ❑Yes ❑No

Do you have a uterus? .... ❑Yes ❑No ❑Don't know

Do you have both ovaries? .... ❑Yes ❑No ❑Don't know

Do you have a cervix? .... ❑Yes ❑No ❑Don't know

If not still having periods, what was your age when you had your last period? ______

If still having periods, how often do they occur? ______

How many days does your period last? ______

Are your periods painful? ❑Yes ❑No If yes, how painful? ❑Mild ❑Moderate ❑Severe

Do you have spotting or bleeding between periods? .... ❑Yes ❑No

Is there a recent change in how often you have periods? ❑Yes ❑No

Is there a recent change in how many days you bleed? ... ❑Yes ❑No

Has your period recently become very heavy? .... ❑Yes ❑No

Do you think you have a problem with your period? ...... ❑Yes ❑No

If yes, explain: ______

Do you have any problems with PMS? (PMS is having mood swings, bloating, headaches just prior to your period) ❑Yes ❑No

Do you examine your breasts? .... ❑Yes ❑No If yes, how often? ______

Did your mother take DES when she was pregnant with you? ❑Yes ❑No ❑Don't know

Do you douche? .... ❑Yes ❑No If yes, how often? ______

What is the date and results (if known) of your last test regarding:

Pap smear: ______ Any abnormal Pap tests? ❑Yes ❑No If yes, when? ______

Mammogram: ______ Any breast biopsies? ❑Yes ❑No If yes, when? ______

Thyroid: ______ Any abnormal thyroid tests? ❑Yes ❑No If yes, when? ______

Cholesterol test: ______ Colonoscopy: ______

Blood sugar test: ______ Sigmoidoscopy: ______

Fecal occult blood test: ______ Bone density test: ______

Section 7. OBSTETRICAL HISTORY

Please indicate the method of birth control, if any, that you are currently using or have used previously:

	Using Now	Previously Used		Using Now	Previously Used
None	❑	❑	Implanted hormone	❑	❑
Sterilization (tubes tied)	❑	❑	Diaphragm	❑	❑
Male partner had vasectomy	❑	❑	Foam/gel	❑	❑
Birth control pill, ring, or skin patch	❑	❑	Condoms	❑	❑
IUD	❑	❑	Natural family planning/rhythm	❑	❑
Injectable hormone	❑	❑	Other	❑	❑

How many times have you been pregnant?

How many children do you have? How many were adopted?

How old were you when you first child was born? How old were you when your last child was born?

Please provide the number of your:
Full term births: Premature births: Miscarriages: Abortions: Living children:

Any complications during pregnancy, delivery, or postpartum? ❑Yes ❑No
If yes, please describe:

Section 8. SEXUAL HISTORY

Are you currently sexually active? .... ❑Yes ❑No
If yes, are you currently having sex with: ❑A man (or men) ❑A woman (or women) ❑Both men and women
How long have you been with your current sex partner? ________________
Are you in a committed, mutually monogamous relationship?.... ❑Yes ❑No
If no, do you use condoms (practice safe sex)? .... ❑Yes ❑No
In the past, have you had sex with: .... ❑A man (or men) ❑A woman (or women)
Have you had any sexually transmitted infections? .... ❑Yes ❑No
Do you have concerns about your sex life? .... ❑Yes ❑No
Do you have a loss of interest in sexual activities (libido, desire)? ❑Yes ❑No
Do you have a loss of arousal (tingling in the genitals or breasts;
vaginal moisture, warmth? .... ❑Yes ❑No
Do you have a loss of response (weaker or absent orgasm)?.... ❑Yes ❑No
Do you have any pain with intercourse (vaginal penetration)?.... ❑Yes ❑No
If yes, how long ago did the pain start? ______________________
Please describe the pain: ❑Pain with penetration ❑Pain inside ❑Feels dry

Section 9. ALLERGY INFORMATION

Are you allergic to any medications? ❑Yes ❑No ❑Don't know If yes, please indicate which one(s):

Medication: Rection:

Medication: Reaction:

Medication: Reaction:

Do you have any other allergies? ❑Yes ❑No ❑Don't know If yes, please indicate:

To what? Reaction:

To what? Reaction:

Section 10. MEDICATION HISTORY

Are you currently using hormone therapy for menopause? ❑Yes ❑No
If no, why not?

If yes, for what reasons?

Please indicate the medications and supplements (such as vitamins, calcium, herbs, soy) you are currently using. Include prescription drugs and those purchased without a prescription. Also include all hormone therapy you have used in the past (examples include contraceptives, thyroid hormones, and hormone therapy for menopause).

Medication/ Supplement	Dose	Frequency	Date Started	Date Stopped	Why Stopped

Have you used any other therapy for menopause (such as acupuncture or yoga)? ❑Yes ❑No If yes, please indicate:
Of these, what are you currently using?

Is this therapy helpful? ❑Yes ❑No

Section 11. FAMILY HISTORY

Please list family member (i.e., mother, father, sister, brother, grandparent, aunt, uncle) who currently has or once had the following:

High blood pressure:	Colorectal cancer:
Heart attack (indicate age):	Ovarian cancer:
Stroke (indicate age):	Other cancer:
Blood problems	Depression:
(including sickle cell trait):	Other emotional problems:
Blood clots:	Alzheimer's disease:
Bleeding tendency:	Domestic violence victim:
Glaucoma:	Domestic violence person:
Osteoporosis:	Sexual abuse victim:
Hip fracture:	Sexual abuse person:
Diabetes:	Alcoholism:
Breast cancer (indicate age):	Drug abuse:

Is there anything about your family's health history that concerns you, or that you would like to discuss? ❑Yes ❑No If yes, what?

Section 12. PERSONAL HABITS

Do you consider your health to be: ❑Excellent ❑Good ❑Fair ❑Poor

Exercise

How often do you exercise? ❑Almost daily ❑At least 3x/week ❑Occasionally ❑Rarely ❑Never

If you exercise, what do you do? ___

For how long and how often?

Diet

How many meals do you consume each day? ______________________

Do you try to eat a special diet? ❑Low-fat ❑Low carbohydrate ❑High protein ❑Vegetarian

What dairy products do you consume each day?

❑Milk How much? ______________ ❑Yogurt How much? ______________

❑Cheese How much? ______________ ❑Other ______________

Are you lactose intolerant (diarrhea or gastrointestinal/GI upset after dairy products)? ❑Yes ❑No

How many servings of fruits do you consume each day?

How many servings of vegetables do you consume each day?

How many servings of soy foods do you consume each week?

How many servings of fish do you consume each week?

Tobacco use

Do you currently smoke cigarettes? ❑Yes ❑No

If yes, how many per day? ______________ When did you start? ______________

How do you feel about quitting smoking? ______________________

If you do not currently smoke cigarettes, have you ever smoked? ❑Yes ❑No

If yes, when did you start? ________ How many per day? ________ When did you stop? ________

Do you use any other type of tobacco? ❑Yes ❑No If yes, what?

Caffeine use

Do you consume drinks with caffeine (coffee, tea, soda drinks)? ❑Yes ❑No

If yes, how many drinks each day?

Alcohol and drug use

Do you drink alcohol? .... ❑Yes ❑No

If yes, how many drinks do you have each week? _______

Do you ever have a drink in the morning to get you going? ❑Yes ❑No

Have you ever tried to cut down on your drinking? .... ❑Yes ❑No

Have you ever felt guilty about the amount you drink? ...... ❑Yes ❑No

Have you ever been an alcoholic? .... ❑Yes ❑No

Do you use illegal drugs? .... ❑Yes ❑No

Abuse

Within the last year, have you been hit, slapped, kicked, or physically hurt by someone? .... ❑Yes ❑No

Within the last year, has anyone ever forced you to have sexual activities? .... ❑Yes ❑No

Do you feel you are verbally or emotionally abused by someone? ❑Yes ❑No

Have you had counseling for these issues? ❑Yes ❑No

Stress management

What are the current major stressors or life changes in your life?

Any major changes in the family health during the past year? ❑Yes ❑No

If yes, explain:

How do you handle stress? ❑Very well ❑Moderately well ❑Poorly

What do you do to relax?

Section 13. SYMPTOMS

Please indicate how bothered you are now and in the past few weeks by any of the following:

	Not at all	A little bit	Quite a bit	Extremely
I have hot flashes	□	□	□	□
I have night sweats	□	□	□	□
I have difficulty getting to sleep	□	□	□	□
I have difficulty staying asleep	□	□	□	□
I get heart palpitations or a sensation of butterflies in my chest or stomach	□	□	□	□
I feel like my skin is crawling or itching	□	□	□	□
I feel more tired than usual	□	□	□	□
I have difficulty concentrating	□	□	□	□
My memory is poor	□	□	□	□
I am more irritable than usual	□	□	□	□
I feel more anxious than usual	□	□	□	□
I have more depressed moods	□	□	□	□
I am having mood swings	□	□	□	□
I have crying spells	□	□	□	□
I have headaches	□	□	□	□
I need to urinate more often than usual	□	□	□	□
I leak urine	□	□	□	□
I have pain or burning when urinating	□	□	□	□
I have bladder infections	□	□	□	□
I have uncontrollable loss of stool or gas	□	□	□	□
My vagina is dry	□	□	□	□
I have vaginal itching	□	□	□	□
I have an abnormal vaginal discharge	□	□	□	□
I have vaginal infections	□	□	□	□
I have pain during intercourse	□	□	□	□
I have pain inside during intercourse	□	□	□	□
I have bleeding after intercourse	□	□	□	□
I lack desire or interest in sexual activity	□	□	□	□
I have difficulty achieving orgasm	□	□	□	□
My opportunity for sexual activity is limited	□	□	□	□
My stomach feels like it's bloated or I've gained weight	□	□	□	□
I have breast tenderness	□	□	□	□
I have joint pains	□	□	□	□

Section 14. RISK ASSESSMENT (optional)

The following questions will help determine your risk for disease later on in life. Please check all that apply to you.

Osteoporosis risk

❑Bone density test shows low bone mass
❑Bone density test shows osteoporosis
❑Family history of osteoporosis
❑Small, thin frame
❑Caucasian or Asian
❑Missed menstrual period for 6 months or more (not including when pregnant or breastfeeding) ❑ Menopause at or before age 40 ❑Taking thyroid, antiseizure, anticoagulant, or cortisone medication ❑ Diet low in milk and dairy products ❑Do not take calcium supplements ❑More than 7 alcoholic drinks each week ❑Prolonged bed rest ❑Exercise less than 3 times a week ❑Cannot rise from chair without using arms ❑Cannot rise from floor without difficulty ❑ Frequent falls ❑Previous episodes of severe dieting, bulimia, or anorexia ❑Hemophilia ❑Type I diabetes ❑ Chronic liver or kidney disease ❑Crohn's disease ❑ Rheumatoid arthritis ❑Current smoker ❑Spend little or no time in sunlight and don't take vitamin D ❑Loss of height greater than 1.5 inches ❑Previous fracture ❑ More than one previous fracture ❑Scoliosis ❑Back pain ❑Gum disease or tooth loss

Cardiovascular risk

❑Previous heart attack
❑Previous stroke
❑Previous or current chest pain (angina)
❑Previous or current heart rhythm problem (arrhythmia)
❑Diabetes
❑High blood pressure
❑High total cholesterol
❑Low HDL (good cholesterol)
❑High triglycerides
❑Current smoker
❑Over 65 years old
❑Black skin color
❑My shape is like an apple (waist bigger than hips)
❑Exercise less than 3 times a week
❑More than 30% over ideal weight (e.g., should be 120 pounds, but now weigh 160; should be 150 pounds, but now weigh 200)
❑Have not cut down on fat in my diet
❑Family history of heart disease

Cancer risk

A. Cervical cancer risk

❑Smoking
❑Genital warts (HPV)
❑Abnormal Pap test
❑Sexual intercourse at an early age
❑Multiple sexual partners
❑Sexual partners who have had multiple sexual partners
❑HIV
❑Have unsafe sex (without a condom)

B. Uterine cancer risk

(If you no longer have a uterus, skip to C.)

❑More than 30% over ideal weight (eg, should be 120 pounds, but now weigh 160; should be 150 pounds, but now weigh 200) ❑Unexplained uterine bleeding ❑ Prolonged time spans without menstrual periods (except when pregnant) ❑Have not given birth ❑Began menstrual periods before age 12 ❑Reached menopause after age 53 ❑Diabetes ❑Gallbladder disease ❑Use of tamoxifen ❑Use of estrogen therapy for menopause without adding a progestogen

C. Breast cancer risk

❑Mother or sister diagnosed with breast cancer before menopause ❑Previous breast, uterine, or ovarian cancer ❑Positive *BRCA1* (gene mutation) ❑Reached menopause after age 55 ❑Began menstrual periods before age 12 ❑Had first child after age 30 ❑No children
❑More than 30% over ideal weight (eg, should be 120 pounds, but now weigh 160; should be 150 pounds, but now weigh 200)
❑Drinking more than 7 alcoholic drinks each week
❑Lack of exercise
❑Diet low in vegetables and fruits
❑Have used estrogen therapy more than 5 years

(continued)

Section 14. RISK ASSESSMENT (continued)

D. Ovarian cancer risk

❑No children

❑Previous breast or uterine cancer

❑Family history of ovarian, breast, or uterine cancer

❑Positive *BRCA1* and *BRCA2*

E. Colorectal cancer risk

❑History of colorectal cancer or adenomatous polyps

❑Family history of colorectal cancer or adenomatou polyps

❑Inflammatory bowel disease

❑Diet low in vegetables, fruits, and fiber

❑Smoking

F. Lung cancer risk

❑History of lung cancer ❑Family history of lung cancer ❑Current smoker ❑Previous smoker

❑Smoker in home

❑Work around asbestos, smokers, or talc

❑Work around cancer-causing chemicals (gasoline, diesel exhaust, arsenic, uranium, vinyl chloride, nickel chromates, coal products, mustard gas, chloromethyl ethers)

❑Exposure to radon gas

❑Smoke marijuana

❑History of tuberculosis

G. Skin cancer risk

❑Light skin color

❑Previous skin cancer

❑Family history of skin cancer

❑Severe sunburn(s) when a child

❑Numerous moles and freckles

❑Sunbathe regularly or for longer than 1-hour sessions

❑Visit tanning salons

Section 15. ABOUT MENOPAUSE AND HORMONE THERAPY

How do you view menopause?

❑ **Positively.** For example, menopause means no more periods and no more worry about contraception. Menopause marks a new life phase.

❑ **Negatively.** For example, menopause means a loss of fertility and loss of youth.

❑ Other:

What concerns you about menopause?

(Please continue on back, if needed.)

What are your current views regarding hormone therapy for menopause?

❑ Positive. Hormone therapy is appropriate for some women.

❑ Negative. I don't support the use of hormone therapy.

What concerns you most about hormone therapy for menopause?

(Please continue on back, if needed.)

How would you rate your knowledge about menopause?

❑ Very good ❑ Fair ❑ Moderately good ❑ Little knowledge

How do you get your information about menopause? (Mark all that apply.)

❑ Books ❑ Internet ❑ Magazines ❑ Friends ❑ TV

❑ Healthcare providers

Is there anything else you would like your healthcare provider to know?

(Please continue on back, if needed.)

Thank you! Please note that the information you have provided will be held in the strictest confidence.

The North American Menopause Society has provided this form as a service to the healthcare community based on the best understanding of the science related to menopause at the time of publication, but the form should be used with the clear understanding that continued research may result in new knowledge and recommendations. This form is provided only as a diagnostic assist to practitioners making clinical decisions regarding the health of women in their care. Its contents provide guidance and, as such, it cannot substitute for the individual judgment brought to each clinical situation by the caregiver with respect to any additional data that may be required in order to make appropriate clinical decisions. The North American Menopause Society is not responsible nor liable for any advice, diagnosis, course of treatment, or drug or device application based on the healthcare provider's use of this form.

Risk Calculators (available online)

Breast Cancer Risk Calculator

http://www.cancer.gov/bcrisktool/

FRAX Fracture Risk Assessment

http://www.shef.ac.uk/FRAX/tool.jsp

APPENDIX ❖ C

BILLING AND CODING IN WOMEN'S HEALTH

Diane Marie Schadewald ◆ Catherine Juve

Billing for services provided is done using Current Procedural Terminology (CPT) codes. These codes are developed, maintained, and copyrighted by the American Medical Association (AMA) to communicate with third-party payers about services provided. The CPT codes identify the level of service, procedures performed, counseling and coordination of care, and the time used to complete these activities (AMA, 2011). In other words, CPT codes are utilized to describe what has been done during the visit. In determining billing level, the clinician may include the factor of time spent in order to coordinate care or counsel the patient. If billing for coordination of care or counseling, more than 50 percent of the visit time must have been spent for these endeavors and clinicians must include a statement in their note about the total time of visit and total time spent in counseling or coordination of care. The authors have chosen not to list any of the CPT codes that are utilized for billing and refer the reader to their clinic setting for further information about these codes. Students and clinicians are encouraged to familiarize themselves with the CPT codes that are commonly used in their clinical setting. The remainder of this appendix covers commonly used diagnostic codes. Diagnostic codes identify what problem the patient was determined to have and/or what service the patient needed.

Commonly Used ICD-9 (International Classification of Diseases, Ninth Revision) Diagnostic Codes in Women's Health

Preventive

V65.4x	Advice/instruction
V81.1	Blood pressure check
V76.10	Breast screening, unspecified
V65.3	Diet instruction
V65.41	Exercise counseling
V01.6	Exposure to chlamydia or gonorrhea
V18.0	Family history of diabetes
V16.3	Family history of malignancy breast
V16.41	Family history of malignancy ovary
V67.9	Follow-up exam
V16.82	History of tobacco use
V15.89	Screenig Pap High-risk breast cancer
V72.6	Lab testing
V70.0	Physical routine
V70.3	Physical school/sports
V70.5	Physical (work)
V72.84	Pre-op exam, unspecified
V72.32	Repeat Pap
V76.2	Screening Pap
V15.89	High risk breast cancer
V74.5	Screening for sexually transmitted disease
V77.91	Screening for cholesterol
V77.1	Screening for diabetes
V77.0	Screening for thyroid disorder
V81.2	Screening for hyperlipidemia
V78.0	Screening for iron-deficiency anemia
V10.3	Personal history of breast cancer
V04.81	Vaccination for influenza
V05.3	Vaccination for hepatitis
V04.89	Vaccination again for other viral diseases (can be used for human papillomavirus vaccines)
V06.4	Vaccination for measles, mumps, and rubella
V06.5	Vaccination for tetanus/diphtheria
V05.4	Vaccination for varicella
V72.31	Yearly/Pap/pelvic

Genitourinary

622.9	Abnormal cervix
795.0	Abnormal Pap
626.2	Abnormal bleeding (menorrhagia)
626.6	Abnormal bleeding (unrelated to cycle)
628.0	Absence of menstruation
595.0	Acute cystitis
626.0	Amenorrhea
565.0	Anal fissure
616.2	Bartholin's cyst
622.7	Cervical polyp
616.0	Cervicitis
595.1	Chronic interstitial cystitis
132.2	Crabs/lice
595.9	Cystitis
618.01	Cystocele midline
626.8	Dysfunctional uterine bleeding
625.3	Dysmenorrhea
625.0	Dyspareunia (female)
788.1	Dysuria
621.30	Endometrial hyperplasia, unspecified
621.0	Endometrial polyp
617.9	Endometriosis, site unspecified
617.0	Endometriosis uterus
621.2	Enlarged uterus
455.3	External hemorrhoids without complications
218.9	Fibroid uterus
620.0	Follicular cyst ovary
788.41	Frequency of urination
599.70	Hematuria
218.1	Intramural leiomyoma uterus
182.0	Malignant neoplasm corpus uteri ex isthmus
183.0	Malignant neoplasm of ovary
179	Malignant neoplasm of uterus, part unspecified
627.2	Menopausal symptoms
626.4	Menstrual irregularity
788.33	Mixed incontinence
078.0	Molluscum contagiosum
616.0	Nabothian cysts
626.1	Oligomenorrhea
620.0	Ovarian cyst
789.3	Pelvic mass
625.9	Pelvic pain
614.2	Pelvic inflammatory disease/salpingitis
256.4	Polycystic ovaries
626.7	Postcoital bleeding
627.3	Postmenopausal atrophic vaginitis
627.1	Postmenopausal bleeding
627.0	Premenopausal menorrhagia
625.4	Premenstrual syndrome
698.0	Pruritus ani
618.04	Rectocele
133.4	Scabies
625.6	Stress incontinence
788.30	Urinary incontinence, unspecified
788.63	Urgency of urination

788.41	Urinary frequency
788.31	Urge incontinence
599.0	Urinary tract infection
618.1	Uterine prolapse
623.5	Vaginal discharge
623.9	Vaginal irritation
625.1	Vaginismus
616.10	Vaginitis NS/gardnerella
133.01	Vaginitis trichomonal
112.1	Vaginitis yeast
624.9	Vulvar disorder
625.71	Vulvar vestibulitis

Hormonal Changes/Endocrine and Infertility

783.1	Abnormal weight gain
V26.1	Artificial insemination
V49.81	Asymptomatic postmenopausal status
628.9	Female infertility unspecified origin
628.2	Female infertility tubal origin
628.8	Female infertility other origin
628.0	Female infertility anovulation
V26.21	Fertility testing
611.6	Galactorrhea nonobstetric
704.1	Hirsutism
244.9	Hypothyroidism, unspecified
V07.4	Hormone therapy
783.21	Loss of weight
783.5	Polydipsia
788.42	Polyuria
627.2	Symptoms of menopausal state
627.4	Symptoms of state artificial menopause
242.9	Thyrotoxicosis
783.1	Weight gain

Breast Disorders

611.0	Abscess/mastitis
610.0	Cyst (solitary)
610.2	Fibroadenosis breast
610.1	Fibrocystic breasts
611.72	Mass/lump
611.71	Mastodynia
611.79	Nipple discharge/inversion

General

789.0x	Abdominal pain
706.1	Acne
453.40	Acute venous embolism (deep vein thrombosis)
303.90	Alcohol abuse
995.3	Allergic reaction
285.9	Anemia, unspecified
280.9	Anemia, iron deficiency
307.1	Anorexia nervosa
300.00	Anxiety, unspecified
796.2	Blood pressure elevated without hypertension
466.0	Bronchitis
923	Bruise
304.90	Chemical dependency
564.0	Constipation
799.81	Decreased libido
311	Depression
692.9	Dermatitis
250.0	Diabetes
307.50	Eating disorder
782.3	Edema, lower extremities
692.9	Eczema
780.7	Fatigue
704.8	Folliculitis
784.0	Headaches
785.2	Heart murmur
455.6	Hemorrhoids
455.8	Hemorrhoids bleeding
272.4	High cholesterol
401.9	Hypertension, unspecified
733.90	Hypoactive sexual desire disorder
684	Impetigo
564.1	Irritable bowel syndrome
783.0	Loss of appetite
346.9	Migraines, unspecified
075	Mononucleosis
787.0	Nausea/vomiting
278.00	Obesity, unspecified
278.01	Obesity, morbid
278.02	Overweight
733.90	Osteopenia
733.00	Osteoporosis, unspecified
733.01	Osteoporosis, postmenopausal
380.10	Otitis externa
382.9	Otitis media
785.1	Palpitations
462	Pharyngitis
696.1	Psoriasis
782.1	Rash
706.2	Sebaceous cyst
473.9	Sinusitis
246.9	Thyroid disorder
305.1	Tobacco dependence
V58.32	Removal of sutures

454.8	Varicose veins of lower extremities
454.9	Varicose veins of lower extremities (asymptomatic)
671.1	Varicose veins of vulva
281.1	Vitamin B_{12} deficiency
268.9	Vitamin D deficiency

Family Planning

995.29	Birth control pill problems
V25.41	Birth control pill refill
V25.0	Contraceptive advice/counseling/management
V25.4	Contraceptive surveillance
V25.04	Counseling fertility awareness
V26.49	Counseling, procreative
V25.03	Emergency contraception
V25.09	Family planning education
V25.5	Implanon insertion
V25.43	Implanon check or removal
V25.42	Intrauterine device (IUD) check/removal
V25.1	IUD insertion
996.32	IUD complications
V26.41	Natural family planning
V25.02	Other contraception (barriers, Depo)
V25.49	Other contraceptive maintenance (Depo, diaphragm)
V45.51	Presence of intrauterine contraceptive
V25.01	Prescription oral contraceptives

Sexually Transmitted Infections

099.8	Chlamydia
098.0	Gonorrhea
054.10	Herpes, genital
099.9	Sexually transmitted disease, other
099.40	Urethritis
078.11	Warts, genital
042	HIV
079.4	Human papillomavirus infection

Pregnancy

796.50	Abnormal antenatal screening
648.83	Abnormal glucose tolerance test, antepartum
634.9	Abortion, spontaneous
659.63	Advanced maternal age, antepartum
659.64	Advanced maternal age, unspecified
V28.8	Antenatal screening of Strep B
V28.9	Antenatal screening, unspecified
648.03	Antepartum diabetes
V02.51	Carrier Group B Strep
765.21	< 24 completed weeks of gestation
765.29	37+ completed weeks of gestation
642.03	Essential hypertension, antepartum
648.63	Gentiourinary infection, antepartum
V23.3	Grand multiparity
659.43	Grand multiparity, antepartum
641.9	Hemorrhage
642.90	Hypertension pregnancy, unspecified
V23.7	Insufficient prenatal care
648.20	Maternal anemia pregnancy
648.40	Mental disorder pregnancy, unspecified
V23.9	Other high-risk pregnancy
641.03	Placenta previa, antepartum
656.53	Poor fetal growth
645.10	Post-term pregnancy, unspecified
V72.41	Pregnancy test negative
V72.42	Pregnancy test positive
V22.2	Pregnant state
V23.2	Pregnancy with history of abortion
V23.0	Pregnancy with history of infertility
V23.41	Pregnancy with history of preterm labor
V23.49	Pregnancy with other poor obstetric history
654.20	Previous C-section, unspecified
654.21	Previous C-section, unspecified antepartum
646.93	Pregnancy complications, unspecified antepartum
656.13	Rh isoimmunization, antepartum
V73.3	Screening for rubella
V74.1	Screening for pulmonary tuberculosis
V28.3	Screening for fetal malformation
649.63	Size/date discrepancy, antepartum
634.90	Spontaneous abortion uncomplicated, unspecified
V22.0	Supervision of normal first pregnancy
V22.1	Supervision of other normal pregnancy
V22.8	Supervision of other high-risk pregnancy
779.6	Termination of pregnancy
640.0	Threatened abortion, unspecified
644.03	Threatened preterm labor
644.13	Threatened labor, otherwise antepartum
642.33	Transient hypertension pregnancy
633.1	Tubal pregnancy
651.00	Twin pregnancy
671.0	Varicose veins of lower extremities complicating pregnancy
671.1	Varicose veins of vulva complicating pregnancy
643.83	Vomiting complications pregnancy, antepartum
V23.83	Young primigravida

Postpartum

659.61	Advanced maternal age delivered
675.24	Mastitis postpartum
648.44	Mental disorder postpartum
V24.0	Postpartum care after delivery
V24.1	Postpartum care lactating mother
654.22	Previous C-section, unspecified delivered
V67.59	Postabortion check
V24.2	Routine postpartum follow-up

This list is not to be considered inclusive of all codes used in women's health. Readers are encouraged to consult with the billing and coding department of their agency for more codes that are utilized for various conditions and procedures. The authors would like to acknowledge the assistance of the Family Tree Clinic, Typhon, and the University of Minnesota Physicians Primary Care Clinic in compiling this list of billing and diagnostic codes. An online resource, http://www.icd9data.com/2009/Volume2/default.htm, 2011 ICD-9-CM Volume 2 Index, was also utilized.

REFERENCES

American Medical Association (AMA) (2011). 2011 AMA CPT Professional Coding Book, Chicago, IL: AMA

ICD-9 CM (2011) Volume 2 Index, retrieved from: http://www.icd9data.com/2009/Volume2/default.htm

APPENDIX ❖ D

SELECTED LABORATORY VALUES[a]

Diane Marie Schadewald ◆ Ellis Quinn Youngkin

Comprehensive Metabolic Panel (1,2,3)	
Sodium	135–145 mEq/L (mmol/L)
Potassium	3.5–5.2 mEq/L (mmol/L)
Chloride	96–106 mEq/L (mmol/L)
Carbon dioxide	22–30 mEq/L (mmol/L)
Glucose (fasting)	70–110 mg/dL
Blood urea nitrogen	6–19 mg/dL
Creatinine	0.4–1.0 mg/dL
Calcium	8.8–10.4 mg/dL
Albumin	3.5–5.2 g/dL
Bilirubin (total)	0.3–1.0 mg/dL
Alkaline phosphatase	25–100 IU/L
AST (SGOT)[b]	10–37 IU/L
ALT (SGPT)[b]	7–35 IU/L
Protein (total) (3)	6–8.0 g/dL

Lipid Profile (1,3)	Desirable	Borderline	High Risk
Cholesterol	140–199 mg/dL	200–239 mg/dL	≥ 240 mg/dL
Triglycerides	35–149 mg/dL	150–199 mg/dL	200–499 mg/dL
LDL-C[b]	< 130 mg/dL[c]	140–159 mg/dL	> 160 mg/dL
HDL-C[b]	46–80 mg/dL or greater	36–45 mg/dL	< 35 mg/dL
Cholesterol/HDL ratio (1)	≤ 4.4		
Apolipoproteina (A1/B ratio)	0.94–2.63		

Thyroid Profile (1,4,5)	
TSH[b]	0.4–4.2 μIU/mL
T_3 uptake[b]	25–35%
T_4 (total)[b]	5.4–11.5 μg/dL
FTI (calc)[b] (T_4 total × T_3U/100)	1.5–4.5
Free T_4 (1)	0.7–2.0 ng/dL
T_3 (total)	80–200 ng/dL

Other Values			
Prolactin (1)	4–23 ng/mL (premenopausal)	Testosterone (1)	15–70 ng/dL (adult females)
FSH (3)		Free testosterone (1)	1.0–8.5 pg/dL
Follicular	4.0–30.0 mIU/mL	DHEA-SO_4[b] (6)	12–380 µg/dL (decreases with age)
Luteal	4.0–30.0 mIU/mL	Androstenedione (1)	75–205 ng/dL
Midcycle	10.0–90.0 mIU/mL	17-Hydroxyprogesterone (7)	15–70 ng/dL (follicular phase)
Postmenopausal	40.0–170.0 mIU/mL		35–290 ng/dL (luteal phase)
LH (3)		Cortisol (1,3,6)	
Follicular	5.0–30.0 mIU/mL	8:00 a.m.	5–23 µg/dL
Luteal	2.0–25.0 mIU/mL	4:00 p.m.	3–16 µg/dL
Midcycle peak	50.0–150.0 mIU/mL	10:00 p.m.	< 50% of a.m. value
Postmenopausal	40–100.0 mIU/mL	After ACTH stimulation test, plasma cortisol should increase 2–3 times over baseline at 30 and 60 minutes (6)	
Estradiol (serum) (3)			
Follicular	20–150 pg/mL	Dexamethasone suppression test	5+ µg/dL cortisone = test failure
Midcycle	100–500 pg/mL	Albumin (1,3)	3.5–5.2 g/dL
Luteal	60–260 pg/mL	Vitamin D 1,25 (3,7)	20–76 ng/mL
Postmenopausal	< 30 pg/mL	Insufficiency	20–29 ng/mL
Progesterone (serum) (3)		Optimum level	30–80 ng/mL
Follicular	0.1–1.5 ng/dL	Possible toxicity	> 150 ng/mL
Midcycle	Rising		
Luteal	2–28 ng/dL		

Anemia Workup (1,3)			
Complete blood count		Reticulocyte count	0.5–1.5%
Red blood cells	3.6–5.0 million/mm^3	Iron	50–150 µg/dL
Hemoglobin	12–16 g/dL	Total iron-binding capacity	250–450 µg/dL
Hematocrit	36–47%	Transferrin	200–430 µg/dL
MCV (3)	78–100 μm^3	Transferrin saturation	15–50%
MCH	23–34 µg	Ferritin (3)	10–235 ng/mL
MCHC	31–36 g/dL	Hemoglobin electrophoresis	
White blood cells	5,000–10,000 cells/mm^3 (4.8–10.8 K/mL)	Hgb A1	95–98%
Differential		Hgb A2 (1)	1.5–3.5%
Neutrophils	50–70%	Hgb F	0–2%
Lymphocytes	25–40%	Hgb S	0%
Monocytes	3–7%	Hgb C	0%
Eosinophils	0–3%	Platelet count	140,000–400,000/µL
Basophils	0–1%	Folic acid (3)	3–16 ng/dL
Bands or stabs (young neutrophils)	3–6%	Vitamin B_{12} (1)	280–1500 pg/dL

[a]Values vary from laboratory to laboratory and among clinicians, as well as upon method used for calculation.
[b]AST (SGOT), aspartate aminotransferase (serum glutamic-oxaloacetic transaminase); ALT (SGPT), alanine aminotransferase (serum glutamic-pyruvic transaminase); LDL-C, low-density lipoprotein cholesterol; HDL-C, high-density lipoprotein cholesterol; TSH, thyroid-stimulating hormone; T_3, triiodothyronine; T_4, thyroxine; FTI (calc), free thyroxine index (calculated); FSH, follicle-stimulating hormone; LH, luteinizing hormone; DHEA-SO_4, dehydroepiandrosterone sulfate; MCV, mean corpusacular volume; MCH, mean corpuscular hemoglobin; MCHC, mean corpuscular hemoglobin concentration; Hgb, hemoglobin.
[c]Less than 100 desirable in the presence of cardiac risk factors.

REFERENCES

1. Fischbach, F., & Dunning III, M.B. (2009). *A manual of laboratory and diagnostic tests* (8th ed.). Philadelphia: Wolters Kluwer Lippincott Williams & Wilkins.
2. The basic metabolic panel is comprised of the first seven tests.
3. Kee, J.L. (2010). *Laboratory and diagnostics tests with nursing implications* (8th ed.) Upper Saddle River, NJ: Pearson.
4. Arem, R. (2007). *The thyroid solution*. New York: Ballentine Books.
5. Shames, R.L., & Shames, K.H. (2011). *Thyroid mind power: The proven cure for hormone-related depression, anxiety, and memory loss*. New York: Rodale.
6. Van Leeuwen, A.M., & Poelhuis-Leth, D.J. (2009). *Comprehensive handbook of laboratory and diagnostic tests with nursing implications* (3rd ed.). Philadelphia: F. A. Davis.
7. ARUP Laboratories: National Reference Laboratory, *17-Hydroxyprogesterone: 0070005*. Retrieved October 27, 2011, from www.aruplab.com/guides/ug/tests/0070005.jsp

APPENDIX ❖ **E**

FEDERAL AGENCIES CONCERNED WITH WOMEN'S HEALTH

Diane Marie Schadewald

U.S. DEPARTMENT OF LABOR, WOMEN'S BUREAU

This bureau was established in 1920 and is concerned with women in the workforce. Its mission concentrates on safeguarding the interests of working women, advocating for equality and economic security of women and their families, and promoting quality work environments. Current priority issues include equal pay, workplace flexibility, higher paying jobs for women, and assisting homeless women veterans to return to the workforce (U.S. Department of Labor, 2011).

THE DEPARTMENT OF HEALTH AND HUMAN SERVICES

The Department of Health and Human Services (DHHS) is the federal government's principal agency for protecting the health of all Americans and providing them with essential human services. As a result, both direct and indirect services are of benefit to women. Although the roots of health services can be traced to the earliest days of the United States, the Department of Health, Education, and Welfare (HEW) came into a cabinet-level existence in 1953. Education was made into a separate department in 1979, and HEW became the DHHS in 1980. The department includes over 300 programs.

OFFICE ON WOMEN'S HEALTH

Established in 1991, the Office on Women's Health (OWH) reviewed its strategic plan in 2007 and now has four main goals focused on eliminating disparities for women and girls in the areas of health care promotion, service delivery, public and health care professional development, and career advancement for women in the health professions and science. The OWH goals as listed in its Strategic Plan for FY2010–FY2015 are the following:

1. To develop and impact national health policy as it relates to women and girls.
2. To develop, adapt, implement, evaluate, and replicate model programs on women's and girls' health.
3. To educate, influence, and collaborate with health and human services organizations, health care professionals, and the public.
4. To increase OWH's organizational efficiency and performance.

The OWH has opportunities for internships for undergraduate and graduate students as well as funding opportunities for research related to the health of women and girls (OWH, 2011).

National Women's Health Information Center

An additional service offered by the OWH is the National Women's Health Information Center, which is a national information and referral service designed to provide women and their families with current, reliable, and cost-free health information and materials from federal agencies and respected private-sector organizations. This is accomplished through a comprehensive web site and a toll-free call center number 1-800-994-WOMAN (9662).

OFFICE OF RESEARCH ON WOMEN'S HEALTH

Established in 1990, the Office of Research on Women's Health (ORWH) at the National Institutes of Health (NIH) Division of Program Coordination, Planning, and Strategic Initiatives serves as a focal point for women's health research. The ORWH promotes, stimulates, and supports efforts to improve the health of women through biomedical and behavioral research. It works in partnership with NIH institutes and centers to ensure that women's health research is part of the scientific framework at NIH and throughout the scientific community.

Since its inception, the focus and resources dedicated to research on women have generated considerable new knowledge about women's health. For example, research has led to a better understanding of the interaction between life behaviors and health outcomes. A case in point is that women who take folic acid before pregnancy and especially during the first month following conception reduce the incidence of neural tube defects in their offspring.

FOOD AND DRUG ADMINISTRATION OFFICE OF WOMEN'S HEALTH

The Food and Drug Administration (FDA) has jurisdiction over drugs, medical devices, vaccines, blood and tissue products, foods, and cosmetics used by women and their families on a daily basis. The creation of the Office of Women's Health in 1994 provided for the inclusion of patients of both genders in drug development and analyses of clinical data (women of childbearing potential were excluded from all drug research prior to this time). The Office of Women's Health has established itself as an effective voice for women's health concerns. According to the Office of Women's Health's published description, its mission is to "protect and advance the health of women through policy, science, and outreach and to advocate for the participation of women in clinical trials and for sex, gender, and subpopulation analyses" (FDA, 2011). To meet its goals, the Office of Women's Health coordinates its activities through two program areas: (1) research and development and (2) outreach.

A number of programs have been conducted to meet stated goals. Premier among them is the Take Time to Care (TTTC) campaign that started in 1998 called Use Medicines Wisely. The program provides a medication record keeper that is translated into 14 languages and reaches millions of women of many cultures where they live and work to educate them about using medicines wisely. Other campaigns now included under TTTC are Pink Ribbon Sunday, College Women's Campaign, Diabetes Campaign, and Menopause Hormone Therapy Campaign (FDA, 2011).

AGENCY FOR HEALTHCARE RESEARCH AND QUALITY

The Agency for Healthcare Research and Quality (AHRQ) is another DHHS division that provides evidence-based information on health care outcomes; quality; and cost, use, and access. Information from AHRQ research helps people to make informed decisions and also improve the quality of health care services. In addition, it addresses medical errors. AHRQ research listings are extensive and currently include a variety of topics of concern to women, such as heart disease and stroke, breast and cervical cancer, hysterectomy, urinary incontinence, pelvic inflammatory disease, health care access, preventive services, domestic violence, HIV/AIDS, and alternative medicines. The agency also offers women's health email updates for those interested (AHRQ, 2011).

HEALTH RESOURCES AND SERVICES ADMINISTRATION

Health Resources and Services Administration (HRSA) of the DHHS directs programs that improve the nation's health by providing access to essential health services for people who are poor, uninsured, vulnerable; have special needs; or who live in rural and urban areas where health care is scarce. Working in partnership with state and community organizations, HRSA ensures the availability of quality health services through its key program areas: National Health Service Corps, HIV/AIDS, Health Center Program, Maternal and Child Health, Health Professions Workforce, Rural Health, Donations and Transplants, and Injury Compensation.

Maternal Child Health Bureau

HRSA's Maternal Child Health Bureau is an outgrowth of the 1912 Children's Bureau and the 1935 Social Security Act and is authorized to provide programs and foundations for maternal and child health services. The bureau strengthens maternal child health infrastructures; assures availability of medical homes; and improves health, safety, and well-being of the mother and child population.

ADDITIONAL DHHS DIVISIONS

A number of other divisions under the DHHS offer programs that affect the health and safety of women. A brief list includes the following:

SUBSTANCE ABUSE AND MENTAL HEALTH SERVICES ADMINISTRATION

The Substance Abuse and Mental Health Services Administration works to improve the availability and quality of programs in substance abuse prevention, addiction treatment, and mental health services.

CENTERS FOR DISEASE CONTROL AND PREVENTION

The Centers for Disease Control and Prevention works with states and other partners to monitor disease outbreaks, implement prevention strategies, and maintain national health statistics.

CENTERS FOR MEDICARE AND MEDICAID SERVICES

Formerly the Health Care Financing Administration, the Centers for Medicare and Medicaid Services administers programs that provide health care to about one fourth of Americans. Medicare provides insurance for seniors and the disabled. Medicaid, a joint federal and state program, provides health coverage for low-income persons. The Centers for Medicare and Medicaid Services also administers the new Children's Health Insurance Program through approved state plans.

ADMINISTRATION FOR CHILDREN AND FAMILIES

The Administration for Children and Families administers the state-federal welfare program as a means to promote the economic and social well-being of individuals and families. It also administers the Head Start Program and supports state activities in foster care and adoption services.

ADMINISTRATION ON AGING

The Administration on Aging is the federal focal point for older persons and their concerns. It administers key programs for seniors and works with state and regional agencies to provide services that meet the unique needs of older persons and their caregivers.

NONFEDERAL ORGANIZATIONS

There are many state and local governmental agencies that provide significant services to women in conjunction with and independent of federal programs. Also, nonprofit community and professional organizations make considerable contributions to the health and well-being of women and their families. Women's health has received significant attention since the early 1990s; however, there is a need to continue this directed focus to ensure that women's unique needs are understood and addressed. In addition to the continuation of research and therapeutic and educational efforts, it is vital that special consideration be given to distribution and application of newly derived evidence-based information.

REFERENCES

Food and Drug Administration (FDA). (2011). *Office of Women's Health.* Retrieved November 27, 2011, from http://www.fda.gov/AboutFDA/CentersOffices/OC/OfficeofWomensHealth/default.htm

Office on Women's Health (OWH). (2011). *About us.* Retrieved November 27, 2011, from http://www.womenshealth.gov/about-us/

U.S. Department of Labor. (2011). *Women's bureau.* Retrieved December 4, 2011, from http://www.dol.gov/wb/welcome.html

INDEX

B

C

D

E

F

G

H

M

N

T

U

W

X

Y